BERKOWITZ'S
Pediatrics
A PRIMARY CARE APPROACH

4th Edition

Carol D. Berkowitz, MD, FAAP

Professor of Clinical Pediatrics
David Geffen School of Medicine at
University of California Los Angeles
Executive Vice Chair
Department of Pediatrics
Harbor-UCLA Medical Center
Torrance, CA

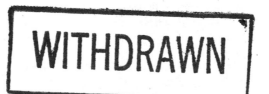

American Academy of Pediatrics
DEDICATED TO THE HEALTH OF ALL CHILDREN™

Editor: Diane Lundquist, MS

Marketing Manager: Linda Smessaert

Production Manager: Theresa Wiener

Copy Editor: Kate Larson

Design and Production: Peg Mulcahy

Library of Congress Control Number: 2011908351

ISBN: 978-1-58110-635-0

MA0615

The recommendations in this publication do not indicate an exclusive course of treatment or serve as a standard of care.
Variations, taking into account individual circumstances, may be appropriate.

Brand names are furnished for identification purposes only. No endorsement of the manufacturers or products mentioned is implied.

Every effort has been made to ensure that the drug selection and dosage set forth in this text are in accordance with the current recommendations and practice at the time of publication. It is the responsibility of the health care provider to check the package insert of each drug for any change in indications and dosage and for added warnings and precautions.

The publishers have made every effort to trace the copyright holders for borrowed material. If they have inadvertently overlooked any, they will be pleased to make the necessary arrangements at the first opportunity.

Berkowitz's Pediatrics: A Primary Care Approach, 4th Edition

Printed in the United States of America.

9-297/1011

Last digit is the print number: 10 9 8 7 6 5 4 3 2 1

Preface

Though many of the "usual diseases of childhood" have been eliminated through expanded immunizations, new and more challenging morbidities confront pediatric patients, their families, and their health care providers. Violence, obesity, genomics, and the Internet and their impact on children are ever-present on the front pages of our newspapers and in our offices and clinics. The world is contracting and diseases once isolated by oceans are now only a plane ride away. This fourth edition of *Berkowitz's Pediatrics: A Primary Care Approach* examines a series of emerging entities that pediatricians are expected to be knowledgeable about and able to address. Because we interface with other disciplines, we must be equipped to understand the principles of their practices and communicate effectively with them. And lastly, our multicultural society includes children from all parts of the world and from all kinds of families, and we need to be prepared to address their needs.

My thanks to all the contributors and to the staff of the American Academy of Pediatrics, especially Diane Lundquist, MS; Kate Larson; Linda Smessaert; Theresa Wiener; and Peg Mulcahy, and my assistant, Mary Magee, for all their help.

Carol D. Berkowitz

Contributors

Sudhir K. Anand, MD
Professor of Clinical Pediatrics, David Geffen School of Medicine
at University of California Los Angeles; Chief, Division of Pediatric
Nephrology, Harbor-UCLA Medical Center, Torrance, CA

David Atkinson, MD
Associate Professor of Clinical Pediatrics, David Geffen School of
Medicine at University of California Los Angeles; Division of Pediatric
Cardiology, Harbor-UCLA Medical Center, Torrance, CA

Sarah Atunah-Jay, MD
Academic General Pediatrics Fellow, Division of General Pediatrics,
Department of Pediatrics, University of Minnesota, Minneapolis, MN

Justine Bacchetta, MD, PhD
Visiting assistant researcher, Pediatric Nephrology, David Geffen
School of Medicine at University of California Los Angeles

Martin Baren, MD†
Attending Physician, Developmental and Behavioral Pediatrics,
Children's Hospital of Orange County, Orange County, CA

Andrew J. Barnes, MD, MPH
Assistant Professor of Developmental-Behavioral Pediatrics,
Division of Academic General Pediatrics,
University of Minnesota, Minneapolis, MN

Lindsay S. Baron, MD
Resident, Department of Radiology, Montefiore Medical Center
of The Albert Einstein College of Medicine, Bronx, NY

Maneesh Batra, MD, MPH
Assistant Professor of Pediatrics
University of Washington School of Medicine, Seattle

Andrew K. Battenberg, BS
Medical Student, David Geffen School of Medicine
at University of California Los Angeles

Carol D. Berkowitz, MD
Professor of Clinical Pediatrics, David Geffen School of Medicine at
University of California Los Angeles; Executive Vice Chair, Department
of Pediatrics, Harbor-UCLA Medical Center, Torrance, CA

Iris Wagman Borowsky, MD, PhD
Associate Professor of Pediatrics and Director, Academic General
Pediatrics Fellowship, Division of Academic General Pediatrics,
Department of Pediatrics, University of Minnesota, Minneapolis, MN

†Deceased.

Paul Bryan, MD
Attending Physician, Department of Emergency Medicine, Children's
Hospital Central California, Madera, CA

Casey Buitenhuys, MD
Clinical Instructor of Medicine
David Geffen School of Medicine at University of California Los Angeles
Fellow, Pediatric Emergeny Medicine, Harbor-UCLA Medical Center,
Torrance, CA

David B. Burbulys, MD
Director, Emergency Medicine Residency Program,
Harbor-UCLA Medical Center; Associate Professor of Medicine,
David Geffen School of Medicine at University of California
Los Angeles, Torrance, CA

Kelly Callahan, MD, MPT
Assistant Professor of Pediatrics, University of California Los Angeles
School of Medicine; Harbor-UCLA Medical Center, Torrance, CA

Gangadarshni Chandramohan, MD, MS
Associate Professor of Pediatrics, David Geffen School of Medicine at
University of California Los Angeles; Division of Pediatric Nephrology,
Harbor-UCLA Medical Center, Torrance, CA

Grant P. Christman, MD
Assistant Professor of Clinical Pediatrics,
Keck School of Medicine of the University of Southern California
Division of Hospital Medicine, Children's Hospital Los Angeles,
Los Angeles, California

Noah Craft, MD, PhD
Los Angeles Biomedical Research Institute, Torrance, CA
Medicine-Pediatrics Resident, University of Minnesota, Minneapolis, MN

Alejandro Diaz, MD
Categorical Pediatrics Resident (PGY-3)
Harbor-UCLA Medical Center
Torrance, CA

Sabrina D. Diaz, MA
Los Angeles Biomedical Research Institute at Harbor-UCLA, Torrance, CA

Robin Winkler Doroshow, MD, MMS, MEd
Associate Professor of Pediatrics, The George Washington University
School of Medicine and Health Sciences; Pediatric Cardiologist, Children's
National Medical Center, Washington, DC; Associate Professor of
Pediatrics, Georgetown University School of Medicine; Director, Division
of Pediatric Cardiology, Georgetown University Hospital

Elizabeth A. Edgerton, MD, MPH
Division of Emergency Medicine, Department of Pediatrics, Children's National Medical Center, Washington, DC

Melissa K. Egge, MD
Chief Resident, Department of Pediatrics,
Harbor-UCLA Medical Center, Torrance, CA

W. Suzanne Eidson-Ton, MD, MS
Health Sciences Associate Clinical Professor of Family and Community Medicine, University of California, Davis School of Medicine, Sacramento, CA.

George Gershman, MD
Professor of Pediatrics, University of California Los Angeles School of Medicine; Chief, Division of Pediatric Gastroenterology and Nutrition, Department of Pediatrics, Harbor-UCLA Medical Center, Torrance, CA

Rick Goldstein, MD
Attending Physician in Pediatric Palliative Care, Dana-Farber Cancer Institute, Children's Hospital Boston, Harvard Medical School, Boston, MA

H. Mollie Greves Grow, MD, MPH
Assistant Professor of Pediatrics, University of Washington Research Faculty, Seattle Children's Research Institute

Geeta Grover, MD
Attending Physician, Developmental and Behavioral Pediatrics, Children's Hospital of Orange County, Orange, CA; Associate Clinical Professor of Pediatrics, University of California, Irvine, Irvine College of Medicine, Irvine, CA

Thomas R. Hawn, MD, PhD
Associate Professor, Department of Medicine,
Division of Allergy and Infectious Diseases
University of Washington School of Medicine
Seattle, WA

Kenneth R. Huff, MD
Professor of Pediatrics and Neurology, University of California Los Angeles; Chief, Division of Neurology, Department of Pediatrics, Harbor-UCLA Medical Center, Torrance, CA

Wendy T. Hui, MD
Pediatrician, Long Beach Comprehensive Health Center,
Long Beach, CA

Lynn Hunt, MD
Clinical Professor of Pediatrics,
University of California, Irvine, Santa Ana, CA

Stanley H. Inkelis, MD
Professor of Pediatrics, University of California Los Angeles School of Medicine; Director, Pediatric Emergency Medicine, Harbor-UCLA Medical Center, Torrance, CA

Walter Jiminez, MD
Research Fellow, Division of Pediatric Nephrology, David Geffen School of Medicine at University of California Los Angeles

Jesse Joad, MD, MS
Professor of Pediatrics
Associate Dean Diversity and Faculty Life Emerita
University of California, Davis

Doron D. Kahana, MD
Assistant Clinical Professor of Pediatrics, Division of Pediatric Gastroenterology, Hepatology & Nutrition,
Harbor-UCLA Medical Center, The David Geffen School of Medicine

Elaine S. Kamil, MD
Clinical Professor of Pediatrics, David Geffen School of Medicine at University of California Los Angeles; Clinical Director, Pediatric Nephrology, Cedars-Sinai Medical Center, Los Angeles

Jane S. Kim, MD
Resident, Department of Radiology,
Montefiore Medical Center, Bronx, NY

Kathy K. Langevin, MD, MPH
Private Practice, Tucson, AZ

Steve L. Lee, MD
Chief of Pediatric Surgery at Harbor-UCLA
Associate Professor of Surgery and Pediatrics,
David Geffen School of Medicine at UCLA

Charlotte W. Lewis, MD, MPH
Associate Professor, Department of Pediatrics,
Divisions of General Pediatrics and Craniofacial Medicine,
Adjunct Associate Professor, Pediatric Dentistry,
University of Washington School of Medicine, Seattle, WA

Lenna Liu, MD, MPH
Professor, Department of Pediatrics, Odessa Brown Children's Clinic
Physician Lead, Seattle Children's Obesity Program
Seattle, WA

Catherine S. Mao, MD
Associate Professor of Clinical Pediatrics, David Geffen School of Medicine at University of California Los Angeles; Division of Pediatric Endocrinology, Harbor-UCLA Medical Center, Los Angeles Biomedical Research Institute, Torrance, CA

ChrisAnna M. Mink, MD
Clinical Professor of Pediatrics,
David Geffen School of Medicine at University of California Los Angeles School of Medicine; Department of Pediatrics, Harbor-UCLA Medical Center, Torrance, CA

Julie E. Noble, MD
Clinical Professor of Pediatrics, The David Geffen School of Medicine, University of California Los Angeles School of Medicine; Director, Pediatric Managed Care, Director, Low Risk Nursery, Harbor-UCLA Medical Center, Torrance, CA

Suzinne Pak-Gorstein, MD, PhD, MPH
Assistant Professor, Department of Pediatrics, University of Washington
Co-Director, Global Health Pathways, Seattle Children's Hospital

Bonnie R. Rachman, MD
Associate Professor of Clinical Pediatrics,
David Geffen School of Medicine at University of California Los Angeles
Division of Pediatric Critical Care, Harbor-UCLA Medical Center,
Torrance, CA

Christian B. Ramers, MD, MPH
Assistant Professor, Departments of Medicine (Infectious Diseases)
and Global Health
University of Washington School of Medicine, Seattle, WA

Nasser Redjal, MD
Professor of Clinical Pediatrics and Allergy/Immunology,
University of California, Los Angeles School of Medicine; Director,
Allergy/Immunology Managed Care, Harbor-UCLA Medical Center,
Torrance, CA

Katherine E. Remick, MD
Clinical Instructor of Pediatrics
David Geffen School of Medicine at University of California Los Angeles
Fellow, Pediatric Emergency Medicine, Harbor-UCLA Medical Center,
Torrance, CA

Teresa Rosales, MD
Clinical Professor of Ophthalmology, University of California Los Angeles
School of Medicine, Jules Stein Eye Institute; Pediatric Ophthalmologist,
Private Practice, Long Beach, CA

Isidro B. Salusky, MD
Professor of Pediatrics, University of California Los Angeles School
of Medicine; Director, Pediatric Dialysis Program, Program Director,
General Clinical Research Center, University of California Los Angeles

Jeremy Screws, MD
Assistant Professor of Pediatrics, University of Tennessee College of
Medicine, Chattanooga Unit, Chattanooga, TN

Erica Sibinga, MD, MHS
Assistant Professor of Pediatrics, Johns Hopkins School of Medicine,
Baltimore, MD

Monica Sifuentes, MD
Professor of Clinical Pediatrics, David Geffen School of Medicine at
University of California Los Angeles; Associate Program Director, Vice
Chair of Education, Department of Pediatrics, Harbor-UCLA Medical
Center, Torrance, CA

Lynne M. Smith, MD
Professor of Clinical Pediatrics, David Geffen School of Medicine at
University of California Los Angeles; Department of Pediatrics,
Division of Neonatology, Harbor-UCLA Medical Center, Torrance, CA

Blanca Solis, MD
Associate Physician
Primary Care Network
University of California, Davis

Robin Steinberg-Epstein, MD
Director of Developmental and Behavioral Pediatrics and
Clinical Professor of Pediatrics University of California,
Irvine School of Medicine and Children's Hospital of Orange County
Developmental Behavioral Pediatrician at the For OC Kids
Neurodevelopmental Center

Kenneth W. Steinhoff, MD
Associate Clinical Professor, Department of Pediatrics, University of
California, Irvine, CA; Child Psychiatrist, Child Development Center,
Department of Pediatrics, University of California, Irvine, CA

Miriam T. Stewart, BA
Johns Hopkins School of Medicine
Balimoe, MD

Sara T. Stewart, MD
Harbor-UCLA Medical Center, Torrance, CA

Ki-Young Suh, MD
Assistant Clinical Professor, Division of Dermatology,
Department of Medicine, David Geffen School of Medicine at the
University of California, Los Angeles

Benjamin H. Taragin, MD
Assistant Professor of Radiology and Pediatrics
Director Pediatric Radiology
Division of Radiology
Montefiore Medical Center of The Albert Einstein College of
Medicine, Bronx, NY

Wendy Y. Tcheng, MD
Pediatric Hematology-Oncology
Children's Hospital of Central California

Alan Tomines, MD
Assistant Clinical Professor of Pediatrics and Health Services,
David Geffen School of Medicine at University of California Los Angeles
and UCLA School of Public Health; Harbor-UCLA Medical Center,
Torrance, CA

Hendry Ton, MD, MS
Health Sciences Associate Clinical Professor
of Psychiatry and Behavioral Sciences
University of California Davis School of Medicine

Derek Wong, MD
Assistant Professor of Clinical Pediatrics, David Geffen Medical School at
University of California Los Angeles; Division of Medical Genetics, UCLA
Medical Center, Los Angeles, CA

Jennifer K. Yee, MD
Assistant Professor of Pediatrics, David Geffen School of Medicine at
University of California Los Angeles; Division of Pediatric Endocrinology,
Harbor-UCLA Medical Center, Torrance, CA

Kelly D. Young, MD, MS
Health Sciences Clinical Professor of Pediatrics
David Geffen School of Medicine at UCLA
Harbor-UCLA Medical Center Department of Emergency Medicine

David P. Zamorano, MD
Assistant Professor, Department of Orthopaedic Surgery, California
School of Medicine, Irvine, CA

Contents

SECTION II

Health Maintenance and Anticipatory Guidance

SECTION III

Acute and Emergent Problems

SECTION IV

Head, Neck, and Respiratory System

SECTION V

Hematologic Disorders

SECTION VI

Cardiovascular System

SECTION VII

Genitourinary Disorders

SECTION VIII

Orthopedic Disorders

SECTION IX

Gastrointestinal Disorders

SECTION X

Neurologic Disorders

SECTION XI

Dermatologic Disorders

SECTION XII

The New Morbidity

SECTION XIII

Chronic Diseases of Childhood and Adolescence

Primary Care: Skills and Concepts

CHAPTER 1

Primary Care: Introduction

Julie E. Noble, MD

Primary care is defined as the comprehensive health care that patients receive from the same health care provider over a longitudinal period. The term was first used in the 1960s to designate the role of the primary care physician in response to the abundance of subspecialists and lack of generalists among practicing physicians. It is generally accepted that primary care physicians include pediatricians, family physicians, and internists. In 1966 the Millis Committee Report to the American Medical Association on graduate medical education recognized the importance of primary care and recommended a national commitment to educating primary care physicians. Primary care was further defined in 1974 by Charney and Alpert, who separated it into component parts: first contact, longitudinal care, family orientation, and integration of comprehensive care. To understand the depth of primary care, the component parts should be explored.

First contact occurs when a patient arrives for medical care at the office of a primary care physician. The visit includes an intake history, complete physical examination, and an assessment of problems with treatment (if indicated). Of great importance is the establishment of the physician–patient relationship. Physicians become the primary medical resource and counselors to these patients and their families and the first contacts when successive medical problems arise.

Longitudinal care, the second component of primary care, implies continuity of care over time. Physicians assume responsibility for issues concerning both health and illness. In pediatrics, such care involves monitoring growth and development, following school progress, screening for commonly found disorders, making psychosocial assessments, promoting health, and preventing illness with immunization and safety counseling programs.

Family orientation is the third component of primary care. Patients must be viewed in the context of their environment and family. Otherwise, practitioners cannot adequately care for patients. In pediatrics, a child's problems become the family's, and the family's problems become the child's. This has become increasingly apparent with the recognition that problems of poverty, drug use, HIV exposure, teenage pregnancy, and gang involvement directly affect a child's health and quality of life. The psychosocial forces in a particular child's life are intricately interwoven into their health care, and their assessment is an essential component of the primary care of that child.

As pediatric medical problems become more complex, many health and educational resources may be used to supplement care.

Primary care physicians integrate and coordinate these services in the best interest of patients, thus providing **integration of comprehensive care,** the fourth component of primary care. Working with social service agencies, home care providers, educational agencies, and government agencies, physicians can use multiple resources for the benefit of patients. Understanding the resources of the community is an important part of a primary care physician's education.

Medical Home

When patients select a primary care provider, they have identified a medical home. That home incorporates the physical, psychological, and social aspects of individual patients into comprehensive health care services, thus meeting the needs of the whole person. This concept of the medical home was first documented by the American Academy of Pediatrics (AAP) in 1967 in the book *Standards of Child Health Care,* which noted that a medical home should be a central source of all the child's medical records. The idea of a medical home developed into a method of providing comprehensive primary care and was successfully implemented in the 1980s by Dr Calvin Sia in Hawaii. He is considered to be the "father" of the medical home. In policy statements published in 1992 and 2002, the AAP defined the characteristics of a medical home to be "accessible, continuous, comprehensive, family-centered, coordinated, compassionate, and culturally effective." To make that home work for patients, geographic and financial accessibility are key elements. The most important aspect of a home is that it is a place where patients feel "cared for."

Since its implementation in pediatrics in 2004, the medical home model was adopted by the American Academy of Family Practice and American College of Physicians. Its definition was expanded to include use of electronic information services, population-based management of chronic illness, and continuous quality improvement. The concept has been accepted as a form of high-quality health care. Cost and quality benefits have been well documented. Recognizing these benefits, large corporations with providers formed the Patient-Centered Primary Care Collaborative to promote the idea of designated medical homes. As part of that collaborative, the National Committee for Quality Assurance adopted eligibility criteria for a practice to define itself as a medical home. Requirements for the designation include the adoption of health information technology and decision support systems, modification of clinical practice patterns, and ensuring continuity of care. With the advent of health care reform in the United States, as part of the effort to control the rising cost of health care, the federal government has endorsed the concept of the medical home model. The Academic Pediatric Association has defined the family-centered medial home to delineate the dependency of the child to the family and community in the medical home model.

Role of the Primary Care Pediatrician

As a primary care physician, the role of the pediatrician has not only included the care of acute illnesses and injuries, but also the preventive aspects of well-child care with its focus on immunizations, tracking growth and development, and anticipatory guidance. Now there is a renewed emphasis on the importance of the role of the pediatric primary care provider in assessing the psychosocial aspects of pediatric patients. Termed the *new morbidity* by Robert Haggerty, MD, in the 1970s, recognizing these social issues including family dysfunction; developmental problems, including learning disabilities; and behavioral problems, including emotional disorders, have become a significant part of the role of the provider. In 1993 the AAP stated that pediatricians are obliged to have knowledge of physical and environmental factors and behaviors affecting health, normal variations of behavior and emotional development, risk factors and behaviors affecting physical health, and behavior problems. The focus of the pediatrician should be detection, evaluation, and management, with referrals if needed. Newer morbidities secondary to the increasing complexity of our society were outlined in 2001 by the AAP. These include school problems, mood and anxiety disorders, adolescent suicide and homicide, firearms, school violence, drug and alcohol abuse, HIV, obesity, and the effects of the media on children. Other psychosocial factors such as poverty, homelessness, single-parent families, divorce, working parents, and child care necessitate that pediatricians work with social service agencies to deliver appropriate care to their patients. The role of the primary care physician is continually expanding in an effort to deliver comprehensive care to each patient.

Subspecialist Care

Medical knowledge and technology have made amazing advancements in the past several decades. Total knowledge of all fields is impossible for individual physicians. As a result, the role of the subspecialist physician has developed as an adjunct to that of the primary care physician. New fields of subspecialties, such as child abuse pediatrics, have arisen as a response to the increased knowledge. Primary care physicians should seek subspecialist consultation when the suspected or known disease process is unusual or complicated, when it demands specialized technology, or when they have little experience with the disease. Generally, subspecialists evaluate patients and concentrate on the organ system or disease process in their area of expertise.

Primary care physicians can use a subspecialist for either a consultation or referral. When initiating a consultation, primary care physicians seek advice from the consultant regarding workup or management of the patient. Consulting physicians assess the patients with a history and physical examination, focusing on their specialty. They then recommend possible additional laboratory tests, offer a diagnosis and treatment plan, and send the patients back to their primary care physicians for coordination of further care.

Use of the subspecialist is termed **secondary care.** For example, an 8-year-old girl with weight loss and persistent abdominal pain has an upper gastrointestinal radiograph series that reveals a duodenal ulcer. She is sent by her primary care physician to a pediatric gastroenterologist for **consultation,** with a request for an endoscopy to allow definitive diagnosis and up-to-date management guidelines. The girl then returns to the primary care physician with recommendations for treatment and further care.

Primary care physicians can also generate a referral to a subspecialist, which differs from a consultation. A **referral** requests that the subspecialist assume complete care of the patient. This transfer of a patient to a tertiary care site establishes a subspecialist as the coordinator of further health care for the patient. For example, a 4-year-old boy with recurrent fevers, hepatosplenomegaly, and blasts on peripheral blood smear is referred to a pediatric oncologist for diagnosis, the latest treatment, and ongoing medical care.

When requesting advice from subspecialists, whether on a consultative or referral basis, primary care physicians should outline specific questions with a probable diagnosis to be addressed by the subspecialist. For example, a consultation requesting evaluation of a child with hematuria is inappropriate. The primary care physician should perform a basic diagnostic evaluation and should make the most likely diagnosis. The child can then be referred appropriately. For example, a child diagnosed with nephritis should be sent to a pediatric nephrologist, whereas a child diagnosed with Wilms tumor should be sent to a pediatric oncologist.

When primary care physicians and subspecialists function cooperatively and offer the 3 levels of care (primary, referral, and consultative), patients receive the highest-quality medical care. In general, care provided by subspecialists is characterized as being more expensive and procedure driven. Laboratory studies are ordered with increased frequency by subspecialists, further inflating the cost of medical care. If patients have no longitudinal health care and see multiple providers, repeat laboratory studies are often ordered. Primary care is believed to deliver more cost-effective, improved medical care. With the spiraling cost of medical care, there continues to be a nationwide movement to produce more primary care physicians. However, it should be remembered that the role of the subspecialist is an essential supplement to the primary care physician when managing complicated disease. A balance between generalists and subspecialists needs to be maintained in the education process.

Laboratory Tests

For most conditions, the diagnosis is revealed by the history and physical examination in more than 95% of cases. Thus good communication skills are a basic tenet of primary care. Patients' complaints often concern unnecessary laboratory tests, which increase the cost of medical care, and the prescription of unnecessary medications. To lessen these problems, the primary care physician should use laboratory tests and medications discriminatingly, recognizing their value as well as their potential iatrogenic effects.

In primary care, laboratory tests should be used to help confirm a condition suspected on the basis of the history or physical examination or diagnose a condition that may not be apparent after a thorough history and physical assessment. In pediatrics especially, the value of each test result should be weighed against the inconvenience, discomfort, and possible side effects in children. Tests can also be used as screening tools to prevent disease or to identify a disease early so that treatment can begin and symptoms can be minimized. Laboratory studies can provide a variety of other information, including data to establish a diagnosis, knowledge necessary to select therapy or to monitor a disease, and information about the risk of future disease. Organ function, metabolic activity, and nutritional status can also be assessed, and evidence of neoplastic or infectious disease can be provided. In addition, laboratory studies can be used to identify infectious and therapeutic agents or poisons.

Screening laboratory tests are used when the incidence of an unsuspected condition is high enough in a general population to justify the expense of the test (see Chapter 11). Subclinical conditions, such as anemia, lead poisoning, and hypercholesterolemia, are part of some health maintenance assessments.

Physicians must remember that there is variability in test results and that laboratory error can occur. Laboratory results should always be viewed in the context of the patient. The sensitivity of a test, the ability of the test to detect low levels, and the specificity of a test for the substance being measured must also be considered by the physician when evaluating a test result.

Challenges for the Future

As this edition of *Primary Care Pediatrics* is being written, the initial elements of health care reform are being implemented. As with any political initiative, it remains to be seen whether full reform will continue or whether the reform may be modified. But it is apparent that the role of the primary care physician has increased importance in health care delivery. Two of the basic tenets of primary care, accessibility and an ongoing relationship with the provider (both of which are reported by patients to be very important), are now recognized as essential components of the medical home. The challenge continues to ensure continuity in health care funding to preserve the continuity of the medical home. Payment reform promises to improve reimbursement to primary care practices and rewards high performance. Through accountable care organizations as proposed in health care reform, primary care physicians would be the foundation of the organization whose mission is management of the continuum of care and cost, as well as to ensure quality of care.

Access to same-day care, which is part of the obligation of the medical home, can be difficult in the busy schedule of primary care

providers. It will be a challenge for primary care physicians to reorganize their practices to accommodate same-day visits. Walk-in immediate medical care clinics and retail clinics have arisen. Patients like the convenience, but episodic visits in a variety of settings do not deliver comprehensive care for the patient, and these short visits may not take into account the entirety of the patient's medical history. This creates a challenge for the primary care provider and medical home to develop a system to integrate the information from these encounters into the comprehensive medical record.

With the advent of hospitalists providing inpatient care, primary care physicians may not be included in in-patient management. They then face a challenge in retrieving important information regarding the care of their patients.

Medical care reform incorporates accountability, demonstration of quality of care, and standards of medical practice into the medical home model. These have increased the oversight and bureaucracy of medical care exponentially. This business of medicine with redundant oversight of medical care has put a tremendous burden of administrative activities in the lap of the primary care physician. There is a significant challenge to providers to provide care while answering to administrative structures.

The biggest challenge to pediatric primary care providers continues to be ensuring the future of health care funding to provide access and availability in a medical home of health care to all children. This is a priority for child health policy reform at the national level. At this point there are a multitude of programs, varying in each state, to pay for children's health care. Universal health care for children is being advocated. Without a national plan for financing, children's health care will continue to be variable, leading to disparities in children's health.

Selected References

Academic Pediatric Association Task Force on the Family-Centered Medical Home. The family-centered medical home: specific considerations for child health research and policy. *Acad Pediatr.* 2010;10:211–217

American Academy of Pediatrics Committee on Psychosocial Aspects of Child and Family Health. The new morbidity revisited: a renewed commitment to the psychosocial aspects of pediatric care. *Pediatrics.* 2001;108:1227–1230

American Academy of Pediatrics Medical Home Initiatives for Children With Special Needs Project Advisory Committee. The medical home. *Pediatrics.* 2002;110:184–186

American Academy of Pediatrics Retail-Based Clinic Policy Work Group. American Academy of Pediatrics principles concerning retail-based clinics. *Pediatrics.* 2006;118:2561–2569

American Association of Medical Colleges. Policy on the generalist physician. *Acad Med.* 1993;68:1–6

Carrier E, Gourevitch MN, Shah NR. Medical homes—challenges in translating theory into practice. *Med Care.* 2009;47:714–722

Cheng TL. Primary care pediatrics: 2004 and beyond. *Pediatrics.* 2004;113: 1802–1809

Noe DA, Rock RC. *Laboratory Medicine: The Selection and Interpretation of Clinical Laboratory Studies.* Baltimore, MD: Williams & Wilkins; 1994

Rittenhouse DR, Shortell SM, Fisher ES. Primary care and accountable care—two essential elements of delivery-system reform. *N Engl J Med.* 2009;361:2301–2303

Starfield B. *Primary Care. Concept, Evaluation, and Policy.* New York, NY: Oxford University Press; 1992

Tonniges TF, Palfrey JS, Mitchell M, eds. The medical home. *Pediatrics.* 2004;113(5 suppl):1471–1548. http://pediatrics.aappublications.org/content/vol113/issue5/#SUPPLS1

CHAPTER 2

Child Advocacy

Grant P. Christman, MD, and Julie E. Noble, MD

CASE STUDY

A 15-year-old male is brought to the emergency department with a gunshot wound to his left leg. He says he was hanging out at the park with his friends when a random car drove by and shots were fired. He denies being in a gang, but his mom suggests otherwise during a private conversation with the emergency physician. His physical examination reveals a gunshot wound to his left lower leg, with intact sensation, movement, and pulses in the left foot, and no other signs of injury. A radiograph shows a fractured left tibia, and he is admitted for orthopedic surgical treatment.

Questions
1. What does it mean to be a child advocate?
2. Aside from caring for individual patients, what is expected of pediatricians in the community?
3. What is the role of pediatricians in child advocacy?
4. What are the levels of advocacy?
5. How do pediatricians implement advocacy?

An advocate is someone who speaks on behalf of a person or cause. No group in our society has a greater need for advocates than children. Children are ill equipped to face the many threats to their health; they cannot obtain their own health insurance, access available social services, or even take themselves to the doctor when sick. Children also have no voice in our society. They cannot vote, donate money to political campaigns, or speak publicly to advance their interests. The word *advocate* is derived from a Latin root meaning "one who has been called to another's aid." From the beginnings of pediatrics as an independent branch of medicine, pediatricians have answered this call to advocate for the health and well-being of children.

The father of American pediatrics, Abraham Jacobi, MD, spent his career in the late 1800s and early 1900s advocating for children through legislation in New York and Washington, DC. He was a great teacher of pediatrics, introducing the discipline into academic medicine, but truly believed that physicians needed to be involved in public policy. Another founder of American pediatrics, Job Lewis Smith, MD, recognized the need for a clean water supply and decent housing to decrease the high infant mortality rate at that time. He worked through public advocacy to improve conditions not only for his patients but for children in general. The American Academy of Pediatrics (AAP) was founded on federal advocacy principles. In June 1921, the Sheppard-Towner Act on maternal and child health legislation was introduced into Congress. It was the first involvement of the federal government on behalf of children and provided federal matching funds to states for services for pregnant women and new mothers. The American Medical Association (AMA), worried that the legislation would lead to socialized medicine, condemned the act, while the AMA Section on Diseases of Children supported the legislation. When the act was up for reauthorization in 1930 and the AMA still opposed it, the pediatric group left the AMA and founded the AAP. This organization has been advocating for children ever since.

The New Morbidity

Advocacy has become increasingly important because the new morbidities in pediatric medicine are related to community forces. As our society has become more complicated, major health concerns have become even more intertwined with the environments in which children are involved. Child health outcomes improved dramatically in the 1900s with the development of vaccines, antibiotics, and new and improved surgical care to treat the classic morbidities of infectious disease, infant mortality, poor nutrition, epidemics, overcrowding, and chronic disease. But there have emerged new morbidities that are negatively affecting child health outcomes. These morbidities of the 1960s to 1980s, as described by Robert Haggerty, MD, include family dysfunction, learning disabilities, emotional disorders, and educational problems. The face of childhood morbidity continued to evolve in the 1980s to 2000s. Judith Palfrey, MD, documented social disarray; political ennui; the sequelae of high-tech care; and new epidemics of violence, AIDS, cocaine, and homelessness as the new challenges for pediatricians. We have now expanded morbidities in the 2000s to include major health concerns with the increased prevalence of overweight children, increased mental health issues, significant health disparities in cultural groups, and major socioeconomic influences affecting child health.

At the same time, children in America continue to face challenges in obtaining access to quality health care. Over the past several decades, government programs like Medicaid and the Children's Health Insurance Program have expanded the availability of health care to children of limited financial means. As of 2007 there were still 8.1 million children younger than 18 years with no health insurance coverage, representing 11% of that population. Among insured children, 23.5% had inadequate coverage as determined by a survey of their parents.

It is clear that these significant issues affecting child health cannot be adequately dealt with on an individual basis, but require advocacy on a community or national scale to improve child health outcomes and life for children.

Community Pediatrics

Community pediatrics has developed as the vehicle to implement advocacy. Robert Haggerty, MD, first originated the concept in 1968 in an article published in the *New England Journal of Medicine*. In his work as department chair of pediatrics at the University of Rochester, NY, he developed an extensive advocacy agenda for the children of the community of Rochester. Subsequently, the AAP published a policy statement from its Committee on Community Health Services titled, "The Pediatrician's Role in Community Pediatrics." The policy delineates 5 components of community pediatrics: a *perspective* from the individual patient to all the children in the community; a *recognition* that family, education, society, culture, spirituality, economy, environment, and politics all affect the health of children; a *synthesis* of clinical practice and public health principles directed to providing health care to a child and promoting the health of all children; a *commitment* to collaborate with the community to optimize health care for all children, especially disadvantaged children; and an *integral part* of the role of the pediatrician. All of these components are recommended as a part of pediatric practice, and training in advocacy has been instituted in pediatric training programs. Examples of potential involvement in the community include serving as a board member, developing health agendas, working with an existing organization to design and fund a community service project, and being a source of information for the community on child health issues.

Levels of Advocacy

Every pediatrician functions as a child advocate on a daily basis. With every patient encounter the pediatrician advocates for care in the best interest of the patient. This first level of advocacy includes treating the *individual's* immediate medical needs, performing screening tests, giving anticipatory guidance, and coordinating referrals as needed. The pediatrician may step beyond direct medical care to advance the welfare of the child, for example by writing letters to help a patient obtain social services, or visiting a patient's school for an Individualized Education Program meeting. The second level of advocacy is *community* advocacy. Pediatricians are an integral part of the community, and the community directly affects the health of their patients. Thus pediatricians have a responsibility to improve conditions in their community to benefit children. To do this, they must be familiar with the services that are available for children. They can develop relationships with child care centers, schools, community coalitions, city governments, and local organizations to advocate for the best interest of children. On a *state* level, pediatricians

can work to improve health care resources or develop policies to help and protect children. Opportunities for involvement include working on legislation, budgets, regulations, and initiatives or working with the executive branch of local and state government. The next level of advocacy would be the *federal* level, where pediatricians can be involved with their senators and congressmen lobbying for child health issues. Pediatricians may also be involved in testifying before a congressional subcommittee. The final level of advocacy is the *international* level. For example, pediatricians may decide to work with the World Health Organization to improve immunizations for all children worldwide.

Becoming a Child Advocate

To become an effective child advocate, pediatricians must first identify an issue that they want to change or set a goal to improve the lives of children. The more specific the issue or goal, the easier it is to develop a solution. Ideas often come from clinical practice, where repeatedly engaging in individual advocacy efforts on behalf of patients suffering from the same problems suggests the need for a larger solution. The first step is to obtain background information about the problem and to collect objective data that support the need for change, and then to define the nature of the problem and the affected population in clear and precise terms.

Community Projects

The pediatrician may find that the issue would be best addressed through a community advocacy project. In developing such a project, the pediatrician's relationship with the community is of the utmost importance, and the pediatrician should endeavor to become familiar with the community as a whole. Community exploration, potentially as simple as walking or driving through the community and looking around, can reveal areas of need, such as dilapidated housing or unsafe streets. Equally important is the discovery of the community's assets, institutions such as churches, schools, and banks, which give the community strength and could provide support and counsel for the project. Pediatricians should view themselves as members of the community, acting from within and in collaboration with the community, rather than as outsiders bringing about change externally.

The next step is to develop an intervention. After the possible solutions are considered, pediatricians need to collaborate with community stakeholders to develop and implement the solution that is the most practical. Having credibility in the community makes the task of collaboration much easier. Everyone is more effective working with others, but collaboration necessitates the ability to compromise and be flexible in implementation plans. Larger projects may require funding, and grants may be sought from advocacy organizations, the government, or even local corporations. Data should be collected during the intervention to monitor the success of the project. If the project is successful in effecting change, its methods may be adopted by child advocates in other communities.

Legislative Advocacy

Though initially daunting for a physician without political expertise, involvement in the legislative process is often the only way to effect a desired change for children's health. A pediatrician might begin by tracking existing bills that affect child health and contacting legislators by letter, e-mail, or phone to offer a position. It is helpful to become familiar with the process by which a bill becomes a law, both at the state and federal levels; the identities of the important players change as a bill progresses through the various subcommittees and committees, and ultimately to a floor vote.

The pediatrician may also arrange to meet with a legislator or staff member at a district or capital office to discuss the position personally. When meeting with a legislator or staff member, remember to inspire both the heart and the mind. State the problem clearly and explain why a new law is the solution. Present well-researched facts that support your position, and stick to layman's terms, avoiding medical jargon whenever possible. Share a story about a patient encountered in practice who has been affected by the problem. This is especially helpful if the patient is a constituent of the legislator (though the patient's identity must of course never be discussed). After the meeting, leave behind a concise 1-page fact sheet summarizing your position and the pertinent background information.

Be prepared to encounter opposition from some legislators, and avoid responding with angry statements that would alienate a legislator. Effective advocacy requires building relationships with legislators over the long term, and a legislator who opposes your position this year may be a potential supporter next year, when the political climate changes, or may be a potential ally on another important issue. There are a number of other potential pitfalls to avoid. Avoid making or agreeing with partisan statements. Do not claim to represent an organization like the AAP or an institution like a university unless you are authorized to do so. Minimize the appearance of self-interest by focusing on how the proposal will benefit children, rather than how it will benefit pediatricians. Avoid guessing if you do not know the answer to a question; offer to do further research and contact the legislator with the requested information.

When seeking to develop a new legislative proposal from scratch, remember that though the factors contributing to child health may be numerous and complex, legislative proposals must by nature be concrete and limited. Don't be afraid to start small, and to work for incremental change. Identify a clear and, if possible, measurable objective, and define the target population. If the proposal requires funding, consider what the funding source will be. Know which government agencies may be involved in implementation or enforcement. Having a legislator as an ally early on in the process is important, as some of the aforementioned issues will be outside the experience of the average pediatrician, and because a bill must be sponsored by a legislator to be considered for passage. Build a coalition of support within the community, involving important stakeholders such as politicians, businessmen, other health care professionals, educators, and parents.

Again, be prepared to meet opposition and identify potential sources of opposition in advance. If opposition from a powerful interest group is anticipated, meet with a representative of that group to state your case. Potential arguments might include ways in which the proposal is really in the group's self-interest, the moral imperative to help children, or that opposing an initiative to benefit children might generate negative publicity. Consider compromising on aspects of the proposal, when to do so might turn an enemy into an ally. When facing intractable opposition from powerful interests, try to bring even stronger allies into your coalition.

Be aware that the process of turning a policy idea into real legislation may be lengthy. A bill may have to be reintroduced repeatedly over several years before achieving passage. Once a bill becomes a law, advocates must continue working to ensure that the bill is reauthorized when applicable and that regulatory processes develop favorably. Physicians who are recognized as experts in child health policy will be called on to testify before committees in Congress or the state legislature on other policy issues affecting children.

Media Advocacy

The media, including newspapers, magazines, radio, television, and the Internet, are extremely influential in our society. News stories about child health and welfare may not always be written from a child-friendly point of view. Pediatricians play an important role in providing the media with better information and a different angle on a story. For instance, a pediatrician reading a newspaper story about a child who exhibited signs of autism shortly after his 1-year-old physical might write a letter to the editor discussing the lack of scientific evidence for a connection between vaccinations and autism. Over time pediatricians can develop relationships with local journalists, who can then turn to them for information when covering child health stories.

A directed media campaign may also be a key element in an advocacy project. At the community level, the media can help spread ideas, notify the public of events, and bring out potential allies and coalition members. When advocating for legislation, pediatricians can use the media to reach legislators directly and, equally important, to reach thousands of the legislators' constituents all at once, who may in turn help pressure their legislators for change. In such situations, it is essential to plan a media strategy ahead of time by determining the most important target audience, selecting the appropriate types of media to approach, crafting a message appropriate to those media, and preparing thoughtfully for encounters with journalists.

Getting Connected

The AAP is a vital resource for pediatricians interested in child advocacy, with its Federal Advocacy Action Network, as well as the various state chapters advocating at the state level. Other national organizations that are available for involvement by pediatricians include Docs For Tots, Children's Defense Fund, and the Child Welfare League of America. Toolkits for advocacy are available through these organizations.

Improving the health of all children through advocacy is considered to be the responsibility of pediatricians and can be a tremendously rewarding part of pediatric practice.

CASE RESOLUTION

In the case scenario, treating this teen for his orthopedic injury is only the first part of thorough pediatric care. His social history and the environment in which he lives are essential information for the pediatrician to obtain to be an advocate for this patient and prevent a second admission for a subsequent and potentially worse injury. A social work evaluation is performed and reveals that he lives in poverty in the inner city and does indeed belong to a gang. The patient and his family are counseled regarding his high-risk behavior, and he is referred to the police department for their Gang Alternative Program. His pediatrician becomes concerned about the high prevalence of gang activity in the community putting many teens at risk of injury. He explores coalitions in the area that recognize similar concerns. To have an effect on decreasing youth gang activity, a solution is identified to establish high-quality after-school programs to involve teens in productive activities. The Boy's and Girl's Club organization is contacted, and they have an interest in establishing a center in this community. The pediatrician volunteers to be on the board and help develop the after-school programs.

Selected References

American Academy of Pediatrics Committee on Community Health Services. The pediatrician's role in community pediatrics. *Pediatrics*. 2005;115:1092–1094

American Academy of Pediatrics. *AAP Advocacy Guide*. Elk Grove Village, IL: American Academy of Pediatrics; 2009. http://www.aap.org/moc/loadsecure.cfm/advocacyguide/pdf_version/AdvocacyGuide.pdf

American Public Health Association. *APHA Media Advocacy Manual*. Washington, DC: American Public Health Association; 2011. http://www.apha.org/about/news/mediaadvocacy.htm

Anne E. Dyson Community Pediatrics Training Initiative. *Community-based Resident Projects Toolkit*. Elk Grove Village, IL: American Academy of Pediatrics; 2011. http://www.aap.org/commpeds/CPTI/Toolkit-Bod-2005.pdf

Bar-on M. The use of public education in practice. *Pediatr Rev*. 2001;22:75–80

Berman S. Training pediatricians to become child advocates. *Pediatrics*. 1998;102:632–636

Kaczorowski J, ed. Community pediatrics: making child health at the community level an integral part of pediatric training and practice. *Pediatrics*. 2005;115(suppl):1119–1212

Palfrey JS. *Child Health in American: Making a Difference through Advocacy*. Baltimore, MD: Johns Hopkins University Press; 2006

Palfrey JS, Hametz P, Grason H, McCaskill QE, Scott G, Chi GW. Educating the next generation of pediatricians in urban health care: the Anne E. Dyson Community Pediatrics Training Initiative. *Acad Med*. 2004;79:1184–1191

Paulson J. Pediatric advocacy. *Pediatr Clin North Am*. 2001;48:1307–1318

Rudolf MC, Bundle A, Damman A, et al. Exploring the scope for advocacy by paediatricians. *Arch Dis Child*. 1999;81:515–518

Sheehan K, ed. *Pediatr Ann*. 2007;36(10):(entire issue)

Sia CC. Abraham Jacobi Award address, April 14, 1992. The medical home: pediatric practice and child advocacy in the 1990s. *Pediatrics*. 1992;90:419–423

Taylor D, Raman R. Look how far we've come as advocates for children—but consider where we still need to go! *Contemp Pediatr*. 2005;22:54–64

US Department of Health and Human Services, Health Resources and Services Administration, Maternal and Child Health Bureau. *Child Health USA 2008–2009*. Rockville, MD: US Department of Health and Human Services; 2009

CHAPTER 3

Global Child Health

Suzinne Pak-Gorstein, MD, PhD, MPH, and Maneesh Batra, MD, MPH

CASE STUDY

You are watching television when the programming is interrupted by breaking news that a severe earthquake has struck a developing country that you have recently visited. You wonder if and how you could become involved in efforts to help the country respond to the disaster, prevent diseases, and help rebuild its health structure.

Questions

1. What are the global trends in childhood disease and mortality? How does this compare with the United States?
2. What is global health (GH)?
3. What is the role of a pediatrician in GH?
4. What are the key organizations in GH that pediatricians work in?
5. How can pediatricians carry out international work in an ethical and effective manner?

Background

Worldwide, an estimated 7.7 million children younger than 5 years died in 2010, which translates into more than 21,000 children dying each day. This figure actually represents a one-third reduction from the 11.9 million child deaths estimated in 1990. Still, significant disparities in child mortality persist and have become increasingly concentrated in specific regions of the world that bear a disproportionate burden. Africa and Asia combined account for 83% of all child deaths, with one-third of these deaths occurring in south Asia, and half in sub-Saharan Africa. Less than 1% of deaths occur in high-income countries.

Three diseases—pneumonia, diarrhea, and malaria—accounted for 41% of all child deaths worldwide in 2008. Most of these lives could be saved through increased coverage of low-cost prevention and treatment measures, including antibiotics for acute respiratory infections, oral rehydration therapy for diarrhea, immunizations to protect against pneumococcal pneumonia and rotaviral diarrhea, and the use of insecticide-treated mosquito nets and appropriate drugs for malaria.

Undernutrition is an underlying cause of at least a third of all deaths in children younger than 5 years. Reducing both chronic and acute undernutrition will have a substantial impact on reducing child mortality. Furthermore, improved coverage of specific nutritional interventions, such as early and exclusive breastfeeding, are cost-effective and reduce the prevalence of pneumonia and diarrhea.

An estimated 40% of deaths in children younger than 5 occur in the first month of life, and most of these deaths occur at home in the first postnatal week. Hence, improving newborn care is essential to the goal of improving child health. Increased access to basic, inexpensive interventions are needed to reduce neonatal mortality rates globally, including delivery by skilled birth attendants, hygienic umbilical cord care, and training community health workers to assess and begin early treatment for neonatal infections.

In September 2000 world leaders from 190 nations came together to adopt the United Nations Millennium Declaration, committing to reduce extreme poverty through a series of time-bound targets. The 8 Millennium Development Goals (MDGs) range from halving extreme poverty to providing universal primary education, and reducing child mortality by two-thirds—all by the target date of 2015 (Box 3-1). The MDGs form a blueprint ratified by more than 190 nations and have galvanized unprecedented efforts to meet the needs of the world's poorest people.

Though progress has been made toward achieving MDG 4, the pace has been modest and insufficient to meet the goal of two-thirds

---

Box 3-1. Millennium Development Goals (MDGs)

The **MDGs** were developed and signed by all United Nations member countries in September 2000. There are 8 goals with 21 targets and a series of measurable indicators for each target.

Goal 1: Eradicate extreme poverty and hunger.

Goal 2: Achieve universal primary education.

Goal 3: Promote gender equality and empower women.

Goal 4: Reduce the child mortality rate.
> Target: Reduce the under-5 mortality rate by two-thirds between 1990 and 2015.

Goal 5: Improve maternal health.

Goal 6: Combat HIV/AIDS, malaria, and other diseases.

Goal 7: Ensure environmental sustainability.

Goal 8: Develop a global partnership for development.

reduction in childhood mortality by 2015. Enormous gaps in child mortality rates exist between high- and low-income countries, with a rate of 2 child deaths per 1,000 live births in Singapore compared with 257 in Afghanistan in 2008.

Large inequities in child health also exist within countries. For example, in Bolivia and Peru the richest fifth have almost universal access to a skilled attendant at birth, compared with only 10% to 15% among the poorest fifth. Women in poor rural households accounted for two-thirds of unattended births.

How does the United States compare to the rest of the world with respect to child mortality rates and health inequities? While the United States has one of the world's highest expenditures on health ($7,285 per capita in 2007, United Nations Development Programme) it ranks among the poorest among highly developed nations with respect to its under-5 mortality rate (8 deaths per 1,000 live births), which is higher than rates in most of Europe, including countries with far fewer resources, such as Estonia, Croatia, and Hungary. Although the under-5 mortality rate in the United States has improved in recent decades, it is still higher than many other wealthy nations—2.3 times that of Iceland and more than 75% higher than the rate of the Czech Republic, Finland, Italy, Japan, Norway, Slovenia, and Sweden. Great health inequities are also apparent within the United States. Native American children ages 1 to 4 have the highest death rates (49 per 100,000), followed by African American children (46 per 100,000), while non-Hispanic white children have the lowest death rates (28 per 100,000).

It has been projected that policy interventions aimed at country-level inequities would have a major effect on the under-5 mortality rate for the country as a whole, even in low-inequality regions. Worldwide, about 40% of all under-5 deaths could be prevented by bringing rates in the poorest 80% of the population down to those of the richest 20%.

While the Institute of Medicine has defined GH to encompass "health problems, issues, and concerns that transcend national boundaries, and may best be addressed by cooperative actions and solutions," the World Health Organization has emphasized GH to signify health problems that impact global politics and economies, and arise from disparities in sociopolitical and economic status. Inequalities in health within and between countries arise from inequalities within and between societies. These disparities in social and economic conditions impact children's risk of illness as well as the actions that families take to prevent or treat illness when it occurs. Consequently, the emerging field of GH intersects medical and social science disciplines, such as demographics, economics, epidemiology, political economy, and sociology.

Integrating GH into Pediatrician Careers

The most vulnerable groups in a society are children, and the strongest medical advocate for the health of children is the pediatrician. Consequently, pediatricians have been leaders in addressing global and local health disparities, and their collective voice has been powerful. Global health work varies widely in scope and extent. The duration of GH activities ranges from singular short-term medical missions to long-term postings in resource-limited settings. Involvement in GH encompasses the direct provision of clinical services, technical assistance for program development, research, education and training of health care workers, and governmental advocacy for policy changes. The goals of GH activities range from forging novel directions in areas of basic sciences and epidemiological, clinical, and operations research, to addressing the needs of the world's poorest communities. Ideally, GH experiences should be transformative, both for the poor communities of the world, as well as for the clinicians who engage in these experiences.

By committing to a single international site—such as a hospital, rural clinic, or community—and by working with a partner based at that site, the pediatrician can engage in a longitudinal supportive relationship that is sustainable and effective. Pediatricians can also make a sustainable impression by empowering in-country partners through training of trainers, such as community health workers, supervisors, and clinicians responsible for health professional trainees.

Pediatricians have also played an important role in responding to humanitarian emergencies in the United States as well as in other countries, such as the aftermath of the Haiti earthquake. In addition, pediatricians with skills in research and evaluation may contribute to GH through clinical research and program evaluations.

Many GH opportunities do not require an overseas trip. While vulnerable populations and inequities to health certainly exist in low-income countries, significant inequities abound in the United States. Among developed countries, those with the highest health status have the lowest levels of health inequality. The United States ranks at the bottom of this list, with one of the poorest health rankings and the highest inequalities in health. Opportunities to carry out *local* GH work are plentiful and include supporting the care and resettlement of local refugee and immigrant families, supporting international adoptees, serving migrant farm workers, and supporting Native American health issues.

The pediatrician may also work locally for GH by advocating for equity of health care at all levels domestically and globally, working in the home office of a US-based GH organization, and providing expertise to support international organizations dedicated to vulnerable children. Finally, pediatricians can make a significant impact in GH by lobbying the US government for more international relief funding, or supporting corporations with ethical international trade practices.

Beyond the Hospitals—Global Public and Community Health, and Advocacy

As a growing number of US medical students and residents seek training opportunities in developing country settings, most of these trips are spent in a foreign hospital on a pediatric ward providing direct clinical care. In addition to observing and managing tropical diseases and more severe forms of commonly encountered pediatric conditions, visiting physicians and students learn and experience common themes in these low-resource settings: underpaid and under-trained health workers, hospital administration untrained in health management, dilapidated facilities, basic medicine shortage, lack of tools in testing and imaging, and higher mortality rates. Because the needs at such hospitals and clinics are glaring, the clinician instinctively seeks to fill the gaps with what defines quality health care in the United States—more medicines, equipment, clinical staffing (through visiting physicians), and perhaps training. However, the long-term impact of a brief visit, even repeated visits, may be further improved through efforts to prevent disease using public health approaches and focusing on communities.

With further training in areas such as public and community health or health service management, the pediatrician may act as an "agent of change" by undertaking systems-based quality improvement approaches, public health measures, and community-based strategies to have lasting positive impact on child health. Box 3-2 lists some key categories of GH organizations. In collaboration with community groups, the clinician or student can effectively empower community health workers and work within local community-based nongovernmental organizations (NGOs) to contribute to lasting and contextually appropriate change.

"Experiencing" how most of the world lives is a tremendous gift, honor, and burden that accompanies these experiences. Continuing to advocate for the children living in poverty in the world after returning from a short-term medical experience is a fantastic way to enact one's ongoing responsibility. Additionally, though perhaps less glamorous than traveling overseas, working within the US health care and political system to promote awareness for change has the potential to catalyze lasting and significant improvements in child health. Similarly, through work to empower local refugee communities in the United States or to advocate for more equitable access to health care for vulnerable immigrant children, pediatricians can make a significant and lasting difference in the efforts to close the gap in health disparities.

Ethical Issues in GH

The traditional model for medical experiences for US-based physicians presumes that in the United States we possess the knowledge, skills, and resources to improve the conditions of people living in developing countries. However, most students and physicians who have participated in such an experience report that the greatest benefit from such experiences is for themselves.

Though the desire to improve the conditions of children by providing clinical care is well-intentioned and altruistic, there is potential for both short- and long-term harm. In the short-term, caring for children in such settings with conditions that are unfamiliar to the visiting student or physician and out of the scope of their training can lead to errors in diagnosis and management. For students, often there is less supervision of their clinical work in these settings, which can result in harm to the patient and the student's growth as a clinician. In the long-term, provision of clinical care by visiting providers can undermine the existing health system infrastructure.

Box 3-2. Global Health (GH) Organizations— Some Examples
International Health or Multilateral Organizations
World Health Organization (WHO)
UNICEF
Bilateral Government Organizations
US Agency for International Development (USAID)
Centers for Disease Control and Prevention (CDC)
The Peace Corps
International Donor Foundations
Bill and Melinda Gates Foundation
Wellcome Trust
Children's Investment Fund Foundation (CIFF)
US-Based Nongovernmental Organizations (NGOs)
Partners in Health
Global Health Council
Save the Children
International NGOs
Specialized services and/or training—short-term service/training trips (eg, cleft palate repairs)
Emergency relief and rehabilitation
Doctors Without Borders (MSF)
International Committee of Red Cross
CARE International
Consultant Organizations—For-Profit and Not-for-Profit
Family Health International
John Snow International
• GH consultant organizations may take government contracts to provide international support
Faith-Based Organizations
World Vision
Aga Khan Foundation
American Friends Service Committee
Academic Institutions
An increasing number of academic institutions are developing GH programs in partnership with international groups, overseas academic institutions, or ministries of health.
Local and Domestic
GH advocacy organizations
Refugee resettlement agencies
Indian health services
Resources
Global Health Education Consortium (GHEC)
American Academy of Pediatrics Section on International Child Health (AAP-SOICH)
Physicians for Social Responsibility

As the number of US medical students, trainees, and physicians who visit developing countries for short-term training experiences continues to grow, concern for medical tourism and the long-term impact of these training experiences on the under-resourced hosts is rising. Key factors for ensuring effective, sustainable, and ethical international collaborations include forethought, planning, and long-term partnership.

Proper *pre-departure preparation and education* for any overseas medical experience is a critical first step. Proper education entails orientation regarding the country and its sociopolitical context and public health priorities. Knowledge of the key medical problems facing the communities as well as international and local treatment guidelines and strategies to deliver care within the confines of the existing local resources are also important.

Suchdev et al and others have outlined fundamentals for the creation of a meaningful international partnership with a community. The first step is the development of a *mission* or an identified shared purpose with the partners prior to visiting a new international site. Also, it is critical to establish a *collaboration* with a local agency, such as an NGO, governmental agency, or other local organization to promote sustainability and to enhance the effectiveness of the care delivered. Another important component for long-term impact and partnership is to ensure that the *education* of the community members, other physicians, and trainees is a part of the mission and that appropriate educational experiences are structured into the trip and planning. Closely related to this is the appreciation of the reciprocal nature of any education: The visiting physician is in a position to be learning just as much if not more than the local providers about working in the local setting.

A fourth fundamental for meaningful partnerships involves ensuring that *service* is truly being provided to the community by *learning about the health priorities* of the community from the NGO or other local agency. Also, it is important to encourage *teamwork* by working with appropriate supervision, including physicians from the host country. Effective international collaboration also requires sensitivity to the *costs and burden* that a visitor will have on the host. Finally, assurance of the partnership effectiveness requires building an *evaluation* process early on that incorporates the perspectives of all the players, including local officials, health professionals, and community members. This would include assessment of whether the educational objectives are being met for all stakeholders, including the host site.

CASE RESOLUTION

You learn about a US-based NGO with a long history of partnership and work in the earthquake-stricken country. You research that NGO further and find that it is a reputable group with long-term interests in the country. You speak to friends who have recently visited the country and learn more about what skills and resources are needed. You make arrangements to join a team of experienced health workers from the NGO by taking time from work and garnering support from your family to manage with your absence. You undergo an in-depth orientation of the site, the people, the sociopolitical situation, team roles, and expected activities through a series of discussions with all participants.

Selected References

Black RE, Cousens S, Johnson HL, et al. Global, regional, and national causes of child mortality in 2008: a systematic analysis. *Lancet.* 2010;375(9730):1969–1987

Rajaratnam JK, Marcus JR, Flaxman AD, et al. Neonatal, postneonatal, childhood, and under-5 mortality for 187 countries, 1970–2010: a systematic analysis of progress towards Millennium Development Goal 4. *Lancet.* 2010;375:1988–2008

Suchdev P, Ahrens K, Click E, Macklin L, Evanelista D, Graham E. A model for sustainable short-term international medical trips. *Ambul Pediatr.* 2007;7(4):317–320

United Nations Development Programme. *Human Development Report 2010—The Real Wealth of Nations: Pathways to Human Development.* Geneva, Switzerland: United Nations Development Programme; 2010

Victora CG, Wagstaff A, Schellenberg JA, Gwatkin D, Claeson M, Habicht JP. Applying an equity lens to child health and mortality: more of the same is not enough. *Lancet.* 2003;362:233–241

CHAPTER 4

Talking With Children

Geeta Grover, MD

CASE STUDY

The moment you walk into the examination room, the 2-year-old girl begins to cry and scream uncontrollably. She clings to her mother and turns her face away. The mother appears embarrassed and states that her daughter reacts to all physicians this way. After reassuring the mother that you have received such welcomes before, you sit down at a comfortable distance from the girl and her mother. You smile at the girl and compliment her on her dress, but she does not seem to be interested in interacting with you at this point. You begin your interview with the mother and try not to look at the girl. Out of the corner of your eye, you see that her crying is easing a bit and that she is looking at you very carefully. Without moving from your chair, you hand her your stethoscope with a clip-on toy teddy bear attached to it. She accepts it hesitantly and begins to examine it as you and the mother continue talking.

Questions

1. How does children's age influence their understanding of health and illness?
2. Should physicians speak directly with children about their illnesses?
3. At what age can children begin to communicate with physicians about their illnesses?
4. How can positioning and placement of children in the examination room affect the overall tone and quality of the visit?

Effective doctor–patient communication, which is difficult enough when patients are adults, becomes even more challenging when patients are children. In pediatrics, interviewing involves balancing the needs of both parents and children. Whereas parents may be more focused on issues pertaining to disease, treatment, or aspects of parenting, children look to physicians with different needs and concerns, depending on their age. To have a meaningful and satisfying exchange with children, pediatricians must take into account children's age, intelligence, and developmental maturity because all of these factors affect their concepts of health and illness. As children grow and develop, their understanding of health and illness increases.

Developmental Approach to Communicating With Children

An appreciation of the cognitive stages of development helps pediatricians develop a healthy relationship with their patients by allowing them to communicate with the children in an age-appropriate manner. Piaget defined 4 stages of cognitive development, which occur in the same sequence but not at the same rate in all children (Table 4-1). Children in the sensorimotor stage (birth–2 years of age) experience the world and act through sensations and motor acts. They are developing the concepts of object permanence, causality, and spatial relationships. Children in the preoperational stage (2–6 years) understand reality only from their own viewpoint. As egocentric thinkers, they are unable to separate internal from external reality, and fantasy play is important. School-aged children (6–11 years)

Table 4-1. Piaget's Stages of Cognitive Development		
Age[a]	*Stage*	*Characteristics*
Birth–2 y	Sensorimotor	Experiences world through sensations and motor acts
2–6 y	Preoperational	Egocentric thinking; imitation and fantasy play
6–11 y	Concrete operational	Mental processes only as they relate to real objects
>11 y	Formal operations	Capacity for abstract thought

[a] Approximate ages

are capable of concrete operational thinking. These children can reason through problems that relate to real objects. Older children (>11 years) have the capacity for abstract thought, which defines the stage of formal operations.

An appreciation of how children's cognitive development affects their understanding of illness and pain aids physicians in developing therapeutic relationships. Bibace and colleagues have outlined a developmental approach to children's understanding of illness: Children's explanations of illness are classified into 6 categories consistent with Piaget's cognitive developmental stages. Children 2 to 6 years of age view illness as caused by external factors near the body (phenomenism and contagion). Young children engage in so-called magical thinking; proximity alone provides the link between cause and illness. Children 7 to 10 years of age should be able to differentiate between self and nonself. At this stage they begin to understand that although illness may be caused by some factor outside the body, illness itself is located inside the body (contamination and internalization). Children older than 11 years understand physiological and psychophysiological explanations for illness (Table 4-2).

A similar developmental sequence applies to children's understanding of pain. Gaffney and Dunne have outlined a developmental approach to this understanding. Younger children may attribute pain to punishment for some transgression or wrongdoing on their part. They may not understand the relationship between pain and illness (eg, "Pain is something in my tummy."). Children with concrete operational thought can appreciate that pain and illness are related, but they may have no clear understanding of the causation of pain (eg, "Pain is a feeling you get when you are sick."). Older children and adolescents begin to understand the complex physical and psychological components of pain. For example, they realize that although the bone in the arm is broken, pain is ultimately felt in the head (eg, "Pain goes up some nerves from the broken bone in my arm to my head.").

Guidelines for Doctor–Child Communication

A developmental framework that takes into account children's language skills and causal reasoning abilities is essential in providing appropriate health care to children. Successful communication with children depends not only on spoken words but also nonverbal cues and the environment itself. A pleasant, child-friendly environment with bright colors, wall decorations, and toys helps make children feel more comfortable. Health care practitioners should be sincere, because children are extremely sensitive to nonverbal cues. Pediatricians should take a few minutes to enjoy children; this not only gives children a chance to evaluate their physicians, but also allows clinicians to begin assessing areas of development. A general principle of the pediatric examination is to begin with the least invasive portions of the examination (eg, heart, lungs, abdomen) and save the most invasive for last (eg, oropharynx, ears). Pediatricians should maintain their self-control in difficult situations. If they approach their limit, they should step outside for a few minutes or ask someone for assistance. Overall guidelines for communicating with children are provided in Box 4-1. Age-specific guidelines follow.

Birth to 6 Months

Examination of children of this age is usually pleasant. Although verbal interaction is limited, it is important to play with children, hold them, and talk to them. By watching physicians interact with their children, new parents have an opportunity to learn how to behave with their infants. Infants have not yet developed a fear of strangers and can usually be easily examined either in parents' arms or on the examination table.

7 Months to 3 Years

This is perhaps the most challenging age group with regard to developing rapport and performing examinations. After entering

Table 4-2. Children's Concepts of Illness[a]		
Age	**Concept of Illness**	**Example**
	Preoperational	*How do people get colds?*
2–6 y	Phenomenism	"From the sun."
	Contagion	"When someone else gets near them."
	Concrete Operational	*How do people get colds?*
7–10 y	Contamination	"You're outside without a hat and you start sneezing. Your head would get cold—the cold would touch it—and then it would go all over your body."
	Internalization	"In winter, people breathe in too much air into their nose and it blocks up the nose."
	Formal Operations	*How do people get colds?*
>11 y	Physiological/Psychophysiological	"They come from viruses, I guess."
		How do people get a heart attack?
		"It can come from being all nerve-racked. You worry too much, and the tension can affect your heart."

[a]Modified and reproduced with permission from Bibace R, Walsh ME. Development of children's concepts of illness. *Pediatrics.* 1980;66:912–917.

Box 4-1. Physician–Child Communication	
Dos	*Don'ts*
Provide a pleasant environment.	Limit the child's participation.
Pay attention to nonverbal cues.	Threaten the child.
Be sincere and honest.	Compare the child to others.
Enjoy the child.	Get into power struggles.
Speak age appropriately.	
Get down to the child's eye level.	
Examine from least to most invasive.	
Respect the child's privacy.	
Maintain self-control.	
Have a sense of humor.	

the examination room, pediatricians should take a few moments to converse or play with children. Such actions help put children at ease and allow them to get to know their doctors. Children who are 1 to 2 years of age will probably busy themselves, exploring the room during the history taking. By acknowledging them periodically, physicians build rapport that will help later during the examination. Two- to 3-year-old children are usually very apprehensive of the examination. Physicians should get down to children's eye level when speaking to them. Reassurances such as, "You're not going to get any shots today," can help alleviate their fears. Because stranger anxiety has developed, physicians should try to do as much of the examination as possible with children in parents' laps. Distractions such as stethoscope toys, flashing penlights, or keys may be helpful.

3 to 6 Years

Children's expressive capabilities are growing at tremendous rates during this period. Children can usually be engaged in conversation. They should be given repeated opportunities for participation, but they should not feel pressured to take part. Children may doubt physicians' true intentions and will probably only speak once their comfort level has been achieved. Children should be involved; they can be asked simple questions regarding their illness (eg, "Where does it hurt?"). In addition, children should be given some control during the examination (eg, "Should I look in your mouth next or your ears?"), and they should be allowed to handle physicians' equipment. Knowing what to expect next and having some control over the examination can help to decrease fear and increase cooperation.

7 to 11 Years

Examination of children in this age group can be rewarding. Physicians should make a point to speak directly with children and not just with parents concerning the chief complaint and history. Children can usually provide a good history regarding their illness, although their concept of time may be misleading. For example, a "long, long time" may mean hours, days, or months, and parents need to clarify this. Children should be asked about school, friends, and favorite activities. Answers to such questions give physicians an idea of children's social and emotional well-being, which may be affecting their physical health. Physicians sometimes overlook children's need for privacy at this age. Drapes should be used appropriately during the examination, and physicians should be sensitive to the presence of other children or adults in the room.

Physicians should begin to involve older children in the management of their illness. Children's understanding of their illness and its management should be assessed (eg, children with asthma could be asked, "What is this inhaler for? When are you going to use it? Show me how."). Children should be given an opportunity to express their fears and anxieties, and these concerns should be discussed (eg, "Asthma can be scary, especially when you can't catch your breath. Have you ever felt like that? Tell me about it."). Children should be involved in the management of their illness, which allows them to develop a sense of responsibility for their own health and medical care. Active participation in their health care visits leads to greater visit satisfaction, knowledge, and competence of prescribed medical therapies.

Older Than 12 Years

Communication with adolescents is discussed in detail in Chapter 6.

Barriers to Effective Communication With Children

The manner in which adults speak to children is influenced by what they think children can understand. Clinicians tend to overestimate the understanding capabilities of younger children and underestimate those of older children. Lack of appreciation for the cognitive sophistication of children may lead to frustration for all involved.

Younger children are presented with information they may not be able to comprehend, and older children may feel frustrated because they are being spoken to in a childlike manner.

Overestimating children's receptivity to medical information can be particularly problematic in the case of children with chronic illness. It is easy to assume that children with chronic medical conditions or those with more hospitalizations would have more sophisticated understanding regarding illness causation. Although these children may seem more savvy and knowledgeable regarding medical procedures, there is little research to support the assumption that they have more sophisticated understanding of illness causation than would be expected based on their age or developmental level, nor that they are better able to understand and retain medical information than their peers without chronic medical concerns.

Another potential barrier in communicating with children is limiting their participation. Physicians tend to elicit information from children but exclude them from diagnostic and management information. Older children want to know about their illness and are capable of learning about management.

All physicians have been frustrated or pushed to the limit at one time or another when working with children. In such situations, practitioners should remember that children are probably not trying to irritate physicians on purpose. Crying or lack of cooperation generally stems from fear or a sense of lack of control over the situation. Pediatricians should avoid taking part in a battle over power or control with children. Threatening remarks (eg, "If you're not good, I'll have to give you a shot.") or comparisons between children (eg, "Your brother is younger than you, and he didn't cry.") not only are ineffective but may make the situation worse. A clear perspective, empathy, and a sense of humor are much more useful.

CASE RESOLUTION

In the case presented in the opening scenario, you learn from the mother that her daughter has been in good health. The mother has brought in the child for a routine health maintenance visit. You assess that her development is normal and that her immunizations are up to date. As you and the mother talk, the child appears more relaxed and less frightened. She begins to respond to your questions and cooperate with the examination, but she chooses to remain on her mother's lap. Praising a child who is cooperative helps reinforce preferred behavior.

Selected References

Bibace R, Walsh ME. Development of children's concepts of illness. *Pediatrics.* 1980;66:912–917

Croom A, Wiebe DJ, Berg CA, et al. Adolescent and parent perceptions of patient-centered communication while managing type 1 diabetes. *J Pediatr Psychol.* 2011;36(2):206–215

Erickson SJ, Gerstle M, Feldstein SW. Brief interventions and motivational interviewing with children, adolescents, and their parents in pediatric health care settings; a review. *Arch Pediatr Adolesc Med.* 2005;159:1173–1180

Gaffney A, Dunne EA. Developmental aspects of children's definitions of pain. *Pain.* 1986;26:105–117

Ginsburg H, Opper S. *Piaget's Theory of Intellectual Development.* 3rd ed. Englewood Cliffs, NJ: Prentice-Hall; 1988

Myant KA, Williams JM. Children's concepts of health and illness: understanding of contagious illnesses, non-contagious illnesses and injuries. *J Health Psychol.* 2005;10:805–819

Nobile C, Drotar D. Research on the quality of parent-provider communication in pediatric care: implications and recommendations. *J Dev Behav Pediatr.* 2003;24:279–290

Perrin EC, Perrin JM. Clinicians' assessments of children's understanding of illness. *Am J Dis Child.* 1983;137:874–878

Tates K, Meeuwesen L. 'Let Mum have her say:' turn taking in doctor-parent-child communication. *Patient Educ Couns.* 2000;40:151–162

Van Dulmen AM. Children's contributions to pediatric outpatient encounters. *Pediatrics.* 1998;102:563–568

CHAPTER 5

Talking With Parents

Geeta Grover, MD

CASE STUDY

An 8-month-old boy with a 1-week history of cough and runny nose and a 2-day history of vomiting, diarrhea, and fever, with a temperature of 101°F (38.3°C) is evaluated in the emergency department (ED). The mother is very concerned because her son's appetite has decreased and he has been waking up several times at night for the last 2 days.

A nurse interrupts and says that paramedics are bringing a 5-year-old trauma victim to the ED. The appearance of the 8-month-old child is quickly assessed; he seems active and alert. Bilateral otitis media is diagnosed. Before leaving the examination room the physician says to the mother, "Your son has a viral syndrome and infection in his ears. I am going to prescribe an antibiotic that you can begin giving him today. Give him Tylenol as needed for the fever. Don't worry about his vomiting and diarrhea; just make sure that he drinks plenty of liquids and don't give him milk or milk products for a few days. Bring him back here or to his regular doctor if his fever persists, he doesn't eat, he has too much vomiting or diarrhea, he looks lethargic, or if he isn't better in 2 days."

Questions

1. How much information can most parents handle? Did this mother receive more information than she can be reasonably expected to remember?
2. How do you assess parental concerns? Did the physician address the mother's worries sufficiently?
3. How do you know whether a parent has understood all the information? Was this mother given a chance to clarify any questions she had?
4. What are some barriers to effective doctor–patient communication?
5. How does the setting itself influence communication?

Communication is the foundation of the therapeutic relationship between clinicians, patients, and their families. Effective communication in the pediatric setting involves the exchange of information between physicians, parents, and children. In addition, observing the interaction between parents and children gives physicians an opportunity to assess parenting skills and the dynamics of the parent child relationship. The communication needs of both parents and children are quite different; this makes the exchange of information challenging. Parental concerns should be addressed in a sensitive, empathetic, and nonjudgmental manner. A nonthreatening, pleasant demeanor and age-appropriate language help facilitate communication with children (see Chapter 4).

Pediatrics encompasses not only the traditional medical model of diagnosis and treatment of disease but also maintenance of the health and well-being of children through longitudinal care and the establishment of ongoing relationships between physicians and families. Personal relationships between physicians and families create an atmosphere in which information can be exchanged openly. The pediatrician's role in such relationships is to not only diagnose and treat, but also to listen, advise, guide, and teach.

The doctor–patient relationship is truly a privilege. Patients entrust physicians with their innermost thoughts and feelings, allow them to touch private parts of their bodies, and then trust them to perform invasive procedures or administer medications. Mutual respect is essential for the development of a healthy relationship between physicians, parents, and children. Through practice and continued awareness of interpersonal abilities, physicians can develop good communication skills. All physicians eventually develop their own personal interviewing and examination style. What seems awkward and difficult at first soon becomes routine and even enjoyable as physicians become more comfortable with patients.

Parental Concerns

Parents' preconceived ideas and concerns regarding their children's illnesses can greatly influence the exchange of information between physicians and patients. At health maintenance or well-child visits, it is important for pediatricians to address the nonmedical and psychosocial concerns of parents, such as their children's development, nutrition, and growth. Often these questions stem from discussions with other parents or information received through the media. Although such concerns may seem trivial to pediatricians, they may be extremely important to parents. In addition to addressing the needs of the child, the health maintenance visit also gives the pediatrician an opportunity to assess and address parental needs. Parental depression, substance abuse, family violence, or marital discord can all have profound effects on children's health and development. When evaluating children brought in for illness, it is important to ask parents what concerns them the most. Parental fears may be much different than medical concerns. Failure to give parents the opportunity to ask questions or to address these concerns in a sensitive manner may lead to dissatisfaction and poor communication.

The Pediatric Interview

Pediatric interviews are conducted in a variety of settings for many different reasons. The first interaction between the physician and parents may be during the prenatal interview before the birth of the child, in the hospital following the delivery, or in the doctor's office during the well-baby visit. Later, the physician may see children in the office for regular health maintenance visits or in the office, ED, or hospital for an acute illness.

The specific clinical situation dictates the information that needs to be gathered and the appropriate interviewing techniques. During the prenatal visit, physicians should discuss common concerns and anxieties about the new baby with prospective parents. In addition, parents have an opportunity to interview physicians and evaluate their offices and staff.

In the emergency setting, physicians must elicit pertinent information needed to make decisions regarding management within a short period. Absence of long-term relationships can make communication in the ED particularly challenging. Focused, closed-ended questions should be used primarily. The periodic health maintenance visit is at the opposite end of this spectrum. Here the use of broad, open-ended questions is more appropriate; closed-ended questions should be used as needed for clarification.

Communication Guidelines

Overall principles, applicable regardless of the setting, include interacting with the child and family in a professional yet sensitive and nonjudgmental manner. Common courtesies, such as knocking before entering the room, dressing and behaving in a professional manner, introducing oneself, and addressing parents and children by their preferred names, are always appreciated and welcomed. Taking a few moments to socialize with families develops a more personal relationship that may allow more open conversation about sensitive and emotional issues.

Family-centered care is an approach to health care in which the practitioner realizes the vital role that families play in ensuring the health and well-being of children. Family-centered care practitioners convey respect for parents' insight into and understanding of their children's behavior and needs and actively seek out their observations and incorporate their family preferences into the care plan as much as possible. Benefits of family-centered care include a stronger alliance between the practitioner and the family; increased patient, family, and professional satisfaction; and decreased health care costs.

The medical visit may be divided into 3 parts: the interview, the physical examination, and the concluding remarks. Examples of doctor–parent and doctor–child communications for each of these components are given in Table 5-1.

The Interview

The goal of the interview is to ascertain the chief complaint and determine the appropriate medical history. The interview usually begins with open-ended questions to give parents and children an opportunity to discuss their concerns and outline their agenda for the visit. Not uncommonly, the real reason for the visit may not be disclosed until the family believes the physician is trustworthy and honest. Once the issues have been laid out, closed-ended questions can be used to clarify and further define the information presented. It often becomes necessary to guide the interview, especially when parents have several broad issues on their agenda for that visit and time does not permit their discussion.

Physicians should gently acknowledge parental concerns and define time limitations. These actions allow physicians to focus on the most salient issues of that visit. Physicians should limit their use of medical jargon (scientific terms) and be aware of nonverbal communication. Practitioners should empathize with parents; this makes them feel that their situation is truly understood even if physicians can do very little to help them. Pauses and silent periods should be used, especially when discussing emotionally difficult issues, to convey to parents and children that their physician cares enough to listen. Physicians should not underrate their own knowledge, but at the same time they should recognize their limitations and use consultants appropriately. Finally, physicians' understanding of the chief complaint and history should be summarized so parents have an opportunity to clarify points of disagreement.

Today there are increasing demands for primary care practitioners to address not only the physical but also the psychosocial health needs of their patients. Patient-centered care is a comprehensive approach to medical care that encourages communication between physicians, patients, and their families. Clinicians address the immediate pressing medical concerns in the context of each patient's unique environmental circumstances and underlying psychosocial concerns, both of which may directly or indirectly affect health-related outcomes. Empathy, unconditional positive regard, and genuineness are essential clinician characteristics in this collaborative approach. Motivational interviewing (MI) is one such patient-centered, collaborative, and directive interaction style that offers an effective means of addressing these developmental, behavioral, and social concerns within the context of a primary care setting. Motivational interviewing addresses the ambivalence and discrepancies between a person's current values and behaviors and their future goals. In contrast to more traditional medical approaches that rely primarily on authority and education, MI is a collaborative approach that relies on elicitation of the patient's ideas regarding change. Motivational interviewing practitioners understand that trying to move beyond a patient's readiness to change is likely to increase their resistance to treatment (eg, lecturing to an adolescent who is not yet ready to quit smoking about the dangers of smoking is unlikely to be effective and may even produce more resistance). Motivational interviewing requires that the practitioner

Table 5-1. Communication Guidelines and Techniques	
Techniques	*Examples*
The Interview	
Open-ended questions	"How is Susie?"
Closed-ended questions	"Does she have a cough?"
Repetition of important phrases	"She has had a high fever for four days now?"
Clarification	"What do you mean by 'Susie was acting funny'?"
Pauses and silent periods	
Limit medical jargon	"Susie has an ear infection." vs "Susie has otitis media."
Guide the interview	"Right now I am most interested in hearing about the symptoms of this illness."
Be aware of nonverbal communication	Use eye contact and phrases such as "I see."
Acknowledge parental concerns	"Worrying about hearing loss is understandable."
Empathize	"A fever of 104°F can be very frightening."
Remember common courtesies	Knock before entering.
Recognize personal limitations	"I am not an expert in this area. I would like to consult with a colleague."
Summarize	"So she has had fever for four days but the rash and cough began one week ago?"
The Physical Examination	
Show consideration for the child	"It's OK to be afraid."
Inform	"That took me some time, but her heart sounds normal."
Explain procedures	"You may feel a little uncomfortable during the rectal examination."
Avoid exclamations	"Wow! I have never seen anything like this."
Concluding Remarks	
Provide closure	"Our time is over today. May we discuss this at the next visit?"
Minimize discharge instructions	
Be specific	"I am going to treat her with amoxicillin." vs "I'll prescribe an antibiotic."
Praise	"You're doing a great job."
Confirm parental understanding	"Please repeat for me Susie's diagnosis and treatment instructions so I'm sure I've been clear in explaining them to you."

follow 4 principles (Table 5-2). Operationally, open-ended questions (eg, "How do you feel about smoking?"), affirmations (eg, "You are tired of having to monitor your blood sugar every day and stick to your diet."), and reflective listening (eg, "You are worried about your daughter's behavior and are concerned that if it persists, she may be expelled from school.") are important tools of MI. In addition, MI practitioners ask permission before giving advice (eg. "Would it be OK if I shared some information with you?"), or the practitioner may state the facts but let the parent interpret the information (eg, "What does this mean to you?"). Motivational interviewing is not only effective with adults, but research with adolescents has shown MI to be an effective tool to increase self-efficacy to enact change (eg, adolescent smoking cessation).

The Physical Examination

Parents keenly observe physicians' interactions with their children during the examination. It is an important time for physicians to

Table 5-2. Principles of Motivational Interviewing[a]	
Principle	*Example*
Express empathy.	Use reflective listening.
Develop discrepancy between patient's current behavior and his treatment goal.	Patient, not practitioner, presents arguments for change.
Roll with the patient's resistance.	Avoid arguing for change.
Support the patient's self-efficacy.	Patient's own belief in the possibility of change is an important motivator.

[a]Adapted from Miller WR, Rollnick S. *Motivational Interviewing: Preparing People for Change.* 2nd ed. New York, NY: Guilford Press; 2002.

build a therapeutic relationship with children (see Chapter 4). The transition between the history and physical examination can be made by briefly telling children and parents what to expect during the examination. Practitioners should show consideration for children's fears. Clinicians often find it helpful to speak with families at periodic intervals during the examination regarding their observations. Prolonged periods of silence as the doctor listens or palpates may be anxiety provoking for families. Physicians should be sure to explain any procedures that either they or their staff are going to perform at a level that is appropriate for both parents and children. In addition, physicians should try to avoid exclamations or comments to themselves during the examination (eg, "Wow, that's some murmur!"), which may be alarming to families.

Concluding Remarks

This portion of the visit, which is all too easy to rush through, is extremely important. Closure can be provided by either summarizing the diagnosis or outlining plans for the following visit. Parents should be asked to participate by acknowledging closure and helping to develop a management plan. It is important to assess parental readiness for knowledge (especially in emotionally difficult situations) and keep family resources and limitations in mind. Discharge instructions should be minimized; physicians should be specific; and the number of diagnoses, medications, and "as needed" instructions (indications for seeking medical advice such as "return as needed for high fever") should be limited. When complicated discharge instructions are given, additional physician time may be required to ensure parental understanding. Praising parents on their care of their children can boost their self-esteem and confidence and may minimize calls and questions. Parental understanding should be confirmed; parents should be asked to repeat the diagnosis and treatment plan. Simply asking parents if they have understood is not enough, because parents often say "yes" out of respect for the physician's time or embarrassment that they have not understood what has been said. For example, the physician could say, "I want to be sure that I've spoken clearly enough. Please repeat for me [child's name] diagnosis and treatment instructions."

Barriers to Effective Communication

Barriers to effective communication may be divided into systems barriers and interpersonal barriers (Table 5-3). The primary systems barriers are the setting itself and lack of continuity of care. Because of access problems within the health care system (ie, lack of health insurance coverage), many children receive only episodic

care from different physicians in acute care clinics or EDs. Without the benefit of long-term relationships, doctor–patient communication may suffer.

Interpersonal barriers include physician time constraints, frequent interruptions, and cultural insensitivity. Frequent interruptions or apparent impatience on the part of physicians conveys to parents and children that either they do not care or they are too busy for them. Language differences may pose a significant barrier depending on the region in which physicians practice. Ideally, physicians themselves should be able to speak with parents and children. If translators must be used, children should not play this role, if possible, because this places them in an awkward situation. Parents of other patients should not be used because this violates patients' privacy. Physicians should be sensitive to cultural differences (eg, gender issues, views on illness, folk remedies, and beliefs). Suggesting treatments that are not culturally acceptable or are contrary to folk wisdom simply decreases compliance with prescribed treatment plans. For example, many Eastern cultures believe in the concept of "hot" and "cold" foods and illnesses. Suggesting to a mother that she feed primarily "hot" foods to a child she believes to have an illness that is also "hot" may not be acceptable to her. Such information is rarely volunteered and must be elicited through sensitive patient interviewing.

Effective communication is not only essential for accurate diagnosis, but also correlates with improved patient recall of instructions and adherence to prescribed courses of treatment. Poor communication can have negative consequences for both the patient (eg, compromised care) and for the practitioner (eg, medicolegal consequences).

CASE RESOLUTION

The doctor–patient interaction presented in the case history lacks several of the points discussed here. The physician did not acknowledge parental concerns or make sure that the mother had understood the diagnosis and treatment plan. The mother was presented with more information than she could have reasonably been asked to remember. This interaction could have been improved (1) if the physician conveyed to the mother that her concerns were appreciated and (2) then reassured her that her child was going to be all right. Furthermore, the physician could have told the mother the name and dosage schedule of the antibiotic to be prescribed and limited the number of "as needed" instructions.

Table 5-3. Barriers to Effective Communication	
Barriers	*Examples*
Systems	
Lack of continuity of care	Episodic care that is primarily illness driven
The setting itself	Emergency departments and acute care clinics
Interpersonal	
Physician time constraints	Appearing impatient or preoccupied
Frequent interruptions	Beeper goes off or asked to come to the phone
Cultural insensitivity	Suggesting treatments that are not acceptable within the family's belief systems

Selected References

American Academy of Pediatrics. *Bright Futures: Guidelines for Health Supervision of Infants, Children, and Adolescents.* Elk Grove Village, IL: American Academy of Pediatrics; 2008

American Academy of Pediatrics Committee on Hospital Care. Family-centered care and the pediatrician's role. *Pediatrics.* 2003;112:691–696

American Academy of Pediatrics Committee on Psychosocial Aspects of Child and Family Health. The new morbidity revisited: a renewed commitment to the psychosocial aspects of pediatric care. *Pediatrics.* 2001;108:1227–1230

Dixon SD, Stein MT. *Encounters with Children: Pediatric Behavior and Development.* 4th ed. Chicago, IL: Mosby-Year Book; 2006

Erickson S, Gerstle M, Feldstein S. Brief interventions and motivational interviewing with children, adolescents and their parents in pediatric health care settings. *Arch Pediatr Adolesc Med.* 2005;159:1173–1180

Grover G, Berkowitz CD, Lewis RJ. Parental recall after a visit to the emergency department. *Clin Pediatr.* 1994;33:194–201

Korsch BM, Freemon BF, Negrete VF. Practical implications of doctor-patient interaction analysis for pediatric practice. *Am J Dis Child.* 1971;12:110–114

Levetown M; American Academy of Pediatrics Committee on Bioethics. Communication with children and families: from everyday interactions to skill in conveying distressing information. *Pediatrics.* 2008:121:e1441–e1460

Miller WR, Rollnick S. *Motivational Interviewing: Preparing People for Change.* 2nd ed. New York, NY: Guilford Press; 2002

Regalado MG, Halfon N. Parenting: issues for the pediatrician. *Pediatr Ann.* 1998;27:31–37

Young KT, Davis K, Schoen C, Parker S. Listening to parents: a national survey of parents with young children. *Arch Pediatr Adolesc Med.* 1998;152:255–262

CHAPTER 6

Talking With Adolescents

Monica Sifuentes, MD

CASE STUDY

This is a first-time visit for a 15-year-old girl who is accompanied by her mother. The mother is concerned because her daughter's grades have been dropping since beginning high school, and she appears fatigued and irritable. The mother reports no new activities or recent changes in the home situation and no new stressors in the family. Both parents are employed, the girl has the same friends she has always had, and her siblings currently are doing well academically. The girl is healthy and has never been hospitalized. After the mother leaves the room, the girl is interviewed alone.

Questions

1. When interviewing adolescents, what is the significance of identifying their stage of development?
2. What are important areas to cover in the adolescent interview?
3. What issues of confidentiality and competence need to be discussed with adolescents before conducting the interview?
4. When should information be disclosed to others, despite issues of confidentiality?

Adolescence is a time of unique change. Unlike other periods in life when individuals have at least some knowledge or experience to guide them, adolescence can be characterized by feelings of physical awkwardness, emotional turmoil, and social isolation. In addition, the teenage years are dreaded by most parents, who often feel ill equipped to handle the wide range of children's responses. So instead of "taking the bull by the horns," parents choose the route of quiet observation. They fully intend to "be there" for their children but wait to be approached. Hence, many adolescents do not have the guidance or advice of parents during the teenage years and prefer to spend their time alone or in the company of friends or acquaintances. Fortunately, most adolescents pass through this period uneventfully. In fact, many individuals go through this period gladly, finally being permitted to drive a car or go out on a date.

Physicians must use a different approach when interviewing adolescents because information comes directly from the teenager, rather than the parents. Unlike an interview with a younger pediatric patient, the adolescent interview should focus on several psychosocial issues that may be uncomfortable to discuss with the parent present. Each teenager should therefore be interviewed alone. The goal of the interview is to discover any problems that might interfere with a relatively smooth passage through adolescence.

Stages of Adolescence

Adolescents are stereotypically labeled as difficult, complex, time-consuming patients with complicated problems or complaints that lead to uninteresting diagnoses. In addition, they are often accompanied by overbearing, demanding parents, or sometimes no parents at all.

The quality and quantity of information obtained during the medical and psychosocial interview can be greatly enhanced by taking developmental milestones into consideration. Adolescence can be divided into 3 developmental stages: early, middle, and late (Table 6-1). For example, interest in discussing long-term educational goals varies depending on the age of the adolescent. Most 18-year-olds are prepared to discuss college plans, specific vocational interests, and employment opportunities. In contrast, 12-year-olds are still anchored in the concreteness of early adolescence and often are ill prepared to discuss plans for higher education. Current school experiences are much more important to this age group and should therefore be the focus of discussion. Peer pressure is most prominent during middle adolescence; therefore, 14-year-olds with friends who smoke cigarettes and drink beer probably use the same illicit substances.

Table 6-1. Developmental Milestones During Adolescence[a]			
	Early Adolescence (11–13 y)	*Middle Adolescence (14–16 y)*	*Late Adolescence (17–21 y)*
Thought processes	Concrete	± Abstract	Abstract
Parental supervision	+	±	−
Risk-taking behavior	+	±	−
Peer pressure	±	++	+

[a]Modified from March CA, Jay MS. Adolescents in the emergency department: an overview. *Adolesc Med State Art Rev.* 1993;4:1.

Knowledge of these developmental differences allows the interviewer to more effectively explain instructions and diagnoses to teenagers. For example, 19-year-olds can better understand the effects of untreated or recurrent chlamydia cervicitis on long-term fertility than 13-year-olds. This is not to say that physicians should not discuss these possible consequences with a sexually active 13-year-old with chlamydia, but they should use more concrete wording and repeat the information at future visits. Age guidelines are not rigid, however, and each interview should be individually tailored to the particular adolescent and the circumstances surrounding the visit.

Issues of Confidentiality and Competence

A discussion regarding **confidentiality is essential** and can be approached in 2 ways. Each method has distinct advantages as well as disadvantages. Interviewers should use the approach that they find most comfortable; this allows conversation to flow more naturally.

The first approach involves informing adolescents at the beginning of the interview that most issues discussed are held in strict confidence and will not be repeated to anyone. Exceptions are suicidal or homicidal behavior and a history of or ongoing sexual or physical abuse. In any of these instances, other professionals are told of the disclosed information, and parents ultimately are informed of the disclosure. The advantages to this approach are that discussion of these "logistics" at the beginning of the interview is less awkward, making the ground rules clear from the start. This contributes to an atmosphere of trust and honesty. The disadvantage is possible inhibition by adolescents who are unsure about disclosing particular incidents (eg, those concerning sexual abuse); some teenagers are now almost certain not to share this information for fear of involving other professionals or family members. Interviewers should be nonjudgmental, reassuring, and empathetic to reduce the possibility of such an occurrence.

The second, less popular approach to the discussion of confidentiality involves informing adolescents at the end of the interview or when and if one of the exceptions to maintaining confidentiality arises. Proponents of this approach argue that adolescents tend to respond more honestly to questions when they do not believe physicians will inform others, including their parents or legal guardians. Physicians have a legal responsibility, however, to report sexual and physical abuse; in cases of suicidal or homicidal behavior, it is in the patient's best interest to inform other professionals of this disclosure. The disadvantage to this method is that these issues often arise at very emotional times during the interview, and it is difficult to interrupt the patient to discuss mandated reporting. If physicians wait until the end of the interview to inform adolescents about mandated reporting, however, patients may leave the office feeling deceived and probably will not return for future visits. For this reason, most health care providers prefer to inform adolescents at the onset of the interview about confidentiality with the hope that it contributes to the development of a trusting relationship.

An assessment of the adolescent's ability to make health-related decisions is another important aspect of the interview. **Competence** is the ability to understand the significance of information and assess the alternatives and consequences sufficiently to then identify a preference. Various factors besides age must be considered, such as level of maturity, intelligence, degree of independence, and presence of any chronic illness. This last factor is included because adolescents with chronic conditions may have already participated in decisions regarding their health care. Regardless, it can be difficult to assess competence from just one visit. It may not even be necessary to make an assessment emergently, except in certain cases such as with unplanned pregnancy.

Although it is imperative to interview adolescents alone, every attempt should be made to involve parents in all health-related decisions. Although specific state laws allow physicians to treat minors in emergent situations and in cases of suspected sexually transmitted infections (STIs) without parents' consent, physicians should urge adolescents to inform their parents of any problems disclosed during the interview. The ultimate decision, however, rests with the adolescent. Physicians can assist adolescents to discuss delicate issues with their parents by role-playing with the teenager or by sitting in on the conversation between the adolescent and the parent.

Psychosocial Review of Systems

A major part of the adolescent interview involves taking an adequate psychosocial history, which can be completed in 20 to 30 minutes in most cases. The approach, known by the acronym **HEADDSSS** (*h*ome *e*nvironment, *e*mployment and *e*ducation, *a*ctivities, *d*iet, *d*rugs, *s*exual activity/sexuality, *s*uicide/*d*epression, *s*afety), allows interviewers to evaluate the critical areas in adolescents' lives that may contribute to a less than optimal environment for normal growth and development (Questions Box). Questions about sexuality must be asked in a nondirected, nonjudgmental fashion, giving adolescents time to respond. This information is useful to assess risks for conditions such as STIs, including HIV. In addition, an inquiry about both sexual and physical abuse is indicated during this part of the interview.

Since many adolescents now have access to the internet 24/7 via their cellular telephone or home computer, it is important to discuss "screen time" with them and their parents. In addition to reviewing the amount of time actually spent on the computer each day, the health care provider also should inquire about texting, sexting, and whether the patient is a victim of cyberbullying.

Issues That Need Immediate Attention

Many issues discussed during the psychosocial interview can be a source of anxiety for adolescents. Certain problems must be taken more seriously than others, and may demand immediate attention. Suicidal ideation, with or without a previous attempt, definitely requires a more in-depth analysis of the gravity of the problem. Physicians should make sure that adolescents feel they can make

Talking With Adolescents: HEADDSSS[a]

H: Home environment

- With whom does the adolescent live?
- Have there been any recent changes in the living situation?
- How are things between parents?
- Are the parents employed?
- How does the adolescent get along with the parent and siblings?

E: Employment and education

- Is the adolescent currently in school?
- What are his or her favorite subjects?
- How is the adolescent performing academically?
- Has the adolescent ever been truant or expelled from school?
- Are the adolescent's friends attending school?
- Is the adolescent currently employed? How many hours does he or she work each week?
- What are the adolescent's future education/employment goals?

A: Activities

- What does the adolescent do in his or her spare time?
- How much time is spent on the computer and cell phone?
- What does the adolescent do for fun? Is the adolescent ever bored?
- With whom does the adolescent spend most of his or her time?

D: Diet

- What is a typical meal for the adolescent?
- Does the adolescent have any food restrictions?
- What does the adolescent think about his or her current weight and shape?
- Is there a recent history of weight loss?

D: Drugs

- Is the adolescent currently using, or has he or she ever used, tobacco?
- Is the adolescent currently using, or has he or she ever used, any illicit drugs? What about steroids? Alcohol?
- Does the adolescent ever feel pressured by friends to use drugs or alcohol?

S: Sexual activity/sexuality

- What is the adolescent's sexual orientation?
- Is the adolescent sexually active?
- If so, what was the age of the adolescent's sexual debut?
- How many sexual partners has the adolescent had in his or her lifetime?
- Does the adolescent have a history of sexually transmitted infections?
- Does the adolescent (or the partner) use condoms?
- Does the adolescent (or the partner) use other methods of contraception?
- Does the adolescent have a history of sexual or physical abuse?

S: Suicide/depression

- Is the adolescent bored all the time? Ever sad or tearful? Tired and unmotivated?
- Has the adolescent ever felt that life is not worth living or ever thought of or tried to hurt himself or herself? More importantly, does the adolescent have a suicide plan or access to a firearm?

S: Safety

- Does the adolescent use a seat belt and bicycle helmet?
- Does the adolescent participate in high-risk situations, such as riding in the car with someone who has been drinking?
- Does the adolescent feel safe at home? At school? In his or her neighborhood?
- Is there a firearm in the adolescent's home? If so, what does the adolescent know about firearm safety?

For more detailed information, see the Goldenring entries under Selected References

[a] Reprinted with permission from Goldenring JM, Rosen DS. Getting into adolescent heads: an essential update. *Contemp Pediatr.* 2004;21:64. Copyright © Advanstar Communications.

---

verbal contact and call someone if they feel like hurting themselves. Mental health professionals should be involved in the clinical assessment of these situations. Other issues that require immediate attention include possible danger to others, possible or confirmed unplanned pregnancy, and sexual or physical abuse.

Concluding the Interview

The adolescent interview should be conducted at a time when the adolescent is relatively healthy and the interviewer has set aside ample time for a thorough, uninterrupted discussion. However, all topics need not be addressed during the initial interview if time does not permit. Issues that are not covered at this visit can be addressed at the next one. The number of appointments needed to work through or solve a particular problem is unlimited.

At the end of each visit, the interview should be summarized; any difficult topics should be mentioned, and the issue of confidentiality should be reviewed. Adolescents should then be asked to identify a person whom they can trust or confide in should any problems arise before the next visit. In some instances, this issue may already have been discussed during the interview. Adolescents also should be given the opportunity to express any other concerns not covered in the interview and ask additional questions.

Physicians should clearly point out to the adolescent any significant risk factors or risk-taking behaviors that have been identified during the interview and assess the teenager's readiness to change this behavior. For those adolescents who are not engaging in high-risk behaviors, physicians should acknowledge that things seem to be going well, praise them with positive feedback, and review their individual strengths and accomplishments that have been discussed. Available resources, such as teen hotlines and popular Web sites, should be given to the adolescent prior to inviting the parent or guardian back into the examination room. General concerns should then be reviewed with the parent while maintaining the adolescent's confidentiality. The follow-up visit should be arranged at that time.

CASE RESOLUTION

The adolescent in the case history initially should be informed about confidentiality and the specific exceptions to maintaining it. Nonthreatening topics, such as home life, school, and outside activities, should be explored first, followed by questions regarding sexuality, sexual activity, and illicit drug use. Suicidal behavior or depression and safety issues should also be reviewed with the teenager alone. In addition, computer and cell phone use should be evaluated. High-risk behaviors and their consequences should be discussed with the adolescent at the end of the interview, and a plan for future visits should be arranged.

Selected References

Akinbami LJ, Gandhi H, Cheng TL. Availability of adolescent health services and confidentiality in primary care practices. *Pediatrics.* 2003;111:394–401

Bravender T, Price CN, English A. Primary care providers' willingness to see unaccompanied adolescents. *J Adolesc Health.* 2004;34:30–36

Breuner CC, Moreno MA. Approaches to the difficult patient/parent encounter. *Pediatrics.* 2011;127:163–169

Cavanaugh RM. Managing the transitions of early adolescents. *Adolesc Health Update.* 2008;20:1–10

English A, Kenney KE. *State Minor Consent Laws: A Summary.* 3rd ed. Chapel Hill, NC: Center for Adolescent Health and the Law; 2010

Ford C, English A, Sigman G. Confidential health care for adolescents: position paper for the Society for Adolescent Medicine. *J Adolesc Health.* 2004;35:160–167

Ford CA, English A. Limiting confidentiality of adolescent health services: what are the risks? *JAMA.* 2002;288:752–753

Ginsburg KR. Viewing our adolescent patients through a positive lens. *Contemp Pediatr.* 2007;24:65–76

Goldenring JM, Cohen E. Getting into adolescent heads. *Contemp Pediatr.* 1988;5:75–90

Goldenring JM, Rosen DS. Getting into adolescent heads: an essential update. *Contemp Pediatr.* 2004;21:64–90

Green M, Sullivan P, Eichberg C. Avoid a "swiss cheese" history when psychosocial complaints are on the menu. *Contemp Pediatr.* 2002;19:115–125

Gutgesell ME. Issues of adolescent psychological development in the 21st century. *Pediatr Rev.* 2004;25:79–84

Hawkins JD, Smith BH, Catalano RF. Delinquent behavior. *Pediatr Rev.* 2002;23:387–392

Knight JR, Sherritt L, Shrier LA, Harris SK, Chang G. Validity of the CRAFFT substance abuse screening test among adolescent clinic patients. *Arch Pediatr Adolesc Med.* 2002;156:607–614

Kokotailo PK, Gold MA. Motivational interviewing with adolescents. *Adolesc Med.* 2008;19:54–68

Kreipe RE. Introduction to interviewing: the art of communicating with adolescents. *Adolesc Med.* 2008;19:1–17

Ott MA, Labbett RL, Gold MA. Counseling adolescents about abstinence in the office setting. *J Pediatr Adolesc Gynecol.* 2007;20:39–44

Resnick MD. Protective factors, resiliency and healthy youth development. *Adolesc Med.* 2000;11:157–165

Sieving RE, Oliphant JA, Blum RW. Adolescent sexual behavior and sexual health. *Pediatr Rev.* 2002;23:407–416

Van Hook S, Harris SK, Brooks T, et al. The "Six T's": barriers to screening teens for substance abuse in primary care. *J Adolesc Health.* 2007;40:456–461

CHAPTER 7

Telephone Management

Iris Wagman Borowsky, MD, PhD

CASE STUDY

The mother of an otherwise healthy 10-month-old girl calls and tells you that her daughter has a fever. The girl's rectal temperature has been 103°F to 104°F (39.4°C–40.0°C) for the past 2 days. Although she is cranky with the fever, she plays normally after receiving acetaminophen. The girl is eating well and has no runny nose, cough, vomiting, diarrhea, or rash.

Questions

1. How do telephone and face-to-face encounters between physicians and patients differ?
2. What are some general guidelines for effective doctor–patient communication over the telephone?
3. What historical information is necessary for appropriate telephone management?
4. What points are important to cover in-home treatment advice?

Parents frequently call their pediatricians seeking medical advice about their children. It is estimated that pediatricians spend more than 25% of their total practice time engaged in telephone medicine. Telephone medicine serves 2 purposes: (1) it provides a service and (2) it controls costs and overcrowding by reducing unnecessary visits to the office and emergency department (ED). Most calls concern upper respiratory symptoms, fever, rash, trauma, or gastrointestinal complaints—the same problems most commonly seen in the office. In addition to acute illness care, triage, and advice, telephone care services provided by pediatricians include chronic disease management, care coordination, patient education, counseling, test result interpretation, illness follow-up, adherence checks, and medication adjustments.

Telephone management of illnesses differs in that it requires pediatricians to give advice based on history alone and precludes the opportunity to see the child, much less do a careful physical examination. For example, a practitioner in the ED who does not know the patient or family may choose to see the child if questions about the child's general health or the feasibility of continued contact with the family arise. On the other hand, a primary care physician who knows the patient and family and can follow the child's progress by telephone may advise home management for a child with a similar history. Pediatric practice settings, whether in an ED or primary care office, should have an organized approach to telephone care. In addition to physicians, nurse practitioners, and physician assistants, telephone care systems may include trained and supervised nurses and nonmedical office staff using protocols.

Telephone Communication Skills

Parents commonly call their pediatricians because they are worried about their child. The friendly voice of a health care worker who is ready to lend an ear goes a long way toward reassuring an anxious parent. Calls should begin with a "verbal handshake." Staff should identify themselves and the place where the call is received and offer to help. They should learn the caller's name, his or her relationship to the child, and the child's name and gender; these names, as well as the child's gender, should be used in the conversation, thereby creating a more personal atmosphere.

Telephone calls for medical advice are often received in busy environments, such as EDs or clinics, where patients are waiting to be seen. It is easy to be abrupt under these circumstances and not give complete attention to callers. If calls are not emergencies, practitioners can take the caller's telephone number and return the call as soon as possible. If callers do not feel that their concerns have been fully acknowledged, they are likely to feel dissatisfied, even if they are given sound advice. Furthermore, research on doctor–patient relationships suggests that lack of friendliness or warmth in the doctor–patient relationship and patient dissatisfaction are associated with noncompliance with medical advice. Studies show that the length of a patient visit does not correlate with patient satisfaction. Telephone encounters do not necessarily have to be lengthy; the average length of a call is reported to be 3 to 5 minutes, depending on the setting. Calls must be pleasant, however, and they must address callers' concerns. Open-ended questions such as "Tell me about your child's illness" or "Are there any other symptoms?" are useful at the beginning of a call because they give callers an opportunity to explain the situation without interruptions.

Establishing rapport over the telephone is more difficult than in person because the practitioner is limited to verbal communication. In face-to-face encounters, physicians can use words as well as means of nonverbal communication, such as facial expressions, eye contact, gesturing, and touch, to convey warmth and empathy. Practitioners should use various aspects of **verbal communication** to convey sincere interest in callers' concerns, and they should pay attention to these verbal cues in callers. Many components of verbal communication (in addition to words themselves), including vocal expression, pace, articulation, tone, volume, and pauses, affect telephone interactions. Health care professionals should speak clearly and use vocabulary that callers understand; **medical jargon should be avoided.** A friendly yet respectful tone and a calm, professional manner should be maintained.

Careful listening is crucial to obtaining the information necessary to make medical decisions over the telephone. One of the major goals of health care professionals is to recognize and respond to callers' main concerns and expectations. This can be difficult because most callers do not specifically tell their major concerns to their physicians. Researchers have found the following questions useful in the identification of parents' chief concerns: "What worries you the most about [use child's name] illness?" and "Why does that worry you?"

For callers who ramble, health care professionals may need to focus the conversation. Asking the question "What can I do to help?" should clarify the reason for the call. If information needs to be verified, practitioners can summarize what they have heard and ask if they have understood correctly.

Angry callers may elicit defensive or confrontational behavior from health care professionals. Responding to anger with arguments, however, is time-consuming, stressful, and pointless. Practitioners should be warm and understanding so that callers who want to discuss their feelings are comfortable. Acknowledging anger may encourage open discussion and problem-solving (eg, "You sound upset. Is there anything I can do to help?"). Empathizing with callers (eg, "I don't blame you for being upset." "That must have been very frustrating.") may also help.

Practitioners can build confidence in callers by complimenting them on the way they have handled things so far (eg, "You did the right thing by giving [child's name] Tylenol and a lukewarm sponge bath for the fever. That is exactly what I would have done." or "I'm glad that you called about this."). They may even be able to offer reassurance to parents who are not managing their child's illness correctly by commenting that many parents try the same treatment. A different treatment approach can then be suggested.

Before the end of the conversation, callers can be given an opportunity to ask questions and encouraged to call again if additional problems occur.

Telephone History Taking

How much history should be obtained over the telephone? Enough information should be gathered to make an appropriate decision. Questions should be directed at **determining whether an emergency exists** and **making a diagnosis.** For example, if the mother of a 20-day-old girl reports that her daughter has a temperature of 102°F (38.9°C), the infant must be seen immediately. If diarrhea is the chief complaint, some additional information would be helpful before giving advice (eg, "How many bowel movements did the girl have in the last 24 hours? Is there any blood in the diarrhea? Does she have a fever? Is she drinking less than usual? Is there any decrease in urine output?"). An older child with the same chief complaint of fever may be safely managed at home, depending on the answers to other questions about additional symptoms.

Pediatricians typically follow an organized approach to history taking for acute care visits that includes the chief complaint, history of present illness, pertinent review of systems, medical history, and family and social history. A similarly **organized framework** should be used to obtain a history over the telephone (Questions Box). Specific questions should then be asked to clarify the child's condition and obtain all the information necessary to make a good decision. A child's medical history may affect a practitioner's management of the current problem. For example, knowing that a child who has been exposed to chickenpox has asthma and is receiving steroids or has leukemia is crucial in providing the appropriate telephone advice. Practitioners can refer to several texts on pediatric telephone decision-making (see Selected References). These books outline protocols for common chief complaints to serve as guides for history taking and management over the telephone. The most efficient way to provide such medical advice is to obtain critical information that affects decisions about diagnosis and management instead of asking all possible questions. For example, with a child who is vomiting or has diarrhea, the state of hydration is critical; with a cough, the occurrence of breathing difficulty; and with head trauma, loss of consciousness. Methods of teaching telephone management skills include role-playing, listening to mock calls by "simulated" parents, and reviewing tapes of actual calls.

Because most childhood illnesses are mild and self-limited, evaluation of the safety of medical advice obtained over the telephone requires large samples to detect poor outcomes associated with mismanagement. Research has described a "wellness bias" in which practitioners, who primarily see patients with mild, self-limited illnesses, may downplay the severity of reported symptoms and choose the most benign diagnostic possibility. This bias may be more pronounced in a telephone encounter, where the physician cannot see the child. One study reported telephone encounters in which physicians seemed to make a decision early in the conversation and then "shut out" additional information that should have led to the consideration of more serious diagnoses. The safest approach is to always have a high index of suspicion for a serious condition. Questions can then be asked to confirm or dispel those suspicions.

Questions

Telephone Management

- How old is the child?
- What is the child's chief problem? What are the child's symptoms?
- How long has the child had these symptoms?
- How is the child acting?
- Does the child have any chronic illnesses?
- Is the child taking any medications?
- What is the caller most worried about?

Telephone Advice

Pediatricians should formulate an **assessment and management plan** based on the child's history. If the situation is an emergency, this should be explained to the caller, and appropriate follow-up plans should be made (ie, sending an ambulance for life-threatening conditions such as respiratory depression or uncontrollable bleeding, advising the caller to bring the child by car to the ED or physician's office within a specified amount of time for potentially dangerous complaints, such as right lower quadrant pain or possible fracture). If the call is not an emergency, then health care professionals must decide if and when the child should be seen by a physician and the appropriate home treatment.

Research shows that parents need and expect to receive an explanation of their child's illness. Practitioners should clearly state what the child's illness seems to be, what probably caused it, and what the parents can expect (eg, length of time that the child is likely to be sick, additional symptoms that may appear).

Before giving any treatment advice, health care professionals should ask callers the following questions: "What have you done so far?" "Have you given the child any medications?" and "How is this treatment working?" If the therapy seems appropriate, callers should be complimented and encouraged to continue the treatment. The regimen should be modified as indicated. Instructions for home treatment should be clear and as easy to implement as possible. If the instructions are complicated or lengthy, callers may want to write them down. When prescribing medication, ask if the child has any known drug allergies, and give the dose, frequency of administration, and information about possible side effects. Practitioners should verify that the caller can follow the telephone advice (eg, a parent has a thermometer and knows how to use it). If pediatricians plan to check up on children by telephone, they should confirm that callers (or relatives or neighbors) have a telephone and record the number.

Practitioners should confirm that callers understand the information and instructions and agree with the plan. Asking questions such as "What questions do you have?" encourages callers to raise uncertainties and ask for needed clarification. Most importantly, if the decision is to manage at home, callers should always receive specific instructions about when to call back. Caregivers should call if the child's symptoms change, persist, worsen, or cause anxiety. Also, symptoms specific to the child's condition should be followed (eg, child has fever for more than 2 days, irritability, decreased urination). Parents who seem unduly anxious or uncomfortable with home treatment should be given the opportunity to have their child seen by a physician.

Documentation

All calls for medical advice should be documented in a telephone log book or the child's medical record, for both medical reasons (eg, better follow-up, improved continuity of care) and legal purposes. The form used for documentation should include the date and time of the call; the name, identity, and telephone number of the caller; the name and age of the child; the chief complaint; other symptoms; possible diagnoses; advice given; and the name of the person who took the call.

CASE RESOLUTION

In the case history at the beginning of this chapter, the pediatrician learns several facts that lead to the recommendation that the child be seen that day (the next day if the call is made at night). These facts include the child's age, the height and duration of the fever, and lack of any symptoms of localized infection.

Selected References

American Academy of Pediatrics Section on Telehealth Care. http://www.aap.org/sections/telecare

American Academy of Pediatrics Section on Telephone Care and Committee on Child Health Financing. Payment for telephone care. *Pediatrics.* 2006;118:1768–1773

Brown JL, Swiontkowski MF. *Pediatric Telephone Medicine: Principles, Triage, and Advice.* 3rd ed. Philadelphia, PA: J. B. Lippincott; 2003

Bunik M, Glazner JE, Chandramouli V, Emsermann CB, Hegarty T, Kempe A. Pediatric telephone call centers: how do they affect health care use and costs? *Pediatrics.* 2007;119:e305–e313

Kempe A, Bunik M, Ellis J, et al. How safe is triage by an after-hours telephone call center? *Pediatrics.* 2006;118:457–463

Kempe A, Luberti A, Belman S, et al. Outcomes associated with pediatric after-hours care by call centers: a multicenter study. *Ambul Pediatr.* 2003;3:211–217

Lee TJ, Baraff LJ, Guzy J, Johnson D, Woo H. Does telephone triage delay significant medical treatment? Advice nurse service vs on-call pediatricians. *Arch Pediatr Adolesc Med.* 2003;157:635–641

Lee TJ, Guzy J, Johnson D, Woo H, Baraff LJ. Caller satisfaction with after-hours telephone advice: nurse advice service versus on-call pediatricians. *Pediatrics.* 2002;110:865–872

Poole SR. *The Complete Guide: Developing a Telephone Triage and Advice System for a Pediatric Office Practice.* Elk Grove Village, IL. American Academy of Pediatrics; 2003

Reisman AB, Brown KE. Preventing communication errors in telephone medicine: a case-based approach. *J Gen Intern Med.* 2005; 20:959–963

Schmitt BD. *Pediatric Telephone Protocols: Office Version.* 13th ed. Elk Grove Village, IL: American Academy of Pediatrics; 2011

CHAPTER 8

Informatics

Alan Tomines, MD

CASE STUDY

You are a physician in a small pediatric practice. Your hospital is planning to acquire an electronic medical record, which will be made available within the hospital and to the offices of its affiliated practices. The hospital chief of staff asks you to sit on the hospital's informatics committee to participate in the vendor selection process and to assist with the implementation of the selected system. You have previously used the hospital's computer to check patients' laboratory results, and your practice uses computers for billing and scheduling. However, you don't consider yourself a technology expert and express your trepidation to the chief of staff, who asks you to speak with the head of the informatics committee.

Questions

1. What is informatics?
2. What are the important informatics concepts to understand?
3. What are the important drivers of health care information technology?
4. What are the challenges to implementing successful health information systems?
5. What are the special pediatric considerations in health information systems?

To make the best possible clinical decisions, physicians must have information about their patients' health that is current, accurate, complete, and reliable. This information should be available wherever and whenever it is needed. Where possible, the physician should be presented with information that will encourage an evidence-based approach to decision-making, and the decisions made should be communicated to other health care providers in a manner that is clear and error-free. The physician should also be able to receive feedback on the quality of care provided. Health care information technology (HIT) holds the promise of increasing access to patient health information, improving patient safety, reporting and measuring desired health outcomes, and making health care more efficient; at the same time, it holds the promise of decreasing health care expenditures. However, the implementation of HIT is not without challenges.

Basic Concepts

Although the terms *data, information,* and *knowledge* are sometimes used interchangeably, these concepts are distinct. Data are mere observations or facts (eg, hemoglobin equal to 9 g/dL). Information is data placed in meaningful context (eg, hemoglobin equal to 9 g/dL in a breastfed 3-month-old infant). Knowledge is the understanding of information, including an assessment of its completeness (eg, hemoglobin equal to 9 g/dL in a breastfed 3-month-old infant may represent a physiological nadir, but may also represent blood loss, increased destruction of red blood cells, or decreased production of red blood cells). Any structured collection of data may be referred to as a *database.*

Information technology refers to any hardware or software that support the acquisition, storage, retrieval, transformation, interpretation, and dissemination of data and information. An *information system* is the sum of the people and work processes that are supported by information technology. Depending on the degree to which technology is applied, the processes of an information system may be automated, manual, or a combination of both.

What Is Informatics?

Medical informatics is the science that deals with the appropriate application of information technology to health care work processes. To apply information technology appropriately, specialists in informatics (referred to as *informaticians* or *informaticists*) focus first on improving the quality of data and the efficiency of workflow in the patient care setting; it is in this optimized environment that technology may be applied most effectively. Medical informatics places great emphasis on non-technological considerations that can influence the successful implementation of health information systems, including information science, cognitive psychology, project management, organizational and change management, health care policy, and ethics.

As a field, medical informatics can itself be subdivided into specific clinical domains, such as nursing, pharmacy, veterinary medicine, dentistry, and imaging. *Biomedical informatics* is a term of broader scope that encompasses medical informatics, bioinformatics (having the primary domain of genomics and bioengineering), and public health informatics. Outside of the United States, *health informatics* is the term more frequently used to convey the same breadth.

Electronic Health Information Systems

Although all electronic health information systems ultimately deal with managing some aspect of patient care, they are divided here into 4 coarse groupings: electronic records of patient care, administrative systems, ancillary clinical systems, and telemedicine. Box 8-1 lists several common abbreviations used in electronic health information systems.

Electronic Records of Patient Care

An electronic medical record (EMR) represents the clinical documentation and legal record of care provided to a patient by a health care provider or organization. An EMR can usually create and store traditional clinical documentation, such as progress notes and consultations. However, a full-fledged EMR represents more than an "electronic version" of the traditional paper-based record. Important components of an EMR include a clinical data repository (CDR), a clinical decision support system (CDSS), and computerized provider order entry (CPOE). A CDR is a real-time database containing all of the clinically relevant patient data in an institution. A CDSS is a special computer program that applies medical knowledge to clinical data to produce patient-specific recommendations, such as differential diagnoses or clinical recommendations. A CPOE is a special computer program that allows providers to write electronic orders that are directed to the appropriate clinical staff or ancillary department. A CPOE can decrease errors due to illegible handwriting, decrease delays in the receipt and execution of orders, allow for orders to be entered away from the care setting, and (in conjunction with a CDSS) provide for error checking (such as appropriate weight-based dosing, drug–drug interactions, or drug–allergy interactions).

An EMR generally operates within the functional boundary of a hospital or practice. However, information about a patient's health is not limited to traditional care settings. A personal health record (PHR) is a summary of an individual's health history, usually self-maintained, that contains information collected from encounters with different providers, medicolegal documents (such as living wills or advance directives), and other health information that may be relevant to the patients (such as regimens for nontraditional remedies or the results of home testing for blood pressure). The concept of a PHR is not new: Patients with multiple medical problems have long maintained paper-based PHRs out of necessity—to have at least one reliable and portable source containing a complete medical history. The electronic PHR is an evolving entity, ranging from scanned paper documents stored on CD-ROM or other removable media to Web-based applications that interface with EMRs and capture data from medical devices. The PHR is not considered a legal record of care.

The electronic health record (EHR) represents the next stage in the evolution of the EMR. An EHR will have all of the desired functionality of a full-fledged EMR, but will capture data from multiple different EMRs to provide the entire longitudinal history of the patient. In addition, the EHR will support functionality related to research and public health, such as identification of patient-appropriate clinical

Box 8-1. Abbreviations Used in Informatics	
ARRA	American Recovery and Reinvestment Act of 2009
CDR	clinical data repository
CDSS	clinical decision support system
CPOE	computerized provider order entry
EHR	electronic health record
EMR	electronic medical record
eRx	electronic prescribing
HIE	health information exchange
HIPAA	Health Insurance Portability and Accountability Act
HIS	hospital information system
HIT	health care information technology
HITECH	Health Information Technology for Economic and Clinical Health Act
IIS	immunization information system or registry
P4P	pay-for-performance
PACS	picture archiving and communication system
PHI	protected health information
PHR	personal health record
RIS	radiology information system

trials, mandatory reporting of notifiable disease, and provision of clinical data (stripped of patient-identifying information) to support clinical and public health research.

A health information exchange (HIE) is an enabling technology that acts as a hub for the secure exchange of data between EMRs. An EMR that is connected to an HIE has the ability to exchange health information with other EMRs that are connected to that HIE, precluding physicians and hospitals from having to establish an interface between their EMR and every other EMR where a patient might have data. While an HIE generally serves a specific geographic region, the interconnection of HIEs provides the capability for an EMR in one region to share data with an EMR in another region, reducing the barriers to accessing a patient's entire longitudinal history of care.

Administrative Systems

A hospital information system (HIS) encompasses all of the clinical and nonclinical information systems of an institution. An HIS may be a single integrated information system or it may represent multiple information systems that are connected with specially designed interfaces. Hospitals and large practices often have separate information systems to manage individual administrative functions, such as appointment scheduling, insurance eligibility, and billing and reimbursement. A practice management system is an information system designed to manage administrative tasks and is considered to be appropriate for small- and medium-sized practices.

Ancillary Clinical Systems

Information systems that support clinical ancillary services focus on a limited set of tasks and data. A laboratory information system manages the entry and reporting of laboratory results, often capturing electronic data directly from laboratory analyzers. A pharmacy information system manages patients' prescription information, checks appropriate dosing and drug interactions, and tracks medical insurance; a related concept is e-prescribing (electronic prescribing or eRx), which uses technology to write and transmit prescriptions electronically to a pharmacy information system. A picture archiving and communication system (PACS) manages the storage and distribution of patients' electronic medical images; a radiology information system incorporates the functionality of a PACS and also manages radiology service activities, such as reporting, scheduling, and billing. An immunization information system (IIS or immunization registry) is used to document and track patient vaccinations. An IIS can send reminder or recall notices, as appropriate, to physicians and parents when vaccinations are due or delinquent. Because these systems are usually maintained regionally by public health entities, they also collect reports on adverse vaccine events and provide summaries of regional vaccination prevalence. These systems are usually able to exchange data with capable EMRs.

Telemedicine

Telemedicine is not an information system, but a related concept of interest in informatics. Telemedicine is the use of information and communication technologies to deliver health care over a distance, often to support patient care in rural or underserved areas. There are many specialties within telemedicine, roughly corresponding to distinct medical specialties, such as teleradiology (the transmission of radiologic images electronically for interpretation) and telesurgery (the use of video and robotic technology to perform surgery). The use of e-mail and Web sites to communicate with patients is also a form of telemedicine.

Drivers

The key health care drivers for the adoption of HIT are the improvement of patient safety, the measurement of health care outcomes, the increased efficiency of workflow in the patient care setting, and the reduction of health care expenditures.

Patient safety, through the reduction of preventable errors, is the primary driver of information technology adoption in many health care organizations. In its report *To Err Is Human*, the Institute of Medicine (IOM) estimated that up to 98,000 US deaths annually are attributable to medical errors. Most errors were noted to be preventable and caused by systems and processes that increase, or fail to prevent, human errors. Computerized provider order entry is an example of information technology that has the potential to improve patient safety—by alerting the physician to errors before an order is submitted.

Changes in the health care marketplace are driving the measurement of health care outcomes. Pay-for-performance (relating reimbursement to measures of the quality of care provided) and "medical report cards" that permit comparison of health care plans and providers are examples of market drivers. Information technology is critical to collecting and analyzing data to calculate these measures. In addition, a CDSS may improve health care outcomes through guideline adherence by reminding physicians and patients about necessary care services that may have been overlooked.

Improvements in efficiency are another driver in the adoption of information technology. The automation of highly repetitive, data-intensive activities, such as billing or scheduling, is an example of where efficiency can be improved. However, introduction of information technology into a clinical setting without thorough consideration of workflow may actually decrease efficiency.

Health care spending is approaching 20% of the gross domestic product of the United States and is increasing at a rate nearly twice that of inflation. Information technology is considered to be a potential source of cost savings by reducing duplication of diagnostic studies and decreasing the time spent on administrative tasks. In addition, in the IOM report *Crossing the Quality Chasm,* the use of e-mail was touted as a method for meeting the needs of patients more quickly and at lower cost than a traditional visit.

Challenges

Despite the significant health care drivers for adopting HIT, there are a number of challenges that prevent the easy implementation of systems.

The ease with which information systems can exchange electronic patient data should not belie the care that must be taken to protect that data. Protected health information (PHI) is any information about a patient (such as name or medical record number) that may be used to identify a patient. Privacy is the patient's right to keep this information a secret. Confidentiality is the assurance made by health care providers that private information will not be revealed. Security involves the policies and technologies that support the assurance of confidentiality. The Health Insurance Portability and Accountability Act defines the measures that must be taken to ensure that PHI is secure and made available only to authorized individuals or organizations. Appropriate concerns exist about breaches of patient privacy when data are stored electronically. Although health information systems often employ sophisticated technical barriers to protect patient data, it is often the case that data breaches are the result of people failing to adhere to policy safeguards. Educating providers and other users of patient data is critical to guaranteeing patient confidentiality.

The cost of implementing health information systems can be prohibitive for health care delivery organizations, particularly small practices. To address this barrier, the Health Information Technology for Economic and Clinical Health (HITECH) Act was included in the American Recovery and Reinvestment Act of 2009. The HITECH Act authorizes Medicare and Medicaid incentives to be provided to clinicians and hospitals that adopt EHRs and demonstrate their *meaningful use* by meeting specific objectives toward improved health care delivery and outcomes. These objectives include using EHRs for fundamental activities, such as recording patient demographics and vital signs; maintaining active problem, medication, and allergy lists; providing patients with summaries of outpatient visits and inpatient discharge instructions; electronic prescribing and ordering; and providing drug–drug and drug–allergy checks. The objectives also include more esoteric or complex functions, such as providing data to public health agencies for disease surveillance, providing data to immunization registries or immunization information systems, generating lists of patients with specific conditions for quality improvement and research, identifying and providing patient-specific education resources, and providing summary of care records and medication reconciliation across health care settings. To assure physicians and hospitals that they are adopting EHRs that allow them to meet meaningful use regulations, the US Department of Health and Human Services has developed a process and criteria for certifying EHRs.

Change management is an important element to consider when implementing an information system. Introduction of technology inevitably results in changes in the workflow of physicians and nurses and may lead to repurposing of administrative staff. Resistance to change should be anticipated; strategies to mitigate resistance should be employed, including involvement of health care professionals in the selection and deployment of HIT.

Human–computer interaction is the study of the interactions between people and information technology. It is important for users to perceive that the technology is useful (supports the work being done) and that the technology is usable (readily learned, efficient, and helps them to avoid and correct errors).

Effects of technology on the patient–physician interaction must also be considered. Constraints on time or location of computers may compel some providers to do electronic documentation during their visits. Physicians should be sensitive to patients who feel that technology is intrusive; where appropriate, physicians should acknowledge the intrusion, and identify potential benefits to the patient (including efficiency of access to information and more efficient communication of prescriptions to pharmacies or orders to ancillary services).

Pediatric Considerations

Although pediatric patients represent approximately one-quarter of the US population, pediatric features are often underdeveloped in electronic health information systems. When considering these systems for pediatric settings, particular attention should be focused on the highly specific data, task, and policy needs of pediatric practice.

The presence of functionality to support clinical tasks that are generally, if not uniquely, pediatric should always be examined. Immunization management, including the ability to assess a patient's status or to exchange data with an immunization information system, is highly desirable. Weight-based dosing and the tracking of growth parameters are other functions that are often overlooked. Age-specific documentation and educational materials can be well-managed electronically.

The data and terminology of an information system should suit the highly specific needs of pediatric practice. Units of measure should reflect the requisite data precision. For example, the age of a patient in hours (rather than years, months, or even days) and weight in grams is critical to appropriate care in the neonatal period. Laboratory values should be accompanied by age-appropriate normal ranges. Patient identification must account for the frequent changes in names and numerical identifiers that may occur in infancy or during change of custody. Pediatric terminology, such as developmental milestones, type of cry, or characterization of stool, are often overlooked in information systems designed for adults.

Pediatric policy issues should also be reflected in the design of an information system. Authorization for the child (or the child's parents, guardians, or other legal authority) to view all, none, or parts of a child's medical record should be enforced electronically as it would be for the paper medical record. Likewise, secondary use of patient data for public health, research, or commercial purposes should be allowed or restricted as appropriate.

At this time, there is no electronic medical home for the care of children. The electronic history of care may be distributed across EMRs, immunization information systems, school health information systems, and specialty registries for rare conditions, trauma, or foster care. With the emergence of health information exchanges as a conduit for data exchange, it may be possible to create a virtual medical home. It is important that pediatricians work toward reducing the legislative, technological, and cultural barriers to linking child health information systems without compromising the security or confidentiality of protected health information.

Pediatricians should be actively involved in the acquisition and development of information technology to ensure that child-specific data and policy needs are addressed. Pediatricians should also be involved in national policy initiatives to ensure that health information systems are certified for pediatric use and integrated to support care that is child-centered.

CASE RESOLUTION

In the case history at the beginning of this chapter, the pediatrician speaks with the head of the informatics committee. The pediatrician learns that she has been asked to participate because of her understanding of physician workflow in the office setting and to advocate for the highly specific data needs and policies associated with the pediatric population. Her expertise will help to identify issues that, if addressed, may contribute to successful acceptance of the information system by pediatricians and other physicians.

Selected References

American Academy of Pediatrics Task Force on Medical Informatics. Special requirements for electronic medical record systems in pediatrics. *Pediatrics.* 2001;108:513–515

Blumenthal D, Tavenner M. The "meaningful use" regulation for electronic health records. *N Engl J Med.* 2010;363:501–504

Committee on Quality of Health Care in America, Institute of Medicine. *To Err Is Human: Building a Safer Health System.* Kohn LT, Corrigan JM, Donaldson MS, eds. Washington, DC: The National Academies Press; 2000

Gerstle RS; American Academy of Pediatrics Task Force on Medical Informatics. E-mail communication between pediatricians and their patients. *Pediatrics.* 2004;114:317–321

Hinman AR, Davidson AJ. Linking children's health information systems: clinical care, public health, emergency medical systems, and schools. *Pediatrics.* 2009;123:S67–S73

Johnson KB. Barriers that impeded the adoption of pediatric information technology. *Arch Pediatr Adolesc Med.* 2001;155(12):1374–1379

Kaushal R, Barker KN, Bates DW. How can information technology improve patient safety and reduce medication errors in children's health care? *Arch Pediatr Adolesc Med.* 2001;155:1002–1007

Kemper AR, Uren RL, Clark SJ. Adoption of electronic health records in primary care pediatric practices. *Pediatrics.* 2006;118:e20–e24

Nielsen J. Usability 101: introduction to usability. useit.com: Jakob Nielsen's Website. http://www.useit.com/alertbox/20030825.html. Accessed November 30, 2010

Shekelle PG, Morton SC, Keeler EB. *Costs and Benefits of Healthcare Information Technology. Evidence Report/Technology Assessment No. 132.* Rockville, MD: Agency for Healthcare Research and Quality; 2006. AHRQ publication 06-E006

Shiffman RN, Spooner SA, Kwiatkowski K, Brennan PF. Information technology for children's health and health care. *J Am Med Inform Assoc.* 2000;8:546–550

Spooner SA; American Academy of Pediatrics Council on Clinical Information Technology. Special requirements for electronic health record systems in pediatrics. *Pediatrics.* 2007;119:631–636

Yasnoff WA, O'Carroll PW, Koo D, Linkins RW, Kilbourne EM. Public health informatics: improving and transforming public health in the information age. *J Public Health Manag Pract.* 2000;6:67–75

CHAPTER 9

Counseling Families About Internet Use

Alan Tomines, MD

CASE STUDY

A 16-year-old girl is accompanied by her mother for a routine visit. The girl is doing well in school, is active in team sports, and has a small circle of friends that are well-known to her mother. The mother describes no new problems at home, nor any changes in behavior, except that she is concerned that her daughter "spends too much time on the computer."

Questions
1. What is the Internet?
2. What are the commonly used Internet services?
3. What are the benefits and risks of the Internet?
4. What strategies may be used to make the Internet safer to use?
5. What signs may indicate that an adolescent is engaging in risky behaviors on the Internet?

The Internet is a worldwide system of interconnected computer networks. At its inception, it was the exclusive domain of the military and academia; today, the Internet is a public gateway to electronic information, communication, and commercial services. The Internet has profoundly changed the way that we learn, work, play, and interact with others. Its influence is so pervasive that it has become an integral part of the education and socialization of children, making it a subject of interest for parents, providers, and researchers. Physicians can provide pragmatic counsel to families that focuses on the benefits and risks of the Internet, strategies for safer use, and the assessment of online behavior in adolescents. Physicians should also be prepared to discuss health information that families find on the Internet.

A Brief History of the Internet

The Internet began in the 1960s as ARPANET (Advanced Research Projects Agency Network), a US Department of Defense project to share government-funded, university-based computer resources across a reliable communications network. Through the 1970s, ARPANET found acceptance with academics and researchers as a conduit for scientific information exchange, due in large part to **e-mail** (electronic mail), a technology for sending and receiving messages.

Recognizing the potential of the ARPANET, the National Science Foundation (NSF) began a separate effort to connect the computer science departments at non-ARPANET universities; initially dubbed CSNET (Computer Science Network) and later renamed NSFNET, this new network further expanded electronic information exchange. In 1990 the ARPANET was retired, with many of its networks being absorbed into NSFNET. The resulting network, renamed the *Internet,* extended its reach into the business sector and to international researchers but remained relatively inaccessible to the general public.

During the early 1990s, the European Organization for Nuclear Research (CERN) developed protocols to facilitate the sharing of physics research data over the Internet. These protocols allowed computer files, on different computers and having different formats (such as text and images), to be shared as single documents that could be viewed using a special computer program (browser). This system of linked documents was collectively dubbed the *World Wide Web* (*WWW,* or simply the Web), with collections of documents referred to as *Web pages* or *Web sites.* In 1993 CERN made their work freely available, leading to the rapid proliferation of commercial and individual Web sites.

Internet Services and Concepts

Today the most commonly used Internet services are e-mail and the Web. A person actively using an Internet service is said to be **online.** Use of the Web is sometimes referred to as *surfing the Web* or *surfing the Net,* and is facilitated by **search engines** (programs that use keywords or topics to find related documents, images, Web sites, or other services on the Internet) such as Yahoo! and Google. Internet services may be accessed by a wide range of computing devices, from personal or laptop computers to smartphones (mobile phones that provide access to Internet services). No matter what technology is used, access is usually provided by an **Internet service provider** or ISP (a company that has an Internet connection that it shares with consumers on a subscription basis).

Due to their popularity in the pediatric age group, there are a few specialized Internet services of which physicians should take special note. Web logs (or **blogs**) are Web-based journals. Like a traditional paper-based diary, a blog can be used to express activities, thoughts, or feelings. Blogs may be public (available for anyone to read) or private (having restricted access); the owner of a blog may allow readers to add comments to the blog. **Social networking** Web sites, such as Facebook, Twitter, and MySpace, are similar in content to blogs, with the added dimension that users are encouraged to create a network of online friends by establishing links to other users' Web pages. Blogs and social networking Web sites are examples of **asynchronous** services (where communication between users does not have to take place in real time) whose content may be moderated by the owner of the service to ensure that content is appropriate. In contrast, **chat rooms** are Internet venues that permit the real-time exchange of text messages between multiple simultaneous participants. **Instant messaging** is similar to a chat room, although it is generally limited to one-on-one exchanges of real-time messages. Although sometimes referred to as *text messaging*, instant messaging is a more inclusive term that better reflects the immediacy of interaction and expansion of content to include images and multimedia (such as streaming audio and video files). Instant messaging is a popular premium service with mobile phone subscriptions, making it possible to have an online presence at all times without a computer. Adolescents have shown an increasing preference for instant messaging—estimated to be used by one-third of all teens.

Internet Benefits and Access

Physicians should be able to identify the benefits of Internet use. The Internet provides access to a wealth of educational resources and cultural experiences through the use of text, images, and multimedia. Access to these resources allows children to exercise their reading, writing, information-seeking, and technology skills. The Internet also provides the opportunity to exchange messages frequently with family and friends. In addition, children with common interests, or even common medical conditions, can use e-mail, chat, blogs, or social networking to communicate, commiserate, and encourage.

Physicians may also take a role in reducing disparities to Internet access. Internet use and access is correlated with socioeconomic status. While nearly 90% of adolescents in the United States are regularly online, millions do not have access. Pediatricians may help families gain access to the Internet by identifying institutions that provide safe online environments, such as libraries, community centers, and schools. In addition, patient-centered Internet-based health interventions are increasingly being studied as a supplement to traditional health care delivery; addressing disparities to Internet access may increase opportunities for these interventions, particularly in underserved communities.

Physicians should also be aware that children with disabilities may have a difficult time using the Internet without **assistive technology** (hardware or software designed to improve the accessibility of computers). Visually impaired or blind children may be aided by the use of special software, including screen magnifiers, Braille embossers, or screen readers (software that uses a computer-generated voice to read e-mail and Web pages); however, it is important to note that many Web sites are not developed to be compatible with screen readers. Hearing-impaired or deaf children may be aided by ensuring that their computers are set to provide visual cues rather than audio prompts; this functionality is usually built into the operating system of a computer. Children with mobility or dexterity challenges may find it difficult to use a traditional keyboard and mouse; alternative keyboards, manual pointing devices, and computer touch screens should be investigated. Pointing devices that employ sound or infrared beams, as well as software that responds to the spoken word, may be viable alternatives where manual control is not possible.

Internet Threats

While the Internet has many benefits, being online does entail some risks. To understand these risks, it is helpful to understand many of the Internet's neutral properties. The Internet is interactive: Unlike traditional media, such as newspapers, radio, and television, the Internet user may have real-time interactions with a person or a sophisticated computer program. The Internet has few restrictions: Anyone can put almost anything on the Internet, without regard to credibility or appropriateness. The Internet is public and permanent: Although information on a Web site may be removed, it is possible for anyone that visits a Web site to make an electronic copy of what is there, and many Web sites are archived historically (www. archive.org) and remain publicly retrievable long after they seem to be gone. The Internet is anonymous: People are not necessarily who they represent themselves to be. These Internet properties do not encourage, but do enable, the most common threats, which include strangers/predators, interpersonal victimization, and pornography, among others (including gaming, gambling, and shopping).

Internet predators are the greatest concern of parents. More than one-half of children online have shared personal information about themselves (including name, address, or phone number) with a stranger. Nearly one-third of children online have "friends" that they have never met in person. Approximately three-fifths of online adolescents have received an instant message or e-mail from a stranger.

Online interpersonal victimization is the receipt of unwanted harassment or sexual attention over the Internet. One-fifth of children have reported being victimized, and a high risk factor was talking about sex with someone online. Cyberbullying is a specific type of online interpersonal victimization involving repetitive contact with electronic messages or images that are harmful or threatening. Cyberbullying may be as prevalent online as "traditional" bullying, with nearly one-fifth of middle school–aged children reporting that they had been cyberbullied at least once in the last couple of months and more than 10% reporting that they had cyberbullied others at least once in the last couple of months.

While children may be individually targeted by strangers or cyberbullies, they may passively encounter undesired Internet content. More than 40% of children reported having been exposed to pornography online, and nearly two-thirds of them described this exposure as unwanted. In adolescents between the ages 15 to 17, more than 70% reported accidentally being exposed to online pornography. A high risk factor for exposure to pornography was the downloading of images.

Sexting is the exchange of sexually explicit text, images, or multimedia, generally via instant messaging. Sexting sits at the convergence of pornography and cyberbullying, with the added danger that some adolescents may not perceive sexting as harmful or threatening. In some jurisdictions, minors that have participated in sexting have been charged with possessing child pornography.

Strategies for Safer Internet Use

The American Academy of Pediatrics (AAP) has provided age-specific guidance for a safer Internet experience: For children through age 14, parents should be actively involved with all online activities, establish rules for safe online behavior, and use Internet safety tools; by age 15, parents may permit Internet access without restriction, but should continue to reinforce rules.

Parents may be actively involved by educating themselves about the Internet and their children's Internet access, sharing time with their children online, and advocating for a safer Internet environment. Some parents may not be technically savvy and may require basic instruction on Internet technology. Classes may be available through libraries, community centers, the local Parent-Teacher Association, or online primers such as "Teach Parents Tech" (www.teachparentstech.org). Parental education on Internet safety can begin with Web-based resources, such as the Federal Trade Commission's OnGuard Online (www.onguardonline.gov), NetSmartz Workshop (www.netsmartz.org), iKeepSafe.org (www.ikeepsafe.org), and INOBTR (www.INOBTR.org). Parents should be aware of other venues where their children may access the Internet, such as schools, libraries, and friends' homes, and they should find out what Internet safety policies and technologies have been instituted in these environments.

By sharing time online, parents can promote and model responsible Internet behaviors. Parents should talk about what they see together on the Internet, and encourage children to share what they have experienced when online alone, whether good or bad. Placing the computer in a public location in the home will encourage the idea that the Internet is a shared experience; however, parents should be aware that laptops and mobile telephones allow covert Internet access. Children should be provided with a separate account to access the Internet, which their parents can also access. Having a separate account will allow parents to directly restrict the software and content that children can access and periodically review Web sites visited and e-mails. Parents should understand that some children may be savvy enough to erase their Web browsing history; absence of a Web browsing history may be a cause for suspicion. Parents should regularly monitor mobile telephone activity for instant messaging activity.

Parents should act as advocates for their children's Internet experience. When a child encounters inappropriate Internet content, or messages that are hurtful or distressing, parents should alert their ISP, as well as the owner of the Web site where the content or messages were discovered. Parents should also contact the appropriate legal authorities and the National Center for Missing and Exploited Children (www.missingkids.com). Commercial Web sites that collect personal information from children younger than 13 are required to follow the Children's Online Privacy Protection Act of 1998, which is enforced by the Federal Trade Commission. According to this law, Internet Web site operators must post their policy indicating what personal information is collected, how that information will be used, and if that information will be shared with a third party. Parents must consent to the collection and use of personal information, and may revoke this consent at any time.

Parents should set and enforce house rules for Internet use. Children should not communicate with nor plan to meet strangers known only to them through the Internet, nor should they respond to unsolicited messages, or any other messages that make them feel uncomfortable. Children should not share personal information or pictures with others on the Internet, nor should they download files from the Internet. Children should be encouraged to be good citizens, including not doing anything that may be hurtful to others or plagiarizing information that they find freely on the Internet. For older children, safety pledges can be used as formal agreements of acceptable use. Time limits should be set and strictly enforced. The AAP recommends not more than 2 hours of total screen time (computer and television) for children older than 2 years. Any activities that are not allowed should be specifically identified.

Even with house rules in place, physicians should recommend the use of Internet safety tools to protect against inappropriate use and external threats. Although not directly targeted at children, parents should be aware of software to protect against malware. Malware generally includes viruses and worms (software programs that can corrupt the information saved on a computer), spyware (software that tracks Internet activity and sends this information to another person), and pop-ups (a new browser window that may contain marketing or other undesired content). Viruses and worms are generally downloaded as attachments in e-mail, whereas spyware and pop-ups are introduced by surfing the Web. Parents should also protect against spam (unsolicited e-mail), which may contain undesired content or solicitations.

Filters are special computer programs that allow acceptable Internet content to be presented and block content deemed to be inappropriate. Filtering may use one or more of the following methods: "black lists" of Web sites that are specifically blocked, "white lists" of Web sites that are specifically permitted, the blocking of specific words or terms, and the maturing technology of blocking suspicious image content. Filters are neither perfectly specific nor perfectly sensitive and may require parental adjustment to achieve an acceptable level of filtering. Parents may contact their ISP to enable filtering of content before it enters the home (server-side filtering). If server-side filtering is too restrictive for some members in the household, or not restrictive enough for others, parents may acquire filtering software that is installed directly on computers in the home (**client-side filtering**). Client-side filters work with standard Web browsers, although special child-oriented Web browsers may be acquired that have client-side filtering built in.

Monitoring software automates parental tracking of Internet usage by creating a reviewable record of Web sites and images viewed, messages sent and received, and even individual keystrokes entered. The potential benefits of monitoring software should be weighed against the invasiveness to the privacy of the child. Monitoring software often includes time-limiting software, which can be set to allow Internet access only during certain hours of the day and can be set to disable access to the Internet after a specified amount of time has elapsed.

Adolescents on the Internet

As with other aspects of their lives, adolescents should feel that they can discuss what they see on the Internet with their parents without imperiling their access to the Internet. Most adolescents have access to the Internet from home, and nearly all have access to the Internet at school or at a friend's house. Parents should be aware that adolescents who have restrictive Internet rules at home are more likely to attempt Internet access outside the home, where their activity may be more difficult to monitor.

Adolescents may engage in risky online behaviors, including communicating with and planning to meet in person strangers met online. From a review of past cases, the Federal Bureau of Investigation has identified specific behaviors that may indicate a child is engaging in risky online behaviors, including spending several hours online, especially at night; having pornographic images on the computer; turning the monitor off, or quickly changing the screen when a parent enters the room; and using unrecognized usernames or accounts. Other non-Internet behaviors that should arouse suspicion include phone calls from unknown adults, outgoing calls to unrecognized phone numbers, gifts or packages received, or unexplained credit card activity.

The physician should consider addressing online activities in the adolescent psychosocial review of systems. Asking adolescents about online activities may unveil risky online behaviors or provide an opportunity to discuss concerns about their health and well-being. Nearly one-third of adolescents have searched the Internet for health information, most often related to sex and sexually transmitted infections, nutrition, and exercise and fitness. Additionally, adolescent girls also search for information on physical abuse, sexual abuse, and dating violence. Online activities worthy of inquiry include health topics searched for on the Internet; maintenance of a social networking (such as a Facebook or MySpace) page; sharing personal information on the Internet; communicating with strangers; meeting people known only via the Internet; and engaging in, or being a victim of, cyberbullying or sexting. Adolescents should also be reminded that the Internet is not private, and that colleges and employers may discover information about the adolescent on what seem to be "private" social networking pages.

Health Information on the Internet

Patients regard physicians as the preferred and most trusted source for health information; however, patients do seek out health information on the Internet prior to, or sometimes in lieu of, consulting with their physician. It is important to remind families that health information on the Internet may be outdated, incomplete, incorrect, intentionally misleading, or easily misinterpreted. When patients have questions about information that they find on the Internet, physicians should take care not to disregard the information outright. Inquiries should be viewed as opportunities to address points of concern. Most often, patients simply want their physician's opinion of the information, as opposed to a specific treatment.

Providing patients with Web sites that provide reliable information can improve the quality of information seen and reduce the overwhelming quantity of information that parents must sort through. Physicians may help support patients by identifying evidence-based health information resources on the Internet, such as the AAP (www. aap.org), the National Library of Medicine's MEDLINEPlus (www. medlineplus.gov), the Centers for Disease Control and Prevention (www.cdc.gov), and the US Department of Health and Human Services' Healthfinder (www.healthfinder.gov). Specialists should be prepared to identify online information sources and support groups, particularly for rare, chronic, or debilitating conditions. Physicians should caution families caring for children with special medical conditions about the characteristics of less reliable online resources or support groups, which may include novel or alternative treatment regimens, advice to stop treatment, or charging of fees for participation or treatment.

CASE RESOLUTION

In the case history at the beginning of this chapter, the pediatrician finds out that the girl uses the computer for 1 to 2 hours every afternoon to complete her homework assignments and is on the Internet for 2 to 3 hours every evening surfing the Web and checking her Facebook page. The pediatrician advises the girl that, for safety reasons, personal information should never be shared over the Internet, adding that colleges and employers often research prospective candidates using the Internet. With the mother and daughter, the pediatrician discusses the option to have a parent–child contract that clearly establishes the rules for acceptable Internet use in and out of the home, including appropriate time limits. The pediatrician also directs the mother to Internet-based resources for safeguarding the home environment, and to a workshop for new Internet users at the local library.

Selected References

Ahmad F, Hudak PL, Bercovitz K, Hollenberg E, Levinson W. Are physicians ready for patients with Internet-based health information? *J Med Internet Res.* 2006; 8:e22

D'Alessandro DM, Dosa NP. Empowering children and families with information technology. *Arch Pediatr Adolesc Med.* 2001;155(10):1131–1136

Diaz JA, Griffith RA, Ng JJ, Reinert SE, Friedmann PD, Moulton AW. Patients' use of the Internet for medical information. *J Gen Intern Med.* 2002;17:180–185

Federal Bureau of Investigation. A Parent's Guide to Internet Safety. FBI Web site. http://www.fbi.gov/stats-services/publications/parent-guide/parentsguide.pdf. Accessed December 1, 2010

Glowniak J. History, structure, and function of the Internet. *Semin Nucl Med.* 1998;28(2):135–144

Hesse BW, Nelson DE, Kreps GL, et al. Trust and sources of health information: the impact of the Internet and its implications for health care providers: findings from the first Health Information National Trends Survey. *Arch Intern Med.* 2005;165:2618–2624

Jimison H, Gorman P, Woods S, et al. *Barriers and Drivers of Health Information Technology Use for the Elderly, Chronically Ill, and Underserved. Evidence Report/ Technology Assessment No. 175.* Rockville, MD: Agency for Healthcare Research and Quality; 2008. AHRQ Publication No. 09-E004

Kowalski RN, Limber SP. Electronic bullying among middle school students. *J Adolesc Health.* 2007;41:S22–S30

Lazarus W, Lipper L. *Parents' Guide to the Information Superhighway.* Santa Monica, CA, and Washington, DC: The Children's Partnership; 1998

Lenhart A, Madden M, Hitlin P. Youth are leading the transition to a fully wired and mobile nation. Pew Internet & American Life Project. July 27, 2005. http://www.pewinternet.org/~/media//Files/Reports/2005/PIP_Teens_Tech_July2005web.pdf.pdf. Accessed December 1, 2010

Mandl KD, Feit S, Pena BM, Kohane IS. Growth and determinants of access in patient e-mail and Internet use. *Arch Pediatr Adolesc Med.* 2000;154:508–511

McClung HJ, Murray RD, Heitlinger LA. The Internet as a source for current patient information. *Pediatrics.* 1998;101:e2

Murray E, Lo B, Pollack L, et al. The impact of health information on the Internet on the physician-patient relationship: patient perceptions. *Arch Intern Med.* 2003;163:1727–1734

OnGuard Online. http://www.onguardonline.gov. Accessed December 1, 2010

Sim NZ, Kitteringham L, Spitz L, et al. Information on the World Wide Web— how useful is it for parents? *J Pediatr Surg.* 2007;42:305–312

Smith PK, Mahdavi J, Carvalho M, Fisher S, Russell S, Tippett N. Cyberbullying: its nature and impact in secondary school pupils. *J Child Psychol Psychiatry.* 2008;49:376–385

Stop Bullying Now. http://stopbullyingnow.hrsa.gov/adults/default.aspx. Accessed December 1, 2010

Teach Parents Tech. http://www.teachparentstech.org. Accessed December 13, 2010

US Department of Education. Parents Guide to the Internet. http://www.ed.gov/pubs/parents/internet/index.html. Accessed December 1, 2010

Wolak J, Mitchell K, Finkelhor D. Unwanted and wanted exposure to online pornography in a national sample of youth Internet users. *Pediatrics.* 2007;119:247–257

CHAPTER 10

Cultural Considerations and Competence in Pediatrics

W. Suzanne Eidson-Ton, MD, MS; Hendry Ton, MD, MS; Blanca Solis, MD; and Jesse Joad, MD, MS

CASE STUDY

You are seeing A.J., a 12-year-old Mexican American boy, for a well-child visit. His mother speaks Spanish and "a little" English, is single, and works full time in motel custodial services. After school and during summers, A.J. is cared for by his older brother (17 years old) and his maternal grandmother, who lives a block away. His weight and body mass index (BMI) are well above the 95th percentile for his age. When discussing his diet, you learn that his mother buys packaged foods that he can make for himself when she is away. She is concerned that he will not eat if she does not buy the processed, high-fat foods that he likes. Further, these types of foods are more readily available than healthier options at the local market where she shops. A.J. sometimes eats at his grandmother's place, but

she is elderly and not cooking much anymore. When discussing physical activity, he states that he wants to play soccer. His mother is concerned about this, however, because he often complains of headaches and stomachaches when it is time for practice, and she does not want to buy the equipment if he will quit after a few weeks, as has happened in the past.

Questions
1. What is meant by culture?
2. What is meant by cultural competence?
3. What constitutes health care disparities?
4. What are some of the social determinants that impact the health of a population?

Culture

Culture is defined as a set of meanings, norms, beliefs, and values shared by a group of people. It is dynamic and evolves over time and with each generation. Culture encompasses a body of learned behaviors and perspectives that serves as a template to shape and orient future behaviors and perspectives from generation to generation and as novel situations emerge. As relates to health, culture shapes how and what symptoms are expressed and influences the meaning that one attributes to symptoms, including one's beliefs about the cause, the impact, and the potential remedies. Culture is considered to be broad, encompassing not only race/ethnicity, but also sexual orientation, gender roles, gender identity, socioeconomic status, nationality, and other group affiliations. The interaction between the culture of the patient and family and that of the provider is often significant, and can lead to bias in assessment and treatment. These biases, in turn, can contribute to health and health care disparities.

Health Disparities

Health disparities are defined as differences in health outcomes across different groups. Health *care* disparities, as defined by the Institute of Medicine in the document *Unequal Treatment: Confronting Racial and Ethnic Disparities in Health Care* are "racial or ethnic differences in the quality of health care that are not due to access-related factors

or clinical needs, preferences, and appropriateness of intervention." Both health disparities and health care disparities exist within the United States and particularly affect minority populations. While health disparities may be due to many social determinants of health, such as class, access to safe neighborhoods and healthy food, as well as access to health care, health care disparities are directly related to what happens to certain patients in the health care system once they have accessed care.

Latino children in the United States face significant health and health care disparities. In particular, as alluded to in the case study, the highest prevalence of overweight children in the United States is in the Latino population. Latino children also have a lower fitness level and watch more television than white children in the United States. The reasons behind these disparities are complex and multifactorial. Latino children also face disparities in the health care they receive. For example, the duration of their routine well-child visits is shorter and they are less likely to receive counseling at these visits compared with white children.

In addition to the lack of access to quality health care, there are many social, political, and cultural elements that contribute to the health care disparities observed in certain ethnic groups. Individual providers may have limited impact on the economic, environmental, and political issues that contribute to poor outcomes. It is nevertheless important to understand these issues and how they may contribute to their patients' health outcomes. For example, lack of access to quality, low-cost foods in one's neighborhood, lack of transportation, advertising practices that target low-income communities, and lack of access to safe playgrounds are examples of social determinants that contribute to obesity. It is also essential to understand the influence of culture on patients' health beliefs, health behavior, and health status.

Finally, acculturation is likely to have an impact on health, health beliefs, and health behaviors as well. Second-generation Latino adolescents are twice as likely as first-generation ones to be obese or overweight. Acculturation across generations in Latinos has been associated with decreased fruit and vegetable consumption, increased soda consumption, and decreased physical activity. However, acculturation is a complex variable in relationship to pediatric obesity. Mexican American mothers who were less acculturated had children with higher BMIs in one study.

Cultural Competence

Providers who strive for cultural competence try to minimize their bias and seek to incorporate cultural assets into their work with patients. Cross and colleagues also describe cultural competence as a continuum. While this continuum was used to characterize organizations, it is also relevant for health care providers (Box 10-1). At the most negative pole, *cultural destructiveness* is comprised of attitudes and practices that are meant to be harmful to cultures and individuals within the particular culture. Clinicians at this level may overtly discriminate against individuals based on their culture (ie, intentionally making homophobic, racist, or sexist remarks to colleagues). Clinicians who have *cultural incapacity* do not overtly discriminate, but lack the ability and willingness to recognize and intervene when discrimination happens. As a result, they ultimately reinforce culturally oppressive behaviors and policies. In the *cultural blindness* phase, culture is believed to make no difference and that all people are the same. This viewpoint ignores cultural strengths, encourages assimilation, and often leads to blaming the victims of racial injustices for their problems. Clinicians at this stage may have difficulty believing in the validity of health disparities, despite the enormous body of evidence supporting this. While they strive to give quality care to everyone, they fail to recognize the culture-specific experiences that impact their patient's health (such as poverty or violence based on race, sexual orientation, or gender), and they miss opportunities to incorporate culturally relevant strengths into the treatment (ie, collaboration with traditional healers, extended family, and/or

Box 10-1. Continuum of Cultural Competence
• Cultural destructiveness
• Cultural incapacity
• Cultural blindness
• Cultural pre-competence
• Cultural competence
• Cultural proficiency

faith-based organizations). *Cultural pre-competence* is characterized by a willingness to deliver quality services and a commitment to civil rights but a lack of knowledge and experience to implement culturally relevant services. Clinicians here often struggle with knowledge that disparities exist, and that they perhaps continue to contribute to them. Yet they are at a loss as to what to do about it. A provider at the stage of *cultural competence*, in contrast, seeks to expand his or her cultural knowledge and resources often in consultation with culturally diverse communities. They also continuously self-assess and adapt traditional service models to enhance care for culturally diverse patients. Finally, a provider with *cultural proficiency* holds cultural diversity in highest esteem and continuously advocates for increased cultural competence throughout the system of care. It is important to recognize that providers move back and forth along this continuum dynamically, influenced by their own experiences. For example, a provider who identifies with being in the culturally competent phase when working with Latino patients may find themselves having cultural incapacity when working with gay or lesbian patients.

Communication

As proposed in the opening case study, communication between the physician, the patient, and the parent may pose unique challenges when dealing with language and cultural differences. Effective communication results in improved patient–doctor relationship, treatment adherence, and health outcomes. Poor communication may have negative consequences. Patients with limited English proficiency (LEP) in particular have greater barriers to health care, poorer quality of health, and poorer health status. In a Joint Commission on Accreditation of Health Care Organizations study involving 6 hospitals, researchers found that patients with LEP were at greater risk for iatrogenic harm. In contrast, use of interpreters is associated with greater follow-up with preventive and primary care services. Ideally, one would have a trained medical interpreter in order to communicate with the patient and their parents. It would be inappropriate for a patient to communicate for his parents, although this happens often in clinical practice. It is clearly a difficult position for a child or teen to interpret health information to his parent. There is no guarantee that the patient understands what the physician is communicating, nor that he is interpreting correctly. It also disturbs the appropriate power balance between parent and child. Strategies to incorporate when using interpreters are noted in Box 10-2.

Unconscious Bias

In addition to ensuring effective communication, it is important to address the unconscious biases that one may have as the provider. While few health care providers intentionally discriminate based on culture, studies suggest that physicians are likely to have unconscious biases that can significantly affect their care of patients. Providers can take steps to decrease unconscious bias. It is essential to first acknowledge that bias really does exist, in the health care system

Box 10-2. Strategies When Using Interpreters in Medical Settings

1. Meet with the interpreter briefly prior to the interview to discuss overall goals for the interview and ground rules (ie, use word for word interpretation).
2. Use nonverbal behaviors, such as eye contact, nodding, or facial expressions, to let the patient know that the provider understands what is being communicated.
3. Speak directly to the patient and address the patient in the first person.
4. Use short, simple statements and stick to one topic at a time.
5. Avoid medical jargon and ambiguous statements.
6. Meet briefly with the interpreter after the interview to confirm pertinent information, ask about cultural information, and discuss feedback.
7. Remember that the interpreters are not medical professionals. Therefore, regard information volunteered by interpreters as reliable as collateral information provided by other non–health professionals.

and within the lived experience of patients as well as providers. It is good practice for health care providers to explore Harvard's Project Implicit Web site (https://implicit.harvard.edu/implicit/) and take the online tests designed to detect bias across various cultural dimensions, including race, gender, and sexual orientation. Most people who take these tests realize rather quickly that they carry biases that they had no idea existed within themselves. For many, acknowledging one's own biases may be the most difficult step. The next step is to work toward replacing one's biases with positive and realistic associations about other groups. For example, seeking out dialogue and companionship with people culturally different from oneself can help to reshape one's negative assumptions with more positive associations. Finally, it is important to be mindful of the potential influence of unconscious bias on medical decision-making, whether treating a patient of similar background to the provider or a patient of a very different background. While it is essential to consider the cultural context, it is also important to keep in mind that each patient is a unique individual. In situations where bias may be present, providers should speak less and listen more, striving to avoid assumptions.

Eliciting the Patient's Perspectives

A patient's and provider's understanding of the health issue is an important part of the overall clinical collaboration. Typically, the patient's history is obtained with limited consideration to the patient's beliefs about the health problem. Difficulties may arise if the patient and/or their family members disagree with the physician's explanations of the illness. Openly disagreeing with a physician's assessment and treatment recommendations is considered disrespectful in many cultures. The patient and their family may instead acknowledge the physician's status by expressing agreement but maintain their own ideas about how to address the issue. The mother in our case study, for example, may report her intention to follow through with his physician's recommendations to change to a healthier diet, but may in fact continue with the ready-made foods because she feels there are

difficulties getting healthier foods given her long work hours and the availability of healthy food in her neighborhood. The provider may characterize the obesity as a primarily biological problem, whereas A.J.'s mother might see it as primarily a problem of access and time.

Further, our patient's mother may not see his overweight status as a problem at all. The relationship of pediatric obesity to cultural ideals and norms around food, eating, and parenting is complex. There is some evidence in ethnographic studies that, in some Latino cultures, feeding children, and especially giving "treats," is a way of showing love. Parents who have children who are "healthy eaters" may not want to limit their children's enjoyment of food. In addition, body size ideals vary across communities, and there is some evidence that in some Latino as well as other communities (Pacific Islanders, some Asian communities), children meeting criteria for being overweight are considered more attractive and healthier than thinner children, who may be considered frail. Further, poverty and the experience of food scarcity can further exacerbate overeating when food is more accessible. Finally, particularly when other friends or family members offer food to children, it may be considered socially unacceptable for the parent to refuse or criticize the type of food being offered. Understanding these types of cultural norms can be helpful in treating individual patients. However, it is important to remember that particular individuals and families have their own cultural norms, which may or may not be consistent with others in their ethnic group.

Conflicts in health beliefs between the provider and patient/family may result in treatment non-adherence and drop out. It is important that the physician and patient/family both discuss their respective health perspectives. The more that the provider understands the patient/family's health beliefs, the more effective he or she will be at addressing differences and building on common ground. Likewise, patients/families may feel a greater level of comfort with the provider's recommendations if their questions and concerns about the provider's perspectives are addressed. Questions can help a provider further understand their patient's health beliefs and facilitate discussions about health issues identified by the provider (Box 10-3).

Box 10-3. Questions to Help Facilitate Discussion About Provider-Identified Issues

1. About which problem are you most concerned?
2. What do you think about my concerns (the provider's identified problems, eg, obesity)?
3. What do you think has caused the problem?
4. What are your concerns about this problem? How does it affect you?
5. What treatments do you think might work for it?
6. What are your goals for treatment?
7. What is your understanding of the treatment offered? What are your concerns about it? What are the barriers for completing or carrying out the treatment?

Decision-making

It is also important to understand how a patient or their family makes medical decisions. Many providers look to the child's parents as the primary decision-makers. This process may be culturally influenced. Parents from strongly collectivistic cultures, in which the needs and priorities of the group supersede those of the individual, may wish to have others, such as family members, spiritual leaders, or clan leaders, be involved in health care decision-making. Failure on the part of the provider to allow the inclusion of these people in decision-making may result in the parents feeling forced into a decision, precipitate conflict within the family, and lead to the family or community blaming the parents if a bad outcome occurs. Again, dialoguing may promote better understanding about health care decisions (Box 10-4).

Box 10-4. Questions to Facilitate Decision-making

1. How do you usually make decisions about health care?
2. Do you involve anyone else in that process? Who, and what are their roles?
3. Who usually makes the final decision?
4. How comfortable are you with using that process to make decisions about your current situation?

CASE STUDY, continued

At a follow-up visit for A.J., you ask to speak with him alone. During your HEADDSSS assessment, you learn that he is attracted to boys, but has not shared this with anyone. He is certain that his brothers will not approve and his mother will be heartbroken. He is sometimes teased at school because he is "not tough enough," and he fears some of the bigger bullies might try to jump him if he hangs around after school to participate in any of the after-school sports activities.

At this visit, it is extremely important to remain nonjudgmental and supportive of this patient's early sexual identity development. See Chapter 41 and Chapter 137 for suggestions in addressing the sexual identity and bullying issues presented here. The Fenway Learning Module is another resource on caring for lesbian, gay, bisexual, and transgendered (LGBT) youth (http://www.fenwayhealth.org/site/PageServer?pagename=FCHC_ins_fenway_EducPro_modules).

There are several other factors to consider with respect to health disparities in this case. In the National Longitudinal Study of Adolescent Health, in which 20,000 adolescents were surveyed in 1995, Latino male and female adolescents were more likely to report same-sex romantic attraction than their white and Asian peers. In addition, both male and female Latino adolescents are more likely than their peers to experience violence. Therefore, both the issues of sexual minorities and that of bullying are important to consider in addressing adolescent health disparities in culturally diverse communities in the United States. It is also important to understand A.J.'s sexual orientation in the context of his family and ethnic community. While there are certainly challenges for LGBT youth in Latino families, such as anti-gay sentiments in some faith traditions, there are also strengths for LGBT individuals with strong cultural identities.

For example, urban young Latino men who have sex with men were less likely to engage in risky sexual behavior if they were connected to their ethnic community. These are some examples of the complicated intersection of sexual identity and ethnic identity in cultural issues in pediatrics.

CASE RESOLUTION

You are supportive of your patient in his early sexual identity development, explore safe adults in A.J.'s life with whom he can explore his feelings and concerns, and identify LGBT community resources. You also discuss A.J.'s and his mother's perspectives around food, his weight, and his activity level, using a medical-trained interpreter for his mother. You identify some of this family's strengths: A.J.'s mother's desire to help him be healthier; A.J.'s relationship with his grandmother, who cooks healthy traditional foods; and A.J.'s supportive relationship with his older brother. After discussion, the patient decides that he would like to learn to cook from his grandmother and will commit to cooking dinner for a family meal once a week, which delights his mother. His brother has also agreed to take him to soccer practice and games for a neighborhood soccer team. The patient likes this idea as he feels safe from bullies around his brother, and he feels that soccer will help him be stronger and more confident. You arrange for a follow-up visit in several months to check in with A.J. and his mother regarding their progress and to brainstorm about further interventions.

Selected References

Caprio S, Daniels SR, Drewnowski A, et al. Influence of race, ethnicity, and culture on childhood obesity: implications for prevention and treatment: a consensus statement of Shaping America's Health and the Obesity Society. *Diabetes Care*. 2008;31:2211–2221

Flores G, Abreu M, Tomany-Korman SC. Limited English proficiency, primary language at home, and disparities in children's health care: how language barriers are measured matters. *Public Health Rep*. 2005;120(4):418–430

Flores G; American Academy of Pediatrics Committee on Pediatric Research. Technical report: racial and ethnic disparities in the health and health care of children. *Pediatrics*. 2010;125:e979–e1020

Gaw AC. *Concise Guide to Cross-Cultural Psychiatry*. Washington, DC: American Psychiatric Press; 2001

Green AR, Carney DR, Pallin DJ, et al. Implicit bias among physicians and its prediction of thrombolysis decisions for black and white patients. *J Gen Intern Med*. 2007;22:1231–1238

Jacobs EA, Shepard DS, Suaya JA, Stone EL. Overcoming language barriers in health care: costs and benefits of interpreter services. *Am J Public Health*. 2004;94:866–869

Kaufman L, Karpati A. Understanding the sociocultural roots of childhood obesity: food practices among Latino families of Bushwick, Brooklyn. *Soc Sci Med*. 2007;64:2177–2188

Kumanyika SK. Environmental influences on childhood obesity: ethnic and cultural influences in context. *Physiol Behav*. 2008;944:61–70

Matsumoto D. *Culture and Psychology*. San Francisco, CA: Brooks/Cole Publishing Co.; 1996

O'Donnell L, Agronick G, San Doval A, et al. Ethnic and gay community attachments and sexual risk behaviors among urban Latino young men who have sex with men. *AIDS Educ Prev*. 2002;14:457–471

Popkin BM, Udry JR. Adolescent obesity increases significantly in second and third generation US immigrants: the national longitudinal study of adolescent health. *J Nutr.* 1998;128:701–706

Russell ST, Truong NL. Adolescent sexual orientation, race, and ethnicity, and school environments: a national study of sexual minority youth of color. In: Kumashiro KK, Lanhan MD, eds. *Troubling Intersections of Race and Sexuality: Queer Students of Color and Anti-Oppressive Education.* Rowman & Littlefield Publishers, Inc.; 2001

Schulman KA, Berlin JA, Harless W, et al. The effect of race and sex on physicians' recommendations for cardiac catheterization. *N Engl J Med.* 1999;340:618–626

Schyve P. Language differences as a barrier to quality and safety in health care: the Joint Commission perspective. *J Gen Intern Med.* 2007;22(suppl 2):360–361

Smedley BD, Stith AY, Nelson AR, eds. *Unequal Treatment: Confronting Racial and Ethnic Disparities in Health Care.* Washington, DC: The National Academies Press; 2003

Stewart MA. Effective physician-patient communication and health outcomes: a review. *Can Med Assoc J.* 1995;152;1423–1433

Sussner KM, Lindsay AC, Peterson KE. The influence off maternal acculturation on child body mass index at age 24 months. *J Am Diet Assoc.* 2009;109:218–225

Timmins CL. The impact of language barriers on the health care of Latinos in the United States: a review of the literature and guidelines for practice. *J Midwifery Womens Health.* 2002;47(2):80–96

CHAPTER 11

Principles of Pediatric Therapeutics

Elizabeth A. Edgerton, MD, MPH

CASE STUDY

An 18-month-old girl who has had a cough, runny nose, and fever for 2 days is brought to your clinic for evaluation. The previous night she awoke from sleep crying and pulling at her ear. The patient has no other symptoms. Her mother states she has had previous ear infections, the most recent occurred 2 months ago. The last time she took amoxicillin she broke out in hives. Otherwise the patient has no significant medical history.

On physical examination, the patient is febrile to 102°F (38.9°C) and has yellow rhinorrhea. The ear examination reveals a red, bulging, nonmobile tympanic membrane in one ear, while the other ear appears normal. The remainder of the examination is benign.

Questions

1. What are the current practice guidelines for antibiotic treatment of otitis media? How does treatment change with the age and symptoms of the patient?
2. How does the previous reaction to a medication influence the antibiotic choice?
3. How do factors such as child care, work, and family plans affect the choice of medication?
4. What role do over-the-counter medications have in the management of the patient's symptoms?
5. What resources are available to obtain information on therapeutic effectiveness, costs, side effects, and drug–drug interactions?

The use of prescription and over-the-counter (OTC) medications is common in pediatrics. The Slone Survey, a random digit–dial survey of medication use, found that families with children reported more than 55% of children younger than 12 years had taken some medication preparation within the last 7 days. Of those taking a medication, 22% were taking at least one prescription medication. Many OTC medications contain multiple active ingredients, raising the concern about their safety profile for children, considering that the use of OTC medications is reported as being so prevalent. Furthermore, it is estimated that only one-third of drugs used to treat pediatric patients have adequately been studied in the populations in which they are being used and have appropriate labeling information. This does not mean that the other two-thirds of medications are unsafe for children but that their use in children is extrapolated from adult studies.

Differences in pharmacokinetics among infants, children, and adolescents can produce significant differences in drug efficacy and toxicity. Body composition, the rate of drug binding, and metabolism change with development. The consequences of not fully studying the clinical effectiveness and safety profile of therapeutics can lead to potentially harmful outcomes. Significant medical tragedies in the past include the use of sulfonamides in the newborn period leading to kernicterus, chloramphenicol causing gray syndrome, and in utero exposure to thalidomide leading to birth deformities. Recently, the US Food and Drug Administration (FDA) removed OTC cough and cold preparations for infants and toddlers due to safety concerns. Poison control centers managed 750,000 calls due to cold and cough medications, and the FDA is investigating the deaths of 123 children associated with these types of medications. Factors believed to contribute to the harm associated with OTC cough and cold medications included inappropriate dosing by caregivers, use of more than one product, and use of adult product formulations.

Since 1962 the FDA has required drugs to be proven safe and effective before they can be marketed. The FDA can only regulate the safety, effectiveness, and labeling of medication and is not authorized to regulate a physician's use of a medication. When data are not sufficient for a specific population or age group, it will be specified in the product labeling that use in that population has not been established. Using a medication for a condition or specific population not specified by the product insert is referred to as **off-label prescribing.** Depending on the practice setting, off-label prescription rates range from 11% to 80%, with the highest rates among younger patients and hospitalized settings. Pediatricians rely on the published literature, adult studies, and knowledge of pediatric physiology and pharmacokinetics for prescribing. While off-label prescribing is not illegal, it does put children at greater risk of unexpected adverse reactions as well as lack of optimal treatments. Through the Best Pharmaceuticals for Children Act in 2002 (Public Law 107-109) and again in 2007 (Public Law 10-85) and the enactment of the Pediatric Research Equity Act (Public Law 108-155), the FDA has been mandated by Congress to increase the level of pediatric research prior to approval and during the post-marketing phases. Even with increased regulation, implementation of pediatric clinical trials faces critical issues, such as the ethics of parental consent, multiple age groups to be tested, and the unknown long-term effects in a developing child. The pediatric population lacks the autonomy to fully give consent and understand the implications of studies, thus the American Academy of Pediatrics Committee on Drugs and Committee on Pediatric Research developed guidelines to address the special issues of drug research among children.

Principles of Therapeutics

A drug or therapeutic can be defined as any substance that is ingested, absorbed, or injected that alters the body's function. This includes OTC medications, homeopathic substances, illicit substances, and prescription drugs. Each drug has a different safety profile and level of regulation depending on its category. The most regulated and standardized drugs are those requiring a prescription. Homeopathic substances often lack any standardization, safety testing, and regulation, and illicit drugs such as heroin or cocaine receive no quality testing. Choosing the most appropriate therapeutic is a complex process involving a number of factors: patient characteristics, disease epidemiology, safety profile, patient compliance, and cost-effectiveness (Box 11-1).

Box 11-1. Factors in Choosing the Appropriate Therapeutic	
Patient Characteristics	**Patient Compliance**
Age	Taste
Medical history	Purpose of treatment
Allergies	Storage
Use of other medications	Side effects
Diagnosis	**Cost-effectiveness**
Epidemiology	Drug availability
Age-specific factors	Formulary restrictions
Safety Profile	
Therapeutic index	
Black box warning	

Patient Characteristics

The organs of infants and children are growing and maturing, which can affect how a medication is absorbed, distributed, and excreted. Neonates have immature liver and kidney function compared with older children and adults. For example, similar microgram per kilogram doses of fentanyl can result in a 2- to 3-fold higher plasma concentration in the neonate compared with an adult. Knowledge of the age of the patient is critical to account for developmental pharmacokinetic differences for age-appropriate as well as weight-based dosing.

The choice of an appropriate therapeutic is influenced by a patient **medical history.** Depending on the type of clinical conditions or surgeries a patient has, the absorption, metabolism, or clinical effectiveness of the therapeutic may be altered. Children with short bowel syndrome can potentially have difficulty absorbing oral medications depending on which portion of the bowel was removed. Children with mental retardation who are given central nervous system–altering medications can be difficult to monitor for changes in mental status seen with systemic infection. In addition, children with glucose-6-phosphate dehydrogenase deficiency can suffer from drug-induced hemolytic anemia when given certain drugs such as sulfonamides. Malnourished children are at a greater risk for drug toxicity because low serum albumin levels decrease the amount of bound drug and result in increased levels of unbound drug in circulation. While not an exhaustive list of medical conditions that can alter medication delivery, these demonstrate the need to consider underlying medical conditions in choosing the most appropriate therapeutic.

Before prescribing any medication, physicians need to ask patients and their families about any previous reactions to drugs and obtain detailed information about the symptoms and class of medications involved in these reactions. **Drug allergies** are those reactions that have an immunologic basis. Of the 4 types of immune mechanisms associated with drug allergies, immunoglobulin E–mediated reactions are of greatest concern because they can result in anaphylaxis, a life-threatening condition. **Adverse reactions** can be idiosyncratic or non–immune-mediated. A **side effect** is an expected but undesirable consequence of taking the medication. Families often attribute any symptom the patient suffered while taking the medication to a drug allergy. It is therefore important to know which side effects are associated with a medication to determine whether an allergy is present. Any medication that has been associated with an allergic reaction (eg, skin eruptions, swelling, urticaria, or respiratory difficulty) should not be used again without consulting a specialist.

Finally, knowing what other medications a patient is taking can affect the choice of therapeutic. The mechanism of metabolism of one drug can affect the metabolism of another. Drug metabolism is divided into 2 types: phase I reactions include oxidation, reduction, and hydrolysis; phase II reactions involve adding subgroups to a drug. Other drugs can affect reactions during either phase. For example, the enzyme activity of the P-450 system involved in oxidation can be induced or inhibited depending on the other medications being taken, resulting in an altered rate of metabolism. Common drugs used in pediatrics that inhibit the P-450 system include cimetidine and erythromycin, while phenobarbital and phenytoin induce the system. Drug interactions are not a contraindication to the use of a therapeutic, but the dose and serum levels may need to be closely monitored. Referencing the package insert, the *Physicians' Desk Reference (PDR)*, or a pharmacist can aid in determining potential drug-to-drug interactions. Handheld devices that provide formulary information often have drug compatibility functions that allow a provider to enter a patient's medication list and screen for potential drug interactions.

Diagnosis

Choosing the appropriate medication depends on understanding the condition being treated as well as the epidemiology of the disease for a specific age group. Etiologies of pneumonia for an infant, child, and adolescent can be completely different, thus requiring a different type of antibiotic. Even when a potential organism is identified, the profile of the medication needs to be reviewed. For a patient with group A streptococcal pharyngitis, a gram-positive organism, penicillin G, penicillin V, erythromycin, or a first-generation cephalosporin is an acceptable choice. Although tetracycline and sulfonamides can be effective in treating patients with gram-positive infections, tetracycline is contraindicated in young children, and sulfonamides do not eradicate group A streptococcal infection. Treatment duration can also vary depending on the age of the patient. An adult with a simple urinary tract infection may receive only a 1- to 3-day course of treatment, while a child may receive 7 to 10 days of treatment because of the high recurrence of infection that has been observed with a shorter duration of treatment.

Safety Profile

The safety profile of a medication is the balance between its benefits and its potential risks. The risks can be dependent on the duration of treatment, dose, or interactions with other medications. Using the **therapeutic index** is one way to quantify the risk associated with a specific dose. The therapeutic index is the difference between the dose that provides a desired effect and the dose that provides an undesired effect. For example, a medication with a wide therapeutic index is one in which a desired effect is achieved with a dose much lower than that required to produce a toxic effect. In general, a medication with a wide therapeutic index, such as ibuprofen, is considered safer than a medication with a narrow therapeutic index. The higher the morbidity and mortality associated with a condition the smaller the accepted therapeutic index can be. Food–drug interactions and drug–drug interactions are other risks that can be anticipated. These are best delineated in pharmacologic references. There are also risks that are independent of the dose of the therapeutic called idiosyncratic effects. These are unexpected and usually unavoidable risks associated with the medication.

In the United States, a **black box warning,** also known as a **black label warning,** is a type of warning that appears on prescription drugs that may cause serious adverse effects. Named for the black border that usually surrounds the text of the warning, it means that medical studies indicate that the drug carries a significant risk of serious or even life-threatening adverse effects. The FDA can require a pharmaceutical company to place a black box warning on the labeling of a prescription drug or in literature describing it. It is the strongest warning that the FDA requires. Psychotropic medications, selective serotonin reuptake inhibitor antidepressants, stimulants for attention-deficit/hyperactivity disorder, and the long-acting β-agonist salmeterol are a few of the medications that have a black box warning for use in the pediatric population. A complete list of medications with black box warnings can be found at www. fda.gov. This warning does not preclude the use of the medication, but requires the physician and family to evaluate the risks and benefits of its use.

Patient Adherence

Patient adherence is dependent on the convenience of administering and taking the medication, the patient's and caregiver's comprehension of the medication's purpose, and any potential discomfort caused by side effects. Because children are dependent on their caregivers to administer medications, it is crucial that caregivers know why the drug has been prescribed, how it should be dispensed, and why it must be given for a specific length of time. For a child with tinea capitis, a fungal infection of the scalp and hair follicles, parents may think that a topical antifungal is sufficient to treat the infection. Explaining the difference between a fungal skin infection (tinea corpus) versus the fungal scalp infection can facilitate adherence with the treatment. To eliminate the fungal infection in the hair follicles, a systemic medication is needed. Furthermore, because of the slow growing cycle of both the fungus and the hair, patients need to take the medicine for up to 6 weeks. To ensure accurate dosing, a staff member should demonstrate how to dispense the medication and then ask the parent to repeat the process. Such a simple intervention can make an important difference in obtaining adherence and influence the effectiveness of the therapeutic.

The taste and texture of a medication are also important considerations in pediatrics. Children may not be able to understand the importance of taking a medication and refuse to take it because they don't like the taste. Physicians should be familiar with the taste and consistency of medication and be prepared to find alternatives. Prednisone is a commonly used medication for the treatment of acute asthma. It comes in both a pill and suspension form. For children requiring a suspension, a vast difference exists in taste depending on the preparation prescribed. Children are known to vomit the less palatable version. Knowing in advance what is acceptable to children may prevent complications with noncompliance.

Cost-effectiveness

Cost-effectiveness is defined as the best outcome per unit cost. The outcome is the treatment of a condition or alleviation of a symptom; the cost includes the price of the medication and the time spent by the physician and family. For instance, a specific medication may cost less but be less effective, so that in the long run it costs more to the patient in return visits to the doctor. Many physicians practice in settings where the pharmacy has a set inventory or formulary of medications, limiting the selection of medications for each condition. Thus the physician's choice of a cost-effective drug might depend on which are available in the formulary. From the patient perspective, many families may have limited or no health insurance coverage and may have to incur the total cost of a medication. The cost of an antibiotic for a course of otitis media can differ by 10-fold depending on the medication prescribed. Thus an appropriate drug of choice is influenced by the out-of-pocket cost to the family. The perceived cost-effectiveness of a therapeutic is different for each situation and depends on the external factors affecting the physician and the family.

Drug Dosing

Most medications used in the adult population are based on a standard dose for an individual regardless of age or body size. In pediatrics, a patient's size and metabolism vary with age such that dosing is usually based on weight or body surface area. When drug dosing is determined by weight, it represents a proportion of the adult dose; when a child reaches a weight of 40 to 50 kg, the dosing is often changed to a standard adult dose. With the increasing prevalence of obesity of children, many school-aged children weigh more than 50 kg, thus it is important to know the maximum daily adult dose of a medication because calculating milligrams per kilogram doses can easily exceed this amount. For drugs with narrow therapeutic indexes, such as immunosuppressive medications, body surface area is used to determine appropriate dosing.

Once a drug is identified, the appropriate dosing schedule must be determined. Dosing guidelines can be presented as a total dose per 24 hours or an amount per dose. Usually a range is given per unit weight, and then the physician must determine the amount of medication based on the concentration of therapeutic agent. An example for dosing acetaminophen for a 1-year-old child is given in Box 11-2.

Medication Errors and Adverse Drug Events

Increasing data demonstrate that a significant number of errors can occur in the delivery of medications. Pediatric patients are at greater risk because most of the dosing needs to be calculated based on weight or surface area, and pharmacists may need to prepare solutions or suspensions rather than use manufacturer-produced pills. These medication errors can lead to potential or actual adverse drug events. It is estimated that 5 medication errors occur per 100 dispensed medications, of which 0.21 per 100 go on to non-preventable adverse drug events. More than half of these errors occur during the prescribing stage, the phase where the medication dose is calculated. Referencing a pediatric drug manual and consulting a pharmacist can be used as steps to reduce medication errors.

The American Recovery and Reinvestment Act of 2009 provides additional momentum toward widespread electronic health records, which include e-prescribing. Patient safety initiatives demonstrate that computerized systems can decrease mediation errors. Specifically, systems that use computerized physician orders or e-prescribing can reduce medication errors by having alerts for inappropriate dosing, improved legibility, warnings for drug interactions, and just-in-time information on the most appropriate drug choice.

Box 11-2. Dosing

A 1-year-old is suffering from a fever and the family wants to know how much acetaminophen to give her. She weighs 11.2 kg. The recommended dose of acetaminophen is 10 to 15 mg/kg every 4 to 6 hours. Acetaminophen drops are sold in a concentration of 80 mg/0.8 mL or as a suspension with the concentration of 160 mg/5 mL.

1. Determine the amount of medication needed by multiplying the weight of the child by the recommended dose.

$$11.2 \text{ kg} \times 10 \text{ mg/kg} = 112 \text{ mg acetaminophen}$$

2. Determine the volume of medication based on the concentration of acetaminophen to be used. Either the dropper or the suspension can be used.

Dosing volume =
(amount of medication) ÷ (concentration of medication)

Dropper

$$
\begin{aligned}
\text{Dosing volume} &= 112 \text{ mg} \div 80 \text{ mg/0.8 mL} \\
&= (112 \times 0.8)/80 \\
&= 1.12 \text{ mL}
\end{aligned}
$$

(This can be rounded to 1.2 mL because the lower range of 10 mg/kg was used to calculate the dose.)

Suspension

$$
\begin{aligned}
\text{Dosing volume} &= 112 \text{ mg} \div 160 \text{ mg/5mL} \\
&= (112 \times 5)/160 \\
&= 3.5 \text{ mL}
\end{aligned}
$$

The family can be instructed to give their daughter either 1.2 mL using the drops or 3.5 mL of the suspension of acetaminophen orally every 4 to 6 hours as needed for fever.

Therapeutic References

Various resources provide information on drug uses, dosing, side effects, and costs. The *PDR* is a comprehensive listing of FDA-approved prescription and commonly used OTC drugs that provides a description of the drug, pharmacology, indications and contraindications, adverse reactions, drug interactions, and manufacturer name. The *Medical Letter* is a periodical that reviews drugs, citing current research on risks and benefits as well as cost comparisons of newly released drugs with those already approved for similar indications. Pocket manuals that are specific to pediatrics include the *Pediatric Dosage Handbook* and *Harriet Lane Handbook*. *Epocrates* is another therapeutic formulary specifically designed for handheld devices that also provides pediatric-specific dosing and side effects. Due to the lack of standardization between the various resources, caution still needs to be used by the clinician when prescribing medications.

CASE RESOLUTION

After obtaining the history and performing a physical examination, the pediatrician determines that the patient has acute otitis media. Depending on the age of the child and the severity of symptoms, the American Academy of Pediatrics clinical practice guideline* suggests a stratified approach to therapeutics. For children younger than 2 years, pediatricians can treat with antibiotics if the diagnosis is certain or observe the patient without antibiotics if the patient is otherwise healthy. In this case the pediatrician discusses the options with the family and, because of the severity of pain and previous ear infections, chooses to treat the infection. The antibiotic of choice for treatment of otitis media is amoxicillin at a dose of 80 to 90 mg/kg/d. The mother stated that her daughter had hives with amoxicillin, a type I hypersensitivity. Other antibiotic choices would include azithromycin 10 mg/kg on day 1 followed by 5 mg/kg for the remaining 4 days or clindamycin at 30 to 40 mg/kg/d. The treatment of pain is essential with otitis media. The patient can take oral acetaminophen or ibuprofen or use otic benzocaine drops.

The mother raises concern about her daughter's cough and runny nose and would like to use an OTC cough medication. The FDA does not recommend use of cough preparations in this age group. Educating the mother about conservative therapies, including nasal suctioning, humidification, and nasal saline, to treat her respiratory symptoms is more appropriate.

If the patient were not allergic to amoxicillin, it would have been the drug of choice. It is inexpensive, has a narrow microbiological spectrum, and is palatable. Amoxicillin does require refrigeration, which would be of concern if the family were traveling. While this case illustrates several obvious constraints, it is important to emphasize that choosing the appropriate medication is dependent on both the intrinsic needs of the patient and the extrinsic factors that can affect adherence and ultimately the effectiveness of treatment.

---

* American Academy of Pediatrics Subcommittee on Management of Acute Otitis Media, American Academy of Family Physicians. Clinical practice guideline: diagnosis and management of acute otitis media. *Pediatrics.* 2004;113:1451–1465.

Selected References

American Academy of Pediatrics Committee on Drugs and Committee on Pediatric Research. Clinical Report: guidelines for the ethical conduct of studies to evaluate drugs in pediatric populations. *Pediatrics.* 2010;125:850–860

Bell EA, Tunkel DE. Over-the-counter cough and cold medications in children: are they helpful? *Otolaryngol Head Neck Surg.* 2010;142(5):647–650

Gerstle RS, Lehmann CU; American Academy of Pediatrics Council on Clinical Information Technology. Technical report: electronic prescribing systems in pediatrics: the rationale and functionality requirements. *Pediatrics.* 2007;119(6);e1413–e1422

Hughes RG, Edgerton EA. Reducing pediatric medication errors: children are especially at risk for medication errors. *Am J Nurs.* 2005;105:79–80

Pollock M, Bazaldua OV, Dobbie AE. Appropriate prescribing of medications: an eight-step approach. *Am Fam Physician.* 2007;75:231–236

United States Health and Human Services Federal Drug Agency. Science and Research Special Topics: Pediatrics. http://www.fda.gov/ScienceResearch/SpecialTopics/PediatricTherapeuticsResearch/default.htm. Accessed November 20, 2010

Vernacchio L, Kelly JP, Kaufman DW, Mitchell AA. Medication use among children <12 years of age in the United States: results from the Slone Survey. *Pediatrics.* 2009;124(2):446–454

CHAPTER 12

Pediatric Pain and Symptom Management

Rick Goldstein, MD

CASE STUDY

You are caring for a 5-year-old girl with stage 4 neuroblastoma who is at home receiving palliative care. Her tumor is refractory. She receives oral chemotherapy and transfusions as an outpatient to offset the bone marrow depletion caused by her tumor. Pain from her metastases is becoming increasing problematic, most especially in her chest wall and right femur. Her spine is also involved but she does not experience weakness. Though fatigued, she derives great pleasure from attending school and being surrounded by friends and family members, playing as she is able. She hates the hospital and her parents have chosen to avoid it, intending to keep her comfortable at home until she dies. Her pediatrician has remained closely involved throughout her illness and would like to help with the management of her symptoms.

Questions

1. What is the approach to pain management children?
2. How does one assess the level of pain in children?
3. What is meant by adjuvant therapy?
4. What is the role of distraction in pain management?
5. What are non-pain symptoms that can cause distress?
6. What is the management of non-pain symptoms?

When children are ill or injured they experience distressing physical symptoms. This is particularly true when the illness or injuries are chronic or serious. The optimal management of such symptoms is fundamental to minimizing their suffering and optimizing their quality of life. A child experiencing poorly controlled pain will withdraw and be unable to engage in the activities that make life, however limited, meaningful. Pain can not only diminish a child's physical well-being, but also impact her psychological, social, and spiritual health. Similarly, a child troubled by nausea will experience distress from the symptom while also losing the simple pleasure of eating and other satisfying comforts. Symptom management is especially important in improving the lives of medically fragile children.

Studies of dying children have noted that distressing symptoms are often untreated. Wolfe et al, in landmark research investigating the symptoms and suffering of children dying from cancer, found that most of the children experienced fatigue, pain, dyspnea, anorexia, nausea and vomiting, and constipation in the last month of their life (Figure 12-1). Similar findings are noted in other children. Neurologically impaired children are particularly difficult to assess because their verbal skills are limited and their responses to pain may be atypical. Research on parents has found that the greatest parental concerns are about symptoms that cannot be satisfactorily controlled. Symptom management of seriously ill children has been improved significantly since these early studies. As more children with chronic and serious illnesses are cared for, and sometimes die at home, their management will increasingly involve their primary care pediatrician.

This chapter will review the basic medical approaches to pain and symptom management in children, particularly those with serious diseases. In addition to pain, approaches to nausea, anorexia, fatigue, and secretions will be presented. The focus will be on the medical management issues a primary care pediatrician should be able to manage in the community setting. When the primary care pediatrician is insufficiently familiar with such treatment, consultation with pain or palliative care specialists is appropriate.

Pain

Pain is an integrated biophysical and "existential" construct. It involves complex mechanisms of nociception modulated by biochemical factors, plasticity, genetic and familial factors, and one's past experience with painful events. Children experience pain in unique ways and quickly develop learned behaviors related to it. As such, there is not a linear association between the objective degree of injury and the experience of pain. More accurately, physical, psychological, interpersonal, and existential factors all contribute in important ways to the experience of pain. A comprehensive approach to pain will address all of these elements.

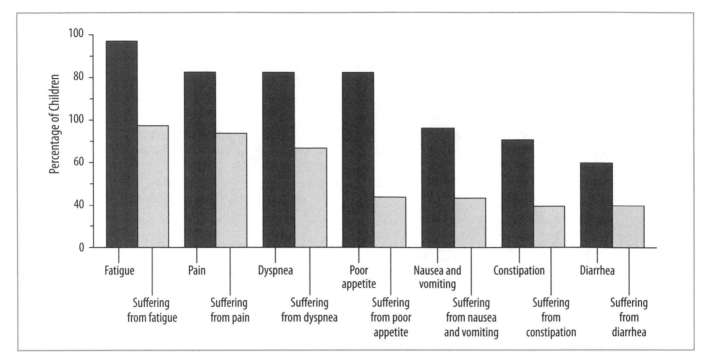

Figure 12-1. The presence and degree of suffering from specific symptoms in the last month of life. (From Wolfe J, Grier HE, Klar N, et al. Symptoms and suffering at the end of life. *N Engl J Med.* 2000; 342:326–333. Reprinted with permission.)

Assessment

Pain is often divided into 2 basic types: nociceptive and neuropathic. An understanding of their presentations can help differentiate the source of pain in children. Nociceptive pain is the activation of peripheral nerve receptors by noxious stimuli causing tissue damage, and its intensity is generally related to the location and the amount of damage. Somatic pain refers to nociceptive pain from musculoskeletal, bony, or superficial sources (skin, mucosa). Deep somatic pain tends to be localized and concentrated, and described as stabbing, aching, or throbbing. Bone pain is deep and aching. Superficial somatic pain is sharper and can be burning or pricking. The source of nociceptive pain can also be visceral. Visceral pain is usually poorly localizable; can be described as cramping, gnawing, or pressure; and may follow daily patterns of varying intensity.

Neuropathic pain is due to injury or dysfunction of the central nervous system (CNS) or peripheral nerves. It can be described as burning, tingling, shooting, or scalding. Its presence points to neuropathies, CNS insult, or evolving damage to the nervous system. Understanding whether the source of pain is somatic, visceral, or neuropathic helps guide treatment choices.

Pain has been referred to as the "fifth vital sign" and should be a part of the medical evaluation of every child. Pain is phenomenological and, thus, while its existence is "real" and "objective," it can only be experienced by the affected person. Though it is not a completely subjective experience, it can only be truly articulated by the person in pain and, fundamentally, the patient's report of the presence or severity of pain is the key to the assessment. In children, and especially children with developmental issues, objective assessment tools may be useful to identify the presence of pain and quantify its severity. In most patients these scales are also helpful in understanding the symptom of pain over time.

Pain scales assess the intensity of pain. Analog pain scales (Figure 12-2), generally scoring intensity on a scale of 1 to 10, have some reliability when used in the same patient over time. Younger children may have difficulty with the concept of quantity or the meaning of greater intensity. An important modification of the analog scale for children with impaired communication skills or cognition is an individualized numeric rating scale, where parents' observations of their child's facial expression, body movements, activity and interaction, cry, and consolability as they experience worsening pain are used to label the points of the scale.

For young children older than 3 years, the Wong-Baker Faces Pain Scale (Figure 12-3) is often used. After showing the child the faces, they are instructed that Face 0 is happy because he has no pain but Face 5 is sad because he has a lot of pain. The child is then asked to choose the face that best describes how he is feeling. More comprehensive pain assessment tools are available that also assess function and mood, but these scales are used most widely. In addition, the perspective of parents and others familiar with the child is crucial to any assessment of a child's pain.

Obviously, the child in pain must be relieved of it. However, it is advantageous to make a strong effort to understand the source of the pain and treat conditions amenable to non-pain medication. For example, chest pain may be due to candidal esophagitis or abdominal pain to constipation. Thinking clearly about the source of pain and not simply providing analgesic agents in a reflexive manner has the benefits of preserving alertness, sparing side effects, and sustaining the least impaired quality of life. It also can permanently eliminate the pain by eliminating the underlying condition responsible for it.

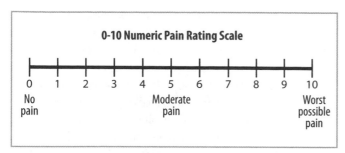

Figure 12-2. **Visual analog pain scale. (From McCaffery M, Pasero C. *Pain: Clinical Manual.* St Louis, MO: Mosby;1999)**

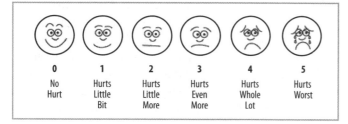

Figure 12-3. **Wong-Baker FACES Pain Scale. (From Wong DL, Hockenberry-Eaton M, Wilson D, Winkelstein ML, Schwartz P. *Wong's Essentials of Pediatric Nursing.* 6th ed. St Louis, MO: Mosby; 2001:1301.)**

Medical Management

Opioids are the mainstay of pain management. Familiarity with the basic principles of treatment with these agents is fundamental to care for children with both serious acute and life-limiting illness. In cases of complex pain or those involving daunting polypharmacy, it may be best to seek guidance from pain or palliative care specialists. Certain medications (ie, methadone or selective norepinephrine reuptake inhibitors) or invasive approaches (ie, intrathecal pumps, regional blocks, and surgical or radiotherapeutic approaches to pain control), as well as the management of chronic pain, particularly in adolescents, often requires consultation with or referral to pain and palliative care specialists. The optimal management of pain includes addressing psychosocial and spiritual distress and making efforts at enhancing a child's function.

Opioids have no ceiling doses. Dose escalation should proceed until the pain is controlled, provided that there are no unacceptable side effects. Children on long-term opioid treatment often receive surprisingly high doses yet, provided the treatment is successful in controlling pain, are comfortable and functional. Intolerable pain is more easily prevented than relieved, and efforts should be directed at "staying ahead of the pain." Anticipated side effects of opioids include constipation, pruritus, and nausea/vomiting. The pruritus and nausea and vomiting are usually short-lived, disappearing in a week, but constipation persists. All patients on opioids should receive scheduled doses of stool softeners and stimulant laxatives. As a general rule, infants younger than 6 months should be started at one-third the general pediatric dose.

Barriers exist in both patients and providers that prevent the optimal use of opioids. Foremost is the concern about respiratory depression. In opioid-naïve patients, this risk is minimized by appropriate

dosing. Even in patients requiring dose escalation, the risk is low and respiratory depression is preceded by sedation rather than an abrupt event. When needed, naloxone can be used to reverse a worrisome respiratory effect, though at the cost of the return of pain. Providers may also be unfamiliar with appropriate dosing, may not view pain control as a priority of care, or may be worried about difficulties ensuring follow-up and ongoing assessment. Families, for their part, may believe that pain is an inevitable part of the child's disease, may worry about the "symbolism" of starting a morphine drip thereby hastening death, or may worry about addiction or the stigma of having their child on such medications. Cultural and religious factors may also elicit reluctance. When these concerns arise, they should be addressed directly. In truth, the greatest concern should be to minimize suffering due to inadequately treated pain.

Parents and some providers may overestimate the benefit of distraction in pain management. Distraction is best thought of as an assessment tool and maybe an adjunct, but not a treatment, for pain. If a child can be substantially distracted from their pain for a significant period, the pain need not be managed with medication. But if their distress is apparent despite the distraction, the pain needs pharmacologic intervention. What must be avoided is a distressed child engaging in the distraction to please adults while their pain goes unabated. Similarly, there is no place for the use of placebos in the treatment of pain.

The World Health Organization Pain Relief Ladder (Figure 12-4) is the most important guide to pain management in children. It presents a step-wise and additive approach to "capture" a child's pain as well as to augment the pharmacologic treatment of pain. The model is premised on the slogan "by the ladder, by the clock, by the appropriate route, and with the child." "By the ladder" means that a child's treatment is guided by their place on the ladder as determined by the intensity of their pain and their response to previous medications. "By the clock" advises that pain needing ongoing attention should be treated with scheduled doses every 3 to 6 hours and not on an as-needed (prn) basis. "By the appropriate route" means by

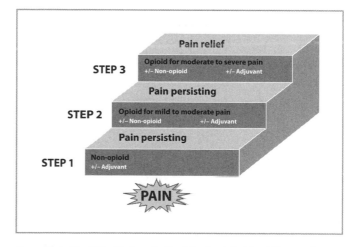

Figure 12-4. **World Health Organization's Analgesic Ladder: A Systematic Approach to Pain Management at End of Life. From World Health Organization, 1992. Available at http://www.who.int/cancer/palliative/painladder/en/.**

the least invasive route necessary to ensure control of a child's pain. Generally, this can be achieved with oral medications, though intravenous (IV) or subcutaneous medications may be required at times. Intramuscular medications are to be avoided because they are painful and erratically absorbed. "With the child" means that regular assessment of the child, the many aspects of their pain, and their response to treatment must be ongoing.

Children with mild or moderate pain, or those who have not been on any analgesic medication, are managed with acetaminophen and ibuprofen or intravenously with ketorolac (Step 1). Adjuvants may be added if appropriate (see below). Acetaminophen can be given orally or rectally. An IV form of acetaminophen is currently being introduced into the US market. Compounded ibuprofen can be given rectally, though its efficacy is still under study. The topical application of these agents in ketoprofen cream or aspirin cream may also be of benefit. All nonsteroidal anti-inflammatory drugs (NSAIDs) have ceiling doses and gastrointestinal toxicities. Except for acetaminophen all affect platelet function.

Adjuvants are non-analgesic medications that are helpful in the management of a child's pain. For example, a medically fragile child's anxiety may potentiate their pain and distress even at Step 1. A benzodiazepine may be helpful in such cases. A lidocaine patch can help with some somatic pain. Certain forms of mild to moderate pain (ie, neuropathic pain) may be adequately addressed with gabapentin or pregabalin and can spare opioids either in part or completely.

Step 2 addresses children with moderate to severe pain and involves the addition of opioids to the treatment plan (Table 12-1). It recommends "weak opioids," which is controversial since codeine is the agent generally intended. There is a growing body of literature to suggest removing codeine from consideration. Research has shown that codeine may be a weaker analgesic than a standard dose of many NSAIDs and it has a ceiling effect. Its oral bioavailability is widely unpredictable at 15% to 80%. Most importantly, codeine is a prodrug, which must be metabolized by the liver into morphine. This is problematic because it is estimated that 35% of children do not metabolize codeine in the anticipated way, leading to great uncertainties in a calculated effect. As an alternative, tramadol has been shown to be effective and safe in children, though it should not be used in children with seizures. Often, Step 2 involves the use of oral oxycodone with a non-opioid analgesic.

When pain persists or worsens, Step 3 advocates for a strong opioid. Hydromorphone, morphine, or oxycodone is a typical initial choice. Doses are escalated until pain is controlled, using the least invasive form of administration necessary. This step may involve the addition of controlled-release preparations of opioid or methadone, while using shorter-acting agents for breakthrough pain. To calculate the prn dose for breakthrough pain, a rule of thumb is that the prn dose is 10% to 15% of the 24-hour total opioid dose or its equivalent, given every 1 to 2 hours.

An in-depth discussion of methadone and fentanyl exceeds the scope of this chapter, but it is worth making several points about them. Neither have active metabolites, making them important options for patients with renal failure where accumulated metabolites from other opioid agents can cause myoclonus, confusion, or hyperalgesia. Fentanyl, a potent analgesic, is available in a transdermal patch, which is an important non-IV, non-oral option for children having difficulty swallowing. They must have adequate body fat, because the drug is deposited across the rate-limiting membrane into fat reservoirs and is absorbed from that reservoir into the child's bloodstream. Methadone has some distinct analgesic advantages. It

		Table 12-1. Dosing of Selected Step 2 and 3 Analgesic Medications		
Drug Name	*Initial Oral Dosing*	*Initial IV Dosing*	*Preparations*	*Comments*
Tramadol	(<50 kg): 1–2 mg/kg PO q 3–6 hours (>50 kg): 50–100 mg PO q 3–6 hours	Not available in US	50- or 100-mg tablets, can be compounded into suspension	Maximum dose of 8 mg/kg/day or if >50 kg 400 mg/day May be administered PO or PR
Oxycodone	0.1–0.2 mg/kg q 4–6 hours	NA	1-mg/mL and 20-mg/mL solutions; 5-, 10-, 15-, 20-, or 30-mg tablets	Available in controlled-release tablets (OxyContin) May be administered PO, sublingual, or PR
Morphine	0.15–0.3 mg/kg q 4 hours	50–100 µg/kg q 2–4 hours Continuous infusion 10–30 µg/kg/hour	2-mg/mL, 4-mg/mL and 20-mg/mL solution 10-, 15-, 30-mg tablets 5-, 10-, 20-, 30-mg suppository	May be administered PO, IV, sublingual, or PR Available in controlled-release tablets (MSContin)
Hydromorphone	60 µg/kg q 3–4 hours	15–20 µg/kg q 4 hours Continuous infusion 5 µg/kg/hour	1-mg/mL oral solution 2-, 4-, 8-mg tablets, 3-mg suppository	May be administered PO, IV, sublingual, or PR Controlled-release tablets not available in US

Abbreviations: IV, intravenous; PO, orally; PR, far point of accommodation; q, every.

is inexpensive, its half-life allows for more convenient twice-a-day or 3-times-a-day dosing, and it is especially helpful in treating neuropathic pain. It is complicated to dose, however, and its long and variable half-life make it a more complicated choice for those not familiar with its use.

The management of moderate and severe pain over time can lead to the development of difficult unintended effects, including sedation, nausea and vomiting, pruritus, or urinary retention. At high doses or when metabolites accumulate, patients may develop delirium, myoclonus, or hyperesthesia. Opioid rotation can be very helpful in these situations. This method involves converting one form of opioid to an equivalently analgesic dose of another. Doses can be calculated using equianalgesic dosing charts (Table 12-2). A critical concept in the conversion is allowing for incomplete cross tolerance.

Rotation of the opioid agent (ie, using a different opioid) holds the promise of maintaining analgesia with lesser amounts of the newly introduced drug and eliminating side effects. Tolerance is the term used to describe the need over time for greater amounts of a specific opioid to achieve the desired analgesic effect. While there is no ceiling dose for opioids, with higher doses there may be an accompanying increase in adverse effects (ie, the emergence of the intolerable side effects noted above, the accumulation of toxic metabolites, or high costs due to the required amounts of the drug). Because of differences in receptor binding between opioids, the cross tolerance from one opioid to another is not complete. An equianalgesic dose of another opioid will require less of the medication and achieve a more favorable balance between analgesia and side effects.

The reduction in equianalgesic dosing for cross tolerance is between 25% and 50%, usually about one-third. In cases of poorly controlled pain, a lesser reduction is appropriate. The steps in a rotation are (1) calculating the daily dose of current opioid in oral morphine equivalents, (2) determining the equianalgesic dose of the agent to be introduced, (3) reducing the calculated amount by one-third to allow for cross tolerance, and (4) dividing the total daily dose into the units of bolus dosing or continuous infusion.

For example, a child is receiving 120 mg oxycodone and 80 mg total prn morphine orally each day. He vacillates between barely adequate pain control and over-sedation. He is no longer able to walk. The decision is made to rotate his opioid to IV hydromorphone. A dosage of 120 mg oxycodone is equivalent to 180 mg oral morphine (oxycodone is 1.5 times more potent than oral morphine) and, when added to the 80 mg oral morphine being used prn, the equivalent daily dose of oral morphine is 260 mg. Parenteral hydromorphone is 20 times as potent as oral morphine, so the equianalgesic amount of parenteral hydromorphone is 13 mg. Reducing by one-third for cross tolerance but rounding up given the barely adequate pain control, the total daily equianalgesic dose of parenteral hydromorphone is 9 mg. That can be divided by 24 to determine the hourly infusion rate of a continuous IV infusion (375 µg/hour) or divided by 6 to determine the bolus dose to be given every 4 hours (1.5 mg). Finally, to determine a prn dose, 10% to 15% of the daily hydromorphone dose is 1 mg, offered every 1 to 2 hours.

Physicians lacking experience in pain management often worry about the difficulty of addressing uncontrolled pain. In addition to feeling distress about their patients' discomfort, physicians are concerned that an escalation in medication will make the child apneic and unnecessarily hasten death. Because expert and effective management is a critical skill in the care of seriously ill children, especially those facing the end of life, the primary care physician may choose to consult with palliative care or pain treatment specialists to

Table 12-2. Opioid Equivalency[a]				
Drug	Oral/Rectal Route	Parenteral Route	Conversion Ratio to Oral Morphine	Equianalgesic Dose of Oral Morphine
Morphine sulfate	30 mg of oral morphine	10 mg of parenteral morphine	Parenteral morphine is **3 times** as potent as oral morphine.	30 mg
Oxycodone	20 mg of oral oxycodone	NA	Oral oxycodone is **roughly 1.5 times** more potent than oral morphine.	30 mg
Hydrocodone	20 mg of oral hydrocodone	NA	Oral hydrocodone is **roughly 1.5 times** more potent than oral morphine.	30 mg
Hydromorphone	7 mg of oral hydromorphone	1.5 mg of parenteral hydromorphone	Oral hydromorphone is about **4–7 times** as potent as oral morphine. Parenteral hydromorphone is **20 times** as potent as oral morphine.	30 mg
Fentanyl	NA	15 µg/hour	Transdermal fentanyl is **approximately 80 times** as potent as morphine (This is based on studies converting from morphine to fentanyl. Currently, there are no empirical studies converting fentanyl to morphine.)	30 mg

[a]Adapted from http://endoflife.stanford.edu/M11_pain_control/equivalency_table.html. © End of Life Curriculum Project, a joint project of the US Veterans Administration and SUMMIT, Stanford University Medical School. Used with permission.

ensure that the child's needs are adequately addressed. Alternatively, hospice medical directors can provide palliative care consultations if hospital-based teams are not available.

The risk of respiratory depression while using an accepted escalation rationale is actually quite small. Patients may fall asleep when their pain is "captured," but this is generally due to exhaustion related to the pain. Even in mild to moderate pain, patients do not notice a change in dose increases when they are less than 25% above baseline. In cases of moderate to severe pain, a dose escalation of 50% to 100% is appropriate. Research has shown that pain relief can be achieved quickly with a rapid medication escalation under close supervision. The recommended approach is to provide doses every 10 minutes, increasing by 50% every third dose, until the symptom is relieved. For instance, using the previous example, 1 mg hydromorphone would be given, then repeated 10 minutes later, then followed 10 minutes later by 1.5 mg hydromorphone, then repeated 10 minutes later, etc, until the pain is adequately controlled. The pain is generally "captured" within 30 to 40 minutes.

The management of neuropathic pain presents a considerable challenge. The source of neuropathic pain is the insult or dysfunction of the central, peripheral, or autonomic nervous system. Pediatric patients may experience this pain due to degenerative CNS processes or injury, as well as treatment-related injuries to the nervous system from drug toxicities, radiation therapy, or surgery. Infection may also cause neuralgia. Children describe neuropathic pain as jolts of burning, stabbing, or shooting. It also causes allodynia, dysesthesia, and hyperalgesia. The results of various approaches to the treatment of neuropathic pain are mixed, and a multimodal approach, including an emphasis on physical therapy and more than one therapeutic agent, is recommended. Adjuvant medications are offered as a first line in children, with gabapentin beginning at 10 mg/kg/day divided 3 times a day and titrating upward to doses as high as 60 mg/kg/day. Strong opioids may be included in an appropriate regimen. Tricyclic antidepressants tend to be used less for children in the management of neuropathic pain due to concerns of arrhythmia risk.

Dystonia and neuroirritability, while not properly neuropathic pain, present similar challenges in children with neurodegenerative conditions. Generalized dystonia is a condition in which there are sustained, erratic, painful muscle contractions that cause twisting and repetitive movements or abnormal postures. Neuroirritability is a term used to describe the difficulty in settling and persistent crying seen in some cognitively impaired children with metabolic and neurodegenerative conditions. These symptoms are distressing and often occur in children whose impairments make an assessment of their experience difficult. Benzodiazepines, typically diazepam, are the first line for dystonia (Table 12-3). Trihexyphenidyl is also commonly considered, as is valproate, baclofen, carbamazepine, or tetrabenazine. In severe, intractable cases, the implantation of deep brain stimulators is being increasingly considered, although the empiric basis for that decision is most unclear. Anticonvulsants are the mainstay in the treatment of neuroirritability. Phenobarbital is often the first medication tried. The treatment of these conditions is generally determined in consultation with a child neurologist.

Management of Non-Pain Symptoms (Table 12-3)

Dyspnea

There are many similarities between the treatment of severe dyspnea and severe pain. Dyspnea is caused by increased work of breathing, hypoxia, and hypercapnia, and the driving desire of the brain to relieve them. Experientially, it may cause a feeling similar to being under water too long and needing to surface. Like pain, it has a physical basis but the distress is potentiated by psychological, interpersonal, and existential aspects. After oxygen, opioids are the treatment of choice and they are dosed at one-third of the dose for pain treatment. While this is another situation where inexperienced physicians are typically worried about worsening the patient's condition by causing respiratory depression, there is strong evidence for its effectiveness in alleviating dyspnea. Due to the anxious state dyspnea often causes and the fact that anxiety worsens dyspnea, an appropriate dose of a benzodiazepine is also helpful, although never as the principal medication. Simple environmental measures, such as the breeze from an electric fan on the patient's face, also cause relief.

Nausea and Vomiting

Nausea and vomiting are common symptoms in children with complex illnesses or facing the end of life, and a significant source of distress and discomfort. They can have different etiologies, principally gastrointestinal, CNS, or treatment-related. Children with neurologic impairments can suffer from retching, and many of their medications have nausea among their side effects. Children are especially vulnerable to anticipatory nausea, a conditioned behavioral response in anticipation of a medication or procedure that has caused nausea and vomiting in the past. Anorexia can be a symptom of low-grade nausea. An approach to nausea and vomiting based on an understanding of the cause of the symptom exacerbation and understanding the symptom mechanism can prove valuable. A careful history and physical examination, with special attention to medications and procedures, is crucial.

While a patient's presentation may be complex, there are 4 pathways to nausea and vomiting. The vomiting center, which lies in the brain stem, receives input from the chemoreceptor trigger zone (CTZ), the cerebral cortex, peripheral pathways in the gastrointestinal tract, and the vestibular system. The CTZ responds to toxins (and medications) in blood and spinal fluid; the cerebral cortex responds to sensory input, anxiety, meningeal irritation, and elevated intracranial pressure; peripheral pathways are stimulated by mechanical stretch in obstruction and by mucosal injury; and the vestibular system is affected by motion and labyrinth disorders. Each pathway involves different neuroreceptors for mechanism-based therapy to target.

The CTZ can be suppressed by the blockage of dopamine type 2 receptors with haloperidol, prochlorperazine, chlorpromazine, or metoclopramide. Peripheral pathways can be addressed by identifying the underlying cause and with the blockage of 5HT3 receptors by

Table 12-3. Medications Used for Common Symptoms in Pediatric Palliative Care[a]

Symptom	Medication	Starting Dose	Comments
Dystonia	Diazepam	0.5 mg/kg/dose IV/PO q 6 hours prn; initial dose for children <5 years is 5 mg/dose, for children ≥5 years dose is 10 mg/dose	May be irritating if given by peripheral IV
	Trihexyphenidyl	0.1 mg/kg/day PO	Would initiate in consultation with child neurologist; not for children <3 years; 2 mg/5 mL liquid available
	Phenobarbital	3 mg/kg/d PO	Helpful with neuroirritability; many liquid concentrations
	Baclofen	5 mg PO tid, increase by 5 mg/dose prn	Helpful with neuropathic pain and spasticity; abrupt withdrawal may result in hallucinations and seizures; not for children <10 years
Nausea	Metoclopramide	0.1–0.2 mg/kg/dose q 6 hours, up to 10 mg/dose (prokinetic and mild nausea dosing) For chemotherapy-associated nausea 0.5–1 mg/kg q 6 hours prn PO/IV/SC, give with diphenhydramine	Helpful when dysmotility an issue; may cause extrapyramidal reactions, particularly in children following IV administration of high doses; contraindicated in complete bowel obstruction or pheochromocytoma
	Ondansetron	0.15 mg/kg/dose q 8 hours to max of 8 mg/dose Some institutions also use daily dosing for chemotherapy	Significant experience in pediatrics; good empiric therapy for nausea in palliative care population; higher doses used with chemotherapy; oral dissolving tablet contains phenylalanine
	Lorazepam	0.025 mg/kg up to 2 mg IV/PO q 6 hours	May be given sublingually; particularly helpful with anticipatory nausea; avoid use in neonates
	Scopolamine patch	1.5 mg patch, change q 72 hours	Good for motion-induced nausea/vomiting; handling patch and contacting eye may cause anisocoria and blurry vision; may fold patches but do not cut them
	Prochlorperazine	0.4 mg/kg/day PO/PR divided q 8 hours	Available in suppositories and 1 mg/mL syrup; not for children <2 years
Anorexia	Megestrol acetate	10 mg/kg/day in 1–4 divided doses, up to 15 mg/kg/day or 800 mg/day.	For children >10 years; acute adrenal insufficiency may occur with abrupt withdrawal after long-term use; use with caution in patients with diabetes mellitus or history of thromboembolism; may cause photosensitivity
	Cyproheptadine	0.25–0.5 mg/kg/d PO divided q 6 hours	
Respiratory secretions	Glycopyrrolate	0.04–0.1 mg/kg po q 4–8 hours	Excessive drying of secretions can cause mucus plugging of airways; anticholinergic side effects possible
	Scopolamine patch	1.5-mg patch, change q 72 hours	Excessive drying of secretions can cause mucus plugging of airways; handling patch and contacting eye may cause anisocoria and blurry vision; may fold patches but do not cut them
	Atropine 1% ophthalmic drops	One drop sublingual, titrate to effect	
Fatigue	Methylphenidate	Norms not established Begin with a fraction of a 0.3 mg/kg/day	Daytrana patch can be helpful

Abbreviations: IV, intravenous; PO, orally; PR, far point of accommodation; prn, as needed; q, every; SC, subcutaneous; tid, 3 times a day.

[a]Modified from Wolfe J, Ullrich C. Pain and symptom control in pediatrics. In: Walsh et al, eds. *Palliative Medicine.* Philadelphia, PA: Saunders Elsevier; 2008, with permission.

ondansetron. The cortex can be addressed with anxiolytics; attention to sensory stimuli (smells, tastes); and, in cases of elevated intracranial pressure, high-dose steroids. Dronabinol may also be helpful. The vestibular system is managed by blocking muscarinic acetylcholine and histamine receptors with scopolamine, hyoscyamine, and diphenhydramine. (Promethazine is useful in adults but is to be avoided because of its implication in sudden death in some children.)

The causes of nausea and vomiting are often not pure but involve multiple pathways. For instance, opioid-induced nausea and vomiting may be due to constipation or gastroparesis, stimulation of the CTZ, or sensitization of the labyrinth. Choices must be made about how to approach the possible causes in a step-wise manner. The literature suggests that mechanism-based therapy is more effective, employs a systematic approach that identifies all possible contributors, and encourages the treatment of underlying causes. It uses medication in a targeted manner, lessening the risk of untoward effects and oversedation. Finally, it is worth remembering that the risk of extrapyramidal side effects is greater in children, and when using high doses of metoclopramide or the phenothiazines, premedication with diphenhydramine is recommended.

Anorexia

Anorexia is an anticipated symptom at the end of life. Some parents have great difficulty with this symptom and can feel overwhelmed by the loss of a concrete expression of their nurturing. They want their child to eat to be better able to fight their illness. Food preparation and feeding them is something concrete they can do for their child. Dying children want to please their parents as much as healthy ones, maybe more so. It is important to acknowledge the feelings behind the desire of parents for their child to eat. Small portions of the child's favorite foods or new favorites he asks for may be comforting to all.

There are times earlier in an illness when it may be appropriate to improve appetite. Cyproheptadine has a long history of safe use in children and has been shown to be helpful in some cases. Megestrol acetate has been shown effective in increasing weight, but not muscle mass, and may be considered in children older than 10 years. Cannabinoids, while stimulating appetite, have not been demonstrated to increase weight. Steroids, while likely to improve appetite, often come at an unacceptable cost of irritability and immunosuppression.

One other consideration related to feeding is whether children are starving when they no longer have the desire to eat. Research comparing the "anorexia-cachexia syndrome" with starvation shows 2 very different metabolic states. Differences in energy expenditure, protein synthesis and proteolysis, glucose metabolism, and hormonal levels reinforce the view that anorexia-cachexia is a hypermetabolic state, while starvation in healthy individuals is an effort by the body to conserve itself. An understanding of this difference enables physicians to explain to parents how the disease is robbing the child's energy and that it is not the fault of their efforts or the lack of food. In fact, research on adults dying of advanced cancer found that even the patients who ate the most lost weight.

Respiratory Secretions

Respiratory secretions are a common symptom in seriously ill children. Children with neuromuscular diseases and neurologic impairment can have problems managing secretions. The presence of a tracheostomy can further complicate matters. The use of suction and cough assist machines is important, particularly in the setting of acute respiratory illnesses that cause increased secretions. In children

at this stage of illness, drying agents (eg, glycopyrrolate, atropine, scopolamine, or hyoscamine) are sometimes helpful, but they may increase the risk of acute obstruction by thickening secretions and causing mucus plugging.

Terminal secretions (the "death rattle") are understandably very distressing to parents. The child does not typically notice them. They are not relieved by suctioning, but sometimes respond to repositioning. Drying agents are usually prescribed in this setting. There is not much advantage to switching between agents if the effect is not substantial, though more than one agent should be tried. Glycopyrrolate stands alone among these agents as the only one that does not cross the blood–brain barrier and thus is the least likely to cause CNS effects.

Fatigue

Fatigue is a highly prevalent symptom at the end of life. In one study of children with terminal cancer, 96% were found to have experienced fatigue in their last month. This symptom is especially disheartening because fatigued children may have the desire to do things that provide a quality of life, but not be up to the task. Fatigue may be due to illness, treatments, stress, isolation, poor sleep hygiene and circadian disorientation, mood, or the lack of pleasure or activity. The sedative effects of some medications certainly contribute. Sleep, exercise, nutrition, anemia treatment, increased interactions, and activity all have been shown to have a beneficial effect in decreasing fatigue. Medical therapy with methylphenidate or modafinil may be helpful, dosed at lower amounts than typically prescribed for attention-deficit/hyperactivity disorder.

CASE RESOLUTION

The patient lived for 4 more months, was never again admitted to the hospital and, until her last days, remained engaged and as playful as her fatigue allowed. Her primary care pediatrician teamed with the pediatric palliative care team at the closest children's hospital, and was assisted with many of the symptom management decisions. In her last days, she was on methadone, morphine boluses, lorazepam, citalopram, gabapentin, ondansetron, Miralax, senna, and prn methylphenidate. Her pediatrician made home visits and remained available for evolving symptoms. She was in the child's home at the time of her death, ensuring comfort, declaring the death, and affirming the value of her life.

Selected References

Breau LM, Camfield CS, McGrath PJ, Finley GA. The incidence of pain in children with severe cognitive impairments. *Arch Pediatr Adolesc Med.* 2003; 157:1219–1226

Pritchard M, Burghen EA, Gattuso JS, et al. Factors that distinguish symptoms of most concern to parents from other symptoms of dying children. *J Pain Symptom Manage.* 2010;39:627–636

Solodiuk J, Curley MAQ. Pain assessment in nonverbal children with severe cognitive impairments: the Individualized Numeric Rating Scale (INRS). *J Pediatr Nurs.* 2003;18:295–299

Ullrich CK, Dussel V, Hilden JM, et al. Fatigue in children with cancer at the end of life. *J Pain Symptom Manage.* 2010;40:483–494

Wee B, Hillier R. Interventions for noisy breathing in patients near to death. *Cochrane Database Syst Rev.* 2008;(1):CD005177

Williams DG, Hatch DJ, Howard RF. Codeine phosphate in paediatric medicine. *Br J Anaesth.* 2001;86:413–421

Wolfe J, Grier HE, Klar N, et al. Symptoms and suffering at the end of life in children with cancer. *N Engl J Med.* 2000;342:326–333

Wood GJ, Shega JW, Lynch B, Von Roenn JH. Management of intractable nausea and vomiting in patients at the end of life: "I was feeling nauseous all of the time…nothing was working." *JAMA.* 2007;298:1196–1207

World Health Organization. *Cancer Pain Relief and Palliative Care in Children.* Geneva, Switzerland: World Health Organization; 1998

CHAPTER 13

Complementary and Alternative Medicine in Pediatric Primary Care

Miriam T. Stewart, BA, and Erica Sibinga, MD, MHS

CASE STUDY

A 14-year-old girl is brought to your office to follow up on her migraine headaches. She has no other significant medical history, but has experienced intermittent migraine headaches over the past few years. The headaches occur approximately weekly in the evenings, do not wake her from sleep, and improve with ibuprofen 400 mg, as had been previously prescribed at your office. At this visit, the girl states that she wishes she didn't have to take medicine for her headaches. Her mother reports that a family friend has suggested acupuncture or herbs for the headaches and asks whether there are other "complementary and alternative medicine" (CAM) approaches that they could try.

Questions

1. What are CAM therapies?
2. How does a provider explore if there are any CAM approaches that are appropriate for the treatment of chronic or recurrent conditions such as headaches in a child or adolescent?
3. What is the best way to determine if a family is using CAM?
4. What is the best way to communicate with a family about CAM therapies?
5. What is the best way to monitor the safety of CAM approaches?

Complementary and Alternative Medicine

Complementary and alternative medicine (CAM) refers to a wide variety of therapies that are not typically part of "conventional" medical approaches. Conventional medicine (also called allopathic or Western medicine) is the general approach of medical doctors (MDs), doctors of osteopathy (DOs), and the allied health professionals. The specific therapies thought of as CAM versus allopathic may change over time, as CAM practices may be incorporated into allopathic medicine.

Complementary and alternative medicine therapies may be used in a number of different ways. When CAM therapies are used in addition to allopathic care, they are termed "complementary"; this is by far the most common way CAM therapies are used. "Alternative" medicine refers to therapies used instead of allopathic care. A small but growing number of practitioners are using both allopathic and non-allopathic approaches, a practice referred to as "integrative medicine."

Epidemiology

The use of CAM has risen steadily over the past several decades and now comprises a significant subset of health-related visits and expenditures. In 2007 more than one-third (38.3%) of American adults surveyed reported having used some form of CAM in the previous 12 months. As of 1997 the number of visits to CAM providers exceeded those to primary care physicians, and out-of-pocket expenditures for CAM, estimated at $33.9 billion per year. These statistics demonstrate the importance of physician awareness of CAM and support the routine inclusion of questions about CAM in the medical history.

A growing body of evidence reveals that the pediatric population is also using CAM. A large-scale survey of caregivers found that 1 in 9 children use CAM (11.8%). Higher prevalence, up to 60%, has been found in certain populations, such as children with cancer, epilepsy, sickle cell disease, and other chronic diseases. Adolescents are more likely to use CAM than younger children, and CAM is more often used in the Western United States than in other regions of the country. Other factors associated with CAM use in children include parental education beyond high school; higher household income; coverage by private health insurance; use of prescription medications; and number of health conditions, doctor visits, or school days missed for illness in the past year. Non-Hispanic whites are more likely to use CAM than Hispanics or blacks, though the strength of this association diminishes when data are adjusted for confounding factors. When worry about cost delays or prevents the receipt of conventional medical care, children are more likely to use CAM. The strongest predictor of CAM use in children is CAM use by a parent; children whose parents use CAM are 5 times more likely to use CAM. When discussing CAM with families who are using it for their children, pediatricians need to be aware that parents may also be using CAM.

Motivations for Using CAM

Complementary and alternative medicine can be used for health maintenance, for symptomatic relief, as an adjunct to curative conventional medical care, for relief from side effects of conventional medical care, or in place of conventional medical care. Families choose to use CAM for many reasons. Word of mouth and belief in the efficacy of the treatment can be strong motivators. Some parents express a desire for more options and feel a sense of empowerment in their parental role as a result of CAM use. Complementary and alternative medicine may also be more congruous with a family's values, philosophies about health, and understanding of the basis of disease. Parents may fear the side effects of conventional medicines or be dissatisfied with the care their child receives in conventional medical settings. Families may seek the additional personal attention afforded by CAM providers. For some families, CAM offers additional hope when conventional medical care fails. Underlying all these motivations is the desire for the child's health and well-being and the quest for safe and effective treatments for disease. Physicians and families can find common ground in this most basic of motivations, which can inform conversations about both CAM and conventional medical care.

CAM Categories

Complementary and alternative medicine therapies can be thought of as falling into one of 5 categories: whole medical systems, mind–body therapies, biomechanical therapies, bioenergetic therapies, and biochemical therapies (Table 13-1). Besides whole medical systems, these categories are chosen to reflect purported similarities in underlying mechanism of effect. A particular therapy may be used as part of a whole medical system approach or on its own. For example, acupuncture may be part of an individualized, comprehensive traditional Chinese medicine (TCM) treatment approach, also consisting of herbs and lifestyle recommendations. Or a standardized acupuncture treatment may be used without evaluation and treatment by a TCM provider, in which case it can be thought of as a bioenergetic therapy. Additionally, a particular therapy may belong to more than one category, for example herbal preparations may have both a biochemical and a placebo (mind–body) effect.

Whole Medical Systems

Whole medical systems, including allopathic medicine, are whole-system approaches to treatment, consisting of an underlying theory of healing, standardized training, and diagnostic and treatment approaches reflective of the underlying theory. For instance, TCM is based on the theory that illness and symptoms result from yin-yang energy imbalances. These energy imbalances are diagnosed through history and physical examination and treated by altering the energy balance using acupuncture (or other mechanical or thermal stimuli), herbs, and lifestyle changes (diet, sleep, physical activity).

Mind–Body Therapies

These therapies are intended to enhance the mind's ability to benefit health. A number of mind–body therapies are integrated into allopathic treatment, such as psychotherapy, group therapy, imagery, and biofeedback. Others are still considered CAM, such as meditation and hypnotherapy.

Biomechanical

Biomechanical therapies aim to improve health through physical manipulation of the body. This may involve working with muscles, as with massage, or spinal alignment, as with chiropractic and osteopathic approaches. Massage therapies range from relatively light muscle work to deep tissue massage, as well as physical therapy to work with muscles and joints. Spinal manipulation therapies are used commonly in the United States and are most often practiced by chiropractors or DOs.

Bioenergetic

Bioenergetic therapies are directed at improving health through altering the body's energy as it runs through, on, or around the body. As allopathic training does not include the concept of energy in this way, bioenergetic therapies tend to draw skepticism from allopaths. With increasing scientific evidence for its beneficial effects, acupuncture is purported to affect the body's vital energy (*qi*) as it courses through energy channels, called meridians. In 1997 a National Institutes of Health (NIH) consensus panel declared the evidence sufficient for integration of acupuncture into a number of allopathic treatments, including the treatment of chemotherapy-associated nausea and emesis, anesthesia-associated nausea and emesis, and pain syndromes. Homeopathic remedies are theoretically bioenergetic therapies, as the "ingredients" are successively diluted beyond the point of significant molecular presence; therefore, it is the resulting change in the energy of the diluents (sometimes called the "memory of the molecule") that is responsible for the therapeutic effect. Additionally, a number of therapies aim to affect energy at or near the surface of the body, including therapeutic touch and Reiki, which involve a trained practitioner identifying the energy imbalance and directing his or her own energy to improve the patient's energy balance and promote healing.

Table 13-1. Selected Examples of Complementary and Alternative Medicine Therapies by Category[a]

	Modality	Description: At a Glance	Licensure and Regulation
Whole Medical Systems	Traditional Chinese medicine (TCM)	• Originated in China more than 5,000 years ago; rooted in the Taoist philosophy. • Views the human body and mind as an integrated whole in which tissues, organs, and parts function interdependently. • Yin-yang theory—the concept of 2 opposing but interdependent forces that shape the world—is a core principle. Health and disease relate to balance between yin and yang in the body. • Treatments to restore balance include herbs, massage, acupuncture (see page 72), diet, and exercises such as tai chi (see page 72) and qi gong.	• Most states license acupuncture, but vary in their inclusion of other TCM treatments in licensure. • Acupuncture and TCM schools are accredited by the federally recognized Accreditation Commission of Acupuncture and Oriental Medicine.
	Ayurveda	• Originated in India several thousand years ago and is still used by 80% of the population either exclusively or in combination with Western medicine. • Health and disease are thought to relate to a person's constitution (prakriti), which is composed of a unique combination of the 3 life forces (doshas). Imbalances between the doshas can lead to disease. • Treatments are tailored to the individual's unique constitution and are aimed at eliminating impurities, reducing symptoms, increasing resistance to disease, reducing worry, and increasing harmony in the patient's life. • Treatments include herbs, vitamins and minerals, massage, yoga (see page 70), enemas, and specialized diet and lifestyle recommendations.	• Ayurvedic medicine is not accredited in the United States, though several states have accredited ayurvedic schools. • In India, ayurvedic medicine can be studied at the bachelor's and doctorate level.
	Naturopathy	• Developed in Germany and the United States in the late 19th—early 20th centuries. • Central belief is that nature has healing power and practitioners view their role as supporting the body's inherent ability to restore health. • Naturopathic practitioners strive to use the most natural and the least invasive approach to restore and maintain health • Treatment modalities used by naturopaths include nutrition, vitamins and minerals, herbal medicines, homeopathy (see page 72), therapeutic massage and joint manipulation, hydrotherapy, exercise, and lifestyle counseling.	• Naturopathic physicians (ND or NMD degrees) complete a 4-year graduate-level program at a naturopathic medical school accredited by the Council on Naturopathic Medical Education, which is recognized by the US Department of Education. States vary in their licensing of naturopathic physicians and the scope of naturopathic practice, including the ability to prescribe drugs, perform minor surgery, and assist in childbirth. • The American Association of Naturopathic Physicians (www.naturopathic.org) is the national professional society of naturopathic physicians.
	Native American healing	• Broad term that encompasses the healing traditions of hundreds of indigenous tribes. Has been practiced in North America for more than 40,000 years. • Can combine religion, spirituality, herbal medicine, shamanic healers, purification activities, and symbolic rituals in the treatment of medical and emotional problems. Treatments may be individual or may involve the entire community. • Treatment is often a slow process that is spread over days and weeks. There is a strong belief in the therapeutic value of the relationship with the healer.	• There is no government oversight of education or licensure for Native American healers.

Table 13-1. Selected Examples of Complementary and Alternative Medicine Therapies by Category^a, continued

	Modality	Description: At a Glance	Licensure and Regulation
Mind–Body Therapies	Meditation/mindfulness	• There are many types of meditation, most of which originated in ancient religious and spiritual traditions. Some of these include mindfulness meditation, transcendental meditation, and Zen Buddhist meditation. • In meditation, a person learns to focus attention. Some forms of meditation instruct the practitioner to become mindful of thoughts, feelings, and sensations and to observe them in a nonjudgmental way. • Meditation is believed to result in a state of greater calmness, physical relaxation, and psychological balance, and can change how a person relates to the flow of emotions and thoughts. • Meditation has been studied in a variety of populations and is used for general wellness and for various health problems, including anxiety, pain, depression, stress, insomnia, and physical or emotional symptoms that may be associated with chronic illnesses such as AIDS and cancer.	• There is a broad diversity of meditation practices, each of which may have its own training programs and certification policies. • There is no national or state-based accreditation for meditation practitioner education or licensing. However, meditation programs may be eligible for continuing education credits toward licensing for health professionals. • The University of Massachusetts Center for Mindfulness in Medicine, Health Care, and Society (www.umassmed.edu/cfm) is the oldest and largest mindfulness program associated with an academic institution and is a source for training and research on mindfulness and mind–body medicine.
	Hypnotherapy	• Hypnotherapists use exercises that bring about deep relaxation and an altered state of consciousness, also known as a trance. • Through hypnosis, people learn how to master their own states of awareness. By doing so they can affect their own bodily functions and psychological responses. • Hypnotherapy has been studied for a number of conditions, including state anxiety (eg, before medical procedures or surgeries), headaches, smoking cessation, pain control, hot flashes in breast cancer survivors, and irritable bowel syndrome. It is also used in managing pain during childbirth.	• Most hypnotherapists are licensed medical doctors, registered nurses, social workers, or family counselors who have received additional training in hypnotherapy. • Several national bodies provide training certificates. • The American Society of Clinical Hypnosis (www.asch.net) is the largest organization of health professionals using clinical hypnosis and provides hypnotherapy training.
	Biofeedback	• Technique that trains people to improve their health by controlling certain bodily processes that normally happen involuntarily, including heart rate, blood pressure, muscle tension, and skin temperature. • Biofeedback practice involves attaching the patient to electrodes (or other monitoring device) that monitor the desired process (eg, muscle tension, skin temperature). The therapist leads the patient in exercises designed to assist them in controlling the desired variable, while the electrodes provide real-time feedback on the patient's success. • Biofeedback is used in a variety of conditions, including high blood pressure, headaches, chronic pain, and urinary incontinence.	• The Biofeedback Certification International Alliance (BCIA) certifies individuals who have met their educational and training standards, which include didactic training, supervision hours, patient sessions, and case presentations. • Pelvic floor muscle dysfunction is a subspecialty within biofeedback that provides specialized training. Only licensed health care providers may apply for certification in this specialty.
	Yoga	• Yoga practice was developed in ancient India, with fully developed practice appearing around 500 BC. There are numerous branches or paths of yoga. • Derived from the Sanskrit word meaning "union," yoga strives to connect the body, breath, and mind with the goal of energizing and balancing the whole person. • Yoga practice can be individual or class-based and consists of physical postures (asanas), breathing exercises, and meditation. • Yoga is used for maintaining health and has also been studied in a wide variety of conditions, including anxiety, arthritis, asthma, cancer, back pain, diabetes, heart disease, pregnancy (when modified for pregnancy), and chronic headaches.	• There is no government oversight of yoga training or practice. • There are numerous organizations and training programs in the United States and worldwide that offer training. • The Yoga Alliance is the most widely recognized educational and professional organization for yoga in the United States. It accredits yoga training programs based on a minimum training standard. Teachers who complete Yoga Alliance accredited training are eligible to register as Registered Yoga Teachers (RYT).

Table 13-1. Selected Examples of Complementary and Alternative Medicine Therapies by Category[a], continued

Modality	Description: At a Glance	Licensure and Regulation
Biomechanical		
Chiropracty	• Developed in the United States at the end of the 19th century. • Based on the notion that the relationship between the body's structure—most notably the alignment of the spine—and its coordination by the nervous system affects health. • People most often seek chiropractic care for musculoskeletal complaints (back, neck, and shoulder pain), headaches, and extremity problems. • Hands-on spinal adjustment and manipulation is a core treatment in chiropractic care, but treatment can also include heat and ice; electrical stimulation; exercise; and counseling about diet, exercise, and lifestyle.	• Chiropractic practitioners must meet the licensing and continuing education requirements of the states where they practice. • All states require chiropractors to complete a Doctor of Chiropractic degree at an accredited college. • The American Chiropractic Association (www.acatoday.org) is the largest professional organization representing chiropractic doctors.
Osteopathy	• Developed in the United States at the end of the 19th century. • Core principle is that disease and illness begin with structural problems in the spine and resulting abnormalities in the function of the nervous system. • Doctors of osteopathy receive conventional medical training, but are also trained in osteopathic manipulation techniques and craniosacral therapy, both of which involve hands-on manipulation of bones and tissues. • People seek care from osteopathic doctors both for conventional medical care and specifically for musculoskeletal conditions.	• Doctors of osteopathy (DOs) complete a 4-year training program in conventional medicine and osteopathy and also complete medical residencies in their specialty of choice. • DOs are recognized for full practice rights in all 50 states once they are licensed. • The American Osteopathic Association (www.osteopathic.org) is the primary professional organization and accreditation agency for osteopathy in the United States.
Massage therapy	• Massage therapy has been in use for thousands of years in diverse cultures, including China, Japan, India, Egypt, and Europe. • The term "massage therapy" encompasses more than 100 distinct techniques, but the core practice is manipulation of the muscles and soft tissues of the body using the hands and fingers. • People use massage for general wellness, as well as in the treatment of a wide range of conditions including sports injuries, stress, pain, musculoskeletal complaints, anxiety, and depression.	• Most states have laws regulating massage therapy and typically require a minimum number of training hours and passage of a national exam. Massage training can be accredited by state boards or by an independent agency. • The National Certification Board for Therapeutic Massage and Bodywork certifies massage practitioners who pass a national examination. • The American Massage Therapy Association (www.amtamassage.org) is the nation's largest professional organization for massage practitioners.
The Feldenkrais Method	• A method of somatic education that uses gentle movement and directed attention to movement patterns in order to expand movement options and improve functioning. • Treatment can be carried out via verbal guidance in a class setting or with hands-on gentle manipulation. • People use Feldenkrais to maintain well-being and enhance performance in performing arts and athletics, as well as in the treatment of a variety of conditions including multiple sclerosis, stroke, cerebral palsy, and repetitive stress injuries.	• Feldenkrais practitioners must complete 700–800 hours of training over 3–4 years in order to apply for certification. Certification and training is governed by the Feldenkrais Guild of North America (www.feldenkrais.com). • There is no government oversight of training or licensure.
Alexander Technique	• Educational method whose emphasis is on changing faulty postural habits in order to improve mobility and performance. • Treatment has 2 components: table work (hands-on manipulation) and guided activity, in which the practitioner observes the person in action and gives verbal, visual, and physical cues to help the person perform the activity with greater ease. • People use the Alexander Technique for improved performance in performing arts and sports as well as in the treatment of musculoskeletal problems, repetitive stress injuries, and chronic pain.	• In order to be certified by the American Society for the Alexander Technique (www.amsatonline.com), practitioners must complete 1,600 hours of training over 3 years. • There is no government oversight of training or licensure.

Table 13-1. Selected Examples of Complementary and Alternative Medicine Therapies by Category[a], continued

Modality	Description: At a Glance	Licensure and Regulation
Acupuncture	• Acupuncture is a modality of TCM (see page 69). The earliest recorded use of acupuncture dates from 200 BCE. • The core principle of acupuncture is the belief that a particular type of life force or energy (*qi*) circulates through the energy pathways (meridians) in the body. *Qi* maintains the dynamic balance of yin and yang. An imbalance of *qi* can cause symptoms and disease. • Acupuncture treatment involves stimulation of specific points along the meridians using pressure (acupressure), thermal energy (moxibustion), or very fine acupuncture needles. • Acupuncture has been studied in a variety of conditions, including chronic pain, post-surgical recovery, chemotherapy-related nausea, musculoskeletal problems, headaches, addiction, asthma, and menstrual problems.	• Most states require a license to practice acupuncture, though licensing and education standards vary from state to state. Licensure confers the title of LAc. • In 1997 the National Institutes of Health recognized acupuncture as a mainstream medicine healing option with a statement documenting the procedure's safety and efficacy for treating a range of health conditions. • The American Academy of Medical Acupuncture (http://www.medicalacupuncture.org/) maintains a database of licensed physicians who are also trained to perform acupuncture.
Tai chi	• Originated in ancient China as a component of TCM. • Rooted in the principles of yin-yang balance and the balanced flow of a vital life force or energy (*qi*). • There are many different styles, but all involve slow, deliberate movements that flow into each other. Meditation, deep breathing, and maintenance of good posture during continuous movement are foci of the practice. • People use tai chi to improve overall fitness, balance, coordination, and agility. It is also used for chronic pain, gout, heart disease, high blood pressure, arthritis, osteoporosis, diabetes, headaches, and sleep disorders.	• No licensing or government accreditation exists for the training or practice of tai chi. • There are a variety of organizations that offer training programs and certification for tai chi.
Reiki	• Developed in Japan in the early 20th century. • Based on the idea that there is a universal energy that supports the body's innate healing abilities. Practitioners seek to access this energy, allowing it to flow to the body and facilitate healing. • During treatment, the practitioner's hands are placed lightly on or just above the client's body, palms down, using a series of 12–15 hand positions to promote the flow of energy. Each position is held for 2–5 minutes. • People use Reiki for relaxation, stress reduction, symptom relief, and general well-being. It can also be used to help promote peace at the end of life.	• No licensing or government accreditation exists for the training or practice of Reiki. • Multiple organizations offer training programs and certifications.
Homeopathic remedies	• Developed by a German physician at the end of the 18th century. • Based on 2 core principles: (1) the principle of similars ("like cures like") states that a disease can be cured by a substance that produces similar symptoms in a healthy person and (2) the principle of dilutions ("law of minimum dose") states that the lower the dose of the medication, the greater its effectiveness. Homeopathic remedies are so dilute that few or no molecules of the healing substance remain in the diluent. It is believed that the substance has left its imprint, which stimulates the body to heal itself. • Homeopathic remedies are derived from natural substances that come from plants, minerals, or animals.	• Homeopathic remedies are prepared according to the guidelines of the *Homeopathic Pharmacopeia of the United States*, which was written into federal law in 1938. • The US Food and Drug Administration requires that homeopathic remedies meet legal standards for strength, purity, and packaging, but since they contain little or no active ingredient, they do not have to undergo the same safety and efficacy testing as other over-the-counter medications. • If a homeopathic remedy claims to cure a serious disease such as cancer, it needs to be sold by prescription.

Bioenergetic

Table 13-1. Selected Examples of Complementary and Alternative Medicine Therapies by Category^a, continued

	Modality	Description: At a Glance	Licensure and Regulation
Bioenergetic	Therapeutic touch	• Developed in the 1970s in the United States. • Based on the belief that problems in the patient's energy field that cause illness and pain can be identified and rebalanced by a healer. • The technique consists of using the hands to release harmful energy and direct healthy energy for healing purposes. During a session, the hands are held 2–6 inches away from the body and there is no direct physical contact between practitioner and patient.	• No licensing or government accreditation exists for the training or practice of therapeutic touch. • Multiple organizations offer training programs, including some hospitals. • Many therapeutic touch practitioners are nurses or other licensed health professionals.
Biochemical	Herbal medicine	• Herbal medicine refers to using a plant's seeds, berries, roots, leaves, bark, or flowers for medicinal purposes. • Plants have been used for medicinal purposes since long before recorded history in a wide range of human cultures. • According to the World Health Organization, 80% of the world's population relies on herbal medicines for some part of their primary care. Nearly one-third of Americans use herbs. • The most commonly used herbal supplements in the United States include echinacea, St John's wort, gingko, garlic, saw palmetto, ginseng, golden seal, chamomile, feverfew, ginger, valerian, evening primrose, and milk thistle. • Herbal remedies are used in conventional medicine as well as in a variety of complementary and alternative medicine practices, including naturopathy, TCM, ayurveda, and Native American healing. Many people also use herbal remedies on their own, without the advice of a health practitioner.	• In the United States, herbal supplements are classified as dietary supplements and thus can be sold without being tested to prove they are safe and effective. They must be made according to good manufacturing practices. • In the United States, no organization regulates the manufacture or certifies the labeling of herbal preparations.
	Dietary supplements	• Dietary supplements contain one or more dietary ingredients, including vitamins, minerals, herbs, or amino acids, or their constituents. Herbal medicines are considered a subset of dietary supplements in the United States. • Some dietary supplements have been proven to prevent or treat disease (eg, folic acid in the prevention of neural tube defects, and calcium and vitamin D in the prevention of osteoporosis), while other claims about dietary supplements are unproven. • The most commonly used dietary supplements are fish oil, echinacea, flaxseed, ginseng, multivitamins, vitamins E and C, calcium, and B-complex vitamins.	• In the United States, dietary supplements can be sold without being tested to prove they are safe and effective. They must be made according to good manufacturing practices. • In the United States, no organization regulates the manufacture or certifies the labeling of dietary supplements.

^aInformation in this table is adapted from the Health Topics pages at the National Center for Complementary and Alternative Medicine Web site (http://nccam.nih.gov/health/atoz.htm), the University of Maryland Alternative Medicine Index (www.umm.edu/altmed), and The American Cancer Society's Complementary and Alternative Medicine Index (http://www.cancer.org/Treatment/TreatmentsandSideEffects/ComplementaryandAlternativeMedicine/index).

Biochemical

These therapies are intended to improve health through their biochemical effects. Conceptually related to the biochemical mechanism of effect of allopathic medications, herbal remedies and dietary supplements have a few important differences. First, herbal remedies are by nature complex mixtures of chemicals, so their effects are likely due to multiple biochemical reactions. Second, there is currently no federal regulation or oversight of the production of herbs or supplements in the United States, as there is with pharmaceuticals, so quality control is extremely variable. Third, safety concerns are not addressed before they are available commercially to consumers, as with pharmaceuticals, but only after products are on the market and adverse events are reported to the US Food and Drug Administration (FDA). Because of the lack of oversight of both production and premarket safety, it is important for practitioners to research not only the evidence for an herb's effect and potential adverse effects, but also the particular formulation's production and quality control.

Approaching CAM Use From an Allopathic Perspective

As with any treatment option, the safety (risks) and efficacy (benefits) of a CAM modality must form the basis for therapeutic decision-making about its use. Table 13-2 can be a helpful guide in directing physician responses to a particular CAM therapy.

Table 13-2. Guide to Complementary and Alternative Medicine Treatment Recommendations			
		Is the therapy effective?	
		Yes	No
Is the therapy safe?	Yes	**Recommend**	**Tolerate**
	No	**Monitor closely or discourage**	**Discourage**

If there is insufficient evidence to assess safety or efficacy
- Establish a plan with the family for monitoring response to treatment.
- Discourage if adverse reactions develop.
- Tolerate if no adverse reactions develop.

Assessing Efficacy

Data on the efficacy of CAM treatments are increasingly available as CAM becomes a greater focus of research effort and funding in the United States and worldwide. When searching the medical literature for CAM evidence, international and foreign-language articles can be useful, as certain CAM modalities may have been studied in greater depth or over a longer period in other countries. As with any research data, it is important to consider study design, outcome measures, sources of bias, methods of data analysis, and applicability of results for a given indication, patient, or patient population. With herbal remedies and supplements, it is also important to acknowledge that

formulations differ, so efficacy as reported in a clinical trial may be altered if a different formulation is used.

Assessing Safety

The huge diversity of CAM makes it difficult to discuss safety in general terms. Each CAM modality has its own unique risk profile. However, awareness of broad categories of risk can help physicians prevent bad outcomes.

- *Delay of allopathic care:* In studies of CAM risks in the pediatric population, the risk associated with the highest morbidity and mortality is delay of allopathic care. This delay can come about for a number of reasons, including a family's perception that care from a CAM provider obviates the need for allopathic care, a family's inability to afford allopathic care, or a family's belief that allopathic care will be harmful. It may be helpful to contract with families that they will seek allopathic care prior to or in conjunction with CAM care for a new symptom or acute illness to rule out disease processes that require allopathic treatment.

- *Drug–drug interactions:* Certain supplements and herbal remedies may interfere with or alter the effects of conventional medicines. Particular attention has been given to substances that are inhibitors or inducers of hepatic drug metabolism by the cytochrome P-450 enzyme, with St John's wort (used for depression) and grapefruit juice being the most well-known examples. See Resources at the end of this chapter for online resources for checking drug–drug interactions with herbal remedies and supplements.

- *Adverse reactions:* Allergic reactions, side effects, and idiosyncratic reactions are possible with CAM therapies as well as conventional therapies. Close follow-up is helpful in monitoring response to therapy.

Regulation and Licensure

Licensure and accreditation for CAM providers varies from state to state. Chiropractic care, massage therapy, acupuncture, naturopathy, and homeopathy have licensing bodies in some states. In states where licensing exists for a CAM modality, it is incumbent on the physician to ensure that any referrals are made to licensed practitioners. None of these licenses authorizes the practitioner to practice medicine. Other CAM modalities may have a national organization that supervises training and certifies practitioners. Though these are not subject to government oversight, there still may be value in preferentially seeking out providers who are approved by their national organization, as these providers have had to meet a standard established by their colleagues.

Regulation of herbal remedies and supplements is the subject of ongoing scrutiny and debate. Currently, the FDA does not regulate production or marketing of these products, so it is often difficult to verify their composition, safety, or efficacy unless they have been independently studied. The burden of researching products and manufacturers falls to the consumer.

Communication About CAM Use

Most caregivers of children who use CAM do not disclose this use to their pediatrician despite the fact that most report a desire to discuss it. The high rate of nondisclosure is alarming, as it places patients at risk for drug–drug interactions with conventional medications, robs physicians of the opportunity to monitor for adverse reactions, and interferes with the development of trust in the doctor–patient relationship. Reasons cited by patients and caregivers for nondisclosure include

- Negative experiences with past disclosures to physicians
- Fear of disapproval or judgment on the part of physicians
- Belief that physicians do not need to know
- Lack of time with physician
- The physician does not ask

Many of these barriers can be improved by the health care provider.

Physicians may be reticent to discuss CAM, as evidenced by the fact that CAM discussions are patient-initiated in most cases. Physicians may worry about legal liability if there is a bad outcome. They may fear conflict with families over use of CAM. They may be afraid to reveal their lack of knowledge about CAM and may worry that this lack of knowledge will threaten a family's trust in their abilities. They may feel pressured by time constraints and overwhelmed by the need to acquire new knowledge. There is often a disconnect between the meaning that patients and families attribute to CAM use—more options and a greater sense of empowerment—and the meaning that physicians may attribute to it—irrationality given lack of evidence and the threat of interference with conventional medical care. This disconnect can influence both patients and physicians to avoid the subject of CAM.

Communication Tips

- Make questions about CAM use a routine part of the medical encounter.
- Pose questions about CAM use in an open and nonjudgmental way.
  - Suggested opening: "In order for me to take the best possible care of your child, it is helpful for me to know about all the ways your family manages health and illness. Are there any treatments, medications, herbs, or supplements that your child uses that we have not talked about yet? Does your child see any other providers for health-related care or treatments?"
- Explore details of CAM use. Ask families not only what CAM modalities they are using, but also why they chose the treatment, how it works, whether they have noticed a difference, and if there have been any downsides to the treatment.
- Validate the family's desire for health and well-being for their child.
- Do not be afraid to acknowledge the limits of your knowledge. If asked to provide a recommendation about an unfamiliar CAM modality, offer to do further research and revisit the question at a follow-up visit.

- Seek out information about CAM, including literature on safety or efficacy.
- Involve families in the thinking process regarding risks versus benefits of a CAM intervention or modality. Provide evidence-based advice when possible. If there is little or no evidence to support or discourage use of a CAM modality, share this information with families.
- Make a plan with families to monitor the child's response to treatment, including measurable outcomes (eg, symptom relief, increased quality of life) and any adverse effects.
- Encourage families to share information about CAM use on an ongoing basis, even if they choose to continue a treatment about which you have raised concerns.
- Document CAM-related discussions in the medical record.

Effective communication about CAM use is a wonderful opportunity to improve rapport and better understand a patient and his or her family. Communication can be a powerful tool for ensuring safety and reducing harm, as well as for broadening physician knowledge and building trust with families. Even if they do not initiate or recommend a CAM treatment, pediatricians can play an important role by monitoring a child's response to the treatment over time and engaging the family in a discussion about risks and benefits if adverse reactions arise. Discussion about CAM may also bring about a greater understanding of families' explanatory models of illness as well as their expectations of health care providers and their beliefs about conventional medicines. Deeper insight into a family's health beliefs and values can facilitate more successful patient–physician partnership and better patient care.

CASE RESOLUTION

Explaining that this is not your area of expertise, you ask the family to return in 1 week to discuss this further. After consulting the National Center for Complementary and Alternative Medicine Web site and a brief review of the medical literature, you find that there are data on efficacy and safety of CAM therapies for migraine headache prevention, including acupuncture and self-hypnosis. At the follow-up visit, you discuss these options with the family. The girl is interested in both modalities but decides to try acupuncture first. You offer her support for this choice and ask that she keep close track of her headaches and return in 1 month to let you know how she's doing with the acupuncture treatments and her headaches.

Resources

National Center for Complementary and Alternative Medicine (NCCAM) at NIH

http://nccam.nih.gov/

NCCAM is the federal government's lead agency for scientific research on CAM. The Web site provides information about CAM modalities for both providers and patients, results of clinical trials supported by NCCAM, lists of ongoing trials, and information about training and funding opportunities in the field if CAM.

University of Maryland Medical Alternative Medicine Index

http://www.umm.edu/altmed/

Provides information on CAM therapies, which is searchable both by modality name and by symptom/disease. Also provides information on drug–drug interactions and side effects of herbal remedies.

Georgia Health Sciences University Robert E. Greenblatt, MD Library

Complementary and Alternative Medicine Resources

http://www.lib.mcg.edu/resources/links/cam.php

A list of helpful links to governmental, university-based, and nonprofit sources for information on research, training, policy, regulation, and integration of CAM.

CAM on PubMed

http://nccam.nih.gov/research/camonpubmed/

NCCAM provides a link to a PubMed search box that is limited to the CAM subset of PubMed.

Cochrane Reviews

http://www2.cochrane.org/reviews/en/subtopics/22.html

Link to more than 700 Cochrane Reviews on CAM interventions. The Cochrane Collaboration is an independent, international network of leaders in the health care field who are committed to helping health care providers make evidence-based decisions. Subgroups devoted to specific topic areas produce systematic reviews of available evidence for health-related interventions. The CAM-related subgroup is coordinated through the University of Maryland Center for Integrative Medicine.

Longwood Herbal Task Force

http://www.longwoodherbal.org/

Detailed, evidence-based monographs on individual herbal remedies including a review of available evidence, contraindications/cautions, and safety information. Administered by a group of faculty from the Boston Children's Hospital, the Massachusetts College of Pharmacy and Health Sciences, and the Dana Farber Cancer Institute.

The Natural Standard

http://naturalstandard.com/

Subscription-based site that includes evidence-based information on CAM modalities as well as online tools to check for drug–drug interactions.

Consumer Lab

http://www.consumerlab.com/

A for-profit organization that carries out independent testing of dietary supplements and herbal remedies, both by request of manufacturers and for the benefit of the public. In either case, samples for testing are not obtained directly from the manufacturer, but from the consumer marketplace. The use of the "CL seal of approval" image that appears on vitamin bottles can be purchased by manufacturers once their product has been tested by Consumer Lab.

Selected References

Barnes PM, Bloom B, Nahin RL. Complementary and alternative medicine use among adults and children: United States, 2007. *Natl Health Stat Report.* 2008;12:1–24

Eisenberg DM, Kessler RC, Foster C, Norlock FE, Calkins DR, Delbanco TL. Unconventional medicine in the United States—prevalence, costs, and patterns of use. *N Engl J Med.* 1993;328:246–252

Kabat-Zinn J. *Full Catastrophe Living: Using the Wisdom of Your Body and Mind to Face Stress, Pain, and Illness.* New York, NY: Delta; 1990

Kemper K. *The Holistic Pediatrician.* 2nd ed. New York, NY: Harper Collins; 2002

Kemper KJ, Vohra S, Walls R; American Academy of Pediatrics Task Force on Complementary and Alternative Medicine and Provisional Section on Complementary, Holistic, and Integrative Medicine. The use of complementary and alternative medicine in pediatrics. *Pediatrics.* 2008;122:1374 1386

Kligler B, Lee R. *Integrative Medicine, Principles for Practice.* New York, NY: McGraw-Hill; 2004

Rakel D. *Integrative Medicine.* 2nd ed. Philadelphia, PA: Saunders; 2007

CHAPTER 14

Principles of Pediatric Surgery

Steven L. Lee, MD

CASE STUDY

A 4-month-old male infant is evaluated by his pediatrician for swelling in the groin and diagnosed with a right inguinal hernia. The parents are told that their child will be referred to a pediatric surgeon. The parents are concerned about surgery in so young an infant and ask their pediatrician multiple questions. Is he big enough to have surgery? Will he be able to eat before the surgery? Will he be in pain? Will he need to have blood drawn? Will he need to be hospitalized? Will he be put to sleep for the procedure?

Questions

1. What are the typical questions parents ask if their child is undergoing surgery?
2. What is the role of the primary care provider in advising patients/parents about surgical procedures?
3. What is the role of the operating surgeon in advising patients/parents about the surgery?
4. What are general guidelines for feeding infants and children prior to surgery?
5. What are the risks of general anesthesia in infants and children?
6. How long is the hospitalization following surgery?
7. What should parents do before meeting with the surgeon?
8. How do you prepare children who are about to undergo surgery?
9. What laboratory studies are needed prior to surgery?

No matter what the age of the patient, the prospect of surgery is generally anxiety-provoking for both the patient and the patient's parents. As with any stressful patient encounter, communication is the key to educating, calming, and reassuring both patients and their parents. This is particularly true when patients are being referred even initially for surgical consultation. Pediatricians can make a significant impact by providing basic information to parents regarding surgical care. It is also important for primary care physicians and surgeons to communicate with each other in order to provide the highest level of care.

Preoperative Care

Initial Consultation

The first task of the primary care provider is to initiate a referral to the pediatric or general surgeon. The initial surgical visit will be to confirm the diagnosis and discuss surgical and nonsurgical options for treatment. Typically, no surgical procedures are performed during this consultation. This point must be clarified as many children and parents mistakenly think that surgery will occur at the time of the first encounter and are therefore unduly anxious. Some parents will even schedule time off unnecessarily, expecting to have to care for their postoperative child. They become disappointed and even angry when the surgery is not performed. Sometimes the diagnosis of the primary care provider is incorrect, and the surgeon can reassure the parents about the correct diagnosis obviating the need for any surgery.

A significant amount of information is given to parents and children during the surgical consultation. The diagnosis is confirmed and a decision is made whether the patient will require an operation. The operation is described in detail to the parents and to the patient when age-appropriate to do so. In addition, a thorough review of the risks of the operation is performed. The surgeon also gives a time estimate on how long the procedure will take. There is also a general discussion on the expected recovery, such as whether the procedure will be as an outpatient versus as an inpatient, where hospitalization occurs, how long the child will miss school, and whether there are any activity restrictions.

To avoid confusion, parents are encouraged to make a list of questions prior to this first encounter and make sure each question is answered. Parents should also write down the answers to refer to them at a later time. Once parents agree to proceed with surgery, the surgeon starts the process and paperwork. Often, this will be the only visit required before the date of the operation. However, some hospitals require patients to be seen by the surgeon within 30 days of a procedure, thus a return visit may be required if the date of surgery is beyond the time frame. Also, some centers require patients to have a preoperative evaluation with the anesthesia team prior to surgery.

Anesthetic Preparation in Infants and Children

Anesthesia is extremely safe in infants and children. The risk of a poor outcome from general anesthesia is less than 1%. In most institutions, pediatric anesthesiologists provide the anesthetic care for infants and young children. If pediatric anesthesiologists are not available, the anesthetic care for infants and children is often limited to a set of experienced general anesthesiologists.

There are many types of anesthetics that can be used, including moderate sedation ("conscious sedation"), regional anesthesia, and general anesthesia. Typically, the type of anesthesia will be determined by both the surgeon and anesthesiologist; however, the anesthesiologist makes the final decision. Although the least amount of anesthesia is desired, all patients must be treated as if they may need to undergo general anesthesia in case moderate sedation or regional anesthetic is inadequate.

To minimize the risk of aspiration with general anesthesia, the stomach must be empty of food and liquids. Although each hospital has its own policies, Box 14-1 lists frequently recommended guidelines for the time interval between meals and the surgery. In general, most infants and children will have to miss one meal prior to surgery. Often this meal can be replaced with clear liquids.

Laboratory Studies

Laboratory studies should be performed if indicated by the patient's underlying comorbidities or current disease process. Blood products may be needed during or after surgery if there is blood loss. If blood loss is anticipated, the parents or other family members will be given the option of directly donating blood prior to the procedure. However, directly donating blood takes time (days to weeks depending on the specific blood bank) and may not be an option for urgent and emergency operations. In addition, the cost of directly donating blood is often the responsibility of the patient.

Patients Requiring Urgent/Emergency Surgery

Patients with acute conditions will often present to their pediatrician or primary care provider. Common conditions include abdominal pain consistent with appendicitis, abscess requiring drainage, incarcerated hernia, or vomiting due to pyloric stenosis. Such patients will need to be directed to the emergency department (ED) for further management, and the pediatric surgeon should be notified. Any time a patient is sent to the ED, it is essential to remind the parents to keep the patient NPO, that is, not to give them anything to eat or drink. If parents feed patients en route to the ED, this will delay treatment due to anesthetic concerns. The NPO guidelines (Box 14-1) will still be enforced even in urgent conditions; only in life-threatening emergencies will the NPO guidelines typically be disregarded. In most acute situations, patients are often dehydrated, either from vomiting, poor oral intake, or third space fluid losses. Thus, prior to surgery, it is essential that patients are adequately resuscitated. Standard intravenous (IV) fluid resuscitation of 20 mL/kg of lactated Ringer's solution or normal saline should be administered followed by continuous administration of maintenance (or higher) fluids. Appropriate antibiotics should also be administered as indicated. Patients with acute appendicitis should be started on single, double, or triple agent broad spectrum antibiotics depending on their symptoms and the

> **Box 14-1. Guidelines for Time Interval Between Eating/Drinking and Surgery (NPO [Nothing by Mouth] Interval) in Infants and Children**
>
> **<6 months old**
> 4 hours breast milk/formula
> 2 hours clear liquids[a]
>
> **6 months–36 months old**
> 8 hours solids
> 6 hours breast milk/formula
> 2 hours clear liquids[a]
>
> **>36 months old**
> 8 hours solids/milk
> 2 hours clear liquids[a]
>
> [a]Formula, milk, orange juice, and colas are *NOT* considered clear liquids. Clear liquids include any liquid that you can see through (water, sugar water, apple juice, Jell-O, broth).

preference of the surgical team. Patients with abscesses should be administered antibiotics with excellent gram-positive coverage, with special attention to methicillin-resistant *Staphylococcus aureus*, given its high prevalence. Pain medication should also be given as needed, even if the surgeon has not evaluated the patient. It is rare that a true surgical condition will be masked by an appropriate dose of pain medication. Finally, basic laboratory studies, such as a complete blood cell count and electrolyte panel, should be obtained.

Perioperative Care

The final operating room schedule for elective cases is made the day before. Thus the specific time of an elective procedure is not known until 1 day prior to surgery. Often the surgeon can give parents an estimated start time. Families will be called the day before surgery to confirm the time of the procedure and when and where to arrive. Often, patients are asked to arrive 1.5 to 2 hours before the scheduled start time. This extra time is to ensure patient safety by completing all of the necessary steps before the actual operation.

In general, patients are put under anesthesia in the operating room. For infants and young children, an IV line is placed after the patient is asleep. To minimize anxiety, preanesthetic sedation is administered orally before proceeding to the operating room. Once in the operating room, patients are often administered an inhalational anesthetic, followed by placement of the IV line, and then intubation. Some institutions allow parents to accompany their child to the operating room and see the child put to sleep with the inhalational anesthetic.

Once the operation is complete, patients are brought to the recovery room. Parents typically are allowed in the recovery room until the time of discharge. Criteria for discharge from the recovery room are listed in Box 14-2. For children who have undergone surgery as outpatients, careful written instructions are provided to the parents along with follow-up appointments and telephone numbers in case problems should arise. Children who are inpatients are discharged

<table>
<tr><th colspan="2">Box 14-2. Criteria for Discharge After Outpatient Surgery</th></tr>
</table>

Box 14-2. Criteria for Discharge After Outpatient Surgery

Stable and appropriate-for-age vital signs
Age-appropriate ambulation
Ability to tolerate oral fluids
No bleeding
No respiratory distress
No pain that cannot be controlled by oral medication
Age-appropriate alertness

from the recovery room to the pediatric inpatient service, along with appropriate orders for the nursing personnel.

There continues to be controversy over the postoperative management of former premature infants following general anesthesia. Ex-premature infants are at higher risk of postoperative apnea. Reasonable recommendations for typical outpatient operations include overnight admission with apnea monitoring for ex-premature infants who are less than or equal to 50 weeks' postconception. However, each institution has its own specific policy and the exact age for required admission varies. The decision for admission is also based on the patient's current health and comorbidities and should be made by the surgeon, anesthesia team, primary care physician, and the patient's parents. Table 14-1 lists the most common elective and urgent/emergency operations and the anticipated postoperative hospitalization stays.

Postoperative Care

Parents will often call their pediatrician with questions postoperatively, thus the pediatrician should be knowledgeable about routine postoperative care. Most children recover from anesthesia and surgery faster than adults. Unless otherwise specified, such as following an appendectomy for perforated appendicitis, a normal diet can be resumed as soon as the patient desires. If patients are not tolerating a normal diet, a bland diet and plenty of fluids are recommended. Furthermore, patients should resume taking all of their preoperative medications the evening after surgery or the next morning.

Nearly all surgical wounds are closed with absorbable sutures and covered with steristrips. Additional dressings can be removed in 1 to 2 days or as needed. Again, unless otherwise specified, most wounds can get wet (shower or quick bath) 48 hours after surgery. Dressings, except for steristrips, should be removed prior to bathing. Wounds do not need to be covered, unless they are open or there is drainage.

The surgeon will provide details regarding activity limitations and returning to school. Often heavy physical activity, such as physical education in school or with organized sports, should be avoided until the surgeon sees the patient following discharge. While heavy physical activity is to be avoided after surgery, patients should be encouraged to walk as well as to cough and to deep breathe many times a day. Patients can return to school when they are feeling up to it and have no more than minimal pain.

Table 14-1. Common Elective and Urgent/Emergency Operations and the Anticipated Postoperative Hospitalization

Procedure	Length of Hospitalization
Elective	
Inguinal hernia repair	Outpatient
Umbilical hernia repair	Outpatient
Cyst excision	Outpatient
Central venous catheter insertion/removal	Outpatient
Orchidopexy	Outpatient
Laparoscopic cholecystectomy	Outpatient
Lymph node biopsy	Outpatient
Ostomy takedown	3–4 days
Lung resection	3–4 days
Imperforate anus repair	3–4 days
Pectus excavatum repair (Nuss procedure)	4–5 days
Urgent/Emergency	
Laparoscopic or open appendectomy for non-perforated appendicitis	1–2 days
Laparoscopic or open appendectomy for perforated appendicitis	5–7 days
Pyloromyotomy	1 day
Intussusception reduction	1 day
Bowel resection	5–7 days
Bowel obstruction	5–7 days
Tumor resection (Wilms or neuroblastoma)	7 days
Choledochal cyst or portoenterostomy	5–7 days
Pull through for Hirschsprung disease	5–7 days

Main reasons to contact the surgeon after the operation are for fever greater than 101.5°F (38.6°C), worsening or persistent pain, persistent emesis, and any wound drainage or redness. Additional instructions specific to the operation are also provided.

CASE RESOLUTION

In this case, the pediatrician reassured the parents that she has referred many patients to this surgeon. The parents were assisted by the pediatrician in crafting their questions for the surgeon. The surgeon subsequently confirmed the diagnosis of an inguinal hernia and recommended surgery. All of the details were provided and the parents had their questions answered. The patient was scheduled for outpatient surgery and everything went smoothly. Postoperatively, there were no concerns and the patient saw both the surgeon and pediatrician in follow-up.

Selected References

Landsman IS, Vustar M, Hays SR. *Pediatric Anesthesia in Pediatric Surgery.* 6th ed. Grosfeld JL, O'Neill JA Jr, Fonkalsrud EW, Coran AG, eds. Philadelphia, PA: Mosby; 2006:221–256

Malviya S, Swartz J, Lerman J. Are all preterm infants younger than 60 weeks postconceptional age a risk for post-anesthetic apnea? *Anesthesiology.* 1993;78:1076–1081

CHAPTER 15

Image Gently™: Approach to Pediatric Imaging

Jane S. Kim, MD; Lindsay S. Baron, MD; and Benjamin H. Taragin, MD

CASE STUDY 1

A 15-year-old boy comes to your office complaining of 1 week of back pain after exertion. He reports no significant recent trauma. He does play varsity basketball, but has not had any recent falls during games. He is otherwise healthy with no significant medical history.

The pain does not prevent him from playing sports or from going to school. He has no history of prior episodes of back pain. He says the pain is relieved by nonsteroidal anti-inflammatory drugs (NSAIDS). On physical examination, he has left-sided paraspinal focal tenderness in the L3–L4 region. He has limited range of motion twisting to that side.

CASE STUDY 2

A 10-year-old girl is brought to your office with runny nose, congestion, cough, and headache. You saw this patient 4 months ago as well as 6 weeks ago, when she had similar complaints. Her mother reports full compliance with the antibiotic regimen you prescribed, but states that her daughter's symptoms have never fully resolved. On physical examination, the child is afebrile with purulent nasal discharge. There is tenderness to palpation over the cheeks and forehead.

Questions

1. What, if any, is the appropriate imaging for each patient?
2. How does one decide the appropriate imaging studies to obtain on a patient?
3. What is the ALARA principle?
4. What information is available for counseling patients regarding the risks of diagnostic radiation?
5. Where can one find appropriate imaging recommendations for pediatric patients?
6. Does the history influence the choice of imaging studies?
   a. What imaging would be appropriate for the patient in Case Study 1 if there was recent significant trauma?
   b. What imaging would be appropriate for the patient in Case Study 2 if her symptoms were new and started last week?

Overuse of medical imaging is a growing problem in the United States that has both financial and medical repercussions. The primary care provider must often decide what, if any, is the proper imaging for patients with common complaints. In many situations, clinical assessment and physical examination are adequate for diagnosis. In some instances, however, imaging provides vital information that cannot be adequately obtained from other sources. Often, patients and their families insist on diagnostic imaging and can be under the impression that the more technologically advanced the evaluation, the better the care.

Currently approximately 370 million studies that use diagnostic radiation are performed yearly in the United States (Figure 15-1). The most dramatic increase has been in the use of computed tomography (CT) scans. In 1982 there were 1 million CT scans performed in the United States. In 2006 there were 67 million CT scans performed, and of this number it is estimated that 4 to 7 million of these were performed in children. In response to this, many concerned health care professionals and radiologists gathered to create the national *Image Gently*™ campaign, focusing on minimizing the use of diagnostic radiation and using appropriate pediatric imaging for children in the United States.

Basic Concepts

Diagnostic radiology examinations that use ionizing radiation include plain radiography, fluoroscopy, CT, and nuclear medicine. Ionizing radiation causes damage to DNA molecules and may lead to cell death or a mutation. The induction of cancer takes several years, and the effects are hereditary (may be passed down to the next generation).

One of the most common ways to measure radiation dose is by the effective dose (unit: Sieverts), which takes into account all of the exposed tissues and each organ's relative radiosensitivity. Certain organs are more radiosensitive than others and, in particular, children are at an increased risk for breast cancer, thyroid cancer, and leukemia. It is important to note that children are more

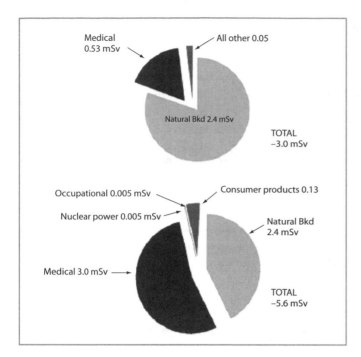

Figure 15-1. US annual per-capita effective radiation dose from various sources. Left: Chart for 1980. Right: Chart for 2006. BKD, background. (From Mettler FA, Bhargavan M, Faulkner K, et al. Radiologic and nuclear medicine studies in the United States and worldwide: frequency, radiation dose, and comparison with other radiation sources—1950–2007. *Radiology.* 2009;253[2]:520–531, with permission.)

Table 15-1. Average Effective Dose in Millisieverts of Different Imaging Studies			
Diagnostic Procedure	**Typical Effective Dose (mSv)[a]**	**Number of Chest X-rays (PA film) for Equivalent Effective Dose[b]**	**Time for Equivalent Effective Dose From Natural Background Radiation[c]**
Chest x-ray	0.02	1	2.4 d
Skull x-ray	0.1	5	12 d
Lumbar spine	1.5	75	182 d
IV urogram	3	150	1.0 y
Upper GI examination	6	300	2.0 y
Barium enema	8	400	2.7 y
CT of head	2	100	243 d
CT of abdomen	8	400	2.7 y

Abbreviations: CT, computed tomography; GI, gastrointestinal; IV, intravenous; PA, posteroanterior.

[a]Average effective dose in millisieverts (mSv) as compiled by Mettler FA Jr, Huda W, Yoshizumi TT, Hahesh M. Effective doses in radiology and diagnostic nuclear medicine: a catalog. *Radiol.* 2008; 248:254–253.

[b]Based on the assumption of an average "effective dose" from chest x-ray (PA film) of 0.02 mSv.

[c]Based on the assumption of an average effective dose from the natural background radiation of 3 mSv per year in the United States.

radiosensitive than adults, secondary to their growth of rapidly proliferating cells. The effective dose also provides a way to compare radiation dose across different imaging modalities. For example, a single CT scan imparts an effective dose that is equivalent to 100 to 250 chest radiographs in children (Table 15-1).

ALARA Principle (As Low As Reasonably Achievable)

Over the last 10 years, there has been increasing attention and research into the radiation imparted to patients from diagnostic imaging. Much of this concern stems from data derived from the atomic bomb survivors of World War II. Based on the distance of survivors from ground zero, the radiation dose to each individual was calculated. More than 50,000 of these patients were followed for more than 50 years. The data showed an increased cancer risk for many of the survivors. Based on this observation, a mathematical model was created, indicating that the risk of cancer proceeds in a linear fashion without threshold (Figure 15-2). Therefore, even a small amount of radiation increases the risk of cancer. Current estimates vary regarding diagnostic radiation and cancer. Based on research by multiple radiation biologists, the American College of Radiology estimates that for adults, one fatal cancer will be induced for every 1,000 CT scans performed. That risk is increased in children, with one fatal cancer occurring for 500 to 1,000 CT scans performed. This is superimposed on the national cancer incidence of 42%.

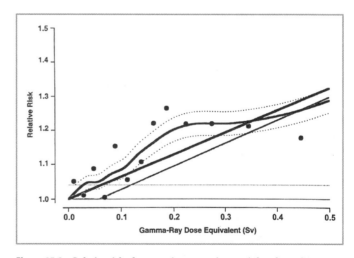

Figure 15-2. Relative risk of contracting cancer in atomic bomb survivors. (Reprinted with permission from Pierce DA, Preston DL: Radiation-related cancer risks at low doses among atomic bomb survivors. *Radiat Res.* 2000; 154:178-186.)

On the basis of this research, the *Image Gently*™ campaign was founded, which stresses a multifaceted approach intended to minimize radiation exposure to children. The campaign has brought together 60 medical and professional organizations representing more than 700,000 imaging specialists from the fields of pediatrics, radiology, physics, and radiology technology. The ALARA principle is based on the notion that any amount of radiation exposure, no matter how small, can increase the chance of negative biological effects. The aim of the ALARA principle is to balance the goals of minimizing the amount of radiation and obtaining sufficient imaging quality, leading to accurate diagnostic information.

Role of the Radiologist

Another guiding principle requires communication and coordination between medical specialties. When in doubt, a call to the local radiologist, whether they are a dedicated pediatric radiologist or not, will often be helpful in determining which test is reasonable for a specific patient. All practicing radiologists have been made aware of the *Image Gently™* campaign and are trying to effectively care for pediatric patients while minimizing diagnostic ionizing radiation. There are many ways that the radiologist can tailor examinations to minimize radiation. The first step often involves asking whether nonionizing diagnostic examinations, such as ultrasound or magnetic resonance imaging (MRI) can be performed to answer the same diagnostic question. In particular, ultrasound can often be used as a screening examination to evaluate conditions that can be clarified with other studies if needed. Radiologists are also focusing on monitoring equipment and protocols for studies. All US commercial CT scanners include multiple methods to adjust the imparted radiation dose. A low dose technique should be used whenever it is appropriate. Breast and gonadal shielding offer additional protection to children.

Available Resources

The American College of Radiology (ACR) has established appropriateness criteria for imaging of specific medical conditions and presentations, coauthored by clinicians and radiologists. They are available free online and can be downloaded as a free mobile application (http://www.acr.org/SecondaryMainMenuCategories/quality_safety/app_criteria.aspx).

Lastly, the *Image Gently™* Web site (http://www.pedrad.org/associations/5364/ig/) offers educational materials for parents to help them understand the risks and benefits of diagnostic imaging and the associated radiation. The site also has printable child imaging history cards so parents can keep track of all the diagnostic radiation examinations performed on their child (Figure 15-3).

Determining the Appropriate Imaging Study

Case Study 1: The Importance of the History

Back pain is a common complaint in active adolescent patients. Many studies have evaluated the use of imaging in patients with non-traumatic back pain. In the absence of significant trauma, most studies have found that there is little value in imaging otherwise healthy adolescents complaining of musculoskeletal pain. If this patient had significant trauma or had focal neurologic findings suspicious for significant cord or disc injury, MRI would be the most appropriate examination. Plain films of the spine are not helpful in

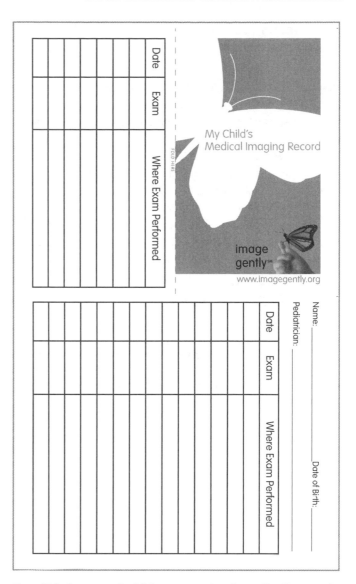

Figure 15-3. Log to record a child's exposure to imaging studies. (Courtesy of Imagegently.org.)

assessing disc disease or intra–central nervous system injury. Plain films are helpful in older patients to evaluate the extent of multilevel disc disease. Obtaining a comprehensive history and performing a complete physical examination will help define the differential diagnosis and assist in the determination of the appropriate imaging study. See Resources at the end of the chapter for a link to the ACR Appropriateness Criteria for suspected spine trauma.

CASE RESOLUTION
Case Study 1
The physician should recommend rest, NSAIDS, and stretching exercises for 4 to 6 weeks. If the pain still persists, MRI of the lumbar spine without contrast would be a reasonable next step in the workup of this patient.

Case Study 2: Symptom Duration and Response to Treatment

Imaging should be obtained in cases of chronic sinusitis that do not respond to treatment and persist without resolution for months. Computed tomography of the sinuses is useful in evaluation of the soft tissues, extent of disease, and any potential intracranial complications. Computed tomography also provides important anatomical detail in the event of the need for surgical intervention. Plain radiography has limited utility in evaluation of sinusitis due to the lack of soft tissue and anatomical detail and low sensitivity. This is particularly true in very young children whose sinuses are not yet well aerated. Imaging is not appropriate in the setting of acute sinusitis. See Resources at the end of the chapter for a link to the ACR Appropriateness Criteria for child sinusitis.

CASE RESOLUTION

Case Study 2

The physician should order a CT of the sinuses as the patient has signs and symptoms of chronic sinusitis despite treatment. If the patient was presenting for the first time with signs and symptoms of sinusitis, medical treatment would be indicated. If the patient does not respond to medical management, imaging should be considered.

Resources

ACR Appropriateness Criteria

Main page: http://www.acr.org/SecondaryMainMenuCategories/quality_safety/app_criteria.aspx.

Child sinusitis: http://www.acr.org/secondarymainmenucategories/quality_safety/app_criteria/pdf/expertpanelonpediatricimaging/sinusitischilddoc8.aspx

Suspected spine trauma: http://www.acr.org/SecondaryMainMenuCategories/quality_safety/app_criteria/pdf/ExpertPanelonNeurologicImaging/SpineTraumaUpdateinProgressDoc13.aspx

Radiation dose assessment: http://www.acr.org/SecondaryMainMenuCategories/quality_safety/app_criteria/RRLInformation.aspx

Image Gently™ **Web site**

http://www.pedrad.org/associations/5364/ig/

Selected References

Bulas D, Goske M, Applegate K, Wood B. Image Gently: improving health literacy for parents about CT scans for children. *Pediatr Radiol.* 2009;39(2):112–116

Frush DP. Radiation safety. *Pediatr Radiol.* 2009;39(suppl 3):385–390

Goske MJ, Applegate KE, Boylan J, et al. The Image Gently campaign: working together to change practice. *AJR Am J Roentgenol.* 2008;190:273–274

Voss SD, Reaman GH, Kaste SC, Slovis TL. The ALARA concept in pediatric oncology. *Pediatr Radiol.* 2009;39(11):1142–1146

CHAPTER 16

Pediatric Genomic Medicine

Derek Wong, MD

CASE STUDY

A 4-year-old male with moderate global developmental delay is brought to his pediatrician's office for evaluation. The patient has an unremarkable family history and a normal physical examination. Previous evaluation included a normal karyotype and fragile X DNA test. The patient's parents would like to know if there is anything else that can be done to determine the etiology of the delay. In addition, his mother has recently read about companies that offer multiple genetic tests to consumers, and wonders if these tests will be useful as well.

Questions
1. How is microarray technology useful in pediatric practice?
2. How will next-generation sequencing technology impact future practice?
3. What are the limitations of these new technologies?
4. What is direct-to-consumer genetic testing?

As a result of the Human Genome Project (HGP), the first essentially complete human sequence was published in 2003. Very rapid progress in DNA sequencing technology has decreased the cost of sequencing an individual from $750 billion in the HGP to less than $20,000 per person in 2010. Currently microarray analysis has resulted in dramatically increased yields for patients with developmental delay, autism, and multiple congenital anomalies. Genetic panels for a variety of conditions, such as familial cardiomyopathy and X-linked mental retardation, offer testing for 20 to 100 genes at the same price as sequencing 2 to 4 genes cost a few years ago. Several companies offer direct-to-consumer genetic testing, designed to provide information without physician input. Pharmacogenomics, which promises individualized drug therapy based on genomic data, is moving from specialized disease therapeutics to common diseases. The promise of a $1,000 genome has been hailed as the beginning of a new era of personalized medicine, in which each patient will have a tailor-made set of interventions to optimize his or her health. As with most breakthrough technologies, these advances will be balanced by significant limitations.

Epidemiology—Human Genome Anatomy

Human cells have 2 haploid genomes, each containing 3 billion base pairs with an estimated 20,000 to 25,000 protein encoding genes, plus a variable number of copies of the mitochondrial genome. On average, 2 humans share 99.9% of their DNA. There are at least 10 million single nucleotide polymorphisms (SNPs), which are single base changes that are present in a substantial percentage of the population (>1%). A small percentage of SNPs fall within the coding or regulatory regions of genes, and directly influence gene function. The remaining SNPs have no known effect on protein production,

but may be inherited in recognizable patterns (haplotypes) with other SNPs.

Recently it has become evident that most human genetic variation is not due to SNPs. Instead, copy number variants (CNVs), in which DNA segments containing up to several million base pairs are duplicated or deleted, account for a substantial portion of variation between individuals. Although studies have found that 12% of the genome is subject to CNV (Redon), the impact of this variation on an individual's phenotype is unknown.

Although most autosomal recessive disorders are rare, most humans are carriers of several disease alleles. In a recent study, there was an average of 2.8 recessive mutations per person in 448 genes involved in severe autosomal recessive conditions.

Pathophysiology—The Genotype/Phenotype Correlation and Environment

There are numerous examples of genetic background affecting the presentation of rare genetic disorders. Although most patients with untreated classic phenylketonuria develop mental retardation, some patients with high blood levels have normal IQ on a regular diet. Patients with thalassemia are affected by the alpha to beta globin gene ratio. Therefore, β-thalassemia "carriers" with one mutation may become symptomatic if they have duplicated alpha chains. Understanding susceptibility to common genetic disorders will require an understanding of a complex network of interacting genes.

Genomic data provide information about only one predisposing factor to a disease state. Many diseases are caused by a combination of genetic susceptibility and environmental forces. The first examples of this interaction that were discovered were monogenic conditions such as complement deficiency, which predisposed patients to bacterial meningitis, or cancer susceptibility genes that caused extreme radiation sensitivity. However, the gene–environment connection is known to be much deeper, with certain environmental conditions causing methylation of the genetic code, silencing multiple genes without changing DNA sequence. These epigenetic changes may persist across generations, causing mothers exposed to wartime famine to produce children who are born to conserve energy. If these children are fed a typical American diet, they are prone to obesity and diabetes. Fetal cells that persist in maternal circulation (fetal microchimerism) may play a role in both tumor prevention and susceptibility to autoimmune disease. Finally, our bodies contain more bacteria than human cells. The interaction of the bacterial genomes and human genomes plays an important role in some disease states.

Clinical Presentation/History and Physical

A thorough history and physical examination will continue to be a critical component of patient assessment in the genomic age of medicine. Large databases will need to be created in order to correlate human genotypes to corresponding phenotypes, which are defined by the patient's clinical presentation. Even when genetic and epigenetic sequencing is commonplace, the only way to measure the impact of the disease on the individual is by clinical assessment.

Laboratory Testing

New genetic laboratory techniques have had a dramatic impact on common pediatric conditions such as developmental delay and autism. Microarray testing uses closely spaced DNA probes to detect chromosomal deletions or duplications at 10 to 10,000 times the resolution of a standard karyotype. The diagnostic yield for developmental delay and multiple congenital anomalies has increased from 3% to 4% to 15% to 20% using this technology. For example, patients with autism with normal karyotypes may have microdeletions or microduplications of 16p11.2. The limitations of this technology are that it cannot detect balanced translocations or most chromosomal mosaic patients.

Next-generation sequencing is a phrase used to describe new methods that allow parallel sequencing of billions of base pairs at relatively low cost. Whole exome sequencing concentrates on the 1.5% of the genome that is the protein coding region, and is predicted to become available on a clinical basis during the next several years. A recent trial of this technology identified genetic causes in 6 out of 10 patients with unexplained mental retardation who had negative testing for fragile X, and normal karyotype and microarray analysis. Shortly after whole exome sequencing becomes established, whole genome sequencing is expected to become available, allowing discovery of variation in regulatory elements located outside the coding regions.

Next-generation sequencing technology has significant drawbacks that must be overcome prior to general use. An error rate of 0.001% is acceptable for a single test, but impractical if billions of base pairs are tested at the same time. Resequencing each region

tens or hundreds of times will eliminate most errors. However, some genes, particularly those with high guanine-cytosine content, are not well sequenced with current high-volume technologies. Thus whole exome sequencing may miss 5% or more of the genome.

A patient's next-generation sequencing results may have millions of differences from reference sequences. Until huge databases of genomes from millions of patients are available, bioinformatics algorithms must be used to sift through the data and determine which changes are potentially relevant. Parental testing is often essential for these studies and may not be available. In general, results may be divided into 3 categories: known mutations, SNPs or other alterations that do not cause disease, and variants of unknown significance. The last category may contain tens or hundreds of altered genes, and matching potential mutations to a given phenotype is very difficult. Technology will drive down the price of sequencing over time, but the cost of bioinformatics will dominate the price of these new technologies as the amount of data increases.

Direct-to-Consumer Genetic Testing

Several companies market genetic tests that report disease risk by analyzing multiple SNPs along with common disease mutations. The companies argue that consumers have the right to know their genetic information, and some offer genetic counseling services. However, the tests may lack sensitivity and specificity, because the analysis is based on limited genetic markers without family history or phenotypic information. Many consumers (and their physicians) are ill-equipped to understand the nature of the results, and patients of non-Caucasian ethnicity may have many indeterminate results. In 2010 the US Food and Drug Administration decided to develop regulations regarding the sale of direct-to-consumer genetic tests.

Treatment—Pharmacogenomics

Individualized pharmacologic treatment is one of the ultimate goals of the HGP. Although pharmacogenomics is in its infancy, several tests are available that reduce the risk of an adverse drug reaction. Patients with variant thiopurine methyltransferase alleles may have severe toxicity to drugs, such as azathioprine and 6-mercaptopurine, that are used in multiple disorders. Children with a 1555A>G mutation in the mitochondrial genome are susceptible to aminoglycoside-induced hearing loss, even after the first dose. Pharmacogenomics for common diseases such as asthma is currently under investigation and may allow a more rational choice of multi-drug regimens.

Future Developments

Despite huge potential, the impact of the HGP has yet to be felt in most areas of medicine, including pediatrics. However, during the next decade, genomics will revolutionize the diagnosis of Mendelian disease. The impact of the HGP on common diseases and therapy is less obvious. It is unclear whether consumers will use genomic information to alter their lifestyles, whether the information comes from their physicians or direct-to-consumer testing. In addition, whole exome and whole genome sequencing create a variety of ethical issues. If a patient presents with heart disease, and testing shows an increased risk for Alzheimer disease, should this information be disclosed to the patient? It is certain that pediatricians will need to familiarize themselves with genomic medicine, because the number of tests will overwhelm the available medical genetics specialists and genetics counselors.

CASE RESOLUTION

The patient's microarray testing shows a small microdeletion in chromosome 6. Parental testing indicates that the microdeletion is present in the patient's father, who has had normal development. Further testing includes a "developmental delay" panel, which shows a potential missense mutation in *CASK*, a gene on the X chromosome that may cause developmental delay. This alteration is not found in the patient's mother, implying that it is most likely deleterious. The parents receive genetic counseling about future pregnancies.

Resources

All About the Human Genome Project
http://www.genome.gov/10001772

Copy Number Variation
http://www.nature.com/scitable/topicpage/copy-number-variation-445

Selected References

Bell CJ, Dinwiddie DL, Miller NA, et al. Carrier testing for severe childhood recessive diseases by next-generation sequencing. *Sci Transl Med.* 2011;3(65):65ra4

Bloss CS, Schork NJ, Topol EJ. Effect of direct-to-consumer genomewide profiling to assess disease risk. *N Engl J Med.* 2011;364(6):524–534

Feero WG, Guttmacher AE, Collins FS. Genomic medicine—an updated primer. *N Engl J Med.* 2010;362(21):2001–2011

Hines RN, McCarver DG. Pharmacogenomics and the future of drug therapy. *Pediatr Clin North Am.* 2006;53(4):591–619

Kuehn BM. Inconsistent results, inaccurate claims plague direct-to-consumer gene tests. *JAMA.* 2010;304(12):1313–1315

Li MM, Andersson HC. Clinical application of microarray-based molecular cytogenetics: an emerging new era of genomic medicine. *J Pediatr.* 2009;155(3):311–317

Redon R, Ishikawa S, Fitch KR, et al. Global variation in copy number in the human genome. *Nature.* 2006;444(7118): 444–454

Vissers LE, de Ligt J, Gilissen C, et al. A de novo paradigm for mental retardation. *Nat Genet.* 2010;42(12):1109–1112

CHAPTER 17

Principles of Quality Improvement: Improving Health Care for Pediatric Patients

Bonnie R. Rachman, MD

CASE STUDY

During a routine staff meeting at your group pediatric practice, it was noted that many of the patients followed by your practice are behind in their immunizations. The reasons for this are unclear since you and your colleagues are strong proponents of the timely administration of preventive immunizations. You want to develop a mechanism to determine what factors are leading to a delay in vaccine administration.

Questions

1. What is quality improvement?
2. How does assessing the delivery of recommended health maintenance relate to quality?
3. How is the prevention of medical errors related to quality improvement?
4. What is the difference between harm and error?
5. What factors are associated with medical errors?
6. What is meant by organizational culture?

History

The origin of medical quality improvement lies not in medicine but in industry and dates back to the 1920s. Dr Walter A. Shewhart was an American physicist, engineer, and statistician. In 1924 Dr Shewhart presented a memo where he showed a schematic control chart. The diagram and text set forth all the essential principles and considerations involved in quality control. Dr Shewhart pointed out the importance of reducing variation in a manufacturing process and noted that continual process adjustment in reaction to nonconformance actually increased variation and degraded quality. He went on to develop **data presentation rules,** which continue to be important today: (1) data have no meaning apart from their context and (2) data contain both signal and noise. To be able to extract information, one must separate the signal from the noise within the data.

In the 1950s Dr Shewhart's colleague, W. Edwards Deming, working in Japan taught top management how to improve design and, subsequently, service, product quality, testing, and sales. Deming applying Shewhart's concepts, described the Plan-Do-Study-Act (PDSA) cycle as an approach to quality improvement. He opined,

"The key is to practice continual improvement and think of manufacturing as a system, not as bits and pieces."

In the 1970s Avedis Donabedian, a physician, proposed a model for assessing health care quality by describing 7 pillars of quality: efficacy, efficiency, optimality, acceptability, legitimacy, equity, and cost (Box 17-1). He posited, "Structure is the environment in which health care is provided, process is the method by which health care is provided, and outcome is the result of the care provided." He emphasized the importance of measurement and evaluation of health care quality, ensuring completeness and accuracy of medical records, observer bias, patient satisfaction, and cultural preferences for health care.

In 1991 Drs Paul Batalden and Don Berwick helped form the Institute for Healthcare Improvement (IHI), which has led to the

Box 17-1. 7 Pillars of Quality	
Efficacy	Legitimacy
Efficiency	Equity
Optimality	Cost
Acceptability	

application of quality improvement science to health care in the United States and internationally. The IHI promotes the adoption of measurement and feedback to improve the quality of health care.

Historically, efforts for improving quality focused on "quality assurance." The goal was to minimize "defects" as measured by audits. Now the emphasis is on "quality improvement," which focuses on moving the entire performance curve toward a greater level of performance by adopting best practices instead of simply focusing on low performers. Ongoing measurement is vital to sustaining any improvement. The process of quality improvement requires careful planning, thorough documentation, consistent analysis, and open-mindedness to results.

Introduction

Quality Improvement in Pediatrics

Pediatrics is a specialty that emphasizes health maintenance and disease prevention. Studies have shown that recommended targets are not being consistently realized. Mangione-Smith and colleagues reported that children received only 46.5% of recommended care for preventive services, acute illness management, and ongoing care of chronic conditions. Shaughnessy and Nickel reported that 21% of outpatient prescriptions in a family medicine practice had at least one error. Other investigators found that medication samples were dispensed with inadequate documentation. In a pediatric emergency department in Canada, 100 prescribing errors and 39 medication administration errors occurred per 1,000 patients. In a sample of new prescriptions for 22 common medications in outpatient pediatric clinics, approximately 15% were dispensed with potential dosing errors.

The Learning from Errors in Ambulatory Pediatrics (LEAP) study aimed to learn the scope, range, potential causes, and possible solutions to medical errors in pediatric ambulatory care. The study found that among 14 pediatric practice sites, there were 147 medical errors reported during the 4-month study period. The largest group of errors was related to medical treatment (37%). Of the medical treatment errors, 85% were medication errors. There were also errors associated with patient identification (22%); preventive care, including immunizations (15%); diagnostic testing (13%); and patient communication (8%).

There are many examples of errors in the inpatient arena as well. A study looking at inpatient medication errors found that among 1,000 children in 12 independent children's hospitals, 1 in 15 children was exposed to wrong medications, side effects, or drug interactions. Takata and Currier reported a rate of 11.1 adverse events per 100 pediatric inpatients; 22% of these errors were deemed preventable. In a 2005 Joint Commission on Accreditation of Healthcare Organizations report, the root cause of more than 70% of 2,400 sentinel events was communication failure between providers or between family and providers. In those events, 75% of patients died due to this type of failure.

Kurtin and Stucky describe 5 barriers or challenges to high-quality care in both the pediatric and adult arenas (Table 17-1). The first is widespread unnecessary variation in care.

In order to prevent medical error, one needs to understand how, when, and where it occurs; to look at the system that allowed the error to happen; and to keep the system open and blame-free (Box 17-2).

The factors associated with risk of error are not the individuals who work in the system but rather the system in which the individuals work. To decrease the risk of error, the language of patient safety must be understood, and a deeper understanding of the principles of systems analysis work models and other problem solutions must be developed.

Definitions

In order to understand quality improvement and improve patient safety, one must be familiar with the terminology. The National Patient Safety Foundation defines *patient safety* as the avoidance, prevention, and amelioration of adverse outcomes or injuries stemming

Table 17-1. Barriers to High-Quality Care	
Barrier	**Explanation**
Unnecessary variation in care	Diagnostic or therapeutic interventions performed at the discretion of the ordering physician and not required by the patient's condition
Gap between knowledge and practice	May be many years; time it takes a proven new practice to go from medical literature to routine clinical care
Failure of physicians to understand and work in the hospital's complex systems of care	Challenges to accessing information/data/personnel/materials to facilitate patient care
Need to improve patient safety	No consistent mechanism in place
Slow adoption and routine use of practices that can improve clinical outcomes and patient safety	Use of clinical pathways may mitigate

Box 17-2. Factors Associated With Errors
Communication failures
Frequent distractions and interruptions
Inadequate supervision
Drug ordering issues
Limited access to patient information
Noisy work environment
Lack of 24-hour pediatric pharmacy
Emergency situations

from the processes of health care. The Institute of Medicine (IOM) defines *patient safety* as freedom from accidental injury.

An *adverse event* is defined as injury caused by medical management rather than by the underlying condition. Some are not preventable. One example of a non-preventable adverse event is the person who receives the appropriate antibiotic at the appropriate time and an appropriate dose who has an allergic reaction to the medication. This differs from *medical error,* which is the failure of a planned action to be completed as intended (error in execution) or the use of a wrong plan to achieve an aim (error of planning). *Outcomes* summarize the effectiveness of care, including adverse events.

James Reason, who did extensive work on organization models of accidents, further delineates the terminology. A *slip* is an error in execution; the observable action deviates from what was planned. A *lapse* is an error in execution due to a memory failure. A *mistake* is a knowledge-based failure; the plan is carried out correctly but the planned action was wrong for the situation. An *active error* (sharp end error) typically occurs in a patient care area by a front-line provider; the effects may be felt immediately. A *latent error* (blunt error) is due to system-based problem and may relate to poor design, incorrect installation, look-alike packaging, sound-alike names, faulty maintenance, or bad management decisions. These are more difficult to identify and hard to recognize. Health care workers frequently develop "work-arounds" to bypass the problem. This often leads to the belief that the "work-around" is normal.

A *system* is a set of interdependent human and nonhuman elements interacting to achieve a common aim. In a hospital, it may be a unit or a department. *Processes* are how care is delivered. (Are policies routinely followed? Are evidence-based medicine guidelines implemented? Does the transfer of patients occur in an organized manner?) *Work models* provide a conceptual framework for investigating events and processes so all contributing factors are evaluated. Plan-Do-Study-Act is an example of a conceptual framework. The premise of all work models is that an organized, systematic approach to event investigation results in reliable data that may be used to develop a new *system.*

Continuous quality improvement (CQI) is the continued process of reviewing and improving the processes and procedures associated with providing goods or services. It may evaluate structure, process, or outcome either as independent components of the CQI process or all simultaneously, because considerable overlap exists between the components and quality of care.

When evaluating the quality of health by comparing outcomes, it is important to understand the concept of *risk adjustment. Risk adjustment* allows statistical adjustment of patient differences, such as severity of illness, to make comparisons of outcomes clinically meaningful. This enables the translation of statistically significant tests into clinically meaningful results.

Errors and How They Occur

The pervasiveness of the medical error problem is enormous. In 1999 the IOM published *To Err is Human.* This report stated that medical error accounted for approximately 44,000 to 98,000 deaths annually in US hospitals. This is more deaths than from AIDS, motor vehicle crashes, or breast cancer. The types of events included adverse drug events, improper transfusions, surgical injuries, wrong site surgeries, suicides, and mistaken patient identity. Most errors occurred in intensive care units, operating rooms, and emergency departments. The annual total cost was estimated to be between $17 billion to $29 billion. The cost of additional care was $8 billion. This figure does not account for lost income and productivity. The IOM made many recommendations in this report, including a balanced approach between regulatory and market-based initiatives as well as the establishment of a national focus to create leadership, research, tools, and protocols to enhance the knowledge base about safety. It recommended raising performance standards and expectations for improvements in safety through the actions of oversight organizations, professional groups, and group purchasers of health care. An additional recommendation was to implement safety systems in health care organizations to ensure safe practices at the delivery level. In 2001 the IOM published the follow-up report, "Crossing the Quality Chasm." Safety was deemed the key dimension of quality. Only a systems approach would work; trying harder was inadequate. A stepwise correction of problems in the system is the key to success. The culture of blame must be overcome: Human error was to be expected. Table 17-2 lists types of errors and their definitions.

Medical errors are not usually a single event or done by a single person. Normally there are numerous safe points and double-checks built into the process, but each layer of safety has gaps or "holes." When these "holes" line up, the error reaches the patient. Standardized approaches can reduce variability and improve system efficiency. The goal is to make the holes as small as possible or even make them disappear. There are many factors associated with medical error, including human factors triggered by interruptions, fatigue, time pressures, anger, anxiety, fear, and boredom. Mistakes can result from a wrong plan of action. Mistakes involve misinterpretation of a problem, lack of knowledge, and habitual patterns of thought. A violation is the purposeful rule violation whether reasoned or reckless. The factors associated with risk are not the individuals who work in the system but rather the system in which the individuals work.

Table 17-2 Types of Errors in Health Care	
Error	*Definition*
Diagnosis error	Error of delay in diagnosis; failure to employ indicated tests, the use of outmoded tests or therapy, or the failure to act on results of monitoring or tests
Treatment error	Error in the performance of an operation, procedure, or test; an avoidable delay in treatment or responding to an abnormal test or inappropriate/not indicated care
Medication error	Most frequent type of error; includes an error in the dose or method of using a drug
Prevention error	Failure to provide prophylactic treatment or inadequate monitoring or follow-up of treatment

Harm Versus Error

Our ultimate goal is to reduce patient harm. Early quality improvement efforts targeted the elimination of error. It had been believed that reducing error would decrease harm. This is not true; most medical errors never harm patients and may be clinically insignificant. One example would be the acetaminophen dose that is given 1 hour late. Why do we differentiate? Focusing on harm puts the microscope on the system not the individual.

Quality Improvement and Organizational Culture

"This is the way we do things around here."

Patients expect to receive quality health care without experiencing preventable harm. The IOM has defined quality in health care as "the degree to which health care services for individuals and populations increase the likelihood of desired health outcomes and are consistent with current professional knowledge." One of the things that influence quality in health care is organizational culture.

Many pediatricians are never taught about organizational culture. It is the invisible powerful dictator of how things are done in the organization. It is a latent and often unconscious set of forces that determine both our individual and collective behavior, ways of perceiving, thought patterns, and values. Hospitals have their own cultures. Subcultures also exist among physicians and nurses as well as within departments, such as critical care. It may be challenging to understand all of the hospital's different subcultures.

Promoting change is rarely easy. Some people may adapt and change appropriately while others resist and become dysfunctional. In order to make changes, there must be an environment where teamwork can grow. "Group think" must be avoided. "Group think" is a term coined by Yale psychologist Irving Janis. It is "a way of thinking that people may adopt when they are members of a cohesive or homogeneous group; in particular, a group whose members seek unanimity of thought to the point that they cannot consider alternative ideas." It can prevent critical thinking and debate. Without disagreement, creativity can be lost. Negative effects of "group think" include an illusion of invulnerability, insulated leaders who may be protected from contradictory evidence, and members who accept confirming data and reject data that fails to fit their views. Alternatives are not considered and individuals with conflicting views are discounted or demonized. Talented leaders welcome diversity of thoughts and ideas. Leaders must empower team members to have open discussions and offer ideas.

Communication is a key component of organizational culture. Communication involves 2 parts: message and meaning. Message is stated; meaning is interpreted and may be different between people. Strategies to improve communication are legion. Included in these strategies are methods for remaining calm in high workload, stressful situations. Other strategies include more verbalization, verbalizations that relate to problem-solving, speaking in first person plural, and coordinating tasks to the right person's experience level. Good communication encourages input from team members.

Offering positive feedback builds confidence, reduces stress, and clarifies ambiguities. Team evaluations provide input on how well team members are communicating with each other and the progression toward achieving team goals. Benchmarking against a similar team may provide valuable information. An outside consultant may be used to observe the team and provide feedback. Internally, the use of informal, regular meetings to discuss the team's progress and provide debriefing sessions to discuss the team process may be constructive in moving the team forward toward their goals and ensuring effective communication. Team conflict is experienced by all teams at one time or another. It happens when people come together to resolve a problem, discuss care improvement, or discuss changing processes to improve care. It needs to be managed effectively so issues at hand can be resolved while still providing the best quality patient care.

Teamwork has been defined by numerous organizations. The IOM in 2003 used this definition: "All healthcare professionals should be educated to deliver patient-centered care as members of an interdisciplinary team, emphasizing evidence-based practice, quality improvement approaches, and informatics." The IOM defines a multidisciplinary team as one in which members cooperate, communicate, and integrate care to ensure that patient care is continuous and reliable.

Measuring Quality

Ideally, measurements should evolve from the IOM quality aims: timeliness, efficiency, effectiveness, safety, equity and patient-centeredness (Box 17-3). Improvement measures may not be sufficiently valid and reliable for public dissemination yet may still be useful for benchmarking, to identify best practice, or as part of quality improvement initiatives.

Adult measures may not be appropriate for pediatrics. Pediatrics is unique due to heterogeneity, including age, size, diagnoses, and treatment modalities including medication dosing.

Measures must be reliable. The definition of reliability is the ability of the measure to perform similarly under stated conditions over time. In health care, reliability is often used interchangeably with the concept of precision. Precision is the ability of a measurement process to reproduce its own outcome. To achieve precision, a reliable system requires clear and concise definitions of the data fields to be collected. An effective approach is to train data collectors. There must also be a robust method for data coding and entry. Reliability needs to be intermittently assessed within and between observers over time to ensure consistency.

Measures must also be valid. A measure is valid if it adequately represents the attribute of interest. Internal validity is the soundness of the developed indicator. External validity is the ability of the indicator to be applied to a broader population.

Box 17-3. Institute of Medicine Quality Aims	
Timeliness	Safety
Efficiency	Equity
Effectiveness	Patient-centeredness

Measures must be feasible and usable. Feasibility is the actual ability to gather the measures. For a measure to be usable, the intended audience must be able to understand the findings and use them in an appropriate fashion. It is usable if it is able to uncover meaningful differences between groups.

Three types of measures are essential to quality improvement.

1. Outcomes measures: Address how the health care services provided to patients affect their health, functional status, and/or satisfaction.
2. Process measures: Address the health care services provided to patients.
3. Balancing measures: Evaluate unintended consequences or the stability of the system being changed in the project.

A balanced set of measures for a quality improvement effort should include at least one outcome, one process, and one balancing measure.

Error Metrics

How does one measure harm?

How does one measure safety?

Measuring harm is often done with occurrence reports. This identifies 2% to 8% of all adverse events in an inpatient setting. It may be done with retrospective, concurrent, or trigger-based chart review. There are no standardized methods for reporting, investigating, or disseminating information related to preventable adverse events. In the past, the qualitative concept of patient safety has been translated in quantitative metrics. Three frameworks that have been used include measuring error, measuring patient injuries, and measuring risk.

Error-based patient safety metrics are premised on the idea that the goal of medicine is to successfully implement the correct plan of care. It is an attractive measure of assessing safety because many errors occur and are somewhat easy to find. There are many problems with error metrics as very few measures of error represent the true rate.

$$\text{Error rate} = (\text{identified errors})/(\text{potential opportunities for that error to occur})$$

The numerator (identified errors) may be hard to obtain, since with reported events one only knows the errors reported not the actual number of occurrences. Therefore, it is nothing more than a rate of reporting.

Some other modalities proposed to get the true numerator include chart review. The difficulty with chart review includes the number of steps in the process: error occurs, each error is recognized by a provider, the error is documented by a provider, the chart is reviewed, the reviewer recognizes the event during the chart review, and the error is attributed correctly. Ethnographic study, the direct observation of people, has the same pitfalls.

Other confounders include hindsight bias. For problems to be effectively rectified, the correct understanding and attribution of events that created the error must occur. The retrospective analysis

of error creates the potential for incorrect or simplistic identification of causes for events. "Subsystem" failures are difficult to identify as a contributing cause to an adverse event. The incorrect or inadequate attribution of causality creates the potential for misguided actions to "solve" the wrong problem.

Focusing solely on active errors leaves the latent failures and the whole system more vulnerable to adverse events. Identifying errors is important, but solely focusing on errors may lead to the "blame game." Trends may be a barometer for the organization's culture as it relates to patient safety. Identified errors provide learning opportunities, preventing harm to other patients.

Injury-based patient safety metrics focus on unintended outcomes, such as catheter-related bloodstream infections, ventilator-associated pneumonia, in-hospital cardiac arrest, and deaths. Improvement efforts are more likely to focus on system vulnerabilities with a high potential for adverse events.

Risk-based patient safety metrics are a measurement of hazards or risks. Using a systems view, errors and injuries are the result of hazards or risks within the system of care. The focus is on hazardous conditions that increase the likelihood of downstream errors. Efforts are centered on 3 core areas: (1) systematic risk identification, (2) risk assessment, and (3) risk reduction/elimination. It is proactive and it saves counting errors and injuries (makes it less important). The elimination of risk includes the substitution of less risky alternatives, the development of administrative controls, and individual protection. It incorporates information gathered from the frontline bedside provider. The focus on risk reduction may decrease the need to quantify error rates or injury prevalence. This requires a shift in thinking from counting errors and injuries to proactively identifying risk. The intent is to identify systems-level problems that may be amenable to quality improvement efforts.

Patient Safety/Error Prevention

The Institute for Safe Medication Practices has developed a rank order of error reduction strategies. They range from most effective (forcing functions and constraints) to least effective (education/information). In between are strategies such as (in order from most effective to least effective) automation and computerization, standardization and protocols, checklists and double-check systems, and rules and policies.

Education and information dissemination are important and helpful; they increase awareness. However, lectures are quickly forgotten and signs are often ignored. It is the least effective means to prevent the occurrence of error. Rules and policies are required by several agencies. They are a good resource but not an effective means of preventing a specific event.

Checklists and double-check systems are very effective when they are a routine part of practice but they are not foolproof. The best example of a double-check system is the surgical sponge and instrument counts done at the end of a surgical case. Checklists are also being used for other procedures like central line placement. Standardization minimizes the risk of error, and protocols bring a standard approach to a clinical issue. They are designed to eliminate variation from practitioner to practitioner and patient to patient. Weak points may still exist and be prone to error. Automation and computerization are 2 of the best means to prevent medical error from occurring. They are only as safe and good as the person entering the data. Forcing functions and constraints is the best way to prevent error through safeguards. In this manner, systems and products are engineered to be safer from the ground up.

Plan-Do-Study-Act cycles are one way of developing and implementing change leading to improved patient safety and quality of care. Plan-Do-Study-Act cycles force small-scale, stepwise thinking; allow for making predictions; force thoughtful deliberation on the increased knowledge; and subsequently facilitate change. The use of small-scale change can cause rapid adaptation and implementation of change in various health care settings.

Conclusions

The key elements to a system change are (1) the will to do whatever it takes to make a change to a system, (2) the ideas on which to base the design of the new system, and (3) the execution of the changes to the system. Change is difficult, but sustaining change is even more complex. Hardwiring sustainability into a new system is imperative. The "old way" has to be more difficult or inconvenient to perform. In health care, spreading improvements depends on key individuals; one critical success factor for spread is the role of leadership. Leaders must inspire and communicate a shared vision; model the way; challenge the current process; no longer accept the status quo; and enable others with resources, training, and time. The successes must be celebrated.

CASE RESOLUTION

During your staff meeting, you decide to use a PDSA cycle to examine the practice's vaccine administration practice, identify barriers to timely vaccine administration, and develop a plan to ensure that vaccines are administered in a timely fashion.

Plan: The charts of all patients seen for routine care in the past 3 months are pulled. The charts are audited using a premade check sheet to identify vaccines given, vaccines missed, and barriers to administration. After analyzing the data, it becomes clear that many opportunities for immunization were missed due to inability to get parental consent. This seemed to coincide with a television program that discussed increasing rates of autism associated with vaccination.

Do: At your next routine staff meeting, you present the data to your colleagues. You recommend rebutting the television show with a fact sheet and a discussion with the parents that is done by the physician. Your colleagues agree to implement this change since it is low cost and easy to put into practice.

Study: Three months after implementation, you re-collect data and find there are fewer missed opportunities for immunization and your program has had some success. Some parents are still resistant to immunizing their children for fear of autism.

Act: You present the follow-up data to your colleagues and they agree to implement the current strategy. The data will be reexamined in 3 months to see if the program continues to be effective.

Selected References

Agency for Healthcare Research and Quality. Improving health care quality [fact sheet]. http://www.AHRQ.gov/news/qualfact.htm. Accessed December 18, 2010

Aguayo R. *Dr. Deming: The American Who Taught the Japanese About Quality.* New York, NY: Fireside; 1991:40–41

Association of Public Health Observatories. The good indicators guide: understanding how to use and choose indicators. NHS Institute for Innovation and Improvement. 2008. http://www.apho.org.uk/resource/item.aspx?RID=44584. Accessed January 4, 2011

Best M, Neuhauser D. Walter A. Shewhart, 1924, and the Hawthorne factory. *Qual Saf Health Care.* 2006;15:142–143

Carey RG, Lloyd RC. *Measuring Quality Improvement in Healthcare: A Guide to Statistical Process Control Applications.* New York, NY: American Society for Quality; 2001

Counte MA, Meuer S. Issues in the assessment of continuous quality improvement implementation in health care organizations. *Int J Qual Health Care.* 2001;13:197–207

Dr. Deming's Management Training. http://www.dharma-haven.org/five-havens/deming.htm

Dill JL, Generali JA. Medication sample labeling practices. *Am J Health Syst Pharm.* 2000;57:2087–2090

Dodek P, Cahill NE, Heyland DK. The relationship between organizational culture and implementation of clinical practice guidelines: a narrative review. *JPEN J Parenter Enteral Nutr.* 2010;34:669–674

Donabedian A, Bashshur R. *An Introduction to Quality Assurance in Health Care.* New York, NY: Oxford University Press; 2003

Griffin E. *A First Look at Communication Theory.* http: www.afirstlook.com. Accessed January 4, 2011

Institute of Medicine. *Crossing the Quality Chasm: a new health system for the 21st century.* Washington, DC: National Academy Press; 2001

Institute of Medicine. *Health Professions Education: A Bridge to Quality.* Washington, DC: National Academy Press; 2003

Institute of Medicine. Committee to design a strategy for quality review and assurance in Medicare. In: Lohr KN, ed. *Medicare: A Strategy for Quality Assurance.* Vol. 1. Washington, DC: National Academies Press; 1990

Institute for Safe Medicine Practices. ISMP rank order of error reduction strategies. http://www.ismp.org. Accessed January 4, 2011

Joint Commission on Accreditation of Healthcare Organizations. Sentinel event statistics. http://www.jointcommission.org/SentinelEvents/Statistics. Accessed December 17, 2010

Kenney C. *The Best Practice: How the New Quality Movement Is Transforming Medicine.* New York, NY: Public Affairs; 2008

Kohn LT, Corrigan JM, Donaldson MS, eds. *To Err is Human: Building a Safer Health System.* Washington, DC: National Academy Press; 2000

Kotter JP. *Leading Change.* Boston, MA: Harvard Business School Press; 1996

Kozer E, Scolnik D, Macpherson A, et al. Variables associated with medication errors in pediatric emergency medicine. *Pediatrics.* 2002;110:737–742

Langley G, Nolan K, Nolan T, et al. *The Improvement Guide: A Practical Approach to Enhancing Organizational Performance.* San Francisco, CA: Jossey-Bass Pub; 1996

Leape LL, Lawthers AG, Brennan TA, et al. Preventing medical injury. *Qual Rev Bull.* 1993;19:144–149

Magnetti S, Behal R. Organizational factors and human factors related to harmful medical event outcomes in 23 academic medical centers using electronic medical error-event reporting systems for targeting patient safety programs. Boston, MA: Academy Health Annual Research Meeting; 2005. Abstract 4205

Mangione-Smith R, DeCristofaro AH, Setodji CM, et al. The quality of ambulatory care delivered to children in the United States. *N Engl J Med.* 2007;357:1515–1523

Measure Type Definition. http://www.health.state.mn.us/healthreform/baskets/measurement090609_definition.pdf. Accessed January 4, 2011

McPhillips HA, Stille CJ, Smith D, et al. Potential medication dosing errors in outpatient pediatrics. *J Pediatr.* 2005;147:761–767

Miles P. Health information systems and physician quality: role of the American Board of Pediatrics maintenance of certification in improving children's health care. *Pediatrics.* 2009;123:S108–S110

Mohr JJ, Lannon CM, Thoma KA, et al. Learning from errors in ambulatory pediatrics. In: Henriksen K, Battles JB, Marks ES, et al, eds. *Advances in Patient Safety: From Research to Implementation.* Washington, DC: Agency for Healthcare Research and Quality; 2005. www.ahrq.gov/downloads/pub/advances/vol1/Mohr.pdf. Accessed November 25, 2010

National Patient Safety Foundation. NPSF patient safety definition. http://www.npsf.org/rc/mp/definitions.php. Accessed December 18, 2010

The Porticus Centre. Western Electric—A Brief History. http://www.porticus.org/bell/westernelectric_history.html#Western%20Electric%20-%20A%20Brief%20History

Reason J. *Human Error.* Cambridge: Cambridge University Press, 1990

Reason J. Human error: models and management. *BMJ.* 2000;320:768–770

Shaughnessy AF, Nickel RO. Prescription-writing patterns and errors in a family medicine residency program. *J Fam Pract.* 1989;29:290–295

Smith D, Bell GD, Kilgo J, et al. *The Carolina Way: Leadership Lessons From a Life in Coaching.* New York, NY: Penguin Press; 2004

Takata GD, Mason W, Taketomo C, et al. Development, testing, and findings of a pediatric-focused trigger tool to identify medication-related harm in US children's hospitals. *Pediatrics.* 2008;121:e9927–e935

Takata G, Currier K. Enhancing patient safety through improved detection of adverse drug events. Presented at: 13th Annual Forum on Quality Improvement in Health Care (Institute for Healthcare Improvement); December 2001; Orlando, FL

Health Maintenance and Anticipatory Guidance

CHAPTER 18

Neonatal Examination and Nursery Visit

Julie E. Noble, MD

CASE STUDY

You are performing a newborn examination on a 16-hour-old infant who was born at 39 weeks' gestation to a 28-year-old healthy primigravida via normal spontaneous vaginal delivery. There were no complications at delivery and Apgar scores were 8 at 1 minute and 9 at 5 minutes. The infant weighed 7 lb, 1 oz (3,200 g) and was 19.7 inches (50 cm) long at birth with a head circumference of 34 cm. The mother received prenatal care beginning at 10 weeks' gestation; had no prenatal problems, including infections; and used no drugs, alcohol, or tobacco during the pregnancy. Her blood type is O positive. She is negative for hepatitis B surface antigen, HIV, and group B streptococcus and nonreactive for syphilis. The father is also healthy.

On physical examination, the infant is average size for gestational age with a length and head circumference in the 50th percentile. Aside from small bilateral subconjunctival hemorrhages, the rest of the physical examination is entirely normal.

Questions

1. What parts of the maternal history are important to review before performing the infant's physical examination?
2. What further history is important for a complete newborn assessment?
3. What aspects of the physical examination of newborns are essential to explain to parents?
4. What physical findings mandate a more extensive workup prior to discharge?
5. What is the routine hospital course for a normal newborn?
6. What are important points to cover with parents at the time of discharge for a normal term newborn?
7. What laboratory studies, if any, should be performed prior to discharge?

The newborn physical examination is an important first encounter with the pediatrician, the infant, the mother, and infant's father, if available, all establishing relationships with each other. The key purpose of this examination is to assess the status of the infant and detect any underlying medical problems. Relaying this information to the parents is essential and answers the question foremost in a parent's mind: "Is the baby normal?" By performing a physical examination in the parents' presence during the infant's first 24 hours of life, pediatricians can play a major role in allaying parental anxiety. More than 90% of newborns are normal, but the pediatrician's role includes identifying medical problems or high-risk conditions in the newborn examination and the history. Evaluation and treatment, if necessary, can be initiated before discharge from the nursery.

Pediatric Prenatal Visit

Ideally, the pediatrician has spoken with the parents at a prenatal visit before meeting them in the hospital. The prenatal meeting provides an opportunity for the parents to interview the physician, as well as the rest of the office staff, regarding general policies and procedures for well-child appointments, sick visits, and contacting the physician after hours. It also is a time to discuss what will take place at the hospital and explain the role of allied health care professionals (eg, lactation specialists) in the overall care of the mother and newborn. For pediatricians and other health care practitioners, the prenatal visit is a time to gather vital medical information regarding the current pregnancy, identifying any high-risk conditions, and to inquire about any problems with previous deliveries. The pediatrician should also review any pertinent family history. In addition, the pediatrician needs to note specific needs of the parents, which may include cultural rituals or ceremonies surrounding the birth of an infant, such as circumcision. Whether the infant is born at a birthing center or in the more traditional hospital setting, arrangements should be made to accommodate the wishes of the family. The prenatal visit also allows physicians to assess any psychosocial issues that may negatively influence initial maternal–infant bonding, such as maternal drug use, no paternal involvement, the absence of a supportive social network, or lack of housing. All of these issues will necessitate social service intervention. The social environment that will surround the infant at home will have a great impact on his future.

This appointment is the ideal time to emphasize the importance of breastfeeding and educate the mother to its many benefits. Anticipatory guidance issues, including positioning the infant on his back to sleep, safe bedding, and child passenger safety, can also be discussed.

Neonatal Nursery Visit

At the time of birth, the infant will receive a screening examination and risk assessment by the nursery personnel when he is stable after any needed resuscitation. If there are no noted abnormalities, the pediatrician is notified of the birth, and the recommendation from the *Guidelines for Perinatal Care* notes that he should evaluate the infant within 24 hours. Meanwhile, in the delivery room, the infant is dried and placed skin to skin on the mother's chest, with a blanket placed over both the mother and infant, to facilitate bonding and early breastfeeding.

If there are perinatal or delivery complications, such as maternal fever, meconium aspiration, asphyxia, prematurity, obvious infant malformations, or distress, the infant should be supported as necessary and kept on a radiant warmer for assessment. The physician should promptly be notified to perform the newborn physical, evaluating the abnormality and initiating treatment.

Evaluation

Perinatal History

The perinatal history is the beginning of the infant's medical history and is very significant to the newborn evaluation. To obtain all of the pertinent history, it may be necessary to review the maternal medical record. Results of maternal laboratory tests, such as blood type; rapid plasma reagin status; purified protein derivative; HIV and hepatitis B status; and chlamydial, gonococcal, and group B streptococcus cultures, should be noted (Questions Box). The pediatrician should also obtain triple screen, prenatal ultrasound, and amniocentesis results if performed. Delivery room events and Apgar scores should also be reviewed before performing the physical examination of the neonate. This review helps the physician focus the examination on findings suggested by the previous medical history. The occurrence of any unusual circumstances surrounding the delivery should be explained to the parents at the time of the examination. They may not have understood the need for a vacuum-assisted delivery or emergent cesarean section. It is important to be prepared to discuss the medical implications of such events.

Physical Examination

Every attempt should be made to perform the neonatal physical examination at the mother's bedside. This gives the physician the opportunity to meet with parents and gives parents a chance to have all of their initial questions answered immediately. In certain circumstances, such as when the infant is premature or when the mother is being treated for a medical complication, an initial bedside

Questions

Neonatal Examination

- Did the mother receive prenatal care? If so, since what month of gestation?
- Were all prenatal studies normal?
- Does either parent have a history of sexually transmitted infections, such as syphilis, gonorrhea, or herpes?
- Does either parent have a history of alcohol, tobacco, or illicit drug use?
- Did the mother take any prescribed or over-the-counter medications routinely during pregnancy?
- Did the mother have any complications, such as bleeding or decreased fetal movement, during pregnancy?
- Were there any indications of a complicated delivery?
- Is there a family history of congenital anomalies or diseases?
- Is the mother planning to breastfeed?
- Does the neonate have any siblings? If so, what are their ages?
- Is anyone available to help with the new baby or siblings?

examination may be impossible to perform. In any event, the physician or other health care provider should speak to parents about the results once the examination has been completed.

The neonatal examination should be performed with the infant completely unclothed and the infant's body temperature maintained. The infant should be assessed for evidence of birth trauma and congenital malformations, and an assessment of normal physiology of organ systems should be done. The infant's birth weight, length, and head circumference should be plotted; physicians should keep in mind that these measurements are often made in the delivery room and may be subject to error. The diagnosis of small for gestational age (weight less than 10th percentile) or large for gestational age (weight greater than 90th percentile) can predispose the infant to several medical problems. Temperature, respiratory rate, and heart rate should be reviewed via the nursery record. Feeding, voiding, and stooling patterns are also available in the nursery record.

The infant evaluation should include an expanded Ballard score, which includes parameters for neuromuscular and physical maturity to accurately estimate gestational age. A late preterm or near term infant, from 35 to 38 weeks' gestation, frequently does not have the physiological maturity to feed vigorously and maintain body weight or heat. These infants are at high risk for readmission for treatment of jaundice, dehydration, and hypoglycemia. They should be followed very closely.

The infant's overall appearance should be noted, particularly for the presence of any dysmorphic features. Physicians should determine whether the infant looks normal or has any abnormal facial features, such as low-set ears and widely spaced eyes (see Chapter 69).

Skin

The presence and location of any rashes or birthmarks should be carefully described and pointed out to the parents. The particular location of the lesion as well as the pathology of the epidermal lesion may aid in its specific diagnosis. Skin lesions from birth trauma must be documented and treated as necessary. Bruising should be differentiated from the benign mongolian spots from dermal hyperpigmentation. Skin color should also be noted: Cyanosis may be indicative of congenital heart disease, the presence of jaundice suggests hyperbilirubinemia, or plethora may be a sign of polycythemia.

Head

Head size and shape, including the size of the fontanelles and the position of the sutures, should be evaluated. The head may be significantly molded into a cone deformity secondary to pelvic pressure at the time of delivery. This resolves within days after birth, and with its resolution there may be a significant change in the head circumference. A cephalohematoma, which is a subperiosteal bleed that does not cross the suture line, appears as a unilateral or bilateral discrete lump on the side of the head. This finding may predispose the infant to hyperbilirubinemia, and resolution may take up to 2 months. A cephalohematoma should be differentiated from a caput succedaneum, which is scalp edema that crosses the midline, and may be ballotable. Edema usually resolves rapidly. Skull fractures may occur with birth trauma and may present as a step-off or crepitus on palpation of the skull. All head findings may be a source of concern to parents.

Eyes

The eyes should be evaluated for subconjunctival hemorrhages, colobomas, extraocular movements, and the presence of red reflexes. If it is not possible to elicit a red reflex, an ophthalmologic evaluation is essential. Its absence suggests conditions such as congenital cataracts or retinoblastomas.

Ears

The placement, size, and shape of the ear pinnae should be noted as well, along with any preauricular or postauricular pits or appendages. The presence of a significant auricular abnormality may correlate with hearing loss or suggest a genetic syndrome.

Nose

The nose should be checked carefully for patency of both nares. This can be easily accomplished by occluding airflow from one nare and observing airflow from the other. Choanal atresia is an important condition to rule out because infants are obligate nose breathers until 3 months of age, and choanal atresia may lead to respiratory distress. A nasal fracture can also occur during the delivery process. This presents as an asymmetrical nose. If the physician presses on the nasal tip and the nares are symmetrical, then the diagnosis is a deformity that will resolve. If the nose falls to one side, there is a probable nasal septum fracture that should be evaluated by an otolaryngologist.

Mouth

The oropharynx should be examined closely for any defects in the hard or soft palate. A bifid uvula may indicate a submucosal defect of the soft palate that may be difficult to appreciate without palpation (see Chapter 70). Common normal findings in the oropharynx, including Epstein pearls located at the midline on the hard palate and epithelial cysts along the gum line, should also be noted. Loose natal teeth should be removed to prevent the possibility of aspiration (see Chapter 71). The tongue should be evaluated for macroglossia or a tight lingual frenulum, which may interfere with effective breastfeeding.

Chest

The neck should be palpated for sternocleidomastoid hematomas and the clavicles for fractures, which are more common in infants who are large for gestational age (LGA) or a delivery complicated by shoulder dystocia. The chest should be inspected for respiratory effort and lungs auscultated to ensure normal breath sounds throughout. The quality of the infant's cry should be assessed. Laryngeal webs or a paralyzed vocal cord may present in the newborn. Chest wall deformities, such as pectus excavatum, should be noted. If an absent rib is suspected, a radiograph is needed. The presence of breast buds is normal, but supernumerary nipples are minor malformations, although no treatment is indicated. Widely spaced nipples are a common minor malformation in patients with Turner syndrome.

Heart

The heart should be auscultated to ensure that it is in the proper position on the left side of the chest. Cardiac murmurs should be appreciated and documented. The presence of a murmur does not always indicate complex congenital heart disease. In the first 24 hours, a murmur may be a closing ductus, and newborns can also have functional murmurs. Peripheral pulmonic stenosis is a common benign heart murmur in the newborn that is characterized by transmission to the back. Every murmur should be evaluated on an individual basis. If assessment is indicated, 4 extremity blood pressures, a pulse oximetry reading, an electrocardiogram (ECG), and a chest radiograph should be obtained. If there are abnormal findings or the murmur is associated with cyanosis, tachypnea, poor feeding, or congenital anomalies there is high suspicion of a pathologic cause. A consult from specialists in pediatric cardiology should be sought and an echocardiogram obtained.

Abdomen

The abdomen is easiest to palpate prior to feeds. It should be assessed for any masses or organomegaly (eg, polycystic kidneys, hepatosplenomegaly, adrenal hemorrhage) that warrant further investigation. Bimanual palpation may be helpful to identify masses. The umbilicus should be examined to identify 3 vessels as well as the quality of the cord. A small, atretic cord can explain a low weight in the infant. Erythema and swelling of the skin around the cord may indicate oomphalitis, a serious infection.

Genitalia

In female neonates, the labia majora may be swollen, but the urethra and vaginal opening should be visualized to ensure patency. It is not uncommon to see hymenal tags. Clitoral size should be noted. Parents should be told that a physiological vaginal discharge and the presence later of a pink or blood-tinged discharge are a normal neonatal response to maternal estrogen withdrawal. In male infants, the penis should be examined for size and length. The foreskin should be retracted sufficiently to reveal the location of the urethral meatus to assess for hypospadius. A testicular examination can rule out hydroceles, inguinal hernias, and cryptorchidism.

Skeleton

The infant skeleton should be assessed for evidence of a skeletal dysplasia. All long bones should be examined for a potential fracture secondary to birth trauma. The infant hip examination is important to detect developmental dysplasia of the hip, seen more commonly after a breech position in utero. The Ortolani test is performed to detect a dislocated hip. The "clunk" felt when performing the examination is the relocation of the femoral head of the affected hip in the joint capsule. In contrast, a "click" may indicate normal perinatal ligament laxity. The Barlow test detects an unstable dislocatable hip. If either test is positive, it is diagnostic for a dislocated or dislocatable hip and warrants an orthopedic consultation. Treatment with a Pavlik harness is initiated until confirmatory testing by an ultrasound is reliable at 6 weeks of age. The spine should be palpated completely to the sacrum. Sacral defects, deep sacral pits, or sacral tufts of hair warrant an investigation for such conditions as spina bifida occulta. Fingers and toes should be counted and assessed for syndactyly. The feet may be turned inward, outward, or up and should be gently moved to a normal position to ensure flexibility. Deformities secondary to intrauterine pressure are common. Clubfoot or equinovarus deformations should receive orthopedic evaluation.

Neurologic Examination

An infant's resting position should be assessed to evaluate tone. All extremities should be flexed. The infant then can be held prone under the shoulder girdle for further evaluation of tone, and extremities should continue flexed. Infants should be observed for motor activity, moving arms and legs symmetrically. Response to sensory stimulation and deep tendon reflexes should be elicited. Facial movements should be closely observed for symmetry. Primitive reflexes, such as suck, rooting, grasp, stepping and, especially, Moro, are an important part of the newborn neurologic examination. The behavior of the infant can also yield information regarding an intact neurologic system. He should respond to sound, fixate on a face, and be capable of attempts at self-consolation.

Normal findings of the nursery physical examination are summarized in Box 18-1. Significant findings that must be addressed immediately when noted at the initial nursery examination include evidence of hydrocephalus, a ductal-dependent cardiac lesion, a diaphragmatic hernia, an abdominal mass, or a possible chromosomal abnormality such as trisomy 13 or trisomy 18, which can all

be life-threatening. The physical conditions associated with trisomy 21 are rarely life-threatening, although suspicion of the diagnosis does warrant a genetics consultation and evaluation for cardiac and abdominal anomalies (see Chapter 37).

Laboratory Tests

Few laboratory tests are needed for the normal newborn. The only test that all US newborns receive is the state mandated newborn screening test prior to discharge from the nursery (see Chapter 20). Heel stick blood usually is evaluated for inheritable conditions, such as phenylketonuria, galactosemia, hypothyroidism, hemoglobinopathies, cystic fibrosis, congenital adrenal hyperplasia, and a panel assessing inborn errors of metabolism. The newborn screen varies by state and depends on the prevalence of a particular disease in a given region (see Chapter 20), but there is a federal effort to standardize testing. In all states, hearing screening is also part of the mandated newborn screening. Screening methods may be by automated auditory brain stem response, otoacoustic emission testing, or conventional auditory brain stem response.

Box 18-1. Common Benign Physical Findings in Newborns

Skin
Milia, erythema toxicum, salmon patch, nevus flammeus, hemangiomas, mongolian spots, lanugo (body hair)

Head
Cephalohematoma, caput succedaneum

Face
Swollen overall appearance, minor malformations

Eyes
Swollen eyelids, subconjunctival hemorrhages

Ears
Preauricular appendages/pits, folded pinnae

Nose
Flattened nose, milia over bridge

Mouth and Throat
Epstein pearls, epithelial pearls, natal teeth, shortened frenulum

Chest
Supernumerary nipples, breast buds, galactorrhea, pectus excavatum or carinatum

Genitalia
Females: swollen labia, hymenal tags, vaginal discharge
Males: hydrocele, undescended testicle (palpated in inguinal canal)

Hips
Click

Extremities
Feet turned up, in, or out, but malleable

Neurologic Examination
Primitive reflexes: Moro, grasp, rooting, stepping

Other laboratory tests that are often performed in a newborn include a serum glucose in infants at high risk for hypoglycemia (which includes infants who are small for gestational age or LGA, infants of diabetic mothers, and infants who are symptomatic). A hematocrit is necessary in jaundiced, pale, or ruddy-appearing newborns and in twins. In cases of ABO or Rh incompatibility, a serum bilirubin and a Coombs test are important to obtain. Screening for hyperbilirubinemia to prevent kernicterus is recommended for all newborns, but recent evaluations of this testing have not demonstrated efficacy. Bilirubin screening can be done easily by a transcutaneous reading followed by a serum level if the transcutaneous reading is elevated (see Chapter 113).

Imaging Studies

Routine radiographs are not indicated in neonates whose examination is normal and should be ordered only if indicated by the examination. Some minor malformations, such as pectus excavatum, do not need radiographs. Vertebral radiographs or ultrasound of the lumbosacral spine is appropriate in the neonate with a deep sacral pit or sacral tuft of hair for the diagnosis of spina bifida occulta. Clavicular radiographs are indicated if swelling or pain is located in the clavicular area or if an asymmetrical Moro reflex is elicited. A chest radiograph and ECG are warranted for a significant murmur. If multiple anomalies are found, a renal ultrasound looking for malformations of the kidneys should be performed. More extensive studies are indicated if an emergent physical finding is discovered.

Management

After stabilization in the delivery room, the infant should be thoroughly dried and given to the mother for breastfeeding and bonding. If mother and baby are healthy, the infant should stay with the mother, receiving an initial bath when the temperature is stable. The administration of intramuscular vitamin K to prevent hemorrhagic disease of the newborn and the application of ophthalmic ointment or silver nitrate in the newborn's eyes to prevent gonorrheal infection is universal. Hepatitis B vaccine is recommended for all infants at birth regardless of mother's serology. Every hospital should encourage rooming-in of the infant with the mother. The infant should feed within 2 hours of birth and continue to feed every 2 to 3 hours to prevent hypoglycemia. The preferred method is breastfeeding, and the mother should receive sufficient postpartum support to ensure success (see Chapter 24). Vital signs should be monitored every 30 minutes until stable during the transition to extrauterine life, then every 4 hours. Daily weights as well as strict documentation of voiding and stooling are necessary to monitor the infant for adequacy of intake and for dehydration. Umbilical cord care remains an area of controversy, and it appears that leaving the cord to dry is a sufficient treatment.

If desired, the circumcision is usually performed on the day of discharge (see Chapter 22). Local anesthesia is now universally recommended for the procedure. Following the procedure, the parents are instructed to leave the gauze or Plastibell in place. It will fall off spontaneously. Petroleum ointment may also be placed on the corona of the penis to prevent its sticking to the diaper. The physician should be notified if excessive bleeding or oozing occurs (eg, soaking of the diaper with blood) after discharge from the nursery.

Discharge Planning and Counseling

In most cases, mother and infant should be discharged home together. The general hospital stay is 48 hours for a vaginal delivery and 96 hours for a cesarean delivery. The physician should examine the infant again within 24 hours of discharge to identify problems that might have developed as well as counsel the mother. Again this examination is best performed at bedside. The infant's physical findings and hospital course should be reviewed with the mother and father. If studies other than routine neonatal screening were performed, the parents should also be informed of the results.

Discharge is the best time to review anticipatory guidance issues. Topics that should be covered at the bedside include feeding patterns and what to expect, sleeping and elimination patterns in the newborn, umbilical cord care, bathing the newborn, and safety issues such as car safety seats and sleeping position. Guidelines regarding symptoms of illness and when to call the office or emergency department should also be addressed. These include a rectal fever of 100.4°F (38.0°C) or greater, respiratory distress, irritability, lethargy, decreased feeding, and evidence of dehydration. If parents have any concerns about their infant, they should be encouraged to call the physician's office. A follow-up visit should be arranged at day 3 to 5 of life for any breastfeeding infant, to give breastfeeding support as well as to assess the infant for evidence of jaundice or dehydration. An early follow-up appointment may also be indicated in an infant with social risk factors and near term infants who are at higher risk for complications. If the infant is delivered by cesarean section or is formula feeding, a follow-up visit at 1 to 3 weeks after discharge is appropriate.

Early newborn discharge is an option if desired by the mother. There are published recommendations from the American Academy of Pediatrics for guidance regarding discharge at younger than 48 hours of age. Generally the history, including social risk factors, physical, and hospital course, should all be low risk and the infant should have been observed for at least 12 hours. If the newborn is stable and sent home at less than 48 hours, a mandatory follow-up appointment should be scheduled in 2 days.

CASE RESOLUTION

In the case presented at the beginning of the chapter, the parents should be told that the weight, length, and head circumference are all normal. The examination is reviewed at bedside and the subconjunctival hemorrhages should be shown to the parents and their benign self-limited nature explained. The infant's blood type from cord blood should be obtained since the mother is O⁺. Routine neonatal screening, feeding, sleeping, elimination, bathing, and safety should be reviewed. Prior to discharge, the infant should receive the hepatitis B vaccine and newborn screening tests. A follow-up appointment should be made in 48 hours after discharge to follow breastfeeding progress.

Selected References

American Academy of Pediatrics Committee on Fetus and Newborn. Controversies concerning vitamin K and the newborn. *Pediatrics.* 2003;112:191–192

American Academy of Pediatrics Committee on Fetus and Newborn. Hospital stay for healthy term newborns. *Pediatrics.* 2010;125:405–409

American Academy of Pediatrics, The American College of Obstetricians and Gynecologists. *Guidelines for Perinatal Care.* 6th ed. Washington, DC: American College of Obstetricians and Gynecologists; 2007

Cohen GJ; American Academy of Pediatrics Committee on Psychosocial Aspects of Child and Family Health. Clinical report: the prenatal visit. *Pediatrics.* 2009;124:1227–1232

Coloherty J, Eichenwald E, Stark A, eds. *Manual of Neonatal Care.* 6th ed. Philadelphia, PA: Lippincott Williams & Wilkins; 2008

Fernoff PM. Newborn screening for genetic disorders. *Pediatr Clin North Am.* 2009;56:505–513

Maisels MJ, Bhutani VK, Bogen D, Newman TB, Stark AR, Watchko JF. Hyperbilirubinemia in the newborn infant ≥35 weeks' gestation: an update with clarifications. *Pediatrics.* 2009;124:1193–1198

Rademacher R, Kliegman R, eds. Common issues and concerns in the newborn nursery, part II. *Pediatr Clin North Am.* 2004;51(4):xv–xvi

Ramachandrappa A, Jain L. Health issues of the late preterm infant. *Pediatr Clin North Am.* 2009;56:565–577

Sayers SM. Indigenous newborn care. *Pediatr Clin North Am.* 2009;56:1243–1261

Stellwagen L, Boies E. Care of the well newborn. *Pediatr Rev.* 2006;27:89–98

US Preventive Services Task Force. Screening for hyperbilirubinemia to prevent chronic bilirubin encephalopathy. *Pediatrics.* 2009;124:1172–1192

Wagner CL, Greer FR. Prevention of rickets and vitamin D deficiency in infants, children, and adolescents. *Pediatrics.* 2008;122:1142–1152

CHAPTER 19

Peripartum Depression: The Role of the Pediatrician

Carol D. Berkowitz, MD

CASE STUDY

You are evaluating a 3-week-old infant who is the product of a 39-week gestation to a 30-year-old gravida I para I mother who has been breastfeeding the infant. The birth weight was 3,650 g, and the baby now weighs 3,380 g. The mother expresses concern about her ability to breastfeed. She also admits to being exhausted and feeling detached from the baby and overwhelmed by being a mom, something she had looked forward to since she was a little girl. She has difficulty concentrating and has no appetite. She asks you if it is normal to feel this way.

Questions

1. What are the signs and symptoms of peripartum depression?
2. What are the risks to infants of mothers who experience peripartum depression and other mood disorders?
3. What is the role of the pediatrician in assessing mothers for peripartum depression?
4. What screening instruments are available to assist in assessing mothers for peripartum depression?
5. What resources are available to offer to mothers who may be experiencing peripartum mood disorders?

Peripartum depression is the term used to encompass a cadre of mental health problems that mothers may experience either during pregnancy or following the birth of a baby. Despite public disclosures and open discussions by celebrities such as Brook Shields and Gwyneth Paltrow, the condition is under-recognized, and many mothers go undiagnosed and untreated. The pediatrician is in an ideal position to assess a mother for the presence of these symptoms following the birth of a baby since the pediatrician usually sees the mother–infant dyad prior to the obstetrical postpartum visit at 6 weeks following the baby's birth. The recommended time points for screening for postpartum depression coincide with well-baby checks: 2 weeks, 2 months, and 6 months. In addition, women are likely to follow up with their child's physician appointments more than their own. While fatigue is a common complaint of new mothers as well as new fathers, other symptoms, particularly those of impaired functioning and diminished ability to care for the infant, may suggest a more significant disturbance.

Epidemiology

The incidence of peripartum depression varies with the population studied, with the estimated range being from 5% to 25%. Between 14% and 23% of pregnant women experience depressive symptoms while pregnant, and approximately 13% of women take an antidepressant at some time during their pregnancy. The prevalence is felt to be much higher at 40% to 60% in certain groups, including low income women, certain ethnic minorities (including Latina and African American), pregnant and parenting teenagers, mothers of multiple births, and women who served in the military in Iraq and Afghanistan. The World Health Organization notes that depression is the fourth leading cause of disease burden in the world. In spite of the high prevalence across all groups, fewer than 50% of cases of maternal depression are identified.

Often there is reluctance on the part of obstetricians or psychiatrists to treat pregnant women with antidepressants because of concerns about the potential effects of the medications on the developing fetus. These effects include fetal malformations, cardiac defects, pulmonary hypertension, and reduced birth weight. However, untreated depression and anxiety in pregnancy also increase the risk of preterm delivery, low birth weight, and infants' own ability to regulate emotions and stress. The American College of Obstetricians and Gynecologists and the American Psychiatric Association have issued joint guidelines on the management of pregnant women with depression, which discuss the indications for psychotherapy as well as psychopharmacology in the pregnant woman. Pediatricians are usually not involved in this part of the decision-making process but should be knowledgeable about the possible complications that the infant may experience following birth from either exposure to antidepressants or to untreated maternal mental illness. Approximately 6% to 10% of fathers experience peripartum depression, with the highest rates seen between 3 and 6 months following the birth of the baby. Paternal rates of depression are higher when there is maternal depression, and the impact on the infant is greater than if the father is not affected. Depressed fathers have a higher rate of substance abuse.

There is a wide range of symptomatology that can be categorized under peripartum mood disorders (Box 19-1). **Baby blues** or **maternity blues** is used to describe the very common experience of new mothers, said to affect 50% to 80% of postpartum women in the first few days after delivery. There is no *Diagnostic and Statistical Manual of Mental Disorders, Fourth Edition Text Revision (DSM–IV-TR)* categorization of "baby blues." Generally symptoms improve over 1 to 2 weeks, and functioning is not impaired, though "baby blues" may herald later depression. Mothers experience sadness, crying, mood swings, anxiety, and worrying.

A diagnosis of **postpartum depression** meets the criteria of depression according to *DSM–IV*, which include a depressed mood, diminished pleasure (anhedonia), changes in appetite and sleep, psychomotor agitation or retardation, fatigue, feelings of worthlessness or inappropriate guilt, decreased ability to concentrate, and recurrent thoughts of death or suicide. Suicide is the leading cause of death in mothers during the first year postpartum. Technically, symptoms of depression must begin within 4 weeks of delivery and may persist

for 1 year, though the onset is often insidious and doesn't come to attention until much later than a month postpartum.

Postpartum psychosis is less frequent, occurring in 1 to 3 per 1,000 deliveries also within the first 4 weeks after delivery. There is severe impairment, with paranoia, mood shifts, hallucinations, delusions, and suicidal and homicidal ideation. Sometimes there is a history of a preexisting bipolar disorder. Affected mothers require hospitalization, in part because the infanticide rate is 4% to 5%.

It is estimated that 400,000 infants are born to mothers who are depressed. These infants are at risk for a host of adverse physical and developmental consequences.

Pathophysiology

The precise pathophysiology of maternal depression has not been elucidated, but sleep deprivation related to the demands of caring for a new infant and hormonal changes are felt to be contributing factors. While there are rapid decreases in the levels of estrogen, progesterone, and cortisol, the changes noted in mothers who experience peripartum depression do not differ from women who do not experience peripartum depression. Perhaps more significantly, there are a number of risk factors that have been associated with its development. These include prior history of depression in general, but especially during a previous pregnancy; mood disorders, including premenstrual dysphoric disorder; substance abuse; alcohol dependence; low socioeconomic status; lack of social support or community network; unintended or unwanted pregnancy; or a family history of depression. Other social/familial factors include marital discord, divorce, and violence.

Evaluation

Mother

Screening for peripartum mood disorders is felt to be within the scope of the pediatric practice. Studies have shown that mothers are comfortable being queried by pediatricians about how they are doing. Some pediatricians express concern about the appropriate strategies for screening and what to do if they determine that a mother has symptoms of depression.

It is important to couch any depression screening in language that makes a new mother feel comfortable and not judged in any way. Postpartum Support International has developed the "Universal Message" to share with depressed new mothers: (1) You are not crazy; (2) you are not alone; and (3) with the right help, you will get better.

There are several instruments that help screen for postpartum depression. A simple tool, called the Parent Health Questionnaire-2, consists of 2 questions. The questionnaire begins with a background statement related to depression as a common and treatable condition that often goes unrecognized. There follows justification citing the recommendation of the US Preventive Services Task Force that all adults be checked for depression. The questions then are as follows: Over the past 2 weeks, you have felt down, depressed, or hopeless (true or false). Over the past 2 weeks, you have felt little interest or

---

Box 19-1. Peripartum Mood Disorders Symptomatology

"Baby Blues"
- Sadness
- Crying
- Mood swings
- Anxiety
- Worrying
- First few days after delivery
- Resolves in 1–2 weeks

Postpartum Depression
- Meets *Diagnostic and Statistical Manual of Mental Disorders, Fourth Edition* criteria for depression
- Depressed mood
- Diminished pleasure
- Change in appetite
- Change in sleep
- Fatigue
- Feelings of worthlessness or guilt
- Inability to concentrate
- Recurrent thoughts of death or suicide

Postpartum Psychosis
- Severe impairment
- Paranoia
- Mood shifts
- Hallucinations
- Delusions
- Suicidal/homicidal ideation
- Usually requires hospitalization

pleasure doing things (true or false). If true, have you felt this way for (several days, more than half the days, or nearly every day)? If either of these questions is positive, a more extensive assessment is indicated to make the diagnosis of depression.

A second instrument is the Edinburgh Postnatal Depression Scale (EPDS). A sample question from the scale is given in Box 19-2. The scale was developed in 1987 and consists of 10 questions completed by the mother. The mother is asked to check the response that comes the closest to how she has been feeling in the previous 7 days, with there being 4 choices ranging from "often" to "never." All items must be completed, and the mother must respond by herself, without the assistance of another unless she has limited English skills. The maximum score is 30. A score greater than 10 indicates risk for depression. A positive response to question 10, which asks about suicidality by itself, is considered a positive screen. The instrument is available in more than 40 languages.

Infants and Children

Infants and children may experience a number of problems as a consequence of maternal depression. These children may develop disorders of attachment, particularly insecure attachment, and they are at risk for the subsequent development of conduct or other behavior disorders. Language development may be adversely affected since depressed mothers speak fewer words and have fewer social interactions with their children. Maternal depression has also been associated with the decision not to breastfeed or the early cessation of breastfeeding. Classic environmental failure to thrive can be related to maternal depression and reduced mother–infant interactions. The effects of maternal depression can be detected in 2-month-old infants who regard depressed mothers less frequently, have poorer state regulation, interact with objects less frequently, and have lower levels of overall activity than infants of nondepressed mothers. Long-term effects of maternal depression on child development have been demonstrated in the magnetic resonance imaging of the brain of such children and increased cortisol level at the time of school entry. Children are characterized as anxious, wary, and withdrawn. Social skills are noted to be poor. Early diagnosis and intervention may prevent the development of these problems.

Management

The major role of the pediatrician is to assist in the early identification of mothers who are experiencing peripartum depression and to make the appropriate referral for more definitive management. Support for this recommendation comes from a number of sources, including the 1999 and 2000 Report of the Surgeon General, *Bright Futures*, the American Academy of Pediatrics (AAP) Medical Home Initiative, and AAP policy statement on family-centered care. Practices that include the presence of social workers or mental health specialists can avail themselves of these individuals to assess, counsel, and refer these mothers as appropriate. The mother may be referred back to her obstetrician for a visit prior to the 6-week checkup. Alternatively, mothers may be referred to local mental health specialists when such resources are known and available.

Box 19-2. Sample Question From Edinburgh Postnatal Depression Scale[a]

As you are pregnant, or have recently had a baby, we would like to know how you are feeling. Please check the answer that comes closest to how you have felt IN THE PAST 7 DAYS, not just how you feel today.

Here is an example, already completed.

I have felt happy:

☐ Yes, all of the time

☒ Yes, most of the time

☐ No, not very often

☐ No, not at all

This would mean: "I have felt happy most of the time" during the past week. The other questions should be completed this way.

[a] Modified with permission from Cox JL, Holden JM, Sagovsky R. Detection of postnatal depression: development of the 10-item Edinburgh Postnatal Depression Scale. *Br J Psychiatry.* 1987;150:782–786.

There are a number of Internet sites that are very helpful in providing information about community resources. Postpartum Support International (www.postpartum.net and 800/944-4PPD) provides geographically specific information. The site can be accessed even while the mother is in the pediatrician's office. To get the needed information, one goes to the site, clicks on get help, clicks on the map for one's specific location, clicks on e-mail for region, and one will get a reply within 24 hours. It is also important to have an "emergency protocol" in place, such as calling 911 or a psychiatric emergency team, should the woman endorse suicidality while in the pediatrician's office. Having such resources and protocols in place can go a long way toward reducing pediatricians' anxiety about screening for depression and suicidality.

Some perinatal programs offer home visitation or the use of doulas (women who support other women through labor, delivery, and after the birth of an infant in a nonmedical capacity), which assist mothers-to-be as well as recent mothers with the demands of birth and parenting. Such programs may offer a preventive and early intervention approach to peripartum depression by offering help and emotional support to the new mother.

When older children have been affected by maternal depression, there are other treatment modalities that focus on both the mother and the child to help address attachment disorders. Research on these dyadic interventions has demonstrated they are associated with decreased psychiatric symptoms and significant improvement in functioning of both the mother and the child. Both internalizing and externalizing child behaviors are reduced when maternal depression is addressed. Some programs include parent–child interactive therapy and parent–child psychotherapy. A program called Circle of Security involves video-based intervention that focuses on strengthening caretaker giving.

Prognosis

The prognosis for peripartum depression and its effects on infants and children is contingent on early recognition and appropriate intervention. Promoting screening is critical to ensuring a positive outcome. Unfortunately, pediatricians still face barriers, which include the need to screen for a number of other conditions (eg, parental smoking, interpersonal violence), insufficient time, inadequate training, lack of appropriate resources, and lack of reimbursement. A number of models have demonstrated that screening for peripartum depression can be successfully undertaken in a pediatric practice. The Assuring Better Child Health and Development Project has been implemented in 28 states and involves the AAP chapters in those states. Pediatricians in Illinois can be paid through Medicaid if they administer the EPDS. *Bright Futures,* the health maintenance guidelines developed by the AAP and Health Resources and Services Administration, endorse assessing parental social and emotional well-being. Incorporating questioning into the well-child visits at 1-, 2-, 4-, and 6-month visits is recommended and can be billed for using the *Current Procedural Terminology* code 99420. Additional information about individual state initiatives can be found at www.abcdresources.org and www.nashp.org (National Academy for State Health Policy).

CASE RESOLUTION

While many of this mother's symptoms are common, her self-assessment that she is unable to function suggests that she is experiencing postpartum depression rather than "baby blues." You ask her if it is all right to contact her obstetrician to see if she could be seen sooner. She agrees. When you reach her obstetrician, she schedules the mom to come in the following morning. The obstetrician tells you she has a therapist in her office who will be able to meet with the mother at that time.

Selected References

Choi Y, Bishai D, Minkovitz CS. Multiple births are a risk factor for postpartum maternal depressive symptoms. *Pediatrics.* 2009;123:1147–1154

Earls MF; American Academy of Pediatrics Committee on Psychosocial Aspects of Child and Family Health. Clinical report: incorporating recognition and management of perinatal and postpartum depression into pediatric practice. *Pediatrics.* 2010;126:1032–1039

Mattocks KM, Skanderson M, Goulet JL, et al. Pregnancy and mental health among women veterans returning from Iraq and Afghanistan. *J Womens Health (Larchmt).* 2010;19:2159–2166

Olson l, Dietrich AJ, Prazar G, Hurley J. Brief maternal depression screening at well-child visits. *Pediatrics.* 2006;118:207–216

Yonkers KA, Wisner KL, Stewart DE, et al. The management of depression during pregnancy: a report from the American Psychiatric Association and the American College of Obstetricians and Gynecologists. *Obstet Gynecol.* 2009;114:703–713

CHAPTER 20

Newborn Screening

Derek Wong, MD

CASE STUDY

A 1-week-old male infant is brought to his pediatrician's office for a positive newborn screening test for congenital adrenal hyperplasia. The baby was a product of a 38-week gestation and was born by normal spontaneous vaginal delivery to a 30-year-old gravida II para II woman with an unremarkable pregnancy. Birth weight was 3,300 g, and the baby is feeding and acting appropriately. Family history is unremarkable, and the physical examination is normal.

Questions

1. What are the proposed benefits of newborn screening?
2. Which newborn screening tests are most commonly performed?
3. How are the results of newborn screening tests reported to physicians?
4. How should a patient with an abnormal newborn screening result be managed?
5. What are the most common causes of false-positive and false-negative results?
6. What are the ethical issues and future challenges surrounding newborn screening?

Newborn screening programs are designed to identify infants at risk for catastrophic outcomes from treatable illnesses. During the past 40 years, technological advances such as tandem mass spectrometry have made it possible to test for more than 50 metabolic disorders from a single blood spot. New techniques in molecular biology allow for rapid diagnostic testing of conditions such as cystic fibrosis.

From the inception of newborn screening in the 1960s until 2005, each state chose a different set of conditions for their newborn screening programs based on disease prevalence, cost, availability of treatment, and false-positive rate. Recently, the American Academy of Pediatrics (AAP) and other agencies produced a series of articles that outlined a strategy to move toward a uniform national newborn screening panel. In 2005 an expert panel from the American College of Medical Genetics recommended 29 core disorders for which newborn screening was most effective (Table 20-1), as well as 25 secondary disorders that are in the differential diagnosis of a core disorder. In 2010, severe combined immune deficiency (SCID) was added to the list of core disorders. By the end of 2010, all states offered testing for the 29 original core disorders, although screening for secondary disorders and SCID was variable. Most infants born in Europe, Japan, and Australia undergo similar screening, and other nations are actively exploring similar technologies.

Primary care physicians have 3 crucial roles in the newborn screening process. First, they provide education to parents about the newborn screening process. Second, they ensure that specimens are drawn under proper circumstances and that the results are promptly followed up. Finally, they provide medical follow-up and referral in positive cases. Providers need to have contact information for state newborn screening programs and local pediatric subspecialists. The following Web sites link to contact information for these groups:

1. State newborn screening programs—http://genes-r-us. uthscsa.edu/
2. Geneticists, metabolic and clinical—The Society for Inherited Metabolic Disorders (www.simd.org) and The American College of Medical Genetics (www.acmg.net)
3. Pediatric endocrinologists—The Lawson Wilkins Pediatric Endocrine Society (www.lwpes.org)
4. Pediatric hematologists—The American Society of Pediatric Hematology/Oncology (www.aspho.org)
5. Pediatric pulmonologists—The Cystic Fibrosis Foundation (www.cff.org) (under "Care Center Network")

Epidemiology

More than 4 million infants are screened each year in the United States. The National Newborn Screening 2006 Incidence Report shows that as a result of newborn screening, 1 in 3,200 newborns were diagnosed with a metabolic disorder, 1 in 2,200 were diagnosed with congenital hypothyroidism, 1 in 2,200 were diagnosed with sickle cell disease or a related hemoglobinopathy, and 1 in 29,000 infants were diagnosed with congenital adrenal hyperplasia. Several disorders are more common in particular ethnic groups: Cystic fibrosis has an incidence of 1 in 2,500 in whites, and sickle cell disease has an incidence of 1 in 400 in African Americans.

Table 20-1. Core Newborn Screening Disorders[a]	
Disorder	*Possible Signs and Symptoms in Neonates[b]*
Organic Acid Disorders	
Glutaric aciduria type I	Macrocephaly
Biotinidase deficiency	
Multiple carboxylase deficiency	
HMG-CoA lyase deficiency	Vomiting, lethargy, tachypnea
Cobalamin A,B deficiency	Seizures, coma, anion gap acidosis
Isovaleric aciduria	Hyperammonemia
Methylmalonic acidemia	Anemia, neutropenia, thrombocytopenia
Propionic acidemia	
3-methylcrotonyl-CoA carboxylase deficiency	
β-ketothiolase deficiency	Asymptomatic[c]
Fatty Acid Oxidation Disorders	
Medium-chain acyl-CoA dehydrogenase deficiency	Lethargy, coma, sudden death, hypoketotic hypoglycemia
	Reye-like syndrome
Very long-chain acyl-CoA dehydrogenase deficiency	Lethargy, coma, sudden death, hypoketotic hypoglycemia
Long-chain L-3-OH acyl-CoA dehydrogenase deficiency	Cardiomyopathy, arrhythmias
Trifunctional protein deficiency	Cholestasis, Reye-like syndrome
Carnitine uptake defect	Asymptomatic[c]
Amino Acid Disorders	
Maple syrup urine disease	Poor feeding, vomiting, lethargy, seizures, coma, maple syrup odor
Citrullinemia	Hyperammonemia, vomiting, seizures, lethargy, coma
Argininosuccinic aciduria	
Tyrosinemia type I	Hepatomegaly, increased PT/PTT, liver failure, boiled cabbage odor
Homocystinuria	Asymptomatic[c]
Phenylketonuria	Asymptomatic
Hemoglobinopathies	
Sickle cell disease (Hb SS)	Dactylitis
Sickle β-thalassemia	Asymptomatic[c]
Hemoglobin C sickle cell disease	
Other	
Congenital hypothyroidism	Umbilical hernia, enlarged fontanelle, macroglossia, jaundice
Congenital adrenal hypertrophy	Virilization in females; salt wasting crisis
Galactosemia	Cataracts, jaundice, poor feeding, sepsis
Cystic fibrosis	Meconium ileus, intestinal obstruction
Severe combined immune deficiency	Recurrent infections

Abbreviations: HMG, 3-hydroxy-3-methylglutaryl; CoA, coenzyme A; PT, prothrombin time; PTT, partial thromboplastin time.

[a] Most of these conditions may not be asymptomatic outside of the neonatal period.

[b] Many neonates with these disorders are completely asymptomatic.

[c] "Asymptomatic" covers the first month of life and does not exclude very rare case reports of neonatal presentation.

Clinical Presentation

Most infants with disorders detected by newborn screening are clinically asymptomatic in the first 2 weeks of life, but the remainder may have significant signs and symptoms (see Table 20-1). The presence of such features may lead to a more urgent workup and/or hospitalization. Unfortunately, severe forms of some metabolic disorders may cause coma and encephalopathy by 48 hours of age. In these cases, the newborn screening results are critical, for they will suggest a probable diagnosis and will allow early optimization of therapy.

Differential Diagnosis

While newborn screening techniques are continually improved, both false-positive and false-negative errors occur. Mislabeled specimens, technical errors, and reporting errors can occur in any laboratory. Any specimen collected before 12 hours of age is at risk for a false-negative metabolic result or a false-positive hypothyroidism result. Premature infants have a reduced metabolic capacity and therefore exhibit higher metabolite levels and increased false-positive results compared with term infants. Anemia or polycythemia can affect the amount of serum per blood spot and increase false-negative results, and transfusion may alter galactosemia and hemoglobinopathy testing. Infants on hyperalimentation may have increased amino acid and lipid levels, especially if the newborn screen is drawn from a central line. To ensure accurate and uniform testing, it is imperative to communicate relevant clinical information to the state newborn screening office.

Newborn Screening Practices

Parental Education and Consent

All parents should therefore be informed of the state screening program either at the prenatal visit or during the initial newborn examination. Written materials that explain the screening program are available from the state screening office, and online materials explaining abnormal results are available on fact sheets at Web sites such as http://pediatrics.aappublications.org/cgi/content/full/118/3/e934. Health care providers are responsible for educating parents regarding the method for obtaining the blood specimen, the risks and benefits of the screening tests, the conditions to be screened, and the implications of positive results.

It is important to tell parents that positive results do not necessarily mean that their infant has a particular disorder; the results must be confirmed by more specific tests. In addition, parents should know that disorders in some children are missed either because of sampling errors, faulty testing, or inadequate accumulation of the abnormal metabolite at the time of testing.

Newborn screening is mandatory in all states, although many states allow exemptions for religious beliefs or other reasons. In most states, parents have given informed consent if practitioners have discussed the state-mandated program with them and they have agreed to participate. A few states require signed consent to opt into the newborn screening program, and several more require consent to disclose identifiable information. Providers should document parental refusal regardless of state laws.

Specimen Collection and Handling

Proper specimen collection and handling are essential components of a successful screening program. All newborns should be screened before discharge from the hospital, ideally between 48 to 96 hours of age. Early screening increases the chance of a false-negative metabolic result or a false-positive hypothyroidism result. For this reason,

some states have a mandatory second screen between 1 and 6 weeks of age, while others require a second screen only if the first screen is obtained before a specified time (12–48 hours depending on the state). Late screening increases the sensitivity of metabolic testing, but also increases the chances for a delay in diagnosis of life-threatening conditions such as galactosemia. If possible, blood samples should be obtained prior to any transfusions or dialysis. Otherwise, screening tests should still be performed as outlined previously, and arrangements should be made to have them repeated at an appropriate time. It is likely that guidelines that recommend screening premature and/or sick newborns at birth, 48 to 72 hours, and 28 days/discharge will be considered for implementation into state newborn screening programs in the near future.

Only a few drops of blood are needed for each disk on the filter paper, but the sample must saturate the paper evenly. The use of needles and glass capillary tubes for blood collection is discouraged because they may cause hemolysis or microtears in the filter paper. The specimens must be individually air-dried in a horizontal position, thus avoiding contamination and excessive exposure to heat. They should be mailed to the laboratory within 24 hours of collection. Inadequate specimen collection and handling can lead to test inaccuracies, delays in reporting results to physicians, and unnecessary repetition of screening tests. Therefore, all individuals who are involved in the newborn screening process should adhere strictly to the procedures set forth by their state program.

Reporting of Results

In most states, all results of neonatal screening tests, whether normal or abnormal, are reported to the physician of record. Normal results are mailed to the physician for placement in the patient's medical record. Abnormal results are usually reported by telephone or letter, depending on the severity of the potential condition. Results are also sent to the hospital where the infant was born for inclusion in the medical record. The physician of record is responsible for contacting the parents regarding the need for confirmatory testing and, if necessary, referral to an appropriate subspecialist. If a newborn is no longer under the care of this physician or if the family cannot be located, state and local public health departments can be called on to assist in the search for the infant and family.

Diagnostic and Therapeutic Considerations

A health care team consisting of a primary care physician and staff, state newborn screening office personnel, the state newborn screening laboratory, local laboratories, and subspecialty physician is responsible for care and follow-up of patients with positive newborn screening results. All infants with abnormal results, whether borderline or clearly significant, should be evaluated by the primary care physician. A complete history and physical examination as well as a family history should be obtained. Abnormal results for some newborn screening tests, such as very long-chain acyl–coenzyme A (CoA) dehydrogenase deficiency, may normalize with a second screen. Therefore, most follow-up evaluation centers on targeted diagnostic tests. Depending on the nature of the suspected disorder, initiation of treatment before confirmatory laboratory results are known may be appropriate. For example, prophylactic antibiotics should be administered if sickle cell anemia is suspected. After confirmatory results have been received, the treatment can be modified or halted.

Potentially life-threatening conditions in the newborn period, such as galactosemia, maple syrup urine disease, and congenital adrenal hyperplasia, are particularly important to evaluate and treat emergently. Depending on the clinical picture, the suspected disorder, and the experience of the practitioner, telephone consultation with a specialist or immediate referral to a regional medical center may be necessary.

Nearly all of the diseases in the current newborn screening panels are inherited in an autosomal recessive manner. Families of affected infants should be offered genetic counseling for future pregnancies, in addition to written information about the newly diagnosed condition. Depending on the condition, older siblings may need to be evaluated. In some conditions, such as 3-methylcrotonyl-CoA carboxylase deficiency, a positive newborn screen may reflect an affected asymptomatic mother whose metabolites have passed to her infant.

Current Issues and Future Challenges

Protecting patient privacy is of the utmost importance, and nearly all programs have laws to protect a patient's personal information, blood spots, and genetic information. There is great concern amongst parents and providers that insurance companies will use newborn screening information to discriminate against children and their families.

There is no dispute that newborn screening saves lives. Additionally, the cost of newborn screening programs is outweighed by the reduction in morbidity and mortality from a purely economic standpoint. However, some diseases under consideration for newborn screening, such as lysosomal storage disorders, have extremely costly treatments, which may total several million dollars over the lifetime of the patient and produce significant morbidity. Cost-benefit analysis will be crucial to shaping future newborn screening panels. Pediatricians and other health professionals need to advocate for insurance coverage for newborn screening panels because patients may be charged up to $130.

Currently a large percentage of false-positive results occur in premature infants, in part due to the lack of age-specific laboratory values for all metabolites. In several states, a lack of appropriate cutoff values led to a large number of false-positive results among babies in neonatal intensive care units that strained the state programs. In the future, careful pilot testing of new tests in infants of all gestational ages will be needed to improve the screening process.

There is debate about the benefit of early detection of disorders such as cystic fibrosis. While recent studies have suggested that patients benefit from early therapy, it is unclear how much early detection improves the long-term pulmonary or nutritional status

of affected children. Some disorders, such as short-chain acyl-CoA dehydrogenase deficiency, are asymptomatic in most individuals and have a high rate of false-positive tests due to the presence of common polymorphisms in the population. The lifelong treatment of patients who would otherwise remain asymptomatic, the added burden of a genetic diagnosis, and family stress caused by a false- or true-positive result have led several countries to remove this disorder from their newborn screening panels. Fortunately, there has been a large amount of progress made in reducing false-positive results using new algorithms for second-tier testing.

Several newborn screening tests detect asymptomatic carrier status in infants. While the knowledge of a patient's carrier status may be of some advantage for childbearing, it has no immediate benefit for the infant and may lead to discrimination and stigmatization. Parents of affected infants (who are usually asymptomatic carriers) face the same dilemma and should be given the option to refuse testing for carrier status.

New challenges will emerge as genetic technology advances toward the ultimate goal of sequencing a patient's entire genome. Practitioners will have to weigh the decision of whether to inform parents about non-treatable or late-onset conditions. The AAP Committee on Bioethics advises against screening for such conditions, but the debate has been reopened as testing for spinal muscular atrophy has been developed. Finally, some conditions that are caused by a complex interaction between genetics and environment, such as celiac disease, may require screening at school age. Pediatricians should be involved in decisions concerning the addition of new disorders to existing newborn screening programs because they are key players in the implementation of these programs.

CASE RESOLUTION

This patient should have a full evaluation, including an electrolyte panel, due to the possibility of salt wasting congenital adrenal hyperplasia. Confirmatory testing, including measurement of precursor hormones such as 17-hydroxyprogesterone and subsequent molecular testing, and glucocorticoid therapy should be considered in consultation with a pediatric endocrinologist.

Selected References

American Academy of Pediatrics Committee on Bioethics. Ethical issues with genetic testing in pediatrics. *Pediatrics.* 2001;107:1451–1455

American College of Medical Genetics. Resources: ACT Sheets. www.acmg.net

American College of Medical Genetics Newborn Screening Expert Group. Newborn screening: toward a uniform screening panel and system—executive summary. *Pediatrics.* 2006;117:S296–S307. www.acmg.net/resources/policies/NBS/NBS-sections.htm

Fernhoff PM. Newborn screening for genetic disorders. *Pediatr Clin North Am.* 2009;56(3):505–513

Hewlett J, Waisbren SE. A review of the psychosocial effects of false-positive results on parents and current communication practices in newborn screening. *J Inherit Metab Dis.* 2006;29:677–682

Kaye CI; American Academy of Pediatrics Committee on Genetics. Introduction to the newborn screening fact sheets. *Pediatrics*. 2006;118:1304–1312

Kaye CI; American Academy of Pediatrics Committee on Genetics. Newborn screening fact sheets. *Pediatrics*. 2006;118:e934–e963. www.pediatrics.aappublications.org/cgi/content/full/118/3/e934

Lipstein EA, Vorono S, Browning MF, et al. Systematic evidence review of newborn screening and treatment of severe combined immunodeficiency. *Pediatrics*. 2010;125(5):e1226–e1235

Matern D, Tortorelli S, Oglesbee D, Gavrilov D, Rinaldo P. Reduction of the false-positive rate in newborn screening by implementation of MS/MS-based second-tier tests: the Mayo Clinic experience (2004-2007). *J Inherit Metab Dis*. 2007;30(4):585–592

National NBS Resource Center. http://genes-r-us.uthscsa.edu/

CHAPTER 21

Caring for Twins and Higher-Order Multiples

Sabrina D. Diaz, MA, and Lynne M. Smith, MD

CASE STUDY

An expectant mother visits you. She has been advised by her obstetrician that an ultrasound shows she is pregnant with twins. She asks about care of twins and what special considerations she should keep in mind as she looks forward to the delivery. In particular, she is concerned about the feeding schedule and whether she will be able to breastfeed.

Questions

1. What is the incidence of multiple births?
2. What is the difference between fraternal and identical twins?
3. What major medical problems may affect twins and higher-order multiples?
4. What developmental and behavioral problems are associated with raising multiples?

With the advent of artificial reproductive therapy, the incidence of twins and higher-order multiples is increasing. Counseling the parents of multiples provides a unique opportunity for pediatricians. Much of what is known about caring for multiples comes from work with twins. Many societies have been fascinated with twins, and many myths and superstitions surround their birth. Some people believe that a mother of twins must have been unfaithful to her husband because a father cannot sire 2 children. Native Americans of the Iroquois nation believed that one twin was good and the other was evil. To prevent the recurrence of twins, the Khoikhain removed one of the father's testicles.

Parents of multiples often have many questions regarding the care of their children, but they rarely pose them to health care providers. In one study where 18 out of 29 mothers breastfed their twins, only 3 received information about breastfeeding from their physicians. One mother had been told by her obstetrician that she could not breastfeed her twins. Physicians should become knowledgeable about caring for multiples and the unique challenges they present to parents related to feeding, sleeping, and behavior.

Epidemiology

Since 1980 there has been a 101% increase in twin deliveries in the United States, and the number of higher-order multiples has increased 5-fold. Twinning rates have also increased in Finland, Norway, Austria, Sweden, Australia, Hong Kong, Japan, Canada, Singapore, and Israel. A major contributor to the increase in multiple births is that women are starting their families later than in previous generations. Because of the increased risk of infertility with advanced maternal age, more couples are choosing to conceive with assisted reproductive technologies, including ovulation-stimulating drugs, in vitro fertilization (IVF), and intracytoplasmic sperm injection. Assisted reproductive technology results in multiple gestations in approximately 50% of pregnancies and accounts for 18% of all multiple births nationwide. Single embryo transfer has lower success rates than multiple embryo transfer, increasing the likelihood of multiple births. In addition, advanced maternal age is associated with increased follicle-stimulating hormone levels and the release of multiple eggs by the ovary, increasing the chance of multiple births.

The overall natural incidence of twin births is about 1 in 87. Twins account for just slightly more than 1% of all births, and 20% of infants born under 30 weeks' gestation are twins. The average incidence of monozygotic or identical twins, which is the same for all women regardless of race and age, is about 1 in 300 births. The incidence of dizygotic or fraternal twins varies among different groups and method of conception. In the United States, African Americans and whites have comparable incidences of live-born twin deliveries and both have significantly higher rates than Hispanic women. A maternal family history of dizygous twins correlates most strongly with an increased incidence of twinning. A family history of monozygous twins or a paternal family history of dizygous twins does not increase the risk of twins.

Pathophysiology

Higher-order multiples, conceived either naturally or via artificial reproductive technology, may be fraternal or a combination of monozygotic twins and fraternal siblings. Monozygotic twins result from the splitting of a single egg. They may share a placenta (monochorionic, Figures 21-1A and 21-1B) and in rare cases may

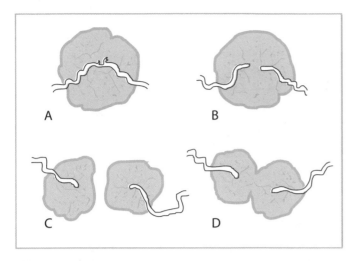

Figure 21-1. **Variations in placentas in twin births. A. Monochorionic placenta, cords close together. B. Monochorionic placenta, cords farther apart. C. Dichorionic placentas, separate. D. Dichorionic placentas, fused.**

also share an amniotic sac (monoamniotic). When splitting occurs early (after several cell divisions of the zygote), each fetus develops its own chorion and amnion, leading to dichorionic and diamniotic placentas. Dizygotic twins result from 2 eggs, and each egg is fertilized by a different sperm. Dizygotic twins have 2 placentas (Figure 21-1C). Although these placentas may fuse together like 2 pancakes, they are almost always dichorionic and diamniotic (Figure 21-1D). Sonography at 14 weeks or less has been found to be 96% predictive of monochorionicity, and can also predict amnionicity, anomalies, and syndromes.

Following the birth, many parents want to determine whether twins are monozygotic or dizygotic. Different sex twins are almost always dizygotic, although monozygotic twins of different sexes have been reported in the literature. This occurs when one twin loses a Y chromosome and becomes a phenotypic female with Turner syndrome (XO). Occasionally the male twin may be XXY and have Klinefelter syndrome.

To determine whether twins are monozygotic or dizygotic after birth, a number of procedures can be undertaken. Visual or pathologic examination of the placenta is helpful. About two-thirds of monozygotic twins have a common chorion and share one placenta. Finding a single chorion usually means the twins are monozygotic, unless the placentas of dizygotic twins have fused together. DNA testing is the preferred method for determining zygosity. Most commercially available testing involves examining DNA obtained from buccal swabs from each child. Identification of short tandem repeats via polymerase chain reaction is typically accurate 99% of the time and is similar to techniques used in forensic medicine. Commercial laboratory charges range from $150 to $500, though prices vary significantly.

Differential Diagnosis

Diagnosing multiples is not difficult, but physicians should be aware of the problems these newborns may experience.

Perinatal Complications

Multiple births are associated with a significantly higher risk for perinatal complications relative to singleton births. The maternal complication most commonly reported with multiples is pregnancy-induced hypertension. Maternal preeclampsia rates are higher in twins and increased nearly 5-fold with triplets. In addition, mothers of twins who conceived via IVF have a higher rate of preeclampsia than mothers of twins who conceived naturally. Other maternal complications include placenta previa, antepartum hemorrhage, gestational diabetes mellitus, anemia, uterine atony, and maternal death.

Neonatal mortality is 4-fold higher in twins and 15-fold higher in higher-order multiples. Neonatal morbidity is much higher in multiple births because of the increased incidence of prematurity and growth restriction. The risk for these complications increases with the number of fetuses. The perinatal mortality of monozygotic twins is 8 times that of singletons and 4 times that of dizygotic twins. Twins and higher-order multiples are also at increased risk for cerebral palsy.

Monozygotic twins are at greater risk for death and cerebral palsy because of complications such as severe birth weight discordance and twin-to-twin transfusion syndrome (TTTS). Twin-to-twin transfusion syndrome is seen in 10% to 15% of monochorionic pregnancies and results from unbalanced blood flow due to vascular anastomoses within the shared placenta. The diagnosis is suspected by ultrasound when one fetus is growth restricted with oligohydramnios and the other fetus has evidence of volume overload with polyhydramnios. Both twins are ultimately at risk to become hydropic and/or die. Without treatment, TTTS-induced death of at least one twin is as high as 80% to 100%. Of additional concern, the death of one twin is associated with neurologic damage or subsequent death of the surviving twin, with 1 in 10 surviving twins developing cerebral palsy.

Until recently the treatment was drainage of amniotic fluid in the twin with polyhydramnios to reduce the risk of preterm delivery. Endoscopic laser ablation of placental anastomoses is emerging as the treatment of choice. Laser ablation addresses the primary pathology and results in an average gestation at delivery of 33 weeks, which is a significant improvement from the average 29 weeks with serial amniotic fluid reductions. Laser ablation is not without risks, however; reported complications include premature rupture of membranes, amniotic fluid leakage into the maternal peritoneal cavity, vaginal bleeding, and chorioamnionitis.

One percent of monozygotic twins are monochorionic–monoamniotic. Although monoamniotic twins have a lower risk of TTTS, they are at very high risk for cord accidents. Monoamniotic pregnancies are monitored closely, and once the fetuses reach viability, emergent delivery is indicated if fetal distress is noted to avoid fetal death. Because fetal death significantly increases the risk of cerebral palsy and other neurologic disorders in the surviving twin, it is no longer recommended to allow fetal death in one monoamniotic twin to lengthen the gestation of the non-distressed twin.

Congenital Malformations

Twins and higher-order multiples have an increased risk of anomalies. Monochorionic twins have a higher risk of cardiac anomalies than dichorionic twins, increasing their need for fetal echocardiograms. Multiples conceived via IVF or intracytoplasmic sperm injection have increased risk for anomalies and aneuploidy. Disorders of genetic imprinting (eg, Beckwith-Wiedemann, Angelman syndrome) are also increased with intracytoplasmic sperm injection. These genetic complications are thought to be secondary to the underlying cause of the infertility instead of artificial reproductive technologies. Because the costs associated with infertility treatments are substantial, many couples choose not to obtain a comprehensive chromosomal analysis looking for deletions or translocations on themselves prior to using reproductive technologies. Nuchal translucency and chorionic villus sampling can be used to detect and confirm suspected aneuploidy as early as the first trimester. Chorionic villus sampling is not widely available and ranges from $1,000 to $2,000; however, many insurance companies will cover the procedure in women over 35 years of age or in women with risk factors that may increase the baby's likelihood of having a serious health problem.

In addition to the increased risks for malformations, multiples are at risk for deformations secondary to crowding, including torticollis, hip dislocation, plagiocephaly, and foot deformities. Monochorionic twins are also at risk for conjoined twinning, estimated to occur in 1:50,000 to 200,000 gestations, with more than 50% dying in utero or stillborn and 35% dying within the first 24 hours. Although monochorionicity is more common in males, conjoined twins are often female. Conjoined twinning occurs due to incomplete splitting of the embryo or after a secondary fusion between 2 previously separate embryos. Prenatal ultrasound is commonly used to diagnose this condition, and more recently prenatal magnetic resonance imaging has been used to evaluate the specific anomalies. Due to recent surgical advances, some parents continue the pregnancy with hopes the live-born infants can be separated, while others often terminate the pregnancy.

Postnatal Complications

Approximately 60% of twins and 90% of triplets are born prematurely, increasing the risk of morbidity and mortality. Though growth in twins tends to be normal until 30 to 34 weeks, growth restriction is commonly associated with multiple births. Twins conceived by IVF are more likely to be born low birth weight than spontaneously conceived twins. Smaller twins have an increased incidence of hypoglycemia in the newborn period and have higher rates of targeted learning deficits and school failures during childhood. In addition, children born growth-restricted have an increased risk for obesity and diabetes in later life. Selective intrauterine growth restriction

(IUGR), when only one twin is affected by IUGR, occurs in 10% of monochorionic twins. This occurs when the twin with IUGR has reversed flow or persistent absent flow in the umbilical artery.

Evaluation

History

A general medical history should be obtained, including a history of the pregnancy. Any specific medical complaints should also be addressed (Questions Box).

> **Questions**
>
> ## Caring for Twins
>
> - Did the mother have any problems during the pregnancy?
> - How long did the pregnancy last?
> - Did the mother take any medications, including fertility drugs?
> - Did the children have any problem after the delivery or in the newborn nursery?

Physical Examination

The initial evaluation of newly born twins involves assessment of gestational age and determination of the presence of any medical problems or anomalies (see Chapter 18). Older twins may undergo health maintenance visits where routine as well as specific complaints are addressed.

Laboratory Tests

Newborns should be assessed for the presence of anemia or polycythemia with a hemoglobin determination. Hypoglycemia may occur in the newborn period and should be assessed frequently until glucose levels are stable. If the twins are premature, they may have many of the problems seen in preterm infants, such as respiratory distress syndrome and necrotizing enterocolitis.

Older children should receive an appropriate evaluation for age, with a specific focus on any behavioral concerns.

Management

The focus of the management of multiples involves counseling the parents about issues related to routine care and the anticipated stress of caring for more than one newborn simultaneously. Parents often care for 2 or more children at the same time, but multiples present unique issues related to multiple children who are developmentally and chronologically at the same point. Many parents experience anxiety regarding the upcoming challenges they will face. Baby care books that specifically deal with birthing and raising multiples are available. Support groups and Web sites also provide information for families of multiples.

Feeding multiple newborns is often an exhausting challenge for parents, and consultation with a lactation expert is recommended.

The physical demands of feeding multiple newborns are often compounded by women recovering from prenatal complications such as preeclampsia. Because prematurity is common, the newborns may have an immature suck reflex, making feeding more challenging. Few multiples are still receiving human milk by 3 to 4 months of age, and common reasons cited for unsuccessful breastfeeding of multiples include maternal stress, depression, fatigue, perceiving they were producing insufficient milk, and time burden. Despite these obstacles, parents should know that breastfeeding is possible even for triplets and understand the benefits of breastfeeding to the newborns' health.

Some options for breastfeeding twins are as follows:

1. Feed both infants *at the same time,* with one on each breast. This method is recommended only after adequate breastfeeding has been established in each twin, typically not until after 1 week of age. It is advised that the baby having fewer problems latching be placed on the breast first so that the milk ejection reflex is already established for the poorer-feeding baby. Because the babies may not drink the same amount, it is important that they feed on the opposite breast for the next feeding to maximize milk production.

   The infants may be put in a number of positions. The mother can be sitting and cradling one infant while holding the other infant like a football. Alternatively, the mother may cradle both infants, so that they are cross-positioned over one another, or she may have both infants under her arms in a football position. Breastfeeding pillows designed for feeding multiples are helpful, and electric breastfeeding pumps are essential.

2. Feed the infants *at different times.* The mother breastfeeds one infant and then the other. The mother starts with the more vigorous feeder. This approach may pose a problem; both infants may be hungry at the same time and maternal fatigue may inhibit success because the chance for sleep is diminished with this method.

3. *Breastfeed one infant and bottle-feed the other,* which gives the mother a free hand. Most parents use a combination of breastfeeding and bottle-feeding. A mother can let the first infant feed on demand but wake up the second one when the first one is done. Eighty percent of parents of twins acknowledge that they prop the bottle instead of holding it, and they should be counseled against this. There are several effective feeding positions that do not require bottle propping, and parents should be encouraged to adopt one of these positions.

   Breastfeeding triplets and higher-order multiples is even more challenging than breastfeeding twins. Mothers of triplets exclusively breastfeeding report they feed 2 children, one on each breast, and the third follows on both breasts. Because the hindmilk has higher fat content, it is important to rotate the feeding order of the children. Another popular option is to breastfeed 2 and have the third bottle-feed simultaneously.

Feeding twins or higher-order multiples may decrease the amount of sleep a mother gets. Because sleep deprivation is associated with maternal depression and exclusively breastfeeding mothers of multiples report more sleep problems compared with mothers who do not breastfeed or who formula-feed and breastfeed, these factors should be discussed when offering feeding options to the parents. Encouraging paternal involvement with feeding may alleviate some maternal stress and sleep deprivation.

Sleeping in the same crib is no longer recommended because of concerns regarding cosleeping. It is important to counsel parents about **car safety seats.** Parents who cannot afford the cost of multiple car safety seats may resort to placing one child in the car safety seat and the others on the seat of the car, a dangerous practice that is illegal throughout the United States. Parents should be advised about the need for car safety seats for all infants.

Bathing should be done separately in the interest of safety until infants can sit up.

Toilet training is reportedly easier with some twins because one twin learns from the other via modeling and/or peer pressure.

Maintenance of individuality for multiples may be challenging. Researchers suggest that mothers can bond to only one infant at a time, a concept called *monotropy.* In addition, mothers bond more strongly with the twin who leaves the hospital first. Twins are often dressed alike and given similar names as this may facilitate the bonding process. To help with individual development, physicians are encouraged to obtain history and examine each child individually. Physicians should attempt to distinguish the children from one another independent of parental reminders. Twins should not be referred to as "the twins" but by their respective names. As multiples get older, issues related to classrooms and birthday parties frequently arise, and they should be consulted concerning their preferences. Individual birthday parties and gifts should be considered. (Some multiples comment on their disappointment at receiving the same present for birthdays and holidays. There is no surprise in opening gifts if the other twin opened a gift first.)

Whether multiples should be placed in the same or different classrooms is unclear. Placement in different classrooms is advocated to support each child's individual development. However, there are no data to support separate classroom placement. It is currently recommended that school districts have a flexible policy regarding school placement of twins. A checklist has been created to assist families and schools determining the best school placement for twins (available at www.twinsandmultiples.org). Families with higher-order multiples are more likely to have children in separate schools because of the higher risk that some of the children will have developmental delays.

Sibling rivalry is common among co-multiples as well as other siblings within a family. Older siblings may resent the attention paid to the new babies, so family and friends should be reminded to shower attention on the older siblings. Because twins often exclude siblings and peers socially, parents are encouraged to schedule times when one twin and sibling are with one parent and the other twin is alone with another family member. Isolating twins (or 2 triplets from a third) fosters more sibling interaction and less dependency between the twins. These separations are encouraged to begin early in development because the later in development isolation is introduced, the less agreeable they are to the separations.

Developmental differences among multiples may also contribute to sibling rivalry. The smaller or more delayed child may become jealous of their co-multiple. Conversely, typically developing children may become frustrated when the sibling with special needs receives more attention than they receive.

Until age 3 years, **language development** is delayed in twins relative to singletons. Contributing factors to language delay include less time for individual facilitated play, which is helpful for language development. If twins communicate with a private language they have an increased risk of language and cognitive delays. Language delays usually become much less pronounced by mid-childhood.

The risk for **cerebral palsy** is increased with higher multiples because of the increased rates of prematurity and IUGR. Fetal death of a co-multiple and monochorionic placentas are the biggest risk factors for developing cerebral palsy.

Attention-deficit/hyperactivity disorder is more common in twins. The temper tantrums multiples display can be severe and are understandable given the heightened need to gain parental attention from their sibling. Having twins in the home is a risk factor for **child abuse,** either to a twin or to their siblings.

Prior to delivery, parents should be made aware that **maternal depression** is frequently reported after the birth of multiples. The physical stress of caring for multiple newborns can be overwhelming, and the parents often feel isolated at home. The incidence of depression is higher in mothers of twins than of singletons, with sleep deprivation being a cited contributing factor. It is important to suggest that parents of multiples obtain outside aid, including help from high school students after school and family members to decrease fatigue and increase their ability to experience respite even for short periods.

In addition to exhaustion and isolation, the increased financial demands that accompany multiple newborns can strain the parents' relationship. Mothers often have to leave work earlier in the pregnancy than women with singleton pregnancies, adding financial burden. The medical costs associated with prematurely delivered newborns can be substantial. To cover for the loss of income at a time of increasing family expenses, the father is often required to work more hours. This increased occupational stress comes at a time when child care demands at home have increased significantly. Financial burdens are especially difficult with multiples conceived artificially because of the cost associated prior to birth. This may be a contributing factor to why parents of twins conceived artificially reported less satisfaction than parents of twins conceived naturally.

Grief is another significant contributor to parental depression. Approximately 15% of children from multiple births grow up as a singleton survivor. Birthday celebrations serve as reminders to the parents of the death of the other child. Parents grieving the loss of one of their twins have comparable grief to those grieving the loss of a singleton pregnancy. It is imperative that physicians caring for the family acknowledge the parents' grief because family and friends often do not acknowledge the parents' pain if there is a surviving newborn.

Surviving children born prematurely and/or small for gestation are at increased risk for developmental delays. The stress of raising a child with special needs is also a source of grief because parents mourn the loss of their dreams of having a normal child.

Prognosis

Although multiples have a higher incidence of perinatal problems, appropriate anticipatory guidance and routine health maintenance can help families optimize their children's outcome.

CASE RESOLUTION

The mother in the case scenario is advised that breastfeeding is not only possible but recommended. She is told about the options for timing and positioning of the infants. The issues of family history and child passenger safety are also discussed, and anticipatory guidance regarding the potential stress of raising multiples is given.

Selected References

Physicians

Chauhan SP, Scardo JA, Hayes E, Abuhamad AZ, Berghella V. Twins: prevalence, problems, and preterm birth. *Am J Obstet Gynecol.* 2010;203:305–315

Cowan JM, Demmer LA. Assisted reproductive technology and preimplantation genetic diagnosis: impact of the fetus and newborn. *Neoreviews.* 2007;8:e127–e132

Flidel-Rimon O, Shinwell ES. Breast feeding twins and high multiples. *Arch Dis Child Fetal Neonatal Ed.* 2006;91:F377–F380

Hansen M, Kurinczuk JJ, Bower C, Webb S. The risk of major birth defects after intracytoplasmic sperm injection and in vitro fertilization. *N Engl J Med.* 2002;346:725–730

Hay DA, Preedy P. Meeting the educational needs of multiple birth children. *Early Hum Dev.* 2006;82:397–403

Klock SC. Psychological adjustment to twins after infertility. *Best Pract Res Clin Obstet Gynaecol.* 2004;18:645–656

Moore JE. Q&A's about multiple births. *Contemp Pediatr.* 2007;24:39–55

Pharoah POD, Dundar Y. Monozygotic twinning, cerebral palsy and congenital anomalies. *Hum Reprod Update.* 2009;15:639–648

Shinwell ES, Haklai T, Eventov-Friedman S. Outcomes of multiplets. *Neonatology.* 2009;95:6–14

Siegel SJ, Seigal MM. Practical aspects of pediatric management of families with twins. *Pediatr Rev.* 1982;4:8–12

Sutcliffe AG, Derom C. Follow-up of twins: health, behavior, speech, language outcomes and implications for parents. *Early Hum Dev.* 2006;82:379–386

Thorpe K. Twin children's language development. *Early Hum Dev.* 2006;82:387–395

Parents

Center for Loss in Multiple Birth, Inc. (CLIMB). www.climb-support.org

Luke B, Eberlein T. *When You're Expecting Twins, Triplets, or Quads, Revised Edition: Proven Guidelines for a Healthy Multiple Pregnancy.* New York, NY: HarperCollins Publishers Inc.; 2004

Mothers of Supertwins (MOST). http://MOSTonline.org

Neifert M. *Dr. Mom's Guide to Breastfeeding.* New York, NY: Penguin Group; 1998

CHAPTER 22

Circumcision

Lynne M. Smith, MD

CASE STUDY

An expectant mother visits you prenatally. She talks about circumcision in addition to issues relating to breastfeeding and car passenger safety. Her husband is circumcised. She is unclear about the medical indications for circumcision and asks your opinion about circumcision in the newborn period.

Questions

1. What are the benefits of circumcision?
2. What are the indications for circumcision in older children?
3. What are the techniques used to perform circumcision?
4. What are the complications of circumcision?

Male circumcision, a procedure in which the foreskin of the penis is removed, has been performed for more than 4,000 years. It is routinely performed in certain groups, most notably among Jewish and Muslim people. In many other cultures (eg, Abyssinian, Australian [aborigine], Polynesian), circumcision is presumably performed to facilitate intercourse. Circumcision can be viewed as a ritual procedure, but its role as a medical one is open to greater controversy.

The benefits of male circumcision have been debated for years. Over the past 20 years, even the American Academy of Pediatrics (AAP) has changed its official position on the medical indication for circumcision. In 1999 the AAP stated and then reaffirmed in 2005 that there are potential benefits to circumcision, though the procedure is not medically indicated. Disadvantages of routine circumcision in infants concern cost-effectiveness and the risk of complications. The procedure is sometimes viewed as an archaic and maiming ritual. Female circumcision, which may involve clitorectomy or resection and closure of the labia minora or majora, is infrequently practiced in Western culture and is not discussed here. There are no medical benefits attributable to female circumcision.

Circumcision in newborns has been performed in a routine and preventive manner, much the same way immunizations are administered. Primary care physicians should be aware of the risks and benefits of the procedure to be able to counsel parents and make referrals to consultants when certain medical conditions arise.

Epidemiology

The prevalence of neonatal circumcision, a procedure that became increasingly popular in the United States in the 1950s and 1960s, once ranged from 69% to 97% depending on cultural mores. Changing cultural patterns have resulted in a lower frequency of circumcision to 56% in 2005, which reflects, in part, state Medicaid programs no longer covering circumcision. Rates also vary by race, religion, and geographic region. In 2005 the circumcision rate in the western

United States was 31%, compared with 75% in the Midwest, 65% in the Northeast, and 56% in the South. The higher Hispanic birth rate in the West contributes to these regional differences because Hispanic neonates are less likely to receive a circumcision. The prevalence of neonatal circumcision for Australian-born men is reported to be 69% (though only 32% in those aged 16–20); in Canada, 35%; and in the United Kingdom, 4%. Circumcision is the second most common surgical procedure after vasectomy in adult males. It is the most commonly performed operation in children.

A reported 10% of uncircumcised males ultimately require circumcision as adults because of complications of phimosis and balanitis. Uncircumcised males with diabetes are particularly prone to these complications.

Clinical Presentation

Most often parents will query their pediatrician about the advisability of a circumcision and the infant will not have any clinical symptomatology. Older infants and children in need of a circumcision can present with symptoms of phimosis, in which the foreskin balloons out on urination; paraphimosis, in which a retracted foreskin cannot be returned to its normal position; or recurrent problems of infection or inflammation of the foreskin (posthitis), glans (balanitis), or both (balanoposthitis).

Pathophysiology

In uncircumcised males, the foreskin adheres to the glans until about the age of 6 years. A gradual, normal lysing of the adhesive bands connecting the foreskin to the under portion of the glans then occurs. Non-physiological phimosis occurs as a result of scarring of the preputial wing. Lysing of adhesions in an effort to treat the phimosis usually leads to further adhesions. If the foreskin is retracted and remains in that position, paraphimosis develops.

Differential Diagnosis

The differential diagnosis relates to conditions that may be managed with a circumcision. Such conditions include phimosis, paraphimosis, and infection and inflammation of the penis. Conditions such as hypospadias may be mistaken for a partially circumcised penis because the condition is associated with absence of the ventral foreskin. A careful history will differentiate hypospadias from a circumcision.

Evaluation

History

In cases involving newborn infants, a history should include the presence of any coagulopathies involving family members, which would preclude the performance of a circumcision. In older infants and children, the history should include problems relating to voiding, such as ballooning of the foreskin or difficulty initiating the urinary stream.

Physical Examination

The physical examination should assess the genitalia, particularly to determine if there is evidence of hypospadias, in which the urethral orifice is not located at the tip of the glans. In such a situation, circumcision should be delayed because the foreskin is used to reconstruct the urethra. In cases of phimosis, the degree of phimosis should also be assessed.

Laboratory Tests

Routine laboratory tests are not indicated, although a urinalysis may be obtained in children with a history of prior urinary tract infection. Coagulation studies would be appropriate if there is a family history of a bleeding disorder.

Imaging Studies

Imaging studies are not indicated in most children undergoing a circumcision. Such studies would be relevant if there was concern that the urogenital anatomy was abnormal.

Prognosis

The prognosis is excellent with complications being exceedingly rare.

Benefits

It has been stated that circumcision facilitates penile hygiene by removing the foreskin, which may serve as a repository for bacteria, smegma, and dirt. Retractability of the foreskin increases with age (Table 22-1) and, thus, penile hygiene is easier to achieve in older children. The term **phimosis** refers to inability to retract the foreskin. In male infants beyond the newborn period, phimosis is the major indication for circumcision. Phimosis is normal in children up to about 6 years of age but is non-physiological if urination results in ballooning of the foreskin, regardless of age. When the retracted foreskin acts as a tourniquet in the midshaft of the penis, **paraphimosis**

Table 22-1. Retractability of the Foreskin in Boys (by Age)	
Age	*Percentage With Retractable Foreskin*
Birth	4%
6 mo	15%
1 y	50%
3 y	80%
6 y	90%

occurs, preventing the return of lymphatic flow. Paraphimosis is commonly related to traumatic retraction of the foreskin, typically during cleaning or by medical personnel during bladder catheterization. Because of this, parents are no longer advised to retract the foreskin in an effort to lyse adhesions. The incidence of paraphimosis is increasing in adults secondary to body piercing. Newly placed penile rings can cause enough pain to prevent foreskin retraction.

Balanitis, or inflammation of the glans, is not uncommon in young infants. It is frequently associated with *Candida* infection, and the glans is swollen and erythematous. Posthitis, or inflammation of the foreskin, is also often secondary to *Candida* infection. Other organisms, including gram-negative microbes, may be associated with balanitis. The presence of recurrent balanitis is an indication for circumcision. In older males, indications for circumcision include phimosis, paraphimosis, balanitis, posthitis, and balanoposthitis.

Urinary tract infections (UTIs) reportedly occur 10 times more often in uncircumcised (1:100) than in circumcised infants (1:1,000). In young uncircumcised boys, UTIs are directly related to colonization of the foreskin with urotoxic organisms. Pyronephritogenic, fimbriated *Escherichia coli* bind to the inner lining of the foreskin within the first few days of life. Other bacteria preferentially bind to this mucosal surface, including fimbriated strains of *Proteus mirabilis* and non-fimbriated *Pseudomonas, Klebsiella,* and *Serratia* species. The incidence of UTIs has increased as the rate of circumcision has decreased. In addition, complications associated with UTIs, particularly bacteremia, meningitis, and subsequent death, have occurred.

In Western countries, penile cancer is reported in 0.7 to 0.9 per 100,000 men, but is as great as 4.2 per 100,00 men in Paraguay. These regional differences are thought to be related to lack of circumcision of the penis. Only a few isolated cases of cancer of the penis occur in circumcised men. The estimated lifetime risk of penile cancer is 1 in 600 in uncircumcised males compared with 1 in 50,000 to 1 in 12 million in circumcised males. From 1930–1990, 10,000 men died from penile cancer; there were 1,280 new cases found in 2007 with 290 deaths. The reported mortality of invasive penile cancer is 25%. Phimosis is strongly associated with invasive penile cancer, with other cofactors such as human papillomavirus (HPV) infection and poor hygiene possibly contributing. Smoking is consistently associated with penile cancer and is further reason to strongly advocate for smoking cessation programs.

Cervical carcinoma among the partners of uncircumcised men has been reported with increased incidence. In addition, current partners of circumcised men with a history of multiple sexual partners have a decreased risk of cervical cancer compared with partners of uncircumcised men. Circumcision in adolescent boys and men in Uganda found a significantly decreased incidence of HPV and herpes simplex virus type 2 (HSV-2) infection. Circumcision has also been associated with a lower risk of HIV infections. Three randomized controlled trials conducted in South Africa, Kenya, and Uganda confirmed findings in observational studies that circumcision is protective against HIV infection. In addition, circumcision was not associated with increased HIV risk behavior. Based on these findings, in 2007 the World Health Organization stated that male circumcision should be part of a comprehensive strategy for HIV prevention. It remains critical, however, to promote the practice of safe sex as circumcision confers only partial protection from HPV, HSV-2, and HIV.

Risks

The risks related to circumcision are related to complications from the procedure. These are listed in Box 22-1 and discussed under Management.

Box 22-1. Complications Associated With Circumcision	
• Bleeding	• Inclusion cysts
• Infection	• Penile lymphedema
• Repeat circumcision	• Urethrocutaneous fistulae
• Phimosis	• Penile cyanosis
• Skin bridges	• Penile necrosis
• Urinary retention	• Wound dehiscence
• Meatitis	

Parent Counseling

Parents of Newborns

In the newborn period, proper counseling of the parents, including a discussion of the risks and benefits of circumcision, is important. Opponents to neonatal circumcision cite psychological trauma to neonates from so painful a procedure. Local anesthesia minimizes this effect. Parents should be informed about the benefits of circumcision, including a reduction in occurrence of UTIs, sexually transmitted infections, and cancer of the penis and cervix. Problems related to the foreskin itself, such as phimosis, paraphimosis, posthitis, and balanitis, should also be discussed.

It is appropriate to tell parents that boys who are not circumcised in the neonatal period may need to be circumcised later in life. Parents should be informed about the risks associated with circumcision in newborns, which are discussed in greater detail in the following text. In older individuals, risks include hemorrhage, infection, and injuries to the penis and urethra. In addition, parents should be told that approximately 2% of circumcised neonates require a second circumcision due to inadequate foreskin removal.

Research has shown that parents are more influenced by the circumcision status of the father, religion, and race than by physician attitude regarding their ultimate decision about circumcision. Counseling during the second trimester of pregnancy results in no change in parents' decision about circumcision.

Parents of Older Infants

The need for circumcision in young male infants who present with UTIs is problematic. The evaluation usually tries to determine the existence of other predisposing conditions that could lead to the UTI. Investigators disagree on the need for circumcision following the initial UTI in uncircumcised boys. No clear-cut evidence indicates that circumcision at this time decreases the incidence of future UTIs, so the decision is parental rather than medical. In older children who present with significant phimosis or paraphimosis, circumcision is usually recommended to prevent recurrences of these problems. Medical management, including the use of topical steroids for phimosis, may obviate the need for surgery in some children. Such treatment involves the daily external application of betamethasone cream from the foreskin tip to the corona glandis for 4 to 6 weeks. A history, including the duration of symptoms and whether the child has had similar episodes in the past, helps formulate the appropriate management.

Management

The medical attitude toward circumcision has changed over the last 40 years, with an initial inclination toward circumcision, followed by a move away from circumcision. The present position on circumcision as described by the AAP Task Force on Circumcision suggests that newborn circumcision has potential medical benefits and advantages as well as disadvantages and risks. When circumcision is considered, the benefits and risks should be explained to the parents, and informed consent should be obtained. Parents should be advised that the frequency with which third-party payers reimburse for circumcisions, particularly for routine circumcisions in the newborn period, has decreased.

Contraindications

Circumcisions should only be performed in completely healthy neonates. Contraindications to circumcision are well defined. Any abnormalities of the penis, such as hypospadias, absence of any portion of the foreskin, or chordee, preclude circumcision. Ambiguous genitalia and prematurity are contraindications. Circumcision should be delayed in premature and ill term newborns until they are ready for discharge. Patients with a personal or family history of bleeding diathesis should not be circumcised. Infants from such families should be assessed for evidence of coagulation problems. If these are present, circumcision should not be carried out.

Circumcision Procedure

Numerous techniques are used to perform circumcisions. These procedures may involve clamp techniques with Gomco, Mogen, or Plastibell clamps. Any of these techniques is believed to give comparable results in the hands of trained, experienced operators. Formal surgical excision may also be carried out, usually in older children and adults. Three guidelines should be followed to decrease the incidence of complications: (1) marking of the coronal sulcus in ink, (2) dilation of the preputial wing, and (3) retraction of the foreskin so that the urethral meatus is visualized. This prevents cutting the meatus. Electrocautery should never be used in conjunction with metal clamps because of the danger of extensive injury.

Appropriate anesthesia in newborns undergoing circumcision is the standard of care. The pain and stress of circumcision is evidenced by changes in infant state and behavior. Local anesthesia is the preferred method of pain management. Dorsal penile nerve block, the subcutaneous injections of local anesthetic at the base of the penis, is effective at reducing pain responses during circumcision. Ring block, the subcutaneous circumferential injection of a local anesthetic around the midshaft of the penis, has been shown to be effective and avoids the potential complication of injecting local anesthesia toward the dorsal vessels. Topical application of lidocaine/prilocaine cream (EMLA) or oral sucrose solution on a pacifier also reduces pain and its associated stress, but to a lesser extent than local anesthesia. For older, prepubertal children requiring formal surgical excision, sutureless circumcision using tissue glues has been associated with reduced operative time and an improved cosmetic result.

Complications

A number of complications are associated with circumcision in newborns (see Box 22-1). The most common complication is **bleeding,** which may occur in 0.2% to 8% of cases. Bleeding can usually be controlled using local pressure. More significant bleeding may require local pressure with 1:1,000 adrenaline-soaked gauze or with the use of other topical agents such as Surgicel. The second most frequently seen complication is **infection,** reported in up to 8% of circumcised infants. Plastibell clamps are associated with a higher incidence of infection than Gomco clamps. Most infections usually respond to local treatment, though intravenous antibiotics should be considered because neonatal sepsis and necrotizing fasciitis may occur secondary to infections following circumcision.

Poor cosmetic outcome is also a complication of circumcision. **Phimosis** may occur if removal of the foreskin is insufficient. If the foreskin is inadequately freed up from the inner preputial epithelium, a concealed penis, with the shaft retracted backward into the abdominal wall, may develop. **Skin bridges** may form between the glans and the shaft, leading to accumulation of smegma or the tethering of the erect penis. Most post-circumcision adhesions are reported to resolve at the time of puberty with the onset of masturbation or sexual activity.

In the immediate postsurgical period, urinary retention may occur secondary to tight surgical bandages. This complication can be prevented by applying local pressure rather than tight bandages to obtain hemostasis. Meatitis and meatal ulcers possibly caused by irritation from ammonia or damage to the frenular artery at the time of circumcision are also reported in circumcised males. Inclusion cysts that represent implantation of smegma are also seen. Additional injuries following circumcision may include penile lymphedema, urethrocutaneous fistulae secondary to misplaced sutures, penile cyanosis, and necrosis secondary to tight Plastibell clamps. Wound dehiscence, which involves separation of the penile skin from the mucous membrane, and denudation of the penile shaft may occur more frequently with Gomco than Plastibell clamps.

CASE RESOLUTION

In the case history at the beginning of this chapter, the risks and benefits of circumcision should be discussed with the mother. The father should be encouraged to participate in the decision-making process.

If the parents elect not to have their son circumcised, they should be instructed on the appropriate care of the uncircumcised penis, which involves gentle external washing without retraction of the foreskin.

Selected References

Alanis MC, Lucidi RS. Neonatal circumcision: a review of the world's oldest and most controversial operation. *Obstet Gynecol Surv.* 2004;59:379–395

American Academy of Pediatrics Task Force on Circumcision. Circumcision policy statement. *Pediatrics.* 1999;103:686–693

Anderson JE, Anderson KA. What to tell parents about circumcision. *Contemp Pediatr.* 1999;16:87–103

Binner DS, Mastrobattista JM, Day MC, et al. Effect of parental education on decision-making about neonatal circumcision. *South Med J.* 2002;95:457–461

Brady-Fryer B, Wiebe N, Lander JA. Pain relief for neonatal circumcision. *Cochrane Database Syst Rev.* 2004;4:CD004217 (affirmed 2009)

Castellsague X, Bosch FX, Munoz N, et al. Male circumcision, penile human papillomavirus infection, and cervical cancer in female partners. *N Engl J Med.* 2002;346:1105–1112

Fergusson DM, Boden JM, Horwood LJ. Circumcision status and risk of sexually transmitted infection in young adult males: an analysis of a longitudinal birth cohort. *Pediatrics.* 2006;118:1971–1977

Gee WF, Ansell JS. Neonatal circumcision: a ten year overview. With comparison of the Gomco clamp and the Plastibell device. *Pediatrics.* 1976;58:824

Kim, HH, Li PS, Goldstein M. Male circumcision: Africa and beyond? *Curr Opin Urol.* 2010;20:515–519

Lane V, Vajda P, Subramaniam R. Paediatric sutureless circumcision: a systematic literature review. *Pediatr Surg Int.* 2010;26:141–144

Merrill CT, Nagamine M, Steiner C. *Circumcisions Performed in US Community Hospitals, 2005.* Rockville, MD: Agency for Healthcare Research and Quality; 2008. HCUP Statistical Brief #45

Minhas S, Manseck A, Watya S, Hegarty PK. Penile cancer—prevention and premalignant conditions. *Urology.* 2010;76:S24–S35

Schoen EJ. Ignoring evidence of circumcision benefits. *Pediatrics.* 2006;118:385–387

Tobian AA, Serwadda D, Quinn TC, et al. Male circumcision for the prevention of HSV-2 and HPV infections and syphilis. *New Engl J Med.* 2009;360:1298–1309

Van Howe RS. Is neonatal circumcision clinically beneficial? Argument against. *Urology.* 2009;6:74–75

CHAPTER 23

Nutritional Needs

Wendy T. Hui, MD, and Geeta Grover, MD

CASE STUDY

At a routine health maintenance visit, a mother asks if she may begin giving her 4-month-old daughter solid foods. The infant is taking about 4 to 5 oz of formula every 3 to 4 hours during the day (about 32 oz per day) and sleeps from 12:00 am to 5:00 am without awakening for a feeding. Her birth weight was 7 lbs (3,182 g), and her present weight and length (13 lbs [5,909 g] and 25 in. [63.5 cm], respectively) are at the 50th percentile for age. The physical examination, including developmental assessment, is within normal limits.

Questions

1. What are some of the parameters that may be used to decide when infants are ready to begin taking solid foods?
2. Up to what age is breast milk or infant formula alone considered adequate intake for infants?
3. At what age do infants double their birth weight? At what age do they triple their birth weight?
4. What problems are associated with the early introduction of solid foods?

Good nutrition is essential for normal growth and development. The physician plays an important role not only in assessing the growth of children from infancy through adolescence but also in counseling parents regarding the nutritional needs of maturing children. The primary care physician should be knowledgeable about key nutritional concepts in children, including growth patterns and nutritional requirements of normal children and how they vary with age, feeding patterns of infants and children, assessment of nutritional status, and common feeding and nutritional disorders.

Growth Patterns and Nutritional Requirements of Normal Children

Monitoring the growth and nutritional status of infants and children is an integral component of well-child care. The average normal expected increases in weight, height, and head circumference for the first several years of life are listed in Table 23-1.

The energy and nutritional requirements of children vary with age. Postnatal growth is most rapid during the first 6 to 12 months of life. Hence, caloric and protein needs are very high at this time. The average daily energy and protein needs of children from birth to 18 years of age are presented in Table 23-2.

On average, newborns weigh 7.7 lb (3.5 kg), are about 20 in. (50 cm) long, and have a head circumference of 14 in. (35 cm). They lose about 5% to 10% of their birth weight during the first several days of life and usually regain this weight by the age of 10 to 14 days. During the first several months of life, weight gain serves as an important indicator of children's general well-being. Failure to gain weight during this time may be a clue to a wide variety of problems, ranging from underfeeding to malabsorption. Newborns gain about 30 g/day (roughly 1% of their birth weight per day) for

Table 23-1. Normal Expected Increase in Weight, Height, and Head Circumference of Infants and Children	
Normal Weight Gain	
Age	*Expected Weight Increase*
0–3 mo	25–35 g/d
3–6 mo	12–21 g/d
6–12 mo	10–13 g/d
1–6 y	5–8 g/d
7–10 y	5–11 g/d
Normal Height Increase	
Age	*Expected Height Increase*
0–12 mo	10 in/y (25 cm/y)
13–24 mo	5 in/y (12.5 cm/y)
2 y–puberty	2.5 in/y (6.25 cm/y)
Normal Increase in Head Circumference	
Age	*Expected Increase in Head Circumference*
0–3 mo	2 cm/mo
4–6 mo	1 cm/mo
7–12 mo	.05 cm/mo
Total increase	12 cm in the first year

the first 3 months of life, and about 10 to 20 g/day for the rest of the first year. Infants double their birth weight by 6 months of age and triple their birth weight by 12 months of age. On average, children weigh about 10 kg at 1 year of age, 20 kg at 5 years of age, and 30 kg

Table 23-2. Energy and Protein Needs of Children		
Age (y)	*Calories (kcal/kg/d)*	*Protein (g/kg/d)*
0–1	90–120	2.5–3.0
1–7	75–90	1.5–2.5
7–12	60–75	1.5–2.5
12–18	30–60	1.0–1.5

at 10 years of age. A rough rule of thumb that can be used to estimate the expected weight of a child based on age is 2 × (age in years) + 10 = weight (kg).

Feeding Patterns of Infants and Children

Liquid Foods

Breast milk or one of the several iron-fortified infant formulas provides complete nutrition for infants during the first 4 to 6 months of life. During the first month or two of life, infants take about 2 to 3 oz of formula (approximately 10 minutes on each breast) every 2 to 3 hours.

Because human milk is more easily digested than formula, it passes out of the stomach in 1½ hours. Formula may take up to 4 hours. Therefore, during the first 4 to 6 weeks of life, breastfed infants want to feed more frequently (8–12 times in 24 hours) than formula-fed infants (6–8 times in 24 hours), with an increased number of nighttime feedings as well. By about 3 to 5 months of age, breastfed and bottle-fed infants do not differ in the number of nighttime feedings, although some breastfed infants continue to awaken out of habit.

Most infants 6 months of age or younger consume about 4 to 5 oz per feeding every 4 to 5 hours. Under routine circumstances, human milk is preferred to infant formulas because it has emotional, nutritional, and immunologic advantages. Breastfeeding allows infants and mothers to develop a unique relationship that can be emotionally satisfying (see Chapter 24).

The composition of human milk varies over time. Colostrum, the first milk produced after delivery, is high in protein, immunoglobulins (Igs), and secretory IgA. Colostrum gradually changes to mature milk 7 to 10 days after delivery. The nutrient content of human milk of mothers who deliver preterm compared with those who deliver at term may vary considerably. Individual assessment may be necessary to determine the appropriateness of human milk for preterm infants.

Nutritionally, human milk is uniquely tailored to meet the specific needs of infants. Human milk provides approximately 20 kcal/oz, the same as routine infant formulas. Table 23-3 compares the composition of human milk and several infant formulas. Human milk has relatively low amounts of protein compared with cow's milk (1% vs 3%), yet the levels are sufficient to provide for satisfactory growth of infants.

Qualitative differences also make human milk more desirable. The casein-whey ratio in human milk is about 40:60, making it easier to digest than most infant formulas, which tend to have higher casein-whey ratios. Lactose is the major carbohydrate of both human and cow's milk, but it is present in higher concentrations in human milk. Fat is the primary source of calories in human milk. The fat in cow's milk, which contains primarily saturated fatty acids, is not as well digested by infants as human milk fat, which is predominantly composed of polyunsaturated fats. Recently, the long-chain polyunsaturated fatty acids docosahexaenoic acid (DHA) and arachidonic

Table 23-3. Composition of Human Milk and Select Infant Formulas (Calories: 20 kcal/oz)			
Formula	*Protein*	*Carbohydrate*	*Fat*
Human milk (mature)	40% casein and 60% whey	Lactose	Human milk fat
Cow's milk	80% casein and 20% whey	Lactose	Butterfat
Enfamil Lipil	Nonfat cow's milk and whey	Lactose	Palm olein, soy, coconut, and high-oleic sunflower oils; DHA, ARA
Similac Advance	Nonfat cow's milk and whey	Lactose	High-oleic safflower oil, coconut and soy oils, DHA, ARA
ProSobee Lipil	Soy protein and methionine	Corn syrup solids	Palm olein, soy, coconut, and high-oleic sunflower oils
Isomil Advance	Soy protein and methionine	Corn syrup solids and sucrose	High-oleic safflower oil, soy and coconut oils; DHA, ARA
Nutramigen Lipil	Casein hydrolysate, cystine, tyrosine, tryptophan	Corn syrup solids and cornstarch	Palm olein, soy, coconut, and high-oleic sunflower oils; DHA, ARA
Pregestimil Lipil	Casein hydrolysate, cystine, tyrosine, tryptophan	Corn syrup solids, modified cornstarch, and dextrose	MCT, high-oleic safflower and soy oils, DHA, ARA
Alimentum Advance	Casein hydrolysate, cystine, tyrosine, tryptophan	Sucrose modified tapioca starch	Safflower oil, MCT, soy oil, DHA, ARA

Abbreviations: ARA, arachidonic acid; DHA, docosahexaenoic acid; MCT, medium-chain triglycerides.

acid (ARA) have been added to most infant formulas to simulate the higher levels found in human milk. Although research suggests that DHA and ARA supplementation may enhance visual and cognitive development in formula-fed infants, the exact degree of effect remains unclear.

Human milk from well-nourished women should provide adequate amounts of all vitamins and other micronutrients. However, vitamin K, vitamin D, iron, and fluoride are not present in sufficient quantities to satisfy all nutritional needs over a prolonged period, and supplementation should be considered. The American Academy of Pediatrics recommends that all newborns receive a prophylactic dose of 0.5 to 1 mg of parenteral vitamin K in the immediate newborn period to help prevent bleeding disorders. Even though the vitamin D content of human milk is low compared with cow's milk, infants of healthy mothers have generally not been observed to develop rickets if there is sufficient exposure to sunlight. The newborn requires about 1 minute of exposure to sunlight on the face to produce enough vitamin D. However, adequate sun exposure is difficult to assess, and there are increasing concerns over the harmful effects of sunlight. Compared to the previous recommendation of an average intake of 200 IU of vitamin D per day, the 2010 Institute of Medicine recommendation calls for an average intake of 400 IU of vitamin D per day to meet the needs of most infants younger than 12 months. Although human milk contains less iron than iron-fortified formulas (fortified to about 12 mg/L of iron), the bioavailability of the iron in human milk is greater. Breastfed infants do not need iron supplementation until 6 months of age. Exclusively breastfed infants and infants who are fed ready-to-eat formulas or formulas prepared with bottled water should all receive supplementation with 0.25 mg of fluoride per day starting at 6 months of age (see Chapter 26).

Human milk has several immunologic advantages, which are both allergy protective and infection protective, over standard cow's milk–based formulas. Its allergy protective characteristics are attributed, in part, to the decreased intestinal permeability associated with human milk compared with standard formulas. The host defense factors present in human milk include Igs, complement, and cellular components (eg, macrophages, neutrophils, lymphocytes). Studies have shown that the incidences of both viral and bacterial illnesses are lower in exclusively breastfed infants compared with their formula-fed peers.

Breastfeeding is the recommended method of infant feeding during the first 6 months of life, but it is not always possible and is occasionally contraindicated. Although maternal infection is usually not a contraindication to breastfeeding, maternal HIV infection is one exception to this recommendation in the United States. This is not necessarily true, however, in many developing countries, where the risk of death during the first year of life without breastfeeding is greater than the risk of HIV infection. Antibiotics are generally safe during breastfeeding, but certain other drugs are contraindicated.

Solid Foods

Supplemental foods may be added to infants' diets between the ages of 4 to 6 months. Solid foods should be introduced as soon as infants require the additional calories and are developmentally mature (eg, infant can sit and support the head). Early introduction of solid foods has been associated with an increased incidence of food allergy and may contribute to overeating and obesity. Factors that indicate infants may be ready for solid foods include (1) current weight twice that of birth weight, or about 13 lbs; (2) consumption of more than 32 oz of formula per day; (3) frequent feeding (regularly more than 8–10 times per day or more often than every 3 hours); and (4) persistent dissatisfaction due to hunger.

The quantity of formula should be limited to no more than 32 oz to allow for the introduction of solid foods. An iron-fortified infant cereal, most commonly rice cereal because it does not contain gluten, is usually the first solid food offered to infants. Other single-grained cereals, such as barley cereal or oatmeal, are also appropriate early supplemental foods. Fruits and vegetables may be introduced within a few weeks. The order is not as important as the need to add only one new food at a time—no more than 1 to 2 new foods per week. Meats may be introduced after 6 months of age.

Although commercially prepared infant juices are an important source of vitamin C for infants and may provide a smooth transition to solid foods, excessive juice intake may be associated with diarrhea and growth failure. About 2 oz of apple juice can be given at 4 to 6 months of age. This can be gradually increased to about 4 oz/day. Once infants have accepted the juice, juice can be mixed with a small quantity of cereal and offered to infants with a spoon. Solid foods should not be mixed in the bottle; caregivers should wait until the infant can accept spoon feedings. The vitamin C in the juice increases the bioavailability of the iron in the cereal. It is not unusual for infants to reject their first several spoonfuls of cereal because the tastes and textures are new. If they refuse the feeding, it should be stopped. Solid foods should be reintroduced in 1 week.

Precooked infant cereals, such as rice cereal, can be mixed with a variety of liquids, including human milk, formula, infant fruit juices, or water. Initially, the cereal should be mixed to a thinner consistency (eg, about 1 tablespoon of cereal to 2 oz of liquid), and once infants have accepted the new taste and texture, the mixture should gradually be worked to a thicker consistency. By about 7 to 8 months of age, infants should be taking 4 to 6 tablespoons of cereal mixed with enough liquid to give the mixture the consistency of mustard. Mixed cereal grains may be given to older infants.

A wide variety of commercially prepared baby foods designed to be developmentally appropriate and labeled by stage (ie, first, second, third stage) are available. The jars of different stages contain the amount of food that an infant at a given age should be able to eat at one sitting. This is not always the case, however, and opened jars of baby food may safely be stored in the refrigerator for 2 to 3 days. Infants should not be fed directly from the jar, because saliva on the spoon mixes with the remaining food and digests it, causing it to liquefy. Vegetables and meats may be offered at room temperature but should be warmed slightly for greater palatability. Fruits and desserts may be at room or refrigerator temperature.

First-stage foods, for infants 4 to 6 months of age, include strained infant juices; single-grain cereals; and puréed strained fruits and vegetables, such as bananas, carrots, and peas. These foods contain no egg, milk, wheat, or citrus, to which some infants may be sensitive. Second-stage foods, for infants from about 6 to 9 months of age, are smooth, mixed-ingredient foods, such as mixed vegetables, or meat dinners, such as chicken noodle. Third-stage foods, or junior foods, are for infants about 9 to 10 months of age who can sit well without support, have some teeth, and have begun self-feeding. These more coarsely textured foods contain a wider variety of nutrients, such as vegetable and meat dinner combinations. Finger foods, such as crackers, cheese wedges, or cookies, can also be introduced by 9 to 10 months of age, once infants have developed a pincer grasp. Most infants are eating the same meals as the rest of the family (table foods) by about 1 year of age. Foods that can easily be aspirated, such as raw carrots, nuts, and hard candies, should be avoided, however, until children are older than 4 years.

Baby foods can be prepared at home as long as they are finely puréed or strained and contain enough liquid to make them easy for infants to swallow. One danger of preparing foods at home is that sugar, salt, or spices can be easily added to make foods palatable to adults. These ingredients are not necessary for infants. In addition, homegrown, home-prepared vegetables may be contaminated with high levels of nitrates (eg, due to contaminated well water) and nitrites (eg, in vegetables such as carrots, beets, and spinach). Nitrates and nitrites have been implicated in the development of methemoglobinemia, especially in infants younger than 6 months. Methemoglobinemia decreases the oxygen-carrying capacity of the blood, leading to anoxic injury and death.

Weaning from the breast or bottle to a cup usually occurs at 6 to 12 months of age but may be delayed up to 18 months of age in some children. Homogenized, vitamin D–fortified cow's milk may be given at 12 months of age. Skim milk or low-fat milk (2% milk fat) should not be given before 2 years of age.

Diet of Children and Adolescents

The caloric and protein needs of children decrease in the second year of life, paralleling the decrease in growth rate during this time. Milk intake also decreases, and may drop to 16 oz/day by 24 to 36 months of age. Except for increased caloric requirements, the diet of school-aged children and adolescents should be similar to that of normal adults. Evidence that foods eaten during childhood may have long-lasting effects on adult health is increasing, and it is important that children develop healthy eating habits early in life. Atherosclerosis, osteoporosis, and obesity are some of the diseases that may have their beginnings during childhood.

A major revision to the US Department of Agriculture's (USDA) dietary guidelines and food pyramid for ages 2 and older was released in 2005. This new pyramid emphasizes physical activity, moderation, gradual improvement, personalization, portionality, and variety in food groups. A child-friendly version of this pyramid has been incorporated in the highly interactive Web site of these new dietary guidelines.

To promote lifelong heart healthy habits, the American Heart Association (AHA) released a statement of dietary recommendations for children and adolescents. It recognizes that children are often offered nutrient-poor foods that are high in fat and sugar and overly processed. The AHA recommendations support the USDA guidelines and include eating fruits and vegetables daily while limiting juice intake, using vegetable oils and soft margarines low in saturated fat and trans-fatty acids instead of butter or other animal fats, eating whole grain rather than refined grain breads and cereals, using nonfat or low-fat milk and dairy products, eating more fish, and reducing salt intake. The AHA also encourages behaviors for parents/caregivers that promote healthy habits for the whole family. These recommendations ask parents/caregivers to choose mealtimes, to provide a social context for eating by having regular family meals, to lead by example in their own eating habits, and to allow children to self-regulate food intake and not to force them to finish meals if not hungry.

Children who consume a varied diet do not need routine vitamin supplementation. However, children and teens who are considered "picky eaters," as well as children at nutritional risk, may benefit from supplementation. This includes children and teens who are anorexic or those who follow fad diets, those with chronic diseases, those who consume a vegetarian diet, and those with failure to thrive. A standard pediatric vitamin-mineral supplement should contain no more than the dietary reference intakes of its components. Parents should be counseled to teach their children that the supplements are not candy and to keep them out of reach. Serious overdoses can occur, especially with iron-containing formulations.

Bone health is determined by calcium and vitamin D intake, as well as weight-bearing physical activity. Recent data suggest the possibility of other important health benefits throughout life of these key nutrients, in addition to bone growth and development. The 2010 Institute of Medicine Guidelines call for a recommended daily allowance of 600 IU per day of vitamin D for children older than 1 year and 1,300 mg of calcium per day for children 9 to 18 years of age. Unfortunately, calcium intake for most US children, and particularly adolescents, is generally below the recommended levels. Barriers to adequate calcium intake may be due to the preference of sweetened juice and soft drinks over milk as well as lactose intolerance in certain populations. Nondairy calcium sources include salmon, white beans, broccoli, and calcium-fortified foods such as orange juice, breakfast cereals, and soy milk. Adequate calcium intake can be achieved by eating 3 (or 4 for adolescents) age-appropriate servings of dairy products or other calcium-rich food per day. In children and adolescents who do not consume adequate amounts of calcium from dietary sources, a calcium supplement is recommended. This can be in the form of a multivitamin in the younger child or in the form of calcium carbonate tablets with or without vitamin D for the adolescent.

Adolescence is a period of tremendous physical and emotional growth, both of which greatly affect nutritional needs and habits. Although their rapid physical growth requires increased energy and nutrients, the common eating habits of teens do not always support their needs. Teens tend to skip meals, eat outside the home, consume fast food and snacks, and experiment with different restrictive diets that are fad diets or various forms of vegetarianism.

Teen athletes also have their own unique nutritional concerns. They want to maximize performance while maintaining the desired physique for their particular sport or weight class. While there are many nutritional supplements, such as creatinine, carnitine, various amino acids, and dehydroepiandrosterone, that claim to enhance athletic performance, none has thus far been fully evaluated scientifically. Instead, teen athletes should be counseled on the importance of a basic nutrient: water. Proper hydration does enhance performance and prevents heat injury. Approximately 4 to 8 oz of fluid for every 15 minutes of exercise is recommended regardless of actual thirst. Carbohydrate loading before competition is believed to enhance performance; however, this practice has no effects on non-endurance events and may confer only a modest effect for endurance events by prolonging time to exhaustion. In counseling a teen athlete, specific questions should also be directed to elicit any unhealthy practices to maintain or lose weight.

Vegetarianism is gaining popularity among adolescents. Reasons for choosing vegetarianism are varied, including health benefits, means for weight loss, animal cruelty concerns, and religious beliefs. It is important to ask the vegetarian their specific restrictions as these relate to their nutritional risks. Semi-vegetarians are those who avoid red meat but eat fish and chicken in moderation. Lacto-ovovegetarians consume animal products, such as dairy and eggs, but avoid animal flesh. Vegans do not eat any animal products, such as dairy, eggs, honey, or gelatin. Those who follow a macrobiotic diet restrict not only animal products but also refined and processed foods, foods with preservatives, and foods that contain caffeine or other stimulants.

A well planned vegetarian diet can provide for all of the necessary nutrients; however, many teens experiment with vegetarianism in a nonvegetarian household and require guidance. The nutrients that may be deficient in a vegetarian diet are protein, calcium, vitamin D, vitamin B_{12}, iron, and zinc. Protein intake is usually not a concern for lacto-ovovegetarians because eggs and dairy have high-quality proteins. Vegans and macrobiotic followers have a variety of plant-based protein sources from which to choose, such as legumes, cereals, nuts, seeds, and fruits. Since vitamin B_{12} is only found in animal-based foods, vegans and macrobiotic followers must ensure adequate intake by taking supplements or consuming vitamin B_{12}-fortified foods, such as soy and nut beverages and cereals.

Lastly, familiarity with the latest fad diets is an asset for any primary care practitioner. These diets are usually restrictive in certain nutrients and recommend unusual dietary patterns that are inconsistent with current USDA guidelines. Although there are some suggestions that these diets work for some adults, there are almost no

scientific data for children and adolescents. Popular plans include Atkins and other high-fat/low-carbohydrate diets; the Zone Diet, which emphasizes a very specific ratio of protein and carbohydrates; the Ornish diet, which is extremely low fat; the South Beach Diet, which alters the types of carbohydrates for an optimal glycemic index; and the more exotic liquid or detoxification plans. To keep abreast of the latest fads, the reader is referred to the American Dietetic Association's Web site (www.eatright.org), which maintains an annual review of such popular fad diets.

Evaluation

History

Nutritional assessment begins with a complete dietary history. The dietary assessment should emphasize the quantity, quality, and variety of foods in the diet. Any special or restricted dietary habits should be noted (eg, vegetarian diet). A 3-day food record listing the types and quantities of food eaten throughout the day can be very helpful in evaluating the dietary history.

In addition, the child's routine medical, family, and social history all may influence nutritional status. For example, the economic status of families may affect the variety and type of foods that they may be able to purchase, and the level of education of parents influences their ability to understand the concepts of a healthy diet. Poverty and ignorance regarding nutritional needs are among the most common reasons for malnutrition in children. Family access to food can be estimated by asking parents about how often the family skips meals during the average month. Such information assesses food insecurity within a household. Specific cultural food preferences and feeding practices should also be included in the history.

Physical Examination

Weight, length or height, head circumference, weight for length, and body mass index (BMI) should be measured or calculated routinely and plotted on a longitudinal basis on appropriate growth curves. In addition to the charts provided by the Centers for Disease Control and Prevention, additional charts are available for special populations for which growth is altered, such as infants and children with low birth weight and prematurity, Down syndrome, Turner syndrome, William syndrome, and several other chromosomal and genetic disorders. Changes in the rate of growth over time are more useful than a single measurement in time in the assessment of nutritional problems. Calculation of the height age (age for which the child's height is at the 50th percentile), weight age (age for which the child's weight is at the 50th percentile), and ideal weight for actual height may be useful when deviations from normal are noted.

In addition to the overall impression regarding nutritional status, certain findings on physical examination may be characteristic of particular nutritional disorders. The evaluation of the hair, skin, eyes, lips and oral mucosa, dentition, and musculoskeletal system should be emphasized because the examination of these areas is most likely to show the effects of malnutrition. Muscle wasting;

hepatosplenomegaly; skeletal deformities; decayed teeth; rough, dry skin; easily pluckable hair; and irritability may all be clues to inadequate nutrition.

Laboratory Tests

Suspected malnutrition or nutrition-related disorders, based on history and physical examination, can be further investigated with laboratory studies. Tests that may be used in the evaluation of anemia, one of the most common nutrition-related disorders seen in children, include a complete blood cell count, reticulocyte count, serum iron, ferritin, and total iron-binding capacity. Investigation of suspected malnutrition begins with an assessment of protein status, with measures of indicators such as serum albumin, total protein, and prealbumin. Liver function tests and a lipid profile may also be useful in the evaluation of suspected malnutrition. Screening tests that may be used in the evaluation of failure to thrive (FTT) include thyroid function studies, urinalysis, and bone age (see Chapter 129). More specific tests, such as serum vitamin levels (eg, folate or vitamin B_{12} levels in suspected malabsorption) or hormone assays (eg, growth hormone levels in the evaluation of short stature), may be obtained in certain instances.

Common Feeding and Nutritional Problems of Childhood

Several gastrointestinal (GI) problems have been attributed to diet. A small amount of spitting up is seen in most children, especially during the first 6 months of life. However, vomiting can be a sign of several disorders, ranging from viral GI tract infections to more severe illnesses, such as pyloric stenosis, urinary tract infection, and GI obstruction (see Chapter 107). Constipation, which is seen more commonly in formula-fed than breastfed infants, may be due to insufficient fluid intake (see Chapter 111). The simple addition of 4 to 6 oz of water to an infant's diet or temporary use of apple or prune juice may solve the problem. Enemas and suppositories should not be recommended routinely.

Chronic nonspecific diarrhea of childhood, or "toddler's diarrhea," may be seen in infants and children 6 months to 5 years of age with low dietary fat intake and excessive fruit juice consumption (see Chapter 110). Failure to absorb sugars, especially sorbitol and fructose, can lead to an osmotic diarrhea.

Underfeeding or a diet that is not nutritionally balanced may result in FTT (see Chapter 129). The opposite problem, obesity, is one of the most common nutritional problems of children in the United States (see Chapter 135). The prevalence of this condition in children 6 to 11 years of age is estimated to be about 20% to 25%. Finally, the eating disorders anorexia nervosa and bulimia nervosa are estimated to affect about 1 in 100 adolescent females 16 to 18 years of age (see Chapter 133).

The "picky eater" is a common parental concern in the primary care setting. For practitioners who work with the Latino population, the child who "no come nada," literally translated as the child "does not eat anything," is a similar common parental concern. Parents can be reassured by their child's normal weight for height or BMI and

growth velocity. They should be counseled that it is normal for preschoolers to exert their individuality by limiting food preferences, the fact that it may take up to 10 exposures for a child to accept a new food, the difference between child and adult portion sizes, and the concept that children can self-regulate food intake to sustain normal growth and health.

Nutritional disorders include malnutrition and deficiencies of vitamins and minerals. Iron deficiency anemia is one of the most common nutrition-related problems seen in children and adolescents. Malnutrition is one of the leading causes of childhood morbidity and mortality worldwide. Although primary protein-calorie malnutrition (PCM) is rare in most parts of the United States, surveys conducted on pediatric wards have demonstrated that about one-third of pediatric inpatients with chronic disease have evidence of some degree of PCM. The most common deficits were weight for height below 90% of standard (ie, evidence of acute malnutrition) and height for age below 95% of standard (ie, evidence of chronic malnutrition). The 2 forms of PCM are marasmus (severe caloric depletion) and kwashiorkor (inadequate protein intake). Untreated PCM can result in impaired growth, poor intellectual development, and impaired immune functioning.

CASE RESOLUTION

The infant described in the case history is probably ready to begin some solid foods because she is consuming 32 oz of formula per day and continues to be hungry. In addition, she has reached a weight of 13 lbs and has almost doubled her birth weight. The mother is counseled to begin feeding her daughter a single-grain infant cereal mixed with either formula or juice. (The cereal should be fed by spoon, not given in a bottle.) Within a few weeks, once the infant is taking the cereal well, other first foods, such as fruits and vegetables, may be introduced.

Selected References

Abrams SA. Dietary guidelines for calcium and vitamin D: a new era. *Pediatrics.* 2011;127:566–568

American Academy of Pediatrics. *Pediatric Nutrition Handbook.* 5th ed. Kleinman RE, ed. Elk Grove Village, IL: American Academy of Pediatrics; 2004

American Dietetic Association. Food & Nutrition Information. www.eatright.org/

Cahill JB, Wagner CL. Challenges in breastfeeding. *Contemp Pediatr.* 2002;19:94–138

Chandran L. Is there a role for long-chain polyunsaturated fatty acids in infant nutrition? *Contemp Pediatr.* 2003;20:107–124

Chandran L, Gelfer P. Breastfeeding: the essential principles. *Pediatr Rev.* 2006;27:409–417

Fiocchi A, Assa'ad A, Bahna S; Adverse Reactions to Foods Committee; American College of Allergy, Asthma and Immunology. Food allergy and the introduction of solid foods to infants: a consensus document. *Ann Allergy Asthma Immunol.* 2006;97:10–21

Fiorino KN, Cox JM. Nutrition and growth. In: Robertson J, Shilkofski N, eds. *The Harriet Lane Handbook: A Manual for Pediatric House Officers.* 17th ed. St Louis, MO: Mosby; 2005:525–608

Garcia RS. No come nada. *Health Aff.* 2004;23:215–219

Gartner LM, Greer FR; American Academy of Pediatrics Section on Breastfeeding and Committee on Nutrition. Prevention of rickets and vitamin D deficiency: new guidelines for vitamin D intake. *Pediatrics.* 2003;111:908–910

Gidding SS, Dennison BA, Birch LL, et al. Dietary recommendations for children and adolescents: a guide for practitioners: consensus statement from the American Heart Association. *Circulation.* 2005;112:2061–2075

Greer FR, Krebs MD; American Academy of Pediatrics Committee on Nutrition. Optimizing bone health and calcium intake of infants, children, and adolescents. *Pediatrics.* 2006;117:578–585

Heird WC. Progress in promoting breast-feeding, combating malnutrition, and composition and use of infant formula, 1981–2006. *J Nutr.* 2007;137:499S–502S

Kleinman R. Chronic nonspecific diarrhea of childhood. *Nestle Nutr Workshop Ser Pediatr Program.* 2005;56:73–79, discussion 79–84

Larson N, Neumark-Sztainer D. Adolescent nutrition. *Pediatr Rev.* 2009; 12:494–496

Maternal and Child Health Bureau, US Department of Health and Human Services. *Growth Charts Training: Using the CDC Growth Charts for Children With Special Health Care Needs.* http://depts.washington.edu/growth/. Accessed April 11, 2007

Moilanen BC. Vegan diets in infants, children and adolescents. *Pediatr Rev.* 2004;5:174–176

Ogden CL, Kuczmarski RJ, Flegal KM, et al. Centers for Disease Control and Prevention 2000 growth charts for the United States: improvements to the 1977 National Center for Health Statistics version. *Pediatrics.* 2002;109:45–60

US Department of Agriculture. Center for Nutrition Policy and Promotion. MyPyramid for kids. www.mypyramid.gov/kids/index.html. Accessed April 10, 2007

CHAPTER 24

Breastfeeding

Julie E. Noble, MD

CASE STUDY

A 25-year-old female, pregnant with her first child, comes into your office with her husband for a prenatal visit. She would like to know what advice you can give her regarding breastfeeding. She expects a normal delivery, has had no breast surgery, and is not on any medications, but does smoke cigarettes occasionally. She plans to return to work when the baby is 4 months old.

Questions

1. What is the normal physiology of lactation?
2. What are the benefits of breastfeeding?
3. What are the contraindications to breastfeeding?
4. What management maximizes a mother's success at breastfeeding?
5. How do you manage some of the common problems that may arise during breastfeeding?

Human milk is the natural food source for human infants. It is a complete nutritional product made specifically for human infants, and all **formulas** are incomplete attempts to try to replicate it. **Human milk** is made of water, fat, lactose-containing carbohydrates, and protein, as well as vitamins, **immunoglobulins,** enzymes, hormones, and even phagocytes and lymphocytes. It is a dynamic fluid that changes in composition as the infant grows. From the early **colostrum,** which is high in lactose and protein in the form of casein and whey and very immunologically active, it matures through lactogenesis to a substance in much greater quantity with lower protein, but still immunologically active.

Epidemiology

In previous generations, infants were totally dependent on breastfeeding by their mother or a wet nurse for their survival. When formula feeding was attempted at foundling hospitals in Europe and the United States in the 1800s, the infant mortality rate was as high as 85%. Thus the advantages of breastfeeding were recognized and still promoted in the early 1900s. Following the advent of pasteurization, cow's milk formula became much safer. Formula development allowed more mothers to enter the workforce, which became a necessity during World Wars I and II. With poorer urban mothers working outside the home and upper-class mothers choosing not to breastfeed preferring the freedom that formula feeding allowed, breastfeeding rates declined over the course of the 20th century. **Formula** feeding became the norm and formula companies successfully marketed formulas as the better method to feed an infant. But current scientific understanding of the many benefits of breastfeeding for both infant and mother has been the impetus to again promote breastfeeding as the preferred food source for infants.

In the United States today following the **Healthy People 2010 initiative,** which included a national agenda calling for an increase in the rate of breastfeeding, 75% of mothers are initiating breastfeeding. But the rate of mothers sustaining breastfeeding to 1 year of age is only 22%. Rates of breastfeeding are lower in low socioeconomic groups and among women with lower levels of education. The rates also vary with different ethnic groups; in the United States the African American community has the lowest rate of breastfeeding.

Multiple health professional organizations have endorsed breastfeeding. In 1991 the World Health Organization and UNICEF developed the Baby-Friendly Hospital Initiative delineating 10 steps to undertake in the hospital to promote successful breastfeeding. This initiative is used worldwide to improve breastfeeding rates. The American Academy of Pediatrics published its policy statement, "Breastfeeding and the Use of Human Milk" in 2005. This policy endorses breastfeeding and delineates the physician responsibility to promote and support it. In 2011 the US Department of Health and Human Services issued *The Surgeon General's Call to Action to Support Breastfeeding.* There is now an imperative to promote breastfeeding in this country.

Anatomy and Physiology of Lactation

During pregnancy the breast responds to **estrogen, placental lactogen, prolactin,** and **progesterone** by enlarging. There is an increase in breast lobules and alveoli where milk is produced; and the **ductile system** grows, leading to 10 to 15 milk duct openings in the nipple. The nipples develop and the surrounding areolas enlarge. Prolactin from the anterior pituitary is inhibited by progesterone and estrogen. With the drop in these hormones after delivery, the **prolactin** is free to stimulate increased milk production. With the stimulus of suckling, **oxytocin** is released from the posterior pituitary and causes contraction of myoepithelial cells, which squeeze milk from the alveoli. Production of **milk** is dependent on infant suckling. The more the infant feeds and the more the breast is effectively emptied, the more milk will be produced.

Benefits of Breastfeeding

For the infant, the benefits to being breastfed are myriad. Studies have demonstrated that breastfed infants have a decreased incidence and severity of **infectious illnesses,** including diarrhea, respiratory infections, otitis media, bacterial meningitis, and urinary tract infections. The incidence of otitis media is 100% higher in formula-fed infants than exclusively breastfed infants. There have also been studies demonstrating better performance on **cognitive testing** among breastfed infants. Among preterm infants fed human milk, the incidence of necrotizing enterocolitis is also significantly reduced. Breastfeeding in infancy also reduces the later incidence of **atopy, allergies, asthma, childhood obesity, type 2 diabetes,** and even childhood **cancer.** Decreased rates of **sudden infant death syndrome** (see Chapter 59) have also been documented.

For the mother, an immediate benefit to breastfeeding is oxytocin-induced decreased postpartum blood loss and enhanced infant bonding. Lactation amenorrhea may serve subsequently as birth control. Breastfeeding has also been associated with decreased risk of breast cancer, ovarian cancer, and osteoporosis in the mother. There is also some evidence to suggest that breastfeeding decreases the risk of postpartum depression.

Societal benefits from breastfeeding include markedly decreased annual health care costs. An estimated savings of $10.5 billion dollars yearly could be generated if 80% of American families breastfed exclusively for the first 6 months. A decreased incidence of illness among infants would also enable mothers to miss fewer workdays, increasing their productivity and benefiting the workplace. In addition, with an increased breastfeeding rate there would be a reduction in environmental waste from bottles and **formula** containers.

Barriers to Breastfeeding

There have been many studies evaluating the barriers in the United States to breastfeeding. Understanding these barriers is essential to devising strategies for effective interventions to improve breastfeeding rates. With effective physician, nursing, and peer support, most mothers should be able to breastfeed successfully. One of the most important barriers is the lack of knowledge in pregnant women about the benefits of breastfeeding. Education beginning at the first prenatal visit is vitally important. Campaigns encouraging breastfeeding through public health venues can help with education of the general populace.

Some mothers experience embarrassment at breastfeeding. Identifying this issue and helping these mothers become more comfortable with their own body through counseling can be useful for these mothers. Physicians can also counsel the mother and family about ways to preserve privacy while breastfeeding.

Many new mothers have poor family support for breastfeeding, and sometimes the whole family needs to be included in breastfeeding counseling. The mother will not be successful if her mother is negative to the proposal.

Some mothers find that their place of employment does not make accommodations for a breastfeeding mother. It may be that the workplace needs to be reminded of laws promoting breastfeeding in the workplace. The Affordable Care Act provided a provision that the workplace needed to provide a private place for nursing mothers to pump for up to 1 year.

Hospitals may have practices or policies that interfere with successful breastfeeding, including high cesarean delivery rates or no rooming-in policy. Physicians should work with their hospitals to minimize these potential barriers.

Contraindications

The true contraindications to breastfeeding are few but need to be addressed. If an infant has **galactosemia** as detected by newborn screening, and is therefore unable to metabolize lactose or galactose, he may not breastfeed. Infants can also inherit defects in protein metabolism that may call for a special diet, precluding breastfeeding. In most states, newborn screening now includes testing for most of these metabolic disorders.

Maternal infections prohibiting breastfeeding include active, untreated tuberculosis; HIV; and human T-cell lymphotropic virus types I and II. If herpetic vesicles are present on the breast, the mother should not breastfeed.

Many medications are safe for a mother to use while breastfeeding, but each should be reviewed for potential contraindications before administering because most medications pass into **human milk.** Chemotherapeutic agents, antimetabolites, and radioactive isotopes are all contraindicated for breastfeeding. Drugs of abuse are definitely contraindicated in a breastfeeding mother, although a mother with a history of drug use may benefit from breastfeeding as long as her toxicology results are closely monitored and are negative.

Breastfeeding Management

The management of breastfeeding should begin in the prenatal period. The US Preventive Services Task Force endorses promotion and support for breastfeeding at all health care encounters. The pregnant woman should be educated by both her pediatrician and obstetrician on the benefits of breastfeeding. Her history should be reviewed for potential contraindications. If none exist, she should be encouraged to breastfeed. If she commits to breastfeeding before the baby is born, she is more likely to be successful. Involving her partner in these discussions has also been shown to improve breastfeeding success rates.

At the time of delivery if there are no complications, the infant should be dried, assigned Apgar scores and, after a screening physical examination, be placed skin-to-skin on the mother's abdomen or chest for warmth and contact. He will find his way to the breast and latch on. This early breastfeeding experience will greatly facilitate further breastfeeding. The infant should not be separated from the mother except for medical reasons. A hospital policy for rooming-in will greatly facilitate breastfeeding. A healthy full-term infant has no medical need for formula supplements.

During the hospital stay, the infant should breastfeed every 1 to 2 hours on both breasts for as long as he wants. Without pacifiers or supplemental feeds, the infant will learn to breastfeed more quickly. The mother should be counseled regarding appropriate latch-on, positioning of the infant, and manual expression of milk. Breastfeeding support should be available from all involved hospital staff, and a certified lactation consultant can be very helpful. Generally the infant should nurse at least 8 times a day. The infant should be monitored for weight, evidence of jaundice, and urination and stool patterns. A successful breastfeeding infant should urinate 3 to 5 times per day and stool 3 to 4 times per day by 3 to 5 days of age and not lose more than 7% of his birth weight. By day 5 to 7 of life he should urinate 4 to 6 times per day and pass 3 to 6 stools per day.

Vitamin K (1.0 mg intramuscularly) is indicated within the first 6 hours of life to prevent hemorrhagic disease of the newborn. The only supplement to breastfeeding that is needed is vitamin D 400 IU daily after 2 months of age to prevent rickets.

After hospital discharge the breastfeeding infant should be seen by his physician at day 3 to 5 of life and again at 2 weeks of age to support breastfeeding. Early assessment may prevent many breastfeeding problems and will allow the physician to intervene early if problems arise, preventing discontinuation of breastfeeding. New mothers need encouragement and reassurance. At each visit, the infant should be assessed for weight, feeding schedules, voiding and stooling patterns, and jaundice. The mother's breasts should be examined and a feeding observed.

The infant should exclusively breastfeed until 6 months of age. At that time an iron source is needed, and iron-fortified cereal can be given with a gradual introduction of other puréed foods. The recommendation is that breastfeeding continue until at least 1 year of age or as long as the mother and infant are content.

If a mother is returning to work, she should be counseled to initiate breastfeeding and establish a schedule. When breastfeeding is well established, she can introduce a bottle of expressed milk when the infant is about 2 months of age. When separated from the infant, she should pump her breasts at regular intervals. The milk can be saved in the refrigerator for up to 8 days or in the freezer for up to 6 months (ideal) or even 12 months (acceptable) for later use. Milk should be used within 4 to 6 hours if at room temperature. In general milk should be stored in 2- to 4-ounce bags or containers, which are labeled with the date. Many states have legislation to ensure that working mothers have time and an appropriate place in the work environment to pump. When she is back with the infant, she should put the infant to breast at the usual interval. Many mothers can work and breastfeed well past the infant's first birthday.

Sometimes pediatricians will be consulted about weaning the breastfed infant. There is no age at which weaning must occur, and in many cultures toddlers nurse until the age of 3 to 4 years. While some infants readily give up the breast, others are more reluctant to do so. There are no easy solutions to dealing with a reluctant toddler, and some suggestions include the adage, "Don't offer but don't refuse." Lactation consultants may be a valuable resource at this time.

Potential Problems

Attachment

Latching-on is the first step that is essential for successful breastfeeding. An infant with a correct latch will have the nipple and significant portion of the areola under the nipple in his mouth with his lips flanged outward. If an infant is not latching effectively, the mother will experience pain and the infant should be removed from the nipple and attached again. If problems persist, a medical professional should evaluate the mother–infant dyad for problems. Causes can include inverted nipples, flat nipples, ankyloglossia (tongue-tie), small mandible, or nipple confusion. Treatment may consist of help with positioning, nipple shields, frenectomy, or syringe feeding until the infant learns to latch.

Sore Nipples

Breastfeeding should not be painful. If the mother is experiencing pain, the infant is probably not latching correctly and may be chewing on the nipple. This may cause cracked and even bleeding nipples. The infant should be positioned on the breast to get as much of the areola in the mouth as possible. Cracked nipples can be treated with lanolin and/or hydrogel pads and repositioning. Expressed milk left to dry on cracked or bleeding nipples has healing properties. If there is significant bleeding the mother may need to pump that breast for 24 hours, while the nipple heals. The infant can be syringe fed if necessary to avoid nipple confusion. Occasionally sore nipples are secondary to a candidal infection and should be treated with an antifungal medication, such as nystatin.

Engorgement/Mastitis

When there is milk stasis for any reason, a mother may become **engorged.** The breast will appear full, firm, lumpy, and tender. Treatment is to empty the breast, and the infant is the most effective breast pump. Warm packs or a hot shower before feeding can be helpful. Sometimes an electric breast pump expedites emptying, softens the breast, and facilitates infant latching.

If a mother develops **mastitis,** a breast infection with erythema and fever, she should continue to breastfeed. Again, emptying the breast is important. Oral antibiotics and rest are mandatory. There are isolated reports of breastfed infants acquiring a bacterial infection if the mother has mastitis. Mastitis involves a cellulitis of the breast, and the organisms are usually not in the ducts or **milk.** Infants may refuse to breastfeed on an affected breast if the taste of the milk is affected. The mother may then elect to breastfeed the infant on the unaffected side and pump the affected breast. Ineffective treatment of mastitis may cause it to progress into a breast abscess. Treatment may include intravenous antibiotics and surgery. If there is frank pus coming from the nipple, the infant should not breastfeed until the discharge has resolved. The mother should pump the affected breast to empty the milk supply.

Hyperbilirubinemia/Dehydration

If infants lose more than 7% of their birth weight, they are at risk for becoming significantly dehydrated and have a higher likelihood of significant jaundice. Increased intake is necessary, and the frequency of feeds should be increased. If infants are not latching on well, expressed **milk** can be given by syringe. Infants should be closely monitored, and **formula** can be offered after breastfeeding if milk supply is insufficient. The mother should be assisted in increasing her milk supply. This may be accomplished using a breast pump because increased demand increases supply. If the infant appears significantly jaundiced, blood levels of bilirubin should be obtained. Physiological jaundice is related to hepatic immaturity with decreased conjugation of bilirubin as well as decreased excretion and mild dehydration. Breastfeeding infants tend to have higher levels of unconjugated bilirubin. Increased feeding will frequently resolve the problem as hydration status improves and frequency of stooling increases. Occasionally, especially in late preterm infants, treatment with phototherapy is needed. The infant should be evaluated for any other causes of jaundice and should be followed closely (see Chapter 113) and treated as indicated.

Resources for the Breastfeeding Mother

Many hospitals and health care organizations have lactation specialists who can assist nursing mothers and answer questions related to lactation. Health facilities may loan **electric breast pumps** to new mothers to help establish a good supply of milk. Some mothers may choose to purchase such pumps, especially if they are planning to continue to breastfeed after returning to work or to have additional children. Recent legislation has designated breast pumps as medical devices that are covered by health insurance.

Access to information can also be obtained through community agencies or national organizations such as the **La Leche League** (www.lalecheleague.org) or the Special Supplemental Nutrition Program for Women, Infants, and Children (WIC) program. Such agencies provide a resource to the clinician in assisting mothers with breastfeeding.

CASE RESOLUTION

In the case presented, the mother should be informed of the many benefits of breastfeeding to the baby, herself, and society. She should be encouraged to breastfeed because she has no contraindications. You recommend she stop cigarette smoking completely for her own health as well as the baby's. In the hospital she should request she be given her infant to breastfeed in the delivery room and continue to room-in to breastfeed every 2 hours. Reassure her that both the hospital and your office will give her support and guidance with breastfeeding. Even though she is anticipating going back to work, she should initially breastfeed exclusively. She can begin to introduce the bottle with pumped milk at 2 months of age. Her workplace should provide an area for nursing mothers to pump and refrigerate the milk. You encourage her to explore the lactation policies at her place of work.

Selected References

American Academy of Pediatrics. Policy statement: breastfeeding and the use of human milk. *Pediatrics.* 2005;115:496–511

American Academy of Pediatrics, American College of Obstetricians and Gynecologists. *Breastfeeding Handbook for Physicians.* Schanler R, Dooley S, Gartner LM, Krebs NF, Mass SB, eds. Elk Grove Village, IL: American Academy of Pediatrics; 2005

American Academy of Pediatrics, American College of Obstetricians and Gynecologists. *Guidelines for Perinatal Care.* Elk Grove Village, IL: American Academy of Pediatrics; 2007

Brenner M. You can provide efficient, effective, and reimbursable breastfeeding support—here's how. *Contemp Pediatr.* 2005;22:66–76

Chandran L, Gelfer P. Breastfeeding: the essential principles. *Pediatr Rev.* 2006;27:409–417

Chung M, et al. Interventions in primary care to promote breastfeeding: an evidence review for the US Preventive Services Task Force. *Ann Intern Med.* 2008;149:565–582

Feldman-Winter LB, Schanler RJ, O'Connor, Lawrence RA. Pediatricians and the promotion and support of breastfeeding. *Arch Pediatr Adolesc Med.* 2008;162:1142–1149

Gartner LM, Morton J, Lawrence RA, et al. American Academy of Pediatrics Section on Breastfeeding. Breastfeeding and the use of human milk. *Pediatrics.* 2005;115:496–506

Lawrence RA, Lawrence RM. *Breastfeeding: A Guide for the Medical Profession.* Philadelphia, PA: Saunders; 2010

US Department of Health and Human Services. *The Surgeon General's Call to Action to Support Breastfeeding.* Washington, DC: US Department of Health and Human Services, Office of the Surgeon General; 2011

US Preventive Services Task Force. Primary care interventions to promote breastfeeding: US Preventive Services Task Force recommendation statement. *Ann Intern Med.* 2008;149:560–564

Wellstart International. *Lactation Management Self-Study Modules, Level I.* 2nd ed. San Diego, CA: Wellstart International; 2004

CHAPTER 25

Sleep: Normal Patterns and Common Disorders

Geeta Grover, MD

CASE STUDY

During a routine 6-month health maintenance visit, a mother states that although her 6-month-old son falls asleep very easily at about 10:00 pm every night while breastfeeding, he wakes every 2 to 3 hours and cries until she nurses him back to sleep. A review of the dietary history reveals that the infant is breastfed about every 3 hours and was begun on rice cereal 2 weeks ago. His immunizations are current. The boy has no medical problems, and his physical examination is normal.

Questions

1. How old are most infants when they can begin to sleep through the night (at least 5 hours at a stretch) without a feeding?
2. What factors contribute to frequent nighttime wakings during infancy?
3. What advice can be given to parents to facilitate an infant's sleeping through the night?
4. What are sleep disturbances experienced by older children and adolescents?

Sleep disorders are common during infancy and childhood. Getting children to go to bed, fall asleep, stay asleep, and stay in bed can be no small challenge. Parents frequently ask pediatricians about sleep-related problems at routine health maintenance visits. Age-appropriate suggestions on how to help children sleep well are usually welcomed by parents.

Epidemiology

Sleep problems are one of the most common concerns seen in pediatric practice. Bedtime struggles and frequent night wakings occur in 20% to 25% of children younger than 3 years. In preschool-aged children, nighttime fears (eg, fear of noises, fear of the dark) or separation anxiety often contributes to these problems. Estimates of parent-reported sleep problems in school-aged children range between 11% and 40%. As children get older, nightmares and night terrors may contribute to night wakings. About 5% of individuals experience nightmares, which usually begin before the age of 10 years and are seen more often in girls than in boys. Night terrors are a specific form of partial night waking from deep sleep that may begin during the preschool years. The incidence in children is reported to be between 1% and 4%, with the greatest frequency between 5 and 7 years of age. Such terrors are more common in boys than in girls, and a familial tendency has been reported. Febrile illness and obstructive sleep apnea may be predisposing factors.

In most Western countries, children are expected to sleep in their own beds. However, in many cultures, it is not uncommon for infants and young children to sleep in their parents' bed (the "family bed"). Bedsharing in infants younger than 10 to 12 weeks is associated with a higher incidence of sudden infant death syndrome, especially if the mother smokes. Accidental asphyxia from overlaying or the presence of soft bedding or overheating may contribute to bedsharing-related deaths. Parents should always be advised about safe sleeping practices (see Chapter 39). In older infants and children, cosleeping is not a problem in and of itself, and the decision to cosleep, like the decision to breastfeed or bottle-feed, is an entirely personal one. Most infants who share a bed with their parents have sleep onset associations to facilitate falling asleep. Therefore, parents who share a bed with their young children commonly have to lie down with them for 20 to 30 minutes to get them to fall asleep. Several studies have shown that cosleeping infants are 2 to 3 times more likely to have night awakenings than those who sleep alone. Furthermore, infants who are both breastfeeding and bedsharing sleep the shortest periods prior to awakening. Parents who only plan on cosleeping with their infants for a limited period will need a clear transition plan, such as ending this practice by 5 to 6 months of age, before the infants are old enough to object excessively. For children with sleep problems, bedsharing is not a good solution. However, in the absence of any preexisting sleep problems or psychological concerns, cosleeping, as a lifestyle choice, has not been associated with any long-term developmental, behavioral, or psychological problems in the cosleeping children.

Clinical Presentation

Parents may raise concerns about their child's sleep pattern during a routine health maintenance visit. Because some parents may be reluctant to "bother" their physician with such seemingly minor concerns, the physician should routinely question parents about their children's sleep patterns and offer anticipatory guidance as appropriate.

Pathophysiology

To understand disturbances associated with sleep, the physiology of normal sleep and the development of normal sleep behavior in children must be understood.

Sleep States

Normal sleep has 2 distinct states, **rapid eye movement (REM)** and **non–rapid eye movement (NREM)** sleep. Rapid eye movement sleep develops at about 29 weeks' gestation and then persists throughout life. It is an active, lighter stage of sleep that occurs in association with rapid eye movements. Other features of REM sleep include suppression of muscle tone; rapid, irregular pulse and respiratory rate; and body twitches. Dreams occur during REM sleep. The electroencephalogram (EEG) pattern of REM sleep is very similar to stage 1 NREM sleep.

Non–rapid eye movement sleep begins at about 32 to 35 weeks' gestation. During NREM sleep, pulse and respiratory rates are slower and more regular, and body movements are minimal. Most of the restorative functions of sleep occur during this state. After the first several months of life, NREM sleep may be divided into 4 stages ranging from drowsiness to very deep sleep. Each stage represents a progressively deeper state of sleep and has a characteristic EEG tracing: stage 1 has low-voltage, fast activity; stage 2 is notable for the presence of sleep spindles and K complexes against a low-voltage background; and stages 3 and 4 are identified by varying amounts of high-amplitude, slow waves known as delta waves.

The Sleep Cycle

Rapid eye movement and NREM sleep together make up the sleep cycle. Typically, the deepest sleep takes place during the first several hours of the night, with lighter stages of NREM sleep and REM sleep occurring during most of the rest of the night. Although sleep stages are the same in both infants and adults, several differences concerning the onset and duration of REM and NREM sleep between infants and adults exist. First, the sleep cycle is shorter in infants (50–60 minutes) than in adults (90–100 minutes), which means that infants have more periods of active REM sleep compared with adults. Second, the total amount of time spent in REM sleep decreases with increasing age. Term newborns spend about 50% of their total sleep time in REM sleep (up to 80% in premature infants); this decreases to about 30% by 3 years of age and to 20% by adulthood. Third, infants may have very little REM latency, entering their first REM cycle very shortly after falling asleep. Adults, in comparison, generally enter their first REM period about 90 minutes after the onset of sleep.

Sleep-Wake Patterns

Sleep patterns follow a normal developmental sequence in children; the amount of sleep children need changes with maturation (Figure 25-1). Healthy term newborns sleep 16 to 17 hours per day. Because they are unable to sleep for more than a few hours at a time, sleeping and waking periods are fairly evenly distributed throughout the day and night. Many infants are able to sleep through the night (at least 5 hours uninterrupted) by the age of 3 months; most infants are capable of this by 4 months. Brief arousals are a normal part of the sleep cycle at all ages, but children should be able to return to sleep on their own without requiring parents' attention. Children should definitely be able to fall asleep on their own by the age of 4 to 6 months. Otherwise, parental participation to fall asleep becomes required at every awakening throughout the night.

By 12 months of age, infants sleep about 14 hours per day, divided into 2 naps during the day, and a period of about 10 hours at night. During the second year of life, most children stop napping in the

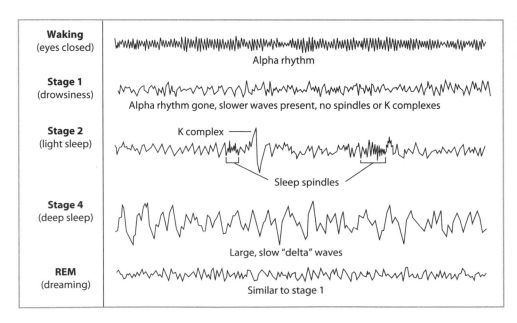

Waking (eyes closed)	
	Alpha rhythm
Stage 1 (drowsiness)	
	Alpha rhythm gone, slower waves present, no spindles or K complexes
Stage 2 (light sleep)	K complex
	Sleep spindles
Stage 4 (deep sleep)	
	Large, slow "delta" waves
REM (dreaming)	
	Similar to stage 1

Figure 25-1. **Typical sleep patterns in childhood.** (Reproduced with permission from Ferber R. *Solve Your Child's Sleep Problems.* New York, NY: Simon & Schuster; 1985:19.)

morning. By 2 years of age, they require about 13 hours of sleep per day (1–2 hours in an afternoon nap and 11–12 hours at night). Most children take an afternoon nap until 3 years of age, and some children continue this until 5 years of age. The amount of nighttime sleep children need gradually continues to decline, decreasing from about 12 hours during the preschool years to about 8 to 9 hours during adolescence.

Sleep Abnormalities

The etiology of sleep disorders can be complex, involving the interaction of children's temperamental characteristics, psychosocial stressors in the home, parental childrearing philosophies, and the developmental nature of normal sleep states and sleep cycles.

Differential Diagnosis

The differential diagnosis of sleep disorders may be distinguished by problems associated with falling asleep or frequent night wakings (Box 25-1). Falling asleep may present 2 types of difficulties: problems associated with settling children to sleep and bedtime refusal.

In infants, **inappropriate sleep-onset associations** are the most common reason for difficulty settling to sleep. These infants require parental participation (eg, holding, rocking, feeding) to fall asleep. They have not learned the critical skills of self-calming and initiating sleep on their own. Because these infants do not have the self-soothing behaviors necessary to fall back asleep after normal nighttime arousals, they may also have nighttime wakings. Brief arousals are a normal component of sleep. Nighttime wakings are different, because parents' participation is needed to resettle children. The difficulty that the children experience falling back to sleep on their own, not the waking itself, is the problem.

An example of an inappropriate sleep-onset association is the child who needs to be breastfed or bottle-fed to fall asleep. The term **trained night feeder** has been coined to describe children who need to be fed before going back to sleep after normal nighttime awakenings. Although they are developmentally old enough to receive all nutrition during the day, they have become conditioned to require nighttime feedings. These children are often breastfed or bottle-fed until they fall asleep and only then placed in the crib. They are conditioned to require feeding to initiate sleep, and when they experience normal nighttime arousals, they require the breast or bottle to go back to sleep.

The term **trained night crier** refers to children who, like trained night feeders, lack the self-comforting and self-initiating skills necessary to fall asleep on their own. Trained night criers awaken; cry; and want to be held, comforted, or entertained before they can go back to sleep.

Acute illness may also be a cause of sleep disturbances. Children with otitis media may awaken at night because of pain. They may continue to experience awakenings after the infection has resolved, however, and require comforting or some sort of attention to fall asleep again.

Box 25-1. Practical Approach to the Differential Diagnosis of Sleep Disorders in Children

Difficulty Falling Asleep

Circadian and sleep schedule disturbances
- Irregular sleep-wake patterns
- Advanced sleep phase
- Delayed sleep phase
- Regular but inappropriate sleep schedules without phase shifts (eg, late evening naps)

Habits, associations, and expectations
- Inappropriate sleep-onset associations
- Bedtime refusal/bedtime struggles
- Poor or inconsistent limit setting

Overstimulation

Psychosocial
- Separation anxiety
- Nighttime fears (eg, fears of the dark, monsters)
- Family and social stresses

Medical
- Acute illness
- Underlying medical problems
- Medications (eg, antihistamines, stimulants, codeine, anticonvulsants)

Nighttime Waking

Normal variation (eg, breastfed infant)

Habits, associations, and expectations
- Inappropriate sleep-onset associations (eg, age-inappropriate night wakings for feeding)

Psychosocial
- Nighttime fears
- Family and social stresses

Medical
- Acute illness
- Underlying medical problem
- Medications

Nightmares

Arousal disorders (eg, night terrors, sleepwalking, and sleep talking)

Miscellaneous Sleep Disorders

Intrinsic sleep disorders
- Narcolepsy
- Sleep apnea (obstructive or central)
- Restless leg syndrome
- Periodic leg movements

Sleep-wake transition disorders (eg, head banging, rocking)

In children between the ages of 9 and 18 months, **separation** and **separation anxiety** may also affect sleep patterns. Children may cry when parents leave the room and have difficulty settling to sleep. Ability to climb out of the crib or bed can be associated with night-time wakings in older toddlers. The transition from a crib to a bed is usually made between 2 and 3 years of age. Children who can climb out of their cribs or beds may come out of their rooms repeatedly for drinks of water, trips to the bathroom, or to sleep in the parents' bed. Such factors as nighttime fears of the dark influence sleep behaviors during the preschool years (3–5 years of age). Children's growing needs for autonomy and control over their environment may lead to bedtime refusals during both the toddler and preschool years.

Disorders of the sleep-wake cycle may contribute to sleep schedule irregularities. Circadian rhythms govern the regularity and degree of wakefulness and sleepiness. The circadian clock inherent in humans is not an exact 24-hour pattern but can be modified or entrained onto one by environmental cues. Regular and consistent structure needs to be provided by parents because development of children's sleep-wake rhythms depends on an interaction of the child's inherent biological rhythms with the environment. Entrainment requires predictable occurrence of time cues such as light and dark, mealtime, and bedtime. A consistent waking time in the morning is one of the most important of these cues.

Irregular sleep-wake cycles may be seen in children living in chaotic environments with irregular mealtimes and sleep-wake schedules. A delayed sleep phase and regular but inappropriate sleep-wake schedule are the most common forms of sleep rhythm disturbance. Children with **delayed sleep phase** have a resetting of their circadian rhythm; they are not sleepy at bedtime and have excessive morning sleepiness. This is a common problem because the inherent circadian clock has a cycle closer to 25, not 24, hours. This clock has not been entrained to a 24-hour schedule in these children.

Examples of **regular but inappropriate sleep-wake schedules** include children who nap at the "wrong" time (eg, a child who regularly naps at 7:00 pm for 1 hour and then has trouble going to bed at 9:00 pm) and infants who seem to have day and night confused. These children sleep most of the day and stay up most of the night.

Night terrors (pavor nocturnus), **sleepwalking** (somnambulism), and **sleeptalking** (somniloquy) are all forms of partial awakenings that occur during deep or stage 4 NREM sleep, most often during the transition from stage 4 NREM sleep to the first REM sleep period. Sleepwalking and sleeptalking usually occur during the school-aged years, whereas night terrors begin during the preschool years.

Both nightmares and night terrors may begin during the preschool years and may continue throughout childhood. Night terrors are different from nightmares and occur during a different stage of the sleep cycle (Table 25-1). With night terrors, children usually sit up in bed and cry or scream inconsolably for up to 15 minutes. They may appear dazed and have signs of autonomic arousal, such as tachycardia, tachypnea, and sweating. These children cannot be consoled. When they finally go back to sleep, they do not remember

Table 25-1. Nightmares Versus Night Terrors		
Characteristic	**Nightmare**	**Night Terror**
Time of night	Late	Early, usually within 4 hours of bedtime
Sleep stage	Rapid eye movement sleep	Partial arousal from deep non–rapid eye movement sleep
State of child	Scared, but consolable	Disoriented, confused, and inconsolable
Memory of event	Clear recall of dream	Usually none
Return to sleep	Reluctant because of fear	Easily, unless fully awakened
Management	Reassure child	Reassure parents

the event in the morning. Because parents are often frightened by the experience, they may think the child is having a seizure or is suffering from an emotional disturbance and may seek medical advice. Although attacks may be precipitated by stressful events or fatiguing daytime activities, night terrors do not indicate excessive stress or emotional disturbance in children's lives unless they recur.

Nightmares usually occur during the last third of the night during REM sleep, whereas night terrors more often take place during the early part of the night. Nightmares are scary dreams that may awaken children, who can often remember them. Children can usually be consoled by parents but are reluctant to go back to sleep because of their fears.

Excessive daytime sleepiness can be a symptom of medical problems such as depression, sleep apnea, narcolepsy, or illness. Viral illness is perhaps the most common medical cause of such sleepiness in children. Inadequate sleep at night may also be a potential cause of sleepiness during the day. Screening for daytime impairments (eg, decline in academic performance or inattention) is important in children suspected of having sleep disorders. Primary sleep disorders, such as obstructive sleep apnea, have been shown to be associated not only with excessive daytime sleepiness, but also with cognitive deficits and impaired attentional capacity.

Narcolepsy, a disorder of excessive sleepiness, is characterized by an overwhelming desire to sleep during the daytime despite adequate sleep at night. Its symptoms include excessive daytime sleepiness, cataplexy, sleep paralysis, and hypnagogic hallucinations. Cataplexy is an abrupt loss of muscle tone that is usually precipitated by an emotional reaction, such as laughter or anger. Sleep paralysis is an inability to move or speak that occurs as patients fall asleep or awaken. Hypnagogic hallucinations, which can be visual or auditory, occur while falling asleep. Narcolepsy affects about 0.05% to 0.1% of the general population. The prevalence increases to 50% of family members when the family history is positive. The exact genetic basis of inheritance is unknown. The age of onset is usually between 10 and 20 years. The diagnosis is often delayed or missed for months to years in some cases because not all symptoms may be present initially. Diagnosis is important because pharmacologic therapy with central nervous system (CNS) stimulants may provide some symptomatic relief.

Sleep-related breathing disorders (SRBD) occur across a spectrum with habitual snoring as the least severe form and **obstructive sleep apnea syndrome (OSAS)** as the most severe form. Risk factors associated with the development of SRBD include obesity, presence of chronic sinus problems, recurrent wheezing, nasal allergies, family history of obstructive sleep apnea, and certain disorders that present with craniofacial abnormalities (eg, Down syndrome and Prader-Willi syndrome). Obstructive sleep apnea syndrome in children is a disorder of breathing during sleep. It is characterized by prolonged partial upper airway obstruction and/or intermittent complete obstruction (obstructive apnea) that disrupts normal gas exchange and normal sleep patterns. Risk factors for OSAS include adenotonsillar hypertrophy, obesity, craniofacial anomalies, and neuromuscular disorders. Obstructive sleep apnea syndrome is thought to be secondary to a combination of adenotonsillar hypertrophy and reduced neuromuscular tone of the upper airway during sleep. Large tonsils and adenoids alone do not necessarily indicate that the child has OSAS. Symptoms include nightly snoring (often with intermittent pauses or gasps), disturbed sleep, and daytime neurobehavioral problems. Obstructive sleep apnea syndrome should be distinguished from **primary snoring,** which is defined as snoring without obstructive apnea, arousals from sleep, or abnormalities in gas exchange. Obstructive sleep apnea syndrome can not only disturb the quality of sleep but can also cause potentially serious complications, such as failure to thrive and, in severe cases, cor pulmonale.

Restless leg syndrome, or periodic leg movements, is a recently described condition characterized by uncomfortable creeping or crawling feelings, mainly occurring in the lower extremities, when the child is resting or inactive and relieved by movement. The condition may be attributed to growing pains in younger children (see Chapter 103) and can be associated with delayed sleep onset.

Evaluation

History

Evaluation of children with sleep difficulties begins with a thorough, detailed sleep history taken from both parents and children, if old enough (Questions Box). The use of a specific screening questionnaire, such as the Children's Sleep Habits Questionnaire by Judith Owens, MD, may facilitate the evaluation. It is designed to screen for the most common sleep problems in children aged 4 to 12 years and is available online at www.kidzzzsleep.org. It is not intended to be used to diagnose specific sleep disorders, but rather to identify children possibly needing further evaluation. Dr Owens has also developed a simple screening acronym, "BEARS" (bedtime resistance/sleep onset delay; excessive daytime sleepiness; awakenings at night; regularity, patterns, and duration of sleep; and snoring and other symptoms), which can be useful as an initial screen to determine if further assessment may be necessary.

Questions

Sleep

- Does the child have regular nap times and bedtimes, or do these depend on changing parental schedules?
- What time does the child go to bed?
- What does the child do in the hour before bedtime? Is there a consistent bedtime routine?
- Where does the child sleep (eg, ask about cosleeping, noise, temperature)?
- Is the child able to fall asleep on his or her own, or does he or she require the parent's participation?
- Does the child require feeding or fluids at night?
- When does the problem occur relative to bedtime and what does the child do (detailed explanation)?
- How often does the problem occur?
- How long has the child been having sleep problems?
- How does the parent respond?
- Does the child snore?
- When does the child wake up in the morning? Is the child difficult to awaken?
- Is the child sleepy during the day?
- How much caffeine does the child consume (eg, in coffee, tea, soda, chocolate)?
- Is the child taking any medications?
- Is there a family history of sleep disturbances?
- Is there any stress within the home due to marital or financial difficulties that may affect the home environment and cause the child to be anxious or stressed?

Evaluation should also include an assessment of children's temperament and psychological well-being. Children's developmental status and level of function should also be evaluated. Children with developmental, neurologic, and psychological concerns have higher rates of sleep disturbances. For example, it is estimated that 25% to 50% of children with attention-deficit/hyperactivity disorder seen in clinical practice will have sleep problems, especially difficulties in initiating and maintaining sleep.

Physical Examination

Physical examination is important to rule out organic causes of sleep difficulties. Special attention should be paid to the airway and nervous system. Acute illness (eg, otitis media), obstructive sleep apnea resulting from adenoidal or tonsillar hypertrophy (most commonly), colic, gastroesophageal reflux, and any CNS disease or abnormality may all alter the sleep-wake cycle.

Laboratory Tests

In most cases, a detailed history and physical examination should be sufficient to establish the reason for the sleep disturbance. Laboratory assessment is usually not necessary. Further evaluation, when warranted, should be tailored to the child's clinical presentation. An EEG may be useful if a central abnormality, such as a seizure disorder, is suspected. Polysomnography, the simultaneous monitoring of EEG, electrocardiogram, chin muscle tone, eye movements, and respirations during a night of sleep in a sleep laboratory, may be very useful in certain children when significant sleep disturbances, such as nocturnal seizures, narcolepsy, or OSAS, are suspected. Any child suspected of a sleep-related breathing disorder (eg, history of snoring or abnormal breathing during sleep) should be evaluated for OSAS.

Management

The goal of management is to help children develop a healthy pattern of sleeping, not simply eliminate the immediate problem. Healthy sleep associations include providing a consistent schedule of naps and bedtime, along with a pleasant bedtime routine. It is important to put infants in their cribs while they are relaxed and drowsy but not already asleep. This gives them the opportunity to develop skills to put themselves to sleep. If they become accustomed to being fed or rocked until they fall asleep, they will seek the same means of falling asleep every time they normally wake up during the night. In addition, overstimulation in the evening may make settling to sleep difficult for toddlers or young children. Instead, a routine such as a bath followed by a story in the child's bedroom with a clearly defined endpoint when the parent leaves the child in the crib or bed sleepy but awake may help facilitate sleep. Children must learn to fall asleep on their own.

Trained night feeders and trained night criers are infants who have not learned to fall asleep on their own. The basic treatment for these children is to put them in their cribs when they are sleepy but awake and ignore the subsequent crying. Their last memory before falling asleep should not be of their mothers holding or feeding them. If the crying persists, the contact with the infants should be brief and boring. Scheduled awakening is a technique in which infants are slightly aroused by the parent 15 to 60 minutes before an expected spontaneous awakening in an effort to prevent spontaneous awakening. Scheduled awakenings may be an effective treatment alternative for some trained night criers. If infants awaken for a feeding, parents should try to stretch the interval between waking and feeding so that children have an opportunity to practice self-calming techniques. Specific sleep disorders can be addressed individually. Older toddlers and preschoolers who delay going to bed or refuse to stay in their rooms at night need clear, firm limits. It is important that these children have consistent bedtime routines and nighttime interventions for when they awaken. A gate may need to be installed in the bedroom doorway to prevent children who refuse to stay in their rooms at night from moving about the house and potentially hurting themselves or disturbing others. Parents of children who have night terrors may require reassurance that their children are not suffering from significant emotional problems or stressors. A night-light may help alleviate the anxieties of preschoolers who are unable to sleep at night because of their fears of darkness. Disturbances of the sleepwake schedule can be corrected over time by gradually shifting children's schedules in the desired direction. For example, children with a delayed sleep phase who go to bed very late can have their morning wake-up time progressively advanced about 15 minutes per day; this is followed by a progressive advancement in their bedtime until the desired schedule is reached.

Implementation of good sleep hygiene practices is an important first step for school-aged children and adolescents who are experiencing sleep problems, especially sleep-onset problems. Sleep hygiene refers to the establishment and maintenance of schedules and conditions conducive to healthy, restorative sleep. Good sleep hygiene practices are outlined in Box 25-2. It is important to remember that adolescents require at least as much sleep as they did as preadolescents—about 9 hours of sleep per night. Referral to a sleep specialist may be necessary for some children, especially when significant sleep disturbances, such as narcolepsy, nocturnal seizures, or OSAS, are suspected.

Prognosis

Unfortunately, infants with sleep problems tend to grow into children with sleep problems. Researchers have found that about 40% of infants with sleep problems at the age of 8 months still had a problem at 3 years. It is to the parents' advantage to help their children develop healthy sleep habits rather than ignore the problems and hope that the children outgrow them.

Box 25-2. Good Sleep Hygiene
Environment
• Dark
• Quiet
• Comfortably cool
Schedule
• Regular bedtime
• Regular waking time
• Naps, if needed, should be early in the day with consistent time and duration
General
• No frightening/stimulating television or stories and no vigorous physical activities in the hour before bedtime
• Limit caffeine, especially after lunchtime
• Consistent and calming bedtime routine
• Consistent soothing methods
• Children put to bed drowsy but awake

CASE RESOLUTION

The 6-month-old infant described in the case history has disordered sleep associations. He has been conditioned to nighttime feedings, although he is old enough not to require them for nutrition. The physician suggests several things the mother can do to try to solve her son's sleep problem. She can begin by gradually lengthening the interval between daytime feedings to 4 to 5 hours. When he cries at night, she can wait progressively longer before feeding him and can then eventually eliminate the feedings altogether. He will learn to fall asleep on his own without requiring feeding.

Selected References

Ferber R. *Solve Your Child's Sleep Problems: New Revised and Expanded Edition.* New York, NY: Fireside; 2006

Givan DC. The sleepy child. *Pediatr Clin North Am.* 2004;51:15–31

Howard BJ, Wong J. Sleep disorders. *Pediatr Rev.* 2001;22:327–341

Moturi S, Avis K. Assessment and treatment of common pediatric sleep disorders. *Psychiatry.* 2010;7:24–37

Okami P, Weisner T, Olmstead R. Outcome correlates of parent-child bedsharing: an eighteen-year longitudinal study. *J Dev Behav Pediatr.* 2002;23:244–253

Owens JA. The ADHD and sleep conundrum: a review. *J Dev Behav Pediatr.* 2005;26:312–322

Owens JA, Dalzell V. Use of the 'BEARS' sleep screening tool in a pediatric residents' continuity clinic: a pilot study. *Sleep Med.* 2005;6:63–69

Owens JA, Moturi S. Pharmacologic treatment of pediatric insomnia. *Child Adolesc Psychiatr Clin N Am.* 2009;18:1001–1016

Pohl CA, Renwick A. Putting sleep disturbances to rest. *Contemp Pediatr.* 2002;19:74–96

Shamseer L, Vohra S. Complementary, holistic, and integrative medicine: melatonin. *Pediatr Rev.* 2009;30:223–228

Sheldon SH. Parasomnias in childhood. *Pediatr Clin North Am.* 2004;51:69–88

Wilson TA. Infant sleep—have you slept lately? *Pediatr Rev.* 2007;28:163

CHAPTER 26

Oral Health and Dental Disorders

Charlotte W. Lewis, MD, MPH

CASE STUDY

The parents of a 9-month-old girl bring her to the office because they are concerned that their daughter has no teeth yet. Growth and development have proceeded normally, and the physical examination is unremarkable.

Questions
1. What is the mean age and range for the eruption of the first tooth?
2. What is meant by *mixed dentition?*
3. When should oral hygiene using a toothbrush begin?

Dental caries comprises the most common chronic disease of childhood. Pediatricians and other health care providers often see young children multiple times before children have their first dental visit. Primary care providers are thus in a prime position to counsel families on preventive oral health and to identify early signs of dental decay so that timely treatment can occur. In 2003 the American Academy of Pediatrics issued a recommendation that pediatricians and other pediatric health care providers begin regular oral health anticipatory guidance and risk assessment before patients are 6 months old. This recommendation affirms the essential need for clinicians to educate themselves on normal and abnormal patterns of dental eruption and occlusion, early and advanced signs of dental caries and its complications, and appropriate preventive oral hygiene practices. Establishing collaborative partnerships with community dentists is helpful in promoting ongoing clinician and family education and appropriate patient referrals.

Epidemiology

Among 5- to 17-year-olds, dental caries is 5 times more common than asthma. Sixty percent of children have at least one or more filled or decayed primary teeth by the age of 5 years and three-quarters of all 17-year-olds have experienced at least one carious lesion in their permanent dentition. Certain groups are at increased risk for earlier and more severe dental caries. Both individual and population risk factors for caries are listed in Box 26-1. Toothache, a complication of dental caries, afflicts millions of US children; in 2007, 14% of 6- to 12-year-olds had experienced a toothache within the previous 6 months. Toothache disproportionately affects children who are poor, minority, and have special health care needs. Occlusal abnormalities are also common in children. At least 30% of the population is estimated to have moderate to severe orthodontic needs.

Box 26-1. Population and Individual Risk Factors for Dental Decay

Population Risk Factors
- Low socioeconomic status
- Recent immigrant
- Latino, Native American, and other non-white race/ethnicity
- No dental insurance or limited access to professional dental care

Individual Risk Factors
- Currently active decay or history of decay in patient
- History of high amount of dental decay in mother or siblings
- Frequent and/or prolonged intake of foods containing fermentable carbohydrate (or frequent/ongoing use of liquid medications prepared with sucrose)
- Presence of visible plaque on the teeth
- Exposed root surfaces
- Impaired ability to maintain oral hygiene (eg, developmentally disabled or otherwise handicapped individuals)
- Inadequate exposure to fluoride
- Reduced salivary flow
- History of radiation therapy to head and/or neck
- Wearing of orthodontic appliances or prostheses

Clinical Presentation

Dental development begins in utero. Subsequently, the teeth erupt into the upper or **maxillary** jaw and into the lower or **mandibular** portion of the jaw. Teeth have a crown and root section (Figure 26-1). The **crown** is the visible portion of the tooth. The **root** is that part contained within the socket of the alveolar bone. The outer, hard coating of the crown is the **enamel.** Beneath the enamel is the

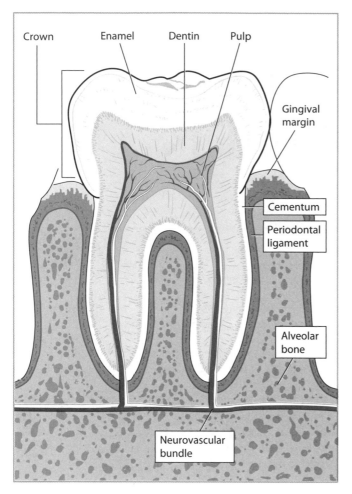

Figure 26-1. **Tooth anatomy.**

dentin, composed of microtubules for transport of nutrients from the pulp to the outer portions of the tooth. The **pulp** contains nerves and vascular structures critical for the health and viability of the tooth. Teeth are anchored to the jaw through **periodontal ligaments.**

There are 20 **primary or deciduous teeth,** which erupt between approximately 6 and 36 months of age (Figure 26-2). The first primary teeth to erupt typically are the lower **central incisors.** These teeth erupt on average at 6 to 10 months of age. A simple but not always precise rule of thumb is that the first tooth erupts at 6 months of age and then one tooth per month erupts until all primary teeth have erupted by about 24 to 30 months of age. In the normal pattern of primary tooth eruption, the incisors erupt followed by eruption of the first molars, then canines (cuspids), and finally the second molars (hence the helpful mnemonic for primary eruption order in each quadrant of the mouth: forward-forward-back-forward-back for incisor-incisor-first molar-cuspid-second molar). There is variation in the timing of tooth eruption in the population, and normal tooth eruption can vary by 6 to 12 months from average. The eruption process may occasionally be preceded by a bluish discoloration to the gum, called an **eruption hematoma,** a benign process. More often eruption of the primary teeth is associated with more generalized symptoms, such as fussiness and drooling. These symptoms are commonly referred to as *teething.* **Teething** does not cause diarrhea, respiratory infections, or true fever, although these entities may be present coincidentally with tooth eruption in infants.

The primary teeth are replaced by the **permanent teeth** (Figure 26-2), which begin eruption at approximately 6 years of age. Both permanent and primary teeth are present during the **mixed dentition phase,** which occurs between 6 and 13 years of age. Early mixed dentition is sometimes referred to as the "ugly duckling" stage

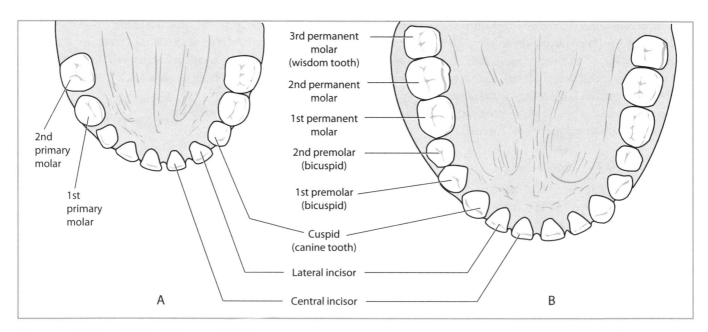

Figure 26-2. **A. Primary dentition. B. Permanent dentition.**

because the permanent dentition looks large and awkward relative to the remaining primary teeth and because there may be transient malpositioning of the teeth. There are normally 32 permanent teeth; the last to erupt are the **third molars,** commonly known as **wisdom teeth,** at about 17 to 21 years of age.

Variations from the normal in number of teeth are not uncommon. **Hypodontia** refers to fewer than normal teeth. The most common teeth to be congenitally absent are the third molars, second premolars, or maxillary lateral incisors. Congenital absence of a central incisor is distinctly uncommon and should raise concern for the presence of other midline defects. Several teeth may be missing in disorders such as **Down syndrome** or **ectodermal dysplasia. Anodontia** is the congenital absence of teeth. Extra teeth are called **supernumerary teeth.** Children may be born with teeth already erupted, known as **natal teeth.** Teeth that erupt shortly after birth are referred to as **neonatal teeth** if their eruption occurs in the first month of life. These teeth are usually incisors, and at least 90% represent normal dentition, rather than supernumerary teeth. The presence of natal or neonatal teeth may be familial, and on rare occasion may suggest an underlying syndrome. In addition to variations in number of teeth, teeth may also demonstrate variations in color and structure due to abnormalities in the tooth development, trauma, or extrinsic factors.

Caries may occur anytime after eruption of the teeth. **Early childhood caries** (ECC), a more general term referring to what in the past was called *baby bottle tooth decay or nursing bottle caries,* affects a substantial portion of children. The pattern of decay seen in ECC is different from that seen in the teeth of older children and adults. Typically ECC first affects the maxillary incisors and spares the lower incisors. This pattern of decay is hypothesized to result from prolonged and frequent exposure of the teeth to sweet liquids, for example, falling asleep with a juice bottle in the mouth, whereby the beverage pools around the upper incisors but the lower teeth are protected by the overlying tongue. The **pit and fissure surfaces** of the molars are more likely sites of decay in older children. Fermentable carbohydrates, particularly those of a sticky nature, become embedded in these surfaces and are not easily reached by the bristles of a toothbrush. This allows for prolonged action of acid-producing bacteria and subsequent caries formation.

In its earliest stages, caries appear on physical examination as white, opaque areas at the gum line **(white spot lesions).** At this early stage the lesion is potentially reversible if remineralization can occur. However, once the decay has eroded the enamel, irreversible damage has occurred. Symptoms differentiate the degree and depth of caries involvement; however, young children often have difficulty localizing dental pain. A cavity into the dentin may produce intermittent pain, especially on exposure to temperature change or pressure on the affected tooth. Once cavitation has extended into the pulp, the resulting pulpitis may cause severe, persistent, often throbbing pain in the affected tooth, possibly awakening the child from sleep. Eventually the pulp undergoes necrosis and pain may disappear. However, the infection is still present and may spread around the tooth apex, forming a periapical abscess or fistula. Dental infection

can progress to involve the maxilla or mandible and then move into the fascial planes of the head and neck, producing facial cellulitis, abscess, and airway obstruction.

The relationship of the maxillary to the mandibular dentition has both functional and aesthetic implications. **Malocclusion** is an abnormal relationship between the upper and lower teeth and may be developmental, genetic, or environmental in etiology. Children with craniofacial disorders often have significant occlusal problems and facial asymmetries necessitating early referral for craniofacial team care. Other children may have milder malocclusion that needs orthodontic care. Normal occlusion occurs when the maxillary incisors are slightly in front of the mandibular incisors and the posterior molars interdigitate (Figure 26-3). This is called **Class I occlusion. Class II occlusion** occurs when the maxillary teeth project too far anteriorly from the mandibular teeth. This may be associated with an **overjet,** commonly known as *buck teeth,* which can predispose to dental injury when children fall. **Class III occlusion** occurs when the mandibular teeth are anterior to the maxillary. This is also commonly referred to as an *underbite.* Other common forms of malocclusion include an **anterior open bite,** whereby the posterior teeth come together but there is an opening between the top and bottom anterior teeth. A **crossbite** occurs when some of the upper teeth are located inside of the lower teeth during occlusion.

Pathophysiology

Hypodontia may be familial or occur secondary to an underlying syndrome. However, failure of one tooth to erupt is also commonly caused by another tooth in the path of eruption or insufficient space in the dental arch. Defects of tooth structure have a variety of causes. Medications, infection, jaundice, metabolic disorders, and irradiation may adversely affect normal tooth formation or mineralization. The permanent teeth begin to develop in utero and mineralize after birth, making them susceptible to both prenatal and postnatal exposures. **Intrauterine infection** with rubella, cytomegalovirus, or syphilis may adversely affect tooth structure. Local oral infection, for example, a periapical abscess involving a primary tooth in early childhood, can damage the developing permanent tooth bud resulting in a malformed permanent tooth.

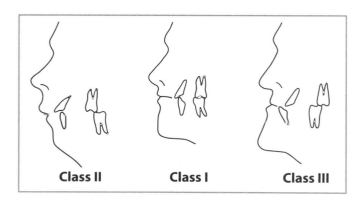

Figure 26-3. **Classes of occlusion. Class I (middle) is considered most desirable from a functional and aesthetic perspective.**

Discolored teeth may be due to intrinsic or extrinsic factors. Tetracycline given to pregnant or lactating women or children younger than 8 years can cause intrinsic staining of the permanent teeth. Exposure to high levels of fluoride during early childhood can cause **fluorosis** of the permanent dentition. Fluorosis, when it occurs in the United States, is usually mild, characterized by white striations on the permanent teeth. Children with mild fluorosis have teeth that are less prone to dental decay. Teeth more severely affected by fluorosis may display hypoplastic enamel.

Inherited enamel or dentin defects may cause abnormal color of the teeth. These conditions may be isolated to the teeth, as in the case of **dentinogenesis imperfecta,** or as part of a systemic disorder, such as porphyria or osteogenesis imperfecta. A single dark tooth is usually non-vital or has bled within the tooth structure after dental trauma. Extrinsic staining is superficial and is usually due to poor oral hygiene; smoking; chewing tobacco or betel nuts; certain beverages such as coffee, tea, or wine; or medications such as liquid iron supplements.

Malocclusion can be caused by tooth crowding, an underlying craniofacial condition, abnormal jaw growth relationship, or malpositioning of the teeth, most commonly as the result of digit (usually the thumb) sucking. The most common types of malocclusion associated with digit sucking are **anterior open bite,** overjet, or posterior crossbite.

Dental decay is the most common disorder of the teeth and is a transmissible infectious disease. Caries results from bacterial action on teeth. Bacteria coat the teeth in the form of plaque or biofilm. Cariogenic bacteria are acquired early in life, usually before 2 to 3 years of age, through transmission from caregivers via contact with and transfer of oral fluids. *Streptococcus mutans,* believed to be one of the cariogenic bacteria, produce acid as the end-product of metabolism of carbohydrates. These acids dissolve the calcium-phosphate mineral of the tooth enamel or of the dentin in a process called *demineralization*. If not reversed or halted, this process results in formation of a carious lesion.

Differential Diagnosis

It can be difficult to differentiate tooth staining from a carious lesion, particularly when there are small areas of discoloration on the pit and fissure surfaces. If the lesion disappears with cleaning, staining is the etiology; however, staining is not always readily removed and examination by a dentist and radiographs can help evaluate such lesions. White spots on the teeth also can have multiple etiologies. When the white spot is chalky in appearance and located along the gingival margin, one needs to consider demineralization that could progress to frank decay. On the other hand, small intrinsic defects of the enamel may also appear as white spots; however, these are usually located throughout the crown and not just along the gingival margin and they also reflect light like the rest of the teeth (ie, not chalky).

Evaluation

History

Dental pathology is diagnosed primarily through history and physical examination. Many physicians have not traditionally included the teeth and supporting structures as part of their routine physical examination. However, pediatricians and other health care providers caring for children are generally the first, and often the only, health care providers to examine a child during the early years of life and therefore play a key role in identification of dental pathology. This is particularly true in settings where access to professional dental care is limited. Early diagnosis facilitates timely referral to dental specialists who provide definitive management.

Physical Examination

During each well-child visit, the medical provider should closely assess the mouth and its structures for the pattern of eruption and dental development; the presence of caries, plaque, gingivitis, and other oral lesions (see Chapter 71); and malocclusion. Physicians should examine the gingiva of children, particularly those with dental decay and/or toothache, to assess for evidence of periapical abscess, which may need antibiotic therapy and/or incision and drainage.

The oral cavity of a young child can be examined most easily with the caregiver and examiner in a **knee-to-knee position,** with the child's head in the examiner's lap and the legs wrapped around the caregiver's waist. Older children can be examined on the examination table or while seated in a chair. It is useful to have a disposable mouth mirror and a good light source. A toothbrush can be used to prop the mouth open to allow for examination of the teeth and oral cavity. The toothbrush can later be used to demonstrate good tooth brushing techniques.

A child's occlusion is best examined by looking at the child face from the anterior and lateral perspectives and watching the child's front and back teeth as the child opens and then bites down. Having the child bite down on a tongue depressor placed horizontally between the child's upper and lower teeth will demonstrate if there is a cant or asymmetry of the occlusion. The lateral profile of a child's face can be particularly revealing. Constructing an imaginary line between the bridge of the nose, the base of the nose, and the tip of the chin defines the shape of the lateral profile. In preschool and older children, a slightly convex profile is preferable both from a functional and aesthetic perspective. A concave profile is never normal and may be due to midface underdevelopment or from protrusion of the mandible. These children usually have a class III malocclusion. An overly convex profile may be due to an overjet or to mandibular retrusion. These children usually have a class II malocclusion.

Laboratory Tests

An ill-appearing child with a dental abscess or facial cellulitis of odontogenic etiology should have a complete blood cell count and a blood culture obtained.

Imaging Studies

Dental radiographs are useful in evaluating for the presence and extent of dental decay. They can also aid in determining whether a tooth that has not erupted as expected is absent or prevented in some way from erupting. Finally, when there is concern for pathology, imaging, particularly a Panorex or computed tomography scan, can be useful in evaluating the facial skeleton.

Management

Much of the definitive management of dental disorders falls to dental professionals. However, physicians play an important role in educating families about prevention, identifying pathology, and in facilitating dental referrals. Some dental conditions commonly fall into the realm of the primary care practitioner. For example, teething symptoms can be alleviated by giving the child a cold teething toy to suck on or with acetaminophen or ibuprofen given orally. Over-the-counter topical anesthetic agents often contain alcohol and are not recommended.

The American Academy of Pediatric Dentistry recommends the first professional dental care visit by 12 months of age. This is particularly important for children at high risk for dental caries. Occasionally, very young infants require a dental consultation. For example, if the natal/neonatal teeth interfere with feeding or are so loose as to pose an aspiration risk, they should be extracted; otherwise they require no intervention. When no teeth have erupted by 18 months of age, a dentist may choose to take radiographs to determine the status of the child's future dentition. If few developing teeth are seen, this can point to other diagnoses where hypodontia or anodontia occur. Most superficial extrinsic tooth stains can be removed during professional cleaning. Intrinsic stains can be treated by a dentist with abrasion and bleach techniques or application of a composite veneer. Malocclusion, when not reversible or self-limited, often is treated with orthodontics. More severe cases may require orthognathic surgery.

In some communities it may be difficult to find a dental provider who will care for a child younger than 3 years, and this further emphasizes the importance of medical providers in monitoring children's teeth and surrounding structures. Publicly insured children may also encounter difficulty accessing professional dental care. Clinicians should be aware of the closest source of specialized pediatric dental care if it is not within their own community. Dental schools or pediatric dental residency training programs generally offer specialized dental care for children, including sedation or anesthesia that may be needed to provide appropriate care.

Particularly in settings of limited access to dental care, physicians play an important role in educating families about the prevention of caries through advice about cariogenic food and beverages, regular tooth cleaning, and appropriate use of fluoride. Although physicians commonly advise parents not to allow their child to take a bottle to bed, it is particularly important that the child not take a bottle with **juice** or other sweetened beverages to bed. The evidence that breast milk, formula, or cow's milk causes caries is equivocal.

Physicians can also actively intervene if early caries lesions or white spots are identified. Application of **fluoride varnish** to the teeth can help to remineralize and reverse early caries lesions. When a child has more advanced caries, prompt referral to a dental provider is indicated. Pulpal involvement and abscess formation may result if a carious lesion is ignored. If dental care is not immediately available, antibiotics (penicillin V or clindamycin) and analgesics (eg, ibuprofen) may alleviate symptoms temporarily; however, more definitive treatment (**root canal** or extraction) is necessary to remove the source of infection and prevent resurgence of symptoms and further complications. When an abscess has spread to involve the cheek, face, or neck, admission to the hospital for intravenous antibiotics and surgical drainage is usually indicated.

Prevention

Prevention of dental disorders and promotion of good oral health are the combined responsibility of the primary physician, child, family, and dentist. Protection against virtually all decay is theoretically possible. Important preventive practices include regular home oral hygiene; access to routine dental care; sound dietary practices, including avoiding frequent and/or prolonged exposure to fermentable carbohydrates, especially sucrose; sealant application; and, importantly, regular use of **fluorides.** Increasing availability of fluoridated water and fluoride-containing toothpaste has dramatically decreased the prevalence of decay in the United States and other developed countries over the last 50 years. Nevertheless, for many in the lay public, fluoride evokes controversy and undue concerns for adverse health effects. Pediatricians have an important role to play in educating families about the safety, effectiveness, and appropriate use of fluoride. Fluoride can reverse or arrest early carious lesions through (1) enhancement of tooth mineralization and (2) reversal of tooth demineralization. The composition of the fluoride-containing enamel, fluoroapatite, is harder and less acid soluble than the original enamel that it replaces. Fluoride works best at remineralizing teeth when it is provided in a topical rather than systemic form (eg, fluoride drops are a systemic form of fluoride). Topical exposure to fluoride occurs through drinking fluoridated water and other beverages manufactured with fluoridated water, using fluoride toothpaste, and professional applications. There have been 2 recent changes to fluoride policies in the United States. First, the optimal fluoride level in drinking water to prevent tooth decay has been decreased to 0.7 mg of fluoride per liter of water (or parts per million [ppm]), which replaces the previous recommended range of 0.7 to 1.2 mg/L. This change has been enacted because of expanded availability of fluoride from sources other than community water fluoridation and concerns for increasing incidence of dental fluorosis. Second, the American Dental Association will now recommend fluoride supplements only for children who are at high risk for caries instead of for all children living in communities without optimal water fluoridation.

Tooth cleaning should begin with first tooth eruption. By the age of about 7 years, most children have developed sufficient fine motor skills to begin flossing and brushing their teeth independently. Until then, parents should help their children brush and floss. It is not necessary to floss while there are still spaces between a child's teeth, as is the usual case in young children with only primary teeth. As additional teeth erupt and become closely approximated, flossing is important in order to remove plaque between the teeth that can contribute to gingivitis and later periodontal disease. The right age to begin using fluoride toothpaste depends on whether a child is at risk for caries. Parents of high-caries-risk children should use a small amount (small pea or rice grain sized) of fluoride toothpaste beginning at first tooth eruption. Parents of low-caries-risk children should wait until after 2 years of age before starting fluoride toothpaste to avoid excessive fluoride intake that can contribute to fluorosis. **Sealants** placed on the pit and fissure surfaces of the permanent molars can also be an important defense against caries in these surfaces. Children should be seen by a dentist for evaluation for sealant placement within 6 to 12 months of eruption of their first permanent molars.

Certain types of malocclusion are preventable. Because caries and trauma can both lead to premature tooth loss and subsequent loss of spacing and overcrowding, prevention of these entities will minimize the need for later orthodontic treatment. Prolonged digit sucking contributes to malocclusion. If children can discontinue these practices before age 4, digit-associated malocclusion is usually reversible. Dentists can employ specific devices and treatment to help stop digit sucking if other methods, including behavior modification, are unsuccessful (see Chapter 51).

Prognosis

Many dental disorders are preventable. Early identification and prompt referral can prevent complications. In the past, edentulism in adulthood resulting from dental decay and periodontitis was common. Fluoride use and increased attention to preventive oral hygiene have reduced this condition as well as the incidence of permanent teeth caries; however, substantial disparities continue to adversely impact the oral health of low-income, minority, and special needs children and adults in the United States.

Selected References

Acad Pediatr. 2009;9(6). Multiple articles on oral health

American Academy of Pediatrics. Protecting all Children's Teeth (PACT): an oral health training program. www.aap.org/oralhealth/pact/index.cfm

Centers for Disease Control and Prevention. Community Water Fluoridation: Questions and Answers. http://www.cdc.gov/fluoridation/fact_sheets/cwf_qa.htm

Holt R, Roberts G, Scully C. ABC of oral health. Oral health and disease. *BMJ.* 2000;320:1652–1655

Lewis CW, Johnston BD, Linsenmeyar KA, Williams A, Mouradian W. Preventive dental care for children in the United States: a national perspective. *Pediatrics.* 2007;119:e544–e553

Lewis CW, Milgrom P. Fluoride. *Pediatr Rev.* 2003;24:327–336

Lewis C, Stout J. Toothache in US children. *Arch Pediatr Adolesc Med.* 2010;164:1059–1063

CHAPTER 27

Normal Development and Developmental Surveillance, Screening, and Evaluation

Geeta Grover, MD

CASE STUDY

The parents of a 12-month-old child are concerned that she is not walking yet. They report that she sat independently at 7 months and began crawling at 8 months. She can pull herself up to stand while holding on but is not cruising. Her birth and medical history are both unremarkable. The physical examination is within normal limits, and review of your records reveals no concerns on a developmental screening test administered at 9 months of age.

Questions

1. What are the major areas in which development is assessed?
2. What are the gross motor, fine motor, and personal/social milestones for a 12-month-old child?
3. What developmental screening tests could you administer to further assess her development?
4. How is developmental delay in children defined?

Development refers to the acquisition of functional skills during childhood. Monitoring the growth and development of children is an integral part of the assessment of pediatric patients. Recording the acquisition of developmental milestones provides a systematic approach by which to observe the progress of children over time. For ease of monitoring, these developmental milestones may be divided into 5 major domains or areas: gross motor, fine motor/adaptive, personal/social, language, and cognitive. This chapter discusses these major areas of development and the principles that govern them.

Four principles apply to all aspects of development. First, motor development is a continuous process that proceeds in the cephalocaudal direction and parallels neuronal myelination; therefore, developmental milestones reflect the maturation of the nervous system. Second, the sequence of development is the same in all children, but the rate of development may vary from child to child (eg, all children must walk before they run, but the age at which children walk or run varies from child to child). Third, the rate of attainment of milestones in one area may not parallel that in another. Fourth, certain primitive reflexes must be lost before corresponding voluntary movements can be attained (eg, the asymmetrical tonic neck reflex must disappear before children can roll over).

Pathophysiology

Development is influenced by both biological and environmental factors. Biological factors such as prematurity, exposure to drugs in utero, or the presence of chronic disease may place children at increased risk for developmental problems and delays. Environmental factors influencing development include parental attitudes and actions, sociodemographic factors, and cultural and societal influences. The quality of parental stimulation may influence the rate of acquisition of certain skills, especially cognitive and language abilities in preschool-aged children. Poverty and other socioeconomic factors may make it difficult for parents to provide their child with an optimal environment for growth and development.

Development in Newborns and Infants

Normal, full-term newborns enter the world capable of responding to visual, auditory, olfactory, oral, and tactile stimuli. They can be quieted and can even soothe themselves. Newborns can signal needs (eg, crying when hungry or wet), but they have a limited ability to respond to caregivers, primarily exhibiting disorganized and seemingly purposeless movements when stimulated. The newborn's reflexive generalized symmetrical movements (eg, arm waving and kicking) in response to environmental stimuli are eventually replaced by cortically mediated voluntary actions in older infants and children. Additionally, in newborns, certain primitive reflexes can be elicited by appropriate peripheral stimuli. Eventually, primitive reflexes are replaced by reactions that allow children to maintain postural stability in response to a variety of sensory inputs (proprioceptive, visual, and vestibular).

Primitive reflexes are mediated by the brain stem; they are involuntary motor responses that are elicited by appropriate peripheral stimuli. They are present at birth and disappear during the first 6 months of life. Normal motor development seems to be related to the suppression of these reflexes (Figure 27-1). Persistence or reappearance of these reflexes may indicate the presence of brain damage. **Postural reactions,** which are ultimately smoothly integrated into adult motor function (Figure 27-1), appear between 2 and 9 months of age. These reactions help maintain the orientation of the body in space and the interrelationship of one body part to another. The 3 major categories of postural reactions are righting, protection, and equilibrium.

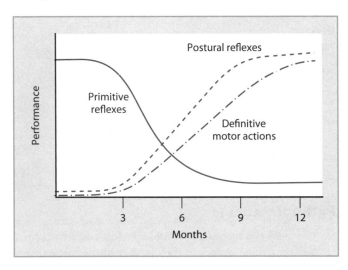

Figure 27-1. Primitive reflex profile. (Reproduced with permission from Capute AJ, Accardo PJ, Vining EPG, Rubenstein JE, Harryman S. *Primitive Reflex Profile*. Baltimore, MD: University Park Press; 1978:10.)

The profile generated by combining primitive reflexes and postural reactions can be used to monitor the course of normal development and identify cases of problematic development. Persistence of primitive reflexes or failure of development of postural reactions can signal developmental problems. Authorities estimate that there are more than 70 primitive reflexes and postural reactions. Researchers do not agree on which of these reflexes or reactions are the most useful in the monitoring of development. The 7 most commonly used primitive reflexes are described in Box 27-1, and selected postural reactions are presented in Box 27-2.

Normal Development

A developmental assessment should include an evaluation of milestones in each of the 5 major areas. **Gross motor skills** are overall movements of large muscles (eg, sitting, walking, running). **Fine motor–adaptive skills** involve use of the small muscles of the hands, the ability to manipulate small objects, problem-solving skills, and

---

Box 27-1. Selected Primitive Reflexes
Moro Reflex
Allowing the infant's head to drop back suddenly results in abduction and upward movement of the arms followed by adduction and flexion. This reflex disappears by 4 months of age.
Rooting Reflex
Touching the corner of the infant's mouth results in lowering of the lower lip on the same side and movement of the tongue toward the stimulus.
Sucking Reflex
Placing an object in an infant's mouth causes vigorous sucking.
Grasp Reflex
Placing a finger in an infant's palm causes the infant to grasp it; the infant reinforces the grip as the finger is drawn upward. A similar response is seen in the foot grasp. Both of these reflexes disappear by 2 to 3 months of age.
Placing Reflex
Stroking the anterior aspect of the tibia against the edge of a table results in the lifting of the infant's leg to step onto the table.
Stepping Reflex
Holding the infant upright and slightly leaning forward produces alternating flexion and extension movements of the legs that simulate walking. This reflex disappears by 5 to 6 weeks of age.
Asymmetrical Tonic Neck Reflex
With the infant lying supine, turning the head to one side results in extension of the extremities on that side and flexion of the opposite extremities (fencer position). This reflex disappears by 3 to 4 months of age.

Box 27-2. Selected Postural Reactions
Righting Reactions
These allow the body to maintain normal postural relationships of the head, trunk, and extremities during all activities. The different reactions appear at different ages, beginning shortly after birth and ranging up to 12 months of age.
Protection and Equilibrium Reactions
Protective Equilibrium Response
When gently pushed toward one side while in a sitting position, infants increase trunk flexor tone toward that side to regain their center of gravity and extend the arm on the same side to protect against falling. This response usually emerges at about 4 to 6 months of age.
Parachute Reactions
When held in ventral suspension and suddenly lowered (downward parachute), infants extend their arms as if to protect themselves from a fall; similar reactions are seen with forward and backward stimulation. These reactions appear at 8 to 9 months of age.

eye-hand coordination. **Language skills** include hearing, understanding, and use of language. **Personal–social skills** involve socialization and ability to care for personal needs. **Cognitive skills** involve the ability to use higher mental processes, including comprehension, memory, and logical reasoning.

Table 27-1 outlines the normal pattern of development with regard to each of these skills. The table lists the average age of attainment of these skills as well as the normal ranges where available. Development is an orderly and sequential process, and children must proceed through several stages before any given milestone is attained. Therefore, the physician should document not only *what* children can do but *how* they do it. For example, to sit without support, children first achieve head control. Several stages later they are able to sit in a "tripod" position with arms extended in front for support, and finally sit with the head steady and back straight without support (Figure 27-2).

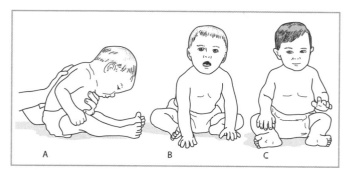

Figure 27-2. Stages in the development of sitting. A. Head control. B. "Tripod sitting." C. Head steady and back straight without support.

Gross Motor Skills

During the first year of life, the ultimate goal of gross motor development is walking. The first step toward this goal is head control. By 6 months of age, children are able to sit without support for a few seconds. At 9 to 10 months of age children are able to pull themselves to a standing position, and by 12 to 17 months of age they are able to walk. Children then learn to run, negotiate stairs, hop on one foot, and skip—in that order.

Fine Motor Skills

Development of the 2-finger pincer grasp is the major goal of fine motor development during the first year (Figure 27-3). The hands primarily remain in a fisted position until 3 months of age. Infants

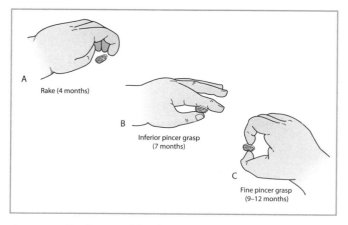

Figure 27-3. Development of the pincer grasp. A. Rake (4 months). B. Inferior pincer grasp (7 months). C. Fine pincer grasp (9–12 months).

also discover the midline at this age, and shortly thereafter they may play with the hands in the midline. Four-month-old children begin reaching for desired objects; by 6 months of age they are able to transfer objects from one hand to the other. By 7 months they have a 3-finger pincer grasp, and by 9 to 10 months they have developed the 2-finger grasp, which allows them to manipulate small objects such as raisins and pencils. By 14 months they begin to scribble, and by 3 to 5 years they are able to copy geometric shapes. Children with early preference for the use of one hand over another, especially prior to about 18 months of age, should be assessed for the presence of paresis or other neuromuscular problems. Handedness may develop by 3 years but often is not firmly established until the age of 4 to 5 years.

Language Skills

The development of normal speech and language skills is discussed in Chapter 28.

Personal–Social Skills

These skills enable children to interact and respond to the surrounding world. Deficits in the development of age-appropriate social skills/social relatedness (eg, social orienting, social referencing, joint attention, and pretend play) are a defining feature of the autism spectrum disorders (ASDs). For children within this spectrum, the development of social skills is characteristically "out of sync" with their overall level of functioning. Joint attention is the inclination to share enjoyment, interests, or achievement with other people, and like other developmental skills, seems to develop in graduated stages (early skills include reciprocal smiling at the sight of a familiar person followed by later emerging skills like the ability to isolate one's index finger and point by 12–15 months of age). Lack of joint attention seems to be a core deficit in ASDs; it also seems to be specific to ASDs. (ASDs are discussed fully in Chapter 124.)

Cognitive Skills

These abilities allow children to think, reason, problem solve, and understand the surrounding environment. The concept of object permanence or object constancy, the realization that objects may exist even if they cannot be seen, develops at approximately 7 to 9 months of age. The understanding of time comes much later. Children develop the concept of "today" at 24 months of age, "tomorrow" at 30 months, and "yesterday" at 36 months. It is extremely important that health care providers realize that children's perception and understanding of pain, disease, and illness are guided by their stage of cognitive development. The psychologist Jean Piaget generated complex generalizations by observing what children did and how they did it; his theories are the cornerstone of knowledge in this area. Piaget's 4 stages of cognitive development are presented in Box 27-3.

Developmental Delay

Children are said to be developmentally delayed if they fail to reach developmental milestones at the expected age. This age ranges widely because of the wide variation among normal children. Individual children may be delayed in one area or several areas of development.

Table 27-1. Normal Pattern of Development[a]		
Skill	*Mean Age*	*Normal Range*
Gross Motor Skills		
Reflex head turn; moves head side to side	Newborn	0–3 mo
Lifts head when prone	1 mo	1–4 mo
Lifts shoulders up when prone	2 mo	1–4 mo
Lifts up on elbows; head steady when upright	3 mo	2–5 mo
Lifts up on extended hands; rolls front to back; no head lag when pulled to sitting from supine position	4 mo	3–6 mo
Rolls back to front	5 mo	4–7 mo
Sits independently (≥30 s)	6 mo	5–9 mo
Crawls on hands and knees	8 mo	6–11 mo
Pulls to stand	9 mo	6–12 mo
Cruises	11 mo	9–14 mo
Walks	12 mo	9–17 mo
Walks backward	15 mo	13–17 mo
Runs	15 mo	13–20 mo
Kicks a ball	24 mo	18–30 mo
Walks up and down stairs (taking one step at a time and holding on)	24 mo	
Stands on one foot	30 mo	
Walks up stairs alternating steps	30 mo	28–36 mo
Peddles a tricycle	3 y	30–48 mo
Walks down stairs alternating steps/hops on one foot	4 y	
Skips	5 y	
Fine Motor-Adaptive Skills		
Tracks horizontally to midline	1 mo	
Tracks past midline/tracks vertically	2 mo	1–3 mo
Unfisted for >50% of the time; tracks 180 degrees; visual threat; discovers midline	3 mo	3–4 mo
Reaches for bright object; brings object to mouth	4 mo	
Transfers object from one hand to the other	6 mo	4–7 mo
3-finger pincer grasp	7 mo	6–10 mo
Neat pincer grasp	9 mo	7–10 mo
Bangs cubes in midline	9 mo	7–11 mo
Tower of 2 cubes; scribbles spontaneously	14 mo	14–20 mo
Tower of 4 cubes	18 mo	17–24 mo
Copies vertical and horizontal line; tower of 6 cubes	2 y	
Copies circle	3 y	
Copies cross (†)	4 y	
Copies square; draws person with 3 parts	5 y	
Copies triangle; draws person with 6 parts	6 y	
Personal-Social Skills		
Regards face	Newborn	
Spontaneous social smile	6 wk	1–3 mo
Discriminates social smile; relates to parent with real joy	6 mo	
Displays stranger anxiety; plays peek-a-boo	7 mo	7–9 mo

Table 27-1. Normal Pattern of Development[a], continued

Skill	Mean Age	Normal Range
Personal-Social Skills, continued		
Orients to name, uses gestures to get needs met	12 mo	
Drinks from a cup	15 mo	10–18 mo
Uses a spoon, spilling a little	15 mo	12–18 mo
Uses sounds, pointing, or other "showing" gestures to draw attention to object of interest	15 mo	12–15 mo
Simple pretend play (eg, feeding doll)	18 mo	
Imitates housework	18 mo	14–24 mo
Helps with undressing	2 y	22–30 mo
Washes and dries hands	2 y	
Parallel play; enjoys being next to other kids	2 y	12–30 mo
Undresses self	3 y	30–40 mo
Toilet training		24–36 mo
Imagines self as different characters	3 y	
Cooperative play	3 y	24–48 mo
Dresses without assistance	5 y	
Language Skills		
Alerts to bell	Newborn	
Searches with eyes for sound	2 mo	
Cooing	3 mo	1–4 mo
Turns head to voice or bell; laughs	4 mo	3–6 mo
Babbles	6 mo	5–9 mo
Mama/Dada nonspecific	8 mo	6–10 mo
Understands the word "no"	10 mo	
Mama/Dada specific	10 mo	9–14 mo
Follows 1-step command with gesture; 3–5-word vocabulary	12 mo	10–16 mo
Follows 1-step command without gesture	15 mo	12–20 mo
Can point to several body parts	18 mo	12 24 mo
50-word vocabulary	2 y	
2-word sentences; pronouns indiscriminately	2 y	20–30 mo
States first name	34 mo	30–40 mo
250-word vocabulary; 3-word sentences; speech intelligible to strangers 75% of time	3 y	
Uses pronouns appropriately	3 y	30–42 mo
Cognitive Skills		
Sensorimotor		Newborn–2 y
Preoperational		2–6 y
Concrete operational		6–11 y
Formal operations		>11 y
Miscellaneous Cognitive Milestones		
Concept of today	24 mo	
Concept of tomorrow	30 mo	
Concept of yesterday	36 mo	
Concept of right and left	7 y	

[a]Detailed language milestones are presented in Chapter 28, Table 28-1.

Box 27-3. Stages of Development of Piaget
Sensorimotor (Birth–2 Years) Children approach the world through sensations and motor actions. They develop a sense of object permanence, spatial relationships, and causality.
Preoperational (2–6 Years) Children's mental processes are linked to their own perception of reality. They do not separate internal and external reality.
Concrete Operational (6–11 Years) Children can perform mental operations in their heads if they relate to real objects. They develop concepts of conservation of mass, volume, and number.
Formal Operations (>11 Years) Children develop the capacity for abstract thought.

Differential Diagnosis

Three factors are involved in the differential diagnosis of children with developmental delays: (1) determination of the area or areas of development in which delay is apparent; (2) if motor delay is evident, determination of whether the condition is progressive or nonprogressive; and (3) assessment to see if developmental milestones previously achieved are lost or if age-appropriate milestones were achieved at all.

Children with an early history of normal development who subsequently experience a slowing of developmental progression, often associated with cognitive delays or seizures, may have a metabolic defect. Children who attain developmental milestones and subsequently lose them may have a neurodegenerative disease (eg, multiple sclerosis, adrenoleukodystrophy) or a lesion of the spinal cord or brain. The presence of habitual rhythmic body movements (eg, body rocking, head banging) may be a sign of a pervasive developmental disorder such as autism.

Cerebral palsy, the classic example of nonprogressive motor abnormality, is a form of static encephalopathy characterized by abnormal movement and posture. The type of cerebral palsy depends on which area of the brain is injured. Spastic cerebral palsy, seen most commonly, is secondary to upper motor neuron injury. The ataxic form of the disease is related to lesions of the cerebellum or its pathways. Dyskinetic cerebral palsy manifests as uncontrolled and purposeless movements that often result from a basal ganglia lesion (eg, athetosis following bilirubin deposition in the basal ganglia [kernicterus]). The onset of symptoms is either in infancy or early childhood. The key factor in making the diagnosis is establishing that the motor deficits are static and nonprogressing.

Evaluation

When evaluating children for possible delays in development, it is important to remember that there is a great deal of variation in the age of attainment of milestones. In addition, the rate of acquisition of milestones in one area of development may not parallel that in another. Routine and ongoing assessment of a child's level of development at all periodic health maintenance visits through observation, history, physical examination, and screening tests allows the physician to form a longitudinal view of the child. The physician is thus able to identify and differentiate true deficits and delays from temporary setbacks.

History

Evaluation of children for suspected delays in development includes a complete history (Questions Box). Family history is important because other family members may have relatively delayed attainment of milestones. Perinatal factors that place children at high risk for developmental difficulties include a history of maternal drug or alcohol use during pregnancy, prematurity in the infant, and congenital infections. Other historical risk factors for developmental delay include history of seizures, sepsis or meningitis, exposure to lead or other toxins, and poor feeding or growth. Environmental factors, such as stressful home conditions, history of abuse or neglect, and lack of stimulation, may also contribute to delayed development.

Physical Examination

Both height and weight should be checked. Abnormal growth (ie, height or weight <5th percentile or head circumference either <5th percentile or >90th percentile) may be a marker for developmental delay. The presence of congenital anomalies (eg, cataracts, hypertelorism, spina bifida) or neurocutaneous lesions (eg, café-au-lait spots) may be suggestive of chromosomal anomalies or other genetic diseases. Neuromuscular examination should emphasize age-appropriate milestones. Abnormalities in muscle tone (eg, hypotonia, hypertonia), bulk, or strength may be clues to the presence of neuromuscular disease (eg, muscular dystrophy), cerebral palsy, or Down syndrome.

Laboratory Tests

Age-appropriate assessment of the child's vision and hearing should be performed if signs of motor, cognitive, or language delays are apparent. Chromosomal studies may be conducted if dysmorphic features are noted on the physical examination. Evidence of cognitive or motor delays may warrant metabolic studies (eg, organic and amino acids).

Questions

Normal Development

- Has anyone in the child's family had developmental problems or delays?
- Did the mother use any drugs or alcohol during pregnancy?
- Was the child premature?
- Does the child have a history of seizures?
- Has the child had meningitis or sepsis?
- Does the child have any history of not feeding well or poor growth?
- Is the child's home environment characterized by any stresses (eg, divorce, limited financial resources)?

Imaging studies of the head, such as magnetic resonance imaging scans or electroencephalograms, may be necessary if the child has a history of seizures or an abnormal neurologic examination.

Developmental Surveillance, Screening, and Evaluation

Early detection of developmental delays is a responsibility of all pediatric health care professionals. Unfortunately current detection rates of developmental disorders are lower than their actual prevalence. About 20% of children between the ages of 3 to 17 years will have one or more developmental, learning, or emotional disorders, with 4% to 5% having developmental delays. Without the use of specific developmental screening tools, only about 30% of developmental disabilities are identified, but with the use of tools this identification rate increases to 70% to 80%.

Developmental surveillance, the ongoing process of monitoring individual children's developmental status, should be incorporated at each health maintenance visit. Surveillance involves eliciting and attending to parental concerns about their children's development and usually involves age-specific queries, such as whether the child is walking, talking, or pointing. Surveillance has been referred to as a kind of developmental growth chart. Recognition of children who may be at risk of developmental delays is the goal of developmental surveillance.

Developmental screening is the administration of a brief standardized tool to identify children at risk of a developmental disorder. Box 27-4 lists frequently used developmental screening tools. A formal developmental screening should be performed when developmental surveillance elicits a risk factor for developmental delay; in the absence of established risk factors or parental concerns, the administration of a general developmental screening tool is recommended by the American Academy of Pediatrics (AAP) at the 9-, 18-, and 30-month (or 24-month) health maintenance visits (AAP, 2006). The AAP further recommends that in addition to a general developmental screening tool, an autism-specific screening tool should also be administered at the 18-month visit. (See Chapter 124 for a listing of autism-specific screening tools.) Periodic screening is necessary to detect emerging disabilities as children grow. Screening instruments should have a broad developmental focus and should be brief, inexpensive, valid, and reliable. Screening tests are not diagnostic. A failed screening test should lead to a referral for a further developmental evaluation.

Developmental evaluation (developmental assessment) is performed when surveillance or screening identifies a child as being at high risk of a developmental disorder. The aim is to identify the specific developmental disorder or disorders affecting the child. Developmental evaluation is performed by trained examiners. Unlike developmental screening, which is not diagnostic, developmental evaluation is diagnostic.

The Bayley Scales of Infant Development II, first published in 1933 by Nancy Bayley, is one of the most commonly used developmental evaluation tools. It has 3 sections: mental, psychomotor, and a behavior rating scale. The Bayley II may be used for children 1 to 42 months of age. Developmental tests, like the Bayley II (emphasizing sensorimotor-based skills), have a poor correlation with later measures of intelligence (emphasizing language and abstract reasoning), especially before 24 to 30 months of age. As such, developmental tests are best used as measures of current developmental functioning, rather than as predictors of future functioning. Intelligence tests, achievement tests, personality tests, or behavior rating scales may be used for preschool- and school-aged children having behavioral or emotional concerns, learning disabilities, or developmental disabilities.

Management

Children with identified developmental delays in one or more areas should be referred to the appropriate specialist, agency, or state program for further testing and assessment. Detailed neurologic examination may be necessary if gross motor delays are identified. Language delays may warrant formal hearing and speech assessment by an audiologist or speech pathologist. Cognitive impairment requires formal psychometric assessment, which in some cases can be performed through the child's school.

Prognosis

The early identification of children with developmental delays is critical. Early identification of developmental problems allows for early intervention, thereby making it possible for individual children to reach their maximum potential. Identification and treatment of underlying disease (eg, hypothyroidism or infection) prevents further damage. Removal of children from adverse home environments or placement of children from impoverished home environments in early intervention programs can greatly stimulate their developmental potential. The prognosis for children with mild developmental delays can sometimes be improved greatly from participation in such infant stimulation programs.

Box 27-4. Frequently Used Developmental Screening Instruments

Developmental Screening Instruments Relying on Information From Parents
- Child Development Inventories
- Child Development Review—Parent Questionnaire (CDR-PQ)
- Infant Development Inventory
- Ages and Stages Questionnaire (ASQ)
- Parent's Evaluation of Developmental Status (PEDS)

Screens Relying on Eliciting Skills Directly From Children
- Bayley Infant Neurodevelopmental Screen (BINS)
- Batelle Developmental Inventory Screening Tool, 2nd Edition
- Brigance Screens—II
- Denver Developmental Screening Test II (Denver II)

CASE RESOLUTION

The parents of the child described in the case history may be reassured that their child is developing normally for her age. Although most children begin walking at about 12 months of age, commencement of walking anywhere up to the age of 17 months is considered to be within normal limits. The AAP recommends that standardized developmental screening should be performed when developmental surveillance identifies high risk factors and routinely at the 9-, 18-, and 30-month health maintenance visits. Administration of a formal screening tool is probably not necessary at this visit, but can be considered again at the 15-month visit if there is a lack of progression in her gross motor skills or if any other risk factor is identified at that time.

Selected References

American Academy of Pediatrics Committee on Children With Disabilities. Developmental surveillance and screening of infants and young children. *Pediatrics*. 2001;108:192–195

American Academy of Pediatrics Committee on Children With Disabilities. Technical report: the pediatrician's role in the diagnosis and management of autistic spectrum disorder in children. *Pediatrics*. 2001;107:e85

American Academy of Pediatrics Council on Children With Disabilities, Section on Developmental Behavioral Pediatrics, Bright Futures Steering Committee, Medical Home Initiatives for Children With Special Needs Project Advisory Committee. Identifying infants and young children with developmental disorders in the medical home: an algorithm for developmental surveillance and screening. *Pediatrics*. 2006;118:405–420

Glascoe FP. Early detection of developmental and behavioral problems. *Pediatr Rev*. 2000;21:272–279

Glascoe FP, Macias MM. How you can implement the AAP's new policy on developmental and behavioral screening. *Contemp Pediatr*. 2003;20:85–102

Hamilton SS, Glascoe FP. Making developmental behavioral screenings work for school-aged kids. *Contemp Pediatr*. 2010:63–87

Roberts G, Palfrey J, Bridgemohan C. A rational approach to the medical evaluation of a child with developmental delay. *Contemp Pediatr*. 2004;21:76–100

Shevell M, Aswal S, Donley, et al. Practice parameter: evaluation of the child with global developmental delay: report of the Quality Standards Subcommittee of the American Academy of Neurology and the Practice Committee of the Child Neurology Society. *Neurology*. 2003;60:367–380

Sices L, Feudtner C, McLaughlin J, Drotar D, Williams M. How do primary care physicians manage children with possible developmental delays? A national survey with an experimental design. *Pediatrics*. 2004;113:274–282

CHAPTER 28

Speech and Language Development: Normal Patterns and Common Disorders

Geeta Grover, MD

CASE STUDY

The parents of a 3-year-old girl bring her to see you. They are concerned because their daughter has only an 8- to 10-word vocabulary, and she does not put words together into phrases or sentences. They report that she seems to have no hearing problems; she responds to her name and follows directions well.

In general, she has been in good health. Her development, aside from delayed speech, is normal. During the physical examination, which is also normal, the girl does not speak.

Questions

1. What language skills should children have at 1, 2, and 3 years?
2. Approximately how many words should 3-year-olds have in their vocabulary?
3. By what age should children's speech be intelligible to strangers at least 75% of the time?
4. What factors may be associated with delayed speech development?
5. What tests are used to assess children's hearing, speech, and language development?

The ability to communicate through language is a uniquely human skill. Speech refers to the production of sounds, whereas language involves both comprehension and expression; it is the use of words, phrases, and gestures to convey intent. **Receptive language** refers to the ability to understand others, while **expressive language** is the ability to produce communication to convey meaning to others. Normal hearing is essential for the development of speech and language.

Speech disorders include problems in the production of speech sounds. Speech disorders may affect articulation (phonological disorders), fluency (stuttering), or voice (tone, pitch, and volume). The development of language skills in a normal sequence but at a slower pace than normal is referred to as language delay; language delays may affect only receptive or expressive language or both (eg, a mixed receptive-expressive language delay). An atypical sequence of language skill acquisition is referred to as a language disorder. Children with developmental language disorders have persistent and significant limitation in their ability to receive and/or express language.

The development of normal speech and language skills is an extremely important developmental milestone that is eagerly awaited by parents. Normal patterns of language development should be as familiar to pediatricians as all other aspects of child development (see Chapter 27). It is important that children with suspected language delays be referred to specialists as early as possible. Children with delayed speech or language development should be suspected of having a hearing deficit. Diminished hearing is an important cause of delayed language development. Delays in language development can also be seen in the context of global developmental or cognitive delays, or associated with autism spectrum disorders (ASDs).

Epidemiology

The prevalence of specific language impairment in school-aged children, who have no hearing loss, or obvious genetic or neurologic condition, is about 7%. Speech and language disorders are more common in boys than in girls, and are more common in children who have a family history of language, speech, or reading disorders. There is good evidence now that early language impairment is associated with later difficulties learning to read.

Clinical Presentation

Lack of response to sound at any age, failure to achieve age-appropriate expressive language skills, and parental concern regarding a child's hearing are the most important signs of hearing or language impairment. Deaf infants coo normally and may even babble; therefore, an infant's vocalizing does not preclude a hearing loss.

Pathophysiology

The left hemisphere of the brain is responsible for language skills in 94% of right-handed adults and approximately 75% of left-handed adults. Peripheral auditory stimuli are transmitted to the primary auditory areas in both temporal lobes. Sounds then undergo a series of analyses, primarily in 3 main areas in the left cerebral cortex: Wernicke area (or auditory association area), which is responsible for the comprehension of language; Broca area (or motor encoding area), which is responsible for the preliminary conversion of language into motor activity; and the primary motor cortex and supplementary motor cortex, which control the movements necessary for speech. This complex process is responsible for the comprehension and production of language.

Speech and language develop in a predictable, orderly sequence. Language skills can be either receptive or expressive. Early receptive milestones refer to ability to hear and respond to sound, whereas later milestones reflect ability to understand spoken words. Early expressive milestones relate to speech production; later, children use language to convey their intent to others. In the first year of life, receptive skills are more advanced than expressive skills.

Knowledge of normal receptive and expressive language skills (Table 28-1) is essential to recognition and identification of developmental delays. Box 28-1 lists "danger signals" that indicate possible delays and serves as a guide for referral to specialists. It is most important to remember that by the age of 3 years, 75% of children's speech should be intelligible to strangers.

Differential Diagnosis

The various causes of delayed language development include hearing loss, disorders of central nervous system (CNS) processing, anatomical abnormalities, and environmental deprivation (Box 28-2). Although birth order (eg, the belief that younger children speak later than first-born children because older siblings speak for them), laziness (eg, "Don't give him what he wants when he points. Make him ask for it"), and bilingualism are commonly believed to lead to speech and language delay, their contributory role has never been proved. For a complete discussion of hearing loss, refer to Chapter 73.

Disorders of CNS processing include global developmental delay, mental retardation, ASDs (see Chapter 124), and developmental language problems. Developmental language disorders produce speech or language delays in children in the absence of hearing loss, anatomical abnormalities of the vocal tract, mental retardation, or global developmental delay. "Late talkers," or children who have normal comprehension but simply begin speaking late, have mild developmental language problems. Children who are completely nonverbal have more severe problems.

Anatomical abnormalities may also result in both speech and language delays. Cleft palate is the abnormality most commonly associated with difficulties in speech production. Children with cleft palate characteristically have hypernasal speech secondary to velopharyngeal incompetence (eg, dysfunction of the soft palate). In

Table 28-1. Receptive and Expressive Language Milestones (Birth to 3 years)		
Skill	*Mean Age*	*Normal Range*
Receptive Milestones		
Alerts to sound	Newborn	
Orients to sound/turns to voice	4 mo	3–6 mo
Responds to name	4 mo	4–9 mo
Understands "no"	10 mo	9–18 mo
Follows 1-step command with gesture	12 mo	10–16 mo
Follows 1-step command without gesture	15 mo	12–20 mo
Points to several body parts	18 mo	12–24 mo
Follows 2-step command with gesture	24 mo	22–30 mo
Expressive Milestones		
Cooing (vowel sounds)	3 mo	1–4 mo
Laughs	4 mo	3–6 mo
Babbling (consonants added to vowel sounds)	6 mo	5–9 mo
Dada/Mama nonspecifically	8 mo	6–10 mo
Dada/Mama specifically	10 mo	9–14 mo
3–5 word vocabulary	12 mo	
Immature jargoning (gibberish with inflection)	13 mo	10–18 mo
Mature jargoning (gibberish with occasional word)	18 mo	16–24 mo
50-word vocabulary	24 mo	
2-word phrases	24 mo	20–30 mo
Uses pronouns indiscriminately	24 mo	22–30 mo
States first name	34 mo	30–40 mo
Uses pronouns appropriately	36 mo	30–42 mo
250-word vocabulary	36 mo	
75% of speech intelligible to strangers	36 mo	

Box 28-1. Danger Signals in Language Development
• Inconsistent or lack of response to auditory stimuli at any age
• No babbling by 9 months
• No intelligible speech by 18 months
• Inability to respond to simple directions or commands (eg, "sit down," "come here") by 24 months
• Speech predominantly unintelligible at 36 months
• Dysfluency (stuttering) of speech noticeable after 5 years
• Hypernasality; inappropriate vocal quality, pitch, or intensity at any age

---

Box 28-2. Causes of Delayed Language Development

- Hearing impairment
- Perinatal risk factors leading to hearing impairment
- Disorders of central nervous system processing
  — Global developmental delay
  — Mental retardation
  — Autism spectrum disorders
- Developmental language disorders
- Disorders of language production
  — Articulation disorder
  — Dysarthria
  — Verbal apraxia
- Presence of anatomical abnormalities (eg, cleft lip, cleft palate)
- Environmental deprivation

Questions

Language Development

- Are the child's language capabilities appropriate for age?
- Do the parents feel that their child has difficulty hearing?
- Is there any family history of childhood deafness?
- Has the child been exposed to any ototoxic agents (eg, aminoglycoside antibiotics)?
- Is there a history of neonatal asphyxia, hyperbilirubinemia, or low birth weight?
- Has the child ever had bacterial meningitis?
- Did the mother have a TORCHS infection (toxoplasmosis, rubella, cytomegalovirus, herpes simplex, syphilis) during pregnancy?

---

addition, conductive hearing losses may result from chronic serous otitis media, which is common in these children. The presence of a submucous cleft palate, characterized by a bifid uvula, diastasis of the muscles in the midline of the soft palate with intact mucosa, and notching of the posterior border of the hard palate, should be considered in children without an overt cleft palate who have recurrent symptomatic serous otitis media and phonation difficulties.

Environmental deprivation is another cause of delayed language development, especially in families where children are not spoken or read to. Sometimes there is additional historical or physical evidence of deprivation (eg, profound failure to thrive, physical or sexual abuse) or emotional trauma (eg, domestic violence).

Evaluation

History

When evaluating children younger than 3 years, pediatricians must rely primarily on parental reports of children's language capabilities (Questions Box). Children who are 3 years of age and older can usually be engaged in conversation during the visit, but younger children are more likely to be uncooperative or remain silent when confronted by strangers or new situations. Historical factors, such as a family history of childhood deafness, exposure to ototoxic agents (eg, aminoglycoside antibiotics), neonatal asphyxia, hyperbilirubinemia, maternal cocaine abuse, or low birth weight, provide valuable information in the identification of high-risk infants (see Boxes 28-1 and 28-3).

Physical Examination

Examination should include a thorough assessment of the head and neck region. Microcephaly may indicate the presence of mental retardation or structural abnormalities. Abnormalities of the external ear (eg, microtia) may be associated with sensorineural hearing loss. Otoscopic examination of the ear is essential. Presence of a middle ear effusion may be associated with a conductive hearing

---

Box 28-3. High-Risk Indicators for Hearing Loss in Children (Birth–24 months)[a]

Neonatal Period (Birth–28 days)

- Family history of sensorineural hearing loss (SNHL)
- In utero infection associated with SNHL (eg, TORCHS infections [toxoplasmosis, rubella, cytomegalovirus, herpes simplex, syphilis])
- Anatomical malformations of the head and neck region
- Hyperbilirubinemia at a level requiring exchange transfusion
- Low birth weight (<1,500 g)
- Bacterial meningitis
- Low Apgar scores
- Respiratory distress (eg, meconium aspiration)
- Mechanical ventilation for 10 days or more
- Exposure to ototoxic medications (eg, aminoglycoside antibiotics) for more than 5 days or in combination with loop diuretics
- Stigmata of syndromes known to be associated with hearing loss (eg, Down syndrome)

Infants and Children (29 days–24 months)

- Parental concern about hearing, speech, language, or developmental delay
- Recurrent or persistent otitis media with effusion for at least 3 months
- Severe head trauma (associated with fracture of the temporal bone)
- Infections associated with SNHL (eg, bacterial meningitis, mumps, measles)
- Neurodegenerative disorders or demyelinating diseases
- Any of the newborn risk factors listed above

[a]Adapted with permission from Joint Committee on Infant Hearing, American Academy of Audiology, American Academy of Pediatrics, American Speech-Language-Hearing Association, Directors of Speech and Hearing Programs in State Health and Welfare Agencies. Year 2000 position statement: principles and guidelines for early hearing detection and intervention programs. *Pediatrics.* 2000;106:798–817 and Cunningham M, Cox EO; American Academy of Pediatrics Committee on Practice and Ambulatory Medicine and Section on Otolaryngology and Bronchoesophagology. Hearing assessment in infants and children: recommendations beyond neonatal screening. *Pediatrics.* 2003;111:436–440.

loss. The tympanic membrane should be examined for evidence of scarring or perforation, often secondary to recurrent otitis media. Pneumatic otoscopy provides subjective assessment of tympanic membrane mobility (compliance) when it is subjected to a pulse of air. Tympanometry (impedance audiometry) performed in the office can provide objective information regarding the mobility of the tympanic membrane and the presence of middle ear effusions (Figure 28-1). Tympanometry is not a hearing test but rather an assessment of middle ear functioning that uses sound energy to determine the compliance of the tympanic membrane and pressure in the middle ear. Physical stigmata of any syndromes that may be associated with deafness (Box 28-4) should be noted.

Laboratory Tests

The advantages of early identification of hearing loss cannot be over-emphasized. The Joint Committee on Infant Hearing's Year 2000 Position Statement, which was endorsed by the American Academy of Pediatrics, endorses universal hearing evaluation of all infants prior to 3 months of age. High-risk indicators for hearing loss (see Box 28-3) serve 2 purposes. First, they help identify infants, living in areas where universal newborn hearing screening is not yet available, who should receive an audiological evaluation. Second, these risk indicators help identify infants who require ongoing medical and audiological monitoring because normal hearing at birth in these children may not preclude the development of later hearing loss (eg, delayed onset).

The evaluation of any child with delayed language development or suspected hearing loss begins with a hearing assessment. Various techniques are available, depending on the child's age and the degree of sophistication required. (A detailed discussion of the various tests used to evaluate children's hearing is presented in Chapter 73.) In addition to a hearing evaluation, a full speech, language, and communication assessment (eg, assessment of pragmatic language skills) should be performed on children with suspected language delays. In the pediatric office, parent report inventories may be used to validate parental concerns, and office-based language assessment may be aided by the use of screening tests such as the Clinical Linguistic and Auditory Milestone Scale or the Early Language Milestone Scale. These tests are used to supplement the clinical history of a child's language abilities. Children, who in addition to speech or language impairments also have signs of possible cognitive or social skills impairments, should receive a comprehensive, multidisciplinary developmental assessment.

Management

The first 3 years of life are extremely important to language development. Hearing impairment is one of the most common causes of delayed language development in young children. The history, physical examination, and initial screening can be used to suggest referral to various specialists (eg, audiologists, speech pathologists, child psychologists, otolaryngologists) for further clarification of hearing, speech, or language deficits and treatment. Early identification of hearing impairment and its degree of severity allow for early

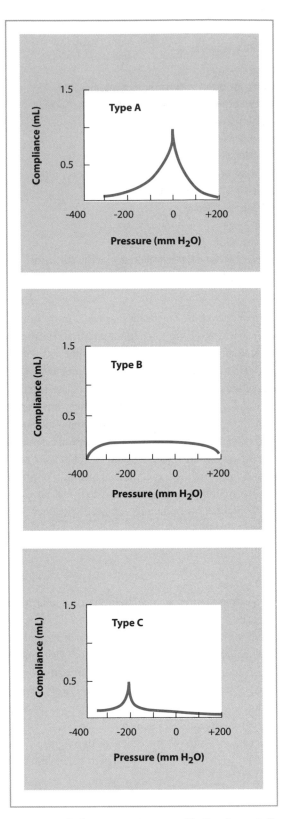

Figure 28-1. **Basic tympanometry curves. The Type A curve indicates a normally compliant tympanic membrane (TM). The Type B curve indicates little or no motion of the TM and can be seen with middle ear effusion, a scarred TM, or a cholesteatoma. The Type C curve indicates negative middle ear pressure and may be seen with a resolving middle ear effusion or eustachian tube dysfunction. Other variations can occur in these basic curves that are not illustrated here.**

Box 28-4. Syndromes Commonly Associated With Hearing Impairment

Autosomal-Dominant Conditions
- Brachio-otorenal syndrome
- Goldenhar syndrome (facioauriculovertebral dysplasia)
- Stickler syndrome
- Treacher Collins syndrome
- Waardenburg syndrome

Autosomal-Recessive Conditions
- Alport syndrome
- Jervell and Lange-Nielsen syndrome
- Pendred syndrome
- Usher syndrome

Chromosomal Disorders
- Trisomy 13 syndrome
- Trisomy 18q syndrome

Miscellaneous Disorders
- CHARGE association (coloboma, congenital heart disease, choanal atresia, growth and mental retardation, genitourinary anomalies, ear anomalies, and genital hypoplasia)
- TORCHS syndrome (toxoplasmosis, rubella, cytomegalovirus, herpes simplex, syphilis)

---

intervention in the form of amplification of sound, special education for children, and counseling and support services for the families with affected children. (See Chapter 73 for further information on management of hearing impairment.)

Special education is of prime importance in the management of children with language difficulties. The Education for All Handicapped Persons Act, federal legislation passed in 1975, and its subsequent more comprehensive reauthorization as the Individuals with Disabilities Education Act (IDEA) in 1990 requires that public schools provide individualized and appropriate education for all children with disabilities. Knowledge of available community resources (eg, special schools) can aid pediatricians in providing **support services** such as special community agencies and support groups for disabled children and their parents. Children with language delay in the context of global developmental or cognitive delays, or ASDs, require prompt referral to early intervention services.

Prognosis

Children with a history of speech and language delays should be monitored carefully for the emergence of reading difficulties. Reading is a language-based skill that requires the appreciation of subtle differences among speech sounds (eg, phonological awareness) and the ability to link these sounds to written symbols. The emergent literacy model of reading development assumes that reading, writing, and oral language develop concurrently from interactions in social contexts.

Children with speech and language delays require long-term monitoring of academic, emotional, and behavioral functioning.

Treated early, speech and language delays and disorders generally improve over time. The final prognosis is dependent on the nature and severity of the underlying cause and the interventions provided.

CASE RESOLUTION

The child described in the case history has delayed development of expressive language skills. At the age of 3 years, she should have a 250-word vocabulary and speak in 3-word sentences; in addition, her speech should be primarily intelligible to strangers. Because of the delay, she should be referred immediately for a hearing assessment and speech and language evaluation. Hearing loss is an important diagnosis to rule out. Simply because her parents report no hearing problems does not mean she does not have a deficit. She may have learned to respond to nonverbal cues, or she may hear only some things.

Selected References

Cunningham M, Cox EO, American Academy of Pediatrics Committee on Practice and Ambulatory Medicine and Section on Otolaryngology and Bronchoesophagology. Hearing assessment in infants and children: recommendations beyond neonatal screening. *Pediatrics.* 2003;111:436–440

Feldman HM. Evaluation and management of language and speech disorders in preschool children. *Pediatr Rev.* 2005;26(4):131–142

Fierro-Cobas V, Chan E. Language development in bilingual children: a primer for pediatricians. *Contemp Pediatr.* 2001;18:79–98

Grizzle KL, Simms MD. Early language development and language learning disabilities. *Pediatr Rev.* 2005;26(8):274–283

Joint Committee on Infant Hearing, American Academy of Audiology, American Academy of Pediatrics, American Speech-Language-Hearing Association, Directors of Speech and Hearing Programs in State Health and Welfare Agencies. Year 2000 position statement: principles and guidelines for early hearing detection and intervention. *Pediatrics.* 2000;106:798–817

Tierney CD, Brown PJ, Serwint JR. Development of children who have hearing impairment. *Pediatr Rev.* 2008;29(12):e72–e73

Zebrowski PM. Developmental stuttering. *Pediatr Ann.* 2003;32:453–458

CHAPTER 29

Literacy Promotion in Pediatric Practice

Lynn Hunt, MD

CASE STUDY

You are seeing a 6-month-old boy for the first time for a well-child visit. The child has a completely negative history and seems to be thriving. The patient's mother works part-time as a housekeeper and his father is a seasonal worker in agriculture. The infant is up to date on his immunizations except for his 6-month shots. The family history is noncontributory, but his mother mentions that her 6-year-old daughter needs to repeat kindergarten. Teachers have advised the mother that her oldest daughter is cooperative, but she has not mastered letters and early reading yet. They feel with "a little more time" she will be fine. The mother does not seem terribly concerned.

Early literacy promotion in the office setting is now recognized as an essential part of pediatric primary care. Both the American Academy of Pediatrics and the Canadian Paediatric Society encourage providers to include literacy promotion in the routine clinical care of toddlers and young children.

Literacy promotion should begin well before a child is ready to learn to read. Eventual mastery of reading will depend on skills such as language ability, imagination, and familiarity with books and the reading process. Children develop many of these skills in the first few years of life before they go to school or even to preschool. In fact, a child's language ability at 3 years of age is strongly correlated with later academic performance. Parent–child interactions are crucial, and guidance for parents regarding literacy promotion activities at home should begin before a child learns to speak.

Reading aloud to children on a regular basis is one of the most effective ways to promote early literacy and language development. Language skills are the foundation for later reading ability and are dependent largely on the amount and quality of language exposure. The architecture of a developing brain is physically altered by experiences during infancy. At birth a baby's brain contains 100 billion neurons, which go on to form trillions more connections. Those connections that are stimulated by frequent use will persist, while less-used synapses will be eliminated as the brain matures. Reading aloud and book sharing may help ensure the preservation of brain connections associated with skills such as memory, creativity, comprehension, and language.

Reading aloud exposes children to vocabulary they don't hear in daily conversations (3 bears, beanstalks, etc). Reading aloud also stimulates the imagination (cows jumping over the moon). Over time, children learn that the abstract letters on the page represent words, and they become aware of different smaller sounds making up words. All of these experiences lead to reading readiness.

Consequences of Low Literacy

There are significant consequences to low literacy as children get older. Poor academic skills are consistently linked with higher dropout rates, entrance into the juvenile justice system, and unemployment. One-third of all juvenile offenders are reported to read below the fourth-grade level and more than 80% of adult prison inmates are high school dropouts.

Literacy level and health outcomes are also intimately related. Health literacy is defined as the degree to which individuals can obtain, process, and understand the basic information they need to make appropriate health decisions. Multiple studies have demonstrated that low literacy impacts health and well-being negatively. Individuals with limited health literacy are more likely to engage in risky behavior and less likely to receive the care they need. Adolescents with low reading ability are more likely to smoke, use alcohol, carry a weapon, and be in a physical fight requiring medical treatment. Conversely, higher levels of literacy are associated with positive health outcomes such as appropriate use of inhaled asthma medication or choosing to breastfeed an infant.

Promoting literacy is good medicine not only for the individual but also for society. Besides the societal impact of school failure, individuals with limited literacy incur medical expenses that are up to 4 times greater than patients with adequate literacy skills. Low literacy costs the health care system billions of dollars every year in preventable visits and hospital stays.

Literacy Promotion in the Medical Office

The model of literacy promotion supported by Reach Out and Read is widely used in many pediatric settings. The Reach Out and Read model has 3 main components.

1. *Anticipatory guidance:* During regular well-child visits, health care providers encourage parents to read aloud to their young children at home. The advice is age-appropriate, and concrete examples are provided or modeled by the provider.
2. *Books:* A new developmentally and culturally appropriate book is given by the doctor at each well-child visit so that parents have the tools to follow their provider's advice.
3. *Waiting rooms:* Literacy-rich waiting rooms contribute to the literacy message. Gently used books for parents to read to their child while waiting and displays or information about local libraries are encouraged. When possible, community volunteers read aloud in the waiting rooms, modeling for parents the pleasures and techniques of reading aloud to very young children.

Reach Out and Read had its origins in an urban clinic serving a high proportion of low-income families and has always had a special focus on children growing up in poverty. For complex reasons, poverty is a powerful predictor of children's exposure to language. Children in low-income homes are 40% less likely to be read to on a daily basis than other children. Pioneer researchers Hart and Risley estimate that by age 4, children living below the poverty line will hear 30 million fewer words in total than those growing up in higher-income households.

Providing advice to parents is easiest and most effective when the book is brought in at the beginning of the visit. That way, physicians can naturally weave in guidance that is appropriate to the age of the child (see Box 29-1 and Table 29-1). Advice should be brief and to the point, supportive, and part of a general conversation about the child's development and behavior.

Another advantage of presenting the book early in the visit is the amount of developmental and relationship information that can be observed. The book is a tool that can speed informal developmental surveillance. If a 2-year-old exclaims, "doggie says wow-wow!" there is no doubt she is putting 2 words together. If a 1-year-old uses an index finger to point and looks to see if his mother is watching, the provider can gain information about fine motor ability and the child's social interaction in only a few moments.

Children benefit from storytelling and book time in whatever fashion is most comfortable for the parent. Ideally books should be in the family's preferred language or bilingual. It is best for parents to use the language that is easiest for them because it is more important for children to hear a language with rich vocabulary and complex sentences than to learn English first. If no book is available in the appropriate language or the parents are not confident with their own reading skills, the primary care provider should encourage parents to look at books, name pictures, and talk about what is going on in the pictures with their children. Provider knowledge of

---

Box 29-1. Anticipatory Guidance for Parents[a]

Specific guidance can help parents with age-appropriate expectations for how their children will handle books and respond to stories.

- ***Newborns and very young babies*** need to hear a parent's voice as much as possible: talking, singing, and telling stories are all good.
- ***6-month-olds*** may put books in their mouths; this is developmentally normal and appropriate and is why we give them chewable board books. It is not in any way an indication that the child is too young for a book!
- ***12-month-olds*** may point with one finger to indicate interest in a picture; parents should see this as developmental progress.
- ***18-month-olds*** may turn board book pages and may insist on turning back again and again to a favorite picture.
- ***2-year-olds*** may not sit still to listen to a whole book, but will still enjoy looking at individual pages, or having parents read them stories bit by bit
- ***3-year-olds*** may retell familiar stories and may memorize their favorite book.
- ***4- and 5-year-olds*** may start to recognize letters or their sounds. They can understand and follow longer stories.
- ***School-aged children*** will start to be able to read to you—but don't stop reading to them, and enjoy taking turns.

[a]Adapted from Reach Out and Read® Provider Training 2010. Used with permission.

---

local programs for adult literacy and English as a second language is often useful because parents may ask for resources when literacy is discussed in the examination room.

Primary Care Providers Can Make a Difference

The primary care setting is the ideal venue for literacy promotion for several reasons. First, almost all parents will bring in their child for immunizations, so there is an opportunity to reach a broad group, not just those seeking learning experiences for their children. In fact, 96% of all children younger than 6 years see their doctor at least once annually. Second, each child is seen for multiple visits from a very young age, providing repeat opportunities to discuss reading aloud during the critical first years. Further, suggestions supporting literacy-focused activities are a logical extension of the advice about growth and development parents are already receiving at these visits. And, when parents trust and value the advice from their primary care provider, early literacy messages assume greater credibility.

The effectiveness of this primary care model to promote reading aloud to young children has been demonstrated in multiple research studies. Parents who received even one book were much more likely to read aloud to their children and report reading as a favorite activity of their child. The effect was greatest for the poorest families, an important finding for children who may need this intervention the most. The outcome was similar for non–English-speaking families, and the findings held even if the book was given in English. Finally, and most encouraging, toddlers and preschoolers who had received

Table 29-1. Developmental Milestones of Early Literacy[a]		
Motor	*Cognitive*	*What Parents Can Do*
6–12 Months		
• Reaches for books • Book to mouth • Sits in lap, head steady • Turns pages with adult help	• Looks at pictures • Vocalizes, pats pictures • Prefers pictures of faces	• Hold child comfortably; face-to-face gaze • Follow baby's cues for "more" and "stop" • Point and name pictures
12–18 Months		
• Sits without support • May carry book • Holds book with help • Turns board pages, several at a time	• No longer mouths right away • Points at picture with one finger • May make same sound for particular picture (labels) • Points when asked, "where's…?" • Turns book right side up • Gives book to adult to read	• Respond to child's prompting to read • Let child control the book • Be comfortable with toddler's short attention span • Ask "where's the …?" and let child point
18–24 Months		
• Turns board pages easily, one at a time • Carries book around the house • May use book as a transitional object	• Names familiar pictures • Fills in words and familiar stories • "Reads" to dolls or stuffed animals • Recites parts of well-known stories • Attention span highly variable	• Relate books to child's experiences • Use books in routines, bedtimes • Ask child "what's that?" and let child answer • Pause and let child complete the sentence
24–36 Months		
• Learns to handle paper pages • Goes back and forth in books to find favorite pictures	• Recites whole phrases, sometimes whole stories • Coordinates text with picture • Protests when adult gets a word wrong in a familiar story • Reads familiar books to self	• Keep using books in routines • Read at bedtime • Be willing to read the same story over and over • Ask "what's that?" • Relate books to child's experiences • Provide crayons and paper
3 Years and Older		
• Competent book handling • Turns paper pages one at a time	• Listens to longer stories • Can retell familiar story • Moves finger along text • "Writes" name • Moves toward letter recognition	• Ask "what's happening?" • Encourage writing and drawing • Let child tell story

[a] Adapted from Reach Out and Read®. Available at www.reachoutandread.org/parents/milestones. Used by permission.

care in clinics applying the Reach Out and Read model had higher scores on language and vocabulary assessments than children not served by the program.

Literacy promotion and the Reach Out and Read model of giving books along with advice provide benefits for all concerned. Medical providers have a tool to assist with development surveillance and a way to build stronger bonds with families. Parents receive important information about reading aloud and advice tailored to the age of their child. And most importantly, children receive the benefits of reading aloud as well as beautiful, developmentally appropriate books.

CASE RESOLUTION

You speak to the mother about the value of reading aloud to her children. You give the 6-month-old a board book with pictures of baby faces. You demonstrate, showing how the 6-month-old is interested in the pictures and watches intently as you turn the pages. At the end of the visit you also find a gently used rhyming book that the mother can take home for her 6-year-old.

Selected References

AMA Foundation—Health Literacy
www.ama-assn.org/ama/pub/category/8115.html

Leyendo Juntos: Spanish Language Literacy Promotion for
Pediatric Primary Care Providers
http://www.reachoutandread.org/FileRepository/
LeyendoJuntosProviderGuide.pdf

Reach Out and Read
www.reachoutandread.org

Summary of studies of relationship between health services,
outcomes, costs, or disparities and literacy
www.ncbi.nlm.nih.gov/books/bv.fcgi?rid=hstat1a.table.32324

What Children Like in Books
www.reachoutandread.org/FileRepository/WhatChildrenLikeinBooks.pdf

CHAPTER 30

Gifted Children

Iris Wagman Borowsky, MD, PhD

CASE STUDY

A 3-year-old girl is brought to your office for well-child care. Her parents believe that she may be gifted because she is much more advanced than her sister was when she was the same age. The parents report that their younger daughter walked at 11 months of age and was speaking in 2-word sentences by 18 months. She is very "verbal," has a precocious vocabulary, and constantly asks difficult questions such as, "How do voices come over a radio?" The girl stays at home with her mother during the day but recently began going to a preschool program 2 mornings a week. She enjoys preschool and plays well with children her own age. She also likes to play with her sister's friends from school.

The girl is engaging and talkative. She asks questions about what you are doing during the examination and demonstrates impressive knowledge of anatomy. The physical examination is normal.

Questions

1. How are gifted children identified?
2. What characteristics are associated with giftedness?
3. What are the best approaches for dealing with the education of gifted children?
4. What is the role of the pediatrician in the management of gifted children?

Giftedness has been defined in several ways. The psychometric definition of giftedness is based on scores obtained on standardized intelligence tests. The 2 most frequently used cutoff points are 2 standard deviations above the mean (IQ = 130–135) and 3 standard deviations above the mean (IQ = 145–150). Children with these scores are in the upper 2% and 0.1% of the IQ distribution, respectively. IQ, which is considered to be fairly stable after the age of 3 or 4 years, is the best single predictor of scholastic achievement at all levels, from elementary school to college.

A second definition of giftedness is based on real-life achievements or performance of exceptional skills rather than on test scores. Children with special talents (other than general intelligence) in areas such as music, mathematics, ice skating, chess, or drama fit this description. Other definitions of giftedness recognize motivation, commitment, perseverance, high self-esteem, and creativity as personality traits that allow children with above-average ability to develop exceptional talents.

Epidemiology

The prevalence of giftedness depends on the somewhat arbitrary definitions of giftedness and the varied approaches for identification of gifted children. Traditional screening systems identify 3% to 5% of students for participation in gifted programs in schools. Some schools use an alternative system, where 10% to 15% of children are recognized as above average. In an effort to foster giftedness in these children, schools offer them enriched programs.

Intellectual giftedness in children has been associated with the social, economic, and educational background of their families. Factors that correlate with higher IQ scores in children are more years of parental education, higher IQ scores of mothers, increased family income, smaller family size, and longer intervals between siblings. Children from low-income and minority backgrounds are less likely to be identified as gifted than other children. African American, Hispanic, and Native American students are underrepresented by 30% to 70% in gifted programs in the United States.

Larger head size at 1 year of age and greater height and weight at 4 years of age have also been reported in children with high IQs. Although researchers have found that academically gifted children, as a group, begin to walk, verbalize, and read earlier, such factors are not useful for predicting giftedness in individual children.

Evaluation

One of the primary goals of child health promotion is **developmental monitoring.** The early identification of developmental delays, which allows for prompt intervention, is one of the primary purposes of such monitoring. Techniques for developmental assessment include **review of developmental milestones** with parents and discussion of parental concerns, **informal observation** of children in the office, and **formal screening with standardized tests,** such as the Denver II.

Identification of Gifted Children

Although parents' first concern is usually to confirm that their child is developing normally, it is not uncommon for parents to ask if their child is gifted. Such questions are typically motivated by parents' desire to optimally encourage their child's development. Sharing information and observations with parents during developmental monitoring may facilitate parent–child interaction and child development. In a competitive society, the pediatric provider should look for signs that above-average abilities are the result of undue pressures placed on children, such as incessant teaching or over-scheduling of time.

Infancy and early childhood may not be the best time to determine whether a child is gifted. Age of attainment of developmental milestones and performance on standardized tests (eg, Bayley Scales of Infant Development) during the first 2 years of life are both unreliable predictors of intellectual giftedness. Reasons for this lack of reliability may include weaknesses in the tests and variable rates of child development that result in transient precocity or delay. Tests that focus on visual memory tasks in infants may be better predictors of later academic intelligence; this possibility requires more research. In addition, many special talents that comprise giftedness, such as creativity or artistic or musical ability, may not manifest themselves until children are older.

The determination of giftedness in older children may involve several factors (Box 30-1). The early identification of giftedness allows for the development of an appropriate educational program that is optimally matched to a particular child's ability to learn. Without early identification and intervention, intellectually gifted children may become disillusioned with school, lose interest in learning, fail to develop study skills because they are never challenged to think and work hard, and develop a pattern of underachievement that may be difficult to reverse by the middle grades.

Special Groups of Gifted Children

Giftedness is harder to identify in some children. In **physically disabled children,** giftedness is often obscured by their obvious physical disability, which demands attention. These children may participate in special programs where their physical needs are the major concern at the expense of their academic or artistic potential. In addition, poor self-esteem associated with the disability may prevent these children from realizing their potential. To identify giftedness in physically disabled children, parents and teachers must make a concerted effort to search for potential and encourage its

development. Strengthening a child's capacities may involve training in the use of a wheelchair or computer or taking frequent breaks to prevent fatigue.

Giftedness also commonly goes unnoticed in children who are **learning disabled.** It is quite possible for exceptional and poor abilities to coexist in a given child. In fact, an estimated 10% of gifted children have a reading problem, reading 2 or more years below grade level. Albert Einstein, Auguste Rodin, and John D. Rockefeller are famous examples of brilliant individuals who had reading and writing problems. An extreme example of the occurrence of both extraordinary and deficient abilities together in one individual is the child savant. Affected children possess amazing abilities in one area (eg, music, drawing, mathematics, memory), but they are delayed in other respects. In addition, they have behavioral problems that resemble autism, such as repetitive behavior, little use of language, and social withdrawal.

Learning disabilities may obscure children's talents, thus preventing awareness of their potential. Conversely, children's giftedness may mask their weaknesses, depriving them of needed help. Worst of all, gifted children who are learning disabled may manage to barely "get by" in the regular classroom setting and fail to receive recognition for strengths or weaknesses. Large differences on intelligence and achievement tests between scores in different areas, such as language and spatial abilities, may indicate both giftedness and a learning disability. Attention should be given to both weaknesses and strengths. Research suggests that programs that focus on strengths, not deficits, however, enhance self-esteem in gifted children who are learning disabled and can be extremely beneficial in their academic development.

The identification of giftedness is also difficult in **underachieving children.** Parents may approach the pediatrician with the following frustrating problem: Their child is doing poorly at school, although they believe that the child is bright because of the child's abilities and participation in advanced activities at home. Underachievement may result from a learning disability; poor self-esteem; lack of motivation; or the absence of rewards, either at home or at school, for succeeding in academics.

As previously stated, giftedness is less likely to be recognized in children from low-income or ethnically diverse families. Many of the tests used to identify giftedness have been "normed" on white, English-speaking, middle-class children. In the absence of tests that are sensitive to socioeconomic differences, other means for identifying giftedness, such as assessment of creative work and teacher and student nominations, should be stressed. Schools with students from low-income or minority backgrounds tend to use their limited resources to help students who are doing poorly in school, rather than gifted students. Research has shown that programs for gifted children from such backgrounds benefit all students by creating positive role models and promoting the school as a place for the cultivation of excellence.

Box 30-1. Factors Used in the Identification of Giftedness in Children

- Intelligence tests
- Standardized achievement tests
- Grades
- Classroom observations
- Parent and teacher rating scales
- Evaluation of creative work in a specific field (eg, poems, drawings, science projects)

Management

At Home

Loving, responsive, stimulating parenting should be encouraged for all children, including gifted children. Parents of gifted children may feel inadequate, fearing that their child is smarter than they are. The pediatrician can provide **parental reassurance** by telling parents, "You must have been doing something right for your child to have been identified as gifted." Children's librarians, periodicals written for parents and teachers of gifted children (eg, *The Gifted Child Today*), and the local chapter of the National Association for Gifted Children are good resources for parents.

Parents are often overwhelmed with complex questions from their precocious preschool children about issues ranging from homelessness and world hunger to theology and the creation of the universe. The pediatrician should tell parents that they (1) should not be afraid to admit that they do not know all the answers and (2) should work together with their child to find the answers.

The pediatrician may need to warn parents about putting too much pressure on their gifted children. For example, enrolling children in multiple classes often leaves little free time for unstructured play. Play affords many opportunities for self-learning, interaction with peers, and development of creativity and initiative. Parents of infants, toddlers, and preschoolers should be encouraged to take cues from their children. If children have a rich environment with plenty of objects and books to explore, diverse experiences, and stimulating interactions, they will develop their own interests. Other educational materials and special instruction can then be provided in a particular area of interest.

Gifted children are often mistakenly considered to fit the stereotype of troubled, socially awkward "nerds." With the exception of children at the genius extreme (IQ>180), gifted children are generally more sociable, well-liked, trustworthy, and emotionally stable than their peers, with lower rates of mental illness and delinquency. Nevertheless, they have the same emotional needs as other children. Gifted children may prefer to play with older children whose interests and abilities are closer to their own. This should be allowed as long as these relationships are healthy.

Parents should be encouraged to treat gifted children the same way they do their other children. Siblings of gifted children may become resentful if attention is centered on their brother or sister. They may feel inferior, particularly if gifted children surpass them in school. Tensions may be magnified if gifted children become friends with their older sibling's friends. To preserve a sense of self-worth and competence in siblings, the pediatrician should recommend to parents that they set aside special time to spend with each of their children. Parents should encourage other talents (eg, musical or athletic abilities) in siblings. Older siblings should receive the special privileges and responsibilities that come with age, such as staying up later or doing different chores. Any tensions within the family should be openly discussed and addressed.

At School

Parents often seek advice from their pediatrician about educational planning for gifted children. A learning environment with the optimal degree of challenge—hard enough to require new learning and stave off boredom, but not so hard as to be discouraging—is the goal for all children. Parents of young children should look for preschools with flexible programs and capable teachers to accommodate children with precocious skills. Parents of school-aged children must decide whether **acceleration** (starting school earlier or skipping grades) or **enrichment** (staying in the same grade but supplementing the regular curriculum) is more appropriate (Table 30-1). The choice depends on the particular child.

Parents and teachers of gifted children are usually concerned that children in accelerated programs may have problems with social adjustment if their classmates are older. Existing evidence, however, suggests that gifted children benefit socially from acceleration. Gifted children in accelerated programs participate in school activities (except contact sports) more often than gifted children placed with classmates of the same age. Even when gifted children are placed with children their own age, they tend to make friends with older children with whom they share more interests. Gifted children also make up any curricular content missed by grade skipping. Because the process may be difficult to reverse, acceleration may not be the best option when the decision is a borderline one.

Table 30-1. Acceleration Versus Enrichment in Gifted Education		
	Advantages	*Disadvantages*
Acceleration	May provide suitable academic challenge	Difficult to reverse
	May have social benefits	May have to skip more than one grade to be properly challenged
	Can be offered by all schools	
	Inexpensive	
Enrichment	Classmates are same age	May be expensive
	May expose children to subjects they would not otherwise learn	Inadequate for highly gifted children
	Appropriate for mildly gifted children	May isolate gifted from non-gifted children and encourage "elite" label
		May lead to excessive homework if children have to make up work of regular class

Enrichment involves keeping gifted children with same-age class-mates, but supplementing the regular curriculum. Regular class placement with a teacher who is willing to offer extra work (eg, special projects) in addition to grade-level assignments, part-time programs to supplement regular class work (eg, field trips, foreign language classes), honors classes that group bright children together for their basic curriculum, and independent study by the family at home are all examples of enrichment programs. These programs may work well for some gifted children, depending in large part on the resources and funding available and the experience, creativity, and enthusiasm of the teachers involved.

Some enrichment programs may isolate gifted from non-gifted children, however, and encourage labeling of the gifted students as elite. If children are required to make up the regular class work that they miss when they are involved in the enrichment program, they may find themselves overloaded with homework.

Often a **combination of acceleration and enrichment** programs is the best option. Either acceleration or enrichment alone may not be enough for the brightest children. Acceleration may not be suffi-cient for markedly advanced children who would have to skip 2 or 3 grades to be appropriately challenged. The pediatrician should rec-ommend that parents work closely with teachers to achieve the best learning environment for their children. Some factors that should be considered are age, physical size, motor coordination, emotional maturity, personality, and particular areas and degrees of giftedness of the child. Acceleration may be a better option for a large, outgo-ing child than for a small one. Gifted children should be asked what they would like to do.

When evaluating the suitability of an educational situation for their gifted child, parents should watch for some warning signs. Excessive homework should neither be expected nor tolerated because it cuts into the child's time to play and develop socially. The emphasis in gifted education should be on broadening perspectives, not increasing busy work. If gifted children are developing a sense of elitism or peer animosity, the nature and philosophy of the pro-gram should be questioned. Boredom with schoolwork, not need-ing to study, signs of depression, or symptoms suggestive of school phobia, such as recurrent abdominal pain or headaches on school mornings, should prompt investigation into the suitability of the child's program.

Home schooling, either partial to complement classroom curri-cula or full time, is an educational alternative. To decide if this is the best choice for their family and gifted child, recommend that parents who are considering home schooling gather as much information as possible, including talking to other parents who are home schooling their children, reviewing sample curricular materials, and contact-ing school districts and state departments about requirements and specific steps.

Prognosis

Gifted children are a diverse group, comprising children with excep-tional academic, artistic, or other abilities, combined with the cre-ativity and commitment to achieve their potential. Gifted children may be gifted in one area and average or even below average in another area. The purpose of identifying gifted children is to pro-vide them with an educational environment to help maximize their potential. The prognosis for gifted children is excellent. Pediatricians can serve as a resource for parents in raising their gifted child, and help the child and family to obtain appropriate evaluation, educa-tional programs, and supportive resources.

CASE RESOLUTION

In the case presented, the physician should reaffirm the parents' observations that their child is gifted. The parents should be encouraged to explore programs in which their daughter's talents may be fostered, but at the same time, they should under-stand that even gifted children need time for play and unstructured activities.

Selected References

Davidson Institute for Talent Development. www.davidsoninstitute.org

Jaffe A. The gifted child. *Pediatr Rev.* 2000;21:240–242

Liu YH, Lien J, Kafka T, Stein MT. Discovering gifted children in pediatric prac-tice. J *Dev Behav Pediatr.* 2005;26:366–369

Lovett BJ, Lewandowski LJ. Gifted students with learning disabilities: who are they? *J Learn Disabil.* 2006;39:515–527

Morawska A, Sanders MR. Parenting gifted and talented children: what are the key child behaviour and parenting issues? *Aust N Z J Psychiatry.* 2008;42:819–827

National Association for Gifted Children (NAGC). www.nagc.org

National Research Center on Gifted and Talented (NRC/GT). www.gifted.uconn.edu/

Pfeiffer SI. The gifted: clinical challenges for child psychiatry. *J Am Acad Child Adolesc Psychiatry.* 2009; 48:787–790

Plucker JA, Callahan CM, eds. *Critical Issues and Practices in Gifted Education: What the Research Says.* Waco, TX: Prufrock Press; 2007

Robinson NM, Olszewski-Kubilius PM. Gifted and talented children: issues for pediatricians. *Pediatr Rev.* 1996;17:427–434

Rosenberg MD, Robokos D, Kennedy RF. The gifted child. *Pediatr Rev.* 2010;31:41–43

Shaunessy E, Karnes FA, Cobb Y. Assessing potentially gifted students from lower socioeconomic status with nonverbal measures of intelligence. *Percept Mot Skills.* 2004;98:1129–1138

Winner E. The origins and ends of giftedness. *Am Psychol.* 2000;55:159–169

CHAPTER 31

Children and School: A Primer for the Practitioner

Martin Baren, MD, and Geeta Grover, MD

CASE STUDY

An 8-year-old boy is brought in by his parents in early April because his third-grade teacher informed them that he is currently failing in school and may not be promoted to the fourth grade. Review of his medical, developmental, and school histories reveals that he was a very colicky infant and continued to be difficult as a toddler. His language skills were somewhat delayed, although not enough to warrant a full evaluation. His preschool teacher felt that he was easily distracted when doing seat work. In kindergarten he had some difficulty learning all of his letters, numbers, and sounds. Early reading was difficult in kindergarten and first grade, but improved by the end of the year. Second grade was fairly good except for continued concerns regarding inattention and distractibility. By third grade he was struggling more, especially with writing, and not reaching grade level in several areas. He also continued to be inattentive and distractible in his classroom.

Examination reveals a well-developed and well-nourished boy whose growth parameters are within normal limits for his age. He appears somewhat anxious in the examination room, and when asked about school he tells you that he feels he is just not as smart as the other children in his class.

Questions

1. Should grade retention be considered when a child is failing in school?
2. What are the advantages and/or disadvantages of grade retention?
3. What is the differential diagnosis of school failure?
4. What steps should be taken at this time by the parents and the school for the boy in the opening scenario?

Pediatricians, because of their routine contact with young children and their families, are often the professionals most knowledgeable about child development. Pediatricians' longitudinal perspective on their patients' lives places them in a unique position to evaluate, diagnose, and manage not only children's medical needs, but also their developmental, social–emotional, behavioral, and educational ones. Traditionally, the 5-year-old health maintenance visit has been regarded as the "school readiness" visit. However, waiting until this date to address concerns regarding educational readiness is too late. **School readiness** must be promoted from infancy through early childhood.

During the school-aged years, pediatricians should continue to monitor children's school progression by inquiring about academic, social–emotional, and behavioral development. Parents often turn to pediatricians for advice regarding their children's behavioral or academic difficulties at school, which may be leading to **school failure.** The evaluation and management of school failure requires a multidisciplinary approach under the guidance, support, and advocacy provided by pediatricians. It is important that pediatricians have an understanding of the evaluation and management of both children's school readiness needs and school difficulties, should such arise.

Epidemiology

School readiness is the term used to describe those qualities and traits that are considered prerequisites for a child to be ready to be successful in school. According to national surveys of kindergarten teachers, about one-third of children are not ready for school when they enter, and of these children, 25% will repeat either kindergarten or first grade. Language deficiencies and problems with emotional maturity are cited most often as the factors that most restrict school readiness.

School failure is a multifaceted issue and epidemiologically complex. Overall, about 20% of children have one or more developmental, learning, behavioral, or emotional disorders. Only 10% to 15% of children in the United States are receiving special education services because of difficulties with school performance. Finally, we know that children with concerns such as these are 2 to 3 times more likely to drop out of school than children without any of these concerns.

Approximately 10% to 15% of school-aged children repeat or fail a grade in school. Children who have disabilities are nearly 3 times more likely to repeat a grade than children without disabilities. About 1 in 5 children who repeat a grade in school has some identifiable disability. Grade failure is also more common among boys, children living in poverty, minorities, and those in single-parent homes.

Given that the average child in the United States spends nearly 50% of his or her waking day in a school or a similar learning situation for approximately 12 or 13 years, it follows that a lack of success in these settings will lead to difficulties for much, or all, of adult life. Undetected school difficulties can create a lifelong pattern of frustration and failure. Children with **attention-deficit/hyperactivity disorder (ADHD)** are 2 to 3 times more likely to drop out of high school than their peers without ADHD; children with ADHD who attend college are less likely to graduate than their non-ADHD peers (see Chapter 125). About 40% of all juvenile offenders have learning disabilities; many have never received any help for their disabilities. Even more alarming is that 85% of juvenile delinquents and 75% of adult prisoners are functionally illiterate—somehow these children slipped through the cracks of our educational system.

Clinical Presentation

Defining **school readiness** is not an easy task because the intellectual, physical, social, and emotional development among kindergarten-aged children varies tremendously. Generally school readiness means that children are adequately prepared to participate in formal schooling. It is the term used to describe those traits that are considered prerequisites for a child to be ready to succeed in school (Box 31-1). Readiness implies not only adequate pre-academic skills, but also adequate physical, developmental, language, social–emotional, and behavioral skills to allow children to be successful in the formal schooling environment.

With regard to **school failure,** the non-specificity of children's presenting signs and symptoms and of parental complaints make it challenging to determine a specific etiology. For instance, parental concern regarding a child's inability to focus could suggest an attention disorder, learning disability, mood disorder, or perhaps all 3. Parental concerns can be categorized into 3 broad areas: learning (eg, learning disability or problems with higher-order cognition including mental retardation), attention (eg, ADHD), and emotional/behavioral (eg, anxiety, depression, or serious emotional disturbance). Signs of school failure are presented in Box 31-2. It is important to look not only at academic skills, but also at other components of the educational experience, such as social and emotional experiences. Finally, it is important to ascertain the basis for the perception that a child is failing. Does the problem exist in the eyes of the student, parent, teachers, or everyone?

Academic achievement across subjects must be assessed, especially in the areas of reading, mathematics, and writing. In addition, it is also important to evaluate students who have good skills but fail to perform satisfactorily in the areas of writing, planning, organization, project completion, test taking, or classroom participation. Difficulty with academic performance may lead to school failure in spite of satisfactory academic skills.

In addition to academic skills and performance, the development of good social skills and peer relations is equally important. Some

---

Box 31-1. Kindergarten Readiness Skills

Academic
- Counts to at least 10
- Recognizes some printed letters and perhaps a few words (eg, name)
- Beginning to understand connection between oral and written language (evidence of phonological skills)
- Recognizes and matches shapes and colors that are the same/different, etc

Personal, Social, Emotional, and Developmental
- Able to separate from parents for several hours at a time
- Takes care of personal hygiene and toileting
- Verbally communicates personal needs
- Able to relate personal experiences, ideas, thoughts, and feelings with words
- Sustains attention to task for 10 to 15 minutes
- Able to understand and follow directions with 2 or 3 steps
- Able to communicate and play cooperatively with other children (eg, shares and takes turns)
- Copes with anger and frustration

Motor
- Uses pencil, crayon, and scissors
- Runs, jumps, hops, skips, and throws ball
- Draws a person and basic shape

Box 31-2. Signs of School Difficulties

- Grade retention
- Loss of self-esteem
- Short attention span/hyperactivity
- Not able to follow directions, pay attention, or finish a task
- History of speech-language problems
- Not able to carry thoughts or ideas to paper
- Not able to read, write, or spell appropriate to age and educational level
- Requires excessive time to complete homework/excessive parental involvement with homework
- Previously tested but not eligible for special education (eg, child may be a "slow learner")
- Child hates school/psychosomatic symptoms
- Child has few, if any, friends or change of friends
- Sudden change in behavior
- Depression
- Substance use

---

students have difficulties "fitting in," which leads to a disappointing educational experience in spite of academic excellence.

Pathophysiology

Developmentally there is support for the concept of promoting **school readiness** from a young age. The developing brain continues to make new synaptic connections and "prune" away underused connections from birth to about age 5—well before formal schooling begins. For example, we know that children who grow up without being read to and with little exposure to books or printed language during the first 5 years of life are at an increased risk of developing reading failure and subsequent school failure (see Chapter 29). School readiness must be promoted from infancy throughout early childhood—waiting for the 4- to 5-year-old well visit is too late. Most children with learning disabilities experience language, motor skills, or behavior problems well before they encounter difficulties in the classroom.

School failure is a complex issue with a wide variety of causes. Both intrinsic, or child-related causes, and extrinsic, or environmental-related causes, relating either to the home or the school setting must be considered (Box 31-3). In most cases, school failure is the result of a complex interaction between child, family, and school-related variables, and not simply the result of a single factor (eg, ADHD). Before looking for specific learning disabilities or disorders or intellectual problems, investigate any type of external situation that may be causing the problem. Medical problems should always be considered. Neurologic, psycho-emotional, and behavioral disorders based in the central nervous system may be responsible for school failure.

Unrecognized ADHD, learning disorders, and learning disabilities are common causes of school failure. Learning disorders are defined problems within the central nervous system that prevent children from learning to their full potential. The brain has difficulty handling information (processing skills), which therefore affects the child's ability to learn and/or perform in school. Some of these processes include memory, language, attention, and coordination. A specific learning disability is a particular type of learning disorder that is defined as a significant difference between a child's natural ability (intelligence—IQ) and his level of achievement, as defined by federal and state laws. This difference is determined by psychoeducational testing performed by psychologists and educators.

Federal law (Public Law 101-476: Individuals with Disabilities Education Act [IDEA]) defines specific learning disability as "a disorder in one or more of the basic psychological processes involved in understanding or in using language, spoken or written, that may manifest itself in an imperfect ability to listen, think, speak, read, write, or to do mathematical calculations, including conditions such as perceptual disabilities, brain injury, minimal brain dysfunction, dyslexia, and developmental aphasia." Operationally, specific learning disabilities are characterized by a discrepancy between ability (as measured by intelligence tests) and actual academic achievement (as measured by school performance). However, specific learning disability does not include children who have "learning problems that are primarily the result of visual, hearing, or motor disabilities, mental retardation, emotional disturbance, or environmental, cultural, or economic disadvantage."

Another important reason for school failure is an unsatisfactory student/teacher relationship. A poor "fit" with either teacher or classroom placement may cause major damage to a child's program.

Finally, there are students who are labeled "lazy" by school personnel. These students are usually found to have one or more of the previously mentioned school difficulties but have never been properly diagnosed. Rarely a student is found who has no major identifiable problem but just isn't motivated to take part in the educational experience. Alternative placement or home schooling may be an answer for these students.

Box 31-3. Causes of School Failure

Intrinsic
- Low cognitive skills (intellect)
- Learning disorders
- Specific learning disabilities
- Attention-deficit/hyperactivity disorders
- Speech and language disorders
- Mood and anxiety disorders
- Low self-esteem
- Social–emotional difficulties
- Neurodevelopmental delays
- Motor coordination disorders
- Chronic or serious medical illness (eg, seizure disorders, cystic fibrosis, asthma)
- Vision, hearing, or speech difficulties
- Poor nutrition
- Sleep problems
- Substance use/abuse
- Genetic history (eg, family history of school problems)

Extrinsic
- Language/cultural differences
- Serious psychosocial concerns: parental depression, history of abuse or neglect
- Disruption in the family (eg, many moves)
- Poor school readiness/absence of enrichment prior to school entry (eg, early book exposure)
- Parental or school expectations not commensurate with child's abilities
- School, classroom placement (poor "fit" or poor teaching)

Evaluation

History

In the past, pediatricians assessed **school readiness** during the 5-year-old health maintenance visit. Clinical approaches to early identification of children at risk for school failure include risk assessments and developmental surveillance and screening. Children most at risk for school problems are those from economically and socially disadvantaged backgrounds. Developmental surveillance and screening (see Chapter 27) allows pediatricians to identify children with developmental, behavioral, and emotional delays, and to provide appropriate anticipatory guidance, as well as referral to early intervention programs.

Historical factors associated with an increased risk of school-related problems include **prematurity; low birth weight; small** for gestational age; and **maternal history of tobacco, alcohol, or illicit substance abuse** during pregnancy (Questions Box: School Readiness). Developmental risk factors especially include delays in the acquisition of language skills. Medical factors that may impact school readiness include lead poisoning, iron deficiency anemia, and failure to thrive. The presence of chronic medical conditions (eg, asthma, diabetes mellitus, and seizure disorders) may impact school readiness either directly or indirectly via absenteeism, medication effects, or self-esteem issues. Environmental risk factors include poverty and lower socioeconomic status, parental depression, domestic violence, substance abuse, or a family history of school problems or learning disabilities.

School Failure

When evaluating for **school failure,** historical information should be sought from parents, schools, teachers, and the children themselves (Questions Box: School Failure). A review of present and past report cards not only provides information regarding academic progress, but also the behavioral and social–emotional assessments. Teacher behavior rating forms and evaluations and results of any psychoeducational evaluations should also be reviewed.

Physical Examination

With regard to **school readiness,** the most important aspect of the 5-year-old health maintenance physical examination includes careful hearing, vision, speech, and language assessments.

The physical examination in the evaluation of **school failure** has a limited but important role. Signs of short attention span, distractibility, overactivity, sadness, or anxiety should all be noted. Special attention should be paid to head circumference, minor congenital anomalies, abnormal facies, and skin lesions suggestive of neurocutaneous disorders (eg, multiple café-au-lait spots or ash leaf spots). The pediatrician should assess for vision, hearing, speech and language, and other appropriate evaluations as suggested by the history.

Neurodevelopmental Assessment

School readiness assessment begins with routine pediatric surveillance and screening (see Chapter 27). Several brief school readiness tests have been developed for use by pediatricians (eg, The Pediatric Examination of Educational Readiness). However, because their reliability and ability to detect subtle learning disabilities or arrive at more complicated diagnoses is not established, it is difficult to recommend any of them for routine use. If a specific school readiness evaluation is warranted, it is best to make a referral either to the school district or to an independent specialist (eg, developmental and behavioral pediatrician or educational psychologist) for a full evaluation.

Neurodevelopmental assessment can help identify the etiology of **school failure.** Neurodevelopmental assessment surveys a child's abilities across the different areas of development (eg, fine motor, language, visual–spatial, and memory skills) and helps to identify areas of strength and weakness. Such an assessment can be performed by professionals such as a developmental and behavioral pediatrician

---

School Readiness — Questions

- Has the child had any preschool or group child care experience and how has the child responded in these settings?
- Were any behavioral, developmental, or emotional concerns raised during those group care experiences?
- Does the child play well with age-appropriate peers or does the child seem to consistently prefer to play with younger or older children/adults?
- Is the child's speech understandable to strangers and can the child hold a conversation about everyday topics of interest?
- Can the child sit and listen to stories or sustain attention to a quiet activity for 10 to 15 minutes?
- Can the child identify colors, shapes, and some letters and numbers?

School Failure — Questions

- How many days of school has the child missed?
- Have any behavioral or attentional concerns been raised by the classroom teacher?
- Is the child having problems in all academic areas or are there particular subjects that are especially difficult for the child?
- Has any testing (eg, psycho-educational evaluation) been performed either by the school district or privately?
- Is the child receiving any special services (eg, speech therapy) or accommodations at school?

---

or a psychologist. Psycho-educational assessment is also critical in the evaluation of children with school failure. Such an assessment includes an evaluation of the children's cognitive abilities, academic achievement across subjects (eg, reading, writing, and mathematics), and assessments of perceptual strengths and weaknesses and social and emotional functioning. This can be accomplished either through the public school system via the **Individualized Education Plan (IEP)** process, as mandated by federal law (**IDEA**) or privately by an educational psychologist.

Management

The first aspect of management is the counseling or demystification of parents and children. Empowering parents with knowledge gives them the confidence to interact positively with their children's schools and allows them to advocate effectively for their children's educational needs. For children, the process of demystification should begin with the assurance that all people have strengths and weaknesses—mentioning one's own weaknesses or citing famous or successful people that have dealt effectively with their own learning concerns helps "humanize" and destigmatize the situation for children. It is important to use an optimistic tone. In addition to addressing the needs of families and children, the physician also serves an important advisory role for the school regarding behavioral consequences of a child's disorder (eg, Should this child have a seizure or a behavioral outburst in the classroom, how should the situation be managed?) or the educational implications of chronic medical conditions.

Early intervention is the key to success with regard to children's **school readiness.** For many at-risk children, early childhood education programs such as Head Start and other preschool compensatory programs may come too late. Programs for younger children and their families (eg, Early Head Start) that promote good parenting, language stimulation, and learning through play are valuable and available in some communities.

Reading aloud to children is one of the most important parental interventions that physicians can promote, and it builds the child's skills required for eventual success in reading (see Chapter 29). Reading promotes language mastery, and language mastery, in turn, is one of the keys to school readiness.

The pediatrician can assist families with children who have clear developmental disabilities, such as mental retardation, cerebral palsy, or autism, to access special education services as mandated by the **IDEA of 1990 and the Amendments of 1997** and **2004.** These laws require public schools to provide a free and appropriate education in "the least restrictive environment" for all children with a disability and require schools to use the IEP process (or Individualized Family Service Plan for children <3 years of age) to identify and evaluate the educational needs of children in order to develop an appropriate educational program to meet each child's needs. Pediatricians should be familiar with their local laws so that they can advocate for these children at the time of school entry if needed.

Children who are at increased risk for school readiness problems because of medical, social–emotional, behavioral, or environmental concerns should be monitored carefully. If these children do not appear to demonstrate age-appropriate skills, they should be referred for further evaluation. Despite early intervention, some children may still not be ready for school at the age-appropriate time. Options for these children include delaying school entry or special educational programs. Delaying school entry may not be the best solution if children remain in the same environment that failed to produce readiness in the first place. In addition, studies have shown that students who are older than their classmates because of delayed school entry have higher rates of behavior problems, substance abuse, and other health risk behaviors in adolescence. An alternative is for these children to enter school along with their same-aged peers, and provide special classrooms or programs for those having difficulties.

The management of school failure requires a multidisciplinary approach. Information from the school, including school reports, teacher conferences and notes, testing that has been completed, and input from other school officials, if appropriate, should be requested. The primary care physician can assist the child and family to work with the school system to obtain the appropriate services. The primary physician may also refer to appropriate resources in the community (eg, educational psychologist or developmental and behavioral pediatrician).

Not infrequently, external factors such as social, family, and school-based issues may be very difficult to alter. Knowledge of the educational laws and community services, as well as ongoing developmental surveillance and screening by the primary care physician, is necessary to build a base from which the prevention of failure in school is possible.

Grade retention is often suggested as the treatment for school failure. At the end of each school year, from kindergarten through 12th grade, the question of promotion is addressed. Though school personnel may regard this decision as "business as usual," the impact of this decision can be far-reaching. Evidence that retention in kindergarten or first grade is helpful in affording mastery of critical reading and other skills is lacking. Retention in higher grades has not been shown to be effective because educational gaps (eg, lack of mastery of first-grade skills) are not readdressed by retention in a higher grade. It is unlikely that "more of the same" will ensure mastery of needed skills.

In fact, data suggest the effect of grade retention on most students is adverse. Most retained students do not improve and many are worse after retention. Self-esteem problems, evident in many cases, often lead to self-destructive behavior and, in later grades, problems such as substance abuse, behavior difficulties, sexual promiscuity, and early drop out from school. In addition, children characterize retention as bad as losing a parent.

To minimize the adverse effects of grade retention, each child's needs and strengths should be addressed and educational programs individualized. Educational alternatives to retention include extra support in the form of classroom accommodations (**section 504 of the Rehabilitation Act of 1973** and also the **Americans with Disabilities Act**) or special education services (**IDEA**). In addition, educational therapy, counseling, or one-on-one tutoring may be beneficial for some children. Equally as important as remediating the areas of weakness is recognizing the child's areas of strength (eg, the idea of using a child's strengths to leverage his weaknesses).

Finally, the pediatrician's role in advocacy can never be underestimated. Examples of advocacy roles for physicians include involvement with the assessment team processes at children's schools, consulting with local school districts, and participation in local or state early intervention interagency councils.

Prognosis

In most cases, most children who show signs of school failure fall into the group of mild to moderate learning and/or neurobehavioral disorders with average cognitive skills. With proper support from educational, medical, family, and psychological sources, most of these students should be able to overcome their particular problems and enjoy successful school careers. Students who may have endured major socioeconomic upheavals will often continue to struggle unless changes in their entire support system are instituted early in their lives. The progress of children who have significant cognitive and/or neurobehavioral or psychological processing problems depends on the severity of their problems and the intensity and timing of the interventions they receive.

Irrespective of its cause, school failure can have lifelong consequences if not properly diagnosed and addressed. Failing students are more likely to drop out of school and/or engage in behaviors that are dangerous to their health as adolescents. Pediatricians can make a significant difference in outcomes by helping families advocate for their failing students to receive appropriate assessment and intervention services.

CASE RESOLUTION

The pediatrician should advise the family to request in writing a psycho-educational evaluation from the school. The pediatrician can also institute an evaluation for ADHD by gathering information from both the family and the school. All of this information should then be discussed with the parents so that formal diagnostic procedures and interventions may be instituted. Ideally the pediatrician will have the time, interest, and training to guide the family through this entire process. However, if this is not possible, referral to an appropriate professional is indicated. With the data from the educational evaluation and the medical workup, an appropriate plan of treatment can be developed.

Selected References

Byrd RS. School failure: assessment, intervention, and prevention in primary pediatric care. *Pediatr Rev.* 2005;26(7):233–243

Byrd RS, Weitzman M, Auinger P. Increased behavior problems associated with delayed school entry and delayed school progress. *Pediatrics.* 1997;100:654–661

Dworkin PH. School failure. In: Parker S, Zuckerman B, Augustyn M, eds. *Developmental and Behavioral Pediatrics: A Handbook for Primary Care.* 2nd ed. Philadelphia, PA: Lippincott, Williams & Wilkins: 2005:280–284

Green M, Sullivan P, Eichberg C. Helping academic underachievers become achievers in their own right. *Contemp Pediatr.* 2005;22:29–36

Levine M. *A Mind at a Time.* New York, NY: Simon and Schuster; 2002

McInerny TK. Children who have difficulty in school: a primary pediatrician's approach. *Pediatr Rev.* 1995;16:325–332

Reiff MI. Adolescent school failure: failure to thrive in adolescence. *Pediatr Rev.* 1998;19:199–207

Rief SF. *Ready-Start-School! Nurturing and Guiding Your Child Through Preschool and Kindergarten.* Paramus, NJ: Prentice Hall Press; 2001

Robinson NM, Olszewski-Kubilius PM. Gifted and talented children: issues for pediatricians. *Pediatr Rev.* 1996;17:427–434

Shaywitz SE, Shaywitz BA. Dyslexia (specific reading disability). *Pediatr Rev.* 2003;24:147–152

CHAPTER 32

Immunizations

ChrisAnna M. Mink, MD

CASE STUDY

A 20-month-old boy who emigrated with his family from Botswana is brought in for a checkup. He has his World Health Organization Expanded Immunization Programme card from his homeland showing that he received a bacille Calmette-Guérin (BCG) vaccine at birth; 3 diphtheria, tetanus, and pertussis vaccines; 3 doses of live oral poliovirus vaccine at 2, 3, and 4 months of age; 3 doses of hepatitis B vaccine at birth and 2 and 9 months of age; and a monovalent measles vaccine at 9 months of age. It is August and his parents plan to enroll him in child care and have brought him for a checkup. His parents report that he is a healthy boy with no immune problems. They report that his uncle, who is infected with HIV, lives with them. The boy has had a 3-day history of a runny nose, cough, and tactile fever. His examination is normal other than mild clear coryza and a rectal temperature of 37.9°C (100.3°F). What immunizations may be given?

Questions

1. What are the different kinds of vaccines?
2. What are the mechanisms of action for live and inactivated vaccines?
3. What are the routinely recommended immunizations for *healthy* pediatric populations?
4. What are the considerations for immunizing selected pediatric populations, such as preterm infants, immunocompromised children, immigrants, international adoptees, and travelers?
5. What are reliable resources for up-to-date information about immunizations?

The Centers for Disease Control and Prevention (CDC) considered immunizations among the top 10 greatest health accomplishments of the 20th century, and vaccines continue to play a major role in the improvement of the health of the world's population. In the United States, almost all of the pathogens for which there are routine vaccinations have decreased in incidence by 95% to 100% since the early 1900s. The only exception to this is pertussis, which has had approximately an 80% reduction. In 2008 the immunization rates for children in the United States remained stable at high levels, with nearly 80% of children aged 19 to 35 months immunized for the 4:3:1:3:3 series [4 diphtheria, tetanus, and acellular pertussis (DTaP): 3 polio: 1 measles, mumps, and rubella (MMR): 3 *Haemophilus influenzae* type b (Hib): 3 hepatitis B virus (HBV)]. Worldwide, the percentage of children immunized with 3 doses of diphtheria, tetanus, and pertussis (DTP) and oral polio vaccines and a measles-containing vaccine is approaching 70%, which is nearly a 3-fold increase in the past 20 years. Since 1990 there has been a decline in the mortality rate for children younger than 5 years in every region in the world, and this is directly related to increased immunizations. Generally, immunizations are safe, well tolerated, and cost-effective, with range of $5 to $16.50 saved for every dollar spent.

Another less recognized benefit of vaccinations is that the schedule has essentially provided the backbone for routine pediatric care in the United States, with regular visits scheduled around the recommended intervals for immunizations. These visits have afforded health care providers opportunities for serial evaluation of infants and young children, as well as education and anticipatory guidance for parents. Increasing availability of new vaccines targeted for older children and adolescents should permit opportunities for improved health care delivery to these older age groups, who have often been medically underserved. Additionally, health care practitioners for adults have a growing appreciation of the critical role of vaccinations for protecting their patients, as well as all members of the family.

General Principles

When considering providing immunizations for an individual, 2 important factors to consider are the health status of the recipient and the type of immunization to be given. The risks and benefits of using the vaccine in the specific host should be weighed carefully. Vaccines are intended for a host who is capable of mounting an appropriate immune response, who will likely benefit from the protection provided and ideally incur little or no risks.

Types of Immunizations

The 2 major types of immunizations are passive and active.

Passive Immunization

Passive immunization refers to the delivery of preformed antibodies, usually as immune globulin (Ig), which may be a general formulation or hyperimmune Ig developed with high concentrations of antibodies against a specific disease, such as HBIg for hepatitis B.

Delivery of Ig may be useful in 3 settings.

1. A host is not able to make antibodies (eg, congenital immunodeficiency).
2. Preventive (pre-exposure or postexposure), especially when the host may not be able to mount an antibody response (eg, immunocompromised child with an acute exposure to hepatitis A [HAV]).
3. Treatment—Ig may be used to ameliorate symptoms when disease is already present (eg, intravenous Ig for Kawasaki disease).

Active Immunization

With **active immunization,** all, part, or a modified product (eg, toxoid or purified antigen) of a microorganism is given to the host to elicit an immune response. The intact organisms may be inactivated (killed) or live-attenuated (weakened). The elicited immune response usually mimics the response to natural infection and, ideally, this occurs with little or no risks to the recipient.

Inactivated Vaccines

Inactivated vaccines may contain **inactivated or killed organisms,** purified components (subunit), or inactivated toxins (toxoids) of the organism. These vaccines are not capable of replication in the host. Most inactivated vaccines are delivered by the intramuscular injection. Generally, inactivated vaccines may be administered simultaneously with other inactivated vaccines, as well as live viral vaccines.

A few viral vaccines are inactivated, including trivalent influenza (TIV), HAV, HBV, inactivated polio (IPV), and human papillomavirus (HPV), and rabies vaccines. Toxoid vaccines that are used routinely include tetanus and diphtheria toxoids alone or in combinations with whole-cell or acellular pertussis components (eg, DTaP, DTP, Td, and Tdap). The acellular pertussis vaccines are composed of one or more purified antigens of *Bordetella pertussis*, in contrast to the whole-cell pertussis vaccines, which are made with killed, whole *B pertussis* organisms. Diphtheria and tetanus toxoids combined with whole-cell pertussis (DTP) vaccines are no longer marketed in the United States, but are used in most developing areas of the world. Other inactivated bacterial vaccines include capsular polysaccharide (CPS) vaccines, such as the 23-valent pneumococcal vaccine and tetravalent meningococcal CPS vaccine.

Conjugate Vaccines

Capsular polysaccharide antigens have been chemically linked to a protein carrier, which converts the T-cell independent polysaccharides to T-cell dependent antigen that can trigger an immune response, even in young infants. The first CPS-protein conjugate vaccine available was for Hib. The Hib bacterium is covered with a CPS, polyribitol-phosphate (PRP). Children younger than 2 years are not efficient at mounting antibodies to the PRP CPS, but with linkage to a protein carrier, the CPS is immunogenic. Since licensure for infants of the Hib conjugate vaccines in 1991, there has been a more than 95% reduction in Hib disease. With the success of the Hib CPS-protein conjugate vaccines, conjugation techniques have been used

for other CPS pathogens including *Streptococcus pneumoniae* and *Neisseria meningitidis.*

Live-Attenuated Vaccines

Live-attenuated vaccines are infectious agents that replicate in the host to elicit an immune response. The administration is generally not IM but by other delivery routes, such as oral, intranasal, or subcutaneous. The live vaccines are often viral, including MMR, varicella-zoster virus (VZV), rotavirus, live-attenuated influenza virus (LAIV, FluMist), oral polio (OPV), and yellow fever (YF) vaccines. Two live bacterial vaccines are available including oral typhoid (Ty21) and BCG used against *Mycobacterium tuberculosis.*

Following measles vaccination, there is a transient suppression of T-cell immunity in the 2- to 4-week postvaccination period. Because of this, when vaccinating with live viral vaccines, give 2 or more live vaccines at the same time or wait at least 4 weeks between vaccines. This principle is also true for tuberculosis skin testing; place the purified protein derivative at the same time as a live viral vaccine or wait at least 4 weeks to avoid a false-negative skin test because of the T-cell suppression. Although this has not been extensively studied with live viral vaccines other than measles, following the same guidelines with other live viral vaccines is recommended.

Vaccination Schedule

Factors for developing the schedule include
- Host ability to respond (eg, lost maternal antibody)
- Need for multiple doses (eg, IPV)
- Minimal intervals needed between serial doses
- Available products (eg, combination vaccines)

A synchronized immunization schedule is posted annually from the American Academy of Pediatrics (AAP) Committee on Infectious Diseases (*Red Book: 2009 Report of the Committee on Infectious Diseases*), American Academy of Family Practitioners, and the Advisory Committee for Immunization Practices of the CDC. Since 2007, 2 immunization schedules have been posted for the pediatric age groups: one for children younger than 7 years and one for individuals 7 through 18 years of age. A separate schedule is available for adults older than 18 years. The US schedules are posted each January at http://www.cdc.gov/vaccines/recs/schedules/child-schedule.htm. Schedules for countries worldwide are available at www.who.int/immunization_monitoring/en.

Vaccine Recipients

Healthy Pediatric Populations

Routine immunizations on the synchronized schedule are targeted for healthy infants, children, and adolescents. All licensed vaccines have undergone review by the US Food and Drug Administration (FDA) and have proven safety and immunogenicity and/or efficacy for the targeted population. However, no vaccine is completely free of adverse events nor will provide 100% protection for every recipient. Every effort should be made to provide immunizations when the recipient is healthy and has the best chance to mount an optimal immune response without delaying vaccination or risking a "missed opportunity."

Special-Risk Pediatric Populations

Although immune responses to vaccinations are likely most favorable in healthy recipients, a growing segment of the pediatric population has underlying health problems. Because of congenital or acquired immune dysfunctions, some individuals should not receive immunizations as directed by the routine schedules. Special accommodations need to be made for immunizing these individuals, such as adjusting the schedule or possibly not administering some agents. There are no indications for giving decreased or partial doses of vaccines. Some of the selected populations for whom special consideration is indicated are discussed below.

Immunocompromised Child

The plan for vaccination of an **immunocompromised** child should be determined by the nature and degree of immunosuppression. The health care practitioner should weigh risks and benefits for each child individually, keeping some general principles in mind. For example, live vaccines should not be given to severely compromised individuals because of the possible risks. Generally inactivated vaccines may be safely administered to nearly all recipients; however, immunocompromised individuals may not mount an optimal immune response. In this setting, try to adjust timing of vaccination to optimize the chance of a good immune response. Guidelines include waiting for 3 to 4 weeks post-chemotherapy and white blood cells greater than 1,000 cells/mm^3 for chemotherapy patients, 4 weeks after stopping high-dose steroids (dose equivalent ≥2 mg/kg/day of prednisone for ≥14 days), and sufficient time after receipt of Ig (see AAP *Red Book*).

Types of Immunodeficiency

Infants and children may have abnormalities of any arm of the immune system, which may affect their ability to receive vaccinations. Weighing the risks (of the disease, as well as vaccine) and benefits of protection is essential. A reasonable approach to developing a vaccination plan for children with immune abnormalities is to consider the pathogenesis of immune defense against the vaccine agents and if the needed defense mechanism is deficient, then immunizing with that agent may not be appropriate. For example, **cellular immunity** is essential in defending against **viral agents.** Thus children with abnormalities of their cell-mediated immunity (primary or acquired) may not be candidates for receipt of live viral vaccines.

Primary immunodeficiencies are generally inherited and secondary ones are acquired, such as infection with HIV, malignancy, illnesses (such as malnutrition and uremia), or related to medications (eg, chemotherapy or immunosuppressive agents), among others. For primary humoral immunity abnormalities (not able to make antibodies), OPV is contraindicated but MMR vaccine may be indicated for some individuals. For cell-mediated abnormalities, generally live viral vaccines should not be used. With complement abnormalities, receipt of live viral vaccines is acceptable for most individuals. For abnormal phagocytic function, live bacterial vaccines should not be given. For individuals with asplenia (traumatic or surgical), vaccination with pneumococcal, meningococcal, and Hib vaccines is indicated and should be considered emergently in the case of trauma. Chemoprophylaxis may also have a role in protection for compromised individuals.

For immunocompromised household contacts of pediatric vaccinees, it is generally acceptable to give MMR, VZV, and oral rotavirus vaccines. Some live vaccines should not be given, including OPV and LAIV in some settings. Additionally, use of some vaccines, such as TIV, is encouraged to protect the vaccinee, as well as the compromised contacts.

Pregnancy

Pregnancy is associated with **some impairment of cell-mediated immunity.** With this decreased immunity, pregnant women may not have protective immune responses to some infectious agents. With this in mind, generally no live vaccines should be administered to pregnant women, though the risks and benefits should be weighed for individual cases. Rubella vaccine should not be given to pregnant women, though there have been no reported cases of rubella embryopathy following inadvertent immunization of a pregnant woman.

Some immunizations are recommended during the second or third trimester to provide protection for the mother (ie, TIV) and possibly the infant (eg, tetanus and diphtheria toxoids combined with acellular pertussis vaccine [Tdap]). Residing with a pregnant household contact is generally not a contraindication for a child to receive live viral vaccines, a question often asked of pediatricians.

Preterm (<37 Weeks) and Low Birth Weight (<2,000 g) Infants

In general, medically stable premature and low birth weight infants may be immunized at the same dose, schedule, and postnatal age as full-term infants.

Special consideration should be given to use of HBV vaccine in infants that weigh less than 2,000 g as follows:

- Hepatitis B surface antigen (HBsAg)-positive or unknown status in mom→Give vaccine and HBIg, then give 3 additional vaccine doses.
- HBsAg-negative mom→Give HBV vaccine at 30 days (sooner if the infant is stable for discharge), and then follow the usual schedule, such that the infant receives a total of 3 doses.

Other Conditions Affecting Immunization Schedule

Egg-Allergic Child

For children with known anaphylactic reactions to eggs or egg components, special consideration is warranted for use of vaccines prepared using egg products. Current measles and mumps vaccines are prepared using chick-derived cell lines, but do not contain significant amounts of proteins that cross-react with egg proteins. Children with egg allergies, including severe hypersensitivity, are at low risk of anaphylaxis from measles- or mumps-containing vaccines.

Additionally, skin testing against these antigens is not predictive of an adverse reaction. Thus, egg-allergic children may be immunized with measles and mumps vaccines alone or in combination preparations (eg, MMR, MMR and varicella) without skin testing. Influenza (TIV, LAIV) and YF vaccines are prepared in eggs and may contain egg proteins, and may rarely induce an immediate allergic reaction. For children with a history of anaphylaxis to eggs or egg components, both TIV and LAIV are generally contraindicated because of the risk of an adverse event and the need for annual immunization. For YF vaccine, skin testing before use is recommended in children with a history of anaphylaxis to eggs.

International Adoptees, Travelers, Immigrants, and Refugees

It is important to remember that travelers are from all socioeconomic strata, so inquiries about foreign travel should be included in routine visits in all clinical settings. First, the health care practitioner should review the child's record to ensure that all routine vaccines are up to date for age. The child should receive vaccinations and other preventive measures (eg, malaria prophylaxis) targeted for his or her destination. There may be a need for accelerated schedule (eg, early MMR for infants 6–12 months of age traveling to a measles-endemic area). Use of Ig prophylaxis should be considered for individuals susceptible to HAV and not candidates for active immunization (eg, too young to receive HAV vaccine or immunocompromised). To help ensure healthy travel, the health care practitioner should check the current recommendations at http://wwwnc.cdc.gov/travel/default.aspx and http://www.who.int/countries/en/.

Immigrants, refugees, and international adoptees may present with additional health concerns. Many of these children have been in poor living conditions and exposed to health hazards of environments like refugee camps and orphanages. Their health status, possible intercurrent illnesses, and need for immunizations should all be evaluated soon after arrival. The United States requires proof of the first dose of vaccines for entry into the country, though there are exemptions for adoptees younger than 10 years and refugees at entry. These high-risk children often have not been immunized or have missing records. Written, dated, and appropriate records (eg, age, dates, interval, and number of doses) may be considered valid, and subsequent immunization may resume according to the US schedule. Another option, especially when documentation is questionable, is to perform serologic studies for vaccine-induced antibodies.

Adolescents

Although the AAP has recommended a routine health visit at 11 to 12 years of age, historically compliance with this visit had been low. Until recently, no immunizations were routinely recommended in this age group. In the late 1990s, hepatitis B catch-up immunization was the first vaccine encouraged at this age and became required for middle-school entry in several states. Now several vaccines are available for protecting teens. One of these vaccines is Tdap for use as a single booster dose in adolescents 11 to 18 years of age who have previously received a series of DTP–containing vaccines.

Two kinds of meningococcal vaccines are available for use in the United States: the CPS vaccine (MPSV4, Menomune) and the CPS-protein conjugate vaccine (MCV4, Menactra and Menveo), with the latter formulation being preferred by the AAP. Both vaccines contain 4 serotypes (A, C, Y, and W135). Meningococcal immunization with MCV4 is recommended routinely at age 11 to 12 years with a booster dose at 16 years of age. MCV4 is also recommended for catch-up dosing for older adolescents who have not been immunized and for individuals 2 to 55 years of age who are at increased risk of meningococcal diseases.

Two HPV vaccines are available in the United States for immunizing females against cervical cancer. Both HPV2 and HPV4 are composed of virus-like particles prepared from recombinant L1 capsid protein of HPV. One of the currently licensed vaccines is HPV2 (Cervarix, GlaxoSmith Kline), containing serotypes 16 and 18, which is available for vaccinating females 10 to 25 years of age. Human papillomavirus 16 and 18 cause about 70% of cervical cancers. The other licensed vaccine is HPV4 (Gardasil, Merck & Co., Inc.), containing serotypes 6, 11, 16 and 18, which is licensed for females aged 9 to 26 years and also for males aged 9 to 26 years for protection against genital warts and anal and penile cancers. Both HPV2 and HPV4 are given in a 3-dose regimen at day 0, 1 to 2 months, and 6 months, and are recommended for routine use in adolescents at 11 to 12 years of age, ideally before their sexual debut.

In addition, at the adolescent visits (including precollege visits), the provider should review the teen's records to ensure that he or she has received all recommended vaccines, inquire about household contacts of infant or compromised host, and provide anticipatory guidance for safe and healthy living for the teen and the parent.

Immunizations Received in Other Countries

Most vaccines used worldwide are produced with adequate quality control and may be considered reliable. Healthy individuals immunized in countries outside of the United States should receive vaccines according to the recommended schedule for age in the United States. In most cases, only written documentation should be accepted as proof of previous vaccination. Written, dated, and appropriate records (eg, correct age, dates, interval, and number of doses, etc) may be considered as valid, and immunizations may resume according to the US schedule.

Although most vaccines are acceptable, there may be some concerns for vaccine potency due to unsuitable storage and handling. Other concerns include inaccurate documentation and possibly inadequate response in some children due to other factors (eg, malnutrition or underlying illnesses). If vaccination status is uncertain, the options include vaccinating with the antigen in question or checking serologic testing against the vaccine antigen, if testing is available. Generally, receipt of additional doses of diphtheria and tetanus toxoids alone or in combination with a pertussis-containing vaccine (ie, DTP, DTaP, Td, and Tdap) may lead to an increase in reactions (especially injection site reactions), and checking antibody titers against diphtheria and tetanus toxoids is encouraged. At this time, no FDA-approved assays for pertussis antibodies are available, and testing for pertussis antibodies is not recommended. For other vaccines, if the status is unknown, vaccination may be performed because extra doses are generally well tolerated. Most developing countries do not have VZV, conjugated pneumococcal, or Hib vaccines, and these should be given as indicated per the US schedule.

Adverse Events and Vaccine Information

Adverse Events

As noted previously, no vaccine is completely free of adverse events, and the known adverse events should be discussed with vaccinees (non-minors) and/or parents/legal guardians. In addition to discussing the risks and benefits of vaccination, the health care practitioner should include education about the risks associated with the natural disease. This is especially important in current times, when many individuals have not seen the diseases for which vaccines have been successful in controlling or eradicating.

In addition to safety information from the AAP and CDC, the manufacturer's package insert provides information about the rates of adverse events and contraindications for the specific vaccine. Most adverse events observed following routine immunizations are local injection site reactions such as erythema, swelling, and pain, and systemic reactions such as fever or fussiness. Although most of these adverse events are mild and self-limiting, some may be associated with significant dysfunction for the child (eg, not using a limb due to pain).

Rarely, serious adverse events may occur following immunization, and these may be associated with permanent disability or life-threatening illness. The occurrence of an adverse event after immunization does not prove a cause-and-effect relationship of the vaccine and the event, but a temporal relationship. If a vaccine recipient experiences a serious adverse event, a complete evaluation for all plausible causes, including the role of the vaccine antigen, should be performed. Additionally, all clinically significant adverse events should be reported to the Vaccine Adverse Event Reporting System (VAERS) at http://vaers.hhs.gov/, which is maintained by the CDC and FDA. Adverse event reporting is important because it helps identify possible unexpected events that were not observed in the prelicensure clinical trials.

Precautions and Contraindications

The Vaccine Information Statement (VIS) and package insert provide information for health care practitioner, vaccinees (non-minors), and parents/legal guardians about the precautions and contraindications for specific products.

A **precaution** suggests that careful analysis of risks and benefits of the vaccine should be done, and if benefits outweigh risks, the vaccine may be given. A **contraindication** means that a vaccine should not be administered. An example of a contraindication is known anaphylaxis to any component of the vaccine. Breastfeeding does not interfere with oral immunization with rotavirus or OPV vaccines and is not a contraindication.

Minor illness without fever (temperature ≤38°C [100.4°F]) should not be considered a contraindication to vaccination. Fever above 38°C (100.4°F) may not be a contraindication, depending on the physician's assessment of the child, the illness, and the vaccine to be given. If the child is early in the disease and the course is not predictable or the illness is moderate to severe, delaying immunization is reasonable. Deferring immunization without appropriate justification can cause a missed opportunity and may lead to inadequate immunization of the child.

Informing Vaccine Recipients and Parents

Vaccine recipients and parents should be informed about the risks and benefits of vaccination and about the disease for which the vaccine is designed. The National Childhood Vaccine Injury Act of 1986 requires that parents receive a VIS each time a child receives a vaccine covered under this legislation, whether the vaccine was purchased with public or private funds. The VISs are available from the CDC at the National Immunization Program site at http://www.cdc.gov/vaccines/pubs/vis/default.htm. The health care practitioner should document in the patient's chart the vaccine manufacturer, lot number, and date of administration and that VISs were provided and discussed with the vaccinee (non-minor) and parent/legal guardian.

Vaccine Information

Information about current immunizations for health care practitioners and for laypersons is available from many resources, including the CDC, AAP, FDA, and the World Health Organization, among others. A list of Web sites is provided in Table 32-1.

Table 32-1. Internet Sources of Vaccine Information	
Source	*Web Site*
American Academy of Pediatrics (AAP)	www.aap.org
Centers for Disease Control and Prevention (CDC)	www.cdc.gov
National Immunization Program	www.cdc.gov/vaccines/pubs/ACIP-list.htm
Morbidity and Mortality Weekly Reports (MMWR)	www.cdc.gov/mmwr/preview/mmwrhtml/rr5102a1.htm
Food and Drug Administration (FDA)	www.fda.gov/cber/vaccine/licvacc.htm
Vaccine Adverse Event Reporting System (VAERS)	http://vaers.hhs.gov/
American Society for Tropical Medicine and Hygiene (ASTMH)	www.astmh.org
World Health Organization	www.who.int/en/
Global Alliance for Vaccines and Immunization (GAVI)	www.gavialliance.org

CASE RESOLUTION

The boy was appropriately immunized for Botswana recommendations through the age of 9 months, though now his immunization would be considered delayed for age on the US schedule. He is past due for the fourth dose of DTaP, MMR, and VZV vaccines. Additionally he has not received any conjugate vaccines or HAV vaccine. The dose of monovalent measles vaccine does not change his need to receive 2 doses of MMR and varicella vaccines after the age of 12 months as listed on the US schedule. His uncle's immune status does not affect the use of MMR or varicella vaccines. His current respiratory illness is considered mild, and he does not have significant fever (<38°C [100.4°F]), so this is not problematic for receiving the needed immunizations.

During this visit, he may receive DTaP, MMRV #1, one dose of Hib conjugate vaccine, dose 1 of 2 of conjugate pneumococcal vaccine (2 months apart), and dose 1 of 2 of HAV (at least 6 months apart). All VISs should be provided. He is scheduled to return in 2 months in October for his next dose of conjugate pneumococcal vaccine and dose 1 of 2 of inactivated influenza vaccine. He may not receive the LAIV because of his young age (LAIV is licensed for children ≥24 months of age), as well as his uncle's immunocompromised status. He will need a fourth dose of inactivated poliovirus vaccine before school age. He is too old to receive the oral rotavirus vaccine.

Selected References

American Academy of Pediatrics. Vaccine information. In: Pickering LK, Baker CJ, Long SS, McMillan JA, eds. *Red Book: 2009 Report of the Committee on Infectious Diseases.* 27th ed. Elk Grove Village, IL: American Academy of Pediatrics; 2009:1–104

Centers for Disease Control and Prevention. *2007 NIP Annual Report. A Global Commitment to Lifelong Protection through Immunization.* www.cdc.gov/nip/webutil/about/annual-rpts/ar2007/2007annual-rpt.htm

Centers for Disease Control and Prevention. FDA licensure of bivalent human papillomavirus vaccine (HPV2, Cervarix) for use in females and updated HPV vaccination recommendations from the Advisory Committee on Immunization Practices (ACIP). *MMWR Morb Mortal Wkly Rep.* 2010;59(20);626–629. http://www.cdc.gov/mmwr/preview/mmwrhtml/mm5920a4.htm. Accessed March 10, 2011

Centers for Disease Control and Prevention. Nation's Childhood Immunization Rates Remain High. http://www.cdc.gov/Features/dsChildImmunization. Accessed March 10, 2011

Centers for Disease Control and Prevention. Recommended immunization schedules for persons Aged 0–18 Years—United States, 2011. *MMWR Morb Mortal Wkly Rep Quick Guide. 2011;*60(5):Q1–Q4. http://www.cdc.gov/vaccines/recs/schedules/downloads/child/mmwr-child-schedule.pdf. Accessed February 14, 2011

Centers for Disease Control and Prevention. Updated Recommendations for Use of Meningococcal Conjugate Vaccines—Advisory Committee on Immunization Practices (ACIP). *MMWR Morb Mortal Wkly Rep.* 2011:60(03);72–76. http://www.cdc.gov/mmwr/preview/mmwrhtml/mm6003a3.htm?s_cid=mm6003a3_e. Accessed March 10, 2011

James JM, Burks AW, Roberson PK, Sampson HA. Safe administration of measles vaccine to children allergic to eggs. *N Engl J Med.* 1995;332:1262–1265

Kroger AT, Atkinson WL, Marcuse EK, Pickering LK; Advisory Committee on Immunization Practices Centers for Disease Control and Prevention. General recommendations on immunization: recommendations of the Advisory Committee on Immunization Practices (ACIP). *MMWR Recomm Rep.* 2006;55:1–48

Losonsky GA, Wasserman SS, Stephens I, et al. Hepatitis B vaccination of premature infants: a reassessment of current recommendations for delayed immunization. *Pediatrics.* 1999;103:e14

Markowitz LE, Dunne EF, Saraiya M, et al. Quadrivalent human papillomavirus vaccine. *MMWR Recomm Rep.* 2007;56:1–24

CHAPTER 33

Health Maintenance in Older Children and Adolescents

Monica Sifuentes, MD

CASE STUDY

Before a 13-year-old girl enters a new school, she is required to have a physical examination. She has not seen a physician in 5 years and has been healthy. Currently she has no medical complaints. Her examination is completely normal.

Questions

1. What are the important components of the history and physical examination in healthy older children and adolescents?
2. What immunizations are recommended for older children and adolescents?
3. What laboratory tests should be performed at health maintenance visits? Why?

Older children and adolescents are generally healthy individuals who infrequently visit physicians. Visits are often for acute complaints, such as upper respiratory infections or sports-related injuries, and are therefore very problem-oriented. Statistics regarding health maintenance visits in this age group are not readily available because patients go to several different sites for health care and often do not receive comprehensive care at any of these places. Older children and adolescents seek treatment for both acute and chronic conditions in private offices, public health clinics, public hospitals, and emergency departments. It is estimated that less than 15% of adolescents consistently go to pediatricians for health care in general, and the same percentage probably applies to older children as well.

This all too common practice contributes to missed opportunities for anticipatory guidance, health education, and screening for preventable conditions. Screening tests also can be used to identify treatable conditions such as hypertension, anemia, and tuberculosis. Ideally, older children and adolescents should receive recommended immunizations beginning at 11 to 12 years of age; counseling concerning sexual activity, contraception, and sexually transmitted infections (STIs), including HIV; reassurance to address their emotional well-being; guidelines for adequate nutrition; education about tobacco, illicit drugs, and alcohol; and information about physical fitness and exercise as well as violence and injury prevention.

Guidelines for preventive child and adolescent health care have been published by the American Academy of Pediatrics (AAP) Committee on Practice and Ambulatory Medicine, the federal Child Health and Disability Prevention Program, the AAP Section on Adolescent Health, and the American Medical Association. Box 33-1 is a brief summary of these guidelines for older children and adolescents.

The Health Maintenance Visit

The purpose of the health maintenance visit for an older child or adolescent is to assess their general health and well-being and establish a relationship of open communication and trust for future visits. Initial questions asked during this visit should be simple and focus on how the patient feels in general about their health, physical growth, and development, and existing relationships with family and friends. More specific questions can then be formulated depending on the patient's responses. In healthy patients, the medical history can be obtained using a questionnaire that parents and children complete in the waiting room. If this method is used, a separate form should be given to adolescents if he or she is accompanied by one or both parents. The information is then reviewed at the start of the interview. Chronic medical conditions also should be addressed at this time.

Medical History

Older children and adolescents should always be questioned directly about their medical history (Questions Box: Screening in Older Children and Adolescents). Parents should be encouraged to participate only after their child has responded to questions or if invited by the child or adolescent themselves. The degree of parental participation also is influenced by the current cognitive and developmental stage of the patient.

Box 33-1. Guidelines for Adolescent Health Maintenance Evaluation

Screening History	Physical Exam	Universal and Selective Screening Labs/Studies	Anticipatory Guidance and Counseling
Eating disorders	Body mass index	Snellen test	Parenting/communication
Sexual orientation	Blood pressure	Audiometry	Pubertal development
Sexual activity	Comprehensive exam	Hemoglobin or hematocrit	Diet/nutrition
• Consensual and nonconsensual	Genital exam	Tuberculin skin test	Exercise
Tobacco use	Pelvic exam[b]	Cholesterol	Injury prevention
Alcohol use/abuse		• If the patient is obese or there is a significant family history of hyperlipidemia, consider other labs such as fasting glucose, lipid panel	Educational plans/goals
Drug use/abuse (CRAFFT questionnaire[a])		If sexually active,	Lifestyle modifications
School performance		• Urine hCG	• Gender identity
Depression		• Urine NAAT for GC/chlamydia,	• Abstinence
Risk for suicide		• Serum HIV, RPR, hepatitis B and C[c]	• Safe sexual activity
		• Pap smear[b]	• Other reproductive health issues
			• Contraception
			• Avoidance of tobacco, alcohol, and illicit drugs
			• Identifying feelings of sadness/anger

Abbreviations: GC, gonorrhea; hCG, human chorionic gonadotropin; HIV, human immunodeficiency virus; NAAT, nucleic acid amplification testing; RPR, rapid plasma reagin.
[a]See Chapter 132 for CRAFFT questionnaire.
[b]A pelvic examination with a Pap smear is recommended within 3 years of the onset of sexual activity (American Cancer Society) or age 21 (ACOG). Indications for a pelvic examination, see Chapter 40.
[c]If patient engaged in injection drug use or young men having sex with men.

Questions

Screening in Older Children and Adolescents

Questions for both the patient and parent
- How has the child or adolescent been doing lately? Does the parent have any complaints or concerns?
- How does the child or adolescent like school? How are they doing academically and socially? What are their future goals?
- What activities does the child or adolescent currently participate in?
- Does he or she have any hobbies?
- With whom does the child or adolescent live?
- Are there any significant illnesses in the immediate or extended family, such as hypertension, diabetes, or cancer?
- Does the child or adolescent take any medications, herbs, or supplements (prescribed or over the counter) regularly?

Questions for the child or adolescent alone
- Do you have any questions or concerns?
- How are things at home? Are there any problems with parents or siblings? Do you feel safe at home and at school?
- Are you attending school?
- Do you like school? Who do you hang out with at school?
- Have you ever been truant, suspended, or expelled?
- What do you like to do for fun?
- See Chapter 6, Questions Box, for the rest of the interview.

Psychosocial History

The psychosocial component of the interview should be conducted with older children or adolescents alone as well as together with parents after the issue of confidentiality has been reviewed (Questions Box: Screening in Older Children and Adolescents). General questions about school, outside activities or hobbies, and family are often less threatening than inquiries about friends and tobacco use. More sensitive topics relating to drug use/abuse, sexuality, and sexual activity should be addressed after parents have left the room. Subjects initially discussed with parents should be reviewed once again with the teenager alone.

A useful tool for conducting the psychosocial interview has been developed and refined by physicians who specialize in pediatrics and adolescent medicine. Known by the acronym **HEADDSSS**, it reviews the essential components of the psychosocial history: *h*ome environment, *e*mployment and education, *a*ctivities, *d*iet, *d*rugs, *s*exual activity/sexuality, *s*uicide/depression, and *s*afety (see Chapter 6).

Dietary History

A general dietary history should be obtained, with particular focus on eating habits, level of physical activity, and body image. Dietary restrictions, if any, should be investigated. Daily calcium, vitamin D, and iron intake also should be reviewed, especially in adolescent females. Adolescent males should be asked about nutritional supplements.

Family History

Significant illnesses, such as hypertension, hyperlipidemia, obesity, and diabetes, in first- and second-degree family members should be reviewed. Family use of alcohol, tobacco, and illegal as well as prescribed substances also should be determined. Age and cause of death in immediate family members should be recorded.

Medications and Allergies

Prescription as well as nonprescription (over-the-counter) medications, herbs, and supplements should be reviewed along with the indications and frequency of usage.

Physical Examination

The height and weight of patients should be plotted on a growth curve, with particular attention paid to the velocity of growth and the body mass index (BMI = weight (kg) /[height (m)]^2). The blood pressure also should be noted and compared to age- and height-related normative values.

Aspects of the physical examination that are influenced by puberty should be emphasized. The skin should be carefully inspected for acne and hirsutism; clinicians should offer treatment whether or not patients acknowledge that they have skin problems. Tattoos, piercings, and signs of abuse or self-inflicted injury (cutting) also should be noted. The oropharynx should be examined for any evidence of gingivitis or other signs of poor dental hygiene or malocclusion. The neck should be palpated for adenopathy and the thyroid gland for hypertrophy or nodules, especially in adolescent females. The back should be examined for any evidence of scoliosis, which is important to diagnose during this time of rapid growth.

Assessment of the pubertal development of the breasts and genitalia in preadolescent or adolescent females and the genitalia, including presence of pubic hair, in adolescent males is essential. The sexual maturity rating (SMR) (Tanner stage) can then be correlated with other signs of puberty, such as the appearance of acne and body odor. For example, the adolescent female with SMR 4 breasts and immature pubic hair distribution may have an underlying problem, such as testicular feminization syndrome.

The abdomen should be palpated for organomegaly and the testicles for masses, hydroceles, hernias, or varicoceles. Lesions such as warts or vesicles also should be documented. The external female genitalia should be inspected for similar lesions and to document Tanner stage development. A speculum examination should be performed in females who are sexually active and complain of vaginal discharge, unexplained vaginal bleeding, or lower abdominal pain. (See Chapter 40 for additional indications for a pelvic examination.) In general, virginal girls do not require a speculum examination; gentle inspection of the external genitalia is adequate in most cases, with special attention to hymenal patency. A rectal examination is generally reserved for patients with chronic abdominal pain or other specific acute gastrointestinal complaints.

Immunizations

Many recent additions have been made to the preadolescent/adolescent vaccination schedule (Table 33-1). As always, practitioners should verify that patients have completed the primary immunization series. If not, they should be given catch-up doses according to the latest Centers for Disease Control and Prevention (CDC) recommendations. The newest vaccines, tetanus and diphtheria toxoids and acellular pertussis (Tdap) (Adacel, Boostrix), human papillomavirus (HPV) (Gardasil, Cervarix), and meningococcal conjugate vaccine (MCV4) (Menactra) should be given to preteens at the 11- to 12-year visit. The Tdap vaccine replaces the tetanus/diphtheria booster previously given at this age. Pertussis was added to the booster because immunity to pertussis has been noted to wane 5 to 8 years after vaccination, and there has been an increasing prevalence of pertussis detected in adolescents and adults with chronic cough in many communities. A conjugate vaccine against *Neisseria meningitidis* (MCV4 or Menactra) was also approved by the US Food and Drug Administration in 2005. The Advisory Committee on Immunization Practices now recommends that MCV4 be given to all 11- to 18-year-olds. Finally, 2 different vaccines (Gardasil and Cervarix) are currently licensed in the United States to protect against 2 of the HPV types that cause most cervical cancers, oncogenic types 16 and 18. The quadrivalent vaccine, Gardasil, also protects against genital warts caused by nononcogeic HPV types 6 and 11. While there has been some controversy surrounding the HPV vaccine, current recommendations state that the 3-dose series of the quadrivalent or bivalent vaccine should be given routinely at 11 to 12 years of age and to all young women and girls between the ages of 13 and 26. The vaccine is approved for patients as young as 9 years. The quadrivalent vaccine also may be given to males between 9 and 26 years of age. Ideally the vaccine should be administered before the initiation of sexual activity, but it also may be given to adolescents who are already sexually active.

Table 33-1. Recent Changes to the Recommended Immunization Schedule Affecting Adolescents[a]		
	Recommended Age (y)	
	11–12	*13–18*
Tetanus, diphtheria, pertussis	Tdap	Tdap (catch-up)
Human papillomavirus	HPV (3 doses)	HPV (catch-up) (3 doses)
Meningococcal	MCV4	MCV4 (booster at 16 years)
Varicella	Varicella 2-dose series	
Influenza	Influenza annually	

Abbreviations: HPV, human papillomavirus; MCV4, meningococcal conjugate vaccine; Tdap, tetanus and diphtheria toxoids and acellular pertussis.

[a]Modified from Centers for Disease Control and Prevention. Available at http://www.cdc.gov/vaccines/recs/schedules/default.htm.

Recommendations regarding some of the older traditional vaccines have changed as well. A second dose of the varicella vaccine is now part of the primary vaccine schedule for persons aged 7 through 18 years without evidence of immunity. Therefore, if an adolescent or preadolescent has only received one dose, a second dose should be administered. Similarly, if the adolescent has not had the disease or been vaccinated, he or she should receive the 2-dose series. Routine vaccination against hepatitis B also is recommended, regardless of sexual activity, if it has not been administered previously. The 2-dose hepatitis A series should be given to all teenagers not previously vaccinated if they reside in high-incidence communities. Influenza vaccine should be given annually to all children and adolescents and to those who come into close contact with individuals with high-risk conditions. Pneumococcal vaccine should be offered to high-risk groups as well. In addition, a Mantoux skin test for tuberculosis should be placed. (For complete recommendations, refer to Chapter 32.)

Laboratory Tests

A hemoglobin level should be obtained to evaluate for anemia and a urinalysis performed to assess for protein, blood, and pyuria. Other suggested screening tests include hearing and vision tests, and a cholesterol and lipid profile. Although cholesterol screening remains somewhat controversial, it is important to consider in patients who are overweight or obese or have a positive family history for hyperlipidemia or premature atherosclerotic heart disease.

In addition to the above laboratory tests, sexually active adolescents should be screened for STIs. If a pelvic examination is performed, an endocervical specimen should be obtained for nucleic acid amplification testing (NAAT) for gonorrhea and chlamydia. However, if a pelvic examination is not indicated, routine screening for gonorrhea and chlamydia may be performed with a urine sample alone using NAAT methods. The 2010 recommendations from the CDC state that all sexually active women younger than 26 years should be screened annually. Males should be screened if they are symptomatic or have a history of multiple partners and unprotected intercourse. In addition, a rapid plasma reagin test for syphilis and an HIV test should be obtained, especially if another STI is suspected or confirmed. All of the above tests should be offered in the clinically appropriate setting after patients have received pretest counseling with a follow-up visit scheduled to discuss the results.

Patient Education

At the conclusion of the health maintenance visit, positive as well as negative findings should be reviewed with patients and their parents. Depending on the nature of these findings and the age of the patient, practitioners may initially choose to address these findings with the patient alone keeping in mind issues of confidentiality. All recommended screening laboratory studies and immunizations also should be reviewed before their administration, including the need for further follow-up. Subsequent vaccine doses must be outlined for patients and parents. The timing of the next visit and reasons for this visit should be discussed.

The remainder of the visit should be spent addressing any specific concerns of patients and parents, highlighting health care problems (eg, obesity, high blood pressure), and identifying any factors that may be contributing to high-risk behavior, such as drug or alcohol use. Older children or adolescents who are not participating in any deleterious activities should be praised for their positive behavior as well as provided with information regarding injury prevention.

Preparticipation Physical Evaluation for School-aged and Adolescent Athletes

The preparticipation physical evaluation (PPE) is essentially the "sports physical" that many schools require for participation in organized athletic programs. The primary objective of the PPE is to assess the young athlete's readiness to compete safely and effectively in a given sport. Ideally, it also should identify athletes at risk for injury or sudden death, as well as those with an underlying medical condition that may preclude athletic participation.

Controversy exists about the appropriate location for performance of the PPE. Community physicians are often asked to perform limited en masse examinations at schools, or a group of clinicians is asked to perform the examinations in the gymnasium using "stations." Either way, the patient does not truly receive a complete physical examination or assessment, and neither approach lends itself to privacy. In addition, parents have a false sense of security and believe that their children have received adequate medical care. Ideally, primary care physicians should perform the PPE annually in their office during a scheduled visit at least 4 to 6 weeks before the beginning of the athletic season. Pediatricians can use this required visit as an opportunity to perform an annual comprehensive health maintenance examination on older children and adolescents, including the various screening tests.

History

The medical history for the PPE should primarily focus on previous athletic participation and any injuries that may have occurred (Questions Box: Preparticipation Physical Evaluation). A standard questionnaire codeveloped by the AAP for this purpose may be used in the office setting. In addition, many practitioners record the results of the physical examination as well as their recommendations regarding the degree of athletic participation on this standard form (Figure 33-1).

Questions

Preparticipation Physical Evaluation

- What sport(s) does the child or adolescent wish to participate in?
- Has the child or adolescent ever experienced a sports injury? If so, how much time did the athlete refrain from sports activities as a result of this injury?
- Has the athlete ever suffered a lapse of consciousness or concussion?
- Does the child or adolescent have a significant underlying health problem?
- Is the child or adolescent taking any prescribed or over-the-counter medications?
- Does the child or adolescent have any allergies?
- Has the child or adolescent ever had syncope, palpitations, or angina during exercise?
- Does the child or adolescent have a family history of sudden, early, non-traumatic deaths?

■ PREPARTICIPATION PHYSICAL EVALUATION
HISTORY FORM

(Note: This form is to be filled out by the patient and parent prior to seeing the physician. The physician should keep this form in the chart.)

Date of Exam _____

Name _____ Date of birth _____

Sex _____ Age _____ Grade _____ School _____ Sport(s) _____

Medicines and Allergies: Please list all of the prescription and over-the-counter medicines and supplements (herbal and nutritional) that you are currently taking

_____

_____

_____

Do you have any allergies?   ☐ Yes   ☐ No   If yes, please identify specific allergy below.
☐ Medicines   ☐ Pollens   ☐ Food   ☐ Stinging Insects

Explain "Yes" answers below. Circle questions you don't know the answers to.

GENERAL QUESTIONS	Yes	No
1. Has a doctor ever denied or restricted your participation in sports for any reason?		
2. Do you have any ongoing medical conditions? If so, please identify below: ☐ Asthma ☐ Anemia ☐ Diabetes ☐ Infections Other: _____		
3. Have you ever spent the night in the hospital?		
4. Have you ever had surgery?		

HEART HEALTH QUESTIONS ABOUT YOU	Yes	No
5. Have you ever passed out or nearly passed out DURING or AFTER exercise?		
6. Have you ever had discomfort, pain, tightness, or pressure in your chest during exercise?		
7. Does your heart ever race or skip beats (irregular beats) during exercise?		
8. Has a doctor ever told you that you have any heart problems? If so, check all that apply: ☐ High blood pressure ☐ A heart murmur ☐ High cholesterol ☐ A heart infection ☐ Kawasaki disease Other: _____		
9. Has a doctor ever ordered a test for your heart? (For example, ECG/EKG, echocardiogram)		
10. Do you get lightheaded or feel more short of breath than expected during exercise?		
11. Have you ever had an unexplained seizure?		
12. Do you get more tired or short of breath more quickly than your friends during exercise?		

HEART HEALTH QUESTIONS ABOUT YOUR FAMILY	Yes	No
13. Has any family member or relative died of heart problems or had an unexpected or unexplained sudden death before age 50 (including drowning, unexplained car accident, or sudden infant death syndrome)?		
14. Does anyone in your family have hypertrophic cardiomyopathy, Marfan syndrome, arrhythmogenic right ventricular cardiomyopathy, long QT syndrome, short QT syndrome, Brugada syndrome, or catecholaminergic polymorphic ventricular tachycardia?		
15. Does anyone in your family have a heart problem, pacemaker, or implanted defibrillator?		
16. Has anyone in your family had unexplained fainting, unexplained seizures, or near drowning?		

BONE AND JOINT QUESTIONS	Yes	No
17. Have you ever had an injury to a bone, muscle, ligament, or tendon that caused you to miss a practice or a game?		
18. Have you ever had any broken or fractured bones or dislocated joints?		
19. Have you ever had an injury that required x-rays, MRI, CT scan, injections, therapy, a brace, a cast, or crutches?		
20. Have you ever had a stress fracture?		
21. Have you ever been told that you have or have you had an x-ray for neck instability or atlantoaxial instability? (Down syndrome or dwarfism)		
22. Do you regularly use a brace, orthotics, or other assistive device?		
23. Do you have a bone, muscle, or joint injury that bothers you?		
24. Do any of your joints become painful, swollen, feel warm, or look red?		
25. Do you have any history of juvenile arthritis or connective tissue disease?		

MEDICAL QUESTIONS	Yes	No
26. Do you cough, wheeze, or have difficulty breathing during or after exercise?		
27. Have you ever used an inhaler or taken asthma medicine?		
28. Is there anyone in your family who has asthma?		
29. Were you born without or are you missing a kidney, an eye, a testicle (males), your spleen, or any other organ?		
30. Do you have groin pain or a painful bulge or hernia in the groin area?		
31. Have you had infectious mononucleosis (mono) within the last month?		
32. Do you have any rashes, pressure sores, or other skin problems?		
33. Have you had a herpes or MRSA skin infection?		
34. Have you ever had a head injury or concussion?		
35. Have you ever had a hit or blow to the head that caused confusion, prolonged headache, or memory problems?		
36. Do you have a history of seizure disorder?		
37. Do you have headaches with exercise?		
38. Have you ever had numbness, tingling, or weakness in your arms or legs after being hit or falling?		
39. Have you ever been unable to move your arms or legs after being hit or falling?		
40. Have you ever become ill while exercising in the heat?		
41. Do you get frequent muscle cramps when exercising?		
42. Do you or someone in your family have sickle cell trait or disease?		
43. Have you had any problems with your eyes or vision?		
44. Have you had any eye injuries?		
45. Do you wear glasses or contact lenses?		
46. Do you wear protective eyewear, such as goggles or a face shield?		
47. Do you worry about your weight?		
48. Are you trying to or has anyone recommended that you gain or lose weight?		
49. Are you on a special diet or do you avoid certain types of foods?		
50. Have you ever had an eating disorder?		
51. Do you have any concerns that you would like to discuss with a doctor?		

FEMALES ONLY		
52. Have you ever had a menstrual period?		
53. How old were you when you had your first menstrual period?		
54. How many periods have you had in the last 12 months?		

Explain "yes" answers here

_____

_____

_____

_____

_____

_____

_____

_____

I hereby state that, to the best of my knowledge, my answers to the above questions are complete and correct.

Signature of athlete _____   Signature of parent/guardian _____   Date _____

©2010 American Academy of Family Physicians, American Academy of Pediatrics, American College of Sports Medicine, American Medical Society for Sports Medicine, American Orthopaedic Society for Sports Medicine, and American Osteopathic Academy of Sports Medicine. Permission is granted to reprint for noncommercial, educational purposes with acknowledgment.

HE0503   9-2681/0410

Figure 33-1

■ PREPARTICIPATION PHYSICAL EVALUATION
THE ATHLETE WITH SPECIAL NEEDS: SUPPLEMENTAL HISTORY FORM

Date of Exam _____

Name _____ Date of birth _____

Sex _____ Age _____ Grade _____ School _____ Sport(s) _____

	Yes	No
1. Type of disability		
2. Date of disability		
3. Classification (if available)		
4. Cause of disability (birth, disease, accident/trauma, other)		
5. List the sports you are interested in playing		
6. Do you regularly use a brace, assistive device, or prosthetic?		
7. Do you use any special brace or assistive device for sports?		
8. Do you have any rashes, pressure sores, or any other skin problems?		
9. Do you have a hearing loss? Do you use a hearing aid?		
10. Do you have a visual impairment?		
11. Do you use any special devices for bowel or bladder function?		
12. Do you have burning or discomfort when urinating?		
13. Have you had autonomic dysreflexia?		
14. Have you ever been diagnosed with a heat-related (hyperthermia) or cold-related (hypothermia) illness?		
15. Do you have muscle spasticity?		
16. Do you have frequent seizures that cannot be controlled by medication?		

Explain "yes" answers here

_____

_____

_____

_____

_____

Please indicate if you have ever had any of the following.

	Yes	No
Atlantoaxial instability		
X-ray evaluation for atlantoaxial instability		
Dislocated joints (more than one)		
Easy bleeding		
Enlarged spleen		
Hepatitis		
Osteopenia or osteoporosis		
Difficulty controlling bowel		
Difficulty controlling bladder		
Numbness or tingling in arms or hands		
Numbness or tingling in legs or feet		
Weakness in arms or hands		
Weakness in legs or feet		
Recent change in coordination		
Recent change in ability to walk		
Spina bifida		
Latex allergy		

Explain "yes" answers here

_____

_____

_____

_____

_____

I hereby state that, to the best of my knowledge, my answers to the above questions are complete and correct.

Signature of athlete _____ Signature of parent/guardian _____ Date _____

Figure 33-1

■ PREPARTICIPATION PHYSICAL EVALUATION
PHYSICAL EXAMINATION FORM

Name _____   Date of birth _____

PHYSICIAN REMINDERS
1. Consider additional questions on more sensitive issues
   - Do you feel stressed out or under a lot of pressure?
   - Do you ever feel sad, hopeless, depressed, or anxious?
   - Do you feel safe at your home or residence?
   - Have you ever tried cigarettes, chewing tobacco, snuff, or dip?
   - During the past 30 days, did you use chewing tobacco, snuff, or dip?
   - Do you drink alcohol or use any other drugs?
   - Have you ever taken anabolic steroids or used any other performance supplement?
   - Have you ever taken any supplements to help you gain or lose weight or improve your performance?
   - Do you wear a seat belt, use a helmet, and use condoms?
2. Consider reviewing questions on cardiovascular symptoms (questions 5–14).

EXAMINATION

Height	Weight		☐ Male ☐ Female		

| BP   /   (/   )   Pulse | | Vision R 20/ | L 20/ | Corrected ☐ Y ☐ N |

MEDICAL	NORMAL	ABNORMAL FINDINGS
Appearance • Marfan stigmata (kyphoscoliosis, high-arched palate, pectus excavatum, arachnodactyly, arm span > height, hyperlaxity, myopia, MVP, aortic insufficiency)		
Eyes/ears/nose/throat • Pupils equal • Hearing		
Lymph nodes		
Heart[a] • Murmurs (auscultation standing, supine, +/- Valsalva) • Location of point of maximal impulse (PMI)		
Pulses • Simultaneous femoral and radial pulses		
Lungs		
Abdomen		
Genitourinary (males only)[b]		
Skin • HSV, lesions suggestive of MRSA, tinea corporis		
Neurologic[c]		
MUSCULOSKELETAL		
Neck		
Back		
Shoulder/arm		
Elbow/forearm		
Wrist/hand/fingers		
Hip/thigh		
Knee		
Leg/ankle		
Foot/toes		
Functional • Duck-walk, single leg hop		

[a]Consider ECG, echocardiogram, and referral to cardiology for abnormal cardiac history or exam.
[b]Consider GU exam if in private setting. Having third party present is recommended.
[c]Consider cognitive evaluation or baseline neuropsychiatric testing if a history of significant concussion.

☐ Cleared for all sports without restriction

☐ Cleared for all sports without restriction with recommendations for further evaluation or treatment for _____
_____

☐ Not cleared
    ☐ Pending further evaluation
    ☐ For any sports
    ☐ For certain sports _____
        Reason _____
Recommendations _____
_____

I have examined the above-named student and completed the preparticipation physical evaluation. The athlete does not present apparent clinical contraindications to practice and participate in the sport(s) as outlined above. A copy of the physical exam is on record in my office and can be made available to the school at the request of the parents. If conditions arise after the athlete has been cleared for participation, the physician may rescind the clearance until the problem is resolved and the potential consequences are completely explained to the athlete (and parents/guardians).

Name of physician (print/type)_____   Date _____

Address _____   Phone _____

Signature of physician _____ , MD or DO

Figure 33-1

■ PREPARTICIPATION PHYSICAL EVALUATION
CLEARANCE FORM

Name _____ Sex ☐ M ☐ F Age _____ Date of birth _____

☐ Cleared for all sports without restriction

☐ Cleared for all sports without restriction with recommendations for further evaluation or treatment for _____

_____

☐ Not cleared

　　　☐ Pending further evaluation

　　　☐ For any sports

　　　☐ For certain sports _____

　　　Reason _____

Recommendations _____

_____

_____

_____

_____

_____

_____

I have examined the above-named student and completed the preparticipation physical evaluation. The athlete does not present apparent clinical contraindications to practice and participate in the sport(s) as outlined above. A copy of the physical exam is on record in my office and can be made available to the school at the request of the parents. If conditions arise after the athlete has been cleared for participation, the physician may rescind the clearance until the problem is resolved and the potential consequences are completely explained to the athlete (and parents/guardians).

Name of physician (print/type) _____ Date _____

Address _____ Phone _____

Signature of physician _____ , MD or DO

EMERGENCY INFORMATION

Allergies _____

_____

_____

_____

_____

Other information _____

_____

_____

_____

_____

_____

_____

_____

_____

Figure 33-1

Physical Examination

A complete physical examination should be performed when possible. If circumstances preclude this, specific attention should be paid to the eyes, heart, abdomen, skin, and musculoskeletal system. Height, weight, blood pressure, and visual acuity also should be measured. Examination of the eyes is essential to document physiological anisocoria (different papillary diameters). A thorough cardiac evaluation should be performed for murmurs, abnormal heart sounds, or arrhythmias. The abdomen should be palpated for an enlarged liver or spleen, especially in the adolescent with a recent viral illness that could suggest mononucleosis. In males, the genitalia should be examined for sexual maturity in addition to assessing for abnormalities, such as atrophy, absence of a testis, or presence of a testicular mass or inguinal hernia. The skin should be inspected for lesions, such as tinea corporis, impetigo, or herpes simplex infection.

The 2-minute orthopedic examination consists of a head-to-toe assessment of all muscle groups and joints; any deformities, anomalies, or evidence of previous injuries should be noted (Table 33-2). Recent studies suggest expanding this examination to include a more detailed evaluation of high-risk areas for injury, such as the knee, ankle, and shoulder.

Laboratory Tests

Routine laboratory screening tests, except for those performed during the general health maintenance visit, are not recommended for the PPE. Screening young athletes for anemia or proteinuria has not been found to be particularly helpful. Such screening may be useful with highly competitive professional athletes, however. Although controversial, some groups believe that an electrocardiogram should be a routine part of the PPE as well.

Exclusion Criteria

The most common causes of unexpected death during athletics include cardiomyopathies, anomalous coronary arteries, heart valve defects, primary cardiac rhythm disorders, and pulmonary hypertension, and part of the PPE is geared toward determining if a patient has risk factors for any of these conditions. Medical exclusion criteria for athletic participation are based on information obtained in the medical as well as family history. Significant historical clues include a family history of sudden, non-traumatic death; premature coronary artery disease in a first- or second-degree relative; a history of palpitations, angina, or syncope during exercise; and recent, documented infection with the Epstein-Barr virus. Controversy exists regarding when athletes can return to collision sports after infectious mononucleosis. A history of a recent or suspected concussion or multiple concussions in the past also requires close consideration regarding when the athlete is cleared to participate in a given sport. Current clinical and research data regarding adolescents and concussions support the mantra, "When in doubt, sit them out." Patients with concussions should rest, both physically and cognitively, until their symptoms have resolved at rest and with exertion, according to the AAP Council on Sports Medicine and Fitness. In most cases, typical recovery occurs in 7 to 10 days, although some athletes require weeks to months to completely recover. The long-term effects of concussions in athletes of all ages is still under intense investigation.

Findings discovered during the physical examination, such as stature consistent with Marfan syndrome, a cardiac arrhythmia, or the midsystolic click of mitral valve prolapse, could preclude the adolescent from participation in a particular sport. Specific conditions, such as the athlete with one eye or one kidney, should be evaluated on an individual basis by a physician qualified to assess the safety of the particular sport for the athlete (contact/collision versus limited contact).

Table 33-2. The 2-Minute Orthopedic Examination	
Instructions	*Points of Observation*
Stand facing examiner	Acromioclavicular joints, general habitus
Look at ceiling, floor, over both shoulders; touch ears to shoulders	Cervical spinal motion
Shrug shoulders (examiner resists)	Trapezius strength
Abduct shoulders 90 degrees	Deltoid strength
Full external rotation of arms	Shoulder motion
Flex and extend elbows	Elbow motion
Arms at sides, elbows 90 degrees flexed; pronate and supinate wrists	Elbow and wrist motion
Spread fingers; make fist	Hand or finger motion and deformities
Tighten (contract) quadriceps; relax quadriceps	Symmetry and knee effusion; ankle effusion
"Duck walk" 4 steps (away from examiner with buttocks on heels)	Hip, knee, and ankle motion
Back to examiner	Shoulder symmetry, scoliosis
Knees straight, touch toes	Scoliosis, hip motion, hamstring tightness
Raise up on toes, raise heels	Calf symmetry, leg strength

Special circumstances to consider during the PPE are menstrual disorders and the female athlete; exercise-induced bronchospasm; anabolic steroid use; and eating disorders that may be associated with certain activities, such as gymnastics, ballet, and wrestling.

CASE RESOLUTION

The young adolescent described in the case history should first be interviewed with the parent and then alone. Her medical and psychosocial history should be reviewed. A complete physical examination should be performed as well as a pelvic examination if she is sexually active and has a history of lower abdominal pain, abnormal vaginal bleeding, or discharge. If she is sexually active and asymptomatic or not sexually active, only general laboratory screening tests should be performed and the results reviewed with the patient. The remainder of the visit should be spent discussing issues such as nutrition, exercise, illicit substance abuse, sexuality and sexual activity, and safety. Results of the physical examination and screening tests should then be discussed with the parent who accompanied her to the office. If necessary, a follow-up visit should be scheduled. Otherwise, the adolescent should be seen annually.

Selected References

American Academy of Pediatrics. *The Adolescent Preventive Care Visit.* Elk Grove Village, IL: American Academy of Pediatrics; 2009

American Academy of Pediatrics Committee on Infectious Diseases. Prevention of pertussis among adolescents: recommendations for use of tetanus toxoid, reduced diphtheria toxoid, and acellular pertussis (Tdap) vaccine. *Pediatrics.* 2006;117:965–978

American Academy of Pediatrics Committee on Sports Medicine and Fitness. Athletic participation by children and adolescents who have systemic hypertension. *Pediatrics.* 2010;125:1287–1294

American Academy of Family Physicians, American Academy of Pediatrics, American College of Sports Medicine, American Medical Society for Sports Medicine, American Orthopaedic Society for Sports Medicine, American Osteopathic Academy of Sports Medicine. *Preparticipation Physical Evaluation.* 4th ed. Elk Grove Village, IL: American Academy of Pediatrics; 2010

Centers for Disease Control and Prevention. Recommended Immunization Schedule for Persons Aged 7 Through 18 Years—United States, 2011. http://www.cdc.gov/vaccines/recs/schedules/downloads/child/7-18yrs-schedule-pr.pdf

Daniels SR, Greer FR; American Academy of Pediatrics Committee on Nutrition. Lipid screening and cardiovascular health in childhood. *Pediatrics.* 2008;122:198–208

Edwards SM, Rosseau-Pierre T. Immunization in adolescents—an update. *Adolesc Med State Art Rev.* 2010;21:173–186

Halstead ME, Walter KD; American Academy of Pediatrics Council on Sports Medicine. Sport-related concussion in children and adolescents. *Pediatrics.* 2010;126:597–615

Herman-Giddens ME, Bourdony CJ, Dowshen SA, et al. *Assessment of Sexual Maturity Stages in Girls and Boys.* Elk Grove Village, IL: American Academy of Pediatrics; 2011

Moscicki AB. Human papillomavirus disease and vaccines in adolescents. *Adolesc Med State Art Rev.* 2010;21:347–363

Rice SG; American Academy of Pediatrics Council on Sports Medicine and Fitness. Medical conditions affecting sports participation. *Pediatrics.* 2008;121:841–848

Strasburger VC, Jordan AB, Donnerstein E. Health effects of media on children and adolescents. *Pediatrics.* 2010;125:756–767

CHAPTER 34

Health Care for International Adoptees

ChrisAnna M. Mink, MD

CASE STUDY

Jaxon is a 14-month-old boy adopted from Thailand. His biological mother was a 26-year-old commercial sex worker who entered a maternity house during her pregnancy to receive care and to relinquish the baby for adoption. His mom reported that she was physically and sexually abused as a child and became a street child when she was 14 years old. She used illicit drugs 5 years ago, but none since. She identifies the father as a European customer, but has no other information. Jaxon was born at 32 weeks' gestation and was placed in an incubator but did not have any respiratory problems. He has been in foster care in a Thai family's home with his care supervised by an internationally respected adoption organization. He was selected by his parents at the age of 4 months, and they have received monthly progress reports on his growth, development, and medical status. Reportedly he has had several "colds" and one ear infection but otherwise has been growing and developing well. Before departure to pick up Jaxon, his adoptive parents met with you to prepare for his arrival.

From the Bangkok airport, the parents placed a call to you because Jaxon would not stop crying. They report that on the morning that his foster mom left him with them, he cried quite a bit but had settled by bedtime and seemed to be adjusting well during the week. However, over the past 12 hours he hasn't stopped crying and refuses to eat. They question if his discomfort is related to teething because he has been drooling, but they have not noticed any other symptoms. They are gravely concerned that he doesn't like them and is having attachment difficulties.

Questions

1. What factors influence the prevalence of international adoption?
2. What are some of the potential health problems of international adoptees?
3. What is an appropriate medical evaluation for international adoptees?
4. What is the pediatrician's role in caring for the child and the newly formed family?

From 1998 through 2008, annually approximately 20,000 children were adopted internationally by parents in the United States. Although these children come from a wide range of birth countries, many of their health-related issues are similar. Many of the children have lived in orphanages in impoverished areas of the developing world and have incurred the maladies associated with poverty and deprivation.

Epidemiology

From 1971 to 2001 a total 265,677 children were adopted internationally into the United States. Most of these children (90%) are from Asia (China and South Korea most commonly), Eastern Europe, and South America (Guatemala and Colombia). From 2000–2009, China, Russia, and Guatemala were the 3 leading countries of origin for children adopted into the United States. A decline in the number of international adoptions has been seen since 2009 due to multiple factors, including economic downturn in the United States; ethnic pride in birth countries; and stricter policies governing adoption, such as The Hague Convention (international guidance for standardizing intercountry practices to promote protection of children available for adoption).

Many factors influence adoptive parents to choose international adoption. In the United States, delays in childbearing and associated infertility have increased the demand for adoptable children. At the same time, more readily available birth control and growing acceptance of single motherhood have decreased the number of US infants available for adoption. In addition to the shortage of **adoptable** children in the United States, additional factors for parents choosing international adoptions include real and perceived risks of domestic adoption (eg, failure of birth parents to relinquish rights), fear of adopting a special needs child from the domestic system, and limited availability of children with desired traits (eg, specific age and ethnicity). In addition, prompt termination of rights of birth parents in international adoption is cited as a factor in the choice.

The advent of **intercountry adoption (ICA)** in the United States occurred with World War II and the large number of orphaned children in Europe, many of whom were fathered by American soldiers.

The second, and more formalized, wave of ICA occurred with the Korean War. Because of the need to care for unwanted orphans, primarily of mixed ethnicities also fathered by American soldiers, South Korea established a foster care system and the children became available for adoption to Americans. War and political turmoil are still factors for children becoming available for adoption. For example, the fall of communism was a significant factor for Russia and other states of the former Soviet Union becoming common birth countries for adoptees in the 1990s and the early part of this century. Recently, with worsening poverty and political strife, more children are being adopted from African countries.

Societal values are also factors for influencing adoption practices. China is often the leading birth country for **adoptees** because of the population control initiatives of the government mandating that families have only one child. With this practice and the desire to have a male heir, some newborn girl infants are abandoned and subsequently become available for adoption. In some countries, local laws and/or cultural practices are prohibitive for adoption, especially for foreigners and, thus, these countries are infrequent birth countries. The United States is the birth country for about 500 children adopted into other countries. Absolute statistics for children adopted out of the United States are not available because the government does not track the number of exit visas issued for adopted children. These US children are often males of African American or mixed ethnicity and are adopted by families in Canada and Western Europe. The children are available purportedly due to the low desire for these infants by adoptive parents in the United States.

The status of the country of origin (ie, war, turmoil, poverty, and societal values) aside, there is significant overlap in the reasons that children from foreign countries and from the United States become available for adoption (eg, parental substance use, abandonment, chronic neglect, abuse, and domestic violence).

Until the 1990s, most international **adoptees** were from South Korea, which had in place an excellent **foster care** system and health care. Since the 1990s, nearly two-thirds of **adoptees** come from institutions in poor nations without a developed foster care system, resulting in a significant decline in the health and well-being of the **adoptees.**

Clinical Presentation

Most internationally adopted children are female (64%), in part reflecting the adoption of girls from China, as well as a preference among some adoptive parents (especially single women) to adopt a girl. International adoptees are young, with approximately 46% being younger than 1 year and 43% between 1 and 4 years of age.

Pre-Adoption

Some **adoptees** become known to the US health care provider **"only on paper"** during the **pre-adoption stage.** Adoptive parents may ask their health care provider for help in assessing the child's medical status. Often parents receive a written health report (varying in the quantity and the quality of information) and photos or videos of the child they are considering adopting. The written documents may be in a foreign language or not translated by an experienced medical translator. Some countries prohibit international adoption of healthy children, so diagnoses may be embellished to improve the child's chances for adoption. Additionally, some medical records contain diagnoses that are nonsensical in US medicine but represent terms used in the country of origin. For example, **adoptees** from Russia often have neurologic diagnoses such as **perinatal encephalopathy,** which suggests serious brain injury and would carry a grave prognosis in Western medicine; in Russia this term may reflect a minor deprivation or a lack of prenatal care and not a specific neurologic injury. However, at other times, a term may have the same meaning and intent to Russian physicians as to US physicians. These inconsistencies are therefore quite challenging when trying to evaluate the medical records of potential **adoptees.** Many physicians may not feel comfortable with reviewing medical records given so many limitations; however, even with all of the caveats, review of the records may still provide insight into the health status of the potential adoptee.

Also during the **pre-adoption stage,** the health care provider may provide information for parents and families for preventive health measures to prepare for travel to a developing area of the world. The Centers for Disease Control and Prevention (CDC) traveler's information Web site (www.cdc.gov/travel) is a good resource for health care providers and the parents. Up-to-date information may also be obtained from the World Health Organization and the US State Department (Table 34-1). Additionally, parents should be informed about the possible infections seen in international adoptees, and they should receive appropriate education and vaccinations (eg, hepatitis B because of the increased risk of the child being positive for hepatitis B surface antigen [HBsAg], seen in 1%–5% of adoptees).

Table 34-1. Web Sites for International Health, Travel, and Adoption Information		
Resource	*Information*	*Web Site*
Centers for Disease Control and Prevention	Up-to-date information for travelers' health	www.cdc.gov/travel
US State Department	Up-to-date information for travelers' risk (eg, civil unrest)	www.travel.state.gov
	Intercountry adoption statistics	www.state.gov
	Intercountry adoption procedures	www.travel.state.gov/family/adoption/adoption_485.html
World Health Organization	Health status and recommendations for immunizations for each country	www.who.int/en/
	Assists with interpreting foreign vaccine records	
US Child Welfare	Adoption information and procedures	www.childwelfare.gov

During the Adoption Trip

All internationally adopted children are required by the US State Department to have a **physical examination** before admission into the country; however, this examination is quite limited in scope and performed primarily to rule out severe impairments or certain communicable diseases that may pose a public health threat (eg, active tuberculosis). This examination should not be considered as a complete medical evaluation for an individual child. Some health care providers are able to provide support for families during travel via e-mail or telephone, similar to telephone consultations performed in general practice.

Post-Adoption

After the adoption, the health status of the children on presentation to the American health care provider is quite variable, ranging from well (eg, infants from Korean foster care) to severely ill with acute infections or chronic diseases (eg, malnutrition and tuberculosis). The adopted child should be seen by the physician within 2 to 3 weeks of arrival in the United States, or sooner if he or she has an acute illness. This 2-week period allows for the child (and parents) to recover from jet lag and to become more familiar with each other, permitting a better assessment at the visit. If an acute illness visit is required, a separate appointment for a comprehensive evaluation should be scheduled.

Health Care Issues

In addition to the problems commonly related to **poverty** and **deprivations,** many health issues are specific to the country of origin (eg, increased risk of **fetal alcohol spectrum disorder [FASD]**

in children from Russia, malaria from Africa, etc). Published data regarding health care issues are limited for children from recent countries of origins (eg, Ethiopia, China, and Russia) (Figure 34-1).

Generally, the health care issues for **adoptees** are extensive, including acute illnesses (eg, respiratory infections), chronic illnesses (eg, anemia, malnutrition, poor dental hygiene, tuberculosis, asthma, and parasite infestation), delayed or unknown immunizations, psychosocial challenges, and impaired growth and development.

Some children have assigned birth dates (eg, **abandoned infants** and **street children** for whom the birth dates are not known), and they may have small growth parameters, making it difficult to know their true age and expected development. **Developmental delay,** most commonly language delay, is frequently identified. Assessment of development may be even more difficult in infants and young children who are nonverbal and older children who speak their native language.

Growth delay is common for **adoptees.** Many children are malnourished or have failure to thrive (FTT), and these afflictions are often multifactorial in origin, including poor prenatal environment (maternal stress, malnutrition, drug and alcohol abuse), inadequate calories, inadequate nurturing, unrecognized genetic or congenital disorders (eg, FASD), and untreated chronic illnesses (eg, rickets). Institutionalized children may suffer from **psychosocial dwarfism,** and may lose 1 month of linear growth for every 3 to 4 months spent in the orphanage. Delay in puberty may be observed in adolescents from deprived environments, such as **orphanages.**

Immunization records may not be available, may be incomplete, or may be in a foreign language, which hinders assessing the vaccination status of adoptees. Additionally, many vaccines available in the United States are not available in the developing world

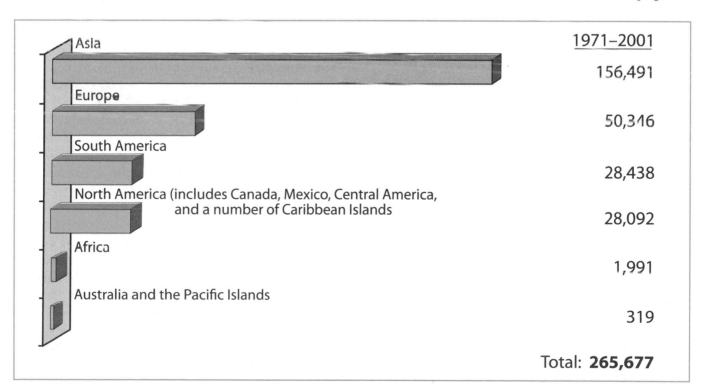

Figure 34-1. **Countries of origin for children adopted by parents in the United States.**

(eg, *Haemophilus influenzae* type b [Hib] and pneumococcal conjugate vaccines) and, thus, children will not have had them. Adopted children immigrating to the United States who are younger than 10 years are exempt from the Immigration and Nationality Act regulations requiring proof of immunizations before arrival; however, adoptive parents are required to sign a waiver that they will comply with US recommended immunizations after arrival.

Psychosocial, emotional, and **mental health problems** are some of the more challenging problems to assess. The spectrum of mental health problems is related to age and previous life experiences for the child. Children may have suffered from physical and/or sexual abuse prior to placement in an institution, where the potential for such abuse also exists. This may be inflicted by adult caretakers or bigger children when supervision is inadequate. Attachment disorders are some of the most concerning abnormalities for adoptive parents, adoption professionals, and health care providers. Because the fundamentals for learning healthy attachments are greatly influenced by early infant–caretaker relationships, many international adoptees have difficulties bonding, in part because they have not had secure caretaker relationships. Issues for attachment and bonding may be especially problematic for children who have resided in an orphanage and/or had multiple caretakers from an early age. Because the children have had multiple caretakers, they may be indiscriminately friendly, which poses risks for their safety. Other common mental health problems include depression, attention-deficit/hyperactivity disorder (ADHD), post-traumatic stress disorder, abnormal behaviors (eg, self-stimulating behaviors, hoarding food, sleep disturbances), and oppositional–defiant disorder. As mentioned previously, communication with the child may be difficult due to language barriers, causing another obstacle to assessing the mental health of the child.

Sensory integration difficulties are increasingly recognized in adoptees. The children may have adverse responses to touch (including new clothing, hugs and kisses, bathing, etc) or textures (such as new foods). Individual or all of the senses (hearing, vision, taste, or smell) may be notably increased or decreased, and some children have decreased sensation to physical pain leading to an increased risk for injuries. Dyskinesia (clumsiness or injury prone) has also been observed.

The most common identified medical issues are **infectious diseases.** These include acute illnesses (eg, upper respiratory infection, bronchitis, otitis, and infectious diarrhea, among others), as well as longer-term infections, such as tuberculosis and parasite infestations (scabies and *Giardia* are common). Because of their biological mother's lifestyle and their time residing in institutions, many adoptees are at increased risk of exposure to infectious diseases such as syphilis, HIV, and hepatitis B and C.

Preventive care considered "routine" in the United States is unlikely to have been part of the child's care and needs to be performed as appropriate for age. This includes newborn screening laboratory studies and assessments of hearing, vision, dental, and mental health. Anticipatory guidance for the new parents should be incorporated into the initial, and all, visits.

Evaluation

The initial office visit with the physician should be scheduled for an extended period because of the complexity of the evaluation and the additional time needed for parental education. If the physician's schedule does not permit extended visits, ancillary staff (eg, nursing, dietitian, and therapists) may perform parts of the evaluation and education.

Observation of the child's behavior, development, and interactions with the adoptive parents and health care provider is a critical element of the evaluation. Most health care providers include such observations in their visits routinely, but particular attention is necessary for new adoptees. Things to notice include the child's behavior. Are they easily engaged or withdrawn? Do they make eye contact with the parent or health care provider? Do they make any vocalizations or words, depending on the child's age? Do they play with toys? Are they too friendly or afraid of strangers? Do they seek comfort from the new parents?

History

Limited medical information is available from most birth countries, though there are some exceptions (eg, from foster care in Korea). Family history and birth history are rarely obtainable for adoptees. Immunization histories are becoming increasingly available. Previously, vaccine records were considered unreliable; however, in recent years, data have emerged to suggest that well-documented immunizations may be considered valid. Written records showing the age of the child when vaccinated, the date of administration, dose given, and proper intervals between dosing that are consistent with the World Health Organization schedules or are comparable to US schedules may be considered acceptable for proof of immunization. (See under Management for guidelines when vaccine records are not available.)

Dietary history is important for assessing the child's nutritional status. Questions to ask include, What food and formula/milk is the child receiving? Has he or she received adequate calories? Is there known or suspected food intolerance (eg, lactose intolerance is more common in Asian ethnicities)? Are there abnormal behaviors associated with food or eating (eg, preoccupation with food, hoarding, food refusal, or gorging)?

An interim medical history may be available because many children are selected by their adoptive parents several months before immigrating to the United States. The interim medical history may be provided from the orphanage or foster care provider through the adoption agency. Parents should be encouraged to solicit as much information as possible from the caretakers of the child. At a minimum, this history should include serial growth parameters, known illnesses, hospitalizations, surgeries, allergies, and immunizations given while the child was under their care. Parents should also ask the caretakers about any food preferences, special fears, toys, or friends from the current placement. If the child has a special "lovey," the parents should request to bring it with the child for a transitional object.

Physical Examination

A complete unclothed physical examination should be performed on infants and children of all ages. However, due to previous trauma, such as sexual abuse, some parts of the examination may have to be done over a series of visits to minimize the possibility of additional trauma from an examination. All aspects of the physical examination are absolutely essential. Accurate measurements of height, weight and, depending on age and size, head circumference should be obtained. Plotting of parameters on the growth curves for the United States (compared with birth country) should be used, with few exceptions. The child should be closely inspected for unusual scars or bruises, evidence of fractures (old or recent), rachitic changes, and genital or rectal scars. The skin should be examined for rashes, lesions, and a bacille Calmette-Guérin (BCG) scar (typically on the upper deltoid). A developmental screen should be performed, and a more complete developmental assessment should be scheduled at a separate visit (when the child is not distressed or acutely ill). A dental examination should be included and referral for a formal dental evaluation will likely be necessary. Screening evaluations of hearing and vision should be performed, and formal testing may be needed depending on the age of the child and ability to cooperate.

Laboratory Testing

Laboratory testing should include complete blood cell count, lead levels, and thyroid function testing (iodine is not in many diets in Asia) (Box 34-1). Additionally, testing for illnesses associated with specific countries of origin, findings on examination (eg, comprehensive metabolic panel for malnourished child), and as directed by the child's age (eg, newborn screening for metabolic disorders in infants) should be performed.

Because of the **increased risks of exposures,** laboratory screening for infectious diseases should be undertaken. Serum samples should be tested for syphilis (non-treponemal and treponemal antibodies), hepatitis B panel (HBsAg, hepatitis B surface antigen antibody [HBsAb], hepatitis B core antibody), hepatitis C antibody, and HIV 1 and 2 antibodies. HIV polymerase chain reaction may be indicated in some children (eg, those who may not make specific antibodies due to malnutrition or immunocompromise). Stool samples should be sent for ova and parasite examination (at least 2 times) and *Giardia* and *Cryptosporidium* antigen testing. Stool for bacterial pathogens (eg, *Salmonella* and *Shigella*) should be sent from children from some regions, such as the Indian subcontinent. Because cytomegalovirus infection is ubiquitous, routine testing is not recommended. Testing for acute infection with hepatitis A virus (HAV) by measuring immunoglobulin M anti-HAV antibodies should be performed for adoptees from HAV-endemic areas, as infants and young children may be asymptomatic but contagious. Administering HAV vaccine, as recommended in the United States, is not problematic for children who may have had previous HAV infection.

Tuberculosis (TB) skin testing (ie, purified protein derivative [PPD]) should be performed on all children; history of receipt of BCG

Box 34-1. Recommended Laboratory Testing for International Adoptees[a]
Hepatitis A IgM
Hepatitis B virus serologic testing • Hepatitis B surface antigen • Antibody to hepatitis B surface antigen • Antibody to hepatitis B core antigen
Hepatitis C virus serologic testing
Syphilis serologic testing • Nontreponemal test (RPR, VDRL, or ART) • Treponemal test (MHA-TP or FTA-ABS)
HIV 1 and 2 serologic testing
Complete blood cell count with differential and red blood cell indices
Stool examination for ova and parasites (3 specimens)
Stool examination for *Giardia intestinalis* and *Cryptosporidium* antigen (1–3 specimens)
Tuberculin skin test[b]
Consider antibody testing to select vaccine antigens (if written records are unreliable)[c]
Additional testing: thyroid function tests, lead level and others as directed by history and physical exam (see text).

Abbreviations: ART, automated reagin test; FTA-ABS, fluorescent treponemal antibody absorption; HIV, human immunodeficiency virus; IgM, immunoglobulin M; MHA-TP, microhemagglutination test for *Treponema pallidum*; RPR, rapid plasma reagin; VDRL, Venereal Disease Research Laboratories.

[a]Adapted from the American Academy of Pediatrics and the Centers for Disease Control and Prevention.

[b]Repeat at 6 months after initial testing.

[c]Children older than 6 months, may check diphtheria, tetanus, and polio; children older than 12 months, may check measles antibodies.

is not a contraindication to skin testing. Bacille Calmette-Guérin vaccinations are usually given at birth in most developing nations, and its influence on skin test status is controversial. Generally, BCG given within the previous 1 to 2 years may contribute to a positive PPD skin test; however, a positive PPD test is more likely reflective of true infection with *Mycobacterium* with or without active disease and merits further evaluation. Latent TB infection has been reported from 0.6% to 30% of international adoptees, which is not surprising because most adoptees come from TB-endemic areas.

Management

Counseling for the Transition

Education and **preparation** for the parents and all family members is a priority. Generally, countries of origin for adoptees are in the developing world, and parents should prepare for healthy travel for themselves by receiving immunizations and following travel guidelines from the CDC and the US Department of State.

Parents should provide consistent structure and boundaries in a loving milieu for the adoptees. A scheduled regimen may be especially important to previously institutionalized children because it has been their way of life, but even noninstitutionalized children benefit from a predictable routine. Parents should maximize their one-on-one interactions with the adoptee, while still allowing time for themselves and other family members (not an easy task with multiple children). Touching and affection may initially need to be tempered as directed by the child's tolerance. Parents should try to enhance bonding and attachment by frequently identifying themselves as "Mom" or "Dad." Other strategies to enhance attachment include initially limiting contact with individuals outside of the family and not "handing" the child to others, including non-household family members, because they are strangers to the child. Frequent verbal reassurances and talking to the child about the people and the new world around them should be encouraged. In caring for the child, parents should be encouraged to "meet the child" at his or her developmental level and not the chronological age.

Growth and Nutrition

When children are identified as malnourished or FTT, a multidisciplinary treatment plan is recommended, including parents, physician, nutritionist, and therapists (eg, occupational therapist for feeding difficulties). The child should be offered familiar foods, if that is his or her preference, and each meal may include a new, more nutritional offering. Children should be offered frequent meals and snacks because they may not be able to eat much at one sitting. Foods should be calorie dense (eg, added butter, cheese, avocado, or peanut butter, depending on age and previous dietary history). Dietary supplements, such as PediaSure, may be indicated.

Precocious puberty has been observed in female international adoptees, more than males, and is thought to be related to the rapid improvement of nutrition. If signs of precocious puberty are observed, evaluation by a pediatric endocrinologist is recommended.

Development

Because developmental delays are so common, most adoptees should have a developmental assessment. Language delays, especially expressive, are frequent and, when identified, formal audiology testing should be part of the assessment. However, performing developmental assessments of language pose difficulties, as most are conducted in English, which is rarely the child's primary language. Repeating the testing after a period of adjustment may be helpful. Language barriers do not preclude audiology testing.

Mental Health

Mental and emotional health problems are common and may manifest early or late, or occur as relapses. Initial problems seen may include sleep disorders, fears and phobias, bizarre behaviors, and self-stimulating behaviors. Unless the behaviors pose a safety risk, the parents should tolerate them because most dissipate with time in a secure environment. At times of emotional distress, parents may observe a relapse of behavior problems. The health care provider may

provide guidance for parents for the milder disorders; however, moderate and severe disorders merit prompt referral to a mental health professional, ideally someone with expertise in adoption.

Immunizations

If vaccinations are considered valid, as described previously, resuming immunizations per the US schedule (see Chapter 32) is appropriate. If immunization status is unknown or incomplete, repeating immunizations or checking antibody concentrations to vaccine antigens is an acceptable option. Most areas of the world routinely administer BCG, polio (oral), and vaccines containing diphtheria and tetanus toxoids with pertussis (often whole-cell) components. Receipt of additional diphtheria, tetanus, and possible pertussis antigens may be associated with an increase in adverse events; measuring antibodies to diphtheria and tetanus is warranted to minimize adverse events. There are no US Food and Drug Administration–approved antibody tests available commercially for pertussis antibodies. Receipt of additional doses of inactivated polio vaccine is not usually associated with adverse events. Testing for HBsAb should be performed on all adoptees, and the results will guide the plan for further immunizations. Hepatitis B vaccine will only elicit HBsAb; the presence of antibodies to other hepatitis B antigens suggests natural infection. For measles, mumps, and rubella (MMR), various formulations and combinations (1- and 2-component more commonly than 3-component) vaccines are available worldwide. Checking antibodies to these antigens is possible, but likely administering a US-licensed combination (eg, MMR) may be necessary to ensure protection against all 3 antigens. Most of the other vaccines available in the United States are not available in the developing world (eg, Hib and pneumococcal conjugates, varicella, HAV, etc), and the child should receive these vaccines as recommended for age per the US schedule.

Infectious Diseases

Any acute identified infectious disease (eg, scabies, otitis) should be treated following standard practice, keeping in mind the possibility that different antibiotic resistance patterns exist in other parts of the world. Thus, if the child does not have the predicted response to treatment, consultation with a pediatric infectious diseases specialist should be considered. For other infectious diseases screening noted previously, additional evaluation and possible treatment should be initiated promptly (eg, penicillin therapy for syphilis) and pediatric infectious diseases consultation may be considered.

For TB evaluation, any positive PPD skin testing merits further investigation for true infection with *Mycobacterium tuberculosis*. A compounding problem is that some children may be anergic due to malnutrition, giving a false-negative PPD test. If malnutrition is suspected, consider a chest radiograph even if the PPD is negative, and consider repeating the PPD when the child's nutritional status has improved. In addition, routinely repeating the PPD 6 months after the child's arrival is advisable if the child is from an endemic area because late exposure to an infected individual is possible.

Prognosis

Being prepared for the complex needs related to international adoption has been identified as the best determinant for parents to consider the adoption experience as positive, regardless of the number or severity of the medical needs of the adoptee.

With improved nutrition and environment, most children have significant catch-up growth; however, up to one-third of adoptees may have unrecoverable loss in linear growth. For intellectual development, by 1 year of age nearly all children in orphanages have one or more areas of delay. However, their prognosis is generally good, with an increase in 2 developmental quotient points per month after arrival in the United States. After 3 years of age in an orphanage, the length of time institutionalized and delays noted at age 11 months correlate negatively with IQ (8 months in orphanage, average IQ = 90; 2 or more years in orphanage, average IQ = 69).

Many children have ongoing mental and psychosocial problems, and some disorders do not manifest until the children are older (eg, ADHD or learning disorders when the child is school-aged). Ongoing attachment disorders seem to occur with greater frequency in children with lower IQs, more behavior problems, and adoptive families with a lower socioeconomic status.

Assessment of the overall outcome for children who spent 8 or more months in institutional care in Eastern Europe, when evaluated at least 3 years after adoption, showed about one-third had multiple serious problems (including IQ ≤85, insecure attachment, and severe behavior problems), about one-third had a few serious problems but were thought to be making progress, and about one-third had progressed very well. The best predictors of major problems were (1) greater length of time in the orphanage, (2) increased number of children adopted at same time, (3) younger adoptive mother, (4) lower socioeconomic status of mother, and (5) father alone selected the child. Although the impact of these risk factors may not be identical for all birth countries, they do provide some insight. Reviewing these risk factors with adoptive parents during the pre-adoption period may aid in their decision-making.

Pediatrician's Role

The pediatrician's role is not to tell the adoptive parent whom to adopt; the parents are essentially choosing life partners, which is an individual decision. Pediatricians, however, can assist the parents in reviewing the available medical information, which may aid them in making an informed decision about proceeding with an adoption.

During the adoption process, the health care provider must assume an active role as a child advocate, as well as parental advocate and educator. This may be the first parenting experience for the adoptive parents and, thus, they need the basics for child care, no matter what the age of the adoptee. This might include feeding and routine care (eg, estimate the number of diapers needed if traveling to an area with no access to supplies), as well as discipline techniques for a traumatized child. Preparation for caring for illnesses is needed because many adoptees are ill at the time of the adoption and

travel. The pediatrician can facilitate emotional preparation because the parents may be isolated from their usual support systems while embarking on the new role of parent.

After returning home, the pediatrician has a role as primary care provider, as well as serving as a referral source for other needed specialists (eg, subspecialists, mental health providers, post-adoption support services, developmental interventions, and nutritionists, among others).

Counseling Adoptive Parents About the Expectations

Parents should be informed that it is unlikely that an institutionalized child will emerge unscathed. With this in mind, parents may make preliminary preparations for treatments and rehabilitation for the child. Families should be counseled that it is OK to say "no" to a potential adoptee. No one has benefited from adoption of children by families that do not have the resources needed to care for them. Most importantly, parents should be reassured that optimism is appropriate. Being prepared matters!

CASE RESOLUTION

In talking with the parents, they report that they have not observed any injuries and no areas seem tender when they examine Jaxon, as you have suggested. They elect to give him some diphenhydramine and take the flight home with the plan to come see you on arrival. Although they are exhausted, they come directly to your office for an acute visit. They report that he remained inconsolable and that the flight home was miserable for him (and everyone around them). On entering the examination room, Jaxon was screaming and noticeably uncomfortable but trying to find comfort in his dad's arms.

His temperature was 38.9°C (102°F) axillary; pulse rate, 144 beats per minute; and respiratory rate, 30 breaths per minute. His examination was notable for extensive oral and pharyngeal vesicular lesions with erythema, but there were not labial lesions. He had multiple shotty cervical nodes, and the rest of the examination was noncontributory. A diagnosis of herpangina was made. He was given a dose of ibuprofen, and 15 minutes later he was quiet, able to swallow electrolyte solution, and was cuddling in his dad's arms. His parents were given reassurance that this was an acute infection and not an indication of poor bonding; in fact he was already seeking comfort from them. Additional testing for infections included obtaining antibodies to HIV, rapid plasma reagin for syphilis, and hepatitis C and a hepatitis B panel, especially with his biological mother's history of being a commercial sex worker. Other testing included complete blood cell count, lead level, and thyroid function tests. He was given an appointment in 2 weeks to complete the assessment, including a developmental assessment, because this was deferred since he was acutely ill.

Selected References

Albers L, Barnett F, Jenista J, Johnson D. International adoption: medical and developmental issues. *Pediatr Clin North Am.* 2005;52:xiii–xv

Ames E. *The Development of Romanian Orphanage Children Adopted to Canada: Final Report.* Burnaby, British Columbia, Canada: Simon Fraser University; 1997

American Academy of Pediatrics. Medical evaluation of internationally adopted children for infectious diseases. In: Pickering LK, Baker CJ, Long SS, McMillan JA, eds. *Red Book: 2009 Report of the Committee on Infectious Diseases.* 27th ed. Elk Grove Village, IL: American Academy of Pediatrics; 2009:177–184

Barnett ED. Immunizations and infectious disease screening for internationally adopted children. *Pediatr Clin North Am.* 2005;52:1287–1309

Cederbald M, Hook B, Irhammar M, Mercke AM. Mental health in international adoptees as teenagers and young adults. An epidemiological study. *J Child Psychol Psychiatry.* 1999;40:1239–1248

Centers for Disease Control and Prevention. Elevated blood lead levels among internationally adopted children—United States, 1998. *MMWR Morb Mortal Wkly Rep.* 2000;11:97–100

Evan B. Donaldson Adoption Institute. *International Adoption Facts.* www.adoptioninstitute.org/FactOverview/international_print.html

Howard CR, John C. International Travel with Infants and Children: International Adoption. CDC Health Information for International Travel 2010, The Yellow Book http://wwwnc.cdc.gov/travel/yellowbook/2010/chapter-7/international-adoptions.aspx

Johnson DE. *International Adoption: New Kids, New Challenges.* www.med.umn.edu/peds/iac/preadoption.htm

Lieberthal JK. Adoption in the Absence of National Boundaries. Paper presented at: 25th Conference of the North American Council on Adoptable Children; 1999, 2003; Vancouver British Columbia, Canada. www.adoptioninstitute.org/policy

Miller LC, Hendrie NW. Health of children adopted from China. *Pediatrics.* 2000;105:e76

Peterson K. Preparing to meet foreign bugs. Travel, immigration, and international adoptions require special precautions. *Postgrad Med.* 2001;110:67–70, 73–74, 77

Saiman L, Aronson J, Zhou J, et al. Prevalence of infectious diseases among internationally adopted children. *Pediatrics.* 2001;108:608–612

Selman P, ed. *Intercountry Adoption: Developments, Trends and Perspectives.* London, England: British Agencies for Adoption and Fostering; 2000:545

Sloutsky V. Institutional care and developmental outcomes of 6- and 7-year-old children: a contextualist perspective. *Int J Behav Dev.* 1997;20:131–151

US Department of State. Immediate Relative Visas Issued. http://travel.state.gov/family/adoption/info/info_458.html.

Weitzman C, Albers L. Long-term developmental, behavioral, and attachment outcomes after international adoption. *Pediatr Clin North Am.* 2005;52:1395–1419

CHAPTER 35

Health Care Needs of Children in Foster Care

Kelly Callahan, MD, MPT; ChrisAnna M. Mink, MD; and Sara T. Stewart, MD

CASE STUDY

A 9-year-old boy is brought to your office by his foster parent for a general physical. The foster parent states that the boy has been living in her home for the past week. When he was initially brought by the social worker, his skin was dirty, and he was wearing dirty clothes. There are no medical records and no immunization records available for your review, and the child states that he "doesn't remember the last time he went to the doctor." The boy states that he sometimes went to school, but that he did not return at the end of the last school break. He gets angry when he is asked about his family, and states that he doesn't want to be in foster care, but that he does not want to return to live with his mother right now. He states he misses his brothers and sisters and wants to live with his father, whom he has not seen in 4 years. The only history known by the foster parent is that the child required some type of special services in school, and that the social worker found drug paraphernalia in his home at the time of his removal. The foster parent also states that 2 nights ago, the patient broke a dish and punched a wall when he became angry.

On physical examination, the patient is alert and refuses to stay in the examination room. His weight is greater than the 95th percentile for his age and his height is in the 25th percentile for his age. He has poor dentition with multiple dental caries. He has a few basilar wheezes on lung examination and has scattered bruises on his anterior shins.

Questions

1. What are the medical, psychological, and behavioral issues that commonly affect children in the foster care system?
2. What is the role of the primary care provider in providing a medical home for the child in foster care?
3. How does a child's legal status as a child in foster care affect how medical care can be delivered?
4. What are the appropriate health care referrals and community resources to access for a patient who is in foster care?

The term **foster care** refers to the **temporary placement** of a child in the home of another caretaker or **foster parent** due to a threat to the child's safety or well-being in the original home environment. Placement of a child in foster care results from an investigation of the child's home environment by **child protective services (CPS)** and may be arranged via voluntary agreement of the parent or through court sanction. The foster parent may be related to the child or may be a nonrelative. For those children in voluntary placement, the biological parent retains the right to terminate the placement at any time. For those placed by **legal sanction,** a series of court hearings give parents, the child, and the CPS agency the opportunity to present their perspectives on the circumstances surrounding the allegations and their respective views on interventions to ensure the child has access to the best home environment.

Children in **foster care** may present to the primary care provider soon after placement in foster care, or may present after having been with a foster parent for a long time. In either scenario, it is recognized that as a subpopulation of pediatric patients, children in foster care have a significant number of **unmet medical** and **mental health** needs and should be considered to be a **"special needs"** patient population. At the time of initial removal, the CPS worker may not be able to obtain a medical history or essential information about medications for the child. Changes in foster care placement may interrupt continuity of care with a health care provider, and frequent changes in the assigned social services caseworker can create barriers to consistent communication among foster parents, health care providers, and caseworkers. These children have rates of medical and mental health disorders that are higher than those of children from equivalent socioeconomic backgrounds who are not in foster care. There has traditionally been a lack of appreciation within the general medical community as to the complexity of the needs of this patient population, and due to low reimbursement rates, there has been difficulty allotting sufficient time in an office visit to complete the comprehensive evaluation needed by these children. For those children with identified mental health needs, there is often a paucity of available psychiatric and psychological resources. This is particularly true for children younger than 5 years.

These unmet needs have long-lasting effects on the well-being of children, even after exiting the foster care system. Because of their complex health care issues and vulnerability to fragmented care, these children merit a medical home, providing comprehensive, multidisciplinary services and medical case management.

Epidemiology

At any point during a given year, between 400,000 and 500,000 children nationwide are in the foster care system. Approximately 300,000 children enter the system annually, and reasons for placement, in descending order of prevalence, include neglect, physical abuse, psychological or emotional abuse, and sexual abuse.

Foster children are of all ethnicities, but there is disproportionate representation of children of color within the foster care population. The age distribution is bimodal, with children younger than 5 years of age and adolescents comprising most of the population. Over the past several decades an increasing percentage of new entrants into foster care are children in the youngest age bracket, particularly infants younger than 1 year. Many of these infants are exposed prenatally to illicit substances and are placed in foster care due to a combination of factors related to the maternal drug use.

Approximately 70% of children leave foster care within 2 years of placement, and more than half of them are reunited with their biological parent or primary caretaker. Thirteen percent remain in foster care for more than 5 years, and approximately 35% of all children leaving foster care reenter the system at some time due to a new report. The number of adoptions from foster care has increased since the late 1990s to account for 17% of those leaving the child welfare system, and an additional 9% of those leaving foster care are emancipating out of the system by reaching 18 years of age without ever attaining a permanent placement. Many of these teenagers later report being incarcerated or homeless at some point after emancipation. Twenty-five percent of the children in foster care will experience 3 or more placements, which leads to further fragmentation of their health care and education. Multiple foster care placements are more common for those children with behavioral, emotional, or coping problems.

As a population, children in the foster care system come from home environments that experience high rates of poverty, parental mental illness, parental substance abuse, low levels of education, high rates of unemployment, and frequent involvement with the criminal justice system. These children have high rates of exposure to domestic violence, and many are victims themselves of physical abuse, sexual abuse, and neglect. Their biological parents often have limited parenting skills, and the children experience inconsistent parenting behaviors along with minimal developmental stimulation and emotional support. All of these factors combine to cause unpredictable, stressful, and unsafe home environments for these children, prompting their removal and placement into foster care.

Clinical Presentation

Medical Issues

Children in the foster care system have been shown to have high rates of both **acute and chronic illness** at the time of their initial medical evaluations after placement (Dx Box). In one study in Utah, more than half of children entering the foster care system had at least one medical problem. Common maladies include obesity; **asthma; vision or hearing problems**; neurologic disorders; **gastrointestinal diseases; dental caries**; and other inadequately treated chronic illnesses, such as **eczema and anemia.** Acute infections are also common, including respiratory tract infections, skin infections, otitis media, sexually transmitted infections (STIs), and intestinal infestations with parasites. Low immunization rates are also a frequent occurrence.

Many children entering foster care have growth delay with a weight, height, or head circumference measurement less than the fifth percentile for age. This may be due to a combination of factors, including inadequate nutrition, environmental deprivation, prenatal alcohol exposure, genetic predisposition, or underlying illness, such as HIV infection. Environments that are chronically stressful or that lack the necessary stimulation and support for a child may also lead to behaviors such as rumination and social withdrawal. (For further discussion of failure to thrive, see Chapter 129.) Overweight (body mass index [BMI] 85th–95th percentile for age) and obesity (BMI >95th percentile for age) are also frequently seen in foster care children. Depression, dysfunctional coping skills, and a lack of family connectedness are thought to contribute to this chronic disease state.

 Common Issues of Children in Foster Care

- Acute infection
- Undiagnosed or inadequately treated chronic illnesses
- Dental caries
- Growth delay and failure to thrive
- Incomplete immunization histories
- Prenatal or perinatal exposure to sexually transmitted infections
- Effects of prenatal substance exposure
- Physical sequelae of physical and sexual abuse
- Developmental delay
- Attention-deficit/hyperactivity disorder
- Post-traumatic stress disorder
- Anxiety
- Depression
- Conduct and oppositional defiant disorders
- Attachment disorders
- Educational disabilities

Many children placed in foster care have a history of **prenatal exposure** to illicit drugs, alcohol, and tobacco. These children have high rates of premature birth and of prenatal or perinatal exposure to infections such as **hepatitis C, hepatitis B, HIV, syphilis,** and **herpes simplex.** This risk of exposure to infectious agents is related to maternal drug use and its frequent association with prostitution, needle sharing, and drug use in sexual partners.

Children who have been placed in foster care may present with physical sequelae of prior physical or sexual abuse. Physical abuse may result in skin trauma, skeletal fractures, head trauma, abdominal trauma, and chest trauma. Sexual abuse may result in genital trauma or symptoms of STIs.

Developmental and Mental Health Issues

A high prevalence of developmental delay, behavioral disorders, and educational difficulties has been noted in foster children of all age groups. These disorders are more common in children with a history of neglect or abandonment than in those who have suffered other forms of child maltreatment. Of children younger than 6 years entering foster care, 23% to 60% have significant developmental delays and 25% to 45% have behavioral difficulties, with 15% of children taking at least one psychotropic medication. Speech and language difficulties, delayed fine motor skills, and poor social–adaptive skills are common, and up to one-fifth of school-aged children entering foster care had been receiving special education services prior to the time of placement.

Common mental health issues in the foster care population include attention-deficit/hyperactivity disorder, depression, anxiety, and suicidal ideation. **Post-traumatic stress disorder** is common and is more prevalent in those who have experienced or witnessed family violence. Adolescents in foster care may "act out" as a manifestation of mental health difficulties, resulting in sexual promiscuity, substance abuse, and truancy, their rates of conduct and oppositional defiant disorders are higher than those in the general adolescent population.

Attachment disorders are seen more frequently in the foster care population and account for a portion of the behavioral difficulties in these children. A secure attachment to a primary caretaker is necessary to the development of emotional security and the sense that one's needs are important. Children who are removed from violent homes, or who may have suffered abuse or neglect, are unlikely to have developed a secure attachment to a primary caretaker in that home environment and, therefore, may have difficulty bonding with a foster parent. This problem is then compounded if the child is moved among multiple foster homes, prohibiting development of a healthy attachment to a caretaker. In addition to their lack of emotional reciprocity, these children may exhibit self-stimulatory behaviors or sleep disturbances.

The behavioral difficulties that children in the foster care system manifest are often due to multiple factors. These children may be predisposed to behavioral disorders by a history of prenatal drug or alcohol exposure or by a history of abuse or neglect. It can also be difficult to determine whether a child's behaviors predate placement in foster care, or whether they are a response to the removal from his or her home. As a result of placement in foster care, children often experience fear, sadness, and a feeling of guilt or responsibility for the family discord that resulted in their removal. Foster placements are invariably sudden and unexpected, involve the loss of a familiar caretaker, and are traumatic for children of all ages.

Evaluation

It is important for a provider to be familiar with the **medical consent legalities** concerning foster children in his or her geographic locale. While specifics vary by locality, generally foster parents have the authority to provide consent for routine medical care. The placement of a child in foster care does not supersede the right of a biological parent to participate in the medical decision-making for his or her child, and many do retain the authority to consent for medical tests and procedures. Any medical procedure or test that requires specific written consent is likely to require **authorization** by the **legally recognized parent** (eg, child welfare agency, the courts, or the biological parent). Two common clinical scenarios that frequently require consent beyond the foster parent's authority are HIV testing and the administration of psychotropic medications.

History

Children in foster care may be brought for medical evaluation by an authorized caregiver, which may include a foster parent, a relative of the foster parent, or the social service caseworker. Often the biological parent is absent from the visit, and the child's medical records are not available at the time of the evaluation. Obtaining past medical records can be difficult, but the caseworker can be of assistance in this process. It is important to ascertain the circumstances that prompted a child's placement in foster care, as this may modify portions of the evaluation.

The biological family history is useful to evaluate for the presence of genetic disorders and communicable diseases. A maternal history regarding drug use or STIs will assist in identifying those children who may have had prenatal exposures to infectious agents.

Birth history should include any history of prenatal care and complications, such as prematurity or drug withdrawal. The results of routine newborn screening (eg, hearing, inborn errors of metabolism, thyroid function, hemoglobinopathies, etc) should also be obtained. The birth weight and gestational age at birth are critical when assessing for growth disturbances.

A complete medical and surgical history should be gathered, including the identification of a regular health care provider if the child has one. Older children and adolescents may be able to provide some of their own histories. Known medications and allergies should be documented, and all available immunization records should be obtained. Documentation of a child's immunization history is frequently unavailable, so all possible sources of records, such as biological parents or school districts, should be identified. Feeding history and nutritional assessments should include the type and amount of formula or breast milk for infants, and types and quantities of foods for older children.

The psychosocial history includes a history of a child's current and prior foster placements or living arrangements, and whether there was exposure to domestic violence, physical abuse, or sexual abuse (Questions Box). Verbal children may also be able to discuss their feelings about their current foster placement. Adolescents should have a confidential screening (eg, HEADDSSS [home environment, employment and education, activities, diet, drugs, sexual activity/sexuality, suicide/depression, and safety] examination) (see Chapter 6) to address drug, alcohol, and tobacco use; issues related to the home and school; sexual activity; violence; and gang involvement.

The **developmental history** should include the results of prior developmental assessments, as well as a listing of therapeutic or early intervention services received. The behavioral history should also include results of prior assessments, mental health services used, and any psychotropic medications prescribed. The foster parent, biological parent, or CPS caseworker may be able to provide useful observations regarding the child's developmental capabilities, behavioral patterns, and social interactions. The biological parent or CPS caseworker may also be able to assist in collecting records from prior assessments.

Educational history is often not available at the time of the medical evaluation. It is helpful, however, to know a child's history of prior evaluations by the school system, special education services provided, or prior therapeutic services (eg, physical therapy, occupational therapy, speech therapy) received through the school district.

Physical Examination

A complete, unclothed physical examination should be performed on each child. Growth parameters, including height, weight, occipitofrontal head circumference (for children <2 years), and BMI (for children ≥2 years) should be plotted on a reference chart, and a close inspection should be performed for signs of prior trauma. The child should be assessed for **dysmorphic features** consistent with prenatal alcohol exposure or other genetic syndromes. The physical examination should include a **genital examination** to also assess for signs of trauma in children of all ages, and sexually active females should have a pelvic examination if there are any reports of abdominal pain, vaginal discharge, or other concerns. (See Chapters 127 through 129 for further descriptions of physical findings.)

Immunizations

Immunizations should be given as appropriate for age, and if immunization records cannot be located, the child should be considered to be unimmunized. In this situation, the options include restarting the vaccination series or checking the antibody titers for selected vaccine antigens (see Chapter 32).

In addition, all children should also receive a purified protein derivative to screen for tuberculosis.

Questions

Psychosocial

- When was the child placed in foster care?
- Why was the child placed in foster care?
- Has the child had prior foster placements? If so, when? Why did placement change?
- Was there prior exposure to domestic violence? Physical or sexual abuse?
- Does the child have siblings in foster care?
- How does the child feel about the current foster placement?
- How has the child integrated into the foster family?
- Has the child previously received mental health services? Therapeutic services for developmental delay or educational difficulties?
- What is the child's social service plan? Parental visits? Reunification? Termination of parental rights?

Additional Assessments

All children should undergo both mental health and developmental screenings and should be referred for comprehensive testing if abnormalities are noted. Vision and hearing screenings should also be performed on all children old enough to cooperate. A referral for expert vision or hearing evaluation should be made if it is indicated by history or physical examination, or the patient is unable to perform the screening procedure (eg, infant or developmentally delayed child).

Laboratory Tests

Routine screening laboratory tests should be performed on foster children just as they are indicated for the general pediatric population. For example, hemoglobin level should be checked annually in all infants, toddlers, and preschool-aged children. Serum lead levels should be checked according to local guidelines but should be checked at least once for a child during the toddler years. A urinalysis should also be recorded at least once in all children at the time of entry into kindergarten and once during adolescence.

For infants with a history of prenatal drug exposure or other known risks for maternal STI, at least a rapid plasma reagin, hepatitis C antibody, hepatitis B surface antigen and surface antibody, and HIV test should be performed.

Adolescents who are considered to have at-risk sexual behaviors, patients with signs or symptoms consistent with an STI, and children with a history of sexual abuse that could result in the transmission of infection should be tested for STIs. Often adolescents are able to sign their own consent forms for evaluations and treatment related to STIs; however, local statutes should be consulted.

Imaging Studies

If a child has a history or physical findings concerning for physical abuse, imaging such as a radiographic skeletal survey, computed tomography and magnetic resonance imaging of the head, or radionucleotide bone scan may be indicated. (For more specific recommendations, see Chapter 15.)

Management

Given the breadth of health-related needs for this patient population, and given the frequency with which they change foster homes, **close case management** is an essential component of their health care delivery. There should be consistent communication with the child's caseworker to ensure that medical and mental health recommendations are incorporated into the child's social service plan. Ideally, a child should have a medical home and continuity with a health care provider over time, but changes in home placements often make this difficult. If continuity of care is broken, incorporation of the health care plan into a child's broader social service plan should ensure that medical history and medical and mental health recommendations are not lost. The use of **electronic health records** is a growing practice in many foster care systems and promotes continuity of care, even with logistical challenges.

Children and adolescents in foster care require frequent health visits. The American Academy of Pediatrics recommends a health screening within 72 hours of placement, a comprehensive medical evaluation within 30 days of placement, and a follow-up medical examination within 60 to 90 days after placement. Because of the prevalence of significant medical, social, and mental health issues affecting children in foster care, additional visits are often advisable. Anticipatory guidance should be provided to the caretaker, and age-appropriate issues should be discussed with older children and adolescents.

Children in foster care often need referral to medical subspecialists, dentists, dietitians, speech therapists, occupational therapists, mental health providers, and other service providers. Case management is necessary to track these referrals and to contact the foster family and/or caseworker if an appointment is missed.

Prognosis

The population of children in foster care has a spectrum of mental health and medical needs, spanning from the needs of a newborn to those of an adolescent emancipating from the child welfare system. Preliminary studies have documented improved physical health status, improved school performance, and improved adaptive functioning of young children after placement in foster care; however, these studies require replication. The strength of the bond between the foster parent and the child, as well as the consistency and predictability of the foster home environment, are significant to the development of that child's sense of safety and well-being.

To date, much of the research on the health status of children in foster care has focused on the delineation and description of the health-related issues that these children face. There has been more limited evaluation of the different models of health service delivery to the foster care population, as well as of the subsequent medical, developmental, and emotional outcomes for the children in these different models.

While there is a need for continued study of health care delivery to the foster care population, it is widely accepted that children in the foster care system benefit from the establishment of medical homes with case management capabilities and providers who are well-versed in the complex medical and mental health issues that affect this vulnerable population.

CASE RESOLUTION

This case illustrates many of the common issues that affect children when they are placed in foster care. Medical and immunization records are frequently unavailable to the medical examiner, and chronic medical needs have often gone unmet. This child's lack of personal hygiene points to a history of parental neglect, and given the presence of drug paraphernalia, his parents were likely involved with substance abuse. This child should have a thorough assessment for behavioral problems, developmental delays, and education-related disabilities. The child is able to state that he does not want to return to his parents' care, but still misses his family members. This may be remedied through his child welfare plan, for example, by arranging for him to remain in contact with his siblings throughout their foster placement. Given his experiences in his prior home environment, he has anger management issues and is likely to have other unmet mental health needs that require referral to a mental health provider. He will also require evaluation by his new school system to determine his specific educational needs and appropriate grade placement.

He is obese and has poor dentition, both of which are common findings in the foster care population. He will require a nutritional evaluation and a referral for dental care. The presence of mild wheezing in a child who otherwise states that he feels fine is a likely marker for untreated reactive airway disease, and may be a reflection of poor continuity of medical care for the boy prior to his placement.

Selected References

American Academy of Pediatrics. *Fostering Health: Health Care for Children and Adolescents in Foster Care.* 2nd edition. Elk Grove Village, IL: American Academy of Pediatrics; 2005

American Academy of Pediatrics Committee on Early Childhood, Adoption, and Dependent Care. Developmental issues for young children in foster care. *Pediatrics.* 2000;106:1145–1150

American Academy of Pediatrics Committee on Early Childhood, Adoption, and Dependent Care. Health care of young children in foster care. *Pediatrics* 2002;109:536–541

American Academy of Pediatrics Committee on Practice and Ambulatory Medicine. Recommendations for preventative health care. *Pediatrics.* 2000;105:645–646

American Academy of Pediatrics Task Force on Foster Care. Healthy Foster Care America. www.aap.org\fostercare. Accessed December 7, 2010

Horowitz SM, Owens P, Simms MD. Specialized assessments for children in foster care. *Pediatrics.* 2000;106:59–66

Jee SH, Simms MD. Health and well-being of children in foster care placement. *Pediatr Rev.* 2006;27:34–36

Racusin R, Maerlender AC Jr, Senqupta A, Isquith PK, Straus MB. Psychosocial treatment of children in foster care: a review. *Community Ment Health J.* 2005;41:199–221

Ringeisen H, Casanueva C, Urato M, Cross T. Special health care needs among children in the child welfare system. *Pediatrics.* 2008;122;e232–e241

Simms MD. Foster children and the foster care system, part I: history and legal structure. *Curr Probl Pediatr.* 1991;21:297–321

Steele J, Buchi K. Medical and mental health of children entering the Utah foster care system. *Pediatrics.* 2008;122;e703–e709

Takayama JI, Wolfe E, Coulter KP. Relationship between reason for placement and medical findings among children in foster care. *Pediatrics*. 1998;101:201–207

US Department of Health and Human Services, Administration for Children and Families, Administration on Children Youth and Families, Children's Bureau. AFCARS report: trends in foster care and adoption FY2006.2008. Available at http://www.acf.hhs.gov/programs/cb/stats_research/afcars/tar/report. Accessed December 7, 2010

CHAPTER 36

Working With Immigrant Children and Their Families

Alejandro Diaz, MD, and Carol Berkowitz, MD

CASE STUDY

A 7-year-old child presents with vomiting and clinical signs of dehydration. The family thinks he has *empacho*. You tell the family that you suspect that he has viral gastroenteritis. You want to draw some blood studies and give him fluids intravenously. The parents are skeptical; they refuse the blood work and want to leave against medical advice.

Questions

1. What are the ways that different immigrant families view illness and health?
2. What are barriers to accessing health care that children in immigrant families face?
3. What questions help the physician understand the health beliefs of immigrant families?
4. What are the considerations when dealing with parents who do not speak English?

Introduction

The United States is described as a nation of immigrants. Out of a population of 310 million, current estimates are that about 40 million, or approximately 10% of the current US population, are either foreign-born citizens or noncitizens. Half of these immigrants are Hispanic and 65% of Hispanics are of Mexican descent. During the 1990s, 70% of the US population's overall growth was influenced by a wave of recent immigrants, mostly from Latin America and Asia, and by the children born to these newcomers. The vast growth in the population of children living in immigrant families, whether foreign-born (first generation) or US-born (second generation), poses a unique set of challenges.

These children are more likely to live in families that live below the federal poverty level and families in which at least one parent did not graduate high school or is not fluent in English. They are also more likely to live in crowded housing (more than one person per room) and in a multigenerational household. While some immigrant children are citizens and eligible for safety net programs, their family's status directly influences whether these children will even access such care. There is also growing concern that the health status of some immigrant children, whether foreign-born or first generation, actually declines after settling in the United States. It is expected that by 2030, Hispanic children will account for most children living in the United States.

Demographics of Immigrant Children

There are 5 general categories of immigrants in this country, each benefiting from specific entitlements and services, and having certain legal rights: lawful permanent residents, naturalized citizens, refugees/asylees, nonimmigrants, and undocumented immigrants (Box 36-1).

In 2007 naturalized citizens made up approximately 32% of immigrants, lawful permanent residents characterized about 29%, undocumented immigrants another 29%, refugees 7%, and nonimmigrants about 3%. From 1980 to 2000, the children of immigrants increased from 5% to 20% of school-aged children, representing approximately 10 million of the estimated 60 million school-aged children in the United States.

By far the largest category of immigrants is nonimmigrants, or temporary visitors. Approximately 3 million children arrive mostly from Asia, Western Europe, and parts of North America, typically accompanying their parents who are seeking work. A smaller percentage are students or exchange visitors. While not technically immigrants, this special group may present for care with similarly unaddressed health issues depending on their country of origin.

The next largest group, almost a quarter-million children, enter the United States as lawful permanent residents, with most eventually becoming naturalized citizens. Although most arrive with or to meet family already residing in the United States, several thousand adolescents immigrate unaccompanied each year; most are female and many are married to a naturalized citizen at the time of

> ## Box 36-1. Categories of Immigrants in the United States
>
> ### Lawful Permanent Residents
> - Carry a green card
> - These are noncitizens with permission to permanently live and work in the United States
> - May apply for naturalization after 5 years (or 3 years if they marry a citizen)
> - Most international adoptees are in this group
>
> ### Naturalized Citizens
> - Born as noncitizens
> - Having met certain English literacy requirements and demonstrating a basic knowledge of civics and a desirable moral character, are granted the same rights as natural born citizens
> - However, are not eligible to hold the office of president or vice president
>
> ### Refugees
> - Granted permission from the US government before entry
> - Fled their country of origin for fear of persecution due to their race, religion, social group, or political opinion
> - Many unable or willing to return to country of origin
> - Those granted permission to remain are deemed asylees
> - After a year, both may apply to adjust their status to lawful permanent residents
>
> ### Nonimmigrants
> - Carry a visa
> - Granted permission to enter for a specified time and a specific purpose (usually to work or study)
>
> ### Undocumented Immigrants
> - Entered the country illegally or even legally but then violated the terms of their stay and remained after their visa expired

immigration. Included in this group are children of refugees or asylees. More than 75,000 arrive each year, most recently from the countries of the former Yugoslavia and former Soviet Union, Vietnam, Somalia, and other war-torn regions. Numbers for the third largest group, undocumented immigrants, are based primarily on estimates. Most are from Mexico or other Latin American states. Some entered the United States legally but have overstayed their visa or lost their status by committing a crime.

Health Care Needs of Immigrant Children

When the child of an immigrant family presents for care, the primary concerns are about the presence of an infectious disease (due to exposures and possible lack of vaccination) or the presence of a hidden genetic or ethnic condition (such as hemoglobinopathies and glucose-6-phosphate dehydrogenase [G6PD] deficiency). Investigating the health status of a child, especially from undocumented immigrant families, is paramount as these children likely have not seen a doctor prior to immigrating. Similarly nonimmigrants, such as tourists and other temporary visitors, from many Western or Pacific

Rim countries are not required to have a medical examination performed as part of their application. Only visas for permanent residency require a health examination to be performed by an approved physician, and even then the focus of the examination is to exclude certain conditions such as active tuberculosis (TB), HIV, and other severe physical or mental handicaps. In children, laboratory testing may be limited and proof of vaccination status may be exempted for certain groups, such as international adoptees.

Lack of education and poverty, which results in relative food insecurity and inadequate, crowded housing conditions, poses an ominous threat to the health of these same children. Noncitizen children must wait at least 5 years before they are able to apply for public assistance. While most refugee children may receive some form of subsidized care, such as Medicaid, many of these benefits are time-sensitive. Even US-born children of undocumented mothers, while legally eligible as US citizens for benefits such as nutritional assistance programs, may not receive these owing to parental fears of detection and deportation. Physicians should ascertain that the family has adequate housing and access to food, 2 basic human needs. Is the food available in the families' neighborhood consistent with the traditional food that the family desires? Is the food healthful or does the family live in a "food desert" where there is a plethora of fast-food restaurants and a paucity of supermarkets or grocery stores (Box 36-2)?

> ## Box 36-2. Risk Factors Affecting the Health of Immigrant Children
>
> ### Social and Economic
> - Inadequate or crowded housing
> - Food insecurity
> - Lack of insurance (due to ineligibility)
> - Lack of access to insurance (eligible but unable or unwilling to apply)
> - Educational level of head of household
>
> ### Cultural
> - Dietary preferences
> - Lack of language fluency or literacy and translation/interpretation issues
> - Disparate ideas regarding the causation and treatment of illness
> - Expectations of the medical system
> - Religious practices with a medical component
> - Lack of access to traditional medical practitioners and treatments
> - Importation drugs not approved in the United States
>
> ### Physical
> - Carriage of infectious disease and the possibility for repeated exposure via travel or living within one's immigrant community
> - Presence of ethnic or genetic conditions
> - Lack of vaccination
> - Poor nutritional status
>
> ### Mental Health
> - Negative past living conditions, including exposure to violence or natural disaster
> - Cultural adjustment (or the process of acculturation and enculturation)

It has traditionally been supposed that immigration itself imposes unique stresses on these children. Mental health challenges (eg, depression, anxiety, and grief) may be related to the reasons for their migration as well as to the inevitable process of acculturation. Stress is compounded by the potential loss of the immigrant's identity and separation from home support systems; inadequate language and literacy skills in a society intolerant of linguistic weakness; disparities between one's country of origin and the United States in economic, social, and professional standards and status; and the psychological and emotional trauma of war, persecution, or exploitation in one's country of origin.

Despite these challenges, epidemiological studies indicate that children in immigrant families experience better outcomes than those in their native countries who did not immigrate, especially in some areas. The most striking example is the lower rate of low-birth-weight children born to foreign-born mothers, especially among Hispanics and non-Hispanic black immigrants, compared with women in their native countries who did not immigrate. This positive effect related to immigration has been studied less in older children due to limited availability of data samples from second-generation children that does not exclude first-generation children.

General Approach to the Initial Medical Evaluation of an Immigrant Child

Ascertaining the "life history" of an immigrant child including any relevant travel history will help determine the extent of the medical evaluation (Box 36-3).

In general, most immigrants from industrialized nations have received comprehensive medical care and the only issues facing these children are routine, such as updating immunization status. In contrast, adoptees, refugees, and undocumented children often have received little or no care. While there is no single approach to the general medical evaluation for all immigrant children, some general principles apply.

Any and all existing medical records should be reviewed. While a complete translation is not always necessary, if an unusual diagnosis or a complicated history exists, use of clinical translational services

---

Box 36-3. Questions to Consider When Evaluating Immigrant Children

1. If parents are not present, does the child's current guardian have any personal knowledge of the child's social and medical history?
2. In which countries has the child resided and under what circumstances?
3. Have the child's living conditions changed dramatically in either the positive or negative recently?
4. Are there verifiable birth and medical records, especially vaccination status, to be reviewed? What age is the child? What quality of care did the child seem to receive in their home country?
5. Has the child undergone any recent procedures or treatments?
6. Was the child exposed to any potentially toxic occupational or environmental risks?
7. What educational level did the child achieve?

---

or a nearby university's academic language department may facilitate the process. Sometimes the records suggest that a diagnosis was considered but not confirmed and it may be appropriate to reevaluate the child for any suspected condition.

It is important to screen for certain infectious diseases. The most common among immigrants are TB, intestinal parasites, hepatitis B, syphilis, and HIV. In fact, the risk for TB is more than 100 times greater in immigrant children than in US children. Fifty percent of all newly identified cases of TB in the United States are diagnosed in immigrants, many within the first 5 years of life. If not clinically apparent (incubation period) or testing is negative but clinical suspicion exists, the TB testing should be repeated in 6 months. Intestinal parasitic infestations may be present without symptoms. Some clinics specializing in immigrant health advocate giving a single dose of albendazole as a more cost-effective approach than screening and diagnosis, but the safety and efficacy of this approach has not been substantiated in children.

Ethnic or genetic conditions should also be considered. Conditions like G6PD in Mediterraneans, Africans, and Southeast Asians may affect the child's health in the short term. Others like hemoglobinopathies and thalassemias, while common among certain ethnic populations, such as Southeast Asians, may not be of immediate importance. Overall, anemia is extremely common among immigrant children and the diagnostic workup of these children may uncover an underlying blood dyscrasia trait or lead intoxication. If iron therapy has been initiated empirically, repeat testing after treatment is paramount to ensure a response and confirm the diagnosis. Also, certain ritual cultural practices, such as female circumcision and tattooing, or the use of certain traditional healing techniques, such as cupping or coining, may have long-term implications. Understanding the risk for nutritional deficiencies based on the country of origin is important. For instance, nutritional disorders, such as rickets and iodine deficiency, are common in ethnic Chinese and children from the former Soviet Union.

Immunizations must be administered as appropriate and following the catch-up recommendations of the American Academy of Pediatrics and the Advisory Committee on Immunization Practices. Records of previous immunizations may be difficult to interpret. Shortened intervals or the administration of a vaccination at too early an age may not be readily apparent. Fraudulent records, especially amongst adoptees and children from institutional settings, often exist. In young children it is generally considered safe and cost-effective to simply give missing vaccines; however, determining serum immunity may be more cost-effective in older children.

Cultural and Linguistic Sensitivity

Bridging language differences using professional interpreter services is required to provide adequate patient care. Such linguistic services are mandated by agencies such as the Centers for Medicare & Medicaid Services for reimbursement from the federal government. The use of children or house maintenance staff is inadequate and potentially violates federal laws, including the Health

Insurance Portability and Accountability Act. Professional interpreters are taught to interpret and not carry on additional conversations with the patient or expound on the questions the physician asks. The physician should address questions directly to the patient, not the interpreter, maintaining eye contact with the patient.

Providing culturally competent care that considers cultural practices and beliefs about child health or illness when coming up with a treatment plan is also critical (see Chapter 10). Does the family access "healers" for medical problems (Box 36-4)? What are their views about medication use? Are there hierarchical structures that influence a parent's acceptance of a physician's advice (eg, father accepting advice from a female physician, or parent accepting advice from a young resident)?

Conclusion

There are numerous barriers that potentially interfere with achieving optimal health status for immigrant children. Trust is a core component of the physician–patient relationship, and establishing trust may be more difficult when the physician and family have different cultural values and expectations. It has been stated that in medicine the sacred trust that develops between a patient and their doctor should never be taken for granted. The development of trust forms the foundation of the therapeutic relationship. It provides credibility to the practitioner. The practitioner must act in a manner that elicits and fosters trust, and being knowledgeable and nonjudgmental about the beliefs and practices of one's patients is pivotal.

Health care providers must work toward creating an atmosphere of trust so that parents feel comfortable revealing their beliefs, concerns, and fears. The threat of deportation should be considered when taking into account whether the patient or their family will follow up or adhere to medical recommendations.

It is unwise not to acknowledge the cultural divide that exists between most pediatric practitioners and the families they serve. Therefore, providers who are less familiar with the enrichment provided by a multicultural patient population may be less inclined to advocate for social reforms that may prove beneficial. We as physicians must approach families with an open mind, respect, and a sense of humility if we are to gain their trust, close the gaps that separate us, and promote the well-being of children.

Children are better served when their families receive information about federal, state, and community programs that provide resources to immigrant families. All children, regardless of their

immigration or socioeconomic status, should receive compassionate, culturally competent, and linguistically effective care services. Such care requires that health care providers incorporate knowledge, attitudes, and skills in cultural and linguistic competence within their professional agenda.

The well-being of all children can be advanced through advocacy, especially on behalf of vulnerable children (see Chapter 2). Such advocacy (1) addresses outreach efforts to children who are potentially eligible for Medicaid and the Children's Health Insurance Program but are not enrolled, (2) simplifies enrollment for both programs, and (3) expands state funding for those who are not eligible. The medical community must collaborate with legislators, families, and organizations representing underserved populations in order to increase the effectiveness of one's own advocacy effort. All children should receive care in a medical home (ie, the establishment of comprehensive, coordinated, and continuous health care services). This is especially critical for immigrant children with chronic health care needs and mental health problems.

Box 36-4. Questions for Understanding Someone's Cultural Concept Regarding the Symptoms of Illness[a]

1. What do you call the problem?
2. What do you think caused it?
3. Why do you think it started when it did?
4. What do you think the sickness does? How does it work?
5. How severe is it? Will it have a long or short course?
6. What are the chief problems the illness has caused?
7. What kind of treatment do you think they should receive? What are the most important results you expect from this treatment?
8. What do you fear most about the illness?

[a]Adapted from Fadiman A. *The Spirit Catches You and You Fall Down*. New York, NY: Farrar, Strauss and Giroux; 1997, quoting medical anthropologist Arthur Kleinman.

CASE RESOLUTION

You reach an agreement with the family that allows a community healer to come and perform a therapeutic massage while allowing you to place an intravenous line and administer fluids. The patient is significantly improved after the massage and intravenous fluids. The family appreciates that you respected their beliefs and agrees to return for a routine well-child visit in 2 weeks.

Selected References

American Academy of Pediatrics Committee on Community Health Services. Providing care for immigrant, homeless, and migrant children. *Pediatrics.* 2005;115:1095–1100

Flores G, Brotanek J. The healthy immigrant effect: a greater understanding might help us improve the health of all children. *Arch Pediatr Adolesc Med.* 2005;159:295–297

Guendelman S, Schauffler HH, Pearl M. Unfriendly shores: how immigrant children fare in the US health system. *Health Aff (Millwood).* 2001;20(1):257–266

Jenista JA. Immigrant, refugee, or internationally adopted child. *Pediatr Rev.* 2001;22:419–429

Mendoza FS. Health disparities and children in immigrant families: a research agenda. *Pediatrics.* 2009;124 (suppl 3):S187–S195

National Immigration Law Center. *Guide to Immigrant Eligibility for Federal Programs.* 4th ed. Santa Monica, CA: National Immigration Law Center; 2002

Virginia Child Protection Newsletter. 2011;90:1–20

CHAPTER 37

Well-Child Care for Children With Trisomy 21

Derek Wong, MD

CASE STUDY

A 6-month-old girl with trisomy 21 whom you have known since birth is brought to your office for well-child care. She and her parents have been doing well, although she has had several episodes of upper respiratory infections. Her medical history is significant for a small ventricular septal defect, which has since closed spontaneously, and one episode of otitis media at 5 months of age. Her weight gain has been good—along the 25th percentile on the trisomy 21 growth chart. She now sleeps through the night and has a bowel movement once a day. She has received all of the recommended immunizations for her age without any problems.

The infant smiles appropriately, grasps and shakes hand toys, and has some head control, but is unable to roll from supine to prone position. Since she was 1 month old, she has been enrolled in an early intervention program. An occupational therapist visits her at home twice a month.

On physical examination, she has typical facial features consistent with trisomy 21, a single palmar crease on each hand, and mild diffuse hypotonia. Her eyes have symmetrical movement, and her tympanic membranes are clear. She has no cardiac murmurs.

Questions

1. What is the prevalence of trisomy 21 (Down syndrome) in the general population? What is the association of maternal age with trisomy 21?
2. What are the clinical manifestations of this syndrome?
3. What medical conditions are associated with trisomy 21 in the newborn period, during childhood, and in adolescence? When should screening tests for these conditions be performed?
4. What is the role of early intervention services for these patients and their families?
5. What specific psychosocial issues should be included in your anticipatory guidance and health education?
6. What is the prognosis for children with trisomy 21?

Trisomy 21, or Down syndrome, is the most commonly known genetic cause of mental retardation in children. The primary care provider is in a unique position to offer affected children routine health care maintenance and anticipatory guidance, follow-up of intercurrent illness and chronic problems, and information on the latest recommendations for screening for conditions associated with trisomy 21. In addition, the general pediatrician has the opportunity to develop rapport with children and families that is particularly important when considering the complex medical and social implications of raising these children. An important goal of the well-child visit is to provide children with trisomy 21 and their families with counseling about educational, social, and financial resources and support to ensure a healthy and productive transition into adulthood.

Epidemiology

The prevalence of trisomy 21 is approximately 1 in 800 to 1,000 live births. It is estimated that trisomy 21 is responsible for up to one-third of all cases of moderate to severe mental retardation. Trisomy 21 has a male to female ratio of 1.3:1.

Ninety-five percent of all cases of Down syndrome are caused by chromosomal nondisjunction, and most of these events occur in the mother. The chance of nondisjunction is determined by maternal age. A 25-year-old woman has a 1 in 1,240 risk of having a live baby with Down syndrome, and the risk increases to 1 in 340 at age 35 and 1 in 98 at age 40. It is estimated that approximately one-half of trisomy 21 embryos abort spontaneously. The risk of recurrence of nondisjunction Down syndrome in subsequent pregnancies is 1 in 100 until age 35, after which the risk determined by age takes precedence. Other family members are generally not at increased risk of bearing children with this type of Down syndrome.

Approximately 3% to 4% of Down syndrome cases are caused by Robertsonian translocations with another acrocentric chromosome (14/21, 15/21, or 21/21). Parental karyotypes should be obtained because balanced translocation carriers have an increased risk of Down syndrome in future children. Approximately 1% to 2% of Down syndrome cases are mosaic. These children are often less severely affected than those with "full" Down syndrome. A small percentage of affected children have a chromosomal rearrangement resulting in 3 copies of a portion of chromosome 21.

Recent advances in first and second trimester screening allow prenatal diagnosis of Down syndrome with a sensitivity of 80% to 90%. If a prenatal diagnosis of Down syndrome is made, and the general pediatrician is asked to participate in counseling the family, the points listed in Box 37-1 should be covered.

> **Box 37-1. Counseling the Family After a Prenatal Diagnosis of Down Syndrome**
>
> - Review the data that established the diagnosis in the fetus.
> - Explain the mechanism of occurrence and risks for recurrence.
> - Review the manifestations of trisomy 21, commonly associated conditions, and the variable prognosis based on the presence of these conditions.
> - Discuss other modalities that confirm the presence of associated anomalies, such as a fetal echocardiogram in the case of congenital heart disease.
> - Explore treatment options and interventions for associated conditions.
> - Offer resources to assist the family with decisions related to completing or terminating the pregnancy.
> - Refer the family to a clinical geneticist or genetics counselor.

Clinical Presentation

Infants and children with trisomy 21 have a characteristic appearance (Dx Box). They may be microcephalic, with flattening of both the occiput and face. The eyes have an upward slant, with prominent epicanthal folds, the ears are low set and small, the nasal bridge is flattened, and the tongue appears large. The feet, hands, and digits are small and stubby, and the fifth digit may be hypoplastic and turned in (brachyclinodactyly). A single palmar crease and wide spacing between the first and second toes may be evident. After the newborn period, diffuse hypotonia and developmental delay are universally seen.

Pathophysiology

Approximately 95% of cases of Down syndrome are caused by trisomy 21 resulting from meiotic nondisjunction. The remaining cases are translocations (3%–4%) and mosaics (1%–2%). The translocations are unbalanced and usually occur with another acrocentric chromosome, usually 14/21 or 15/21. Approximately 75% of these are new mutations, and 25% are the result of a familial translocation. Therefore, if a child has a translocation, the parents must be evaluated for a balanced translocation. Mosaicism implies the presence of 2 cell lines: one normal and one with trisomy 21. As might be expected, children with mosaic Down syndrome are usually affected less severely than children with other types of Down syndrome.

Recent research has focused on the role of individual genes, such as *DYRK1A*, in the pathogenesis of Down syndrome. It is likely that in the near future, pharmacologic agents that mitigate the effects of excess expression of such genes will lead to new treatments for Down syndrome patients.

Trisomy 21

- Microcephaly, with flattening of both occiput and face
- Upward slant to the eyes with epicanthal folds
- Brushfield spots in eyes
- Small ears and mouth (therefore, tongue appears large)
- Low-set ears
- Flat nasal bridge
- Broad, stocky neck, with loose skin folds at the nape
- Funnel-shaped or pigeon-breasted chest
- Small, stubby feet, hands, and digits, with brachyclinodactyly of the fifth digits
- Single transverse palmar crease on each hand
- Wide space between first and second toes
- Fair, mottled skin in newborns; dry skin in older children
- Hypotonia

Evaluation

Routine health care maintenance for infants, children, or adolescents with trisomy 21 should cover the same issues in health education, prevention, and counseling that are discussed with other healthy patients and their families. The schedule of health maintenance visits for infants and young children with trisomy 21 is essentially the same as that recommended by the American Academy of Pediatrics for other children, while older children with Down syndrome should be evaluated annually. The following sections will emphasize additional medical and psychosocial conditions often seen in patients with trisomy 21.

Newborn Period

Verification of the diagnosis of trisomy 21 is perhaps the single most important focus of the initial family visit. Sometimes the diagnosis has been suspected prenatally due to abnormal biochemical markers and ultrasound, and verified by chorionic villus sampling or amniocentesis (Box 37-1). If there is no prenatal testing and the diagnosis is suspected due to clinical findings, a karyotype must be sent from the nursery and reviewed at the 1- to 2-week visit.

Several conditions that are associated with trisomy 21 are important to identify in the newborn period. They include hearing loss, congenital heart disease (most commonly endocardial cushion defect), duodenal atresia, Hirschsprung disease, congenital hypothyroidism, and ocular anomalies (cataracts, strabismus, and nystagmus). Hematologic abnormalities include polycythemia, leukemoid reactions that resemble leukemia but resolve during the first month of life and, rarely, leukemia.

History

A feeding history is critical because hypotonia often leads to swallowing difficulties (Table 37-1). A history of vomiting may be indicative of gastroesophageal reflux, or less commonly a

Table 37-1. Health Supervision for Children With Down Syndrome		
	Initial Evaluation	*Subsequent Evaluations*
History and Physical Exam		
Developmental assessment	Newborn	Same as regular well-child care schedule until age 5, then annual evaluation
Visual and hearing assessment (subjective)		
Laboratory Assessment		
Karyotype	Newborn	None
Thyroid screen	Newborn screen	6 months, 12 months, then annually
Complete blood cell count	Newborn	Same schedule as other children
Celiac screen	2–3 years	Every 5 years[a]
Echocardiogram	Newborn	Depends on condition
Neck radiographs	Age 3–5 years	Sports activities or Special Olympics entry[a]
Audiological evaluation	Newborn	12 months, then annually (if no ear, nose, throat problems)
Consultation		
Genetics	Newborn	As needed[b]
Cardiology	Newborn	Depends on condition
Ophthalmology	6 months	Every 2 years until age 5, then annually
Ear-nose-throat	As needed	As needed
Dental	By 1 year of age	Twice per year

[a] Lack of expert consensus on evaluation.

[b] Depending on experience and comfort level of primary care physician.

gastrointestinal malformation. Constipation may be the first indication of Hirschsprung disease or hypothyroidism. A detailed family and social history should also be obtained if this was not done in the hospital.

Physical Examination

A detailed physical examination should reveal some common features of newborns with Down syndrome (see Dx box). All growth parameters should be recorded and compared with those obtained at birth. The size of the fontanelles should be evaluated because of the increased incidence of congenital hypothyroidism. Bilateral red reflexes and conjugate gaze should be documented to exclude congenital cataracts or strabismus. A careful cardiac examination must be performed, noting any cyanosis, murmurs, irregular heart rates, abnormal heart sounds, or asymmetry of pulses. The abdomen should be palpated for organomegaly or any masses, and patency of the anus should be verified. An Ortolani and Barlow test should

also be performed for hip laxity. Finally, the infant should be evaluated for hypotonia.

Laboratory Tests

A karyotype is an important tool to verify the diagnosis and to assess recurrence risk. Newborn screening laboratory tests must be reviewed, especially hearing evaluations and thyroid screens. In addition, a cardiac evaluation for congenital heart disease should be performed, which may include an electrocardiogram, chest radiograph, echocardiogram, and formal cardiology referral. A complete blood cell count is indicated to look for hematologic abnormalities including leukemoid reaction, transient myeloproliferative disorder (pancytopenia, hepatosplenomegaly, and immature white blood cells), and neonatal thrombocytopenia.

Management

The primary care physician should discuss the increased propensity for respiratory infections in children with Down syndrome. Other important issues to address include those pertaining to available resources for children and families, such as early intervention programs and Down syndrome support groups in the community. Educational materials such as pamphlets and books may also be supplied at this time. Upcoming appointments with other physicians and allied health professionals should be reviewed.

Infancy and Early Childhood

History

Some additional historical issues to address include a detailed developmental assessment focusing on progress made since the last visit because most affected children have motor and speech delays (see Table 37-1). It is important to review any ancillary services, such as physical, occupational, and speech therapy, in anticipation of school entry. The parents should provide their assessment of the child's vision and hearing. A history of recurrent respiratory infections should raise concern about otitis media. Many children at this age develop constipation. A history of snoring and restless sleep may indicate obstructive sleep apnea and require a sleep study. Finally, it is extremely important to document any history of neck pain, gait changes, increased clumsiness, or other neurologic symptoms that would indicate spinal cord compression from atlantoaxial dislocation.

Physical Examination

All growth parameters should be plotted on growth charts for children with Down syndrome (Figures 37-1 through 37-4). Children with trisomy 21 are shorter than other children and may have poor weight gain in their first year. Later in life, obesity unrelated to the syndrome may become a problem, however. As with routine well-child visits in other infants and children, a complete physical examination should be performed at each patient encounter. Noteworthy aspects of the examination in infants and children with trisomy 21 are given in Box 37-2. In particular, the ear canals of these children

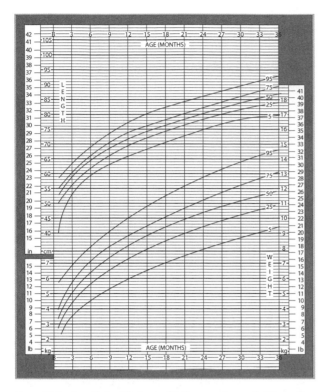

Figure 37-1. Growth chart for boys with Down syndrome: 1–36 months. (Reproduced with permission from Cronk C, Crocker AC, Pueschel SM, et al. Growth charts for children with Down syndrome: 1 month to 18 years of age. *Pediatrics.* 1988;81:102–110.)

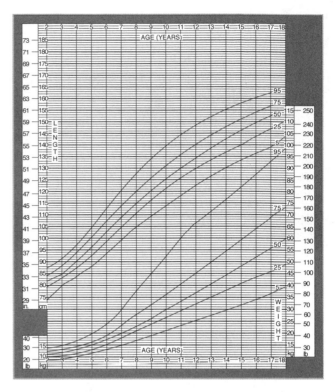

Figure 37-2. Growth chart for boys with Down syndrome: 2–18 years. (Reproduced with permission from Cronk C, Crocker AC, Pueschel SM, et al. Growth charts for children with Down syndrome: 1 month to 18 years of age. *Pediatrics.* 1988;81:102–110.)

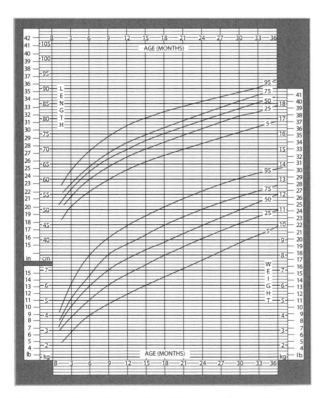

Figure 37-3. Growth chart for girls with Down syndrome: 1–36 months. (Reproduced with permission from Cronk C, Crocker AC, Pueschel SM, et al. Growth charts for children with Down syndrome: 1 month to 18 years of age. *Pediatrics.* 1988;81:102–110.)

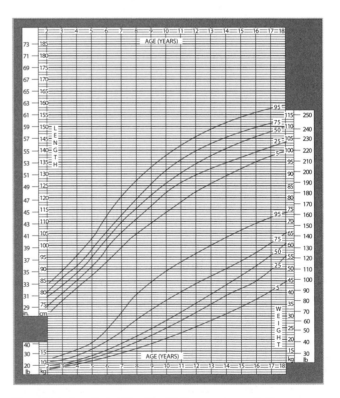

Figure 37-4. Growth chart for girls with Down syndrome: 2–18 years. (Reproduced with permission from Cronk C, Crocker AC, Pueschel SM, et al. Growth charts for children with Down syndrome: 1 month to 18 years of age. *Pediatrics.* 1988;81:102–110.)

Box 37-2. Physical Examination of Children With Trisomy 21

- Look for dry, sensitive skin and alopecia, which develops in approximately 10% of children and resolves spontaneously.
- Monitor the size of the anterior and posterior fontanelles because delayed closure may indicate hypothyroidism.
- Check for visual abnormalities, such as strabismus, nystagmus, cataracts, refractive errors, and blepharitis.
- Document recurrent serous otitis media. It is estimated that 40% to 60% of children with trisomy 21 have significant conductive hearing loss and 20% to 30% have some degree of neurosensory loss.
- Examine the oropharynx carefully for delayed dentition, malocclusion, and caries.
- Perform a thorough cardiac examination and note any evidence of previously unrecognized congenital heart disease.
- Palpate the abdomen for distention or organomegaly. Children with trisomy 21 have a slightly increased risk of developing acute non-lymphoblastic or acute lymphoblastic leukemia.
- Perform a rectal examination in infants or children with a history of constipation.
- Evaluate any musculoskeletal abnormalities such as overall hypotonia and joint laxity (most commonly in the knees and hips) that might contribute to overall gross motor delay.

are easily collapsed, making the tympanic membrane difficult to visualize. In some cases, an otolaryngology referral may be necessary for an adequate otoscopic examination. A complete neurologic examination should be performed at each visit, including an assessment of the degree of hypotonia.

Laboratory Tests

Hearing evaluation should be performed annually, starting with the newborn hearing screen. Developmentally appropriate gross visual screening should be performed in infants between 6 and 12 months of age at each visit, and a formal ophthalmology examination is recommended at 6 months and every 2 years thereafter. Thyroid screening tests should be repeated at 6 and 12 months and then annually.

Children with congenital heart disease should be given antibiotic endocarditis prophylaxis for dental or other procedures. In addition, these children should be considered for monoclonal antibody therapy against respiratory syncytial virus in the winter.

Children with Down syndrome have an increased risk for autoimmune disorders such as celiac disease, Grave disease, and type 1 diabetes. Because the signs of celiac disease may be subtle, most pediatric gastroenterologists recommend measuring tissue transglutaminase immunoglobulin (Ig) A antibodies, as well as an IgA level, at 2 to 3 years of age. Rescreening for celiac disease is currently a topic of debate, but several experts suggest that retesting approximately every 5 years during childhood may be appropriate.

Children with Down syndrome have an increased incidence of atlantoaxial instability when screened with routine lateral cervical

radiographs with flexion and extension views. Any patient with signs or symptoms of cord compression should be evaluated by computed tomography or magnetic resonance imaging and referred to an orthopedic surgeon or neurosurgeon. Symptomatic children should be kept out of any sports that involve contact or neck extension, such as swimming, gymnastics, and soccer. Experts have debated the value of routine radiographs, and most agree that careful neurologic screening at health supervision visits is a much better predictor of serious injury. However, at this time routine radiographs are still recommended at age 3 to 5 years and are required prior to participation in events such as the Special Olympics.

Management

Infants with trisomy 21 should have all routine screening tests and immunizations. Growth and developmental progress should be reviewed with parents at the end of each visit, and any concerns or unmet expectations should be addressed at this time. Often the developmental delay associated with trisomy 21 is not apparent to families until infants are 4 to 6 months of age and not achieving the expected milestones of rolling over or sitting. It should also be emphasized to families that the degree of mental retardation in trisomy 21 is quite variable, ranging from mild to severe. However, social function is not necessarily related to IQ. If the child is not already enrolled in an early intervention program, the positive role of such an experience should be addressed. The availability of support groups for parents and other family members should also be discussed.

In the early childhood years, plans for preschool attendance and future educational opportunities should be reviewed with families. The role of discipline and the presence of common behavioral problems such as temper tantrums and biting should be assessed in preparation for school entry and socialization. Nutrition should be reviewed because children with Down syndrome have a reduced metabolic rate and are at increased risk for obesity. Nutritional supplements and other alternative medicines have not been proven to have any efficacy in the treatment of Down syndrome patients.

A dental referral should be made by the age of 1 year in accordance with the latest recommendation for all children.

Older Childhood and Adolescence

History

School-aged children with Down syndrome should continue to visit their primary care physician at least annually. Educational issues should be discussed, including individual education plans and the transition from school. Specific medical issues to address during the history include visual or hearing deficits, evidence for hypothyroidism (decreased activity, coarse and dry hair, and constipation), skin problems including eczema, and dental problems. A careful nutritional history should also be taken because of the propensity for obesity, and the children should be closely monitored for signs of obstructive sleep apnea.

Physical Examination

Height and weight should continue to be plotted. The skin should be examined closely for xerosis, acne, or syringomas (multiple papules often present on the eyelids and upper cheeks) during adolescence. A cardiac examination is important because of an increased risk of mitral valve prolapse and valvular dysfunction. The sexual maturity rating (Tanner stage) of both males and females should be noted and discussed with the parents. A pelvic examination is not indicated as a part of the routine visit unless there is concern about sexual abuse or a sexually transmitted infection, but a testicular examination is important due to the increased risk of testicular cancer. A complete neurologic examination should also be performed in the patient participating in sports activities to look for signs indicating impending atlantoaxial dislocation.

Laboratory Tests

Annual thyroid screening (thyroid-stimulating hormone, thyroxine) is recommended for all school-aged children and adolescents with trisomy 21, in addition to other routine screening tests. An audiological evaluation should also occur at least once in older children and then annually thereafter. Because of the risk of keratoconus, an annual ophthalmology consultation should be arranged after the age of 10 years. In addition, children with trisomy 21 should be encouraged to continue biannual dental visits because gingivitis, periodontal disease, and bruxism (teeth grinding) are common in these individuals.

Management

The major part of the visit with school-aged and adolescent children should be spent on developmental, educational, and vocational anticipatory guidance. Educational placement and future goals should be both developmentally appropriate for the child and acceptable for the parent. Activities requiring socialization and the development of responsibility should continue to be encouraged; however, these events can be very stressful for parents and other family members. Injury prevention should be highlighted as well, especially because older children are becoming more independent. In early adolescence, prevocational and vocational training within the school curriculum should be reviewed. In addition, brief discussions regarding independent living, group homes, transition of medical care, and financial resources (eg, community-supported employment for young adults) should begin during adolescence.

Puberty, fertility, and contraception are extremely important to address with adolescents and their parents. The patient's psychosocial development and physical sexual maturation should be discussed, including menstrual hygiene and any foreseeable problems with its management. Contraception and the potential for victimization must be addressed as well, particularly with female patients. Males with trisomy 21 are usually sterile, but females have an approximately 50% chance of having children with Down syndrome.

Prognosis

Individuals with trisomy 21 can often live well past the age of 50 unless they are born with a congenital heart lesion, which may limit life expectancy. One major cause of morbidity and mortality is the development of symptomatic Alzheimer disease, which occurs in approximately 15% of adults after the fourth decade. Fortunately, most adults with Down syndrome remain asymptomatic, despite histopathologic evidence of the disease.

CASE RESOLUTION

In the case described at the beginning of the chapter, the family should be encouraged by the healthy progress of their daughter. For this visit, anticipatory guidance should consist of a review of early intervention services, available resources, and general support services for the patient and her family. The increased risk for both upper respiratory infections and otitis media should be reviewed. Medical screening should include thyroid screening, subjective hearing screening, and a formal evaluation by a pediatric ophthalmologist. If the results are normal, the next visit should take place in 3 months.

Selected References

American Academy of Pediatrics Committee on Genetics. Health supervision for children with Down syndrome. *Pediatrics.* 2001;107:442–449

Braganza SF. Atlantoaxial dislocation. *Pediatr Rev.* 2003;24:106–107

Cassidy SB, Allanson JE, eds. *Management of Genetic Syndromes.* 3rd ed. New York, NY: Wiley-Blackwell; 2010

Cohen WI. Current dilemmas in Down syndrome clinical care: celiac disease, thyroid disorders, and atlanto-axial instability. *Am J Med Genet C Semin Med Genet.* 2006;142:141–148

Cohen WI, Nadel L, Madnick M, eds. *Down Syndrome: Visions for the 21st Century.* New York, NY: Wiley-Liss; 2002

Davidson MA. Primary care for children and adolescents with Down syndrome. *Pediatr Clin North Am.* 2008;55(5):1099–1111

Venail F, Gardiner Q, Mondain M. ENT and speech disorders in children with Down's syndrome: an overview of pathophysiology, clinical features, treatments, and current management. *Clin Pediatr (Phila).* 2004;43:783–791

CHAPTER 38

Well-Child Care for Preterm Infants

Lynne M. Smith, MD

CASE STUDY

A 2½-month-old infant girl was discharged from the neonatal intensive care unit 2 weeks ago, where she had been since birth. She was the 780-g product of a 26-week gestation born via spontaneous vaginal delivery to a 32-year-old primigravida. The perinatal course was complicated by premature rupture of membranes and maternal amnionitis. Several aspects of the neonatal course were significant, including respiratory distress that required surfactant therapy and 2 weeks of endotracheal intubation; a grade II intraventricular hemorrhage on head ultrasound at 1 week of life; hyperbilirubinemia, which was treated with phototherapy; several episodes of apnea, presumably associated with the prematurity; and a history of poor oral intake with slow weight gain.

The infant's parents have a few questions about her feeding schedule and discontinuing the apnea monitor, but they feel relatively comfortable caring for their daughter at home. She is feeding well (2 oz of 22 cal/oz post-discharge formula for premature newborns every 2–3 hours)

and is becoming progressively more alert according to the family. She sleeps on her back in a crib.

The infant's weight gain has averaged 25 g/day. The rest of the physical examination is normal, except for dolichocephaly and a left esotropia.

Questions

1. What constitutes well-child care in preterm infants?
2. What are the nutritional requirements of preterm infants in the months following discharge from the hospital?
3. What information must be considered in the developmental screening of preterm infants?
4. What immunization schedule is appropriate for preterm infants? Do they require any special immunizations?
5. What specific conditions or illnesses are more likely to affect preterm infants than term infants?

Premature infants are born at less than 37 completed weeks' gestation and often weigh less than 2,500 g. Providing primary care for these infants is an important and challenging task and often requires coordination of medical, developmental, and social services for multiple chronic conditions. Because preterm infants are at increased risk for both impaired growth and developmental delay, longer visits may be necessary to evaluate the infants' nutritional and developmental progress and to assess how families have adjusted to caring for them at home. Primary care physicians must learn to manage these and many other complex issues while providing families with comprehensive anticipatory guidance.

Epidemiology

In the United States, 1 in 8 newborns is born prematurely, a 30% increase since 1981. The preterm delivery rate is highest for African American women (17.5%) and lowest for white (11.1%) and Asian and Pacific Islander (10.7%) women. Reasons for the increased premature delivery rates include an increased use of artificial reproductive technologies (see Chapter 21) and increased maternal age.

Though most preterm newborns are delivered between 34 and 36 weeks' gestation, these neonates are at increased risk for morbidity and mortality relative to infants born at term. In addition, many neonatologists routinely resuscitate neonates born at 23 weeks' gestation, a gestation that has a survival rate of approximately 25%. Very low birth weight (VLBW, <1,500 g) and extremely low birth weight (ELBW, <1,000 g) newborns are at risk for cerebral palsy, hearing and vision problems, and mental retardation. Further, learning disabilities, attention-deficit disorder, borderline to low IQ scores, and abnormalities in executive function and visuomotor integration occur in more than 50% of VLBW infants, complicating the posthospital care for these children. In 2006 the Institute of Medicine estimated the annual societal cost of prematurity at $26 billion.

Evaluation

The purpose of the health maintenance visit for preterm infants is the same as for other healthy children: to provide consistent preventive health care and education for patients and their parents. Prematurity, however, places children at risk for additional medical and neuro-developmental conditions.

History

At the initial visit, it is imperative to review the entire medical history and hospital course with the family. Ideally, the neonatal intensive care unit (NICU) should provide a discharge summary that includes the following information:

1. Birth weight, gestational age, and significant prenatal and perinatal information
2. An overview of the hospital course, including significant illnesses, events, surgical procedures, and pertinent radiographic studies
3. Nutrition information and present feeding regimen
4. A list of current medications, including dosing intervals and, if appropriate, serum drug levels
5. Immunizations given during the hospitalization
6. Pertinent laboratory data, such as most recent hemoglobin, newborn screening results, ophthalmologic and hearing screening information, neurosonogram and magnetic resonance imaging (MRI) results, and highest serum bilirubin level
7. Discharge physical examination, including most recent height, weight, and head circumference
8. Problems remaining at discharge
9. Follow-up appointments

Any significant complications or concerns should be discussed with the parents as soon as possible to assess their understanding of these issues as well as expectations for improvement.

Specifically, growth, nutrition, and developmental issues should be addressed at each visit (Questions Box). Adequate or desirable weight gain should be explained to the caregivers in terms of the

infant's current weight versus the discharge weight. Infants younger than 6 months should gain, on average, 20 to 40 g/day. To ensure continued weight gain, many preterm infants are discharged from the NICU on a 24-hour feeding schedule, which requires that parents feed infants at least every 3 hours. The necessity for this practice should be reevaluated during the first few weeks following discharge after infants have demonstrated adequate weight gain.

A critical component of the health maintenance visit is the developmental history. Parental expectations and observations should be noted, and any developmental concerns should be evaluated. The adjusted developmental age should be calculated by subtracting the number of weeks the infant was born prematurely from the current chronological age in weeks. The adjusted age should then be used for all formal and informal developmental assessments. The importance of correcting for prematurity until children are 2 years of age must be emphasized when discussing developmental progress and giving anticipatory guidance to parents.

Physical Examination

A complete physical examination should be performed at each visit to monitor the status of associated medical conditions. All growth parameters (weight, height, and head circumference) should be plotted on the growth chart for premature newborns until approximately 50 weeks' postmenstrual age and adjusted for prematurity on standard growth charts until age 2. Because catch-up head growth generally precedes catch-up weight and length, preterm infants may appear to have disproportionally large heads. The onset of accelerated head growth may begin within a few weeks after birth (36 weeks' postconception) or as late as 8 months adjusted age. Average daily weight gain in grams per day should also be calculated.

The size and shape of the head must be evaluated, especially if the infant has a history of intraventricular or intracranial hemorrhage or hydrocephalus. An increase in head circumference of more than 2 cm per week should be cause for concern in these infants. In infants who have been treated neurosurgically for hydrocephalus, ventriculoperitoneal shunt and tubing may be palpated. Visual abnormalities such as strabismus must be carefully ruled out by examination as well as by history because up to 20% of preterm infants may have an ophthalmologic problem (see Chapter 76). Oropharyngeal abnormalities, such as a palatal groove, high-arched palate, or abnormal tooth formation, may occur as a result of prolonged endotracheal intubation. Baseline intercostal, substernal, or subcostal retractions; wheezing; stridor; and tachypnea in former premature babies with moderate-to-severe bronchopulmonary dysplasia (BPD) should be documented.

Chest scars secondary to the placement of chest tubes should be noted. Adult female breasts may be affected if scarring occurs on or close to breast tissue. The umbilicus may appear hypoplastic as a result of umbilical catheter placement and suturing. Multiple scars on the heels from blood sampling or on the distal extremities from intravenous catheters and cutdowns may be evident.

The genitalia of both male and female preterm infants should be examined closely for inguinal hernias. The incidence of inguinal hernias in preterm newborns is up to 30% with incarceration rates of up

---

Questions

Well-Child Care for Preterm Infants

- How much did the infant weigh when discharged from the hospital?
- Is the infant breastfed or formula-fed? Is the infant on any special formula?
- How often and how much does the infant feed? How long do feedings take?
- Does the infant have any feeding problems (eg, pain, vomiting, gastroesophageal reflux)?
- Does the infant take dietary supplementation of vitamins and minerals?
- What developmental milestones has the infant reached? Does the infant roll over? Smile? Sit up?
- Does the infant seem to hear and see?
- Who cares for the infant?
- Where and in what position does the child sleep?
- Do the parents have any concerns regarding growth, development, or nutrition?
- Is the infant on an apnea monitor? Have there been any apneic episodes?

to 31%. If hernias are surgically repaired under general anesthesia, infants should be monitored for apnea for up to 24 hours postoperatively. The male scrotum should be examined for cryptorchidism because only 25% of testes are in the scrotum of prematurely delivered males at term gestation. By 1 year of age, more than 90% of testes are intrascrotal. A careful evaluation for developmental dysplasia of the hip should be performed until children are ambulatory, and a hip ultrasound should be performed at 6 weeks of age for all breech deliveries (see Chapter 100).

A thorough neuromuscular examination is essential in these children. Increased muscular tone, asymmetry, and decreased bulk should be noted along with the presence of any clonus or asymmetry of deep tendon reflexes. Inappropriate reflexes, such as a persistent Moro or fisting beyond 4 months of age, should also be documented. Other abnormalities (eg, scissoring or sustained clonus) in the neurologic examination may become more apparent as infants become older. The detection of subtle early findings is important so appropriate intervention services can begin as soon as possible.

Laboratory Tests

In addition to the standard screening tests performed on all healthy infants and children during health maintenance visits, several laboratory studies are important in preterm infants. Such tests include a complete blood cell count and reticulocyte count to check for anemia; electrolytes in infants with BPD on diuretics to detect abnormalities; and serum calcium, phosphorus, and alkaline phosphatase levels in infants with documented rickets.

Pulse oximetry is indicated for oxygen-dependent infants as well as those presenting with respiratory symptoms greater than baseline. Results from newborn screening tests, including auditory and ophthalmologic examinations, should be reviewed and repeated as indicated. Cranial ultrasound studies should be reviewed with caution because nearly 30% of infants born weighing less than 1,000 g with normal head ultrasound findings develop cerebral palsy or developmental delay. In addition, infants with a grade I or II intracranial hemorrhage have an increased risk for developmental delay. Brain MRI scans should be considered in infants born less than 30 weeks' gestation, or in any infant with a concerning abnormal neurologic examination or abnormal rate of head growth.

Management

Well-child care in relatively healthy preterm infants has 2 components. One is the provision of routine health care maintenance for infants and appropriate developmental anticipatory guidance for parents. The other component involves the incorporation of treatment for chronic conditions into each visit. Health care maintenance should include nutrition counseling, developmental surveillance, immunizations, and assessment of vision and hearing in addition to standard screening tests discussed previously. Outside resources concerning developmental delay can be reviewed with parents (Box 38-1). Care related to chronic conditions includes adjusting medication doses, such as diuretic therapy; weaning from supplemental oxygen; and discontinuing the apnea monitor.

Box 38-1. Physician Support and Education of Parents With Preterm Infants
• Understand parental expectations.
• Legitimize parental fears.
• Be a source of support and encouragement.
• Provide consistent, honest information.
• Assume the role of the overall coordinator of care.
• Provide referrals to outside resources, including respite care.

Parents should be given anticipatory guidance prior to discharge that caring for a NICU graduate is challenging. Premature newborns have poorly organized sleep–wake cycles resulting in more frequent awakening than term newborns. In addition, premature newborns have immature suck–swallow coordination, causing them to feed more frequently and for longer periods. Colic is reported twice as frequently in VLBW infants relative to term newborns, and many are described as having difficult temperament until past their first birthdays.

The medical costs associated with the care of premature newborns often strain the family finances at a time when many women decrease their work schedules. Additional stressors include uncertainty about the long-term outcome of the child, guilt many women feel after delivering prematurely, and anxiety about future pregnancies. The difficulty of caring for these complicated, challenging children results in significant parental stress and can interfere with their ability to properly bond to their newborn.

Nutrition

According to the American Academy of Pediatrics (AAP) Committee on Nutrition, the average daily energy requirement for most hospitalized healthy preterm infants is 105 to 130 kcal/kg/day to achieve adequate growth. Energy requirements vary with individual infants depending on associated chronic conditions, such as BPD or malabsorption. Growth is considered adequate in the newborn weighing more than 2,000 g if weight gain is more than 20 g/day and length and head circumference increase 0.7 to 1.0 cm/week.

At 40 weeks' corrected age, preterm newborns are usually smaller than term newborns. Adequate nutrition in the first year of life is critical because catch-up weight gain is unlikely to occur after age 3. Because breast milk is insufficient for providing adequate protein and micronutrients to preterm newborns, human milk fortifier is added to breast milk.

If not receiving breast milk, children born at 34 weeks or less and/or weighing less than 1,500 g are usually discharged home on a nutritionally enhanced transitional formula (Similac NeoSure Advance, Enfamil EnfaCare LIPIL). The calcium, phosphorous, and caloric content of these 22 cal/oz transitional formulas are between levels found in standard preterm and term formulas. Use of preterm enriched formulas is usually continued until the child reaches the 5th to 10th percentile on the growth chart or is 1 year adjusted age. A meta-analysis, however, failed to demonstrate nutrient-enriched formulas improve growth rates or developmental outcome after discharge relative to standard term formula.

Formula-fed infants require multivitamin supplementation until 750 mL/day of formula is consumed. Breastfed premature newborns may benefit from continuing multivitamin solution as long as human milk is the predominant source of nutrition. Vitamin D supplementation is recommended for all breastfed infants. Because premature newborns are at increased risk for osteopenia of prematurity, soy formulas are to be avoided because of the low phosphate content.

The introduction of solid foods is appropriate once infants have developed acceptable oral–motor skills for swallowing solids. Cow's milk should not be introduced until 12 months' adjusted age.

Developmental Assessment

Both informal and formal developmental surveillance should include referral to an early intervention program, particularly in ELBW infants because routine screening tests are not sensitive enough to pick up subtle neurodevelopmental abnormalities (Box 38-2; see Chapter 27). The Individuals with Disabilities Education Act, Part C guarantees early intervention programs for infants and toddlers with disabilities up to age 3. Children born weighing less than 1,200 g are automatically eligible, but any child suspected of a developmental delay is entitled to an evaluation to determine eligibility for services regardless of a family's ability to pay. Because many developmental issues do not manifest until school age, frequent developmental assessments and enrollment in preschool are especially important for infants born prematurely.

Immunizations

Routine immunization schedules recommended by the AAP Committee on Immunization Practices should be followed. The administration of any vaccine is determined by the chronological or postnatal age, not the gestational age. Standard doses and intervals should also be used (see Chapter 32). Several studies have shown an adequate serologic response despite a history of prematurity. Absolute and relative contraindications to specific vaccine components or to live vaccines for preterm infants are identical to published guidelines for term infants and children. In addition to following the recommendation that all infants 6 months and older be vaccinated against influenza, all household contacts of premature newborns should also be strongly urged to be vaccinated. Two doses of influenza vaccine are administered 1 month apart, with subsequent immunization the following year only requiring one dose. Rotavirus vaccination is recommended for clinically stable premature newborns if they are 6 to 14 weeks' chronological age at discharge or have already been discharged from the NICU.

If adequate weight gain has been established, it is safe to administer hepatitis B vaccine to medically stable neonates weighing less than 2,000 g as early as 30 days of age or at discharge, whichever comes first. All neonates born to mothers who are hepatitis B surface antigen (HBsAg) positive should receive hepatitis B vaccine and hepatitis B immune globulin (HBIG) within 12 hours of delivery. When maternal HBsAg status is unknown, neonates weighing less

---

Box 38-2. Typical Speech, Play, and Physical Development[a]

In addition to standardized tests, the following guidelines provide development milestones useful for early detection:

By 3 months' adjusted age, the infant
- Coos or vocalizes other than crying
- Visually tracks a moving toy from side to side
- Attempts to reach for a rattle held above their chest
- Pushes up on arms
- Lifts and holds head up

At 6 months' adjusted age, the infant
- Begins to use consonant sounds in babbling and uses to get attention
- Reaches for a nearby toy while on their tummy
- Transfers a toy from one hand to the other while lying on back
- Reaches both hands to play with feet while lying on back
- Uses hands to support self in sitting
- While standing with support, accepts entire weight with legs

At 9 months' adjusted age, the infant
- Increases variety of sounds and syllable combinations in babbling
- Looks at familiar objects and people when named
- Explores and examines an object using both hands
- Turns several pages of a chunky book at once
- Imitates others in simple play
- Sits and reaches for toys without falling

At 12 months' adjusted age, the child
- Meaningfully uses "mama" or "dada"
- Responds to simple commands (eg, "come here")
- Produces long strings of gibberish in social communication
- Finger feeds self
- Uses thumb and pointer finger to pick up tiny objects
- Pulls to stand and cruise along furniture
- Stands alone and takes several independent steps

At 15 months' adjusted age, the child
- Has a vocabulary consisting of 5–10 words
- Helps with getting undressed
- Walks independently and seldom falls
- Squats to pick up toy

At 24 months' adjusted age, the child
- Uses 2- to 4-word sentences
- Walks up and down stairs holding on for support
- Builds a tower of 4 blocks or more
- Can identify basic body parts

[a] Modified with permission from Pathways Awareness Foundation. *Assure the Best for your Baby's Physical Development.* Available at: http://www.pathwaysawareness.org/; and Centers for Disease Control and Prevention. Developmental Milestones. Available at: http://www.cdc.gov/ncbddd/actearly/milestones/index.html.

---

than 2,000 g should receive HBIG within 12 hours, neonates weighing more than 2,000 g should receive HBIG within 7 days, and all should be vaccinated for hepatitis B within 12 hours.

Because respiratory syncytial virus (RSV) causes an increased morbidity and mortality in NICU graduates and infants with congenital heart disease, administration of RSV-specific immuno-globulin, palivizumab (Synagis), is recommended every month from November to March (Box 38-3). A documented infection with RSV is not an indication to discontinue passive immunization as multiple strains may circulate during the RSV season.

Assessment of Vision and Hearing

Follow-up visits for visual and auditory sequelae of prematurity must be arranged at the health maintenance visit. An initial ophthalmologic screening examination should have been performed between 4 and 9 weeks of age in infants weighing less than 1,500 g or less than 32 weeks' gestation, irrespective of oxygen exposure. Infants between 1,500 g and 2,000 g or greater than 32 weeks' gestation with an unstable clinical course should also be screened. The frequency and need for repeat examinations are determined based on the initial findings. Preterm infants, regardless of the presence of retinopathy of prematurity, are at increased risk for the development of strabismus, myopia, amblyopia, and glaucoma and need an ophthalmologic examination beginning at 6 months of age.

The AAP recommends universal hearing screening for all newborns. Neonatal intensive care unit graduates account for approximately 50% of all newborn hearing screening failures, and severe sensorineural hearing loss occurs in up to 10% of ELBW infants. Screening is recommended immediately prior to discharge, and repeat testing is recommended if speech delays develop.

Other Possible Problems

Preterm infants with chronic lung disease are at increased risk for respiratory illness, especially during the winter. Parents should be informed of this risk and counseled about symptoms such as tachypnea and wheezing associated with a simple upper respiratory infection. Practitioners should have a low threshold for considering a diagnosis of pneumonia in these infants in the appropriate clinical setting.

Primary care providers should also keep in mind that preterm infants are at increased risk for sudden infant death syndrome (Chapter 59). The AAP recommends that all infants sleep in the supine position. In the NICU, neonates are often placed on their stomachs if they have respiratory difficulties and on their sides if they have symptomatic gastroesophageal reflux. Neonatal intensive care unit personnel need to begin placing these babies on their backs in anticipation of discharge. Parents should also be reminded that cosleeping is not recommended and is highly associated with sudden infant death from accidental asphyxia.

Home apnea monitors are not associated with the prevention of SIDS and should be reserved for infants who are considered to have extreme cardiorespiratory instability. Discontinuation of home monitoring may be considered at 42 weeks' postmenstrual age and when significant apneic events have ceased, whichever comes later.

Preterm survivors who were critically ill can be particularly at risk for developing **vulnerable child syndrome** because their parents often perceive them as fragile and vulnerable. Features of this syndrome include abnormal separation difficulties for both the

Box 38-3. Indications for the Use of Palivizumab for Respiratory Syncytial Virus (RSV) Prophylaxis	
Condition	Age at Onset of RSV Season
Preterm infants with chronic lung disease requiring medical management • Oxygen • Bronchodilator • Diuretics • Chronic corticosteroids	<24 months
Cyanotic or complicated congenital heart disease	<24 months
Significant congenital abnormalities of the airway or neuromuscular disease that compromises handling of respiratory secretions	<12 months
Born ≤28 weeks' gestation	<12 months
Born 29–31 weeks' 6 days' gestation	<6 months
Born 32–34 weeks' 6 days' gestation with at least 1 of 2 risk factors • Attending child care • Sibling <5 years old in the home	<3 months

mother and child, sleep difficulties, parental overprotectiveness and overindulgence, lack of appropriate discipline, tolerance of physical abusiveness by the child toward the parent, and excessive preoccupation with the infant's health. Serious behavioral problems may arise as a result of such parent–child interactions. Primary care providers must be cognizant of early signs of this syndrome and should try to prevent its occurrence by reassuring parents about the infant's well-being. Once vulnerable child syndrome is suspected, connecting the child's history of critical illness with ongoing parent concerns is important as many parents are unaware that current concerns may stem from their unresolved anxiety. Every effort should be made to normalize the family's schedule once the infant is stable and to encourage parent–infant interactions unrelated to health care.

Prognosis

Neurodevelopmental impairment is a concern for physicians who care for preterm infants. Risk factors for developmental delay include postnatal steroid exposure, necrotizing enterocolitis, BPD, and small for gestational age. Chorioamnionitis is a risk factor for cerebral palsy in term infants and possibly in infants born prematurely. Extremely low birth weight infants and those born between 20 to 25 weeks' gestation have significant risk for developmental issues. Surviving infants born at less than 26 weeks' gestation in the United Kingdom in 1995 had median Bayley mental and psychomotor scores at 30 months of age of 80, with comparable cognitive score deficits at age 6.

During adolescence, 50% of former VLBW infants will have an IQ in an abnormally low range, and 30% will have attention-deficit/hyperactivity disorder. Though former premature newborns report more health-related and learning difficulties in adolescence relative to their normal birth weight peers, the VLBW teens rated their quality of life higher than their peers. In addition, increased systolic blood pressure, insulin resistance, and impaired glucose tolerance has also been reported in VLBW adults. Parents should also understand that long-term follow-up information may not accurately reflect the outcome for their child because these adolescents were managed prior to advances in prenatal and neonatal care.

CASE RESOLUTION

In the case presented at the beginning of the chapter, the infant's current feeding schedule should be continued because appropriate weight gain has occurred. Iron and multivitamin supplementation is recommended until 750 mL/day of formula is consumed. Discontinuation of the apnea monitor can be considered after the infant reaches term gestation and has been event-free. The first set of immunizations should be administered at this visit, and any questions that the family has should be answered. A follow-up visit should be scheduled in 3 to 4 weeks. Formal developmental testing should be arranged in 1 to 2 months, and the parents should be encouraged to continue having the child sleep on her back.

Selected References

American Academy of Pediatrics. Pickering LK, Baker CJ, Kimberlin DW, Long SS, eds. *Red Book: 2009 Report of the Committee on Infectious Diseases.* 28th ed. Elk Grove Village, IL: American Academy of Pediatrics.

American Academy of Pediatrics Section on Ophthalmology, American Academy of Ophthalmology, American Association for Pediatric Ophthalmology and Strabismus. Screening examination of premature infants for retinopathy of prematurity. *Pediatrics.* 2006;117(2):572–576

American Academy of Pediatrics Task Force on Sudden Infant Death Syndrome. The changing concept of sudden infant death syndrome: diagnostic coding shifts, controversies regarding the sleeping environment, and new variables to consider in reducing risk. *Pediatrics.* 2005;116:1245–1255

Aylward GP. Neurodevelopmental outcomes of infants born prematurely. *J Dev Behav Pediatr.* 2005;26:427–440

Cortese MM, Parashar UD; Centers for Disease Control and Prevention. Prevention of rotavirus gastroenteritis among infants and children: recommendations of the Advisory Committee on Immunization Practices (ACIP). *MMWR Recomm Rep.* 2009;58(RR-2):1–25

Hack M, Flannery DJ, Schluchter M, Cartar L, Borawski E, Klein N. Outcomes in young adulthood for very-low-birth-weight infants. *N Engl J Med.* 2002;346:149–157

Hamilton BE, Martin JA, Ventura SJ. Births: Preliminary Data for 2008. National Vital Statistics Reports 58 (16), 2008. http://www.cdc.gov/nchs/data/nvsr/nvsr58/nvsr58_16.pdf

Henderson G, Fahey T, McGuire W. Nutrient-enriched formula versus standard term formula for preterm infants following hospital discharge. *Cochrane Database Syst Rev.* 2007;(4):CD004696

Hovi P, Andersson S, Eriksson JG, et al. Glucose regulation in young adults with very low birth weight. *N Engl J Med.* 2007;356(20):2053–2063

Institute of Medicine Committee on Understanding Premature Birth and Assuring Healthy Outcomes. *Preterm Birth: Causes, Consequences and Prevention.* Washington, DC: National Academies Press; 2007

LaHood A, Bryant CA. Outpatient care of the premature infant. *Am Fam Physician.* 2007;76(8):1159–1164

Marlow N, Wolke D, Bracewell MA, Samara M; EPICure Study Group. Neurologic and developmental disability at six years of age after extremely preterm birth. *N Engl J Med.* 2005;352(1):9–19

Moster D, Lie RT, Markestad T. Long-term medical and social consequences of preterm birth. *N Engl J Med.* 2008;359(3):262–273

Tyson JE, Parikh NA, Langer J, Green C, Higgins RD. Intensive care for extreme prematurity: moving beyond gestational age. *N Engl J Med.* 2008;358:1672–1681

Wood NS, Marlow N, Costeloe K, Gibson AT, Wilkinson AR. Neurologic and developmental disability after extremely preterm birth. EPICure Study Group. *N Engl J Med.* 2000;343(6):378–384

Woodward LJ, Anderson PJ, Austin NC, Howard K, Inder TE. Neonatal MRI to predict neurodevelopmental outcomes in preterm infants. *N Engl J Med.* 2006;355(7):685–694

CHAPTER 39

Care of Children With Special Health Care Needs

Julie E. Noble, MD

CASE STUDY

A 5-year-old physically disabled girl is brought to your office for her first visit for a routine physical examination for school entrance. The girl was the full-term product of a pregnancy complicated by an elevated screening α-fetoprotein and a subsequent fetal ultrasound that demonstrated a lumbar myelomeningocele and no hydrocephalus. Delivery was elective cesarean section with Apgar scores of 9 at 1 minute and 9 at 5 minutes to a 25-year-old gravida I para 0–I female. The mother used no illicit drugs, alcohol, or any other medications during pregnancy, but was not on vitamins or folate supplementation at the time of conception. At delivery, a low lumbar spinal malformation was noted without other malformations. The quadriceps muscles were strong but the feet demonstrated a rocker bottom deformity.

Shortly after birth the myelomeningocele malformation was closed by neurosurgery. She has had orthopedic surgical release of Achilles tendon contractions and is ambulatory with ankle–foot orthotics. She has a neurogenic bladder and requires intermittent catheterization.

She has chronic constipation treated with a bowel regimen. Her cognitive function is age-appropriate.

She will be entering a school program for the first time since moving to this community and has not established care with any specialists.

Questions

1. Why is early identification and Intervention important for infants and children with special health care needs (SHCN)?
2. What are the unique needs of infants and children with SHCN?
3. What role do primary care practitioners play in the care of children with SHCN?
4. What are the appropriate referrals and resources for families of children with SHCN?
5. What specific psychosocial issues should be addressed whenever children with SHCN visit their primary care practitioners?

Children and youth with SHCN have disabilities that are defined as abnormalities in body function or structure that interfere with the activities of normal daily life. These disabilities can include physical, sensory, developmental, behavioral, or emotional conditions. They can range from mild to severe, depending on the nature and extent of the condition and its impact on daily living. Frequently the care requirements of both families and medical providers for children diagnosed with a disability are dramatically increased. For parents, the diagnosis of a disability in their child can be initially overwhelming and disappointing. Support of the parents is essential as they transition from disappointment to acceptance and assume the role of facilitator of their child's treatment plans.

Early identification of a disabling condition by physicians can lead to appropriate, definitive treatment for many disabilities. Early intervention can sometimes even prevent secondary conditions (eg, early management of hearing loss with hearing aids may minimize speech abnormalities). Even when such corrective treatment is not available, prompt identification improves children's long-term outcome and allows families to obtain appropriate resources for their children. Through early intervention, infants and children with irreversible conditions can be introduced to medical, educational, and psychosocial services available in the community that serve to help each child maximize and reach full potential.

Epidemiology

The prevalence of children in the United States with SHCN is difficult to assess. Studies report that approximately 17% of children younger than 17 years have at least one disability, including deafness or hearing loss, blindness, cerebral palsy, physical malformations, speech impediments, developmental delay, and other learning problems. Comorbid conditions, such as epilepsy, and secondary conditions, such as behavior problems, have a very high incidence. An estimated 30% of disabled children have more than one disability. A single sensory disability, such as deafness, affects approximately 3.5% of children, and blindness occurs in 1% of children. The prevalence of cerebral palsy is 1.5 to 2 per 1,000 live births. Advances in medical technology, as well as improved survival of low birth weight infants and children with malformations, have increased the number of children living with such disabilities. Environmental exposures have also increased the incidence of chronic medical conditions, such as asthma, which also produces SHCN.

The presence of SHCN has a profound impact on the health and education of affected children. Studies show that children with disabilities have 1.5 times more doctor visits and spend 3.5 more days in the hospital than children without these conditions. Children with disabilities miss twice the number of school days and are twice as likely to repeat a grade compared with children without disabilities.

In addition, numerous associated conditions occur more commonly in children with disabilities. These include mental retardation, growth failure, and nutrition problems. Problems with dentition, respiratory infections, and bowel and bladder continence may also develop. Significant emotional disturbances may occur as the child adapts to his condition.

Clinical Presentation

Children with disabilities can present in a variety of ways depending on their diagnosis. Many physical disabilities may be readily apparent at birth on the newborn examination or through newborn screening. Some diagnoses, such as cerebral palsy, may be detected later, as the motor impairment becomes more evident. Following development at routine health maintenance visits is essential for early detection of developmental delay. Children with disabilities can also present with chronic illness, such as asthma, and diabetes, or with specific complaints, such as poor vision or hearing. Their presentation may be for a more general concern, such as growth failure (Dx Box). Behavioral problems or difficulties in school may precipitate the initial visit.

Dx Children With Physical and Sensory Disabilities[a]

- Growth failure
- Microcephaly
- Abnormal neurologic examination, including hypertonicity, spastic diplegia or quadriplegia, and brisk deep tendon reflexes
- Developmental delay
- Speech or hearing deficit
- Visual deficit
- Physical malformations

[a]May not be present in all children.

Pathophysiology

The pathophysiology of disabilities is totally dependent on the disabling condition. Conditions may be secondary to an embryological defect, such as myelomeningocele, or an infection, such as congenital cytomegalovirus (CMV), which interferes with cochlear development and leads to hearing loss. Etiologies are often multifactorial. For some conditions, autism being an example, the pathophysiology is unknown.

Disabilities may be classified as acquired or congenital, and static or progressive. **Cerebral palsy,** for example, is a group of nonprogressive neuromotor disorders resulting from a central nervous system insult prenatally or in the first 2 years of life. It is characterized by abnormal motor movements and posturing and may be accompanied by other problems. Causes of cerebral palsy include prematurity, low birth weight, asphyxia, prenatal abnormalities (eg, placental insufficiency), congenital infections (eg, toxoplasmosis, CMV), and biochemical abnormalities (eg, severe hyperbilirubinemia). Other causes are environmental (eg, alcohol [maternal alcoholism]) and genetic (eg, inborn errors of metabolism). Severe postnatal injuries or infections can also lead to cerebral palsy (eg, shaken baby syndrome and meningitis). However, an estimated 25% to 50% of cases of cerebral palsy have no discernible cause.

Diagnosis

The term **special health care needs** is used in a broad sense to include conditions that require additional medical care and supervision. The term was defined by the US Department of Health and Human Services Maternal and Child Health Bureau. Children may have significant physical, sensory, or developmental disabilities that may result from prematurity, congenital infections such as CMV, or exposure in utero to alcohol or illicit substances. Some children are born with inborn errors of metabolism that mandate special diets and occupational or physical therapy. Other children with SHCN include those with chronic medical conditions such as asthma and sickle cell anemia. All of these medical conditions alter lifestyle, require increased medical care including subspeciality care, increase medication usage, and use community services beyond the general pediatric population.

Evaluation

History

When initially evaluating children with newly diagnosed disabilities, practitioners should first determine any specific parental concerns. A complete medical history should then be obtained, including information about the pregnancy and birth. The history should also include any possible exposures as well as significant infections. General screening questions about development are also important to ask (Questions Box) so that the child's developmental progress can be assessed. Specific questioning is warranted if parents are concerned about delayed development or if any of their responses indicate that their children are not attaining age-appropriate developmental milestones.

In cases of children with known sensory or physical disabilities, families should be asked directly at each visit about daily activities and the child's ability for self-help skills. Because many children with

Questions

Children With Special Health Care Needs

- Were there any perinatal complications, such as premature rupture of membranes or fetal distress?
- Was the infant born prematurely? If so, how long did the infant remain in the hospital and for what reasons?
- Was the infant exposed to any toxins (eg, alcohol, illicit drugs) in utero?
- Is there any history of infection during the perinatal period or infancy?
- What developmental milestones has the infant or child mastered?
- Is the child attending school or some type of early intervention program?
- How does the child get there?
- What does the child do on returning from school?
- Who feeds and bathes the child?
- Can the older child use the toilet without assistance?
- How is the child sleeping? Does the child take naps at school and at home?
- Has respite care been arranged for the family?
- Does the caregiver seem overwhelmed or excessively tired, especially one who is caring for a child with multiple disabilities?
- Do other family members help care for the child?
- Is the extended family available to help with the siblings?
- Are there any other disabled people in the family?
- Does the family receive any financial assistance for care of the child?

disabilities are also on daily medication for either seizures or other chronic conditions, it is also important to ask about the presence of any side effects of drugs.

Behavioral or emotional problems that the child might be having should be identified. In addition, an overall assessment of family dynamics should be made. It is important to inquire about the relationships between children with disabilities and their siblings, as well as the impact these children have on the parents' marriage.

Physical Examination

In general, a complete physical examination, including a neurologic assessment and neuromotor examination, should be performed at each visit. The height, weight, and head circumference should be plotted on the growth chart and compared with previous measurements. A failure of adequate growth as measured by any of these parameters should be examined closely. For example, microcephaly, nutritional problems, and growth failure are not uncommon in children with cerebral palsy. Depending on the disability, the examination should then focus on physical findings associated with the particular condition. For children with physical disabilities such as congenital or acquired amputations, for instance, assessment of the skin that comes in contact with prosthetic devices is a pertinent aspect of the physical examination. Pressure sores may be found in

non-ambulatory children with cerebral palsy. In children with sensory disabilities such as unilateral hearing loss, the evaluation of a middle ear effusion or infection in the unaffected ear should be a priority. If a child has a tracheostomy or gastrostomy tube, inspection of the site is essential at each visit to look for erosions or skin infections.

Overall, for most children with disabilities, the neurologic examination is extremely important. The following questions should be addressed: Are normal primitive reflexes such as the Moro and rooting reflexes present in neonates? Have all primitive reflexes been extinguished in older children? Do infants appear to visualize and track objects appropriately? Are there any abnormal movements of the trunk or extremities at rest? Is the muscle tone normal? Is any hypertonicity or hypotonicity evident? Is any asymmetry of the upper and lower extremities apparent? Are the deep tendon reflexes normal and symmetrical? Is the gait appropriate for age?

An age-appropriate developmental assessment is also an essential part of the examination at all health maintenance visits.

Laboratory Tests

The laboratory evaluation of infants or children with physical or sensory disabilities depends on the specific condition. Not all patients need a costly array of diagnostic procedures. A **chromosomal karyotype** using peripheral blood is helpful in children with suspected genetic disorders (eg, abnormal facies or a major anomaly and developmental delay). Routine testing for fragile X syndrome in all mentally retarded boys and in girls with a family history should be strongly considered. Other testing should be specific, relating to the suspected diagnosis (see Chapter 69).

Metabolic screening for inborn errors of metabolism should be performed on children with mental retardation and any of the following symptoms: intermittent vomiting or lethargy, loss of developmental milestones, or seizures. Such screening is not needed in the routine evaluation of children with developmental delay and no other symptoms.

A screening test for visual acuity (Snellen test) and hearing (audiogram) should be performed in all children suspected of having sensory deficits, even mild ones. For infants or toddlers, a brain stem auditory evoked response or behavioral audiogram is a more appropriate screening test for hearing. A visual evoked response can be performed to test vision.

Psychometric testing may be helpful in certain school-aged children to assess intellectual function.

An electroencephalogram is indicated in all patients who have a history of seizures or seizure-like episodes.

Imaging Studies

Brain imaging studies, such as magnetic resonance imaging scans of the head, can be informative when intrauterine infection, intraventricular hemorrhage, or genetic disorders with associated developmental delay and even isolated global developmental delay are suspected. An electromyogram can be used to differentiate cerebral palsy from a congenital myopathy.

Management

Caring for children with either a single disability or multiple disabilities can be both a rewarding and challenging task for primary care pediatricians. The pediatrician should be cognizant that the patients will take increased practice time and paperwork to ensure that they receive all services necessary. Case management services are an essential aid to their management. The primary care provider needs to supervise both acute and chronic medical care, provide anticipatory guidance, monitor growth and development, coordinate subspecialty involvement, and offer community services. Sometimes a subspecialist will provide comprehensive care. Although all cases should be handled individually, general guidelines have been developed for the provision of pediatric services for infants and children with SHCN. They include recommendations for establishing a medical home with the primary care provider, medical services, suggestions for parental involvement, assistance from community agencies, and fulfillment of specific federal requirements for educational opportunities for children with disabilities. Pediatricians who care for children with SHCN should be familiar with the principles of care, published by the American Academy of Pediatrics (AAP), and should incorporate these principles into the overall treatment plan. Pediatricians should also be knowledgeable about the rights of such individuals as established by various legislation, including the Americans with Disabilities Act. Coordination of intervention services and the use of adaptive or assistive technology are essential components of management.

General Considerations

The major role of primary care pediatricians who care for children with disabilities is 4-fold: (1) provide primary medical care, (2) serve as the patient and family advocate in evaluating therapeutic options, (3) inform families of available community resources and, most importantly, (4) serve as a proactive coordinator of care. The first task of the pediatrician is to establish the diagnosis and recognize comorbid conditions. Whether the diagnosis is an obvious physical malformation or one that is not readily apparent, physicians are placed in the challenging position of breaking the news to families. Parents should be informed of the diagnosis as soon as possible, but care should be taken to refrain from discussing the prognosis, especially if it is still unknown. The cause of any disability and the possible complications of the condition should be reviewed with the parents. *The primary goal is to help children with disabilities reach their full potential.*

Health care providers are in a unique position to establish a treatment plan with families that includes medical, psychosocial, and educational services. A multidisciplinary team that includes the pediatrician, a member of the school system, a social worker, and a representative of an early intervention program should be identified. Federally funded, nonprofit, regional centers can provide an organized treatment plan and entry into an early intervention program to some children with disabilities. To qualify, children must be diagnosed with an eligible condition, such as cerebral palsy, epilepsy,

autism, or global developmental delay. In addition, infants considered at risk for developing disabilities qualify for assistance (eg, premature infants with bronchopulmonary dysplasia and intraventricular hemorrhage). For children who do not qualify, similar services can be coordinated on an individual basis by the physician's office or the school district.

Children with severe physical and sensory disabilities are often cared for by many medical subspecialists in addition to primary care pediatricians. Referrals to pediatric orthopedic surgeons, plastic surgeons, geneticists, ophthalmologists, otolaryngologists, child neurologists, and psychologists may be necessary. Special comprehensive clinics, such as craniofacial or spina bifida, are established in some children's referral centers to facilitate care of patients, with multiple subspecialists forming a multidisciplinary team in the same clinic setting. In addition, speech and language therapists, occupational therapists, and physical therapists are often an integral part of the medical team. Initial and ongoing therapeutic services provided by each of these individuals must be monitored periodically to assess the progress and overall effectiveness of the treatment plan. Ideally, services should be coordinated so that children as well as parents miss a minimum number of school days and workdays (eg, Saturday and after-school appointments, visits to several providers on 1 day). All information from diagnostic studies and initial evaluations should be shared among each of the health care providers. The AAP has published a Care Coordination Toolkit, which can be very helpful to the primary provider.

The primary care physician should also offer counseling to parents regarding ethical issues as they pertain to the child's condition. These issues include palliative care decisions, decision-making in critical care situations, limiting non-beneficial interventions at the end of life, and advance directives. Because of the pediatrician's relationship with the family, he may be in the best position to engage parents in conversations concerning these topics.

The family has a vital role in caring for the disabled child, and the care can frequently be stressful and emotionally draining. Family support and counseling should be readily available. The sociocultural context of the family and the needs of the other children in the family should to be considered when the care of the child with SHCN is addressed.

With improved medical care and services 90% of children with SHCN reach adulthood. The transition into adult services can be challenging. Preparation for this transition should begin as early as 11 years of age to ensure success. The goal should be independence to the degree that is possible. The individual should be prepared for a work environment if possible and financial independence. The family and child should be evaluated to determine whether the child is capable of independent living, a group home, an institution, or remaining with the family. If necessary, guardianship issues must be addressed. A successful transition to adult health care providers must be ensured, and insurance coverage must be arranged. The Affordable Care Act of 2009 addressed a number of insurance concerns including extending the age of coverage for dependent children until 26 years, preventing exclusion from coverage based on preexisting conditions, and prohibiting lifetime caps on medical expenses.

Economic Concerns

The cost of care for children with disabilities places a significant financial burden for as many as 40% of these families in the United States. Families with an affected child are more likely to have a single income, have a single parent, live in poverty, and have poor-quality housing. Economic evaluation should be performed by the caseworker to determine the eligibility of children with SHCN for financial support through Supplemental Security Income and medical insurance under Medicaid. The caseworker can then assist families to apply for the appropriate assistance or to other programs such as food stamps and the Low Income Home Energy Assistance Program, which can help extend a family's resources.

It is apparent that children with SHCN from low income families have decreased access to health, educational, and social services. Recent studies have been undertaken to determine the best strategy to improve access to services and availability of services for underserved communities.

Specific Medical Conditions

A number of medical conditions commonly occur in children with moderate to severe disabilities. While providing children with comprehensive well-child care, general pediatricians can also address and treat these conditions.

Problems with adequate nutrition, which usually result from insufficient caloric intake, are manifested by growth failure. Depending on the degree of disability and amount of oropharyngeal dysfunction, the placement of a nasogastric or gastrostomy tube may be necessary. Caloric needs may be 10% to 50% higher than normal basal needs to ensure growth.

Respiratory illness is not uncommon among these children. Close observation and conservative treatment of viral illnesses are often necessary. Aspiration pneumonia is likely to occur, especially in children with severe developmental delay because of poor handling of oral secretions or severe oral dyspraxia. To help minimize respiratory infections, influenza vaccine should also be administered during the winter months.

Maintaining good oral hygiene is another challenge because some children with disabilities do not clear oral secretions well and retain food in their mouths, predisposing to cavity development. In addition, many children are treated with anticonvulsants and antibiotics that can cause gingival and enamel dysplasias. Abnormal oromotor coordination, tone, and posturing also contribute to the development of oropharyngeal deformities, such as high-arched palate and overcrowded teeth. As with other children, fluoride supplementation and consistent preventive dental care are recommended.

Bowel and bladder continence is important to attain for several reasons. It allows children to function in a socially acceptable fashion; provides independence; and prevents the development of complications such as recurrent urinary tract infections, diaper dermatitis, and decubitus pressure sores. Behavior modification techniques coupled with positive reinforcement are associated with complete or partial success for bowel training.

Community Resources

Optimal care for children with developmental disabilities depends on maximum use of community agencies and resources. An assessment of parental and patient needs should first be performed and prioritized. The appropriate resources should then be identified for individual children. Early intervention services should be used. Primary care physicians may need to help determine the appropriateness of specific services for patients and families. Emphasis should be placed on integrating each child into support services. Parent-to-parent support and support groups can be very helpful in relieving stress, helping parents to understand the disability, and avoiding feelings of isolation. Support groups for siblings as well as parents are available. Respite care to give parents a break from caregiving and in-home health service programs should also be investigated. Hospice care in the home is now available for children near the end of life. It can be an excellent support for the patient and family. Physicians should act as liaisons between all agencies. Case conferences are occasionally necessary to review the progress of individual children with each member of the health care team.

Education

By federal law, every child with a disability is entitled to an education. Every effort should be made to enroll children with disabilities in conventional schools and to provide opportunities for socialization at an early age. The concept of structured independence and mainstreaming, the placement of disabled children in classes with nondisabled children, can be a very productive setting for the child as well as their schoolmates.

Mainstreaming may not be available in some areas, and the severity of some disabilities may not allow attendance on a regular school campus. Then several other educational possibilities can be considered, and each case should be evaluated on an individual basis. Options include special education classes in designated schools (full- or part-time), special education classes in regular schools (full- or part-time), part-time special education classes and part-time regular classes, or home education. The decision can be facilitated through the development of an Individualized Education Plan by a multidisciplinary team at the school. Parents and primary physicians are encouraged to participate in this evaluation (see Chapter 31).

Prognosis

The prognosis for children with SHCN is dependent on the diagnosis, the severity and extent of any disability, medical and supportive intervention, and the environment of the child. It may be impossible to establish a prognosis at the time of diagnosis. Children can adapt differently to the same disability. It is important to establish realistic goals to determine the best intervention. Most affected children are able to lead productive, independent lives when they receive adequate early intervention and education.

CASE RESOLUTION

Although the girl's medical condition of low lumbar spina bifida seems stable, the physician should inquire about any ongoing problems or concerns. A complete examination should be done. Routine screening laboratory tests and immunizations required for school entry should be performed. The family should be evaluated for financial stability and support services. The mother should be placed on folate supplementation for prevention of recurrence in future children. The patient should be referred to the local spina bifida clinic for comprehensive specialist care by orthopedics, urology, and physical therapy. Integration into the regular classroom should be recommended. The school should be contacted to arrange for adaptive physical education and for intermittent catheterization by school nursing personnel. A follow-up visit is scheduled with the primary care physician in 2 months to review the child's integration into services.

Selected References

American Academy of Pediatrics Council on Children With Disabilities. Care coordination in the medical home: integrating health and related systems of care for children with special health care needs. *Pediatrics.* 2005;116:1238–1244

American Academy of Pediatrics Council on Children With Disabilities. Supplemental Security Income (SSI) for children and youth with disabilities. *Pediatrics.* 2009;124:1702–1708

American Academy of Pediatrics, American Academy of Family Physicians, American College of Physicians-American Society of Internal Medicine. A consensus statement on health care transitions for young adults with special health care needs. *Pediatrics.* 2002;110:1304–1306

Anderson D, Dumont S, Jacobs P, Azzaria L. The personal costs of caring for a child with a disability: a review of the literature. *Public Health Rep.* 2007;122:3–16

Burdo-Hartman WA, Patel DR. Medical home and transition planning for children and youth with special health care needs. *Pediatr Clin North Am.* 2008;55:1287–1297

Cooley W; American Academy of Pediatrics Committee on Children With Disabilities. Providing a primary care medical home for children and youth with cerebral palsy. *Pediatrics.* 2004;114:1106–1113

Davies S, Hall D. "Contact a Family": professionals and parents in partnership. *Arch Dis Child.* 2005;90:1053–1057

Dias MS. Neurosurgical management of myelomeningocele (spina bifida). *Pediatr Rev.* 2005;26:50–60

Kogan MD, Stickland BB, Newacheck PW. Building systems of care for children with special health care needs: findings from the 2005–2006 national survey of children with special health care needs. *Pediatrics.* 2009;124(suppl):S333–S449

Kuo DZ, Turchi RM. Best practices: kids with special health care needs. *Contemp Pediatr.* 2010;27:36–49

Liptak GS, Accerdo P. Health and social outcomes of children with cerebral palsy. *J Pediatr.* 2004;145:S36–S41

McPherson M, Arango P, Fox H, et al. A new definition of children with special health care needs. *Pediatrics.* 1998;102:137–140

Michaud JL; American Academy of Pediatrics Committee on Children With Disabilities. Prescribing therapy services for children with motor disabilities. *Pediatrics.* 2004;113:1836–1838

Okun A. Children who have special health-care needs: ethical issues. *Pediatr Rev.* 2010;31:514–517

Palfry JS, Foley SM, Huntington NL, eds. Children and youth with disabilities and special health care needs from traditionally underserved communities. *Pediatrics.* 2010;126(suppl 3):S107–S196

CHAPTER 40

Reproductive Health[1]

Monica Sifuentes, MD

CASE STUDY

An 18-year-old female college student in good health comes in for a routine health maintenance visit during her spring break. She is unaccompanied by her parents and has no complaints, stating that she just needs a checkup. She enjoys college, passed all of her fall and winter classes, and has some new friends. She denies tobacco use but says most of her friends smoke. She occasionally drinks alcohol and has tried marijuana once. Although she is not sexually active, she is interested in discussing oral contraception. Her last menstrual period, which occurred 2 weeks ago, was normal. She is taking no medications. Her physical examination is entirely normal.

Questions

1. What issues are important to discuss with adolescents at reproductive health maintenance visits?
2. What are the indications for a complete pelvic examination?
3. When is a Pap smear indicated as a part of the reproductive health visit?
4. What methods of contraception are most successful in adolescent patients? What factors regarding each method should be considered?
5. What are the legal issues involved in prescribing contraception to minors in the absence of parental consent?

Adolescent visits to primary care physicians are relatively infrequent by the time teenagers reach puberty. At most, healthy adolescent patients are seen once or twice during high school for preparticipation sports or camp physicals. If adolescents are not involved in athletics or if their schools do not require periodic assessments, these teenagers will probably never visit their health care providers again while in high school. Therefore, it is extremely important to use any interaction with an adolescent as a unique opportunity for anticipatory guidance and health education, particularly reproductive health education.

Reproductive health can be defined as sexuality-related services, screening, and counseling. Such services should be included as a part of the routine health maintenance examination for both male and female adolescents for several reasons. The high incidence of sexually transmitted infections (STIs) in this age group, the risk of acquiring HIV, and the reality of an unplanned pregnancy make reproductive health issues increasingly important for teenagers. In addition, adolescents rarely schedule appointments with health care providers prior to the initiation of coitus. Experimentation with drugs and alcohol at this time in their lives also contributes to early, unplanned sexual experiences (Box 40-1).

Aside from issues of sexual activity, adolescents also may have questions about their progression through puberty. Normal variants in body habitus or certain physical characteristics can be a source of unnecessary anxiety for uninformed teenagers. Health education to alleviate these fears is ideal. Adolescents who come for physical examinations should be allotted extra time so that topics such as puberty, abstinence, sexual activity, STIs, and contraception can be discussed. In addition, during more acute, problem-oriented visits, adolescents should be encouraged to voice any other concerns they may have. Depending on the nature of these issues, follow-up appointments can be scheduled.

Normal Secondary Sexual Development

Puberty begins during early adolescence with the development of secondary sexual characteristics. Because there can be tremendous variation with regard to the age, duration between pubertal stages, and somatic growth of adolescents, a sexual maturity rating (SMR) scale (Tanner staging) is used to describe breast and pubic hair development in females and genital development and pubic hair growth in males (Figures 40-1, 40-2, and 40-3). The average age of menarche in the United States is 12.5 years and for most females occurs during SMR 3 and 4. In contrast, spermarche occurs early in pubertal development in boys, at approximately 13 years of age, with little to no pubic hair development. Full fertility is generally achieved by age 15 years, or mid-adolescence, in most boys and girls.

---

[1] This chapter is largely devoted to a discussion of the reproductive health of adolescent females. However, Evaluation is divided into 2 sections—one for females and one for males. The reader is referred to Chapter 97 for more information regarding male reproductive health.

Box 40-1. Reproductive Health: Sexual Activity

Statistics regarding sexual activity among adolescents in the United States have changed over the last decade. Previously it was reported that 1 in 4 females and 1 in 3 males had had sexual intercourse by 15 years of age. Currently only 13% of teens have ever had vaginal intercourse by age 15 according to the Guttmacher Institute. Most adolescents are now waiting until later to initiate sexual activity; by their 19th birthday, 7 in 10 teens of both sexes have had sexual intercourse. Contraceptive use at first premarital sexual encounter has increased to almost 80% in adolescent females and 87% in adolescent males; however, unintended pregnancy and sexually transmitted infections (STIs) continue to be a major public health concern for this age group. While the pregnancy rate among teenagers has dropped steadily over the past 10 years, each year almost 850,000 adolescent females younger than 20 years become pregnant. Most of these pregnancies are unintended and occur premaritally, especially among certain racial and ethnic minority groups. The outcome of these pregnancies in 15- to 19-year-olds varies. An estimated 50% to 60% of these pregnancies result in live births, 30% end in abortion, and 10% to 15% are miscarried or stillborn.

Unprotected sexual activity among adolescents has several adverse health consequences, the most obvious being teenage pregnancy. Of the adolescents who continue their pregnancies, prematurity (<37 weeks' gestation) and low birth weight (<2,500 g) are 2 of the most frequently reported neonatal complications. Long-term maternal psychosocial sequelae of adolescent pregnancy include undereducation/school failure, limited vocational training and skills, economic dependency on public assistance, subsequent unwanted births, social isolation, depression, and high rates of separation and divorce among teenaged couples.

In addition to unintended pregnancy, the risk of contracting an STI, such as chlamydia, human papillomavirus, herpes, and HIV, is increased. In cases of pelvic inflammatory disease from gonorrhea or chlamydia, future problems with fertility and an increased risk of ectopic pregnancy can occur. Human papillomavirus, which is associated with the development of genital warts, cervical dysplasia, and cancer, accounts for about half of STIs diagnosed in adolescents and young adults. The prevalence rates of other STIs, such as chlamydia and gonorrhea, are still highest among 15- to 19-year-old females compared with older age groups in the United States. More alarming, however, is the relationship between AIDs in young adults aged 20 to 29 and probable exposure to HIV during adolescence.

Many factors have been associated with the initiation of early coitus in adolescents. They include male gender; race/ethnicity; poverty; a large, single-parent family; previous teen pregnancy in the household (either mother or sibling); poor academic achievement; discrepancy between the onset of physical puberty and cognitive development; peer group encouragement; and problem behaviors such as drug use. In addition, religious affiliation and cultural norms probably influence this decision. The role of hormonal changes during puberty and their influence on behavior is yet to be determined.

An estimated 10% to 20% of adolescents have limited typical functioning because of a disability or chronic illness by the age of 20 years. However, most of these adolescents experience normal pubertal development and fertility because of advances in medical treatment for conditions such as diabetes and sickle cell disease. Like their healthy peers, many of these adolescents begin sexual intercourse at an early age. Pregnancy and childbirth can exacerbate some illnesses and increase risks significantly for both adolescents and fetuses. The genetic implications and specific patterns of inheritance of certain chronic conditions must also be considered. For this reason, attention to sexual issues is essential for adolescents with chronic medical illness.

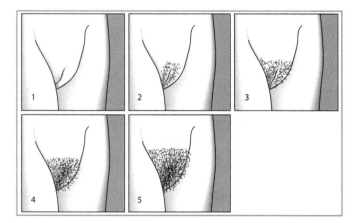

Figure 40-1. Female pubic hair development. Sexual maturity rating 1: prepubertal, no pubic hair. Sexual maturity rating 2: straight hair is extending along the labia and between ratings 2 and 3, begins on the symphysis pubis. Sexual maturity rating 3: pubic hair is increased in quantity; is darker, coarser, and curlier; and is present in the typical female triangle. Sexual maturity rating 4: pubic hair is more dense, curled, and adult in distribution but is less abundant. Sexual maturity rating 5: abundant, adult-type pattern; hair may extend on the medial aspect of the thighs.

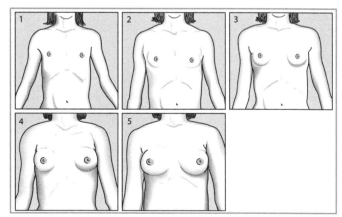

Figure 40-2. Female breast development. Sexual maturity rating 1: prepubertal, elevations of papilla only. Sexual maturity rating 2: breast buds appear, areola is slightly widened and projects as small mound. Sexual maturity rating 3: enlargement of the entire breast with no protrusion of the papilla or of the nipple. Sexual maturity rating 4: enlargement of the breast and projection of areola and papilla as a secondary mound. Sexual maturity rating 5: adult configuration of the breast with protrusion of the nipple, areola no longer projects separately from remainder of breast.

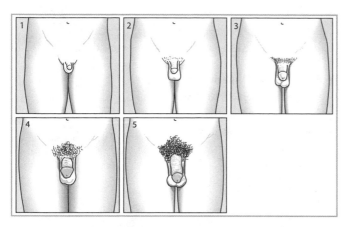

Figure 40-3. Male genital and pubic hair development. Sexual maturity rating 1: prepubertal, no pubic hair, genitalia unchanged from early childhood. Sexual maturity rating 2: light, downy hair develops laterally and later becomes dark, penis and testes may be slightly larger, scrotum becomes more textured. Sexual maturity rating 3: pubic hair is extended across pubis, testes and scrotum are further enlarged; penis is larger, especially in length. Sexual maturity rating 4: more abundant pubic hair with curling, genitalia resemble those of an adult, glans has become darker. Sexual maturity rating 5: adult quantity and pattern of pubic hair, with hair present along the inner borders of the thighs. The testes and scrotum are adult in size.

Evaluation

History

The history obtained at a reproductive health visit should include 2 parts: the medical history, which focuses primarily on the gynecologic history in females, and the psychosocial interview. Regardless of the type of visit scheduled, practitioners should take a few moments at the beginning of the interview to address routine health maintenance issues with the adolescent (Questions Box: Reproductive Health). The provider should find out whether the female adolescent has ever had a genital or pelvic examination. In addition, current methods of contraceptive use, if any, should be reviewed (Questions Box: Contraceptive Use). If the adolescent female takes oral contraceptives, a review of the more emergent complications of birth control pills is warranted, especially at an initial visit. **ACHES** (*a*bdominal pain, *c*hest pain, *h*eadaches, *e*ye problems, *s*evere leg pain) is a useful acronym to remember life-threatening reactions that can be associated with hormonal contraceptive use (Box 40-2), although they occur uncommonly in otherwise healthy adolescent girls.

The rest of the psychosocial history, otherwise known as the **HEADDSSS** interview (*h*ome environment, *e*mployment and education, *a*ctivities, *d*iet, *d*rugs, *s*exual activity/sexuality, *s*uicide/depression, *s*afety), should be completed whether or not the adolescent is currently sexually active (see Chapter 6). Risk factors for an unplanned pregnancy or unintentional exposures to STIs should be kept in mind when formulating health care plans with the teenager.

Questions

Reproductive Health

For males and females

- How is the adolescent feeling overall?
- Has the adolescent had any recent illnesses or conditions that the health care provider should know about?
- When was the last physical examination performed? Did it include a genital or pelvic examination?
- Is the adolescent sexually active?
  — If so, when was the last episode of vaginal intercourse?
  — Was the last episode of sexual intercourse protected or unprotected?
  — Does the adolescent have anal or oral sex?
  — How old was the adolescent when he or she initiated coitus? Was it consensual?
  — How many sexual partners does the patient have currently? How many sexual partners have they had in their lifetime? What gender are they (all contacts may not be heterosexual)?
- Is there any history of physical or sexual abuse?
- Has the adolescent or any of his or her partners ever been treated for a sexually transmitted infection or tested for HIV?

For females only
- What was the age at menarche?
- What was the date of the last menstrual period and the duration and amount of flow?
  — Are any symptoms such as cramping, bloating, or vomiting associated with menses?
  — Are any of these symptoms incapacitating? Do they cause the adolescent to miss school or work?
  — Does the mother or siblings have similar problems? If so, how do they manage them, if at all?

Questions

Contraceptive Use

- Does the adolescent use condoms: never, sometimes, or always?
- Is any other method, such as spermicidal foam or jelly, also used?
- Is the adolescent female currently using oral contraceptives?
  — If so, what particular type is she taking, and how long has she been using this method of contraception?
  — How often does she forget to take the pill? or What does she do when she forgets to take the pill?
  — Does she experience common minor side effects such as breakthrough bleeding or nausea?
- Is the adolescent female using a long-acting progestin, such as Depo-Provera? If so, has she experienced irregular bleeding, weight gain, hair loss, headache, or acne?
- Is there another method of contraception that the adolescent has used or might be interested in discussing and/or starting?
- What does the adolescent know about emergency contraception?

Box 40-2. Danger Signs Associated With Oral Contraceptive Use	
A	Abdominal pain (severe)
C	Chest pain (severe), shortness of breath
H	Headaches
E	Eye problems (visual loss or blur)
S	Severe leg pain (calf/thigh)

Physical Examination

A complete physical examination should be performed on all adolescents, with particular attention paid to their SMR. Chaperones are strongly encouraged, with the permission of the patient, even when the patient and examiner are the same gender, particularly during the breast and genital examination.

Males

The genitalia should be examined closely for penile and testicular size; distribution of pubic hair; and presence of any ulcerative, vesicular, or wart-like lesions. Any urethral erythema or discharge should be noted. Testicular masses require further evaluation. Ideally, clinicians should use this opportunity to teach male adolescents how to perform a testicular self-examination.

Females

Prior to performing the physical examination, the physician should determine whether a full-speculum examination is indicated (Box 40-3). This decision should be based on the details of the individual case and not solely on the basis of sexual activity. With the advent of noninvasive screening methods for STIs, a routine pelvic examination is often unnecessary. Most experts now recommend the use of urine-based nucleic-acid amplification tests (NAATs) to screen for gonorrhea or chlamydia instead of endocervical swabs. However, if a speculum examination is indicated, proper preparation of the adolescent is imperative. This should include an explanation of the procedure and the physical sensations felt while the endocervical specimen is being obtained. The choice of who should be present during the examination (eg, parent or friend who may have accompanied the patient), and a discussion of the desired positioning (ie, supine vs semisitting) are also important points to review. In addition, the speculum, specimen swabs, and other equipment should be shown to the adolescent before she is draped. The goal is to minimize the adolescent's fears, anxieties, misconceptions, and discomfort regarding the examination.

A breast examination should be performed on female adolescents, and any breast tenderness, nodularity, or masses should be noted. Again, this portion of the examination can be used to educate patients about the purpose and importance of breast self-examinations and to document breast SMR.

The external genitalia should be examined in all adolescent females whether or not they are sexually active. The SMR and any congenital anomalies, such as an imperforate hymen, should be identified. In sexually active adolescents, the external genitalia should be carefully examined for warts, ulcers, and vesicular lesions. Any urethral erythema, edema, or discharge that may indicate an otherwise asymptomatic chlamydial infection should be noted. If a pelvic examination is indicated, a vaginal discharge may be appreciated prior to inserting the speculum but, ideally, the cervix should be examined for cervical ectopy, friability, and any lesions or discharge from the os. The vaginal mucosa should also be inspected as the speculum is withdrawn.

During the bimanual examination, the cervix should be palpated for any cervical motion tenderness. Uterine size and position should be appreciated, and adnexal tenderness or masses should be noted. Because normal ovaries are approximately the size of almonds, they are often not palpated by many clinicians. A rectovaginal examination is necessary to rule out fistulas, especially in postpartum adolescents. If the practitioner is unable to perform a vaginal bimanual examination, a rectoabdominal examination can be done to assess uterine size and position and the presence of adnexal masses.

Laboratory Tests

Because most *Chlamydia trachomatis* and *Neisseria gonorrhoeae* infections in adolescents are asymptomatic, screening noninvasive urine-based NAATs should be sent annually in all sexually active adolescents, and more frequently in those who have a history of unprotected intercourse and/or a new sexual partner. If the adolescent has vaginal discharge or cervical friability noted on speculum examination, the specimen should be obtained directly from the cervix and sent for NAAT. A saline and KOH wet mount should also be collected in symptomatic patients. A Pap smear should be performed in sexually active females who are 21 years of age. The Pap smear can also help detect *Trichomonas vaginalis* or the cytological changes associated with human papillomavirus (HPV). A NAAT (eg, polymerase chain reaction) for herpes simplex virus (HSV) should be performed if painful vesicles are noted on examination.

Other laboratory tests include a rapid plasma reagin test for syphilis and an HIV screening test (after appropriate pretest counseling). Baseline complete blood cell count, liver function tests, cholesterol, and fasting glucose may be indicated as part of the health maintenance visit but are not required before starting contraception. A pregnancy test is warranted in sexually active females if the practitioner chooses to begin oral contraceptives or another method of hormonal contraception mid-cycle.

Box 40-3. Indications for a Complete Pelvic Examination
• Pregnancy
• Request by the adolescent
• Unexplained lower abdominal pain
• Persistent abnormal vaginal discharge
• Unexplained vaginal bleeding
• Dysmenorrhea, unresponsive to nonsteroidal anti-inflammatory medications
• Suspected or reported sexual assault
• Perform a Pap test

Management

Reproductive Health Education

All management plans during reproductive health visits should include a frank **discussion of puberty, sexuality, and STIs** regardless of current sexual activity. The adolescent should be counseled about abstinence as an acceptable choice. Ideally, preventive health care measures such as **breast and testicular self-examinations** have been reviewed during the physical examination. It is hoped that by encouraging adolescents' familiarity with these self-examinations, they will continue to perform them throughout their adult lives. The use of posters, plastic models, and electronic or written materials to support the discussion is greatly encouraged. The goal of education should be to assist adolescents in identifying and communicating their thoughts and feelings about sexual abstinence as well as sexual activity and to aid in the prevention of unintended pregnancy, parenthood, and STIs. Prevention programs offered by schools must be supplemented by open parental communication in the home about sexuality.

Legal Issues

The issue of **confidentiality** is important to consider when providing reproductive health care for adolescents. Parental involvement should be strongly encouraged, but health care practitioners are not required to disclose any information to parents except in cases of suicidal ideation, harmful intent to others, and sexual or physical abuse. In most states, contraceptive services can be provided to adolescents of any age without specific parental knowledge or consent. The complex issue of parental consent and pregnancy termination varies from state to state and should be reviewed by the individual health care provider. Of note, all 50 states including the District of Columbia explicitly allow minors to consent for their own health services for STIs and do not require parental consent for STI care. Providing confidential care for adolescents enrolled in private health insurance plans, however, continues to be a difficult issue because many states mandate that health plans provide a written statement to the beneficiary regarding the services covered and received, including clinical services provided confidentially to teens.

Pap Smear

The 2009 recommendation of the American College of Obstetricians and Gynecologists (ACOG) is that cervical cancer screening should begin at 21 years of age in young women. However, the American Cancer Society continues to recommend that young women start cervical screening with Pap tests 3 years after the onset of vaginal intercourse, and no later than age 21 years. After the initiation of screening, a Pap smear for average-risk women aged 21 through 29 years should be performed every 2 years, and every 3 years for women 30 years and older with 3 consecutive normal cervical cytology test results. The rationale for the most recent changes in cervical cancer screening by ACOG is that there seems to be little risk in not treating abnormal cervical cytology in adolescents since 90% to 95%

of low-grade lesions, as well as many high-grade lesions, in this age group regress to normal without treatment. Screening prematurely can lead to an overdiagnosis of cervical dysplasia and an overtreatment of lesions with potentially harmful procedures such as excision or ablation of the cervix. Since the incidence of cervical cancer is very low among adolescents, the benefits of Pap screening are offset by the potential harm of unnecessary treatments in this age group.

Contraceptive Methods

The appropriate method of contraception should be individualized. Barrier methods include condoms (male and female), diaphragms, and cervical caps. Vaginal spermicides such as nonoxynol 9 are available in a variety of forms (foams, gels, films, and suppositories) and should be used with a barrier method since there are general concerns that these products in high doses can increase the risk of genital ulceration and irritation, thereby facilitating STI acquisition. Hormonal contraceptive methods include oral contraceptives, long-acting progestin agents, transdermal methods, and the intravaginal ring. Although previously not recommended for teens, a levonorgestrel intrauterine device may be indicated in postpartum teenagers as well as for the treatment of severe dysfunctional uterine bleeding. The withdrawal method, or coitus interruptus, and natural family planning are ineffective methods for adolescents for protection against pregnancy.

Hormonal Contraception

Combined low-dose oral contraceptives are an effective means of birth control for adolescents, with most pills containing 20 µg to 35 µg of ethinyl estradiol (estrogen) and a progestin. Monophasic pills contain a fixed dose of estrogen and progestin throughout the 21-day pill cycle. Biphasic preparations contain a lower dose of the progestin component during the first 10 days of the cycle, but are rarely used in teens. In triphasic pills, the doses of both estrogen and progestin or the progestin component alone are varied 3 times throughout the cycle. This contraceptive was created to decrease the overall progestin-related side effects, such as hypertension, acne, and lipid abnormalities. Most recently, lower-dose estrogen (20 µg) pills have been developed to minimize estrogen-related side effects and decrease discontinuation rates. Although 20 µg estrogen pills are now considered the "first-line" therapy for most teens, their lower efficacy must be taken into account in patients concurrently receiving medications that increase the metabolism of synthetic steroids, such as anticonvulsants. Other combined oral contraceptive regimens include 3-month continuous hormonal therapy followed by 1 week of withdrawal bleeding for young women who prefer to menstruate only 4 times a year (an extended-cycle pill). To lessen the frequency of breakthrough bleeding often experienced by users of the extended-cycle pill, another product is now available that replaced the placebo pills with 7 days of low-dose estrogen. Progestin-only pills, referred to as the "minipill," also are available and particularly useful in postpartum and lactating teen mothers. Clear benefits associated with oral contraceptive use include prevention of pregnancy, protection against ovarian and endometrial cancers, decreased risk of functional ovarian cysts, and decreased menstrual symptoms, such as dysmenorrhea. The potential risks, which include thromboembolic phenomena, hypertension, and changes in the lipid profile, are minimal in most healthy adolescents compared with the morbidity and mortality associated with teenage pregnancy and childbirth.

The long-acting progestin depot medroxyprogesterone acetate (DMPA) (Depo-Provera) is given intramuscularly every 11 to 13 weeks to inhibit ovulation; a subcutaneous formulation is also available and should be repeated every 12 to 14 weeks. The most common side effect is irregular menstrual bleeding, especially in the first few months, and eventual amenorrhea with prolonged use. Weight gain remains a significant issue for some patients and clinicians, particularly in obese adolescents where exaggerated increases in weight can be seen. Breast tenderness and mood disturbances also can occur, but less frequently. In 2004 the US Food and Drug Administration (FDA) issued a black box warning for DMPA regarding possible irreversible bone loss in women with long-term use of DMPA and a potential reduction in overall bone mineral density (BMD) in teenagers that may contribute to the development of osteoporosis later in life. The FDA therefore recommends that DMPA should not be used in adolescents for longer than 2 years; however, many experts believe that the risk for pregnancy using an inferior method of birth control far outweighs the risk for the development of osteoporosis in a healthy teenager. Ongoing studies suggest that although adolescents may not increase their BMD while receiving DMPA and do experience bone loss, the effects appear to be temporary and reversible with the discontinuation of DMPA.

A subdermal implant (Implanon) received approval by the FDA in 2006 and is available for young women. It is designed to deliver a low, steady dose of continuous progestin for 3 years via a single plastic polymer rod placed below the skin. Formal instruction for insertion and removal is required for the health care professional interested in providing this form of contraception. The subdermal implant is highly effective but, as with other long-acting progestin-only contraceptives, it is associated with bleeding abnormalities, especially during the first year of use.

Other combined hormonal contraceptive methods for the adolescent include the vaginal ring (NuvaRing) and the transdermal patch (Ortho Evra). Approved in 2001, the vaginal contraceptive ring is a soft, flexible device that contains both estrogen and progestin, which is released directly into the vaginal wall. The ring is inserted into the vagina for 3 weeks, and then removed for 1 week to allow for a withdrawal bleed. Systemic side effects are similar to other low-dose combined hormonal methods (headache, breast tenderness, nausea, breakthrough bleeding/spotting); specific local effects include vaginal discharge and discomfort.

The transdermal adhesive patch is a thin, beige, 3-layered plastic patch that contains both estrogen and progestin and is applied weekly to specific areas of the body (lower abdomen, upper torso, upper arm, or buttocks) followed by 1 week off. Although well tolerated, high detachment rates in teens have been documented. In addition, adolescents may have concerns regarding the visibility of the patch. Side effects are similar to other combined hormonal methods of contraception; local effects include skin irritation and rash at the site of application. Recent concerns have been cited by the FDA regarding the risk of venous thromboembolic events associated with the patch, although conflicting data have been reported. The reader is referred to the article by Trenor et al in Selected References for a comprehensive review of this topic.

Emergency Postcoital Contraception

Emergency contraception (EC), or the "morning-after pill," is an effective way to prevent unintended pregnancy in adolescents. It requires, however, that the physician educate teens about its availability and usage and that teens feel comfortable contacting their health care provider within 72 to 120 hours of unprotected or inadequately protected intercourse. Although not meant to be used repeatedly as the sole method of contraception, EC is useful for the "unplanned" sexual encounter, which is often the case with adolescents. The morning-after pill contains a high dose of hormone that is thought to inhibit ovulation, disrupt follicular development, and/or interfere with the maturation of the corpus luteum. Emergency contraception does not interrupt or disrupt an already-established pregnancy and is not an abortifacient.

The original regimen was a combination of high-dose estrogen and progestin, known as the Yuzpe method; however, nausea and vomiting occurred in about 25% to 30% of patients. Plan B is the progestin-only method of EC that is currently available by prescription for adolescents younger than 17 years. It consists of 2 doses of 0.75 mg of levonorgestrel, which should be taken 12 hours apart within 3 days of unprotected intercourse. Based on data reported by the World Health Organization, this regimen has been modified to *take both pills at once up to 5 days after unprotected or inadequately protected intercourse.* Plan B is most highly effective when used within the first 24 hours after unprotected coitus. Although less common than with the Yuzpe method, side effects of Plan B include nausea, vomiting, breast tenderness, and irregular bleeding patterns such as spotting; shortened interval to menses; and lighter or heavier menses. Because EC is both safe and highly effective in preventing pregnancy, physicians should consider providing the sexually active teen with a prescription or advance supply of Plan B at the health maintenance visit.

The patient should be given a follow-up office or clinic appointment 2 to 3 weeks after using EC so that a pregnancy test can be performed, treatment failures can be identified early, STI screening can occur, and issues of contraception can be discussed.

Nonhormonal Contraception

Numerous studies and clinical experience have shown that nonhormonal methods are less effective in adolescents. However, latex condoms in conjunction with a spermicide have become crucial as a method of contraception since the emergence of AIDS. Although they help prevent transmission of some STIs, such as gonorrhea, chlamydia, trichomonas, and HIV, condoms do not protect against HPV and HSV infection overall because the genital area is not completely covered. A few moments, therefore, should be taken during the visit to explain these details and demonstrate proper use of condoms. Risks of condom use are minimal, except for allergic reactions to the spermicide, latex, or lubricants. Although available, the female condom is not widely used by adolescents but may be helpful in situations where a male partner refuses to wear a condom. The inner ring is inserted into the vagina up to 8 hours prior to intercourse, and a prescription or physician visit is not necessary to obtain a female condom. Some teenagers, however, may be uncomfortable with its insertion and the fact that the outer ring remains on the vulva during vaginal intercourse. Similar issues are encountered when considering the diaphragm as a contraceptive method for teens; therefore, it is not recommended as a first-line contraceptive method for most adolescents. Other nonhormonal methods should be reviewed with adolescents as they become available.

Sexually Transmitted Infections

All STIs should be treated according to specific guidelines published by the Centers for Disease Control and Prevention based on current epidemiology. See Chapter 97 for details regarding the diagnosis and management of STIs in adolescents.

CASE RESOLUTION

In the case scenario presented at the beginning of the chapter, a more detailed history should be obtained regarding the adolescent's menstrual history and daily activities (eg, With whom does she spend most of her time? What does she like to do in her spare time?). In addition, the indications for a pelvic examination should be reviewed since most teens are not familiar with the new recommendations to delay the Pap smear until 21 years of age. Since the new indications do not apply in this case, the pelvic examination can be deferred. A discussion should then follow regarding both barrier and hormonal methods of contraception and their role in the prevention of pregnancy and STIs. Emergency contraception should also be reviewed with the teen. Written information as well as useful Web site addresses also should be given to the adolescent.

Selected References

American Academy of Pediatrics Committee on Adolescence. Condom use by adolescents. *Pediatrics*. 2001;107:1463–1469

American Academy of Pediatrics Committee on Adolescence. Contraception and adolescents. *Pediatrics*. 2007;120:1135–1148

American Academy of Pediatrics Committee on Adolescence. Emergency contraception. *Pediatrics*. 2005;116:1026–1035

American College of Obstetrics and Gynecologists. ACOG Committee Opinion No. 415. Depot medroxyprogesterone acetate and bone effects. *Obstet Gynecol*. 2008;112:727–730

Bonny AE, Harkness LS, Cromer DA. Depot medroxyprogesterone acetate: implications for weight status and bone mineral density in the adolescent female. *Adolesc Med*. 2005;16:569–584

Braverman PK, Breech L; American Academy of Pediatrics Committee on Adolescence. Gynecologic examination for adolescents in the pediatric office setting. *Pediatrics*. 2010;126:583–590

Burkett AM, Hewitt GD. Progestin only contraceptives and their use in adolescents: clinical options and medical indications. *Adolesc Med*. 2005;16:553–567

Calderoni ME, Coupey SM. Combined hormonal contraception. *Adolesc Med*. 2005;16:517–537

Cameron CT, Chung RJ, Michelson AD, et al. Hormonal contraception and thrombotic risk: a multidisciplinary approach. *Pediatrics*. 2010;127:347–357

Cavanaugh RM. Screening adolescent gynecology in the pediatrician's office: have a listen, take a look. *Pediatr Rev*. 2007;28:332–342

Centers for Disease Control and Prevention. Summary Chart of US Medical Eligibility Criteria for Contraceptive Use, 2010. http://www.cdc.gov/Reproductivehealth/UnintendedPregnancy/Docs/USMEC-Color-final.doc

Cromer BA, Scholes D, Berenson A, et al. Depot medroxyprogesterone acetate and bone mineral density in adolescents-the black box warning: a position paper of the Society for Adolescent Medicine. *J Adolesc Health*. 2006;39:296–301

Duffy K, Wimberly, Brooks C. Adolescent contraceptive care for the practicing pediatrician. *Adolesc Med*. 2009;20:168–187

Ford C, English A, Sigman G. Confidential healthcare for adolescents: position paper of the Society for Adolescent Medicine. *J Adolesc Health*. 2005;35:160–167

Gold MA, Delisi K. Motivational interviewing and sexual and contraceptive behaviors. *Adolesc Med*. 2008;19:69–82

Greydanus DE, Patel DR, Rimsza ME. Contraception in the adolescent: an update. *Pediatrics*. 2001;107:562–573

Gupta N. Advances in hormonal contraception. *Adolesc Med*. 2006;17:653–671

Gupta N, Corrado S, Goldstein M. Hormonal contraception. *Pediatr Rev*. 2008;29:386–397

Guttmacher Institute. In Brief Fact Sheet: Facts on American Teens' Sexual and Reproductive Health. http://www.guttmacher.org/pubs/FB-ATSRH.html

Guttmacher Institute. State Policies in Brief: An Overview of Minors' Consent Law. http://www.guttmacher.org/statecenter/spibs/spib_OMCL.pdf

Klein JD; American Academy of Pediatrics Committee on Adolescence. Adolescent pregnancy: current trends and issues. *Pediatrics*. 2005;116:281–286

Levine SB. Adolescent consent and confidentiality. *Pediatr Rev*. 2009;30:457–458

Mulchahey KM. Practical approaches to prescribing contraception in the office setting. *Adolesc Med*. 2005;16:665–674

Murphy NA, Elias ER. Sexuality of children and adolescents with developmental disabilities. *Pediatrics*. 2006;118:398–403

Rimsza M. Counseling the adolescent about contraception. *Pediatr Rev*. 2003;24:162–170

Sieving RE, Oliphant JA, Blum RW. Adolescent sexual behavior and sexual health. *Pediatr Rev*. 2002;23:407–416

Trenor CC 3rd, Chung RJ, Michelson AD, et al. Hormonal contraception and thrombotic risk: a multidisciplinary approach. *Pediatrics*. 2011;127(2):347–357

Providing Culturally Competent Care to Diverse Populations: Sexual Orientation and Gender Expression

Lynn Hunt, MD

CASE STUDY

The mother of an 11-year-old boy makes an appointment with you to discuss her son's "behavior problems." He is the youngest of 4 children and is doing well in fifth grade, but she is concerned that her son does not like typical "male" activities. He dropped out of Little League, won't join other sports teams, and prefers riding his bike. In addition he still likes dressing up in costumes and prefers playing with girls rather than boys. She finally mentions that she is worried that he will be gay and is wondering what she can do to help her son develop "normally."

Questions

1. What is meant by gender expression, sexual orientation, and gender identity?
2. What is the role of the pediatrician in counseling parents and patients about gender expression, sexual orientation, and gender identity?
3. What are some of the consequences of discrimination of sexual minority populations?
4. Are there programs that can change sexual orientation?

Every pediatrician and health professional needs a basic understanding of lesbian, gay, bisexual, transgender, and questioning (LGBTQ) populations. Each of us has contact with sexual minority individuals. They are among our teen patients and parents of our patients. Every day we encounter family members of someone who is LGBTQ—whether we are aware of it or not. Furthermore, the Joint Commission on Accreditation of Healthcare Organizations and the American Association of Medical Colleges, among other organizations, call for nondiscrimination and proactive cultural competence as markers of quality, appropriate patient care, and key content for professional education.

Incidence

The US census and other large-scale surveys indicate that approximately 5% of the adult population identifies as LGBTQ or reports same-sex relationships. The prevalence of sexual minority persons is impressively consistent across all ethnic and socioeconomic groups.

The number of adolescents who identify as LGBTQ tends to increase with age. However, in one survey, over twice as many youth reported same-sex sexual experiences as those who eventually identify as gay. These data reinforce the important distinction between sexual orientation and sexual behavior. There is a wide range of sexual behavior in teens, and sexual identity formation is a dynamic developmental process. Teens who eventually identify as gay may have had heterosexual sexual contact and those who identify as straight may have had same-sex partners.

LGBTQ Youth

Despite an increase in public dialogue and a perceptible boost to societal acceptance in recent years, LGBTQ youth continue to suffer stigmatization and its consequences. All too often LGBTQ youth are the objects of bullying, isolation, and family rejection. Additionally, sexual minorities are by far the group most targeted for violent hate crimes in America. According to the Southern Poverty Law Center, gay people are twice as likely to be attacked as Jews or blacks, 4 times as likely as Muslims, and 14 times as likely as Latinos.

Health Consequences of Discrimination

There are data documenting increased suicide attempts, substance use, and risky sexual behavior among LGBTQ youth overall. While it is helpful with all teens to identify those at increased risk, understanding key mediators of risk is also crucial. Youth who have been victimized or who perceive discrimination are more vulnerable to engaging in high-risk behaviors.

Families are particularly important. In one study of family support, LGBTQ young adults who experienced higher levels of family rejection during adolescence were 8 times more likely to report suicide attempts, 6 times more likely to report significant depression, and 3 times more likely to use illegal drugs or report unprotected sexual intercourse compared with those that did not experience family rejection. Conversely, families that are highly supportive are more likely to have children who are resilient and well adjusted. Family acceptance during adolescence is associated with better general health, self-esteem, and social support in LGBTQ young adults.

LGBTQ youth are also significantly overrepresented among homeless youth. Studies estimate that up to 40% of homeless youth identify as sexual minorities. Youth become homeless usually as a result of family conflict regarding their sexual orientation or gender expression. Sexual minority youth are more likely to suffer negative outcomes associated with living on the streets. Physical assault, sexual victimization, substance abuse, and high-risk sexual behavior are all more common for LGBTQ than heterosexual homeless youth.

Important Role of Pediatricians

Pediatric health care providers have a unique opportunity to model acceptance of each patient (Box 41-1) and to provide appropriate risk-reduction counseling, yet studies have shown that many adolescents are reluctant to share information about their sexuality with their health care provider. They are hesitant for various reasons. LGBTQ adolescents want just the same attributes in their health care providers as studies document for other groups of teens: confidentiality, cleanliness, honesty, respect, competence, and a nonjudgmental approach to history taking and guidance.

"Reparative" or Conversion Therapy

Some religiously and politically motivated groups use outdated and discredited medical theories to justify trying to "cure" the natural sexual orientation or gender identity of those who are lesbian, gay, bisexual, and transgender. Reparative therapy does not work and the process can severely damage self-esteem, leading to depression and self-destructive and suicidal behaviors. In 2001 the US Surgeon General's Call to Action to Promote Sexual Health and Responsible Sexual Behavior asserted that homosexuality is not "a reversible lifestyle choice." Reparative therapy is considered inappropriate and dangerous by several professional organizations, including

- American Academy of Pediatrics (AAP)
- American Medical Association
- American Psychiatric Association
- American Psychological Association (APA)

Box 41-1. Ways for Clinicians to Indicate Support for Lesbian, Gay, Bisexual, Transgender, and Questioning (LGBTQ) Youth

Waiting Room or Exam Room Environment
- Signal a welcoming environment with LGBTQ Safe Zone or rainbow stickers.
- Assess the images and literature available in your office. Much available information for teens assumes that the consumer is heterosexual. Consider including some posters or brochures that are not exclusively heterosexual in character.

Office Forms
- Review standard intake and history forms for assumptions that every patient (or parent) is heterosexual and consider modifying them to be more inclusive. Instead of only "single," "married," and "divorced," consider "partnered" and "other." Instead of "mother's name" or "father's name," consider simply using "parent's name."

Patient Interview
- Stress the importance of privacy and confidentiality. Concerns over possible disclosure of sexual orientation or behavior are often reasons mentioned by LGBTQ youth as a reason to avoid seeking health care.
- Use gender-neutral language. Questions like "Are you dating?" or "Are you currently in a relationship?" are more inclusive than "Do you have a boyfriend/girlfriend?" Other approaches, such as "What types of sexual experiences have you had?" or "Have you been attracted to/had sex with boys, girls, or both?" are useful no matter what the self-identified orientation of the patient may be. Discuss "protection" rather than just "birth control."
- As with any adolescent, a nonjudgmental attitude from the provider will help elicit honest and relevant information.

Physical Exam
- General primary care for LGBTQ youth, including examination and laboratory evaluation, should follow the recommendations for all adolescent health care as outlined by the American Academy of Pediatrics *Bright Futures* health supervision guidelines.

- American Counseling Association
- American Federation of Teachers
- National Association of School Psychologists
- National Association of Secondary School Principals
- National Education Association
- The Interfaith Alliance

Children With LGBTQ Parents

LGBTQ parents are raising millions of children across the United States. According to the 2000 census, 33% of female same-sex couple households and 22% of male same-sex couple households reported at least one child younger than 18 living in their home. Children join families with same-sex parents in a variety of ways: adoption, assisted reproductive technologies, and from previous heterosexual contact as step/blended families. It is surprising to some that the "typical" same-sex parent families are not all upper or middle class. Parents in same-sex couples are more likely to be racial minorities;

their children are more likely to have disabilities and to be adopted. And same-sex parents tend to have lower household incomes than opposite-sex couples.

Child Outcomes

Well-crafted longitudinal and cross-sectional studies indicate that children with same-sex parents do well in domains of social, academic, and total competence. In study after study, children in same-sex parent families turn out remarkably similar to children in heterosexual families. The AAP in a 2002 technical report stated, "A growing body of scientific literature demonstrates that children who grow up with one or two gay and/or lesbian parents fare as well in emotional, cognitive, social, and sexual functioning as do children whose parents are heterosexual." That report was reaffirmed in 2010. A meta-analysis of many of the studies found that the sexual orientation of a parent is irrelevant to the development of a child's mental health and social development and to the quality of a parent–child relationship. In spite of the available data, organized opposition to these families remains the law in many states and several myths persist.

Myth #1: Gays are likely to molest children.
Fact: One of the most common arguments against LGBTQ individuals and adoption is that gays are more likely to molest children. The American Psychological Association finds, however, there is no evidence that gays are more likely to molest children than heterosexuals. In fact, when examining percentages, straight men as a group are the most likely to molest children; however, nobody would seriously suggest preventing heterosexual men from adopting children.

Myth #2: Gays recruit young people—or—Children raised by gays will be gay.
Fact: The truth is that being raised in a gay household does not make a child any more or less likely to become gay. In fact, most studies suggest that sexual orientation is biologically determined in a multifactorial way. The percentage of LGBTQ individuals who were raised in heterosexual families would seem to contradict the central role of environmental exposure in influencing sexual orientation.

Myth #3: Children raised in same-sex families are poorly adjusted.
Fact: According to the AAP, the APA, and the National Association of Social Workers, there is no evidence that the sexual orientation of a child's parents or adoptive parents interferes with the child's social adjustment. Children raised in gay households function just as well cognitively, socially, and emotionally as children of heterosexual parents.

How to Be an Ally

An ally is someone straight (or gay) who acknowledges and supports sexual diversity, acts accordingly to challenge homophobic or transphobic remarks and behaviors, and works to understand these forms of bias within oneself.

Following are some concrete next steps providers can take:

- Register as an ally provider in the Gay and Lesbian Medical Association online Provider Directory (www.glma.org). Joining the directory is a great way to signal your support in health care. This is an easy way to let LGBTQ people in your community who are looking for health care providers to know that you're a supportive ally.
- Visit the Parents and Friends of Lesbians and Gays (PFLAG) Web site (www.pflag.org) and review their program for health providers: Straight for Equality in Healthcare.
- Learn more at any of the resources listed at the end of this chapter.

CASE RESOLUTION

This child is displaying behaviors that do not meet his parent's expectation for male gender expression. The pediatrician should let the mother know that gender expression, sexual orientation, and gender identity are separate and distinct, and that there is a broad range of normal for all of these. There is no way to predict sexual orientation or gender identity from the behaviors described.

Many adolescents go through a period of questioning their sexuality. The child's mother should be informed that whether her son grows up gay, straight, transgender, or typically male, a major risk factor for him engaging in unsafe behaviors as an adolescent would be parental rejection. Programs designed to change a person's sexual orientation don't work and are actually dangerous; they are associated with significant depression and thoughts of suicide. For her son to develop normally, he will need supportive adults in his life who accept and love him, ideally his parents.

It would be important to determine if her son has been a victim of bullying at school or on the sports teams. Schedule an appointment for the son. You will have the opportunity to evaluate the child's strengths and note if he is displaying any signs of anxiety of depression. Questions about sexuality would be those appropriate for all children his age and stage of development. An ongoing dialogue with the mother will also help to know if/when referrals to PFLAG or other support and educational groups are appropriate.

Online Resources

For LGBTQ Youth

It Gets Better
www.itgetsbetter.org
See hundreds of videos of encouragement. The Web site is a place where young people who are LGBTQ can see how love and happiness can be a reality in their future. It's a place where straight allies can visit and support their friends and family members.

The Trevor Project
www.thetrevorproject.org
The Trevor Project is a national organization focused on crisis and suicide prevention efforts among LGBTQ youth. Trained counselors are ready 24/7 at 866/488-7386.

The Gay, Lesbian and Straight Education Network
www.glsen.org
GLSEN strives to ensure that each member of every school community is valued and respected regardless of sexual orientation or gender identity/expression.

The National Runaway Switchboard
www.1800runaway.org
Operates 1-800-RUNAWAY, a confidential and anonymous crisis hotline for runaway and homeless youth available 24 hours a day, 365 days a year.

Go Ask Alice
www.goaskalice.columbia.edu
Sexual health information by and for youth.

For Children with LGBTQ Parents

Children of Lesbians and Gays Everywhere

www.colage.org

COLAGE is a national movement of children, youth, and adults with one or more LGBTQ parents.

For Parents and Others

The Family Acceptance Project

http://familyproject.sfsu.edu

A research-based, culturally grounded approach to help ethnically, socially, and religiously diverse families decrease rejection and increase support for their LGBTQ children.

Parents, Families and Friends of Lesbians and Gays

www.pflag.org

PFLAG promotes the health and well-being of LGBTQ persons, their families, and friends through support, education, and advocacy.

For Professionals

Gay and Lesbian Medical Association

www.glma.org

GLMA's mission is to ensure equality in health care for LGBTQ individuals and health providers. The GLMA site features an online provider directory and educational materials.

Fenway Institute

www.fenwayhealth.com

The Fenway Institute is dedicated to advancing the skills, attitudes, and knowledge of clinicians and other health professionals by providing professional development, educational materials, and resources on LGBTQ health topics. There are several online educational modules for clinicians.

Publications

Books

Dibble SL, Robertson PA. *Lesbian Health 101: A Clinician's Guide.* San Francisco, CA: University of California San Francisco Nursing Press; 2010

Kaiser Permanente National Diversity Council and the Kaiser Permanente National Diversity Department. *A Provider's Handbook on Culturally Competent Care: Lesbian, Gay, Bisexual and Transgendered Population.* San Francisco, CA: Kaiser Permanente; 2000. To order: Kaiser National Diversity Department: 510/271-6663

Makadon HJ, Mayer KH, Potter J, Goldhammer H, eds. *The Fenway Guide to Lesbian, Gay, Bisexual, and Transgender Health.* Philadelphia, PA: American College of Physicians; 2007

Glossary	
Sexual orientation	Permanent emotional, romantic, or sexual feelings toward other people. Straight individuals experience these feelings primarily for people of the opposite sex. Gay or lesbian individuals experience these feelings primarily for people of the same sex. Bisexual individuals can experience these feelings for people regardless of sex.
Gender identity	Knowledge of oneself being male or female.
Gender expression	Outward expression of maleness or femaleness.
Gender nonconforming	A person who either by nature or by choice does not conform to gender-based expectations of society. These children and adolescents are among the most vulnerable to bullying and violence.
Sexual behavior	Refers to the way one chooses to express one's sexual feelings. Sexual behavior does not necessarily correlate with sexual orientation. Heterosexually identified individuals may have same-gender sexual experiences and homosexually identified youth may have opposite-gender sexual experiences.
Gay	The adjective used to describe people whose enduring romantic, physical, and emotional attractions are to people of the same sex. Often refers to men, but also used more generically as well.
Lesbian	A woman whose enduring romantic, physical, and emotional attraction is to other women.
Bisexual	A person who develops romantic, physical, and emotional attraction regardless of the other's sex.
Transgender	A term describing a person whose gender identity does not necessarily match his/her assigned gender at birth or, more generally, who experiences or expresses gender differently from what people expect.
Homosexual	An outdated clinical term sometimes considered derogatory or offensive by many gay people.
Queer	Traditionally a pejorative term, queer currently is used by some LGBTQs, particularly among younger people, to describe themselves. Some value the term for its defiance and because it can be inclusive of the entire LGBTQ community, and others find it to be an appropriate term to describe their identities in a less categorical way. Straight health providers should generally avoid using the term.
Intersex	Also known as *disorders of sex development or differences of sex development.* A general term used for the variety of conditions in which a person has atypical external or internal genitalia. These conditions may be apparent at birth and can cause difficulty assigning gender or they may be diagnosed later, due to infertility or other pubertal clues.
Ally	A friend or supporter of the LGBTQ communities.
Partner/spouse	A way to talk about someone's boyfriend, girlfriend, husband, or wife without mentioning gender. Using these words instead of gendered words allows you to be more inclusive, putting LGBTQ patients or parents at ease.

Articles

Gartrell N, Bos H. US National Longitudinal Lesbian Family Study: psychological adjustment of 17-year-old adolescents. *Pediatrics.* 2010;126(1):28–36

Ryan C, Huebner D, Diaz RM, Sanchez J. Family rejection as a predictor of negative health outcomes in white and Latino lesbian, gay, and bisexual young adults. *Pediatrics.* 2009;123:346–352

Reviews

Dowshen N, Garofalo R. Optimizing primary care for LGBTQ youth. *Contemp Pediatr.* 2009;26:58–66

Olson J, Forbes C, Belzer M. Management of the transgender adolescent. *Arch Pediatr Adolesc Med.* 2011;165(2):171–176

CHAPTER 42

Injury Prevention

Sarah Atunah-Jay, MD, and Iris Wagman Borowsky, MD, PhD

CASE STUDY

A 16-year-old girl was brought to the emergency department (ED) after being rescued from her submerged vehicle. The girl was texting a friend while driving and crashed into a pond. After several weeks in the intensive care unit, she was transferred out for rehabilitative care from her drowning injury.

Questions

1. How extensive is the injury problem in children?
2. What are the different methods for injury prevention? How could this particular injury have been prevented?
3. What injury prevention program has been developed by the American Academy of Pediatrics (AAP)?
4. What are some general guidelines for effective injury prevention counseling?

Traditionally, unintentional injuries have been called accidents. The problem with the term accident, however, is that it implies unpredictability, carrying with it connotations of chance, fate, and unexpectedness. The perception that injuries are chance occurrences that cannot be predicted or prevented has been a major barrier to progress in injury prevention and the study and control of injury as a scientific discipline. According to the modern view of injury, accidents must be anticipated in order to be prevented. Specialists in injury prevention have tried to replace the word *accident* with *injury* and have developed the idea of "reducing injury risk." Thus injuries are not random events at all; rather, they occur in predictable patterns determined by identifiable risk factors. For example, if a 16-year-old girl is texting while driving, which has been shown to be a dangerous driving distraction, the resulting injury can hardly be called an accident. On the contrary, the injury is entirely predictable.

Epidemiology

Unintentional injuries are the leading cause of death among people aged 1 to 44 in the United States. In 2007 unintentional injuries claimed the lives of more than 20,000 Americans younger than 24 years. Motor vehicle crashes are the leading cause of unintentional injury–related deaths in people aged 5 to 34. Suffocation and drowning are the leading cause of unintentional injury–related deaths for infants and ages 1 to 4, respectively. Other major causes of unintentional injury death in young people include burns and poisonings.

Intentional injuries are also a major cause of mortality in young people. Homicide ranks second among all causes of death for ages 15 to 24 and third for ages 1 to 4 and 10 to 14. Suicide ranks third for ages 15 to 24 and fourth for ages 10 to 14.

In addition to deaths, in 2009 nonfatal unintentional injuries led to more than 11 million hospital ED visits in persons younger than 24 in this country. In the same year, almost 1 million young

people visited EDs due to a violence-related injury. The most common causes of nonfatal unintentional injuries in people aged 1 to 24 are falls, being struck by or against something, bites, cuttings/piercings, overexertion, and motor vehicle occupancy.

Several epidemiological factors are associated with higher rates of pediatric injuries. These include male gender, low income, and family stressors (eg, death in the family, new residence, birth of a sibling). There is a bimodal age distribution of injuries, with infants and adolescents at greatest risk. Females are most likely to experience rape or assault. American Indian/Alaska Native and black children have higher rates of total injury-related deaths than other racial/ethnic age-matched populations. Geography influences injury rates: Drowning deaths tend to be higher in coastline states (Alaska and California) or states with a higher number of swimming pools (Texas); injury-related deaths are higher in rural areas and may be related to decreased access to emergency medical care; and homicide occurs more frequently in urban areas.

Strategies for Injury Prevention

During this century, efforts to prevent injuries have shifted from changing the behavior of individuals to modifying the environments in which injuries occur. William Haddon, a medical epidemiologist, devised 2 useful frameworks for developing injury prevention strategies.

Haddon Matrix

This matrix relates 3 factors (host, vector, and environment) to the 3 phases of an injury-producing event (pre-event, event, and post-event). The 3 factors interact over time to produce injury. Table 42-1 shows a Haddon matrix of motor vehicle crash injuries. The pre-crash phase describes elements that determine whether a crash will occur, the crash phase describes the variables that influence the nature and

Table 42-1. The Haddon Matrix[a]			
Phase	**Host (Human)**	**Vector (Vehicle)**	**Environment**
Pre-crash	Driver vision Alcohol consumption	Brakes Tires Speed	Speed limit Road curvature Road signs
Crash	Use of safety belts Osteoporosis	Vehicle size	Median barriers Laws about use of car seats and safety belts
Post-crash	Age Physical condition	Fuel system integrity	EMS personnel training

Abbreviation: EMS, emergency medical service.

[a]Adapted from the National Committee for Injury Prevention. Injury prevention: meeting the challenge. *Am J Prev Med.* 1989;5(3 suppl):1–303

severity of the resultant injury, and the post-crash phase describes the factors that determine the degree to which the injury is limited and repaired after the crash occurs. By describing the "anatomy" of an injury, the Haddon matrix illustrates the numerous characteristics that determine an injury and the many corresponding strategies for interfering with the production of an injury.

Haddon also developed a list of **10 countermeasures to prevent injuries** or reduce the severity of their effects.

1. Prevent creation of the hazard (eg, stop producing poisons, toys with small parts, and non-powder firearms; do not participate in dangerous sports; support community centers that engage children in safe after-school activities).

2. Reduce the amount of the hazard (eg, package drugs in nonlethal amounts; reduce speed limits).

3. Prevent the release of the hazard (eg, use child-resistant caps for medications, toilet locks, and safety latches on cabinets and drawers; pass and enforce distracted driving laws; implement restrictions on handgun purchases).

4. Modify the rate or spatial distribution of release of the hazard (eg, require air bags in cars; use child safety seats and seat belts; make poisons taste bad).

5. Separate people from the hazard in space or time (eg, make sidewalks for pedestrians, bikeways for bicyclists, and recreation areas separated from vehicles).

6. Separate people from hazards with material barriers (eg, use bicycle helmets and protective equipment for athletes; install fences around swimming pools; build window guards).

7. Modify relevant basic qualities of the hazard (eg, place padded carpets under cribs; require guns to have safety locks; develop inter-vehicle communication systems).

8. Increase resistance to damage from the hazard (eg, train and condition athletes; make structures more earthquake-proof; use flame-retardant sleepwear).

9. Limit the damage that has already begun (eg, use fire extinguisher; begin cardiopulmonary resuscitation).

10. Stabilize, repair, and rehabilitate injured individuals (eg, develop pediatric trauma centers and physical rehabilitation programs; improve emergency medical services).

Haddon's work serves as a practical guide for thinking about ways to prevent injury. It emphasizes the importance of considering injuries as a result of a sequence of events, with many opportunities for prevention. The shift of emphasis away from changing human behavior to preventing injury is particularly appropriate with regard to injuries in children because inhibiting children's curiosity is impractical as well as undesirable.

Passive and Active Interventions

Interventions to prevent injuries can also be categorized as passive or active. **Passive, or automatic, strategies** protect whenever they are needed, **without the action of parents or children.** An example is the automobile air bag that automatically inflates to cushion the occupants during a crash. Other examples of automatic strategies are water heater temperatures set to 120°F or lower, not having guns in the home, and energy-absorbing surfaces under playground equipment. In contrast, **active interventions require action to become effective.** For example, nonautomatic safety belts are active strategies; every time protection is needed, individuals must "buckle up." Watching children continuously is another example of an injury prevention strategy that requires constant activity.

Some strategies are partially automatic, requiring some action by individuals. Smoke detectors can be very effective in preventing injury and death in house fires, but roughly one-third of smoke detectors do not have working batteries. Batteries should be changed once a year and, ideally, tested once a month. As might be expected, the greater the effort required for children to be protected, the smaller the chance that protection occurs. Therefore, whenever possible, passive measures are preferable because they are the most effective.

Several approaches have been used successfully to prevent childhood injuries, including engineering, education, legislation, and enforcement. An engineering intervention, the car safety seat, is extremely effective (Table 42-2). When used correctly, child safety seats in passenger cars reduce the risk of death by 71% for infants and 54% for toddlers aged 1 to 4 years. Booster seats reduce injury

Table 42-2. Pediatric Car Seat Guidelines[a]		
Age Group	**Type of Car Seat**	**General Guidelines**
Term infant	Rear-facing	Until at least 1 year *and* at least 20 lbs.
Toddlers/ preschoolers	Rear-facing and forward-facing	Should ride rear-facing as long as possible. A full harness should be used as long as they fit.
School-aged children	Booster seat	Usually start at 4 years and 40 lbs. Use until adult belt fits correctly (usually at 4'9").

[a]From American Academy of Pediatrics. *Car Safety Seats: A Guide for Families.* Available at: http://www.aap.org/healthtopics/carseatsafety.cfm.

risk by 59% for children aged 4 to 7 years compared with safety belts alone. Unfortunately, studies indicate that between one-third and two-thirds of car safety seats are used incorrectly. To address this, newborn care units often have car safety seat education programs, and some require possession of an infant car safety seat prior to hospital discharge. Police departments and private motor companies hold free public events to teach and manually check appropriate car seat use. In addition to engineering and education, passage and strict enforcement of child restraint laws are essential to compliance. All 50 states and the District of Columbia have child restraint laws (http://www.iihs.org/laws/restraintoverview.aspx). Nevertheless, loopholes still exist, such as exemptions in some states for seat belt use if older children are riding in rear seats; for car safety seat use in school buses, taxis, or police vehicles; and if all safety belts are already in use. Such exemptions reinforce parental misconceptions, particularly that the lap of an occupant (the "child crusher" position) is a safe position.

Counseling by Pediatricians

Although the existence of significant gaps in parental knowledge about injury prevention has been clearly established, studies have shown that pediatricians spend surprisingly little time counseling parents about childhood safety. One survey found that only 42% of caregivers of children younger than 15 years who had a medical visit in the past year recalled receiving injury prevention information. Another survey found that while 55% of pediatricians responded that they provided injury prevention information, only 19% of their patients recalled receiving this information. Reasons for limited discussion of safety issues may include lack of emphasis on preventive medical care in medical schools and pediatric training programs, inadequate time or reimbursement, and lack of perceived self-efficacy or effectiveness. Research, however, has shown that injury prevention counseling in primary care settings is effective, resulting in increased knowledge and improved safety practices. Parents report that they would listen to physicians much more than any other group regarding child safety.

The Injury Prevention Program (TIPP) was developed in 1983 by the AAP to firmly establish injury prevention as a cost-effective standard of care for pediatricians. The AAP suggests that providers focus their safety counseling on a few topics targeted to individual risk factors (eg, age, gender, location, season of the year, socioeconomic status of family). Table 42-3 shows the age-specific counseling schedule of TIPP, which indicates the minimum topics to cover at each visit. Topics are scheduled for discussion before children reach a particular developmental milestone. For example, a discussion of falls is scheduled for the 2- or 4-week visit, before infants normally begin to roll over, and a discussion of choking is scheduled for 4 months, before they can grasp and put things in their mouths. Specific preventive measures should be reinforced at each visit. Areas of injury prevention guidance recommended for adolescents include (1) traffic safety (eg, seat belts, alcohol use, motorcycle and bicycle helmets), (2) water safety (eg, alcohol use and diving injuries), (3) sports safety, and (4) firearm safety.

Connected Kids: Safe, Strong, Secure is a violence prevention tool introduced by the AAP in 2006 to augment TIPP. Acknowledging that injury and violence prevention are intertwined, it uses an assets-based approach to engage parents in understanding and fostering healthy child development. An emphasis is put on support and open communication to promote emotional and physical safety.

Health care professionals should involve parents and patients in educational efforts (eg, have a bicycle helmet in the office for children to try on). Safety counseling is most effective if limited to 2 or 3 topics per visit. Advice should be well defined and practical rather than general information (eg, write the poison control center number on the phone; never leave children unattended in a bathtub). Advice should be tailored to each family after exploring their individual situation through open-ended questions (eg, "Where does your baby spend awake time during the day?" "What do you think is the biggest safety risk for your child?"). Providers should be aware of different levels of health literacy and should confirm understanding rather than rushing through a prepared statement. Access to interventions should be considered, such as cost and accessibility of helmets and child safety seats. Whenever possible, pediatricians should coordinate their educational efforts with current community injury prevention efforts (eg, bicycle helmet campaigns; handgun regulation).

Recent Recommendations

The AAP has multiple safety recommendations. The following are a few of the newer and revised recommendations.

Motor vehicle crashes are the leading cause of death for children age 5 and older. Comprehensive legislation and education promoting 3-stage graduated driver's license programs should be encouraged. The AAP recommends that pediatricians know their state laws regarding teenage drivers, encourage seat belt use, discourage distractions when driving, encourage restrictions on nighttime driving and limits on the number of passengers, and counsel teenagers about the dangers of driving while impaired (2006). Pedestrian injuries are a significant traffic-related cause of morbidity and mortality. An emphasis should be given to community and school-based strategies to reduce exposure to high-speed and high-volume traffic, to improvements in car engineering, and to driver education to reduce pediatric pedestrian injury (2009). Children between 12 and 24 months should ride in a rear-facing car safety seat until age 2, based on injury statistics showing that they are 5 times safer in rear-facing than in forward-facing seats. Increased efforts should be made to prevent food-related choking among children through federal agency surveillance and regulation, food manufacturer design, and health care provider counseling efforts (2010). Pediatricians should provide general and targeted office-based water-safety counseling, including maintaining 4-sided fences around swimming pools. Body entrapment and hair entanglement in pool and spa drains are potential dangers to children; thus, drain covers and filter-pump equipment should be installed to prevent injuries (2010). Shopping carts with child seats should provide restraints (seat belts)

Table 42-3. The Injury Prevention Program (TIPP) Safety Counseling Schedule for Early and Middle Childhood[a]		
Visit	**Introduce**	**Reinforce**
Prenatal/newborn	Infant car seat, smoke detector, crib safety	
2 d–4 wk	Falls	Car safety seat
2 mo	Burns—hot liquids, choking/suffocation	Car safety seat, falls
4 mo	Water safety—bathtubs	Car safety seat, falls, burns, choking/suffocation
6 mo	Poisonings, burns—hot surfaces	Falls, burns, choking
9 mo	Water/pool safety, toddler car safety seat, firearms	Poisonings, falls, burns
1 y		Water/pool safety, falls, burns
15 mo		Car safety seat, poisonings, falls, burns
18 mo		Car safety seat, poisonings, falls, burns, firearm hazards
2 y	Falls—play equipment, tricycles, pedestrian safety	Car safety seat, water/pool safety, burns, firearm hazards
3 y		Car safety seat, pedestrian safety, falls, burns, firearm hazards
4 y	Booster seat use	Pedestrian safety, falls—play equipment, firearm hazards
5 y	Water/pool safety, bicycle safety	Firearm hazards, pedestrian safety, booster seat
6 y	Fire safety	Bicycle, booster seat, pedestrian, and firearm hazards
8 y	Sports safety, seat belt use	Bicycle
10 y	Firearm hazards	Sports, seat belt use, bicycle safety

[a]Adapted and reproduced with permission from the American Academy of Pediatrics Committee and Section on Injury and Poison Prevention. *TIPP: The Injury Prevention Program, Implementing Safety Counseling in Office Practice.* Elk Grove Village, IL: American Academy of Pediatrics; 2001.

and children should be supervised while in them. Alternatives to shopping carts include strollers, wagons, front/backpack child carriers, or having the child walk (2006). Sports-related concussions are common yet underreported; any pediatric or adolescent athlete who sustains a concussion should be evaluated by a health care professional and receive medical clearance before returning to play (2010). Health care equity is fundamental to child health; children should be protected from injury within the built environment and with access to quality, patient-centered, and culturally effective medical care (2010). Improving pediatric trauma services will decrease injury-related morbidity and mortality. The AAP recommends an integrated public health approach to trauma, starting at preventive care and continuing through long-term follow-up (2008). Additional guidelines can be found at http://aappolicy.aappublications.org/ using keywords "injury prevention."

Pediatricians as Advocates

As advocates for child safety, pediatricians can play a major role in injury prevention outside of the clinical setting. Pediatricians have started community programs or provided support to ongoing programs. Safe Kids (www.safekids.org) is a worldwide organization made up of safety experts, educators, corporations, foundations, governments, and volunteers whose mission is to prevent childhood injury through education and advocacy. Safe Kids and other issue-specific organizations, such as the Children's Defense Fund (www.childrensdefense.org) and Farm Safety 4 Just Kids (www.fs4jk.org), can provide resources to support pediatricians in local or national projects and provide avenues for legislative participation. Through their Community Pediatrics grants programs (www.aap.org/commpeds/), the AAP provides grants to pediatricians and pediatric residents who want to create innovative community projects promoting child health.

Legislative advocacy is an exciting opportunity for health care professionals to effect wide-reaching change. States have enacted laws covering many aspects of injury prevention, including car safety seats, poison control centers, cribs, playgrounds, amusement parks, protective gear for sports, swimming pools, and school buses. Dramatic reductions in injuries often follow safety legislation. For example, infant walker-related injuries have decreased by 76% since the introduction of the American Society for Testing and Materials F977 voluntary infant walker standard in 1997 and the introduction of stationary activity centers as alternatives to mobile infant walkers. Other examples of product-related legislation include federal crib standards of 1974 mandating close spacing of vertical slats to reduce the risk of entrapment, the Child Safety Protection Act of 1995 requiring toy safety labels on any balls with a diameter less than 1¾ inches (4.44 cm), window blinds manufactured with tassels instead of loops and children's clothing without drawstrings to prevent strangulation, and toy boxes manufactured with safer lids and air holes in case of a trapped child. Similarly, in December 2010 the Consumer Product Safety Commission voted to ban drop-side cribs, citing the recall of more than 9 million cribs over the previous 5 years and the entrapment and death of 30 babies over the previous 10 years. The ban went into effect in June 2011 and prohibits the sale of such cribs even at garage sales.

Pediatric practitioners can heighten awareness about the magnitude of childhood injuries through calls or letters to legislators, testifying about the benefits of specific safety legislation, or partnering to introduce new legislation. Pediatrician legislative involvement is critical to ensuring evidence-guided local and national injury prevention.

CASE RESOLUTION

Some of the factors that influenced the injury suffered by the girl in the case history are the age of driver's licensure, the passage and enforcement of laws pertaining to cell phone use in cars, the design of the car, road conditions, and the availability of emergency rescue services and specialized pediatric care. Health care professionals have the opportunity to teach injury prevention to children and their parents as well as to influence the individuals who manufacture the products and pass the laws that affect children's risk of injury.

Selected References

Agran PF, Anderson C, Winn D, Trent R, Walton-Haynes L, Thayer S. Rates of pediatric injuries by 3-month intervals for children 0 to 3 years of age. *Pediatrics.* 2003;111:e683–e692

American Academy of Pediatrics. Connected Kids: Safe Strong Secure. www.aap.org/connectedkids

American Academy of Pediatrics. HealthyChildren Web site. www.HealthyChildren.org

American Academy of Pediatrics. TIPP: The Injury Prevention Program. www.aap.org/family/tippmain.htm

Bernard SJ, Paulozzi LJ, Wallace DL. Fatal injuries among children by race and ethnicity—United States, 1999–2002. *MMWR Morb Mortal Wkly Rep.* 2007;56(SS05):1–16

Chen J, Kresnow MJ, Simon TR, Dellinger A. Injury-prevention counseling and behavior among US children: results from the second Injury Control and Risk Survey. *Pediatrics.* 2007;119(4):e958–e965

DiGuiseppi C, Roberts IG. Individual-level injury prevention strategies in the clinical setting. *Future Child.* 2000;10:53–82

Dowd MD, Keenan HT, Bratton SL. Epidemiology and prevention of childhood injuries. *Crit Care Med.* 2002;30(suppl):S385–S392

Gardner HG; American Academy of Pediatrics Committee on Injury, Violence, and Poison Prevention. Office-based counseling for unintentional injury prevention. *Pediatrics.* 2007;119:202–206

Gittleman MA, Pomerantz WJ, Schubert CJ. Implementing and evaluating an injury prevention curriculum within a pediatric residency program. *J Trauma Injury Infect Crit Care.* 2010;69(4 suppl):S239–S244

Hambridge SJ, Davidson AJ, Gonzales R, Steiner JF. Epidemiology of pediatric injury-related primary care office visits in the United States. *Pediatrics.* 2002;109:559–565

Hunter WM, Helou S, Saluja G, Runyan CW, Coyne-Beasley T. Injury prevention advice in top-selling parenting books. *Pediatrics.* 2005;116:1080–1088

National Center for Injury Prevention and Control, Centers for Disease Control and Prevention. Web-Based Inquiry Statistics Query and Reporting System. www.cdc.gov/injury/wisqars

United States Department of Health and Human Services, Centers for Disease Control and Prevention. Injury Fact Book. www.cdc.gov/Injury/Publications/FactBook

CHAPTER 43

Fostering Self-esteem

Rick Goldstein, MD

CASE STUDY

A 4-year-old girl is brought to the office for her annual physical examination. She has been healthy. Her mother expresses concern that her daughter is shy and does not always play well with other children. She has never participated in a child care program or group activities out of the home. She spends most of her time with her mother, grandmother, and 7-year-old sister, with whom she gets along fairly well. Both parents work outside the home, her father full-time and her mother part-time.

The girl's medical history is unremarkable except for an episode of bronchiolitis at 8 months of age. She has reached all of her developmental milestones at appropriate ages, currently speaks well in sentences, is able to dress herself without supervision, and can balance on one foot with no difficulty.

The physical examination is entirely normal. However, numerous times during the visit, the mother tells her daughter to "sit up straight," "stop fidgeting," and "act your age." The mother rolls her eyes as she tells you "she doesn't know how to act."

Questions

1. What is self-esteem?
2. How do parents or other caregivers affect the development of their children's self-esteem both positively and negatively?
3. What role does discipline play in the development of self-esteem?
4. How does illness affect self-esteem?
5. What suggestions can primary practitioners give parents and other caregivers to help foster positive self-esteem in children?

Self-esteem is a concept that resonates deeply in contemporary American culture. In its casual usage, the term is often used to mean contentment or a sense of agency. Agency is considered the capacity to act in the world, the notion that what the individual thinks, wants, and does matters. Alternatively, poor self-esteem may be used to describe an overly self-critical child with limited confidence. Fundamentally, self-esteem is based on the confidence a child has for success and also the confidence that difficulties, failures, and disappointments are tolerable and can be met while still feeling whole and supported. Self-esteem is grounded in the fact that success with other people is fundamental to a sense of who we are. It is essential to children's health and well-being, and influences the development of relationships and identity during both childhood and adulthood.

Researchers have developed an informative model for understanding self-esteem. In self-determination theory, a child's general self-concept is understood as an organization of complex, hierarchically inter-related components. Self-esteem is the evaluative aspect of self concept, and is linked to and rests on intrinsic motivation. Research has demonstrated that (1) optimal challenges, effectance-promoting feedback, and freedom from demeaning critique; (2) parenting that promotes autonomy rather than control; and (3) a secure interpersonal environment of relatedness are all essential contributions to intrinsic motivation and, by extension, self-esteem.

While self-esteem is a concept in action throughout our lives, it first comes into clear view in the developing internal self-concept of the 4-year-old. In the language of a 4-year-old, the pediatrician or allied health professional can find a child who is learning to know herself and appreciate her abilities. The joy of autonomy and initiative are suffused with a need to live up to expectations—part of feeling she is a big girl is feeling she is a good girl. The first stirrings of conscience and the confidence to manage measured responsibility can be seen. The complex interaction of temperament, developmental stage, the family's security, the parental style of discipline, sibling and peer interactions, and school experiences coalesce in the experience of a uniquely competent child. For her caregivers, the desire to encourage a kind of fearlessness is balanced by the very real need to keep the child safe and appropriate. All of these aspects of her life contribute to the development of her competence, autonomy, and relatedness, and animate her self-esteem.

All parents hope that their children will develop a positive self-concept that will aid them throughout their lives. Unfortunately, discussions related to self-esteem are usually held as a result of a crisis or an observation by worried parents or teachers. Primary care practitioners should bring the parents' focus to this important aspect of the child as a normal part of anticipatory guidance. Pediatricians and child health practitioners are in a unique position to offer specific recommendations for fostering self-esteem that may have a major impact on their patients' lives. During health maintenance visits with the child, they should model respect for the child's self-concept and the fostering of the child's self-esteem in their interactions.

Self-esteem and Growth and Development

While the appearance of what is understood as self-esteem requires the development of certain cognitive abilities, it springs from an accumulated experience with parents and other caregivers. Beginning with the responsiveness of the newborn's environment and continuing onward, distressed infants quickly adapt to the calming influence of a maternal figure. Infants who are 3 to 4 months of age often smile at all individuals for social interaction and protest being left alone. As infants become more verbal and develop more advanced motor skills, they begin to respond consistently to verbal and nonverbal cues from parents (eg, laugh with parents, follow simple commands, are taken aback by a stern voice). If parental figures are warm and loving as well as supportive and consistent, infants learn to trust and enjoy these interactions.

By the time children are toddlers, they have developed a specific relationship with their caregivers and the rest of their environment. As a goal, they are learning to live within consistently set limits and are corrected when they go beyond them in their attempts at exploration. All children, regardless of temperament, exhibit negative behaviors such as temper tantrums and selfish behavior, which elicit some type of response from parents.

Preschool children become much more independent, and they spend more time away from primary caregivers. This newly acquired independence, however, does not remove the need for attention, interest, and approval from their parents. Agency must be nurtured, and not simply controlled, to feed self-esteem. Opportunities to demonstrate the competence of children can be seen in the autonomy that appropriate parenting affords, and heard as a source of pride in parents taking note of it. Preschoolers also enjoy playing alongside other children, although not necessarily in cooperative play (eg, helping each other in addition to playing together).

Much of a child's self-concept is established and reinforced by those around them, especially their primary caregivers. While important activities occur when the child is alone and engaged in individual pursuits, much of a child's self-concept develops in a context of relatedness. This continues into the school years, with peers and teachers eventually assuming a more influential role in the continued development and reinforcement of self-esteem. The development of self-esteem is transactional, built by the responses children receive to their increasing initiative and abilities, resting on a foundation of security.

Optimal Challenges: Encouragement Versus Pressure

Parenting should help promote autonomy, competence, and relatedness. Parents should understand the difference between encouragement and pressure, and should be introduced to the concept of positive communication. To build positive self-esteem, children need encouragement at all levels of their development (Box 43-1). This is communicated both verbally and nonverbally and should be distinguished from overt pressure. For example, a first-grader learning to spell should be praised for his early, if flawed, application of

---

Box 43-1. Encouraging Self-esteem

Don'ts

Have negative expectations.

Focus on mistakes.

Expect perfection.

Overly protect children.

Dos

Show confidence in children's abilities.

Build on children's strengths.

Value children as they are.

Stimulate independence.

---

phonemes when he spells "winter" as "wntur," and may not need criticism at that point. In general, children should be allowed to develop at their own rate and be neither coaxed into activities before they are ready nor judged too harshly for earnest, early attempts.

Successful parenting creates opportunities for the child to safely extend their boundaries while ensuring the child's feeling of personal control. An overly critical or controlling style of parenting constrains the emergence of a child's young sense of competence and, by extension, affects their self-esteem. Being handed a scribble drawing by a preschooler and told what it represents is emblematic. An appreciative, interested, positive response to the disordered marks is sustaining; disinterest or criticism undermines.

When pressure occurs, it is often from parents' having unrealistic expectations of how the child learns and develops, or an improper sense that lack of success is due to laziness or a character flaw. Inadvertent pressure can be detrimental and cause tremendous frustration when, for example, parents try to lead a toddler into toilet training when the child has shown few signs of readiness, even if most of the children in his preschool class are out of diapers. Pressuring young children to give up pacifiers or another security object without giving thought to the child's readiness may also be quite anxiety provoking to them.

While children may not know what is best for their ultimate development, well-intentioned pressure may be equally harmful later in childhood. Forcing children to participate in rigid, structured play, and sometimes classes or lessons, does not foster individual creativity or independence. Children are merely doing what the parents have arranged. Ideally, children should be encouraged to explore and occasionally take risks. They should be helped to build on their "islands of competence." Mistakes should be put into the context of a sincere effort and seen in terms of what can be learned rather than as a humiliation. Pressuring children to do things "right" or "perfectly" discourages normal, healthy, risk-taking behavior and interferes with future efforts by children to participate in activities unless they are certain they can succeed.

A variation on this theme is overprotection, where the parent controls the child's environment so as to reduce any risk of failure or discomfort to the child. This generally comes at the cost of sacrificing the experience of novel achievement and developing the competence to work through frustrations and disappointments. This also has a negative impact on self-esteem.

Communication That Builds Self-esteem

Specific ways to communicate that build self-esteem include active listening, use of positive language, discarding "labels," use of encouragement rather than pressure, and the use of the "I" method of communication (Box 43-2). The pediatrician should coach parents that this is not a rigid code to be followed at all times and at great hazard, but rather that the goal is a "good enough" environment where well-intended parents put up a fairly consistent effort to be mindful of how they deal with their children. A useful way to set the correct tone with parents and caregivers is the use of strength-based counseling, where advice grows out of a focus on what parents are doing right.

The purpose of active listening is to hear the child's message and understand its meaning. Its success rests on a centered approach to important parenting moments: Parents should strive to be attentive and present at these moments. They should stop what they are doing, and look directly at children. They should be aware of nonverbal cues, such as body posture and facial expression. If children are having trouble understanding their feelings, the parent should repeat what they hear them saying ("It sounds like…").

A nonjudgmental response, validating and non-dismissive, should be the goal of communication between primary caregivers and children. The basic message should be stated simply, clearly, and at a level that respects the maturity of the child. Words should be easily understood and spoken in a moderate tone, especially when discipline is necessary. Facial expression and body language should also be consistent with the message parents or caregivers are trying to convey.

The importance of positive language should be emphasized, even when disciplining children (see Chapter 47). For instance, when children are playing kick ball in the house, it is understandable that a parent might yell, "Don't play ball in the house!" or "Haven't I told you before? No ball playing inside!" While emotionally honest parenting in a loving context is the best parenting, practically speaking this rarely occurs 100% of the time and parents need to be aware of when they are speaking in a reprimanding and negative fashion. Parents or other adults should tell children clearly what they can do, what the limits are, and the reason for these rules. For example, they could state: "You have to stop playing ball right now. If you kick the ball inside, you may break a window or hurt yourself or someone else. You may kick the ball outside in the backyard." Communicating

in a clear manner changes the tone of the interaction from a reprimand for being bad to one where rules are clarified to a child who wants to do the right thing.

Parents should praise their children for successes and achievements. Failures should be put into context whenever possible, although the acknowledgment of mistakes can be important. A forgotten jacket or a careless job with homework can be frustrating but are not worthy of demeaning critique. Negative labels have no helpful role. If children hear themselves referred to pejoratively by their primary caregivers, not only is an undesirable behavior modeled, but they will feel undermined and wonder about the truth of such statements, no matter how innocuous they may initially seem to parents.

At the other extreme, parents should be cautioned against always speaking in the superlative to their child and staying blind to any shortcomings. Children are adept at seeing the world as it is. A failure to see themselves reflected realistically by parents or caregivers may feed a kind of insecurity where despite the glowing language of the parents, the child feels uncertain of their actual worth.

Talents and abilities should be recognized and highlighted. Children should know that parents have confidence in their abilities and that any display of effort is appreciated. Even small successes should be noted and not overshadowed by the large ones or the failures. Children thrive on the joy and pride they see in the eyes of their parents. Lack of encouragement can limit their optimism for continued success.

Many parenting courses teach primary caregivers to use the "I" method of communication, which requires that parents explain their feelings to children rather than blame them for their actions. This approach is believed to be less threatening and demeaning for children, especially in situations requiring discipline. The "I" method has 4 recommended steps.

1. Statement of behavior or situation to be addressed (eg, "When you…")
2. Statement in specific terms of how one feels about the effect of the situation on oneself (eg, "I feel…")
3. Statement of reason (eg, "because…")
4. Statement of expectations (eg, "I would like…" or "I want…")

Using this approach, a parent's statement might be: "When you speak so unkindly, I feel upset because I would never speak with you in that way. It makes you seem like the kind of person that you are not. I would like you to speak with me in the way we all try to speak with you, no matter how angry you feel."

Vulnerable Times in a Child's Life

There are instances when a child's self-esteem can be particularly vulnerable. The primary care provider should be cognizant of circumstances where a child may feel shame, confusion, or guilt for problems occurring in them or their family. Negative experiences in school and at home can predispose a child to feelings of shame and worthlessness. Marital conflict, divorce, or the abuse of a parent may negatively influence the self-esteem of children who may feel responsible for the problem. In such circumstances, parents are often

---

Box 43-2. Communication That Builds Self-esteem

Active listening

Use of positive language

Discarding "labels"

Use of encouragement

Use of the "I" method of communication

concerned about the impact on the child, which provides an opportunity to work together to minimize negative effects. Honest, open communication with parents can reinforce the need for sensitive support of the child and help them set priorities or rehearse how they will talk with the child about the matters at hand (see Chapter 136).

Physical and psychiatric illness can challenge a child's sense of competence, autonomy, and relatedness. They can be left uncertain of their standing, expecting failure or feeling they stand apart. It is worth mentioning the challenge of supporting self-esteem that enters the pediatrician's office often when dealing with "new morbidities." The diagnoses of obesity, attention-deficit/hyperactivity disorder, and learning disabilities can have in common the taint of personal judgment and the threat of undermining self-worth. This aspect of a child's care is present in disclosure of diagnosis, the response of the parent and the child, determining a realistic treatment plan, following what can be a frustrating lack of progress, and ultimate outcomes. Parents and patients will benefit from careful modeling when representing the problem and how to talk about it by the pediatrician.

Discipline and Self-esteem

Parents should consider their understanding of the complex relationship between discipline and self-esteem, and they should be questioned about their impressions of their child's independence and competence. Promoting the growth of healthy autonomy should be a goal for all parents. As children grow, so does their ability to act responsibly and their ability to maintain greater self-control. This central insight is an important way to help parents see beyond discipline in simply punitive terms. Children do best when they are provided with clear, consistent guidelines for their behavior while at the same time being encouraged to do well, pursue their interests, and increase their abilities.

They do this even better when they see this modeled in the adults around them. Parents and other caregivers should remember that certain methods of discipline, particularly if harsh or shame provoking, can be very destructive to a child's self-esteem. For instance, making an enuretic child sleep in wet bed sheets or reprimanding a child with physical punishment (eg, spanking) in public places can be demeaning. Several different approaches to discipline have been adapted by various ethnic, cultural, religious, and socioeconomic groups. While a discussion of each of these methods is beyond the scope of this chapter (see Chapter 47), it is important to explore strategies with parents and caregivers.

CASE RESOLUTION

In the case history, the health maintenance visit provides the perfect opportunity for promoting parental support of their child's self-esteem. The shy child should be approached by giving sincere general compliments (eg, "My goodness, you are so big." Or to a carefully dressed girl, "What a beautiful pink outfit!") and, in the interview, inviting her to tell you some things about herself (eg, "What are your favorite things?" "What is your favorite color?"), while employing humor and enthusiasm to engage her in some details. This models interactions, which allows the child to demonstrate her autonomy, with the hope that this approach will be repeated by the parent at home. The health care provider can reassure the girl and her mother that the child's overall health and development are normal. In addition, once the careful, protective experience the parents have managed for their child is appreciated, the practitioner should attempt to normalize the child's behavior for the parent. While it may be important to directly discuss shyness in a developmental context, whether she is shy is not certain and the parent's sense of deficiencies should be challenged by a view of developing competencies. Concrete suggestions should be offered for positive communication, such as minimizing "don't" and "no" phrases and being cognizant of how one speaks about the daughter. The parents should be encouraged to think about the child's temperament when considering involvement in multiple school activities but reminded that they have not yet seen her in an independent setting, where she may negotiate very well and show sociability not yet evident at home.

Selected References

American Academy of Pediatrics Committee on Psychosocial Aspects of Child and Family Health. Guidance for effective discipline. *Pediatrics.* 1998;101:723–728

Briggs DC. *Your Child's Self-Esteem.* New York, NY: Doubleday; 1970

Brooks RB. Self-esteem during the school years: its normal development and hazardous decline. *Pediatr Clin North Am.* 1992;39:537–550

Brooks RB. *The Self-Esteem Teacher.* Circle Pines, MN: American Guidance Service; 1981

Deci EL, Ryan RM. Human Autonomy: the basis for true self-esteem. In: Kemis M, ed. *Efficacy, Agency and Self-esteem.* New York, NY: Plenum Press; 1995:31–49

Howard BJ. Discipline in early childhood. *Pediatr Clin North Am.* 1991;38: 1351–1369

Ryan RM, Deci EL. Self-determination theory and the facilitation of intrinsic motivation, social development, and well-being. *Am Psychol.* 2000;55:68–78

Sieving RE, Zirbel-Donish ST. Development and enhancement of self-esteem in children. *J Pediatr Health Care.* 1990;4:290–296

CHAPTER 44

Sibling Rivalry

Carol D. Berkowitz, MD

CASE STUDY

An 8-year-old boy is brought to the office for an annual checkup. During the course of the evaluation, his mother complains that her son and his 6-year-old sister are always fighting. She says her son hits his sister and pulls her hair, and nothing she does prevents them from fighting. The boy is a B+ student and has no behavior problems in school. The medical history and the physical examination are completely normal.

Questions

1. What is sibling rivalry?
2. What is the physician's role in counseling a family about sibling rivalry?
3. What is the role of anticipatory guidance in preparing older children for the birth of a new sister or brother?
4. What are some practical suggestions to share with parents about sibling rivalry?

Sibling relationships are important in helping children shape peer and later adult interactions. Siblings educate and socialize together, and mediate parental demands. Siblings often spend more time interacting with each other than with either parent. The sibling relationship is characterized by continuity and permanence, but the relationship is not without turmoil.

Sibling rivalry refers to the competitiveness between siblings based on the need for **parental love** and **esteem.** The rivalry is often characterized by jealousy, teasing, and bickering. The term was introduced in 1941 by David Levy who described it as "a common feature of family life." Historical examples of sibling rivalry include relationships between the biblical figures Cain and Abel, Joseph and his brothers, and Jacob and Esau. Sibling rivalry is also noteworthy in pairs of celebrities, such as actresses Joan Fontaine (Academy Award winner for *Suspicion*) and her older sister, Olivia de Havilland (Academy Award winner for *To Each His Own* and *The Heiress*). Their relationship was termed one of the most dysfunctional sibling relationships in Hollywood, and may have had its roots in their simultaneous nomination for an Academy Award in 1942. By 1975 the sisters were no longer in communication with each other.

Sibling rivalry is a **universal phenomenon** occurring even in the animal kingdom. For instance, the firstborn eaglet pushes the other eaglets out of the nest as soon as they are hatched as a way of ensuring an adequate food supply. In humans, the fear of displacement, dethronement, and loss of love occurs with the birth of a new brother or sister, leading to sibling rivalry. Older children fear they are not good enough and need to be replaced. Such feelings lead to a **fear of abandonment.** Jealousy also plays a role, and older children may be angry with younger siblings for displacing them within the family.

Sibling rivalry frequently has a negative effect on parents because it is hard for them to see one of their children hurt, even if it is by a sister or a brother. The challenge for parents is to know when, and when not, to intervene and what strategies to use to minimize conflicts. Physicians can help by offering **anticipatory guidance** to all parents and specific recommendations to parents who are experiencing such individual problems.

Epidemiology

Sibling rivalry is a universal phenomenon, and a number of factors influence its development. Time interval between children affects the degree of rivalry, as does the age of the older children. Toddlers who are entering the **"terrible twos"** may have a particularly hard time mastering independence and tolerating the presence of their younger sibling. Close spacing results in more problems, particularly when the children are fewer than 2 years apart. In such situations, older children still have dependency needs, often feel less secure, and experience a need for maternal attention. They stay closer to mothers, are less playful, and are tenser. Closely spaced children engage in less spontaneous play, seem angrier, and issue sterner commands to their playmates.

Position in the family also influences sibling rivalry. Middle children experience what is referred to as **"middle-child syndrome"**; they lack the prestige of older children or the privileges of younger ones. These children are often least secure and strive hardest to gain affection. Special difficulties may develop if middle children are the same gender as older ones. Middle children grow up to be flexible, adaptable, and good negotiators. In myths and folklore, youngest children are "favorites." They are often the ones defended by parents when there are bouts of fighting.

Twins rarely present a problem of sibling rivalry; instead they have a problem maintaining their individuality. However, sets of twins create problems for older siblings because they are not as unique as the pair of twins.

Step-siblings also present a unique problem in sibling rivalry. Children of divorce frequently feel abandoned by one parent and in competition for the time and love of the custodial parent (see Chapter 136). Competition with step-siblings is especially difficult if the step-siblings are in the same home.

There are also unique considerations when one child has a chronic or potentially terminal illness or long-term disability. Similarly, being the sibling of a gifted child (see chapter 30) places unique challenges on sibling relationships. The unique strengths of each child need to be acknowledged.

Issues of sibling conflict change over time. Toddlers are protective of their toys and belongings and are particularly upset when a younger sibling touches their possessions. Sharing is a challenging theme of the toddler years. Children during their school-aged years are concerned about equity and fairness. They may be upset by what they construe as preferential treatment, for instance when a 1-year-old sibling is not expected to put their toys away. Sibling competitiveness is said to peak between the ages of 10 and 15 years. Adolescents with their additional responsibilities, including minding younger siblings, may resent the siblings for imposing on their time. Sibling rivalry can persist into adulthood, and one-third of adults describe their relationship with a sibling as distant or rivalrous. After age 60 years, 80% of siblings report being close.

Clinical Presentation

Parental complaints related to sibling rivalry consist of fighting between siblings, including physical violence and verbal abuse, bickering, and regression to immature behavioral patterns. Although such immature behavior occurs most often following the birth of a new baby, it may also be apparent if one sibling is receiving more attention, such as during an illness or after a major accomplishment. Regressive behavior includes bedwetting, drinking from a bottle, and wanting to be carried to bed. Substitution behavior, such as nail-biting, in place of biting the new sibling, may occur after the birth of a new baby.

Before the birth of a new baby, parents may complain that their children exhibit temper tantrums, irritability, and solemness. They may mimic the pregnancy by eating a lot and putting a pillow under their clothes. In addition, children may have psychosomatic complaints such as stomachaches or headaches. Risk factors for maladjustment following the addition of a sibling include family discord, physical or emotional exhaustion in parents, and housing insecurity. Conversely, a good marital relationship and family support facilitates the adjustment to new siblings.

Differential Diagnosis

Dilemmas concerning the correct diagnosis of sibling rivalry most often relate to the appearance of behavioral changes, such as regressive or aggressive patterns after the birth of a new sibling. For example, a child who was previously toilet trained may become incontinent of urine. Although urinary tract infection may be considered in the diagnosis, a careful history concerning the birth of the sibling reveals the correct etiology.

Evaluation

The evaluation of children with suspected sibling rivalry involves a history of the problem and parental strategies for dealing with the difficulties. The parent should be particularly queried about one-on-one opportunities between parents and individual children. The physical examination and laboratory assessment are noncontributory.

Management

The focus of management is to allow the parents to recognize the normalcy of sibling rivalry while helping them define the behaviors that are acceptable and not acceptable within the family context. Children fight more often in families when parents condone fighting and aggression between siblings as normal behavior. Likewise, children of parents who are angry may interact with their siblings through anger. Parents should be counseled about this. Parents may not appreciate their child's fear of loss of parental love as the basis of the sibling conflicts. They should be reminded that many children think, "If I am so good, why do I have to be replaced?" Parents should be asked to empathize by imagining how they would feel if their spouse brought home another mate, even if they were reassured about being loved. Physicians can also help parents deal with sibling rivalry by having them consider their treatment of children in terms of uniqueness versus uniformity and quality versus inequality. In general, parents should be advised to set the ground rules for acceptable behavior. Such rules include no hitting, punching, hair pulling, name-calling, cursing, or door slamming. There may be a neutral area in the home that can be set aside for arbitration should disagreements arise. Moving to a neutral area also allows for some time to cool off. Parents should also be reminded that children who are hungry, tired, or bored are more easily frustrated and may start fights more readily.

Birth of New Siblings

Parents may notice the behavioral changes in their children before the birth of the new sibling. These changes depend on the age of the children and the presence of other siblings. Children should be told about the upcoming birth. The timing depends on the children's age; younger children do not need much lead time. Some studies have evaluated the inclusion of older children in the birthing process. The results of these studies vary, but they suggest that children younger than 4 years need their mother for emotional support and are concerned about her physical exertion during the birthing process. Some older children may also want to distance themselves from the actual events.

Physicians should suggest that older children be involved in planning for the arrival of the new baby as a means of minimizing their feelings of exclusion. For example, they can help purchase clothes or prepare the baby's room. Physicians should also suggest that parents purchase a gift for older children that represents a present from the new baby, such as tee shirts that announce the older sibling's new status, such as "big sister" or "big brother." In addition, older siblings may be given a doll to serve as a baby they can care for. Parents should point out the advantages of being older with comments such as, "You can stay up later" or "You can walk and play with all these toys." Frequently, the birth of a new baby is met with regressive behavior in older siblings. Regressive behavior should be handled with tolerance and a realization that symptoms resolve with time.

Once the mother goes to the hospital, she should be advised to maintain contact with older children by telephoning. Many hospitals now allow for visitation by siblings. At present, hospital stays are so brief that this period of separation is much shorter than previously. Household changes that may be necessitated by the birth of the new baby, such as room changes, the substitution of a bed for a crib, and entrance into nursery school, should be made before the arrival of the new baby.

Rivalry Between Older Children

Physicians need to consider individual parenting techniques when counseling parents of older children. Parents who compare one child with the other may foster contentious behavior, and those who strive to treat all children equally may inadvertently perpetuate rivalry. Children need to feel that they are unique rather than ordinary. For example, parents who buy both children the same presents may think they are preventing rivalry from developing, but they are actually depriving each child of a sense of uniqueness. The harder parents try to be uniform, the more vigilantly the children may look for inequality. Each child needs a parent's undivided attention, time alone together. Siblings also need time apart from each other, and they should be encouraged to hold separate play dates and individual activities. Not all children in a family need piano lessons and soccer practice. Individuality and uniqueness are important. The more agreeable a parent–child relationship is, the more agreeable a sibling–sibling relationship is, because each child has good self-esteem. Practitioners should recommend uniqueness and quality in each parent–child relationship.

Parents sometimes have to deal with sibling rivalry between older children. Physicians should reassure parents that these older children should be allowed to vent their negative feelings toward each other. For example, if a girl refers to her brother by saying "I hate him," the parents should respond by validating these emotions and saying something like, "It sounds as if he's done something to really annoy you." Parents should also be advised not to take sides. They should examine how they usually respond to squabbling between siblings. Is one child's name always called first during a fight? Do they perpetuate sibling rivalry by using certain nicknames (eg, "turkey brain") or other derogatory terms? Parents should assume that both parties are at least partially guilty and should not allow themselves to be drawn into the fight as referees. Parents can respond to a request for arbitration with a statement such as, "I wasn't here when

things started, so I don't know who is right or wrong." The parents should also advise siblings that they do not have to be friends with one another, but they should not hurt each other's feelings.

Anticipatory guidance helps parents anticipate conflictual situations, such as who sits where during long car rides and who holds the remote control device. Family meetings can be held to determine the ground rules that may avoid such battles. If conflicts arise, children should be allowed to work out a solution by themselves, with the stipulation that the parents will solve the problem if the children do not reach an agreement. If fights between siblings have recurrent themes (eg, which television shows to watch [who controls the remote] or video games to play), parents can devise a weekly schedule. Failure to abide by the schedule means both children forfeit the activity. If borrowing is the source of disputes, children who borrow from their siblings should leave "collateral," which gets given back when the borrowed item is returned. Box 44-1 lists suggestions for parents who are seeking advice about fighting between children.

Siblings of Children With Special Health Care Needs

Nearly 1 in 5 children in the United States is a child with special health care needs (see Chapter 39). Caring for such children places increased demands on parents and their resources, and there is less parental attention or time available for siblings. Integrating the unaffected sibling into the families' care plan and activities can be empowering for the child and positively influence their self-esteem. As with all children, time alone between the unaffected child and parent should be strongly encouraged. Support groups for siblings of children with special health care needs have been demonstrated to help youngsters cope and to deal with their often conflicted feelings of anger at the special attention their brother or sister receives and their guilt about being healthy.

> **Box 44-1. Coping With Rivalry Between Siblings: Physicians' Advice to Parents**
>
> **Dos**
> - Allow children to vent negative feelings.
> - Encourage children to develop solutions.
> - Anticipate problem situations.
> - Foster individuality in each child.
> - Spend time with children individually.
> - Compliment children when they are playing together.
> - Tell children about the conflicts you had with your siblings when you were children.
> - Define acceptable and unacceptable behavior.
>
> **Don'ts**
> - Take sides.
> - Serve as a referee.
> - Foster rivalry.
> - Use derogatory names.
> - Permit physical or verbal abuse between siblings.

Prognosis

Although sibling rivalry may last for years, most siblings become good friends as adults. Rarely, mental health services are needed, especially if the sibling conflict has lead to marital discord, there is concern about physical or severe emotional harm, or there is evidence of another psychiatric disorder such as depression. Learning how to negotiate with one's siblings enables children to develop skills to collaborate with peers and colleagues as adolescents and adults.

CASE RESOLUTION

In the case history presented at the beginning of the chapter, the mother should be advised not to serve as a referee. She should learn how to validate each child's feelings about the other. The physician can help her by talking to her son about his feelings. She should be advised to have a discussion with her children during which each child has the opportunity to define areas of conflict and the means to resolve them. The mother has the right and responsibility to prohibit physical fighting and encourage verbal dialogue.

Selected References

Adams MM. *Sister for Sale.* Grand Rapids, MI: ZonderKidz; 2002

Alderfer, MA, Lown EA, Marsland AL, Ostrowski NL, Hock JM, Ewing LJ. Psychosocial adjustment of siblings of children with cancer: a systematic review. *Psychooncology.* 2010;19:789–805

Anderson JE. Sibling rivalry: when the family circle becomes a boxing ring. *Contemp Pediatr.* 2006;23:72–90

Dunn J. Annotation: sibling influences on childhood development. *J Child Psychol Psychiatry.* 1988;29:119–127

Goldenthal P. *Beyond Sibling Rivalry: How to Help Your Child Become Cooperative, Caring and Compassionate.* New York, NY: Henry Holt and Company; 2000

Hass E, Light P. Talking about the new baby. *Parents Magazine.* 1983;58:68–70

Leung AK, Robson WL. Sibling rivalry. *Clin Pediatr (Phila).* 1991;30:314–317

Nolbris M, Abrahamsson J, Hellström AL, Olofsson L, Enskär K. The experience of therapeutic support groups by siblings of children with cancer. *Pediatr Nurs.* 2010;36:298–304

Okun A. Ethics for the pediatrician: children who have special health-care needs: ethical issues. *Pediatr Rev.* 2010;31:514–517

Pakula LC. Sibling rivalry. *Pediatr Rev.* 1992;13:72–73

Samalin N, McCormick P. How to cure sibling fights. *Parents Magazine.* 1993;68:147–150

Schmitt BD. Sibling rivalry toward a new baby. *Contemp Pediatr.* 1990;7:111–112

Schmitt BD. When siblings quarrel. *Contemp Pediatr.* 1991;8:73–74

CHAPTER 45

Toilet Training

Sabrina D. Diaz, MA, and Lynne M. Smith, MD

CASE STUDY

A 2-year-old boy is brought to the office for a well-child visit. His mother, who is about to begin toilet training her son, asks your advice. The mother says that by the time her daughter was 2 she was already toilet trained, and she wants to know if training her son will be any different. The boy was the product of a full-term pregnancy and a normal delivery. He has been in good health, and his immunizations are up to date. He is developmentally normal, uses some 2-word phrases, and has been walking since the age of 13 months. His physical examination is normal.

Questions

1. When should physicians begin discussing toilet training with parents?
2. What factors help determine children's readiness to begin toilet training?
3. Is toilet training in boys different from toilet training in girls?
4. What are some of the methods used to toilet train children?

The age at which toilet training is carried out is culturally determined. Some cultures train children at a very early age. For example, in the East African Digo culture, some children between 2 to 3 months of age are conditioned to urinate or defecate when placed in certain positions. Similar conditioning practices are carried out in China. Chinese children are kept without diapers, and when caregivers who are holding them sense a change in their bodies in response to a need to eliminate, they place their children in an appropriate position. In addition, children are dressed in clothing that facilitates toileting. Split pants, with the back and bottom portion missing, are used so that children can squat and eliminate without removing complicated clothing.

American culture has emphasized the learning aspects of toilet training as opposed to the conditioning aspects. This training focuses on the cognitive development of children and children's readiness to learn the complexity of the task. It has been demonstrated that infants as young as 6 months can be trained to signal the need to urinate or defecate and suppress emptying for brief periods.

Toilet training is potentially both a rewarding and frustrating experience for children and parents. Parents may have unrealistic expectations of their children's capability or may be very intolerant of normal accidents that occur in the training process. It is important for physicians to introduce the topic of toilet training early on to prevent these unrealistic expectations. Children's refusal to toilet train or accidents related to toilet training are often cited as a precipitating event for child physical abuse. It is recommended that the issue of toilet training be introduced and anticipatory guidance provided by the age of 18 to 24 months to help parents develop reasonable expectations.

Epidemiology

The age at which children are toilet trained varies depending on social considerations and social pressures. Prior to the 1920s, the American approach to toilet training was permissive. This attitude then changed, and the methods became more rigorous, requiring that children be trained at an earlier age. In 1947 only 5% of children were not trained by 33 months of age, but by 1975, this figure had increased to 42%. Currently approximately 25% of typically developing American children are daytime toilet trained at 24 months and 98% by 48 months, although many parents expect their child to be trained by 18 months. Cultural and socioeconomic factors also influence parental beliefs about toilet training. Horn and colleagues found that white race and higher family income were associated with parents favoring later initiation of toilet training. There has been a renewed interest in earlier toilet training in the United States. This has been attributed to 3 societal factors: the lower cost and increased options for child care and schooling associated with children once toilet trained, concerns about contagious illnesses such as hepatitis and infectious diarrhea in child care facilities where diapers are changed, and the adverse environmental effects of nonbiodegradable disposable diapers. There may be some reversal in these trends related to the development of highly absorbent, biodegradable disposable diapers that are also flushable, and the marketing of nighttime pull-ups to children as old as 4 years.

As a general rule, girls are trained a bit earlier than boys, but only by a matter of a few months. Most children (80%) are trained simultaneously for bladder and bowel control. Approximately 12% are trained first for bowel control and about 8% for bladder control. Girls achieve nighttime continence at a younger age than boys.

Pathophysiology

Toilet training involves the ability both to inhibit a normal reflex release action and then relax the inhibition of the involved muscles. For the process to be successful, a certain degree of neurologic and biological development is essential. Myelinization of the pyramidal tracts and conditioned reflex sphincter control are necessary. Voluntary control is evidenced by myelinization of the pyramidal tracts by the age of 12 to 18 months. Conditioned reflex sphincter control occurs by 9 months of age and voluntary cooperation between 12 to 15 months of age. In assessing the neurologic development of children, walking is viewed as one of the milestones that indicate motor readiness for toilet training.

Toilet training depends on both physiological and psychological readiness. Cognitive development is assessed by a child's ability to follow certain instructions. Two years of age has been suggested as the appropriate age to initiate toilet training in most children. Toilet training usually takes 2 weeks to 2 months to learn, although training may occur in less time using more intense conditioning methods.

Differential Diagnosis

The differential diagnosis of toilet-training difficulties focuses on factors that contribute to a delay in acquisition of skills. Physicians should look for associated symptoms such as dysuria, a weak urinary stream, constantly wet underwear, or fecal soiling when assessing children who continue to manifest signs of either urinary or stool incontinence. In addition, it is important to determine if children are essentially toilet trained but are having intermittent accidents.

Voiding dysfunctions involve an abnormal voiding pattern stemming from a problem with the bladder filling or emptying. They are characterized by urine leakage, an increase in urgency, and an increase in frequency, and often result in frequent urinary tract infections (UTIs). The most common cause of isolated daytime wetting in previously trained children is **UTI** (see Chapter 52). **Chemical urethritis** may also be associated with urinary incontinence. **Stress incontinence,** which has also been called *giggle incontinence,* may result in wetting. **Urgency incontinence** occurs when children delay going to the bathroom and then are unable to hold urine any longer. Some children have ectopic ureters, which can empty into the lower portion of the bladder, vagina, or urethra and cause a constant dribble of urine. **Labial fusion** with **vaginal reflux of urine** may also be associated with daytime wetting. Urine pools behind the fused labia or labia that do not separate sufficiently to allow natural egress during voiding, and when children stand up the urine exits. Children with **neurogenic bladders** may also have symptoms of daytime enuresis.

Stooling accidents may be associated with chronic **constipation** and overflow incontinence or with Hirschsprung disease (see Chapter 53). Stool toileting refusal occurs when a child is trained to urinate in the toilet but refuses to defecate in the toilet for at least 1 month. While many parents view stool toileting refusal as insignificant, it is often associated with developing encopresis, constipation, painful bowel movements, and delayed completion of toilet training.

Children who prefer to stand in a corner to defecate should be commended for recognizing their physiological urge. However, parents should be aware that children who hide while stooling in their diaper are more likely to exhibit stool toileting refusal and be constipated. Successful treatment of constipation may decrease the incidence of toileting refusal.

Evaluation

History

Typically developing toddlers should be assessed for both their physiological and psychological readiness to initiate toilet training, as well as any underlying medical conditions that may affect their ability to learn toileting skills at the customary age. Physicians should provide anticipatory guidance to parents about toileting readiness. Affirmative answers should be obtained to the following 3 questions:

1. Do children exhibit bladder control as evidenced by (1) periods of dryness that last up to 2 hours and (2) facial expressions that show their physiological response to the elimination process?
2. Do children have the motor skills necessary to get around? This essentially involves the children's ability to walk and remove their clothing.
3. Do children have the cognitive ability to understand the task at hand?

Cognitive ability can be assessed by giving children 10 one-step tasks and seeing if they are able to carry out at least 8 of the 10 tasks (Box 45-1). The ability to carry out these tasks does not ensure a willingness to be toilet trained.

Stress in the home may negatively affect a toddler's ability to master the task of toilet training. The physician might counsel a family to delay toilet training if the family has moved recently; the birth of a new baby is expected; or there has been a major family crisis, such as a death or serious illness.

Children who have had difficulties with toilet training need to undergo a similar assessment.

Physical Examination

A physical examination to rule out underlying problems such as spina bifida occulta, which may be associated with a neurogenic bladder, should be performed. A neurologic examination may reveal nerve damage impeding muscles from relaxing or tightening at the right time. A careful examination of the genitalia is important in children who are having urinary incontinence to determine if conditions such as labial fusion, meatal stenosis, or posterior urethral valves are

Box 45-1. Requests or Imperatives Used to Help Assess Toilet-Training Readiness	
Bring me the ball.	Give the pen to your mom.
Go to the door.	Put the ball on the table.
Sit on the chair.	Put the doll on the floor.
Pick up the doll.	Take off your shoes.
Open the door.	Open the book.

evident. In children who are having stooling problems, physicians should check for an abdomen with feces-filled intestines, a sign of obstipation. In addition, a rectal examination should be considered to determine the presence of hard or impacted stools or any other abnormalities in the anal area.

Laboratory Tests

Although a laboratory assessment is not indicated in normal toddlers who are being toilet trained, diagnostic studies may be appropriate in children who are having problems with training. In older children, urinalysis may show evidence of a UTI.

Management

Physicians should help parents understand the appropriate approach to the toilet-training process. Unfortunately, most parents do not obtain the necessary advice from physicians. In one report, no parents attending a clinic and only 7% of parents in a private practice received advice about toilet training from their physicians. Therefore, it is important for physicians to initiate the discussion early enough to prevent the development of any problems.

There are 2 main contrasting styles of toilet training, although reliable efficacy studies are lacking. The first method described by Azrin and Foxx is parent-oriented and uses intense operant conditioning methods and a potty doll to assist with learning. The 5 components of the method include increasing the amount of fluids consumed; regularly scheduled times for toileting starting with 15-minute intervals; positive reinforcement for asking about, approaching, or sitting on the potty chair; grasping pants and successful urinating or defecating in the potty chair; time-out from positive reinforcement/cleanliness training following accidents; and teaching the child to differentiate between wet and dry pants, checking for dry pants every 5 minutes. Though this method has been effective in training children, including those individuals with mental disabilities, it is not recommended for training typically developing children.

The second method, endorsed by the American Academy of Pediatrics (AAP), is a child-oriented approach that stresses the child's physiological and psychological readiness to toilet train. There are 3 versions of this approach: Brazelton, AAP guidelines, and Dr Spock's approach. All versions use the same components, with only minor deviations. This method involves gradual training and emphasizes the use of **rewards,** not punishments. Children with autism who do not understand the social reward system advocated by this method may benefit from the intense conditioning methods described by Azrin and Foxx.

When toilet training typically developing children, parents should be advised to take the following approach:

1. Teach children the **appropriate vocabulary** related to the toilet-training process. This could include words such as "pee," "poop," "urine," "stool," "dry," "wet," "clean," "messy," and "potty."
2. Tell children what the **purpose of the potty** is. Placing the contents of a soiled diaper into the toilet can educate them on the purpose of the potty. In general, a child potty chair should be purchased. The potty chair has a number of advantages over the toilet. Parents can encourage children to decorate the potty and put their names on it. The potty can be kept in a place where children spend much of their time, not necessarily in the bathroom. Children can sit on the potty and have their feet on the floor, which is more physiologically sound and gives them a greater sense of security. Parents should suggest that children stand fully clothed in the bathroom as an initial step in encouraging their use of a potty. Children should be allowed to sit on the potty with their clothes on for about a week before the process of toilet training begins. Then children should sit on the potty without their clothes on, but no attempt to catch either stool or urine should be made. Boys should learn to urinate in the seated position because they may otherwise resist sitting for defecation.

When away from home, the potty chair should be packed to maintain the established routine. It is important that all individuals caring for the child (grandparents, babysitters) understand the parents' plans for toilet training.

Toilet adapter rings can be used if the family is resistant to using a potty chair, or if the transition from a potty chair to the toilet is likely to be stressful, as is true for many children with autism. Adapter rings fit directly onto the toilet and do not require emptying, as do separate potty chairs. They require that the toddler climb up on the toilet, and they need to be removed for others to use the toilet. A stool should be used to aid in climbing onto the toilet as well as to provide more leverage while defecating.

3. Encourage cleanliness and dryness by **changing children frequently.** Parents should ask their children whether they need to be changed using the appropriate vocabulary. This phase is important to continue as the toilet-training process proceeds. Some parents mistakenly do not change their soiled children as a means of punishing them for having accidents. This gives children a confusing message about the need for cleanliness.
4. Explain the **connection between dry pants and going to the potty** to children. Children should understand that dry pants feel good and that they can keep their pants dry by going to the potty.
5. Help children understand the **physiological signals** for using the toilet. Parents can facilitate this by observing children's behavior around the time of elimination and making comments such as, "When you jump up and down like that, Mommy knows you have to go to the bathroom."
6. Children must have the physiological ability to postpone the "urge to go." This usually occurs when children have the ability to delay voiding for at least 2 hours. Parents then can initiate toilet training by taking children to the bathroom at 2 hour intervals. In addition, children should sit on the toilet immediately after naps and 20 minutes after meals. Children should not be left on the toilet for more than 5 minutes and should be permitted to get up if they want. While sitting on the potty, they can be entertained with reading a story or playing games. It is helpful to have designated toys or books enjoyed only when the child is sitting on the potty. Parents are encouraged to rotate the toys so potty training continues to be interesting to the child.

Additional suggestions involve allowing children to have their clothes off and keeping the potty chair near them during play. This facilitates using the potty and is reminiscent of the practice of using split pants in China.

Children who use the potty successfully should be rewarded. Rewards can be in the form of verbal comments such as "Mommy is so proud of you," hand clapping, or the use of star charts that can be redeemed for rewards. Children can be consulted about what rewards they like. The AAP recommends using praise rather than treats for reinforcement. Punishment should not be used, particularly physical punishment. One report indicates that 15% of parents of clinic patients believe that spanking their children for accidents is acceptable. Parental disapproval of accidents can be articulated; however, parents should understand that accidents may continue to occur for months. Regression in a toilet-trained child may also occur with stressors such as a recent move, new sibling, or divorce.

There are 2 additional conditioning methods less commonly used in North America. The first is assisted infant toilet training and begins when the infant is 2 to 3 weeks of age. The infant is placed over a toilet after feeding or if showing signs of elimination, and is rewarded with food or affection for voiding or stooling. The second method focuses on elimination communication and begins at birth. The parent learns infant body language, noises, and elimination patterns. The parent also makes noises, such as the sound of running water, to associate with voiding while the infant is placed in positions to facilitate elimination. Interest in these conditioning methods has increased over the past few years.

If children are trained on a potty chair, they can generally begin using a toilet between 2½ to 3½ years of age. Children should wash their hands following sessions sitting on the toilet. Children can also use training pants, which are thickened underwear, or pull-ups, which are diaper-like underwear, rather than diapers. Pull-ups are now marketed to children as old as 4 to 5 years, and there is anecdotal evidence to suggest that the age of completion of toilet training may be delayed by the use of pull-ups. Regular underwear is promoted as advantageous because it feels different from diapers and encourages the use of the potty. Using a bigger size or snipping the waistband facilitates children's ability to remove their underpants and can be recommended.

If children demonstrate resistance to toilet training, the process should be delayed for 1 to 2 months. Children who learn how to withhold need additional time to learn how to relax their sphincter when sitting on a potty. It is important for parents to avoid an aggressiveness/resistance struggle, because this then may become the source of future bowel problems, including constipation. Children who are regular, particularly those who have a bowel movement at the same time every day, are more easily toilet trained.

Some children seem fearful of certain aspects of the toilet-training process. These include fear of falling into the toilet (this is circumvented with the use of a potty or toilet adapter rings) or fear of the loud noise of the flush. Allowing the child to flush the toilet without using it may dispel the fear. Toilet phobias can cause a child to hold their urine until the last moment, resulting in wetting, or can cause a child to hurry and not fully empty their bladder, resulting in possible infections. Some children become fascinated with flushing or unrolling toilet paper, and parents should discourage children from wasting water or paper.

One of the major components of toilet training children is **modeling.** Children should be allowed to enter the bathroom with the parents and even sit on the potty chair as one or the other parent sits on the toilet. Some children who are very strong-willed and independent, coupled with perfectionist parents, may have problems with toilet training.

Special considerations have to be made for children attending child care. Their teachers should be advised about the toilet training. Children should have "open bathroom privileges," which means that they should be permitted to leave the room to go to the bathroom without raising their hands or other reminders. Child care offers the advantage of peer modeling and peer pressure during the toilet-training process. Potty chairs should not be used in child care settings because of the risk of infectious diseases.

Children with special needs generally encounter more obstacles when mastering toileting. Communication delays, decreased motor skills, sensitivity to stimulation, and preference for routine are just a few of the additional challenges that make it difficult to ascertain whether the child is ready to toilet train. Although incontinence was once thought to be inevitable for children with special needs, it is important for parents to understand that continence can be achieved but that expectations need to modified (may take until age 5 to achieve and standard toilet training methods rarely are successful).

Medications have a limited role in toilet training. Some physicians recommend the use of drugs to increase bladder capacity. Although tolterodine and oxybutynin (Ditropan) increase bladder capacity and decrease the frequency of bladder contraction, they should not be used because they do not assist children with the toilet-training process. However, children who are constipated may require stool softeners, such as mineral oil, or the addition of fiber bulk to their diet and increased fluid consumption to facilitate the stooling process. Physicians should see children who seem to have particularly challenging toilet-training problems on a weekly or biweekly basis until they show improvement.

Parents can also be referred to the many books on toilet training, particularly if problems develop. Many books are geared for children to help them understand their body and the elimination process. Videotapes are also available to help children with toilet training. Children may also have the opportunity to practice with dolls designed to wet or poop after being fed.

Prognosis

All typically developing children are eventually toilet trained. The age when this occurs varies and is significant only if it restricts children from participating in school.

Selected References

Physicians

Blum NJ, Taubman B, Nemeth N. During toilet training, constipation occurs before stool toileting refusal. *Pediatrics.* 2004;113:e520–e522

Choby BA, George S. Toilet training. *Am Fam Physician.* 2008;78:1059–1064

Harris A. Toilet training children with learning difficulties: what the literature tells us. *Br J Nurs.* 2004;13:773–777

Horn IB, Brenner R, Rao M, Cheng TL. Beliefs about the appropriate age for initiating toilet training: are there racial and socioeconomic differences? *J Pediatr.* 2006;149:165–168

Kiddoo D, Klassen TP, Lang ME, et al. *The Effectiveness of Different Methods of Toilet Training for Bowel and Bladder Control.* Rockville, MD: Agency for Healthcare Research and Quality; 2006: No.07-E003

Macias MM, Roberts KM, Saylor CF, Fussell JJ. Toilet concerns, parenting stress, and behavior problems in children with special health care needs. *Clin Pediatr (Phila).* 2006;45:415–422

Mota DM, Barros AJ. Toilet training: methods, parental expectations and associated dysfunctions. *J Pediatr (Rio J).* 2008;84:9–17

Taubman B, Blum N, Nemeth N. Children who hide while defecating before they have completed toilet training. A prospective study. *Arch Pediatr Adolesc Med.* 2003;157:1190–1192

Toilet training guidelines: clinicians—the role of the clinician in toilet training. *Pediatrics.* 1999;103:1364–1366

Toilet training guidelines: day care providers—the role of the day care provider in toilet training. *Pediatrics.* 1999;103:1367–1368

Toilet training guidelines: parents—the role of the parents in toilet training. *Pediatrics.* 1999;103:1362–1363

Vermandel A, Van Kampen M, Van Gorp C, Wyndaele JJ. How to toilet train healthy children? A review of the literature. *Neurol Urodyn.* 2008;27:162–166

Parents and Children

American Academy of Pediatrics. *Guide to Toilet Training.* Wolraich ML, ed. Elk Grove Village, IL: American Academy of Pediatrics; 2003

Azrin NH, Foxx RM. *Toilet Training in Less Than a Day.* New York, NY: Simon & Schuster; 1974

Bennett HJ. *It Hurts When I Poop!: A Story For Children Who Are Scared to Use the Potty.* Washington, DC: Magination Press; 2007

Berger S. *Princess Potty.* New York, NY: Cartwheel Books; 2010

Berry R. *It's Potty Time for Boys.* La Jolla, CA: Penton Overseas Inc; 2009

Brooks JG. *I'm a Big Kid Now.* Neenah, WI: Kimberly-Clark Corporation; 1990

Foote T. *My Potty Reward Stickers for Boys: 126 Boy Potty Training Stickers and Chart to Motivate Toilet Training.* New York, NY: Tracy Trends; 2006

Foote T. *My Potty Reward Stickers for Girls: 126 Girl Potty Training Stickers and Chart to Motivate Toilet Training.* New York, NY: Tracy Trends; 2006

Frankel A. *Once Upon a Potty.* Hauppauge, NY: Barron's Educational Series, Inc.; 1980

Gomi T. *Everyone Poops.* La Jolla, CA: Kane/Miller; 2001

Hochman D. *The Potty Train.* New York: NY: Simon & Schuster; 2008

Katz K. *A Potty for Me!: A Lift-the-Flap Instructional Manual.* New York: NY: Little Simon; 2004

Mack A. *Toilet Learning: The Picture Book Technique for Children and Parents.* Boston, MA: Little, Brown and Company; 1978

Mayer G, Mayer M. *The New Potty.* New York, NY: Golden Book Publishing Company, Inc; 1992

Miller V. *On Your Potty.* Cambridge, MA: Candlewick Press; 1994

Pinnington A. *Big Girls Use the Potty!* New York, NY: DK Publishing; 2008

Rogers F. *Going to the Potty.* New York, NY: Penguin Putnam Books for Young Readers; 1986

Smith DC, McClure D. *Monkey Learns to Potty.* Knoxville, TN: PottyMD LLC; 2004

CHAPTER 46

Crying and Colic

Geeta Grover, MD

CASE STUDY

The parents of a 2-week-old infant bring their son to the emergency department because he has been crying persistently for the past 4 hours. He has no history of fever, vomiting, diarrhea, upper respiratory tract infection, or change in feeding. The infant is breastfed.

On physical examination, the infant appears well developed and well nourished. His weight is 7 lb, 7 oz—7 oz more than when he was born. Although he is fussy and crying, he is afebrile with normal vital signs. The remainder of the physical examination is within normal limits.

Questions

1. What is the normal crying pattern in young infants?
2. What is colic?
3. What conditions are associated with prolonged crying in young infants?
4. What are key factors in the history of crying infants?
5. What laboratory tests are indicated in crying infants?
6. What are a few of the management strategies that can be used by parents to soothe their crying or colicky infants?

Crying, an important method of communication between infants and caregivers, is nonspecific, and many stimuli can produce the same response (eg, hunger, fatigue, pain). Parents report that they can discriminate among various types of cries in their infants. Crying can be divided into 3 categories: (1) normal or physiological crying, (2) excessive crying secondary to distress (eg, hunger) or disease, and (3) excessive crying without an apparent cause.

The difference between normal and excessive crying may be more qualitative than quantitative. Some investigators have used the pneumonic **PURPLE** to characterize crying during early infancy focusing on the qualities that make the crying particularly frustrating to caregivers: **P:** peak pattern (increases weekly until 2 months of age), **U:** unexpected bouts of crying, **R:** resistance to soothing measures, **P:** pain-like facial grimacing, **L:** long periods of crying, **E:** evening clustering. Deciding whether crying is excessive varies with parents' expectations and thresholds. Expressed parental concern about extreme crying or fussiness requires attention. If parents complain that infants cry inconsolably or continuously as well as excessively, the crying may have an underlying organic etiology.

Colic, a poorly understood, benign, self-limited condition, falls into the third category. It manifests as unexplained crying or fussing in infants that usually occurs in the late afternoon or evening. During an episode of colic, infants cry and may either draw the knees up to the chest or rigidly stiffen the legs, flex the elbows, clench the fists, and turn red (Figure 46-1). Although infants may appear to be totally miserable during an episode of colic, they are otherwise healthy, eat well, and demonstrate good weight gain.

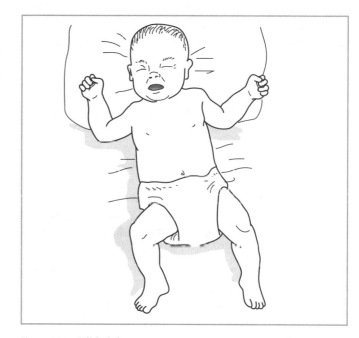

Figure 46-1. Colicky infant.

Epidemiology

Qualitatively, **excessive crying** is any amount of crying that concerns or worries parents. Quantitatively, definitions of excessive crying have been based on the results of Brazelton's study of normal infants. Excessive crying begins at 2 weeks of age (median daily crying time about 2 hours per day), peaks at 6 weeks of age (median daily crying time about 3 hours per day), and then decreases to less than 1 hour per day by 12 weeks of age. Apparently, more crying occurs during the evening hours, especially between the ages of 3 and 6 weeks.

Although many infants exhibit a fairly similar pattern of fussiness that peaks at about 6 weeks of age, infants with colic tend to be inconsolable for longer periods and cry with more intensity. **Colic** affects 10% to 20% of infants younger than 3 months. There is no seasonal variation in its occurrence, and breastfed and formula-fed infants are affected equally. Colic usually begins at 2 to 3 weeks, peaks at 6 to 8 weeks, and resolves by 3 to 4 months of age. In studies of infant colic, the definition of colic that is cited most frequently is the Wessel definition, which describes colicky infants as having unexplained paroxysmal bouts of fussing and crying that last for more than 3 hours a day, for more than 3 days a week, and for more than 3 weeks' duration ("rule of threes").

Clinical Presentation

Colicky infants are otherwise healthy infants younger than 3 months who cry or fuss inconsolably for extended periods, usually during the afternoon or evening. The crying usually resolves within a few hours.

Pathophysiology

Crying is a complex vocalization that changes during the first year of life as infants develop. In the first few weeks of life, crying is a signal that infants are experiencing a disturbance in homeostatic regulation (eg, hunger, discomfort). As infants mature and begin to differentiate internal from external stimuli, crying may also be an indication of too little or too much environmental stimulation. During the second half of the first year, as infants mature neurologically and gain voluntary control over vocalizations, crying can be an expression of different affects (eg, frustration, fear).

A variety of explanations for the etiology of **colic** have been proposed. Some authorities believe that colic may not be a pathologic entity but simply an extreme variant of normal crying. The condition may result from an allergy, cow's milk intolerance, abnormal intestinal peristalsis, or increased intestinal gas, which are some of the more frequently associated factors. Others have proposed that colic is caused by problems in the interaction between infants and their environment, specifically their parents. This interactional theory requires not only excessive crying on the part of the infant, but also an inability of the parents to soothe the crying infant. The "missing fourth trimester" theory of colic posits that infants cry because they are born "3 months too soon" (ie, human gestation should last 3 months longer). There is no scientific evidence to support this hypothesis. Whether maternal anxiety has any role in colic remains a controversial issue. More than one of these factors may contribute to the pathogenesis of colic.

Differential Diagnosis

An acute episode of excessive crying may be secondary to disease (eg, fever, otitis media). An organic etiology should be suspected in infants who present with inconsolable crying of acute onset. Box 46-1 lists the most common causes. Some conditions occur in

Box 46-1. Most Common Causes of Acute Unexplained, Excessive Crying in Infants
Idiopathic[a]
Colic[a]
Infectious
Otitis media
Urinary tract infection
Stomatitis
Meningitis
Gastrointestinal[a]
Constipation
Anal fissure
Gaseous distention
Peristalsis problems
Reflux
Intussusception
Trauma
Corneal abrasion
Foreign body in the eye
Hair tourniquet syndrome
Behavioral[a]
Overstimulation
Persistent night awakening
Drug Reactions
Immunization reactions (previously common: with diphtheria-tetanus-pertussis vaccine)
Neonatal drug withdrawal (narcotics)
Child Abuse
Long bone fractures
Retinal hemorrhage
Intracranial hemorrhage
Hematologic[a]
Sickle cell crisis
Cardiovascular
Arrhythmia (supraventricular tachycardia)
Congestive heart failure
Anomalous left coronary artery

[a]May present as acute or recurrent episodes of excessive crying.

a more chronic or recurrent pattern, particularly if the condition is not treated.

The differential diagnosis of infants who experience recurrent episodes of excessive crying or recurrent night awakenings associated with crying focuses more on behavior and temperament. Colic, neonatal drug withdrawal, or difficult infant temperament (eg, extreme fussiness) may cause recurrent crying. Recurrent night awakening and difficult infant temperament are discussed in Chapters 25 and 48, respectively.

Evaluation

A thorough history and physical examination usually provide clues to the diagnosis in instances of acute onset of crying.

History

The focus of the history should be on determining the presence of any associated symptoms. In addition, the circumstances surrounding the crying (eg, occurrence during day or night) should be ascertained (Questions Box).

Physical Examination

A thorough physical examination is required for accurate diagnosis. Particular attention should be given to the following aspects of the examination:

1. Careful inspection of the skin after all clothing has been removed to look for any suspicious bruises or marks
2. Palpation of all long bones to detect fractures
3. Examination of all digits and the penis to check for hair tourniquets (single strands of hair wrapped around digits or the penis)
4. Examination of the retina to look for retinal hemorrhages (a sign of intracranial hemorrhage)
5. Eversion of the eyelids to check for foreign bodies
6. Fluorescein staining of the cornea to look for corneal abrasion

Laboratory Tests

Except for urinalysis, most screening laboratory tests are probably not useful. Test selection can be guided by the history and physical examination (eg, infants with fever without an apparent cause should have a septic workup, with an examination of blood, urine, and cerebrospinal fluid). Urinalysis, which may provide clues to an underlying metabolic deficiency, is sometimes helpful. Even when the initial history and physical examination are non-diagnostic, infants who persist in crying inconsolably should be suspected of having a serious underlying condition (eg, intracranial hemorrhage, drug ingestion). Such infants may warrant an extended period of observation or a more extensive workup that includes laboratory assessment.

Imaging Studies

Roentgenographic studies such as long bone radiographs may be necessary in some situations (eg, infants with long bone pain on palpation, suspicion of child abuse). Infants with retinal hemorrhages should have a computed tomography scan.

Management

Management and treatment depend on identification of the cause of the crying. Underlying organic conditions (eg, urinary tract infection, fractures) should be treated. Management of colic depends on presumptions regarding its etiology. It is important for practitioners to **reassure** parents regarding the benign nature of colic and its resolution over time. Physicians should provide a caring and supportive environment in which the parents may express their concerns and frustrations. Reassurance along with practical suggestions regarding infant feeding and handling techniques (eg, cuddling, swaddling, or rocking) may often suffice.

Some management strategies have specifically been developed to reduce the risk that an infant will be injured by a frustrated caregiver.

Crying and Colic — Questions

- Is this the first time the infant has cried inconsolably or does this happen on a recurring basis?
- Has the infant had a fever?
- Does the infant have any cold symptoms, vomiting, or diarrhea?
- Is the infant having any difficulty feeding? Is the infant formula-fed or breastfed?
- Has the infant had a recent fall or accident?
- What do you do when your infant cries?

Educational materials in the form of booklets and instructive DVDs have been used to prevent the risk of abusive head trauma.

Management suggestions for colic should be customized for infants and families. The more common management techniques are listed in Box 46-2. Complementary and alternative medicine therapies have been used historically to treat colic. Evidence from recent small clinical trials and pilot studies have shown that some natural health products, nutritional modulation, cranial osteopathy, infant massage, and parental behavioral training have some promise in the treatment of infantile colic, but larger confirmatory trials are needed to address concerns regarding both safety and efficacy.

Changes in sensory input (eg, soothing sounds or motions) may resolve crying and soothe colicky infants. According to the "missing fourth trimester" theory of colic, re-creating the sensory environment of the womb calms infants by triggering a soothing response—the calming reflex—and promotes relaxation. Five maneuvers (swaddling, side or stomach position, shushing, swinging, and sucking—"the 5 Ss") that mimic uterine sensations are noted to activate this calming reflex. It is further recommended by proponents of this theory that 3 to 5 of these maneuvers should be performed simultaneously and vigorously to activate the calming reflex.

Prophylactic measures to prevent the passage of swallowed air through the pylorus can also be useful. Such techniques include feeding in an upright position and limiting the period of sucking at the breast or bottle to about 10 minutes (after this time, greater amounts of air are swallowed relative to the amount of milk ingested). Some infants eat very fast and swallow a lot of air. Burping these infants every 5 to 10 minutes during feeds may help alleviate

---

Box 46-2. Management of Colic

Parental reassurance

Parental education

Alteration in techniques of infant feeding and handling

Alteration of sensory input to infant

Prevention of swallowed air from passing through pylorus

Dietary alterations

Medication

Complementary and alternative medicine therapies

Increased carrying

Responding quickly to crying

discomfort due to excessive air swallowing (aerophagia). Decreasing the size of the opening of a nipple in a bottle-fed infant may reduce the amount of air-swallowing.

Methods to decrease intestinal spasm (eg, abdominal massage, warm baths, avoidance of overfeeding) may be helpful. The use of suppositories or rectal thermometers to break up rectal spasm and thereby release retained gas should be discouraged.

Data regarding **dietary changes,** such as the use of hypoallergenic diets by breastfeeding mothers, have been inconclusive but suggest that there may be some therapeutic benefits. Similarly, the use of soy-based or hypoallergenic infant formulas also seem to have beneficial effects on the symptoms of colic. Generally, these dietary modifications should be reserved for infants with additional symptoms of allergy (eg, wheezing, rash) or intolerance (eg, vomiting, diarrhea, hematochezia, or weight loss).

Various drugs, including anticholinergics, motility-enhancing agents, barbiturates, laxatives, and anti-flatulents, have limited success and are best avoided. Currently, anti-flatulents (eg, simethicone) are prescribed most commonly. Despite lack of scientific evidence to support their efficacy, parents indicate that they are effective.

As long as no adverse effects are evident, limited amounts (eg, 1–2 oz per day) of **herbal remedies** (eg, chamomile tea) can be supported if parents report satisfaction. Over-the-counter homeopathic preparations are also innocuous and have no scientifically demonstrated efficacy, but may be advocated as helpful by some parents.

Finally, the practitioner should encourage parents to respond to the infant's cries quickly and carry the infant as much as possible (eg, at least 3–4 hours daily). Parents should be advised that they cannot "spoil" infants younger than 4 months and that they might actually improve behavior by their own increased responsiveness.

Presently, the best evidence-based approaches to the management of colic include holding, swaddling, and comforting an infant; a trial of dietary modifications; limited amounts of herbal teas; and attempting to minimize environmental stimulation levels.

Prognosis

Fortunately, the natural history of persistent crying during infancy is resolution over time. Long-term sequelae of infant colic that have been identified include possible relationships with irritable bowel syndrome and increased levels of externalizing behavior problems (eg, hyperactivity, conduct concerns, and decreased adaptability) in childhood.

CASE RESOLUTION

The infant described in the case history is experiencing an acute episode of unexplained crying. Despite a normal physical examination, he was observed for 1 hour in the emergency department because his crying persisted. Subsequently, a septic workup was initiated, which revealed that a urinary tract infection was the source of the irritability.

Selected References

Barr RG, Paterson JA, Macmartin LM, Lehtonen L, Young SN. Prolonged and unsoothable crying bouts in infants with and without colic. *J Dev Behav Pediatr.* 2005;26:14–23

Barr RG, Rivara FP, Barr M, Cummings P, et al. Effectiveness of educational materials designed to change knowledge and behaviors regarding crying and shaken baby syndrome in mothers of newborns: a randomized, controlled trial. *Pediatrics.* 2009;123:972–980

Brazelton TB. Crying in infancy. *Pediatrics.* 1962;29:579–588

Garrison MM, Christakis DA. A systematic review of treatments for infant colic. *Pediatrics.* 2000;106:184–190

Herman M, Le A. The crying infant. *Emerg Med Clin North Am.* 2007:25(4):1137–1159

Karp H. The "fourth trimester": a framework and strategy for understanding and resolving colic. *Contemp Pediatr.* 2004;21:94–116

Rosen LD, Bukutu C, Le C, Shamseer L, Vohra S. Complementary, holistic, and integrative medicine: colic. *Pediatr Rev.* 2007:28:381–385

Wessel MA, Cobb JC, Jackson EB, Harris GS, Detwiler AC. Paroxysmal fussing in infancy, sometimes called "colic." *Pediatrics.* 1954;14:421–434

CHAPTER 47

Discipline

Carol D. Berkowitz, MD

CASE STUDY

A 3-year-old boy is being threatened with expulsion from preschool because he is biting the other children. His mother states that he is very active and aggressive toward other children. In addition, his language development is delayed. She is at her wit's end about what to do. The birth history is normal, and the mother denies the use of drugs or cigarettes, but she drank socially before she realized she was pregnant. The medical and family histories are noncontributory, and the physical examination is normal.

Questions

1. What is the definition of discipline?
2. What are the 3 key components of discipline?
3. What strategies can parents use to discipline children?
4. What are the guidelines for using time-out?
5. What is meant by parental monitoring?
6. What is the relationship between corporal punishment and child abuse?

Discipline can be defined as an educational process in which children learn how to behave in a socially acceptable manner. The word is derived from *disciplinare,* meaning to teach or instruct. It involves a complex set of interactions of attitudes, models, instructions, rewards, and punishments. Discipline is not synonymous with punishment. The goal is to help children gain self-control and respect for others and to learn behavior that is appropriate for given situations. It is also to ensure a child's safety in the environment. Proactive discipline is action taken by parents to encourage good behavior, and reactive discipline is parental action following misbehavior. To be effective, child discipline must have 3 components: a learning environment with a positive supportive parent–child relationship, a refined strategy for teaching and reinforcing desired behaviors, and a defined strategy for decreasing or extinguishing undesired behaviors. Children thrive in a supportive environment in which they are praised for socially appropriate behavior and are able to participate in the responsibilities and activities of the household. Parents, however, are more often interested in eliminating unwanted behaviors and may bring these specific concerns to their pediatrician.

Parental monitoring relates to the oversight of children's activities at home, in school, and in the community. The extent and form of parental monitoring varies with the age of the child. Parental monitoring occurs when parents ask their children: "With whom are you going to be? Where are you going? What will you be doing?" Parental oversight involves children's access to and use of the Internet and social media (Chapter 9). Inadequate parental monitoring has long-term sequelae, including a greater incidence of risk-related behaviors. Parental monitoring must be coupled with parental discipline to promote desirable behaviors and eliminate undesirable ones.

Physician–Parent Interactions Concerning Discipline

Practitioners can assist parents by giving them guidelines for appropriate childhood discipline related to both routine and problem development and to counsel about the scope of monitoring. The age and temperament of the child are important factors to consider. In addition, pediatricians can discourage corporal punishment as the major method of discipline. Pediatricians may also have a role in advising against corporal punishment in schools. While most states have banned corporal punishment in the school setting, 21 states still permit it.

It is important to encourage parents to establish a positive interactive environment with verbal communication, monitoring children's behavior and commending desirable behavior, ignoring trivial problems, and consistently applying predetermined consequences for misbehavior. Psychologist Marshall B. Rosenberg promotes the concept of compassionate communication using the analogy of the language of the giraffe, which is a language of requests, versus the language of the jackal, one of demands. Identifying feelings is integral to the language of giraffes. Rules should be simple, clear, and established ahead of time. Frequently physicians fail to inquire about children's behavior. Unless parents bring up the topic, it is not discussed during the physician visit. On average, physicians spend only 90 seconds per visit on anticipatory guidance and counseling. However, one survey of mothers in a physician waiting room showed that up to 90% were concerned about one aspect of behavior. Sixty percent of mothers surveyed found physician intervention quite helpful. The American Academy of Pediatrics recommends anticipatory guidance about discipline at each health maintenance visit between

9 months and 5 years. Such counseling is especially important to help parents understand the value of appropriate discipline in shaping their children's self-esteem. Information about discipline in the media may be confusing and contradictory, and often supports the unfounded approaches of nonprofessionals. Starting when a child is 5 years old, physician–parent discussions should include the notion of monitoring.

Early in the physician–parent relationship, physicians may express their interest in behavioral problems by saying, "I am interested not only in your child's physical well-being, but also in his (or her) growth and development and how he (or she) gets along with friends and family." They may then question parents about how children spend their days. During subsequent visits, pediatricians may say, "Parents of children of (child's name)'s age frequently worry about discipline. I wonder if you have any concerns." In making these inquiries, the physician may establish what factors, such as religious or ethnic beliefs, or family influences are shaping parents' decisions about discipline.

Problem Behaviors

Behavioral problems can be placed in 5 major categories.

1. **Problems of daily routine.** Such problems refer to the refusal of children to go about their daily activities, such as eating, going to bed, awakening at a certain time, and toilet training.
2. **Aggressive-resistant behavior.** This behavior is characterized by negativism and includes temper tantrums and aggressive responses to siblings and peers. Some undesirable behavior can place children or those around them in danger or at risk for injury.
3. **Overdependent or withdrawal behavior.** Such behavior is typical of children who are very attached to their mothers. These clingy children find separation difficult, especially in a preschool setting.
4. **Hyperactivity or excessive restlessness.**
5. **Undesirable habits,** which include thumb sucking, nail biting, throat clearing, and playing with genitals (see Chapter 51).

Some of the behaviors listed above are age-appropriate, and physicians can help parents by counseling them about stage-related behavior, such as oppositional behavior in a 2-year-old and independence-dependence problems in a 3- to 5-year-old. Parents may be more tolerant of a particular behavior if they understand what is normal at a given age. Just because something is normal, however, does not mean that it should be tolerated. Physicians can suggest to the parents ways of dealing with age-appropriate behavior (eg, placing breakable objects out of reach of toddlers).

Certain behavioral problems reflect differences in childhood temperaments. Temperament is the biological predisposition to a style of behavior. Carey has compiled a series of temperament scales

to assess children and adolescents of different ages. For example, some children are shy and have a hard time adjusting to new situations. If parents anticipate such problems, they are often less angry when difficulties arise. Parental expectations can vary with a child's gender. Boys may be permitted to act a certain way ("He's all boy!") that would be disapproved of in girls. Physicians can discuss such expectations at health maintenance visits.

Physicians can also be particularly helpful in detecting and advising parents about disparities in the achievement of different developmental skills. Some children acquire motor skills before verbal skills, yet parents expect their children to be equally versatile in speech and movement.

Psychophysiology

All behaviors are modified by the responses and reactions of other individuals. The basic premise of discipline is to discourage unwanted behavior and to encourage desired behavior. This is accomplished by using techniques that are based on conditioning modalities.

Several factors contribute to an increased incidence of behavioral problems in children. Ten percent to 15% of all preschool children are raised in grossly disrupted family situations. These homes are impacted by divorce, death, separation, violence, parental substance abuse, mental illness, or extreme poverty. Parental insecurity may also be a factor. In addition, families may have fewer social contacts than they once did because of greater mobility within society. As a result, families face greater social isolation.

Differential Diagnosis

In addition to providing anticipatory guidance about discipline, physicians must make 2 diagnostic decisions. First, they must determine whether a specific behavioral problem represents normal childhood behavior or an abnormality in behavior that warrants more specific intervention. Between 8% and 18% of behavioral disturbances may deserve physician intervention. More intensive management may be necessary for problems related to aggressive-resistant behavior and hyperactivity. Hyperactive behavior, which may exist as part of attention-deficit/hyperactivity disorder (ADHD), may be a sign of a significant underlying problem that warrants one-on-one intervention or the use of neuropharmacologic agents (see Chapter 125).

Second, physicians must differentiate between legally permitted corporal punishment and child abuse. Some individuals feel that any form of physical punishment is unacceptable and note studies that suggest that violence in the form of physical punishment is prone to escalate. Despite this, the use of physical punishment remains widely accepted in our society, and is legally condoned in the home setting though there may be guidelines about what exceeds the legal limits. Fractures and bruises are not acceptable, and physical abuse should be suspected in children who present with such injuries.

Evaluation

History

The key component in the evaluation process is the assessment of the means parents use to discipline children (Questions Box). To obtain this information, physicians may simply ask parents, "How do you get your child to mind you?" This question is designed to lead to a discussion of how parents interact with their children. If parents have specific complaints, such as oppositional behavior, they should be questioned about the strategies they have used in their effort to discipline their children.

Physical Examination

Children's behavior should be assessed during the office visit. A general physical examination is useful to check for any signs of physical abuse as well as to evaluate children's well-being. A developmental assessment is also helpful because it may delineate disparities in the achievement of certain skills. Some hyperactive children may warrant a more extensive psychodevelopmental assessment to look for findings consistent with ADHD. Behavioral checklists may be used to evaluate children's temperament.

Laboratory Tests

No specific laboratory or imaging studies are indicated for children with discipline problems. Such studies are indicated if child abuse is suspected (see Chapter 127).

Management

Physicians should assist parents in establishing appropriate guidelines for disciplining their children and reinforce the role of parents as the source of authority (Box 47-1). It is important for parents to realize that total freedom results in uncontrollable anxiety. Children mimic behavior, and **parents should act as role models.** If parents have temper tantrums when they are frustrated, their children may act in a similar manner. **Consistency** is also important. A system with a limited number of enforced rules is better than one with many different rules. In families where both parents are working, especially if they have overlapping time schedules, consistency is sometimes difficult to attain, especially if children are supervised by non-parental caregivers.

Physicians should emphasize to parents that it is best to **avoid power struggles.** Children engaged in a struggle often win because they have final control (eg, refusing to eat). Children should always be given the opportunity to graciously back out of a situation and save face. It is easier to avoid situations that lead to head-on confrontations than to get out of them once the confrontation has occurred. Parents should be the source of information for physicians. This helps strengthen parents' egos and validates their ability to handle their children appropriately.

In the past, specific methods of dealing with children with discipline problems concerned the issues of permissiveness versus over-permissiveness and accommodation versus strict punishment.

Questions

Discipline

- What does the child do that the parents wish he or she would not do?
- What do the parents do to stop unwanted behavior?
- Does the child usually obey the parents?
- When and where does most of the unwanted behavior occur? Does it occur mainly if a child is tired?
- Which parent is responsible for disciplining the child?

Box 47-1. Advice for Parents About Discipline

Set rules.

Set limits.

Define consequences.

Be consistent.

Ignore trivial problems.

Compliment desirable behavior.

Take time out when angry.

Over-permissiveness refers to the allowing of undesirable acts and may exacerbate anxiety and increase demands for privilege.

Physicians should remind parents that preventing many behavioral disorders is easier than treating them. Reasoning is a useful modality, but it is unrealistic to expect infants and toddlers to have the cognitive skills to understand adult reasoning or to consistently respond to verbal commands or reprimands. Discipline should not only discourage bad behavior but also reinforce good behavior. Following are 5 examples of reactive discipline.

Redirection

Redirection is a simple and effective method in which the parent removes the problem and distracts the child with an alternative. This technique is frequently used to remove some object (such as a valued knicknack) from the hands of an infant, replacing it with a toy. Parental patience, ingenuity, and enthusiasm facilitate this approach. This approach is also important in teaching children what is acceptable behavior. For instance, one cannot draw on the wall but can draw on a piece of paper. Children also respond to making tedious routines into a game. For instance, children can be challenged to see who can get their clothes on faster or who can brush their teeth first. Parental creativity and energy often avert confrontations.

Spanking

Spanking involves inflicting physical pain, which is usually successful in bringing about the immediate cessation or a decrease in problem behavior. Spanking is highly prevalent as a form of discipline, with between 70% and 94% of parents reporting using the practice. Spanking is used more often for younger children and for boys and correlates with parental attributes such as age, education, socioeconomic status, and religious orientation. Spanking is often employed when other methods of discipline have failed to abort the unwanted behavior. Spanking tends to clear the air and get the punishment over with rather than producing a lingering guilt. To be truly effective, however, physical punishment must immediately follow the act. The "wait until Daddy comes home" approach is less effective because of the lack of temporal association. In addition, spanking tends to become situation-specific so that children associate a particular action with being spanked. This learning does not generalize to other situations. Spanking can teach children to be afraid of adults rather than to respect them.

Spanking may actually be damaging to the parent–child relationship and have a long-term effect on a child's self-esteem. Many parents feel remorseful after having spanked a child, and some acknowledge that they spank out of anger and frustration and question the efficacy of this modality. Most pediatricians discourage spanking as a means of disciplining children. Differentiation of physical punishment from child abuse is often difficult. In general, punishment with the hands is acceptable, but punishment with objects and spanking on parts of the body other than the buttocks or thighs is unacceptable. Spanking may be an early precursor of later physical violence and subsequent abuse. Again, parents act as role models. Children should never be allowed to hit their parents. This makes children feel extremely insecure.

Devices that are marketed for child discipline and inflict physical pain on a child, such as a sudden sting (modified stun gun), are never appropriate.

Scolding

Scolding involves the excess use of reasoning and explanations and is used by most parents as part of the discipline process. In families where communication or interaction is minimal, scolding or verbal reprimands may result in an initial increase in inappropriate behavior because this is the only way children receive any attention. Verbal reprimands are more effective if used infrequently. Verbal reprimands should not be used during time-outs because they reinforce undesirable behavior.

Scolding, because of its negative focus, can be damaging to children's self-esteem. Scolding would be categorized as "jackal language."

Ignoring

Ignoring represents the opposite of explaining and reasoning. This form of discipline is difficult to use successfully because parents must totally ignore children's behavior. If even the least flicker of recognition occurs, then activity increases. A brief initial increase in unwanted behavior, a so-called response burst, may occur with ignoring. This disciplinary method works better in younger children.

Time-out and Removal of Privileges

Time-out, the form of discipline most recommended, refers to time out from positive reinforcement. In sports, teams call a time-out to rethink what they are doing and to replan their strategies. Children are placed in a neutral or boring environment whenever they engage in inappropriate behavior. The time-out technique can be used to discourage undesired habits. For example, parents may say, "You can suck your thumb, but you may only do it in such and such a room."

This type of discipline is better than ignoring, especially if "ignored" children are receiving attention from siblings and peers. Children should understand the rules ahead of time and why the behavior is unacceptable. Once this is accomplished, time-out may occur without any warning.

A timer should be used, and children should stay in the time-out area for 1 minute per 1 year of age. An appropriate area must be selected. This area should be fairly boring, so children's rooms are often not appropriate. A laundry room, a corner, or a specific chair may be better. If children act unacceptably during the time-out, the timer should be reset. If children have to go to the bathroom during the time-out, they are allowed one trip. After they return from the bathroom, the timer is reset.

The use of the time-out method is sometimes difficult. If the inappropriate behavior occurs in the morning when children are getting ready for school, time-out just encourages children's desire to delay. "Beat the buzzer" is another idea that may be used in such situations. With "beat the buzzer," the timer is set. If children are dressed before the timer goes off, they may be rewarded for the behavior by being allowed to go to bed half an hour later. If the buzzer "beats" them, then they have to go to bed half an hour earlier.

Inappropriate behavior away from home presents the greatest difficulty. These situations can be dealt with in numerous ways, particularly if the behavior problem involves temper tantrums. When children are crying or screaming uncontrollably, it is best to remove them from the embarrassment of the situation. This "manual guidance" often occurs in a supermarket, where children select something that parents do not wish to buy. Parents can often circumvent this problem easily by walking into the supermarket and saying, "If you are a good boy (or girl) during the whole trip, then I will get you something at the checkout counter." If children still have temper tantrums, then they should be removed from the area and brought to a neutral place, such as the automobile or a restroom, and allowed to finish their crying and screaming. It has been said that a glass of cold water splashed in a child's face is sometimes beneficial because it rapidly aborts the behavior. If the inappropriate behavior does not develop into a temper tantrum, then "marking" time-out is helpful. This consists of putting a mark with a colored water-soluble marker on the child's wrist every time he or she engages in an inappropriate behavior. When the child returns home, the marks are totaled, and the time-out method is used.

Removal of privileges is a strategy applied in older children. Classically this involves grounding a child, prohibiting television or video games, or loss of driving privileges. The privilege must be something of value to the child for this method to be effective.

Parents who complain about inappropriate behavior should be asked to keep a record of children's behavior for 1 to 2 weeks. This helps determine if the behavior is really inappropriate and what is motivating it. Parents should be encouraged to talk to their children in a reasonable manner and to verbalize what they think children are feeling. They might say something like this, "It's terrible to be three years old and get so upset. You feel that you can't get the things you want, but some day you will grow up and then you will be in charge.

I am really sorry it is so hard for you right now." Physicians should tell parents that it is important to set limits for children and to avoid threatening, judging, and constantly criticizing children. Frequent threats such as, "If you don't stop hitting your sister, you'll get a time-out" that are not carried out undermine the entire discipline process. To help foster compassionate communication, parents should ask themselves, "If someone said this to me, how would I feel?" Many parents have themselves been disciplined only with spanking and know no other means, and the advice that physicians offer is valuable.

Prognosis

Children raised in a supportive environment that teaches respect for others and self-control grow up as caring adults. Children who have been exposed to excessive physical punishment show aggressive behavior later.

CASE RESOLUTION

In the case presented at the beginning of the chapter, further history should be elicited about the mother's disciplining techniques. It is also significant that the child's speech is delayed. The boy's ability to articulate his feelings may be limited, and a formal speech and hearing assessment is warranted. The preschool should be advised that the evaluation is underway. A report from the preschool concerning the boy's behavior would be appreciated.

Selected References

American Academy of Pediatrics Committee on Psychosocial Aspects of Child and Family Health. Guidance for effective discipline. *Pediatrics.* 1998;101:723–728

American Academy of Pediatrics Committee on School Health. Corporal punishment in schools. *Pediatrics.* 2000;106:343

Barkley RA. *Defiant Children: A Clinician's Manual for Assessment and Parent Training.* 2nd ed. New York, NY: The Guilford Press; 1997

Burke MG. Is a 12-month-old too young to be disciplined? *Contemp Pediatr.* 2006;23:109–110

Carey WB. Pediatric assessment of behavioral adjustment and behavioral style. In: Levine MD, Carey WB, Crocker AC, eds. *Developmental-Behavioral Pediatrics.* 2nd ed. Philadelphia, PA: W. B. Saunders; 1992:609–612

Corwin DG. The fine art of the time-out. *Parenting.* 1996;November:171–172

Regalado M, Sareen H, Inkelas M, Wissow LS, Halfon N. Parents' discipline of young children: results from the National Survey of Early Childhood Health. *Pediatrics.* 2004;113:1952–1958

Rosenberg MB. *Nonviolent Communication; A Language of Life.* 2nd ed. Encintas, CA: Puddledancer Press; 2003

Schmitt BD. Discipline: rules and consequences. *Contemp Pediatr.* 1991;8:65–69

Schmitt BD. Time-out: intervention of choice for the irrational years. *Contemp Pediatr.* 1993;10:64–71

Schmitt BD. When a child hurts other children. *Contemp Pediatr.* 1990;7:81–82

Scholer SJ, Serwint JR. Parental monitoring and discipline in middle childhood. *Pediatr Rev.* 2009;30:366–367

Socolar RRS, Stein REK. Maternal discipline of young children: context, belief, and practice. *J Dev Behav Pediatr.* 1996;17:1–8

Straus MA, Sugarman DB, Giles-Sims J. Spanking by parents and subsequent antisocial behavior of children. *Arch Pediatr Adolesc Med.* 1997;151:761–767

Trumbull DA, Larzelere RE, Wolraich M. To spank or not to spank. *Pediatrics.* 1999;103:696–698

Vittrup B, Holden GW, Buck J. Attitudes predict the use of physical punishment: a prospective study of the emergence of disciplinary practices. *Pediatrics.* 2006;117:2055–2064

Waterson T. Giving guidance on child discipline. *BMJ.* 2000;320:261–262

CHAPTER 48

Temper Tantrums

Geeta Grover, MD

CASE STUDY

During a routine office visit, the parents of a 3-year-old boy express concern about his recent behavior. They report that whenever he is asked to do something he does not want to do, he throws a "fit." He cries fiercely, falls to the floor, bangs his hands, and kicks his feet until his parents give in. He often displays such behavior at bedtime or mealtime if he is asked to turn off the television or eat foods that he does not want. He has 2 to 3 such episodes per week. The parents state that their home life has not changed, and the boy's teacher reports that he displays no such behaviors at preschool.

Questions

1. At what age are temper tantrums common in children?
2. How do parents' reactions encourage or discourage temper tantrums?
3. What appropriate management strategies may help control such oppositional behavior?
4. What factors or aspects of such oppositional behavior indicate underlying pathology?

Temper tantrums are common, normal, age-related behaviors in young children. To a certain degree, oppositional behaviors such as negativism, defiance, and tantrums are part of the normal progression toward self-reliance and independence. Toddlers need to assert their freedom and explore their environment, which often puts them at odds with the limitations imposed by society and well-meaning parents. Young children cannot appreciate that rules and limitations have been established in the interest of their own safety and well-being. They see only that their own desires have been thwarted, and they may react to this disappointment with intense emotions. Children are not simply upset because they cannot have their way. They are angry and frustrated, and they lose control over their emotions. During tantrums children cry and scream uncontrollably. They may fall to the floor, bang their heads, kick their feet, pound their hands, and thrash about wildly. Some children may throw things, try to hit one another, or destroy property.

Such intense displays of anger may be a terrifying experience for both children and parents. Some children use tantrums to gain attention, whereas others use them to achieve something or to avoid doing something. Recurrent temper tantrums may strain relationships among parents, children, and other family members.

Epidemiology

Temper tantrums are noted most often in children who are 2 to 3 years of age, but they may occur any time between the ages of 12 months and 5 years. Parental surveys reveal that about 20% of 2-year-olds, 18% of 3-year-olds, and 10% of 4-year-olds have at least one tantrum per day. Most children are able to express their feeling verbally by 3 to 4 years of age, so temper tantrums begin to taper off. Children who are not able to express their feelings well with words

(eg, children with developmental delays—especially children with speech and language delays or children with autism spectrum disorders [ASDs]) are more likely to continue to have tantrums. Boys and girls are affected equally. Although temper tantrums are unusual in school-aged children, they often reappear in the form of verbal tantrums during adolescence, when autonomy and independence once again become developmental issues.

Pathophysiology

Appreciation of children's level of maturity and the developmental tasks normally associated with the toddler and preschool years, when temper tantrums occur most often, facilitates an understanding of tantrum behavior. Young children who are exploring the world and developing a sense of autonomy think primarily in egocentric terms. They view reality from their own perspective and are unable to appreciate the perspective of other individuals. Only as they mature and enter school do they learn to recognize the position of others and begin to develop a sense of morality, of right and wrong. Toddlers may become frustrated or angry because of their lack of control over the world, inability to communicate, or limitations of their cognitive and motor abilities, which do not allow them to accomplish desired tasks. Unlike adults, who have the ability to verbalize frustrations or simply walk away from unpleasant situations, young children have neither the sophisticated ability to articulate their feelings nor the freedom to walk away. Therefore, they may react to disappointments with temper tantrums.

Temper tantrums may be classified as normal or problematic based on their cause, frequency, and characteristics. Normal tantrums can simply be demands for attention or signs of frustration, anger, or protest. In the interval between tantrums, the child's disposition and mood are normal. The well-behaved 3-year-old boy who has an occasional tantrum following the birth of a sibling, the 2½-year-old girl who throws a tantrum to express frustration because no one understands what she is trying to say, and the 2-year-old boy who cries uncontrollably because he cannot complete the puzzle he has started or run fast enough to keep up with his 4-year-old brother are all examples of normal tantrums. A typical reason for an avoidance-type tantrum is not wanting to go to bed at bedtime. All types of tantrums are more common when children are tired, ill, or hungry, because their ability to cope with disappointment and frustration is limited under these circumstances.

Frequent tantrums (>5 per day) or tantrums that result in destruction of property or physical harm to the child or others are signs of problematic tantrums (Box 48-1). These tantrums result from factors that are beyond the child's control, such as parental problems, school difficulties, or health-related conditions (Box 48-2). For example, the child with unrecognized hearing loss may be performing poorly at school and resort to tantrum behavior in frustration. Marital discord or domestic violence may create anxiety for a child, which may manifest as frequent or destructive tantrums.

Differential Diagnosis

Temper tantrums are readily recognizable because of their classic pattern where a toddler-aged child becomes frustrated, reacts physically, and cries or screams. Sometimes temper tantrums are indicative of more significant problems, such as speech or language delays or ASDs (see Chapter 124).

Evaluation

History

Thorough history taking is essential (Questions Box). The frequency of the temper tantrums, circumstances that provoke them, a description of actual tantrums, and parental reaction must be ascertained. In some instances, this reaction may provide insight as to why the tantrums recur. In addition, parental expectations should be assessed. Expectations that are inappropriate for children's age and developmental maturity may create unnecessary tensions between parents and children and lead to tantrum behavior. Factors associated with problematic tantrums should also be assessed (see Box 48-2).

Tantrums that are frequent (>5 per day), severe, or persist after the age of 5 years may be a sign of underlying conditions, such as depression or low self-esteem. Frequent tantrums may also be associated with attention-deficit/hyperactivity disorder (ADHD). Children with a history of impulsivity, hyperactivity, and inattention that are inappropriate for age should be evaluated for ADHD. Children who hurt themselves or others or destroy property during tantrums may have significant emotional problems. Peer pressure may inhibit tantrum behavior; if tantrums occur frequently at school, the presence of learning disabilities or speech and hearing deficits should be considered.

Box 48-1. Features of Problematic Tantrums

- Tantrums that persist or get worse beyond 5 years of age
- Frequent tantrums (>5 per day)
- Persistent negative mood or behavior in intervals between tantrums
- Recurrent tantrums at school
- Destruction of property during tantrums
- Harm to self or others during tantrums
- Other behavioral problems (eg, sleep disorders, aggressive behaviors, enuresis)

Box 48-2. Underlying Causes of Problematic Tantrums

Parent-Related Factors
- Marital discord
- Abusive behavior toward children
- Domestic violence
- Substance abuse
- Depression
- Inappropriate parental expectations

Child-Related Factors
- Developmental and/or learning disabilities
  — Hearing loss
  — Speech and language delays
  — Autism spectrum disorders
- Mood disorders (eg, depression)
- Attention-deficit/hyperactivity disorder
- Temperament (eg, high persistence and intensity of response and slow adaptability)
- Illness
  — Unrecognized illness (eg, otitis media, sinusitis)
  — Chronic or recurrent illness

Questions

Temper Tantrums

- How often does the child have temper tantrums?
- What circumstances provoke the tantrums?
- How does the child behave during the tantrums? What does the child do?
- How does the child behave in the interval between tantrums?
- How do the parents react to the child during the tantrums? What do they do or say?
- Are parental expectations consistent with the child's developmental stage?
- Have there been any changes at home or school (eg, birth of a sibling, new school)?
- Is the child having any other behavioral or development-related problems (eg, enuresis, sleep difficulties)?

It is important to remember that physicians usually see children whose tantrums are frequent, severe, or cannot be controlled by parents. First, pediatricians must determine whether any underlying pathology may be contributing to the behavior and, if so, what parental or child factors may be provoking it. Second, they must differentiate between normal tantrums and problematic tantrums. Identification and remediation of the cause of problematic tantrums are the first steps toward cure. Children with suspected underlying conditions such as ADHD or mood disturbances should be referred to the appropriate specialist for further evaluation.

Physical Examination

A thorough physical examination is appropriate, as is a developmental assessment to determine if there are findings such as speech delay or behavioral signs consistent with ASDs. Most often, the physical examination is normal.

Laboratory Tests

There are no laboratory tests indicated in the assessment of the child with temper tantrums. Routine tests that are age-appropriate and suggested as part of health maintenance are appropriate.

Management

Punishment is not the solution to temper tantrums (see Chapter 47). Health maintenance visits are an ideal time to provide **anticipatory guidance** regarding tantrums and discuss strategies to prevent or minimize this behavior. Parents typically report that their children become defiant and difficult to manage during the "terrible twos." At the 12- and 15-month visits, physicians should alert parents that this period is approaching and remind them that it is a normal part of development. Preventive strategies, such as **childproofing** the home to minimize unnecessary conflicts, should be discussed. In addition, parents can give young children **frequent opportunities to make choices** (eg, which color shirt to wear or which of 2 foods to have for lunch). These opportunities allow children to exercise independence and autonomy in a positive rather than a negative manner. Physicians can provide **reassurance** that this unpleasant stage will pass; children will eventually become more cooperative and agreeable.

Parents should be told that helping children learn self-control and how to handle anger are keys to management. To expect that children will never get angry is unrealistic. Children should be taught how to **vent their anger and frustration in an acceptable manner** (eg, articulating their feelings or hitting a designated punching bag or pillow). As children mature, their ability to verbalize their feelings increases, but even young toddlers can say "me angry." Physicians should emphasize that it is **important for parents to remain calm** during children's temper tantrums. Shouting and spanking indicate to children that parents are also out of control. Children feel more secure if the adults around them are calm and in control.

Different types of temper tantrums may require specific treatment and management strategies. Parents should **be supportive** of children who are having tantrums resulting from frustration or fatigue by letting the children know that they understand. Children's energy should be redirected into activities they can do well. Parents should be encouraged to **praise positive behavior** (eg, completing tasks properly, handling anger in an acceptable fashion). They should **ignore some tantrums,** such as those for purposes of attention seeking or wanting something. If children have no audience, they have no need to perform. **Time-outs** may also be used in such situations (see Chapter 47). Parents should not give in to children's wishes; this may reinforce tantrum behavior. **Physical movement** of children to where they belong may be necessary if they are refusing to do something (eg, bed for the child who is refusing to go to sleep at bedtime) or in danger of hurting themselves. **Holding children** who are raging may give them a sense of security and help calm them. If temper tantrums occur outside the home, it may be necessary to accompany children to a **quiet, private place,** such as an automobile, until they calm down. Distracting children by suggesting another activity or pointing out something of interest in the environment may also interrupt the unwanted behavior.

CASE RESOLUTION

The child in the case scenario seems to be having normal, age-appropriate tantrums. The boy's tantrums occur when he is asked to do something that he does not want to do. In these situations the parents should try to ignore the tantrums as much as possible and not give in to the child's wishes.

Selected References

Beers NS, Howard B. Managing temper tantrums. *Pediatr Rev.* 2003;24:70–71

Belden AC, Thomson NR, Luby JL. Temper tantrums in healthy versus depressed and disruptive preschoolers: defining tantrum behaviors associated with clinical problems. *J Pediatr.* 2008;152(1):117–122

Degnan KA, Calkins SD, Keane SP, Hill-Soderlund AL. Profiles of disruptive behavior across early childhood: contributions of frustration reactivity, physiological regulation, and maternal behavior. *Child Dev.* 2008;79(5):1357–1376

Needlman R, Howard B, Zuckerman B. Temper tantrums: when to worry. *Contemp Pediatr.* 1989;6:12–34

Potegal M, Davidson RJ. Temper tantrums in young children: behavioral composition. *J Dev Behav Pediatr.* 2003;24:140–147

Potegal M, Kosorok MR, Davidson RJ. Temper tantrums in young children: tantrum duration and temporal organization. *J Dev Behav Pediatr.* 2003;24:148–154

CHAPTER 49

Breath-Holding Spells

Geeta Grover, MD

CASE STUDY

A 15-month-old girl is brought to the office because of parental concern about seizures. In the last month she has passed out momentarily 3 times. Each episode seems to be precipitated by anger or frustration on her part. Typically she cries, holds her breath, turns blue, and passes out. Each time she awakens within a few seconds and seems fine. The medical history and family history are unremarkable, and the physical examination is entirely within normal limits.

Questions

1. What are breath-holding spells (BHS)?
2. What is the differential diagnosis of BHS?
3. What, if any, laboratory studies are indicated in the evaluation of BHS?
4. What measures can be taken to prevent BHS? Are anticonvulsants necessary?
5. What, if any, are the long-term sequelae of BHS?

Breath-holding spells are a benign, recurring condition of childhood in which anger or pain produce crying that culminates in noiseless expiration and apnea. The frequency of BHS, an involuntary phenomenon, is variable and ranges from several episodes a day to only several episodes per year. Although the spells are innocuous, they usually provoke parental fear and anxiety because children often turn blue and become limp. The diagnosis can usually be made on the basis of a characteristic history and description of the episode, but the possibility of seizures should be considered.

Epidemiology

Breath-holding spells occur in about 5% of all children between the ages of 6 months and 6 years, but they are most common in children between 12 and 18 months of age. Most children have experienced their first episode by 18 months and virtually all by 2 years of age. Although BHS have been described in children younger than 6 months, occurrence in such young infants is uncommon. Boys and girls are affected equally. A positive family history is found in about 25% of cases.

Clinical Presentation

The typical clinical sequence of the major types of BHS is described later in the chapter (see Pathophysiology and Dx Box). After the spells, children may experience a short period of drowsiness.

Pathophysiology

Breath-holding spells may be classified as one of the non-epileptic paroxysmal disorders of childhood. These recurrent conditions, which have a sudden onset and no epileptiform focus, resolve spontaneously. Other disorders in this heterogeneous group include

Dx Breath-Holding Spells

- Identifiable precipitating event or emotion
- Brief duration
- Color change, if present, prior to loss of consciousness and rhythmic jerking of extremities
- Rapid restoration of full activity
- Normal neurologic examination

syncope, migraine, cyclic vomiting, benign paroxysmal vertigo, paroxysmal torticollis, sleep disorders (narcolepsy, night terrors, somnambulism), and shudder attacks.

Types of BHS

The 2 major types of BHS are **cyanotic** and **pallid.** The cyanotic type is more common. Approximately 60% of children with BHS have cyanotic spells, 20% have pallid spells, and 20% of affected children have both types. Most commonly, affected children experience several spells per week. Approximately 15% of children with BHS have complicated features. Complicated BHS are defined as typical BHS followed by seizure-like activity or rigid posturing of the body. Unlike the postictal period of epileptic seizures, prolonged periods of lethargy or drowsiness following spells are uncommon.

Pallid spells are similar to cyanotic BHS with some exceptions. Pallid episodes are more commonly provoked by minor injury, pain, or fear rather than frustration or anger; the initial cry is minimal prior to apnea and loss of consciousness; and children become pale rather than cyanotic. In pallid BHS, children often lose consciousness or tone after only a single gasp or cry, whereas in the cyanotic form, the period of apnea prior to loss of consciousness is much longer.

Etiology

Although the spells are triggered by identifiable stimuli, they are involuntary phenomena. It is believed that loss of consciousness in both the cyanotic and pallid forms is caused by cerebral anoxia. The actual mechanisms of the 2 types of BHS are different. The processes involved in cyanotic BHS are not clear. Proposed mechanisms include centrally mediated inhibition of respiratory effort and altered lung mechanics, which may inappropriately stimulate pulmonary reflexes, thus resulting in apnea and hypoxia. In the pallid form, the pale coloration and loss of tone are thought to result from vagally mediated severe bradycardia or asystole. Pallid spells have been spontaneously induced in the electroencephalogram (EEG) laboratory using ocular compression to trigger the oculocardiac reflex. Vagally mediated bradycardia or asystole lasting more than 2 seconds has been produced by this maneuver.

An association between iron deficiency anemia and BHS has been recognized for many years but is poorly understood. It may be related to iron's importance in the function of various enzymes and neurotransmitters in the central nervous system, or may be because children with anemia have decreased cerebral oxygenation making them more susceptible to BHS.

Differential Diagnosis

The differential diagnosis primarily includes seizures and syncope secondary to cardiac arrhythmia or a vasovagal episode. Although vasovagal syncope, like BHS, may be provoked by fear or pain, it is uncommon in children younger than 12 years. Three factors may help differentiate BHS from true epileptic seizure activity. First, spells are usually provoked by some upsetting event or emotion, unlike seizures, which generally do not have a recognizable precipitating event. Second, episodes are brief in duration and followed by rapid restoration of full activity. Third, color change precedes loss of consciousness and rhythmic jerking of the extremities, whereas in the typical epileptic seizure, convulsive activity and loss of muscular tone usually precede change in color. See Box 49-1 for the differential diagnosis of BHS.

Evaluation

History

The history alone may be diagnostic (Questions Box). A family history of BHS should be obtained. It is essential to record a detailed history of the suspected breath-holding episode. The sequence in which the events occurred may help differentiate BHS from epileptic seizures.

Physical Examination

Children should have a complete physical examination, including a thorough neurologic evaluation. Focal neurologic signs or evidence of structural lesions such as meningomyelocele or hydrocephalus may lead the physician away from a diagnosis of BHS.

Box 49-1. Differential Diagnosis of Breath-Holding Spells
Central Nervous System
Seizures (epilepsy)
Occult or overt brain stem lesions (causing dysfunction within the pontomedullary area)
Benign paroxysmal vertigo
Cardiovascular
Cardiac arrhythmia (eg, prolonged QT syndrome)
Syncope (orthostatic or vasovagal)
Miscellaneous
Gastroesophageal reflux/Sandifer syndrome
Cataplexy (transient loss of muscle tone associated with narcolepsy; rare before adolescence)
Central or obstructive apnea
Munchausen syndrome by proxy

Questions

Breath-Holding Spells

- What happened before the episode?
- Was the child crying?
- What was the child's color before and during the episode?
- Was the child lethargic after the episode?
- Does the family have a history of breath-holding spells?

Laboratory Tests

If the history is consistent with BHS and the physical examination is normal, laboratory evaluation is usually unnecessary. Because of the association of BHS with iron deficiency anemia in some children, it is appropriate to determine a hemoglobin level. An EEG may be performed if the physician is concerned about the possibility of epileptic seizures. In both forms of BHS, the EEG shows generalized slowing followed by flattening (a pattern characteristic of cerebral anoxia) during attacks, although it is unusual to record the EEG during BHS. Simultaneous EEG and video recordings can be very useful in helping to distinguish BHS from seizures, especially in children having frequent episodes. The interictal EEG is normal in children with BHS, whereas it may often be abnormal in children with epilepsy. An electrocardiogram may be obtained if there is any question about cardiac arrhythmia (eg, prolonged QT syndrome).

Management

Management of BHS includes **parental support and reassurance.** Breath-holding spells may be extremely frightening for parents to witness, especially if the episodes are routinely associated with loss of consciousness or seizure-like activity. Parents should be told about the involuntary nature of the attacks and be cautioned against reinforcing the spells by giving in to the child's wishes. They should be advised to avoid unnecessary confrontations with the child. Similarly, it is impossible to ensure that the child will never be frustrated or injured. Instead, parents should be encouraged to handle the episodes in a "matter-of-fact" manner and continue age-appropriate discipline. They should be reassured that the long-term prognosis is excellent.

Pharmacologic therapy is usually not necessary, but atropine sulfate may be considered in the management of children with frequent pallid BHS because of atropine's anticholinergic action. Anticonvulsants are not effective. A recent clinical trial showed that iron therapy was effective in the treatment of both cyanotic and pallid BHS, especially in children who were iron deficient. Referral to a neurologist or psychiatrist may be considered at the family's request if the episodes are frequent and associated with loss of consciousness or if there is uncertainty regarding the diagnosis or management.

Prognosis

Breath-holding spells resolve spontaneously in most children by 5 to 6 years of age. About 50% of cases resolve by 4 years of age, and 90% resolve by 6 years of age. Neither pallid nor cyanotic BHS are associated with an increased risk of development of epilepsy, although children with pallid BHS do have an increased incidence of developing syncopal attacks during adulthood.

CASE RESOLUTION

The child presented in the opening case scenario has a history and physical examination suggestive of BHS. The girl's episodes are consistent with cyanotic BHS. The episodes are preceded by an identifiable emotion, are brief in duration, and are followed by a rapid recovery of normal consciousness and activity. Assessment of the hemoglobin level revealed mild iron deficiency anemia. The child received iron therapy, and the parents were reassured about the benign nature of BHS.

Selected References

Anderson JE, Bluestone D. Breath-holding spells: scary but not serious. *Contemp Pediatr.* 2000;17:61–72

Benbadis S. The differential diagnosis of epilepsy: a critical review. *Epilepsy Behav.* 2009;15(1):15–21

Daoud AS, Batieha A, al-Sheyyab M, Abuekteish F, Hijazi S. Effectiveness of iron therapy on breath-holding spells. *J Pediatr.* 1997;130:547–550

DiMario FJ. Prospective study of children with cyanotic and pallid breath-holding spells. *Pediatrics.* 2001;107:265–269

Kelly AM, Porter CJ, McGoon MD, Espinosa RE, Osborn MJ, Hayes DL. Breath-holding spells associated with significant bradycardia: successful treatment with permanent pacemaker implantation. *Pediatrics.* 2001;108:698–702

Mocan H, Yildiran A, Orhan F, Erduran E. Breath holding spells in 91 children and response to treatment with iron. *Arch Dis Child.* 1999;81:261–262

CHAPTER 50

Fears, Phobias, and Anxiety

Carol D. Berkowitz, MD

CASE STUDY

A 5-year-old girl is brought into the office by her mother, who complains that her daughter has been frightened of sleeping alone since the occurrence of an earthquake. The house did not sustain any significant damage, but the entire family was awakened. The mother says that the girl has become more timid. As nighttime approaches, she becomes particularly fearful. She will not stay in her bed, and she is comforted only by sleeping with her parents. In addition, the girl has begun bedwetting since the earthquake, and the mother wonders whether she should put her daughter in diapers. The physical examination, including the vital signs, is normal, except for the observation that the child is very clingy and whiny.

Questions

1. What are normal childhood fears?
2. When do these fears commonly occur?
3. What strategies are used to deal with these fears?
4. What are simple phobias? What are social phobias?
5. What is school phobia, and how is it best handled?
6. What are common anxiety disorders in children and adolescents?
7. How can families deal with childhood disturbances that emerge after natural and man-made disasters?

Fears are normal feelings that cause emotional, behavioral, and physiological changes that are essential for survival. Fears are associated with psychological discomforts, such as a negative, unpleasant feeling. Children may develop fears in response to actual events (eg, earthquakes) or as a result of the temporal association of 2 events (eg, seeing a scary movie on a rainy day and then becoming afraid of rain). Some fears seem to be innate, and others seem to be developmental. Children fear different things at different ages. For example, school phobia is sometimes particularly problematic in young, school-aged children.

Phobias are overwhelming, intense, highly specific, and often irrational fears. The *Diagnostic and Statistical Manual of Mental Disorders, Fourth Edition, Text Revision (DSM-IV-TR)* defines a phobia as excessive anxiety accompanied by worry occurring more often than not, for at least 6 months and associated with one or more of the following: restlessness, easy fatigability, difficulty concentrating, irritability, tense muscles, and disturbed sleep. Childhood phobias can be divided into 5 categories: animals (spiders, snakes, dogs), natural environment (heights), medical related (doctors, dentists, injections), situations (flying), other (loud noises, rain, thunder). Social phobias are specific to social situations that arouse intense concerns about humiliation or embarrassment. Fear of speaking in public may represent a social phobia. Selective mutism involves children who are able to speak but are unable to do so in certain settings, such as school. This probably represents one form of a social phobia. When these fears are combined with avoidance behavior, they may be incapacitating. Anxiety refers to fear without a definable source. It is a vague feeling of uneasiness, apprehension, and foreboding of impending doom. A child may experience an anxiety **problem** where

there is significant but not severe distress and an anxiety **disorder** when the distress is excessive or functioning is impaired. Up to 8% of children and adolescents have anxiety disorders. These may be referred to as generalized anxiety disorders.

Different strategies are useful for dealing with different fears. It is important for parents not to trivialize these fears, nor to reinforce them, but to empower children to deal with them.

It is also important to realize that parents sometimes foster fears by using threats with children such as "the doctor will give you a shot unless you eat your spinach" or "the boogie man will get you." By fostering fears, the parents are also fostering dependency. Parents lack the imagination that children have and find it difficult to understand the degree of fear that children experience.

The opportunities for primary care providers to counsel families about childhood fears has increased over the past 10 years related to a number of catastrophic events, such as the terrorist attacks of 9/11, the tsunami in Asia, hurricane Katrina, and the earthquake in Haiti. Acts of violence such as the shootings at Columbine High School and Virginia Tech also create fear and anxiety in children who witness these events on the television. It is important to recognize the pervasiveness of mental health sequelae following disasters and the factors that influence the prevalence of these disturbances. One percent of children in New York City lost a relative on 9/11. There is a greater risk of mental health sequelae if there are poor social supports, a prior history of psychopathology, or the child is fearful or shy by nature. Natural disasters have less of an impact than intentional ones. While many of the recent disasters have been acute and unexpected, there are children who are continuously exposed to what has been called "process trauma" in the form of war and child abuse.

Epidemiology

Fears follow a developmental pattern. Neonates are believed to have no fear, although young infants whose faces are covered with a blanket struggle to toss off the blanket. Infants who are 6 months of age exhibit what is known as **stranger anxiety** in response to unfamiliar persons, places, or objects. To combat this anxiety, infants seek refuge with a parent. Stranger anxiety becomes equated with separation anxiety and reaches a peak at 2 years of age. Children between 6 months and 2 years of age are also frightened by loud noises and falling or quickly moving objects.

Children between the ages of 2 and 5 years are in what is termed the **age of anxiety.** They fear many things, including animals, abandonment, loud noises, and darkness. Children in this age group are particularly fearful of physicians, hospitals, and getting hurt. Young children are afraid of the physically disabled, who represent bodily injury, and monsters and scary movies. They sometimes displace their anger onto monsters and witches and attribute to these imaginary characters the bad feelings they are experiencing. Children in this age group have strong imaginations, which makes it difficult for them to differentiate fantasy from reality.

School-aged children between 6 years of age and adolescence tend to have more abstract thoughts, and their fears are less relevant to physical immediacy. These children are afraid of the death of their parents or the burning of their home. They also fear war, growing up (expressed as "How will I know what to do?"), going into the next grade, being alone or being kidnapped, and the divorce of their parents. Children in this age group are often reluctant to bother their parents with their fears, and they can easily misinterpret parental concerns when they overhear parental conversations. Childhood anxiety disorders are reported in 6% to 20% of children.

Separation anxiety, which may manifest as school phobia and may be referred to as separation anxiety disorder, may occur in school-aged children. The prevalence is estimated at 3.2% to 4.1%, though up to 50% of third graders report separation anxiety symptoms. Separation anxiety disorder is defined as developmentally inappropriate, excessive anxiety precipitated by actual or anticipated separation from home or family. Affected children develop physical complaints (eg, stomachaches) on school days. The mother–child relationship is often disturbed, and the child is fearful of leaving the parent alone. Childhood school phobia and parental history of panic attacks and agoraphobia may be associated.

Fears during adolescence relate to social functioning, such as public speaking or talking to members of the opposite sex. Older children are also concerned about school failure and physical injury. They have many of the same fears expressed by younger school-aged children, although phobias are uncommon. Phobias, which occur in less than 1.7% of the general population, are reported in 13% of disturbed children.

Anxiety disorders are rare in childhood, but more common during adolescence. They may include panic attacks, which involve the sudden onset of intense fear or discomfort associated with physiological symptoms such as palpitations and shortness of breath.

Fear about a panic attack may lead to agoraphobia, the avoidance of going away from home. Post-traumatic stress disorder (PTSD) involves a set of symptoms that recurs after a person has experienced a traumatic event. Symptoms include intense fear, helplessness, or a sense of horror. The person reexperiences the trauma, avoids circumstances that are reminiscent of the trauma, and is in a state of hyperarousal. It is estimated that 5% of men and 10% of women have a lifetime prevalence of PTSD.

Pathophysiology

Fear has its basis in a series of psychophysiological reactions, which are mediated through a series of neurotransmitters. Elevated levels of certain transmitters, such as γ-aminobutyric acid and norepinephrine, are associated with feelings of anxiety. Excess serotonin has also been related to anxiety disorders. Patients with panic attacks and anxiety disorders have disturbances in neurotransmitter regulation.

Differential Diagnosis

The challenge for physicians is to assess the etiology of the fear and to differentiate normal fears from those that may be signs of unusual stresses or signs of psychopathology. Appropriate fears represent a real reaction to a real danger. As a rule, children are more resilient than adults and recover more rapidly from traumatic events. On the other hand, children are prone to inappropriate fears, which may develop for a number of reasons.

Inappropriate fears may occur because of operant conditioning, in which a conditioned stimulus becomes associated with another object. Fear of the other object becomes reinforced through this association. Inappropriate fears may also develop in a child whose parent has the fear (modeling) or through witnessing a fearful event in the media (informational). True phobias represent neuroses and may occur in more than one family member.

School phobia, also called school refusal, may occur under 3 distinct conditions. Not uncommonly, young children who are entering school for the first time are frightened. This fear is a normal component of separation anxiety, which usually resolves within a few days of starting school. In contrast, older children may experience school phobia because they are truly afraid of a school situation. They may fear a teacher, violence, or a bully. To avoid the problem, children may actually request to change classrooms or schools. It is important to talk to children to find out what is behind their fear of school.

On the other hand, some children who seem fearful of school are actually concerned about parental separation (ie, separation anxiety). Frequently these children enjoy school and miss it when they are absent. Absences occur when feelings of separation from parents are so intense that they do not allow children to function well in school settings. This separation anxiety disorder may result from parental illness or parents' fostering dependency in children. Children then see parents as vulnerable and are uncomfortable about leaving them alone.

School refusal is the third leading cause of school absenteeism after transient illness and truancy. Fifty percent of children with school refusal have other problems, including depression (28%), tantrums (18%), sleep disturbances (17%), obsessive-compulsive behavior (11%), other fears (10%), enuresis (3%), and learning disabilities (3%). Overall, school refusal has a good prognosis, although adolescents do not do as well as younger children, and individuals with a higher IQ have a poorer outcome. Twenty percent of parents of children with school refusal have a diagnosable psychiatric disorder. Issues of mother–child dependency are often a concern.

Another type of childhood fear concerns physicians and hospitals. Children have many concerns about what happens to them at the doctor's office. They are particularly fearful of needles. To children, needles represent possible mutilation. When asked to represent needles in drawings, children often portray needles as larger than themselves and very pointed. They comment that needles are sharp (eg, "Needles can make you pop, just like a balloon." "Needles can also take out all your blood until you die."). In addition, children are preoccupied with what happens to their blood. One youngster commented, "They check out your blood to see if it's good or bad, and if your blood is bad, then it means that you need to have more tests." Another youngster thought that physicians were doing a "blood taste" rather than a blood test.

Hospitalization raises other issues concerning parental separation as well as painful procedures. As children adjust to hospitalization, they progress through 3 stages: protest, during which they complain about the hospital and cry; despair, during which they have given up hope that their parents will return; and detachment, during which they seem to be adjusting but actually have distanced themselves from their parents.

Evaluation

Physicians should explore the area of childhood fears and phobias at routine health maintenance visits, even if parents do not have specific concerns. Sometimes parents are embarrassed by children's fears (eg, the fear of an older child to sleep without a night-light or the fear of dogs, which may preclude the child from visiting certain friends). Parents may not report children's fears unless these fears seem to be unusually intense. Practitioners may ask children, "What is the scariest thing you can think of?" If children are having difficulty providing details, physicians may ask them to name things that other children fear or to complete the sentence, "I feel afraid when…." Alternatively, practitioners may suggest things that other children may fear: "Do the kids you know seem to be worried about kidnapping?"

There are a number of instruments that have been used to assess the level of anxiety in children. These include the Multidimensional Anxiety Scale for Children, Spence Children's Anxiety Scale, and Screen for Child Anxiety Related Disorders. The latter instrument is in the public domain and readily available.

History

The evaluation of children with specific fears demands a careful history that provides information about situations in which children are fearful (Questions Box). Physicians should consider fears within a

Fears and Phobias — Questions

- What fear does the child have? Exactly what does the child fear?
- Under what circumstances was the fear originally expressed? Did any changes in the child's life occur around the time that the fear appeared?
- Under what conditions is the fear currently expressed?
- How long has the child had the fear?
- How does the fear affect the daily living of the child and family?

developmental context because many childhood fears are normal and experienced by all children. It is also important to look at changes in the family situation. Children sometimes develop what seem to be fears but in fact are behaviors designed to manipulate other family members. For instance, young children who sense marital discord may insist on sleeping with their parents as a way of ensuring that the parents are together rather than separate.

Physical Examination

A routine examination is warranted, but findings are usually normal. Such an evaluation, however, is particularly important if presenting complaints include symptoms such as abdominal pain, headache, or palpitations.

Laboratory Tests

As a rule, laboratory tests are not required unless the symptoms suggest an organic etiology, such as hyperthyroidism, as the cause of palpitations.

Management

The management of the fear or phobia is determined by the degree to which children are incapacitated. As a general rule, **children should be empowered to conquer their fears.** Children's books that address the issues of certain fears can help achieve this empowerment. Books such as *The Berenstain Bears in the Dark* (Random House, 1982) discuss specific worries such as fear of lightning and thunder. These books often explain the basis of such natural phenomena in easy-to-understand terms. The books also normalize particular fears and show how one character is fearful. Parents can also re-create some of the sounds that children fear. For example, children who are afraid of the noise the wind makes are shown a teakettle where the hot steam blows through the whistle, creating the same noise as the wind. For fears about nuclear war, empowering children to become active, such as joining a nuclear protest group, may be useful.

Parents may feel helpless because they do not know how to deal with children's fears. Physicians should give them the necessary information. Children's fears should not be trivialized. Even if the **fears** are unfounded, they **should be validated.** In general, children should be questioned about whether they are fearful about a situation. The following 2 examples illustrate the proper handling of fears in children.

If children are visiting the dentist for the first time, it is appropriate for parents to ask, "Are you afraid?" If children reply, "Yes, a little bit," parents can say, "Almost everybody is afraid. Tell me what it is you're afraid of. Fear is a normal emotion, and I'm glad you told me about it."

Parents of children who express fear of imaginary characters can reassure children that they do not exist. In addition, parents can tell children what the parents would do if such characters did exist. For instance, the father of a little girl who was afraid of witches told her, "There are no such things as witches. But if there were, and they came into your room, I would punch them in the nose and punch them in the stomach and beat them up, and then there would be no more witches to hurt you." For those who would opt for a less violent approach, the parent could state: "I would tell any witch who came into your room, 'STOP! Go away. No witches allowed in here.' And the witch would run away and I would slam the door!!" By doing this, parents establish the reality of the situation and then also create a plan to deal with the problem should it actually happen.

Parents can also help to limit or reduce children's fears by **minimizing** their **exposure to fear-provoking situations** such as television shows or scary movies. These programs can be particularly frightening for some children, who should not watch them without adult supervision. Minimizing exposure to television is particularly important following a disastrous event. The recurrent images of planes flying into buildings on 9/11 were interpreted by children as repeated different attacks.

When dealing with children who have school phobia because of problems in school, it is important to determine if a change in school would be appropriate to facilitate their school attendance. This may be particularly appropriate in children whose schools are plagued with violence.

Cognitive-behavioral therapy (CBT) is reported to have the highest rate of success for dealing with anxiety-related conditions. Cognitive-behavioral therapy includes psychoeducation, somatic management (eg, relaxation techniques), cognitive restructuring (modifying negative thoughts), and exposure methods including desensitization. The goal of the therapist is to teach the child alternative ways of viewing the feared object and of coping with the fear itself. Medications such as antidepressants, anxiolytics, sedatives, and β-blockers have an unsubstantiated role in managing phobic disorders in children.

When school refusal is linked to separation anxiety, then a program of **desensitization or habituation (graded exposure)** is recommended. Desensitization may involve the participation of mothers in the classroom for a time. When children acclimate and can tolerate some separation, mothers move to another area in the school, such as the principal's office. Next they go outside the school grounds. As children reestablish a sense of well-being in spite of the separation, the mothers gradually move farther and farther away. This solution is somewhat problematic for mothers who work outside the home. There is some research to suggest that children adjust more readily if they resume school immediately without the gradual withdrawal of their parent. Children with significant school refusal may need the assistance of child psychologists or psychiatrists.

Phobias may be treated using the concept of **flooding,** which consists of rapid, prolonged exposure to the feared item. For example, a child who is afraid of dogs is exposed to a friendly, docile, small dog while in the company of his or her parents. Alternatively, systematic desensitization, during which children are exposed to the feared objects over a series of weeks, coupled with relaxation techniques, is also used. Phobias usually require the help of mental health specialists. Selective serotonin reuptake inhibitors (see Chapter 126) have been found to be beneficial in the management of certain anxiety disorders in children and adolescents. They are noted to be effective for panic disorders, social phobia, generalized anxiety disorder, obsessive-compulsive disorder, and PTSD. Benzodiazepines are safe and generally used on a short-term basis. Sedation is a frequent side effect, and there is the potential for abuse, tolerance, and drug dependence. Propranolol lessens the peripheral autonomic nervous system symptoms of social phobias and may be used for specific instances. Combined therapy involving CBT and medication is beneficial in some patients.

Children who must undergo hospitalization benefit from a prehospital visit, when possible. This visit familiarizes the child with the facilities and explains proposed procedures. Many hospitals have child life specialists who ease the adjustment of children as well as their parents to the hospital stay.

Prognosis

Most childhood fears resolve with time, nurturing, and reassurance. Most fears last only several weeks, and then new fears develop. As a rule, specific fears should not last longer than 2 years, and the younger the child, the shorter the duration of the fear.

Prognosis is good for children with true phobias, with 100% resolution of monosymptomatic phobias. More significant anxiety disorders may persist into adulthood, where similar management involving CBT and medications may be indicated.

CASE RESOLUTION

In the case scenario, the girl's fear of sleeping in her bed was triggered by a significant environmental event. Although earthquakes are uncontrollable, the girl can be empowered to deal with manageable aspects of an earthquake as much as possible. She should be assured that in the same situation, many adults probably would also fear sleeping alone. The parents should stock a box with shoes, flashlight, radio, and water and place the box under the child's bed. In addition, they may also have their daughter get into her bed and then shake it, simulating the jiggling that she would experience during an earthquake. The girl should also practice getting out of bed and standing in the doorway. To combat the child's fear of separation during times of natural disaster, the parents should reassure their daughter that they will all be together.

Selected References

Physicians

American Psychiatric Association. *Diagnostic and Statistical Manual of Mental Disorders.* 4th ed. Text Rev. Washington, DC: American Psychiatric Association; 2000

Benum J, Lewis C, Siegel M, Serwint JR. Fears and phobias. *Pediatr Rev.* 2008; 29:250–251

Bothe D, Olness K. Worried sick. Anxiety among youth. *Contemp Pediatr.* 2007; 24:58–63

Brown EJ. Clinical characteristics and efficacious treatment of posttraumatic stress disorder in children and adolescents. *Pediatr Ann.* 2005;34:138–146

Compton SN, March JS, Brent D, et al. Cognitive-behavioral psychotherapy for anxiety and depressive disorders in children and adolescents: an evidence-based medicine review. *J Am Acad Child Adolesc Psychiatry.* 2004;43:930–959

Emotions and moods. In: Wolraich ML, ed. *The Classification of Child and Adolescent Mental Diagnoses in Primary Care: Diagnostic and Statistical Manual for Primary Care (DSM-PC) Child and Adolescent Version.* Elk Grove Village, IL: American Academy of Pediatrics; 1996:145–149

Hanna GL, Fischer DJ, Fluent TE. Separation anxiety disorder and school refusal in children and adolescents. *Pediatr Rev.* 2006;27:56–62

Jurbergs N, Ledley DR. Separation anxiety disorders. *Pediatr Ann.* 2005; 34:108–115

Kendall PC, Chu BC, Pimentel SS, Choudhury M. Treating anxiety disorders in youth. In: Kendall PC, ed. *Child and Adolescent Therapy: Cognitive Behavioral Procedures.* 2nd ed. New York, NY: The Guilford Press; 2000

Klein RG, Last CG. *Anxiety Disorders in Children.* Newbury Park, CA: Sage Publications; 1989

Sarafino EP. *The Fears of Childhood.* New York, NY: Human Sciences Press; 1986

Walsh KH. Welcome advances in treating youth anxiety disorders. *Contemp Pediatr.* 2002;19:66–82

Williams TP, Miller BD. Pharmacologic management of anxiety disorders in children and adolescents. *Curr Opin Pediatr.* 2003;15:483–490

Parents and Children

Berenstain S, Berenstain J. *The Berenstain Bears and the Bully.* New York, NY: Random House; 1993

Berenstain S, Berenstain J. *The Berenstain Bears in the Dark.* New York, NY: Random House; 1982

Berenstain S, Berenstain J. *The Berenstain Bears Visit the Dentist.* New York, NY: Random House; 1981

Mayer M. *There's a Nightmare in My Closet.* New York, NY: Penguin Books; 1992

Ziefert H. *Nicky's Noisy Night.* New York, NY: Penguin Books; 1986

CHAPTER 51

Thumb Sucking and Other Habits

Carol D. Berkowitz, MD

CASE STUDY

A 5-year-old boy is brought to the office because of thumb sucking. His mother claims that she has tried nearly everything, including tying his hands at night and using aversive treatments on his thumbs, but nothing has worked. She reports that her son has been teased at school and has few friends. He is in good general health, and his immunizations are up to date.

His growth parameters are at the 50th percentile. Except for a callus on the right thumb, the physical examination is normal.

Questions

1. What are common habits in children?
2. What is the significance of transitional objects?
3. What are the consequences of the common habits in children?
4. What are strategies used to break children of habits?
5. How does one differentiate benign habits from self-injurious behaviors?

Habits are defined as somewhat complicated, repetitive behaviors that become automatized, fixed, and carried out easily and effortlessly. They are different from tics, which are rapid, repetitive muscle twitches involving the head, face, or shoulders. Tics are also referred to as habit spasms (see Chapter 117). Children have many socially unacceptable habits, including thumb sucking, nail biting, skin picking, nose picking, hair pulling (trichotillomania), rocking, biting other children, and teeth grinding (bruxism). Some habits, such as pica, are potentially harmful. Children engage in most of these habits because of their soothing potential. In recent years, "cutting," a form of self-injury in adolescents, has received attention. While not a habit in a traditional sense, cutting is described by teens as a way of dealing with stress and alleviating anxiety. One-third of children use transitional objects for comfort. Blankets or favorite toys are traditional transitional objects that represent an age-appropriate coping strategy. Most transitional objects are strokable, and the stroking often occurs in association with thumb sucking. Transitional objects sometimes present a problem because children experience distress if these objects are lost, misplaced, or need cleaning.

Epidemiology

Thumb sucking probably represents the most common habit of children. A reported 50% to 87% of children engage in this habit. The median age for the onset of hand sucking is 54 minutes of life, and 90% of newborns show hand-sucking behavior by the age of 2 hours. Forty percent of children between the ages of 1 and 3 years, 33% of children between the ages of 3 and 5 years, and 25% of children

at the age of 5 years still suck their thumbs. Some children suck their fingers rather than thumbs. Other oral behavior may involve lip sucking, lip biting, and toe sucking. Lip sucking and biting begin at about 5 to 6 months of age and occur in about 90% of infants. It is unusual for these actions to persist as habits. Toe sucking is noted in infants who are 6 to 7 months of age, and it is reported in 80% of normal infants.

Trichotillomania is a disorder once believed to be uncommon but now thought to affect 8 million Americans (about 5 in 1,000). The term, first coined in 1889 by French dermatologist Hallopeau, is derived from the Greek *thrix* (hair), *tillein* (pull), and *mania* (madness). The condition is an impulse control disorder in which alopecia develops from compulsive hair pulling. Hair pulling may involve hair from the head, eyebrows, eyelashes, or pubic area. Although trichotillomania seems to peak during early childhood and adolescence, the disorder is reported from infancy to adolescence. In young children, boys and girls are equally affected, but in older children and adolescents, females outnumber males. The disorder is not associated with comorbid psychopathology, but there may be some association with mood disorders or attention-deficit/hyperactivity disorder. There is a condition in infants, called baby trichs, in which infants pull their mother's hair when they are being held or nursed. This is considered normal exploratory behavior.

Rhythmic habits are stereotypical, repetitive behaviors that usually occur in infants younger than 1 year. These habits are reported in 15% to 20% of the population. Rhythmic habits include rocking (about 19% of infants), when infants rock back and forth; jouncing

(5%–10%), when they move up-and-down on their hands and knees so that the whole crib rocks; head rolling (8%); and head banging (5%). Rhythmic habits are seen more commonly in boys; the male–female ratio is 3:1. These habits usually occur with a frequency of 60 to 80 movements per minute, often when infants are tired, and last for less than 15 minutes before they fall sleep.

Rhythmic movements have been equated with **sleep tics.** These tics are reported in 20% of children, most often between the ages of 6 and 10 years. As a rule, tics are 3 times more common in boys than in girls. They tend to be noted with increased frequency in children who are shy, are overly self-conscious, or have obsessive-compulsive tendencies. Tics usually occur when children are under stress.

Biting, an aggressive habit noted in toddlers, may be related to teething. It occurs more often in children with slow verbal skills.

Nail biting (onychophagia) is usually believed to be a sign of internal tension. The disorder affects 10% to 40% of children. Nail biting begins between the ages of 3 and 6 years , and the peak age is 13 years. One-third of adolescents bite their nails, but 50% of these adolescents break the habit by the time they reach adulthood. Nail biting in adults is regarded as a sign of emotional and social immaturity and regression. The family history for nail biting is often positive. Identical twins are concordant for the condition in 66% of cases. In contrast, the incidence in dizygotic twins is 34%.

Nose picking, noted in children and adults, is reported in more than 90% of individuals. In general, adults and older children limit nose picking to when they are unobserved, but younger children will pick their noses in public. There are no gender-based differences in the incidence of nose picking. Epistaxis is the most common complication of nose picking.

Pica, which is not a normal behavior, is defined as the ingestion of nonfood products. The peak incidence of pica is between the ages of 1 and 3 years. The incidence is increased in children from lower socioeconomic levels, and the behavior occurs in 10% of children who present with lead poisoning.

Teeth grinding (bruxism) is reported in 5% to 15% of children. Boys are more commonly affected than girls, and the disorder seems to regress later in life. It is reported with increased incidence among developmentally delayed children including those with autism spectrum disorder. The cause is unknown, although it may be associated with malocclusion in some children. The disorder may contribute to temporomandibular joint dysfunction and pain.

Self-injury has been reported in up to 20% of mentally retarded adults. Autism and the absence of speech are the highest associated risk factors. Nail biting, head banging, and self-biting are frequently described associated behaviors. Severe self-injury related to biting is seen in Lesch-Nyhan syndrome.

Clinical Presentation

Children with common habits, such as thumb sucking or rhythmic movements, may be brought to the physician with these particular complaints because the parent wants advice about stopping the behavior. Other children may present with consequences of habits,

such as alopecia (trichotillomania), paronychia (nail biting), or lead intoxication (pica). Trichobezoars that can complicate trichotillomania may present with gastric outlet or bowel obstruction. Symptoms then include abdominal pain, anorexia, early satiety, nausea, vomiting, halitosis, and weight loss (Dx Box).

Dx **Childhood Habits**

- History of a habit
- Callus on thumb or fingers
- Short, chewed nails
- Alopecia
- Lead intoxication
- Iron deficiency anemia

Pathophysiology

Children engage in habits to reduce stress and provide comfort. Thumb sucking is related to nonnutritive sucking. Although the initial purpose of sucking is nutritional, the pleasure associated with sucking reinforces the behavior. Infants who are served from a cup from birth develop no interest in sucking. Humans and other primates spend more time in nonnutritive than in nutritive sucking. Monkeys use a 5-point hold, with 2 hands, 2 feet, and mouth (holding on to their mother's nipple) for attachment. Universal thumb sucking is noted even in orphan monkeys, and sucking is thought to be an important aspect of environmental adaptation. Nonnutritive sucking occurs even in the absence of fatigue, hunger, or discomfort, and has a purpose in itself—to provide comfort and be self-soothing. The maximum intensity of sucking occurs at 7 months. For older children (>3 years), sucking is also a way of dealing with boredom.

In bottle-fed infants, thumb sucking seems to commence when feeding stops. Some infants, described as "type A," seem to be satisfied only when their thumb is in their mouth. As infants spend more time engaged in motor activity, they spend less time thumb sucking. Placid infants who cry less also do less sucking. Some studies have shown that thumb sucking is less common in breastfed infants, and that thumb suckers as a group feed less frequently (every 4 hours rather than 3 and for 10 minutes rather than 20).

Nail biting is related to thumb sucking, a form of oral gratification, and children may progress from thumb sucking to nail biting. The pattern of nail biting usually involves placement of the hand in the vicinity of the mouth, tapping of the fingers along the teeth, quick spasmodic bites with the fingers around the central incisors, and the removal and inspection of the hands. Other oral habits, such as pencil gnawing, gum chewing, lip biting, and nail picking, are related activities, as is nose picking. The cause of teeth grinding is unclear.

Rocking habits are believed to be kinesthetically pleasing and soothing and a means of autostimulation. The etiology of hair pulling is less apparent. The *Diagnostic and Statistical Manual of Mental Disorders, Fourth Edition, Text Revision* defines trichotillomania as chronic hair pulling often associated with hair ingestion. In recent years, investigators have linked trichotillomania to disorders of serotonin reuptake and placed it in the category of obsessive-compulsive behavior. Some individuals who engage in trichotillomania have abnormal head positron emission tomography. Although the etiology of trichotillomania is unclear, affected children share certain features, which have been characterized as fiddling SHEEP (sensation, hands, emotion, environment, perfectionism). The overriding factor is a need for tactile stimulation. Pica, which is also considered abnormal, may be associated with mental retardation, environmental deprivation, or inadequate nutrition, particularly iron deficiency.

Differential Diagnosis

The differential diagnosis of most habits is not difficult. Tics or habit spasms should be differentiated from Tourette disorder. This syndrome, which is reported in 1 in 3,000 children, is a neurologic disorder characterized by severe, frequent, and multiple tics. These tics are also often vocal and consist of sounds such as hissing, barking, grunting, or coprolalia (repeating profanities). Some of the rhythmic habits may be mistaken for seizures but can be easily distinguished because of the stereotypical, repetitive nature of the behavior.

Trichotillomania usually has a classic physical appearance that has been referred to as *tonsure Friar Tuck* pattern baldness, with baldness around the vertex of the head. Unilateral temporal baldness is also a consequence of trichotillomania. The differential diagnosis of trichotillomania includes alopecia areata, tinea capitis, syphilitic alopecia, and androgenic alopecia (see Chapter 119). Broken hairs of variable length usually characterize alopecia secondary to trichotillomania. Other disorders in the differential diagnosis include traction alopecia, related to tight braids or hair brushing; atopic eczema; seborrheic dermatitis; hypothyroidism; systemic lupus erythematosus; and dermatomyositis. When trichotillomania is associated with a trichobezoar and signs of gastric outlet obstruction, the differential diagnosis includes neuroblastoma, lymphoma, and gastric carcinoma.

Cutting is not a benign habit, but it can provide stress relief, a feature of many benign childhood habits. It is usually associated with a wide range of psychopathology, including depression; anxiety; eating disorders, especially bulimia nervosa; a history of prior sexual abuse; and obsessive-compulsive symptoms. The mechanism by which cutting alleviates stress and anxiety has not been elucidated, but the role of endogenous endorphins has been suggested. Cutting is felt not to represent suicidal behavior, but some studies differentiate the site of cutting as predictive of suicidality: Wrist cutters as opposed to arm cutters have a higher rate of suicide ideation and attempts. All cutters are at greater risk for suicide than the general population. Management generally involves referral to a mental health specialist and the use of psychotherapy. Other forms of self-injury are reported with increased frequency among children with developmental disabilities, including autism spectrum disorder (see Chapter 124).

Evaluation

History

Children who present with thumb sucking, nail biting, and teeth grinding usually do not require an assessment other than a routine health maintenance history and physical examination. The history should determine the specific circumstances when the habit is manifest. Is the habit more likely to emerge when the child is tired or stressed? Habits must also be evaluated in the context of the child's developmental level and home situation. Understanding the impact of the habit on the child and the family is important. Children who present with movements that resemble tics should be carefully questioned about the frequency and duration of the tics, the effect of the tics on their behavior, and whether coughing is associated with the tics (sign of Tourette disorder). The occurrence of obsessive-compulsive mannerisms should also be noted (Questions Box).

> ### Questions
> **Childhood Habits**
> - What about your child's habit concerns you?
> - Is your child experiencing any adverse consequences (eg, being teased at school) as a result of the habit?
> - Does the habit interfere with your child's routine activities?
> - Can you identify stressors in your child's life?
> - Is your child comforted by the habit?

Physical Examination

A routine physical examination should be performed. The physical examination may reveal the sequelae of the habit, such as thumb calluses, candidal infection of the nails, or evidence of malocclusion with an overbite (Figure 51-1). Children with suspected trichotillomania should have a thorough assessment of their scalp in an effort to differentiate other causes of alopecia (see Chapter 119). A careful neurologic examination should be performed in children with tics, and referral to a child neurologist may be indicated in children with suspected neurologic disorders.

Laboratory Studies

Routine laboratory studies are not needed in children diagnosed with habit disorders.

Children with trichotillomania should be evaluated for the disorders listed previously. An easy evaluation process for trichotillomania involves shaving the hair in the middle of the area of baldness. The growth of these small hairs is uniform because children are unable to pull them out. Head shaving may not be acceptable, however, to the parent or the child. Disorders such as syphilis and collagen vascular diseases can be ruled out using appropriate laboratory studies. Fungal infections can be differentiated by the use of appropriate cultures. A Wood light examination may reveal fluorescence noted with certain fungal infections.

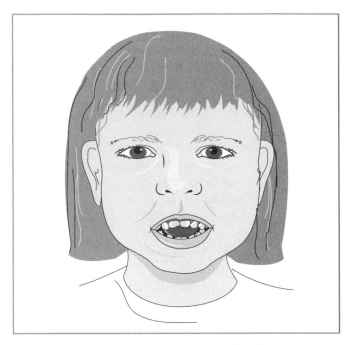

Figure 51-1. Anterior open bite associated with thumb sucking.

Children who present with pica should be evaluated for the presence of iron deficiency anemia and lead poisoning.

Management

The management of childhood habits should be directed at the specific symptoms. For older children, self-monitoring and relaxation training may be helpful as alternative means for dealing with stress. The issue of thumb sucking versus the use of pacifiers can be addressed by anticipatory guidance. **Pacifiers,** which were previously discouraged, are now believed to have some advantages over thumb sucking. A report from the American Academy of Pediatrics noted a decrease in the incidence of sudden infant death syndrome in infants who used a pacifier. With pacifiers, the risk for dental disturbances is lower because the pacifiers are softer and are accompanied by a plastic shield that puts counter pressure on the teeth. Pacifiers are also detachable and cleanable.

Pacifiers can be lost, however. Parents should be advised not to attach a pacifier to the child's shirt with a string because of risk of strangulation. For children who are pacifier-dependent and are unable to go back to sleep if they lose their pacifier at night, multiple pacifiers can be placed in the crib to make finding one easier. For infants who desire pacifiers because they complete their feeding in less than 20 minutes, a nipple with a smaller hole can be used or the cap can be screwed on the bottle more tightly to prolong the time spent in nutritive sucking. Dental problems may develop when pacifiers are used upside down, all day long, or after the eruption of permanent dentition.

It is suggested that parents do not try to stop thumb-sucking behavior until children have reached the age of 4 years. Dental problems in late thumb suckers include anterior open bite, increased overjet (protruding upper incisors), intruded and flared upper

incisors, lingually flipped lower incisors, and warped alveolar ridge. When thumb sucking persists to school age, tongue thrust is noted, as are articulation problems, specifically with consonants s, t, d, n, z, l, and r. The physician should reassure parents that children who stop sucking their thumbs prior to the onset of the secondary dentition are not at risk for poor dentition.

Numerous devices have been proposed to help with the cessation of thumb sucking, but reported success has been variable. The use of arm restraints, particularly at night, is not recommended and may result in rumination. Bitter paints such as Stop Zit seek to reduce thumb sucking by subjecting children to a bitter, aversive taste. This medication consists of 49% toluene, 19% isopropyl alcohol, 18% butyl acetate, 11% ethylcellulose, and 0.3% denatonium benzoate. A three-quarter–ounce bottle is toxic if ingested in its entirety. Nocturnal application is needed if children suck their thumbs during the night. The principle of retraining, where thumb sucking becomes a duty and children are required to suck all 10 fingers one at a time, has also been recommended. Some recommend that elastic bandages be put on the hand of nocturnal thumb suckers. Problems associated with thumb sucking include sore thumbs, calluses, and candidal infections. Dentists may fashion a reminder appliance, called a palatal crib or rake, making it difficult for children to suck their thumbs. Such devices are usually applied for a minimum of 3 months. A fixed appliance is preferable to a removable one and treatment should be initiated in spring or summer when children are engaged in numerous physical activities. Some dental devices are available commercially or online. They may consist of a plastic covering for the thumb and hand. This covering eliminates the pleasurable sensation created by the interaction of thumb, saliva, and mouth. Such devices cost about $80 and success is variable.

Encouragement works better than nagging, as a rule, and a **reward system** is particularly useful in children who are 5 to 6 years of age. Parents may be referred to books such as *Danny and His Thumb* (Ernst KF. Englewood Cliffs, NJ: Prentice-Hall; 1973) and encouraged to talk to their children about how good it feels not to suck their thumbs. A star chart and diary are also useful. Sometimes telling children something like, "Mommy would be so proud of you if you didn't suck your thumb now that you're such a big girl or a big boy" is effective. In addition, the pressure to stop thumb sucking becomes greater during the school years. Children who suck their thumbs are regarded by their peers in first grade as less intelligent, less happy, less likable, and less desirable as friends.

In children who suck their thumbs and twirl their hair at the same time, the hair twirling stops once the thumb sucking ends. The phenomenon is referred to as *habit covariance*. Hair pulling in young children seems to often resolve spontaneously but is more problematic in adolescents and adults. Management of trichotillomania usually involves non-pharmacologic treatments. In children, behavior modification, including putting socks on the hands and the use of time-out for hair pulling, in addition to extra attention for not pulling the hair, is recommended. Substituting behavior is also encouraged. For instance, children should be advised to sit on their hands, wear gloves, pull rubber bands, or squeeze a ball whenever they have an urge to pull their hair. In older individuals, hair pulling may be related to obsessive-compulsive disorders. Trichotillomania may lead to the presence of bezoars (hairballs) from swallowed hair. Sometimes hairballs can extend through the gastric outlet into the small intestine, a phenomenon referred to as Rapunzel syndrome. Gastric hairballs can be dissolved enzymatically or with the installation of Coca Cola through a nasogastric tube. If such maneuvers fail, they are removed endoscopically or through surgery. Pharmacologic therapy for trichotillomania is not routinely recommended for the management of affected children. In adults, selective serotonin reuptake inhibitors, bupropion, and risperidone have been used. Children whose symptoms have not improved with behavioral interventions should be referred to a mental health worker for additional management.

Nail biting also often responds to behavior modification. Olive oil may be put on the nails to make them soft so there are fewer jagged edges to bite. In the children's book, *The Berenstain Bears and the Bad Habit,* collecting pennies is suggested as a habit substitution for nail biting.

Rhythmic habits are less easy to modify. For the most part, reassurance is all that is available. The use of metronome-like devices has had no demonstrable effect. Children older than 3 years who disturb the family's sleep with their rhythmic habits may be given mild sedatives, such as diphenhydramine or hydroxyzine. Medications to reduce head banging include transdermal clonidine and thioridazine (Mellaril). Other maneuvers involve placing the crib or bed on carpeting or bolting the crib to the wall to decrease the amount of noise from movement.

Children who engage in biting behavior should be managed with behavior modification, including praising of good behavior and time-out for inappropriate behavior. Aversive conditioning involves the placement of some non-palatable food, such as a lemon or onion on a necklace, and having the child bite on that object rather than biting another child. Biting behavior is reported to be extinguished with this technique. Another option is the placement of a whistle. The child blows the whistle rather than biting the other child.

Nose picking is a common habit in both children and adults. One suggestion to extinguish or minimize this habit involves letting children look in a mirror and pick their nose or videotaping the child while nose picking. Their reaction is that nose picking looks "gross" and the habit may decrease in frequency.

Iron deficiency related to pica requires iron supplementation. Lead intoxication should be managed with chelation and environmental manipulation.

Prognosis

Most habits are not harmful to children's health. The major problem is social acceptability. Parents should be encouraged to stop a habit before it becomes ingrained. This can often be done by praising good behavior and encouraging activities during which the unwanted behavior does not appear. Habits that do not respond to parental influence often resolve spontaneously under peer pressure.

CASE RESOLUTION

In the case history presented at the beginning of the chapter, it is important for the physician and the mother to empower the boy to stop thumb sucking before he finds himself ridiculed by his classmates. He might be allowed to suck his thumb at certain times and in certain places (eg, "You can suck in your room after school for fifteen minutes."). Books geared at children and parents to help stop the thumb sucking are recommended, and the boy is rewarded for times when he is not sucking his thumb.

Selected References

Blum NJ, Barone VJ, Friman PC. A simplified behavioral treatment for trichotillomania: report of two cases. *Pediatrics.* 1993;91:993–995

Brazelton TB. Sucking in infancy. *Pediatrics.* 1956;17:400–404

Collacott RA, Cooper SA, Branford D, McGrother C. Epidemiology of self-injurious behaviour in adults with learning disabilities. *Br J Psychiatry.* 1998;173:428–432

Davidson L. Thumb and finger sucking. *Pediatr Rev.* 2008;29:207–208

Dimino-Emme L, Camisa C. Trichotillomania associated with the "Friar Tuck sign" and nail biting. *Cutis.* 1991;47:107–110

Flessner CA, Lochner C, Stein DJ, Woods DW, Franklin ME, Keuthen NJ. Age of onset of trichotillomania symptoms: investigating clinical correlates. *J Nerv Ment Dis.* 2010;198:896–900

Friman PC, Barone VJ, Christopherson ER. Aversive taste treatment of finger and thumb sucking. *Pediatrics.* 1986;78:174–176

Friman PC, McPherson KM, Warzak WJ, Evans J. Influence of thumb sucking on peer social acceptance in first-grade children. *Pediatrics.* 1993;91:784–786

Friman PC, Schmitt B. Thumb sucking in childhood: guidelines for the pediatrician. *Clin Pediatr.* 1989;28:438–440

Golomb RG, Vavrichek SM. *The Hair Pulling "Habit" and You: How to Solve the Trichotillomania Puzzle.* Silver Spring, MD: Writers' Cooperative of Greater Washington; 2000

Johnson ED, Larson BE. Thumb-sucking: literature review. *ASDC J Dent Child.* 1993;60:385–391

Koc O, Yoldiz FD, Narci A, Sen TA. An unusual cause of gastric perforation in childhood: trichobezoar (Rapunzel syndrome). A case report. *Eur J Pediatr.* 2009;168:495–497

Peterson JE, Schneider PE. Oral habits: a behavioral approach. *Pediatr Clin North Am.* 1991;38:1289–1307

Repetitive behavioral patterns. In: Wolraich ML, ed. *The Classification of Child and Adolescent Mental Diagnoses in Primary Care: Diagnostic and Statistical Manual for Primary Care (DSM-PC) Child and Adolescent Version.* Elk Grove Village, IL: American Academy of Pediatrics; 1996:269–275

Rosenberg MD. Thumbsucking. *Pediatr Rev.* 1995;16:73–74

Schmitt B. Helping the child with tics (twitches). *Contemp Pediatr.* 1991;8:31–32

Tay YK, Levy ML, Metry DW. Trichotillomania in childhood: case series and review. *Pediatrics.* 2004;113:e494–e498

CHAPTER 52

Enuresis

Carol D. Berkowitz, MD

CASE STUDY

A 9-year-old boy who is in good general health is evaluated for a history of bedwetting. He is the product of a normal pregnancy and delivery, and he achieved his developmental milestones at the appropriate time. The boy was toilet trained by the age of 3 years, but he has never been dry at night for more than several days at a time. Enuresis occurs at least 3 to 4 times a week even if he is fluid-restricted after 6:00 pm. The boy never wets himself during the day, has normal stools, and is an average student. His father had enuresis that resolved by the time he was 12 years old.

The boy's physical examination is entirely normal.

Questions

1. What conditions account for the symptoms of enuresis?
2. What is the appropriate evaluation of children with enuresis?
3. What is the relationship between enuresis and emotional stresses or psychosocial disorders?
4. What management plans are available for enuresis?
5. How do physicians decide which management technique is appropriate for which patients?

Enuresis is defined as involuntary or intentional urination in children whose age and development suggest achievement of bladder control. Voiding into the bed or clothing occurs repeatedly (at least twice a week for at least 3 consecutive months). Urinary continence is reached earlier in girls than in boys, and the diagnosis of enuresis is reserved for girls older than 5 years and boys older than 6 years. The term diurnal enuresis, wetting that occurs during the day, has been replaced by daytime incontinence. The International Children's Continence Society promotes a new standardization for enuresis-related terminology. They prefer the use of the term incontinence to denote uncontrollable leakage of urine, either intermittent or continuous, which occurs after continence should have been achieved. Nocturnal or sleep enuresis refers to involuntary urination or incontinence that occurs during the night. The term **primary nocturnal enuresis (PNE)** is used when children have never achieved sustained dryness, and **secondary enuresis** is used when urinary incontinence recurs after 3 to 6 months of dryness. Monosymptomatic nocturnal enuresis means that nighttime wetting is the only complaint. Children who experience urgency, frequency, dribbling, or other symptoms have polysymptomatic enuresis. Such symptoms may be related to inappropriate muscle contraction, are usually associated with constipation, and are termed dysfunctional elimination syndrome.

Physicians can be particularly helpful by routinely questioning parents about bedwetting during health maintenance visits. Many families are otherwise reluctant to bring up this embarrassing complaint because enuresis is viewed as socially unacceptable. It poses particular difficulties if children wish to sleep away from home. In addition, enuresis may be a marker for other behavioral or developmental problems.

Epidemiology

Enuresis affects 5 to 7 million patients in the United States. It is one of the most common conditions of childhood, affecting 10% to 20% of first-grade boys and 8% to 17% of first-grade girls. By age 10 years, 5% to 10% of boys have enuresis (1% of army recruits are enuretic). Seventy-four percent of affected children have nocturnal enuresis, 10% daytime incontinence, and 16% both. Primary enuresis affects the majority (75%–80%) of children with enuresis, and 80% to 85% of these children have monosymptomatic nocturnal enuresis. Although the overall incidence of secondary enuresis is lower (20%–25%), it increases with age; secondary enuresis makes up 50% of cases of enuresis in children 12 years of age.

Several epidemiological factors have been associated with enuresis, including low socioeconomic level, large family size, single-parent family, low birth weight, short height at 11 to 15 years of age, immature behavior, relatively low IQ, poor speech and coordination, and encopresis (fecal incontinence; 5%–15% of cases). Enuresis has been associated with obstructive sleep apnea where an increased level of atrial natriuretic factor has been reported. Atrial natriuretic factor inhibits the renin-angiotensin-aldosterone pathway, causing diuresis. Correcting the obstructive sleep apnea with tonsillectomy and/or adenoidectomy leads to an elimination of the enuresis. Enuresis occurs more often in institutionalized children. Enuresis has a familial basis, with 44% being enuretic if one parent was enuretic and as many as 77% of children are enuretic if both parents were similarly affected. Concordance for enuresis is reported in up to 68% of monozygotic twins and between 36% and 48% of dizygotic twins.

Clinical Presentation

A history of enuresis may be obtained as a presenting complaint or elicited by physicians during a health maintenance visit. Medical complaints such as encopresis, obstructive sleep apnea (nighttime snoring), or attention-deficit/hyperactivity disorder (ADHD) may be associated with the enuresis (Dx Box). Children with ADHD have a 30% greater risk of being enuretic. The physical examination is usually normal.

Dx **Enuresis**

- Bedwetting
- Old enough to be toilet trained
- Precipitating problem such as diabetes or urinary tract infection
- Encopresis
- Attention-deficit/hyperactivity disorder
- Family history of enuresis

Pathophysiology

Delayed control of micturition has several possible causes (Box 52-1).

1. **Faulty toilet training.** Faulty toilet training may perpetuate both diurnal and nocturnal enuresis but is not expected to selectively perpetuate the latter. Parental expectations are believed to play a role in the toilet training experience. Parents who allow children to sleep in diapers may be delaying the achievement of nighttime dryness, but it is unlikely that the use of diapers causes nocturnal enuresis. Poor toilet habits, particularly infrequent voiding

---

Box 52-1. Causes of Enuresis
Primary Enuresis
• Faulty toilet training
• Maturational delay
• Small bladder capacity
• Sleep disorder/impaired arousal
• Allergens
• Nocturnal polyuria/relative vasopressin deficiency
• Dysfunctional bladder contraction
Secondary Enuresis
• Urinary tract infection
• Diabetes mellitus
• Diabetes insipidus
• Nocturnal seizures
• Genitourinary anomalies
• Sickle cell anemia
• Medication use
• Emotional stress

---

or constipation, may be associated with urinary tract infections (UTIs).

2. **Maturational delay.** The development of the inhibitory reflex of voiding may be delayed in some children, which may contribute to enuresis until the age of 5 years. This is similar to the range with which children achieve other developmental milestones. It is unlikely that maturational delay persists as a cause of enuresis beyond this age. Experts believe that maturational delay is not a reasonable explanation if children can achieve dryness in the daytime but not at night.

3. **Small bladder capacity.** Evidence suggests that some children with enuresis have smaller bladder capacities. Bladder capacity in ounces is estimated as the age in years plus 2. For example, 5-year-old children have a bladder capacity of 7 ounces (210 mL). Adult bladder capacity is 12 to 16 ounces (360–480 mL). Small bladder capacity is associated with diurnal frequency or incontinence.

4. **Sleep disorder/impaired arousal.** It has been suggested that children with enuresis are in "deep sleep" and do not sense a full bladder. This is often the parent's perception of their child's sleep pattern. However, studies have shown that enuresis occurs during all stages of sleep, particularly in the first one-third of sleep and in transition from non–rapid eye movement stage 4 to rapid eye movement sleep. During this period body tone, respiratory rate, and heart rate increase, and erection and micturition occur. Studies suggest that the arousal center in the brain fails to respond (ie, the child does not awaken) to full bladder sensation. Children with enuresis do not seem to sleep more deeply than other children. However, enuretic children may have diminished arousal during sleep. In one study, 40% of enuretic children, compared with only 8.5% of non-enuretic children, failed to awaken to an 80-decibel noise.

5. **Allergens.** No evidence confirms the notion that exposure to certain foods (eg, food additives, sugar) contributes to enuresis. However, some parents believe that bedwetting is decreased if certain foods such as sodas and sweets are eliminated from the diet. The ingestion of caffeine-containing beverages may exacerbate nocturnal enuresis.

6. **Nocturnal polyuria/relative vasopressin deficiency.** Research has shown that although non-enuretic children exhibit a diurnal variation in vasopressin secretion, this rhythm is disturbed in some children with enuresis, resulting in nocturnal polyuria.

7. **Dysfunctional bladder contraction.** In cases of daytime incontinence, contractile disturbances of the bladder affect normal voiding. Children with an "uninhibited bladder" have not learned to inhibit bladder contraction. They may assume a certain posture, called Vincent curtsy, in an effort to prevent micturition. Some children exhibit discoordinated, incomplete voiding and the urine exits the urethra in a staccato stream. Trabeculations or bladder wall thickening may be noted on imaging studies.

Daytime incontinence can be related to problems with bladder filling and storage or to bladder emptying. Each of these functions is under different neurologic control, with filling and storage under the sympathetic nervous system and bladder emptying related to the action of acetylcholine and the parasympathetic system. Effective voiding requires the coordinated effort of these 2 phases. Management of daytime incontinence is dependent of which phase is malfunctioning.

Differential Diagnosis

Primary nocturnal enuresis is usually related to the conditions discussed in Pathophysiology. An organic problem is rarely the cause. However, secondary enuresis may result from an organic problem, such as UTI, diabetes mellitus, diabetes insipidus, nocturnal seizures, genitourinary anomalies (eg, ectopic ureter), sickle cell anemia, medication (eg, diuretics, theophylline), or emotional stress. When primary enuresis is both diurnal and nocturnal, some of these conditions should also be considered. Additional diagnoses include neurogenic bladder, which may occur in association with cerebral palsy; sacral agenesis; or myelomeningocele. Some children experience pollakiuria, a benign self-limited condition characterized by the sudden need to urinate very frequently, often 25 to 30 times a day. Rarely there is nocturia without other urinary symptoms. The condition occurs most often in children between 3 and 8 years, is self-limited, and felt to be stress-related. A urinary diary, noting time and amount of voiding, is sometimes helpful in diagnosing the condition.

Evaluation

History

A thorough history should be obtained when evaluating children with enuresis (Questions Box).

Physical Examination

A general physical examination should be performed, with particular attention to certain areas. The pattern of growth should be plotted. Blood pressure should be obtained. The abdomen should be assessed for evidence of organomegaly, bladder size, and fecal impaction. An anal examination should be performed to evaluate rectal tone.

If possible, physicians should watch children void. Practitioners should determine whether children can start and stop micturition and whether the stream is forceful. Dribbling in girls may indicate an ectopic ureter. A more sophisticated approach involves the uroflow test where the patient voids into an apparatus that electrically senses the rate of flow. A graph is generated that notes the flow rate and quantity. This study is most useful in children with diurnal incontinence. The appearance of the genitalia should be assessed. A rash in the genital area may be secondary to wetness from urinary incontinence. The skin may be macerated, erythematous, or hyperpigmented secondary to persistent moisture and irritation. Labial fusion in girls may trap urine, allow reflux into the vagina, and lead to dribbling. Meatal stenosis, epispadias, hypospadias, or cryptorchidism may be present in boys. Any of these conditions suggests a possible underlying genitourinary anomaly.

Questions

Enuresis

- Is the enuresis primary or secondary?
- Is the enuresis diurnal, nocturnal, or both?
- How old was the child when he or she was toilet trained?
- How old was the child when he or she achieved daytime and nighttime dryness?
- How often does the child urinate and defecate during the average day?
- Is the child's urinary stream forceful or dribbling?
- Does the child dribble before or after voiding?
- Does the child experience symptoms such as polydipsia, polyuria, dysuria, urgency, frequency, or problems with stooling?
- Who changes the bed and who washes the bedclothes after bedwetting occurs?
- Does the child wear diapers or pull-ups, or use incontinence pads?
- Does the child seem to delay using the toilet?
- Does the child assume any unusual or distinct postures to avoid being incontinent?
- What is the attitude of the family toward the child with enuresis? Are family members accepting or ashamed?
- Has the family tried any treatments yet?
- Is there a family history of enuresis?
- Does the child have other symptoms such as encopresis, attention-deficit/hyperactivity disorder, or obstructive sleep apnea?

The neuromuscular integrity of the lower extremities should be evaluated. This may provide a clue to a disorder such as spina bifida occulta. The presence of some anomaly in the sacral area, such as a sacral dimple or a tuft of hair, may also be a sign of this condition.

Laboratory Tests

Only a minimal laboratory evaluation is indicated in most children with primary enuresis. Urinalysis, including specific gravity, is usually indicated. A complete blood cell count, hemoglobin electrophoresis, serum electrolytes, and blood urea nitrogen should also be considered. Studies such as urine culture and blood glucose are more often indicated in cases of secondary enuresis.

Imaging Studies

In cases in which the urinalysis is abnormal, the culture is positive, or genitourinary anomalies are apparent on physical examination, a renal ultrasound and vesicoureterogram may be warranted. Vertebral radiographs or magnetic resonance imaging is appropriate in the diagnosis of spina bifida. Magnetic resonance urography is helpful in girls suspected of having an ectopic ureter. An electroencephalogram is indicated if nocturnal epilepsy is suspected. Urodynamic studies to evaluate bladder contractility are controversial but are recommended by some urologists. They are recommended in children who do not respond to traditional therapy or are suspected of having spina bifida occulta.

Management

Primary Enuresis

Family counseling about enuresis should be part of all management plans. Issues related to psychosocial stress should be explored, particularly in cases of secondary enuresis. Families should be advised that the wetting is not intentional and that punishing children for accidents is inappropriate. However, children may take some responsibility for the consequences of their actions, such as removing soiled bedding or helping with the laundry. They should be rewarded for dry nights. Star charts, in which a sticker or gold star is applied to a calendar for each dry night, have traditionally been used. The exclusive use of these charts without other interventions has limited success, however, and suggests that the enuresis may have a volitional component. Star charts should be used in conjunction with other management strategies.

Two treatment modalities are acceptable for managing enuresis. Most studies do not support the use of fluid restriction as a reliable isolated means of controlling enuresis.

Conditioning therapy involves the use of an alarm that is triggered when children void during the night. Children are awakened by the sounding of the alarm, and further urination is inhibited. Eventually bladder distention is associated with inhibition of the urge to urinate. When conditioning therapy is used for 4 to 6 months, it is associated with a success rate of 70%. If the alarm is used for 4 more weeks with sustained dryness, relapses are uncommon.

Because patient cooperation is needed with the alarm system, its use is reserved for children older than 7 years. A newer system is a transistorized version of the original device that contains a small sensor in the underwear and an alarm on the wrist or collar. Some systems use vibrations so other family members are not disturbed by loud alarms.

Overall, conditioning devices have a cure rate of 70% to 85%, and a relapse rate of 10% to 15%. They incur a one-time cost of $50 to $75. Conditioning devices may be covered by insurance companies if the alarm is prescribed by a physician as a medical device. Conditioning without the use of auxiliary alarms may also be undertaken. One proposed method involves instituting a self-awakening program. Older school-aged children practice lying in bed during the daytime and simulating the experience of awakening, sensing a full bladder, and going to the toilet. Another dry bed training program involves parents' awakening their children first hourly, and then at longer intervals over the period of about 1 week. Children eventually learn to self-awaken. A 92% success rate with a relapse rate of 20% is reported with this program.

Pharmacologic agents include tricyclic antidepressants and desmopressin. Tricyclic antidepressants, especially imipramine, have been successfully used to treat nocturnal enuresis, although the mechanism of action is uncertain. The antidepressant action of the drug, its effect on sleep and arousal, and its anticholinergic properties may all play a role. There is also some evidence that imipramine increases concentrations of antidiuretic hormone. The bladder capacity of individuals with enuresis treated with imipramine may be increased by 34%, which indicates that the anticholinergic effects of the drug may be the most significant.

Imipramine should not be prescribed for children younger than 6 or 7 years because of potential adverse effects. The recommended dosage is 0.9 to 1.5 mg/kg/day. In general, children younger than 8 years are given 25 mg 1 to 2 hours before bedtime, and older children are given 50 to 75 mg. Beneficial results usually occur within the first few weeks of therapy. Medication is usually continued for 3 to 6 months to prevent relapses, which are reported in up to 75% of cases. The drug should be tapered by reducing the dose or using an alternate-night regimen. Side effects are rare and include insomnia, nightmares, and personality changes. Acute overdoses are potentially fatal secondary to cardiac complications. The initial cure rate is 10% to 60% with a relapse rate of 90%. The monthly cost of imipramine is about $5.

Desmopressin, an analog of vasopressin, the antidiuretic hormone, is another pharmacologic agent used for enuresis. Desmopressin probably works to decrease nocturnal urine production. Most patients respond rapidly to desmopressin and become dry within 1 to 2 weeks of the initiation of therapy. The medication is taken orally as 0.2 mg/tablet 1 hour before bedtime. The dose may be increased by 1 tablet at weekly intervals (maximum dose: 0.6 mg). Desmopressin in nasal spray is no longer recommended for the treatment of enuresis because of the risk of severe hyponatremia, seizures, and even death. Hyponatremia has also been reported with oral desmopressin in the face of high fluid intake sometimes associated with habit polydipsia. Fluid restriction is recommended from 1 hour before until 8 hours after desmopressin administration. While some recommend a 6-month course of the medication, others suggest a shorter trial period. If patients achieve a 2-week period of dryness, the dose can be tapered at 2-week intervals. The cure rate is 40% to 50% with a relapse rate of 90% off medication. Desmopressin is expensive, with an average monthly cost of $150 to $250.

Oxybutynin is an antispasmodic, anticholinergic agent used in the management of daytime incontinence or polysymptomatic nocturnal enuresis. The dosage is 5 mg at bedtime for children 6 to 12 years and 10 mg at bedtime for children older than 12 years. The response rate is 33%, and the major side effects include drowsiness, flushing, dry mouth, constipation, and hyperthermia. Hyoscyamine sulfate and flavoxate hydrochloride are 2 other medications used for daytime incontinence.

Treatment of enuresis in children with small bladder capacities includes bladder retention training. Such children are fluid loaded and asked to delay voiding for 5 to 10 minutes. This strategy is generally reserved for children with daytime incontinence.

Associated symptoms, particularly constipation and encopresis should be adequately addressed.

Secondary Enuresis

The management of secondary enuresis should focus on the treatment of the causal disorder, such as a UTI or diabetes mellitus.

Prognosis

The prognosis for children with enuresis is good. The spontaneous cure rate is 15% per year. Medical management results in a reduction in symptoms in more than 70% of affected children.

CASE RESOLUTION

The boy in the case scenario has PNE. The history of childhood enuresis in the father is significant. Two management options, behavior modification and treatment with desmopressin or imipramine, can be discussed with the family. The child's symptoms will probably spontaneously improve over time.

Selected References

Bennett HJ. *Waking Up Dry*. Elk Grove Village, IL: American Academy of Pediatrics; 2005

Graham KM, Levy JB. Enuresis. *Pediatr Rev*. 2009;30:165–173

Joinson C, Heron J, von Gontard A, ALSPAC Study Team. Psychological problems of children with daytime wetting. *Pediatrics*. 2006;118:1985–1993

Mercer R. *Seven Steps to Nighttime Dryness: A Practical Guide for Parents of Children with Bedwetting*. Ashton, MD: Brookeville Media; 2004

Neveus T, von Gontard A, Hoebeke P, et al. The standardization of terminology of lower urinary tract function in children and adolescence: report for the standardization committee of International Children's Continence Society. *J Urol*. 2006;176:314–324

Robson WL. Enuresis. *Adv Pediatr*. 2001;48:409–438

Robson WL, Leung AK. An approach to daytime wetting in children. *Adv Pediatr*. 2006;53:323–365

Treatment of childhood enuresis. *Clin Pediatr (Phila)*. 1993;32:(entire issue)

Robson WL, Leung AKC, VanHowe R. Primary and secondary enuresis: similarities in presentation. *Pediatrics*. 2005;115:956–959

CHAPTER 53

Encopresis

Carol D. Berkowitz, MD

CASE STUDY

A 7-year-old boy presents with the complaint of soiling his underpants. His mother states that he has never been completely toilet trained, and that stooling accidents occur at least 2 to 3 times a week, mainly during the day. The boy rarely has a spontaneous bowel movement without assistance. He sits on the toilet for just a few minutes and passes small, pellet-like stools. His mother has never sought medical care before for this problem.

The boy is very fidgety during the physical examination. The vital signs are normal and the child's height and weight are at the 25th percentile. His abdomen is soft but distended, with palpable loops of stool-filled bowel.

A small amount of stool is present around the anus and in the boy's underpants. Digital examination of the rectum reveals hard stool. The rectal tone is normal as is the rest of the physical examination.

Questions

1. What is the definition of encopresis?
2. What is the difference between retentive and non-retentive encopresis?
3. What are some physiological conditions that contribute to encopresis?
4. What conditions may be mistaken for encopresis?

Encopresis is the repeated passage of stool into inappropriate places (eg, clothing), either voluntary or involuntary, in children who should be toilet trained on the basis of age (usually at least 4 years, the age at which 95% of children have achieved stool continence) and developmental level and who have no primary organic pathology. One such encopretic event occurs each month for at least 3 months. The term *encopresis,* coined in 1926 by Weissenberg and originally used for children with psychogenic soiling, is similar to enuresis. Unlike enuresis, encopresis rarely occurs at night. Now encopresis is used in a broader sense to refer to all types of fecal incontinence.

Retentive encopresis, also referred to as functional fecal retention with encopresis, occurs in the face of constipation (obstipation), in which chronic rectal distention leads to the seepage of liquid stool around hard, retained feces. Sometimes this is called overflow or fecal soiling. The onset of symptoms is usually about 4 years of age. Approximately 95% of cases of encopresis are retentive. **Non-retentive encopresis** is characterized by the passage of soft stool without colonic distention or retention of stool. Some have recognized 2 categories of children with non-retentive encopresis: those who can control defecation but stool in inappropriate places, and those who have true failure to achieve bowel control. Primary encopresis occurs when children have never been completely toilet trained. Secondary encopresis occurs in children who have had a period of complete continence of stool. Most encopretic children have secondary encopresis.

Epidemiology

Encopresis is reported in approximately 1.5% of school-aged children, and boys are reported to be affected 2 to 6 times more often than girls. This gender ratio reverses in the elderly, in which the prevalence of encopresis is twice as high in females as in males. An association between encopresis, enuresis, and attention-deficit/hyperactivity disorder (ADHD) is sometimes present. About 15% of children with enuresis also have encopresis. Family history for encopresis may also be positive; 16% of affected children have one affected parent, usually the father. An association between encopresis and child sexual abuse has been reported in a small number of children. There is no reported relationship between socioeconomic status, parental age, child's birth order, or family size.

Clinical Presentation

Children with encopresis have a history of staining of the underpants, which may be hidden in drawers or under beds by embarrassed children. Occasionally parents are unaware of the problem. Stooling accidents occur more frequently at home than in school. Some children have a history of constipation. Other children may initially be misdiagnosed as having diarrhea and are inappropriately placed on antidiarrheal medications, which then exacerbate their problem. Parents may complain that their children exude a fecal odor, but children are unaware they are malodorous (Dx Box).

Pathophysiology

A history of constipation, often with painful defecation, is associated with retentive encopresis. With time, the colon distends and liquid feces seep around impacted stool (Figure 53-1). In 30% to 50% of children, anal spasm, referred to as animus, occurs and contraction rather than relaxation occurs during evacuation of feces. In another 40%, rectal hyposensitivity is apparent so that the children

Dx Encopresis

- Incontinence of stool
- Constipation
- Hyperactivity
- Distended abdomen
- Stool-filled loops of bowel
- Lax rectal tone
- Soiled clothing or bedding
- Fecal odor

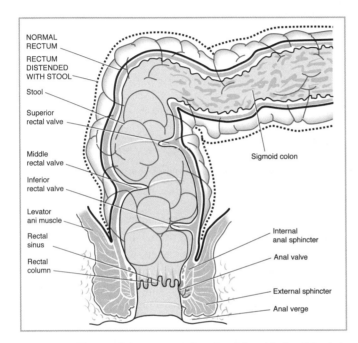

Figure 53-1. Diagram of the rectum, anal canal, and sigmoid colon distended with stool.

are unaware of the presence of the stool. Some children have an evacuation release disorder, in which the presence of the stool does not result in relaxation and stool evacuation. In such cases, the rectum is chronically distended by stool. Water is absorbed and the stool becomes harder and drier. The distended rectum fails to sense the presence of the stool. When evacuation is attempted, the process is painful, leading to further retention (see Chapter 111).

Encopresis has been associated with a short attention span and a high level of motor activity. Affected children are unable to sit on a toilet for more than a few minutes and do not adequately attend to the task of stool evacuation. As a result, they get off the toilet after the incomplete evacuation of only small amounts of stool. In some toddlers, constipation is related to the struggle of toilet training and an unwillingness to sit on the toilet (see Chapter 45).

The pathophysiology of non-retentive encopresis seems to be psychogenic. Some children who have been chronically sexually abused have lax anal tone, which may contribute to the fecal incontinence. Animus, abnormal anal sphincter contraction, has been reported in up to 30% of children with constipation.

Differential Diagnosis

The differential diagnosis of encopresis focuses on organic conditions associated with chronic constipation. Organic conditions account for 5% to 10% of fecal incontinence. These conditions include Hirschsprung disease, disorders of intestinal motility (eg, pseudo-obstruction), disorders of anal tone and anal anatomy (eg, imperforate anus with fistula), disorders of the lumbosacral spine (eg, meningomyelocele), and previous surgeries (eg, repair of imperforate anus). Neurofibromatosis, lead poisoning, and hypothyroidism are also associated with constipation. Congenital anorectal anomalies, which are reported in 1 in 5,000 live births, are rare.

Most of these conditions can be ruled out on the basis of a careful history and physical examination. In some cases, specific testing, such as anal manometry or rectal biopsy, may be necessary to exclude a particular disorder.

Evaluation

History

The age of onset of the problem, as well as the age of initiation of toilet training, should be determined. In general, affected children are 4 years of age and older. A detailed history of the stooling pattern should be obtained (Questions Box). The frequency and consistency of stools as well as quantity of stools should also be noted. In addition, the presence of nocturnal episodes of encopresis should be determined. In cases of secondary encopresis, the duration of fecal continence and the occurrence of any events, such as the birth of a sibling or the start of school, that may have precipitated the

Questions

Encopresis

- At what age was the child toilet trained?
- Does the child have spontaneous bowel movements (without enemas or suppositories)? If so, how frequently?
- Does the child have large, dry, hard stools that clog the toilet?
- Does the child pass blood with the stool?
- Did the child pass meconium within the first 24 hours after birth?
- Has the child had any surgery in the ano-genital area, spine, or bowel?
- Is the child taking any medications, such as aspirin, iron, Ritalin, imipramine, calcium channel blockers, or anticholinergics?
- Does the child seem to resist the urge to defecate (eg, squeeze legs together and rock back and forth)?
- Does the child have a history of enuresis or attention-deficit/hyperactivity disorder?
- What is the pattern of encopresis (ie, is the encopresis primary or secondary)?
- When and where does the child soil (eg, nocturnal, at home)?
- Have there been changes or stresses in the home or family?
- What happens to the child's stained underwear?
- What has the family done to manage the problem?

episodes of encopresis should be noted. Some children experience the onset of encopresis when they start school. Because of "toilet phobia," they are unwilling to use the public toilet in the school setting.

Physical Examination

The next step involves the performance of a comprehensive physical examination, paying particular attention to the abdomen to check for the presence of distended, stool-filled loops of bowel. The rectal area should be assessed for rectal tone, an anal wink, and the presence of hard stool. Rectal prolapse, if present, may be indicative of chronic constipation or another condition, such as cystic fibrosis. Perianal fissures may reflect passage of large, hard stools. Hemorrhoids are unusual in children and can indicate chronic constipation. Location of the anus should also be noted, and anterior displacement may suggest incomplete forms of imperforate anus. Children with retentive encopresis have normal or tight anal tone on rectal examination because they are frequently contracting their external anal sphincter to prevent the seepage of the liquid stool.

Dysmorphic features should be noted and may suggest a syndrome in which constipation is a feature. Abnormalities around the anus, such as fistulas, should also be noted. Fistulas are found in Crohn disease. The underpants should be evaluated for the presence of stool, mucus, or pus. A sensory and motor examination of the lower extremities helps determine if any signs of spinal cord dysfunction are evident. An evaluation of the skin over the spinal area may reveal abnormalities such as sacral dimples or tufts of hair.

Children who do not exhibit abdominal distention may have soft stool on rectal examination, which indicates non-retentive encopresis. If patulous anal tone is noted, spinal cord abnormalities or prior child sexual abuse should be suspected.

Laboratory Tests

Most children with encopresis require few laboratory studies. Studies focus on eliminating organic causes of encopresis, such as Hirschprung disease or spinal cord anomalies. Urinalysis and urine culture are recommended in children with fecal impactions to exclude urinary tract infection. Encopresis is reported to be an independent risk factor for urinary tract infections. Anorectal manometry, which may be used to measure the pressure generated by the anal sphincter, may also reveal abnormalities of anal tone or evidence of aganglionosis. The Child Behavioral Checklist is useful to determine if certain behavior problems exist. Such problems may either potentiate the encopresis or result from it.

Imaging Studies

In most encopretic children, imaging studies are not necessary. If radiographs of the abdomen are taken in children with retentive encopresis, distended, stool-filled bowel may be noted. A barium enema is useful if Hirschsprung disease is to be ruled out. Strictures, which may occur following necrotizing enterocolitis, will also be detected. Electromyogram to determine whether the innervation of the external anal sphincter is intact is recommended for children with encopresis who fail to respond to routine treatment.

Management

The management of encopresis focuses on complete rectal evacuation and patient and parent education and counseling. Regaining muscle tone of the anal canal usually requires 2 to 6 months.

Rectal evacuation requires **pharmacologic management** to ensure an adequate clean-out of retained stools. The decision about which laxatives to use depends on the degree of constipation. If the degree of fecal retention is mild, a high-fiber diet and stool-bulking agents or oral laxatives, such as senna derivatives, bisacodyl, or lactulose syrup, may be used in association with stool softeners or lubricants, such as mineral oil. The amount of mineral oil may be titrated up to ensure success. Some practitioners recommend that mineral oil be given until it oozes from the rectum. The amount may then be titrated back to a lower level. Magnesium sulfate is also recommended to relieve constipation. Magnesium citrate can be used, but should be administered cautiously and with the admonition to drink plenty of fluids to prevent dehydration. Polyethylene glycol 3350 has a very high success rate in the management of constipation and encopresis.

If the degree of retention is more severe, suppositories or enemas may be needed. Occasionally, children have to be disimpacted manually. Alternative methods to manual disimpaction include 2 to 3 sodium phosphate enemas over 1 to 2 days or 8 oz of mineral oil a day for 4 days. Pulsed irrigation–enhanced evacuation involves the insertion of a rectal tube and the installation of pulses of warm irrigating solution, simultaneously draining rectal contents. If the above modalities are not successful, children may need to be admitted to the hospital for oral lavage using polyethylene glycol-electrolyte solution at 30 to 40 mL/kg/hour until successful evacuation has occurred. This procedure often requires insertion of a nasogastric tube and 6 to 8 hours of treatment. Once the fecal accumulation has been relieved, every effort should be made to keep children regular. This can be accomplished with the combined use of toilet retraining, stool softeners or laxatives, and enemas or suppositories. Prokinetic agents such as metoclopramide may also be used.

Dietary manipulation is important to ensure sustained regular stooling. Parents should be told that children require a high-fiber diet with fruit juices, such as pear or peach juice, and decreased milk (≤16 oz/day). It has been suggested that a "team and coach" approach is the most successful route, and that bowel training be likened to fitness training.

The toilet retraining process, sometimes referred to as enhanced toilet training, requires that children sit on the toilet at least 2 or 3 times a day, usually after meals, for about 10 minutes or until they have had a bowel movement. Some practitioners recommend the use of an egg timer to ensure that children spend the appropriate amount of time on the toilet. Children should be requested to maintain a diary of their evacuation, which may take the form of a star chart. Stars or other rewards are given for successful bowel movements in the toilet.

If children skip a day between bowel movements, they may be treated with a suppository, such as a glycerin or bisacodyl suppository.

If they still have not succeeded in having a bowel movement, then an enema may be appropriate. This sequence should be maintained until children are having bowel movements in the toilet and not soiling for at least 1 month. In general, stool softeners are required for at least 3 to 6 months. The regimen may have to be modified, particularly in younger children.

Behavior modification and biofeedback, such as using external anal sphincter electromyography, are 2 other modalities that can be used to help manage encopresis. Consultation with specialists such as pediatric gastroenterologists may be required.

Thirty percent of children with encopresis may need psychological consultation. Psychological intervention in the form of interactive parent–child family guidance has been reported successful when standard gastroenterologic intervention has failed. Children with evidence of child sexual abuse or non-retentive encopresis should be referred to a psychologist early in the course of therapy. The underlying psychosocial problems of children with non-retentive encopresis must be adequately addressed before their condition can improve.

Prognosis

The prognosis for children with retentive encopresis is reportedly good with appropriate intervention. In one study, children who were able to defecate a rectal balloon filled with 100 mL of water within 5 minutes were twice as likely to recover from constipation and encopresis. It is estimated that about 30% to 50% of affected children experience long-lasting remission after 1 year and up to 75% are in remission by 5 years.

The prognosis for children with non-retentive encopresis is less predictable and highly dependent on the underlying psychopathology.

CASE RESOLUTION

In the case scenario, the boy exhibits typical manifestations of retentive encopresis. His condition should be managed with the use of laxatives, stool softeners, and toilet retraining with a star chart. The possible ADHD should be addressed separately but may be contributing to his inability to attend to the task of toileting.

Selected References

Borowitz SM, Cox DJ, Sutphen JL, Kovatchev B. Treatment of childhood encopresis: a randomized trial comparing three treatment protocols. *J Pediatr Gastroenterol Nutr.* 2002;34:378–384

Burket RC, Cox DJ, Tam AP, et al. Are constipated kids just being stubborn? *Develop Behav Pediatr.* 2006;27:106–111

Fishman L, Rappaport L, Cousineau D, Nurko S. Early constipation and toilet training in children with encopresis. *J Pediatr Gastroenterol Nutr.* 2002;34:385–388

Fishman L, Rappaport L, Schonwald A, Nurko S. Trends in referral to a single encopresis clinic over 20 years. *Pediatrics.* 2003;111:e604–e607

Har AF, Croffie JM. Encopresis. *Pediatr Rev.* 2010;31:368–374

Loenig-Baucke V. Encopresis. *Curr Opin Pediatr.* 2002;14:570–575

Loenig-Baucke V. Functional fecal retention with encopresis in childhood. *J Pediatr Gastroenterol Nutr.* 2004;38:79–84

Pashankar DS, Bishop WP, Loenig Baucke V. Long-term efficacy of polyethylene glycol 3350 for the treatment of chronic constipation in children with and without encopresis. *Clin Pediatr (Phila).* 2003;42:815–819

Reid H, Bahar RJ. Treatment of encopresis and chronic constipation in young children: clinical results from interactive parent-child guidance. *Clin Pediatr.* 2006;45:157–164

Setty R, Wershil BK. Fecal overflow incontinence. *Pediatr Rev.* 2006;27:e54–e55

Acute and Emergent Problems

CHAPTER 54

Fever and Bacteremia

Paul Bryan, MD

CASE STUDY

An 8-month-old girl is brought to the emergency department (ED) with a 2-day history of fever and increased fussiness. She is irritable but consolable by parents. Her parents believe that her immunizations are up to date, but they do not have the immunization record with them. On examination, she has a rectal temperature of 39.5°C (103.1°F). The rest of the physical examination is within normal limits, and no source for the fever is apparent.

Questions

1. What are serious bacterial infections in young febrile infants?
2. What has been the impact of conjugated vaccines against *Haemophilus influenzae* and *Streptococcus pneumoniae* on the incidence of bacteremia and meningitis in febrile infants?
3. What are the challenges in differentiating between serious and benign febrile illnesses in young children?
4. What diagnostic studies are recommended in the evaluation of febrile infants and children?
5. When should febrile infants be hospitalized?

Fever is one of the most common chief complaints among pediatric patients seeking medical attention in physician offices, urgent care centers, and EDs and accounts for up to 20% to 30% of these visits. Most of these patients will have a benign, self-limited viral illness. Some patients, however, will have a **serious bacterial infection** (SBI), defined as meningitis, urinary tract infection (UTI)/pyelonephritis, bacteremia, septic arthritis, osteomyelitis, cellulitis, or deep tissue infection. **Bacteremia** is a bacterial infection within the bloodstream. **Occult bacteremia** occurs when there is a bacterial infection in the blood without any apparent source of infection after a thorough physical examination in an otherwise healthy-appearing child.

Epidemiology

Historically, management decisions regarding febrile children have been largely dictated by age. Children have been broken down into age-defined categories: (1) young infants less than 90 days, (2) infants and young children 3 to 36 months, and (3) children older than 3 years. Young febrile infants (ie, <90 days) have higher rates of SBIs than older children and often represent a diagnostic challenge. They have relatively immature immune systems rendering them particularly susceptible to bacterial infections, have not yet received most of their immunizations, and often have limited responses in the face of bacterial infections and, therefore, exhibit relatively nonspecific signs and symptoms. In addition, young infants have different bacterial pathogens that can cause these serious infections, including *Escherichia coli*, *Streptococcus agalactiae* (group B streptococci or GBS), *Listeria monocytogenes,* and other gram-negative organisms (Box 54-1). The prevalence of an SBI among young febrile infants with a fever of 38.0°C (100.4°F) is about 10%, with UTIs being by far

the most common source. A smaller percentage has bacteremia and/or meningitis. Recent studies have demonstrated that young febrile infants with diagnosed viral infections have lower rates of SBI than those without viral infections (4% vs 12%). None of the young febrile infants with viral infections by diagnostic testing had meningitis, but some did have UTIs and, rarely, bacteremia.

Febrile children aged 3 to 36 months are at a higher risk for bacteremia than older children, but less so than young febrile infants. The physical examination, while more reliable than in younger infants, can often be normal without any localizing source of infection. These individuals may in turn have occult bacteremia. Vaccine development and widespread immunization programs have dramatically

---

Box 54-1. Organisms Implicated in Serious Bacterial Infection/Occult Bacteremia in Children

Infants Younger Than 3 Months
- Group B streptococcus
- *Escherichia coli*
- *Listeria monocytogenes*
- *Salmonella* species (infants >1 month)
- *Haemophilus influenzae* type b (Hib)[a] (infants >1 month).

Children Between 3 and 36 Months of Age
- *Streptococcus pneumoniae*
- *Neisseria meningitidis*
- *Salmonella* species
- *Staphylococcus aureus*
- Hib[a]

[a] Hib disease has been virtually eliminated with the routine use of Hib conjugate vaccines.

changed the epidemiology and clinical course of bacteremia among this population within the United States over the last several decades. Prior to the introduction of the *Haemophilus influenzae* type b (Hib) and pneumococcal vaccines, the prevalence rates of bacteremia were around 3%. During this time, *Haemophilus* was considered the most significant organism causing bacteremia because of its invasive ability to cause localized infection, particularly meningitis. In the mid-1980s, the Hib vaccine was introduced, which has now virtually eliminated this particularly invasive organism. In the post-Hib but pre-pneumococcal conjugate vaccine era, the rates of occult bacteremia ranged from 1.6% to 1.9% in children with a temperature of 39.0°C (102.1°F) or higher and no obvious source of infection. More than 90% of the cases of occult bacteremia in this age group were caused by *Streptococcus pneumoniae*, with the remainder being caused by *Salmonella, Neisseria meningitides, Staphylococcus aureus*, and a few other rare organisms. Pneumococcus is not as virulent a microorganism as some other bacteria. Most cases of occult pneumococcal bacteremia resolved spontaneously without any intervention. If untreated, a small percentage (3%–5%) went on to develop pneumococcal meningitis, which has the most serious complication and fatality rate. In 2000 the heptavalent pneumococcal conjugate vaccine was licensed by the US Food and Drug Administration for use within the United States. This vaccine provided coverage against the 7 main serotypes of *S pneumoniae* responsible for approximately 80% of the cases of invasive pneumococcal disease in the United States and Canada at the time. Following the introduction of this vaccine, the rate of invasive pneumococcal disease (including bacteremia) and carriage for the serotypes covered by the vaccine dropped considerably. In addition, there was evidence suggestive of herd immunity in that there was a decline in invasive pneumococcal disease among older individuals who had not received the vaccine. Consequently, there has been a selective pressure that has increased the prevalence of invasive pneumococcal disease caused by strains not covered by the heptavalent vaccine, although the overall magnitude of this effect appears to be relatively small. In addition, other bacteria, such as *E coli, Salmonella,* and *S aureus*, appear to have increased in relative frequency as a source of bacteremia. In 2010 a new 13-valent pneumococcal conjugate vaccine was licensed and is manufactured in the same way as the heptavalent vaccine. This vaccine expanded coverage to include 6 different serotypes that have emerged with increasing frequency as a cause of invasive pneumococcal disease following the introduction of the heptavalent vaccine. The American Academy of Pediatrics and the Advisory Committee on Immunization Practices currently recommends the pneumococcal conjugate vaccine for all infants in a 4-dose regimen to be given at 2, 4, 6, and 12 to 15 months of age. Continued surveillance of invasive disease will be necessary to ascertain what impact the changes in epidemiology of these newer vaccines may have on the diagnosis and management of bacteremia in young febrile children.

Clinical Presentation

In many febrile children, fever is the only complaint or manifestation of disease. These children may look fine and behave normally.

Young children, especially infants younger than 3 months, have fewer and subtler behavioral signs with bacterial infections. Physicians must, therefore, maintain a high index of suspicion for the presence of an SBI even in the absence of localizing signs (Dx Box). Occult bacteremia, by definition, has no abnormal physical manifestations aside from fever.

Dx **Serious Bacterial Illness**

- Lethargy, irritability, or change in mental status
- Tachycardia disproportionate to the degree of temperature elevation
- Tachypnea or labored respirations
- Bulging or depressed anterior fontanelle
- Nuchal rigidity
- Petechiae
- Localized erythema, pain, or swelling
- Abdominal or flank pain
- Fever

Pathophysiology

Fever is an elevation in the thermoregulatory set point of the body. The thermoregulatory center is located in the preoptic region of the anterior hypothalamus, and an elevation in the hypothalamic set point above the normal body temperature initiates the physiological changes that lead to fever. Exogenous pyrogens (eg, bacteria, viruses, antigen-antibody complexes) stimulate host inflammatory cells (eg, macrophages, polymorphonuclear cells) to produce endogenous pyrogens (EPs). Interleukin-1 is currently regarded as the prototypical EP. Endogenous pyrogens cause the hypothalamic endothelium to increase intermediary substances, such as prostaglandins and neurotransmitters, which then act on the preoptic neurons of the anterior hypothalamus to produce an elevated set point. The body uses physiological mechanisms (eg, peripheral vasoconstriction, shivering) and behavioral actions (eg, bundling up, drinking hot tea) to increase body temperature to reach and maintain this higher set point, thus producing fever (Figure 54-1).

In contrast, the thermoregulatory set point of the body is normal in hyperthermia. Due to abnormal physiological processes, heat gain exceeds heat loss, and the body temperature rises in spite of efforts to return to the control set point.

Differential Diagnosis

In most cases, the duration of fever in children is short, and signs and symptoms are localized. Fever without a source involves an acute episode of fever that lasts 1 week or less in children in whom history, physical examination, and preliminary laboratory tests fail to reveal a source. Most affected children are eventually diagnosed with an acute, generally self-limited, infectious illness. Occult bacteremia has been a major concern in young children, primarily in infants younger than 36 months. High risk factors for occult bacteremia are presented in Box 54-2. Fever of unknown origin (FUO) is fever of at least 8

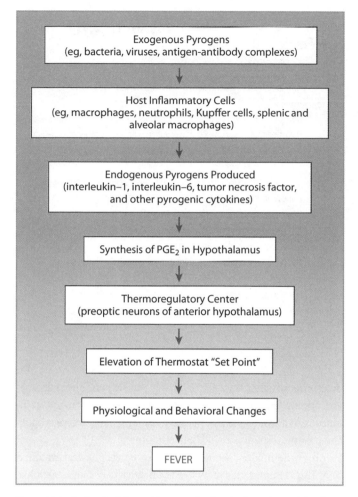

Figure 54-1. Pathophysiology of fever production. Antipyretics work by blocking the synthesis of prostaglandin E₂ (PGE₂).

days' duration in infants or children in whom routine history, physical examination, and laboratory assessment fail to reveal a source.

The differential diagnosis of children with an acute febrile illness is primarily infectious (Box 54-3), including both benign, generally self-limited illnesses such as upper respiratory infections, and less common, more serious illnesses such as meningitis and osteomyelitis. Occasionally a child with a fever without a source turns out to have a noninfectious illness such as a collagen vascular disease or neoplasia. By comparison, the differential diagnosis of children with FUO is quite broad (Box 54-4) and contains both infectious and noninfectious disorders.

Evaluation

History

The medical history can provide a great deal of valuable information in the evaluation of children with fever (Questions Box). The history should focus on the duration and severity of the fever. The presence of associated symptoms that may be signs of specific organ system involvement should also be noted.

Box 54-2. Risk Factors for Occult Bacteremia

- Age 36 months or younger
- Temperature 103.1°F (39.5°C) or higher
- White blood cell count 15,000/µL or higher or 5,000/µL or lower
- Total band cells 1,500/µL or higher
- Erythrocyte sedimentation rate 30 mm/hour or higher
- Underlying chronic disease (malignancy, immunodeficiency, sickle cell disease, malnutrition)
- Clinical appearance (irritability, lethargy, toxic appearance)

Box 54-3. Common Infectious Causes of an Acute Episode of Fever in Children

Upper Respiratory Tract
- Upper respiratory infection (common cold)
- Otitis media
- Sinusitis

Pulmonary
- Bronchiolitis
- Pneumonia

Oral Cavity
- Gingivostomatitis
- Pharyngitis
- Dental abscess

Gastrointestinal Tract
- Acute gastroenteritis (bacterial or viral)
- Appendicitis

Genitourinary Tract
- Urinary tract infection
- Pyelonephritis

Musculoskeletal
- Septic arthritis
- Osteomyelitis

Central Nervous System
- Meningitis

Miscellaneous (including noninfectious causes)
- Bacteremia
- Immunization reaction
- Viral exanthems (eg, chickenpox, measles)
- Neoplasia
- Collagen vascular disease

Physical Examination

Rectal temperatures should be performed in all young infants and children. An elevation in rectal temperature in an infant should not be attributed to overbundling. Vital signs in addition to temperature may provide important diagnostic clues. Tachycardia disproportionate to the degree of temperature elevation may suggest dehydration or sepsis. Tachypnea, which is often the only sign of a respiratory

---

Box 54-4. Common Causes of Fever of Unknown Origin in Children[a]

Infectious Diseases

Bacterial

- Localized infection: mastoiditis, sinusitis, pneumonia, osteomyelitis, pyelonephritis, abscess (eg, abdominal, pelvic)
- Systemic disease: tuberculosis, brucellosis, salmonellosis, leptospirosis, tularemia

Viral

- Hepatitis viruses
- Cytomegalovirus
- Epstein-Barr virus (infectious mononucleosis)
- HIV

Fungal

- Disseminated coccidioidomycosis
- Disseminated histoplasmosis

Miscellaneous

- Malaria
- Rocky Mountain spotted fever
- Syphilis
- Lyme disease

Neoplasia

- Leukemia
- Lymphoma
- Hodgkin disease
- Neuroblastoma

Collagen Vascular Diseases

- Juvenile rheumatoid arthritis
- Systemic lupus erythematosus
- Rheumatic fever

Miscellaneous

- Inflammatory bowel diseases
- Kawasaki disease
- Thyroiditis
- Drugs
- Factitious fever

[a] For a complete discussion of fever of unknown origin, the reader is referred to Lorin MI, Feigin RD. Fever without localizing signs and fever of unknown origin. In: Feigin RD, Cherry JD, eds. *Textbook of Pediatric Infectious Diseases*. 4th ed. Philadelphia, PA: W.B. Saunders; 1998:820–830.

Questions

Fever and Bacteremia

- How long has the child had fever? How high has the temperature been?
- Does the child have any other symptoms, such as rash, vomiting, diarrhea, abdominal pain, or dysuria; cough, rhinorrhea, or other respiratory symptoms; or lethargy, irritability, or change in mental status?
- Is anyone sick at home?
- Has the child's activity level changed (eg, more sleepy than usual) or is the child more irritable?
- What immunizations has the child received?
- Is the child taking any medications?
- Do any pets live in the house?
- Has there been any history of recent travel, especially outside the country?
- Has the child ever been hospitalized for an infectious illness?
- Does the child have any medical problems, especially asthma, sickle cell anemia, congenital heart disease, or immunodeficiency?

---

infection, also occurs in response to metabolic acidosis secondary to sepsis or shock. These changes may suggest an occult focus of infection. Response of the temperature and other vital signs to antipyretics should be noted. The physician must remain cautious because a clinical improvement in response to antipyretics can be seen in younger children and infants even in the face of an SBI. Young infants with recorded fevers at home, but who are afebrile on physician evaluation, should be managed as if they have a fever present.

Observation of the overall hydration and activity of infants and children is extremely important. An attempt should be made to determine whether they are behaving and responding in an age-appropriate fashion. Physicians should look for eye contact, spontaneous motor movements, negative responses to adverse stimuli, and positive responses to pleasant stimuli.

All febrile children should receive a complete physical examination. This is important even when the history may suggest involvement of one organ system. For example, in young children, vomiting and fever may be the only signs of viral illness, or possibly a more serious infection, such as a UTI or central nervous system (CNS) infection. The underlying condition may go undiagnosed unless a thorough examination and diagnostic evaluation are performed.

The anterior fontanelle should be palpated. It may be normal, bulging as a result of CNS infection, or depressed secondary to dehydration. The ears should be examined carefully and pneumatic otoscopy performed. Careful inspection may reveal otitis media as the source of fever, especially in children younger than 3 years. The occurrence of otitis media should not preclude further workup for invasive bacterial disease in children who do not appear well (see Chapter 72). The oropharynx should also be examined carefully. Dry mucous membranes may indicate dehydration. Enlarged, inflamed, or exudative tonsils may signal the presence of a viral infection or group A streptococcal infection in older children. Respiratory symptoms such as retractions, nasal flaring, grunting, stridor, rales, rhonchi, or wheezing may all be clues to respiratory tract infections. Enanthems on the buccal mucosa, or exanthems on the skin, are often signs of viral infections. The presence of petechiae in association with fever may indicate serious underlying infection, such as meningococcemia. The capillary refill time, quality of peripheral pulses, and the general temperature of the extremities assess perfusion. Localized areas of pain, erythema, swelling, induration, or fluctuance may point to cellulitis, septic arthritis, osteomyelitis, or the presence of an abscess. Nuchal rigidity can be an important clue to the presence of meningitis. This is rarely present in infants younger than 15 to 18 months, however, and physicians must maintain an index of suspicion for meningitis in febrile children of this age.

Laboratory Tests

Infants 90 Days or Younger

Because the physical examination alone cannot reliably identify an SBI in all febrile infants 90 days of age or younger with a temperature of 38.0°C (100.4°F) or higher, a thorough evaluation for a bacterial source of infection is required. This evaluation includes a complete blood cell count (CBC) with differential, urinalysis with microscopic evaluation, and blood and urine cultures. Cerebrospinal fluid (CSF) studies and CSF cultures should be performed on all infants younger than 6 weeks, and strongly considered between 6 to 8 weeks. Peripheral white blood cell (WBC) counts, while possibly helpful in older infants and children, do no reliably predict UTIs, bacteremia, or meningitis in young febrile infants. Decisions about whether to send blood and urine cultures, or to perform a lumbar puncture, should not be based solely on the screening peripheral WBC count in this age group. In addition, the standard urinalysis has a sensitivity of only around 85% in this age group and should not be used to determine the need for urine culture. Rapid viral diagnostic techniques that can reliably identify several of the more common viral pathogens (eg, respiratory syncytial virus, influenza, adenovirus, parainfluenza) are also available. The presence of a positive viral test result, however, does not preclude further diagnostic testing in this age group, specifically blood and urine cultures. If empiric antibiotics are to be dispensed, a lumbar puncture must be performed so as not to obscure the possibility of partially treated meningitis should pleocytosis be discovered on a subsequent CSF specimen. Stool analysis and culture should be reserved for those young febrile infants with diarrhea. Routine diagnostic radiographic studies (eg, chest radiographs) are not necessary, and should be reserved for infants with respiratory symptoms (eg, tachypnea, hypoxia, rales, wheezes, increased work of breathing).

Infants 3 to 36 Months

The diagnostic approach to older infants and young children has changed following the introduction of pneumococcal conjugate vaccines. Prior to widespread vaccine use, the standard of care involved an aggressive diagnostic approach looking for occult bacteremia in febrile children 3 to 24 months with temperature higher than 39.0°C (102.2°F), and in those 2 to 3 years with temperature higher than 39.5°C (103.1°F) without any apparent source of infection. The workup included a screening CBC, blood cultures, and empirically treating infants and children with an elevated WBC count greater than 15,000/mm³ or an absolute neutrophil count (ANC) greater than 10,000/mm³ because they were at higher risk for occult bacteremia. The ANC was generally considered to be the best predictor of risk for occult bacteremia. Acute phase reactants such as erythrocyte sedimentation rate and C-reactive protein, while commonly

elevated in serious infections, have not been shown to be better predictors for occult bacteremia than the peripheral WBC count or ANC. Other laboratory tests, including antigen testing, serum cytokine measurements, and polymerase chain reaction, are not particularly useful because of their limited availability, relatively high false-positive rates, and cost. Currently there is no single test that has been able to reliably identify all young febrile children with occult bacteremia.

With the declining prevalence of invasive pneumococcal disease post-licensure of the heptavalent conjugate vaccine, the need for routine screening, culturing, and selective antibiotic use for occult bacteremia has been challenged. The peripheral WBC count is no longer as useful a screening tool in the face of such low rates of invasive disease. In addition, the rates of contaminated blood cultures are now much higher than actual cases of bacteremia, which often results in unnecessary additional testing, hospitalization, antibiotic administration, and family stress. Infants and children who have received at least 2 doses of the vaccine can be safely managed without blood tests because this is no longer a cost-effective strategy. Individuals who are unimmunized, whose vaccine status is uncertain, or who have received only 1 dose of the vaccine may need screening evaluation with CBC, blood, and urine cultures, and expectant antibiotics if they are found to have an elevated WBC count or ANC. The change in epidemiology of bacteremia following the widespread use of the pneumococcal vaccine may warrant reconsideration of this in the future following long-term surveillance of invasive disease. Infants with fever higher than 39.0°C warrant urine testing, especially in girls younger than 2 years, uncircumcised boys younger than 12 months, and circumcised boys younger than 6 months. Chest radiograph should be considered in infants with significant respiratory symptoms or auscultatory findings suggestive of pneumonia. In infants with temperatures higher than 39.5°C and WBC counts greater than 20,000/mm³, chest radiographs should also be obtained to detect occult pneumonias, reported in up to 25% of these patients, even in the absence of significant respiratory symptoms or auscultatory findings.

Children Older Than 3 Years

The laboratory evaluation of children older than 3 years is individualized and influenced by the history and physical examination. Healthy children in this age group are not at high risk for occult bacteremia. In addition their physical examination is more reliable and they are better able to communicate their symptoms than younger children. Routine screening tests are not generally indicated in healthy individuals and should be reserved for those who look toxic or have an underlying disease that puts them at increased risk for bacterial infections (eg, sickle cell disease, cancer, immunodeficiency, nephrotic syndrome).

Imaging Studies

As noted previously, chest radiographs are the most common imaging study done in the routine evaluation of an infant or child with fever and symptoms consistent with lower respiratory infection or with fever and no apparent source. Other imaging studies, such as bone scans, gallium scans, magnetic resonance imaging, and computed tomography scans, are indicated if there are suspected infections such as an occult abscess or osteomyelitis.

Management

Management of children with fever includes both controlling the fever and treating the underlying process causing the fever. There is no evidence that fever itself is harmful. To the contrary, animal studies have suggested that fever may have some survival advantage. Despite the possible beneficial effects of fever, febrile children may still feel uncomfortable. Fever should be reduced to relieve the associated discomfort and malaise. **Antipyretics** such as acetaminophen and ibuprofen can be used. Aspirin should be avoided in children because of the association with Reye syndrome and viral illnesses. **Sponging** or **bathing** with tepid water and **unbundling** children aid in fever reduction. Ice water or alcohol baths should be avoided.

All toxic-appearing febrile infants and children, regardless of age, require hospitalization and administration of broad-spectrum antibiotics. Hospitalization and the initiation of empiric intravenous (IV) antibiotics are recommended for all febrile infants 28 days or younger pending culture results. Ampicillin and gentamicin are the most commonly used initial antibiotics within this age group. Careful consideration must be made to resistance patterns within a particular region. With the onset of standard GBS surveillance during pregnancy and the use of intrapartum antibiotics, more gram-negative organisms and increased gentamicin resistance have been reported, necessitating the use of a third-generation cephalosporin, such as cefotaxime, for initial empiric coverage. Ceftriaxone is generally avoided in this age group, particularly among jaundiced newborns, because of its ability to displace bilirubin from albumin, thereby increasing the risk of kernicterus.

Well-appearing febrile infants aged 29 to 90 days can be managed safely as outpatients either with antibiotics (ceftriaxone 50 mg/kg intravenously or intramuscularly) or close observation alone provided they meet established low risk for SBI criteria (Box 54-5). In addition, parents must have a reliable means of communication and transportation in the event of a positive culture result so that they can be notified to return the infant for reevaluation and possible admission. All febrile infants aged 29 to 90 days need very close follow-up, typically within 24 hours. Most pathogens will be isolated from cultures within the first 24 hours, and hospitalization with IV antibiotics is generally warranted for any young infant with a culture result consistent with a pathogen and not a contaminant. The addition of vancomycin must be considered if resistant pneumococcus is a possibility.

The management of well-appearing febrile infants and children between 3 to 36 months of age is based on the results of any diagnostic studies. Antibiotics should be administered for any bacterial infection identified. Those well-appearing infants who are tolerating oral fluids well and have no significant respiratory distress or hypoxia can be managed as outpatients even if they have a UTI or pneumonia. Clinicians may administer a dose of ceftriaxone for the first 24 hours

Box 54-5. Low-Risk Criteria for Serious Bacterial Infection in Young Febrile Infants
1. Well-appearing
2. No focal bacterial infection on examination
3. Previously healthy term infant with unremarkable neonatal course
4. White blood cell (WBC) count between 5,000 to 15,000/mm³
5. Absolute band cell count less than 1,500/mm³ or a band-to-neutrophil ratio of less than or equal to 0.2
6. Normal cerebrospinal fluid examination with less than 8 WBCs per high-power field and negative Gram stain
7. Normal urinalysis with less than 10 WBCs per high-power field
8. Stool studies with less than 5 WBCs per high-power field (if diarrhea present)
9. Normal chest radiograph (if respiratory signs/symptoms present)

and transition to an oral antibiotic thereafter. Continued close follow-up is necessary, usually within 24 to 48 hours. Infants who have received one dose or less of the pneumococcal vaccine can receive a dose of ceftriaxone pending culture results if the WBC count is greater than 15,000/mm³ or the ANC is greater than 10,000/mm³.

Healthy well-appearing febrile children older than 3 years can be managed as outpatients if they are well hydrated and have no respiratory distress or hypoxia. Children with underlying medical conditions and at risk for bacterial infections may also need hospitalization and IV antibiotics regardless of age.

Children with occult pneumococcal bacteremia who are afebrile and well-appearing at follow-up can probably continue to be managed as outpatients. Additional dosing of ceftriaxone may be necessary or transition to an oral antibiotic can be considered if sensitivity testing has been performed. Repeat blood cultures are probably not necessary if the child is afebrile as the likelihood of persistent bacteremia is low. Those who are younger than 90 days, still febrile at follow-up, or who have clinically worsened warrant hospitalization and IV antibiotics. In addition, a lumbar puncture should be considered if not previously performed in a child with a positive blood culture. All individuals with occult *N meningitides* bacteremia warrant hospitalization and IV antibiotics. A lumbar puncture should also strongly be considered if not previously performed given the substantial risk for meningitis with this particular microorganism. In general, most other cases of occult bacteremia warrant hospitalization and IV antibiotics. Consultation with an infectious disease specialist may be indicated to determine appropriate antibiotic selection and duration of therapy.

Prognosis

Occult bacteremia may resolve without therapy and have no sequelae, but it may persist or produce localized infections such as meningitis or septic arthritis. In children with bacteremia who do not receive antimicrobial therapy, the risk of persistent bacteremia is approximately 20% and the risk of meningitis is about 5% to 10%. These risks vary depending on which organism is isolated from the blood.

In general, the risk of developing serious sequelae is greater with bacteremia caused by *H influenzae* than by *S pneumoniae* (25% vs 5%). Concern about serious bacterial infection related to either of these organisms is now significantly diminished with the introduction of the conjugate vaccines.

CASE RESOLUTION

The infant presented in the case history is irritable and has a high fever of unknown source. Her vaccine status is uncertain. Her physical examination fails to reveal a source of her infection. Because her fever is 39.5°C, she is irritable, and her immune status is uncertain, a complete laboratory assessment, including a lumbar puncture, should be performed. Management should be determined after all laboratory data are available. If laboratory assessment reveals a focus of infection, such as a UTI, she should be managed with antibiotics. If laboratory assessment fails to reveal a source for the fever, and her WBC count is greater than 15,000/mm³ or her ANC is greater than 10,000/mm³, she can receive an intramuscular injection of ceftriaxone as expectant management for occult bacteremia and be reevaluated in 24 hours or be managed without antibiotics.

Selected References

Alpern ER, Alessandrini EA, McGowan KL, et al. Serotype prevalence of occult pneumococcal bacteremia. *Pediatrics.* 2001;108:23–25

American College of Emergency Physicians Clinical Policies Committee and the Clinical Policies Subcommittee on Pediatric Fever. Clinical policy for children younger than three years presenting to the emergency department with fever. *Ann Emerg Med.* 2003;42:530–545

Bachur RG, Harper MB. Predictive model for serious bacterial infections among infants younger than 3 months of age. *Pediatrics.* 2001;108:311–316

Baker MD, Bell LM, Avner JR. Outpatient management without antibiotics of fever in selected infants. *N Engl J Med.* 1993;329:1437–1441

Baraff LJ. Management of infants and young children with fever without source. *Pediatr Ann.* 2008;37:673–679

Bonsu BK, Harper MB. Identifying febrile young infants with bacteremia: is the peripheral white blood cell count an accurate screen? *Ann Emerg Med.* 2003;42:216–225

Brik R, Hamissah R, Shehada N, et al. Evaluation of febrile infants under 3 months of age: is routine lumbar puncture warranted? *Isr J Med Sci.* 1997;33:93–97

Byington CL, Enriquez R, Hoff C, et al. Serious bacterial infections in febrile infants 1 to 90 days old with and without viral infections. *Pediatrics.* 2004;113:1662–1666

Centers for Disease Control and Prevention. Direct and indirect effects of routine vaccination of children with 7-valent pneumococcal conjugate vaccine on incidence of invasive pneumococcal disease—United States, 1998–2003. *MMWR Morb Mortal Wkly Rep.* 2005;54:893–897

Gajdos V, Foix L'Helias L, Mollet-Boudjemline A, Perreaux F, Trioche P, Labrune P. Factors predicting serious bacterial infections in febrile infants less than three months old: multivariate analysis [in French]. *Arch Pediatr.* 2005;12:397–403

Grijalva CG, Poehling KA, Nuorti JP, et al. National impact of universal childhood immunization with pneumococcal conjugate vaccine on outpatient medical care visits in the United States. *Pediatrics.* 2006;118:865–873

Huppler AR, Eickhoff JC, Wald ER. Performance of low-risk criteria in the evaluation of young infants with fever: review of the literature. *Pediatrics.* 2010;125:228–233

Isaacman DJ, Burke BL. Utility of serum C-reactive protein for detection of occult bacterial infection in children. *Arch Pediatr Adolesc Med.* 2002;156:905–909

Isaacman DJ, Zhang Y, Reynolds EA, et al. Accuracy of a polymerase chain reaction–based assay for detection of pneumococcal bacteremia in children. *Pediatrics.* 1998;101:813–816

Joffe MD, Alpern EB. Occult pneumococcal bacteremia. *Pediatr Emerg Care.* 2010;26:448–454

Kaplan RL, Harper MB, Baskin MN, Macone AB, Mandl KD. Time to detection of positive cultures in 28- to 90-day-old febrile infants. *Pediatrics.* 2000;106:e74

Kaplan SL, Mason EO Jr, Wald ER, et al. Decrease of invasive pneumococcal infections in children among 8 children's hospitals in the United States after the introduction of the 7-valent pneumococcal conjugate vaccine. *Pediatrics.* 2004;113:443–449

Krief WI, Levine DA, Platt SL, et al. Influenza virus infection and the risk of serious bacterial infections in young febrile infants. *Pediatrics.* 2009;124:30–39

Kuppermann N. Occult bacteremia in young febrile children. *Pediatr Clin North Am.* 1999;46:1073–1109

Lee GM, Fleisher GR, Harper MB. Management of febrile children in the age of the conjugate pneumococcal vaccine: a cost-effectiveness analysis. *Pediatrics.* 2001;108:835–844

Levine DA, Platt SL, Dayan PS, et al. Risk of serious bacterial infection in young febrile infants with respiratory syncytial virus infections. *Pediatrics.* 2004;113:1728–1734

Newman TB, Bernzweig JA, Takayama JI, et al. Urine testing and urinary tract infections in febrile infants seen in office settings: The Pediatric Research in Office Settings Febrile Infant Study. *Arch Pediatr Adolesc Med.* 2002;156:44–54

Nigrovic LE, Kupperman N, Malley R. Children with bacterial meningitis presenting to the emergency department during the pneumococcal conjugate vaccine era. *Acad Emerg Med.* 2008;15:522–528

Pulliam PN, Attia MW, Cronan KM. C-reactive protein in febrile children 1 to 36 months of age with clinically undetectable serious bacterial infection. *Pediatrics.* 2001;108:1275–1279

Rudinsky SL, Carstairs KL, Reardon JM, et al. Serious bacterial infections in febrile infants in the post-pneumococcal conjugate vaccine era. *Acad Emerg Med.* 2008;16:585–590

Singleton R, Hammitt L, Hennessy T, et al. The Alaska *Haemophilus influenzae* type b experience: lessons in controlling a vaccine-preventable disease. *Pediatrics.* 2006;118:421–429

Strait RT, Kelly KJ, Kurup VP. Tumor necrosis factor-alpha, interleukin-1 beta, and interleukin-6 levels in febrile, young children with and without occult bacteremia. *Pediatrics.* 1999;104:1321–1326

Wilkinson M, Bulloch B, Smith M. Prevalence of occult bacteremia in children aged 3–36 months presenting to the emergency department with fever in the post–pneumococcal conjugate vaccine era. *Acad Emerg Med.* 2008;16:220–224

CHAPTER 55

Emerging Infectious Diseases

Christian B. Ramers, MD, MPH, and Thomas R. Hawn, MD, PhD

CASE STUDY

A previously healthy 8-year-old boy is brought to his pediatrician's office in late August with 2 days of fever, fatigue, headache, myalgias, nausea, and gingival bleeding. On the morning of the visit his mother noted a rash on his legs. He lives with his family in the Northeastern United States but recently returned from a 1-week vacation in Key West, FL. He engaged in extensive outdoor activities, including snorkeling, hiking, and several evening boat trips, and sustained multiple mosquito bites during the trip. He received all routine childhood immunizations, denies any allergies, and takes no medications. No other family members are ill.

On physical examination, his temperature is 101.7°F (38.7°C) and he is generally ill-appearing. He has photophobia and mild meningismus, and a petechial rash is noted on his trunk and lower extremities. Laboratory studies sent from the office reveal microscopic hematuria, leukopenia (white blood cell count 2.8), and thrombocytopenia (platelets 85,000).

Questions

1. What is an emerging or reemerging infection?
2. What pathogens are associated with emerging infections?
3. What are some common or emerging infectious diseases that may cause the clinical syndrome in the case scenario?
4. What types of exposures should be considered when assessing acute febrile illnesses such as that described in the case scenario?
5. How does recent travel influence the differential diagnosis?
6. What are appropriate steps in initial management?
7. What resources can a primary care physician access to help in making a diagnosis?
8. When do isolation and reporting procedures need to be considered?

Introduction

Emerging and reemerging infectious diseases are defined as those whose incidence in human populations has increased in the past 2 decades or threaten to do so in the near future. They may represent the resurgence of an ancient human scourge, a novel zoonosis that has broadened its host range, a common pathogen that has acquired a new antimicrobial resistance profile or, in some cases, a previously unidentified or unknown microorganism. A startling diversity of organisms has met these criteria, including viral, fungal, parasitic, and bacterial pathogens. Likewise, a variety of factors has been implicated in the process of emergence and/or reemergence related to range and susceptibility of human hosts, evolution and antigenic shift of the pathogen, and ecological and environmental changes, such as vector amplification or breakdown of public health measures. Although a select few of these emerging pathogens represent malicious propagation or bioterrorism, most appear spontaneously at ambulatory or emergency health facilities, and are thus relevant to the practicing primary care physician. It has only been through astute clinical observation, targeted outbreak investigation, and a coordinated public health response that many emerging infectious diseases have been identified.

In this chapter we will review the factors involved in the emergence and reemergence of infectious diseases of public health significance, discuss several specific examples that are likely to be most relevant to pediatric practice, summarize regional and global outbreaks of emerging infectious diseases, and provide practical steps for the primary care provider to access local diagnostic and public health support.

Contributing Factors

The spectrum of infectious diseases has always changed and evolved along with societal and environmental changes. Literature supports the supposition that throughout human history, several general driving forces influence the emergence or reemergence of certain infectious diseases. The most important factors are human migration, environmental and ecological changes, changing patterns of human host susceptibility and immunity and, more recently, the use and overuse of antimicrobial agents. Table 55-1 shows some of the mechanisms identified in recent emerging infectious diseases and provides illustrative examples from the United States and abroad. In reality, there are often many simultaneous contributing factors at play, and diseases may emerge or retreat within human populations without clear drivers. Common themes that lead to recognizable emergence events typically couple a vulnerable host population with a pathogen to which that population lacks immunity or prior exposure.

Table 55-1. Factors Contributing to Infectious Disease Emergence/Reemergence[a]

Contributing Factor	Examples	Illustrative Pathogen
Societal change	• Economic impoverishment • Population growth or migration • Globalization of food distribution • Urban decay	Cholera, malaria, salmonella
Advances in health care	• New medical devices • Organ transplantation • Drugs causing immunosuppression • Use of antimicrobial agents	Aspergillosis, cytomegalovirus, methicillin-resistant *Staphylococcus aureus*
Human behavior	• Worldwide travel • Injection drug use • Sexual activity • Outdoor recreation activities	HIV/AIDS, hepatitis C virus, histoplasmosis
Environmental changes	• Deforestation/reforestation • Flood/drought • Global warming	*Cryptococcus gattii*, dengue, *Burkholderia pseudomallei*
Public health infrastructure and control	• Reduction of prevention programs • Inadequate surveillance • Waning immunization rates	*Mycobacterium tuberculosis* (multidrug-resistant and extensively drug-resistant), measles, mumps, pertussis
Microbial adaptation and change	• Antigenic drift/shift • Changes in virulence factors • Development of drug resistance	H1N1 and H5N1 influenza, chloroquine-resistant malaria, vancomycin-resistant enterococci

[a] Adapted from Morens DM, Folkers GK, Fauci AS. The challenge of emerging and re-emerging infectious diseases. *Nature*. 2004;430:242–249

Pediatric populations are particularly susceptible to emerging and reemerging diseases in several of these categories. After immunity from acquired maternal antibody wanes, children develop adaptive immunity on their own and may experience up to 12 upper respiratory and/or diarrheal diseases per year. In some cases an unexplained increase in pediatric mortality from a typical clinical syndrome, such as upper respiratory or flu-like illness, may be the harbinger of an emerging pathogen. Large institutional settings, such as child care centers and schools, place children at high risk for exposure to infectious agents via close contact, respiratory, and droplet spread. Similarly, differing hygiene practices, such as hand washing, cough etiquette, sharing of fomites, and fecal/urinary incontinence, place infants and children at particular risk of exposure.

Antimicrobials are commonly prescribed in primary care settings for otitis media, pharyngitis, or respiratory infections, and overuse of antibiotics in these settings has been associated with a higher risk of colonization and infection with drug-resistant organisms. In many cases, what was once a first-line therapy for a particular clinical syndrome must be reconsidered due to the emergence of altered antibiotic susceptibility patterns. Advances in medical care have expanded the number of vulnerable hosts through increased survival of premature infants, cancer chemotherapy, organ transplantation, and the use of immunosuppressive or immunomodulatory agents. Lastly, due to access, parental belief systems, or personal choice, immunization rates in certain regions remain suboptimal, placing children at risk of acquiring vaccine-preventable disease.

Special Situations

Increasingly, primary care providers find themselves in settings that demand careful consideration of the risks of emerging or reemerging infectious diseases. The following is a collection of some unique clinical settings in which less common or emerging infectious diseases should warrant consideration.

Expanded International Travel

With the increasing accessibility of long-distance international travel, children are more frequently being included in tourist trips or, in the case of immigrant families, visits to friends or relatives back in their home country. Children are less likely to seek pretravel advice and consequently less likely to adhere to recommended travel guidelines. A report from the GeoSentinel Surveillance Network, a large group of worldwide travel clinics, found that only 32% of children visiting friends and relatives in developing countries received recommended travel vaccines or prophylactic medications yet they were more likely to present with illness and require hospital admission after travel. Primary care physicians evaluating returning travelers must consider detailed travel history, prophylaxis or protective measures taken (if any), risk profile of the region visited, and incubation period of the suspected pathogen. Although by far the most common travel-related illnesses are self-limited diarrheal disease, emerging infections, such as dengue, chikungunya, or H5N1 or H1N1 influenza, must be considered along with other infectious diseases, such as malaria or tuberculosis.

Immigration and International Adoption

Increasing rates of international adoption or recent immigration may result in primary care providers evaluating children with unknown or unavailable birth, early childhood, or immunization histories (Chapter 34 and Chapter 36). Vaccine schedules vary by country of origin, including some vaccines that are no longer given in the United States (eg, bacille Calmette-Guérin, oral polio). There is a wide range of reliability among medical reporting in these situations, with some reaching or exceeding developed world standards, but most providing dubious quality. Many providers specializing in "adoption clinics" or working in settings with large immigrant populations obtain serologic evidence of prior immunization (eg, measles, mumps, varicella, polio, diphtheria, tetanus). Providers must also be aware of infections with clinically silent latent phases (viral hepatitis, latent tuberculosis, intestinal helminth infections, and even HIV). Several emerging or reemerging infectious diseases in the United States may be endemic in the countries of origin of adopted or recently arrived immigrant children.

Immune Suppression and Immunomodulation

Therapeutic advances in pediatric oncology, organ transplantation, rheumatology, and care of chronic congenital conditions have resulted in an increasing population of immunosuppressed children. Although typically under the care of specialists, these children may have a medical home in a primary care facility and thus can present with an opportunistic or emerging infectious disease to their primary care provider. The spectrum of risk for infectious diseases varies considerably depending on the type of immunosuppression. For example tumor necrosis factor-α inhibitors, now commonly used in the treatment of juvenile idiopathic arthritis, convey a particularly high risk of fungal and mycobacterial infection. Neutropenia from cytotoxic chemotherapy is associated with an increased risk of bloodstream bacterial infection among others. Similarly, lymphopenia related to solid organ transplantation portends a particular vulnerability to viral infections, ranging from widespread community respiratory viruses to reactivation of common agents such as varicella-zoster virus. Emerging infectious diseases such as human metapneumovirus or H1N1 influenza may have particularly severe clinical manifestations in immunosuppressed children when compared to the general population.

Unvaccinated or Under-Vaccinated Child

Despite the ongoing efforts of public health authorities, some regions have noted a worrisome downward trend in immunization rates. Although the most widely cited study linking autism to measles, mumps, rubella (MMR) vaccination was retracted by the *Lancet* in February 2010, several recent parental surveys indicate persistent beliefs surrounding a suspected vaccine–autism link. In 2004 the Institute of Medicine Immunization Safety Review Committee

published a comprehensive report that found no convincing evidence of a causal link between the MMR vaccine or any thimerosol-containing vaccine and autism. However, in a survey of 1,552 parents conducted in 2009, 25% agreed with the statement, "Some vaccines cause autism in healthy children" (see Freed et al). Decreasing vaccination rates have led to in increased risk for outbreaks of reemerging infectious diseases. In 2008 there were more cases of measles in the United States than any other year since 1997, with more than 90% of cases occurring in unvaccinated individuals or those with unknown vaccination status. Similarly, a 2010–2011 pertussis epidemic in California is the largest since 1955. It is thus crucial for clinicians to include vaccination status and exposure history when evaluating children with an infectious syndrome. Increasingly, the differential diagnosis and diagnostic workup must include emerging and reemerging diseases, some of which may be unfamiliar to the practitioner from their training or clinical experience.

Select Emerging Pathogens

Major emerging and reemerging infectious diseases (Figure 55-1) in the last 20 years are listed in Table 55-2. This table is not meant to be an exhaustive list, but rather a sampling of emerging pathogens most likely to present to a primary care office.

Viruses

Measles

Caused by a virus from the Paramyxoviridae family, measles began to decline as a major threat in the United States after a safe and effective vaccine was developed in 1963. However, a significant resurgence occurred between 1989 and 1991, due largely to a pool of vulnerable unvaccinated preschoolers. Nearly 55,000 cases and 130 deaths occurred in the United States, prompting a renewed effort at prevention through vaccination. A second dose of vaccine for school-aged children was also recommended after this outbreak. Since 2004 there has been another resurgence of new cases, but with new epidemiologic features; 90% of the cases were either directly imported from travelers or immigrants, or were associated with importation from outside the United States. Still, unvaccinated school-aged children make up a large pool of at-risk hosts.

Measles is known as a highly contagious pathogen passed via respiratory droplets. Secondary transmission is thought to be greater than 90% among susceptible household contacts. Roughly 10 days after exposure, clinical illness is characterized by a distinctive febrile prodrome (conjunctivitis, coryza, cough), followed by Koplik spots (blue-gray enanthem on buccal mucosa) and, ultimately, the classic maculopapular erythematous eruption. Diagnosis is usually ascertained on clinical grounds alone given the distinct clinical presentation; however, for confirmatory testing, the immunoglobulin (Ig) M serology is nearly 100% sensitive if performed after the onset of rash. Respiratory droplet isolation should occur until 4 days following appearance of the rash in immunocompetent patients and until the clinical illness resolves in those who are immunocompromised.

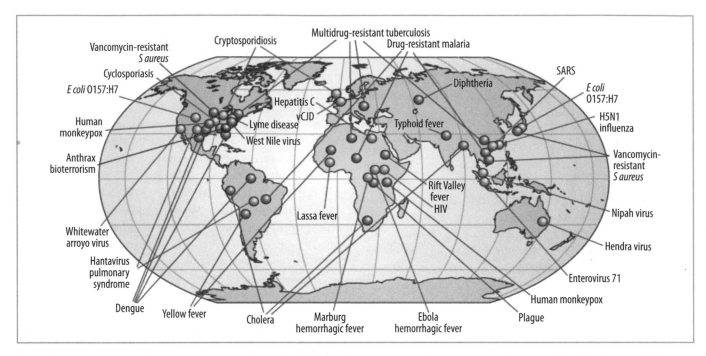

Figure 55-1. **Global examples of recently emerging and reemerging infectious diseases. Does not demonstrate recently increased West Nile virus, methicillin-resistant *Staphylococcus aureus*, and measles. (Reprinted with permission from Fauci AS. Infectious diseases: considerations for the 21st century. *Clin Infect Dis*. 2001;32:675–685.)**

Treatment is largely supportive; however, respiratory and neurologic complications can occur in 6% and 0.1% of patients, respectively. Further control of this reemerging infectious disease will likely depend on renewed attention to domestic vaccination efforts and the roll-out of vaccination worldwide.

Mumps

Although the clinical syndrome of the mumps virus is distinct from that of measles, the 2 members of the Paramyxoviridae family share a similar history of initial control and recent reemergence. A live, attenuated mumps vaccine was licensed in 1967 and incorporated into the Advisory Committee on Immunization Practices recommended schedule by 1977. Due to high vaccination rates, mumps had declined by more than 99% by 2005. However, there have been 2 major resurgences in the United States. In 2005–2006 a total of 6,584 cases were reported in a multistate outbreak in the Midwestern United States. Although numerically most of these cases occurred among college students who had been previously vaccinated, attack rates were considerably higher in unvaccinated individuals. In 2009–2010, an outbreak involving more than 1,500 reported cases occurred in New York and New Jersey.

The clinical presentation of mumps typically involves fever, malaise, and parotitis. Complications are rare, but in some studies up to 10% of patients had aseptic meningitis, of which hearing loss is an important sequela. Up to 37% of adolescent and adult males can present with orchitis, which may result in sterility. Diagnosis is typically made based on a compatible clinical syndrome with confirmation by isolation or polymerase chain reaction (PCR)-based detection of the virus from saliva, cerebrospinal fluid (CSF), urine, or seminal fluid. Immunoglobulin M serology is also a useful confirmatory method.

Treatment is generally supportive, with analgesics used for the pain of parotitis and/or orchitis. For severe cases, intravenous Ig has been used to mitigate immune-mediated post-infectious complications, and interferon-α-2b has been used to alleviate orchitis.

There has been much scrutiny of these outbreaks as indicators of vaccine effectiveness and community vaccination rates. Based on extensive analyses, MMR vaccine effectiveness is still considered 80% to 90% after 2 doses. This, however, leaves a significant portion of the population still vulnerable to sustain occasional outbreaks. No change was made to immunization schedules or interim recommendations after these outbreaks.

Dengue

Dengue fever virus is a member of the Flaviviridae family and is known to occur in 4 serotypes. It is transmitted via a vector, usually *Aedes aegypti,* and is present in more than 100 countries throughout the Americas, Asia, and Africa. Although historically confined to tropical and subtropical regions roughly overlapping with malarial zones, the range of dengue fever virus is expanding. In the United States, there were no cases of locally acquired dengue reported between 1946 and 1980. Since 1980, sporadic cases have been reported along the US–Mexico border, but more recently a small outbreak of locally acquired dengue occurred in Key West, FL, in 2009–2010. The worldwide incidence of dengue has increased at least 4-fold in the past 3 decades for unclear reasons.

Clinical manifestations occur over a wide spectrum, from asymptomatic seroconversion to severe, even fatal disease. Headache and petechial rash are commonly seen. Classically the disease is thought to occur in 3 forms: undifferentiated febrile illness, dengue fever, and dengue hemorrhagic fever. However, in reality clinical manifestations

Table 55-2. A Sampling of Recent Emerging Infectious Diseases			
Pathogen	*Clinical Syndrome*	*Diagnosis*	*Management*

Measles virus	Measles
	  Pneumonia
	  Post-infectious encephalitis
		Clinical
		Confirm with IgM
			Supportive
			Consider antibiotics for bacterial
			  superinfections

Mumps virus	Parotitis
	  Orchitis
	  Encephalopathy
		Serology
		Culture
		PCR
			Supportive
			NSAIDs

Dengue virus	Unspecified febrile illness Dengue fever Dengue hemorrhagic fever	Serology	Supportive Aggressive fluid management
Influenza virus	Fever, respiratory symptoms	PCR or antigen	Oseltamivir, zanamavir, amantadine, rimantadine

Chikungunya virus	Febrile syndrome with arthralgias,
	  rash, conjunctivitis
		Clinical
		Confirm with serology, viral culture,
		  or PCR
			Supportive, NSAIDs

WNV	Asymptomatic
	West Nile fever
	West Nile encephalitis (flaccid
	  ascending paralysis)
		Serology
		WNV antigen or PCR
		IgM in CSF
			Supportive (ribavirin and interferon-
			  α-2b are experimental)

MRSA	Skin and soft tissue infections, bacteremia, pneumonia	Culture and susceptibility	Antibiotics
Resistant gram-negatives	Pneumonia, UTI, bacteremia, sepsis	Culture and susceptibility	Antibiotics
Resistant *Streptococcus pneumoniae*	Pneumonia, meningitis, otitis media	Culture and susceptibility	Antibiotics
Ehrlichiosis/anaplasmosis	Fever, HA, myalgia, rash	PCR or peripheral blood smear	Doxycycline
Cryptococcus gattii	Pneumonia, meningitis	Culture or cryptococcal antigen	Amphotericin, 5-FC, fluconazole

Abbreviations: 5-FC, 5-fluorocytosine; CSF, cerebrospinal fluid; HA, headache; Ig, immunoglobulin; MRSA, methicillin-resistant *Staphylococcal aureus;* NSAIDs, nonsteroidal anti-inflammatory drugs; PCR, polymerase chain reaction; UTI, urinary tract infection; WNV, West Nile virus.

are diverse and may include hepatitis, myocarditis, pericarditis, and encephalopathy. Leukopenia and thrombocytopenia are common laboratory findings and, in severe cases, a coagulopathy and bleeding manifestations seem to be the most dangerous sequelae. Diagnosis can be made with a compatible clinical history and confirmed with serology. Unfortunately, there are no direct-acting antivirals, nor is a vaccine available. Care is generally supportive.

H1N1 Influenza

Although it seemed that bird flu or H5N1 influenza would be the greatest concern to public health in mid-2009, it was a different strain, an H1N1 swine flu, that led to a global pandemic. Influenza viruses have a segmented genome and thus are able to adapt and evolve quite rapidly to evade slower adaptive immune responses. Through antigenic drift, small changes occur in cell surface genes through time, resulting in subtle structural changes to the cell surface proteins (neuraminidase and hemaglutinin) and less recognition by the immune system. In antigenic shift, genome segments from diverse strains recombine in a single new virus particle, creating abrupt and substantial changes in antigenic variation. Typically,

shifts are more likely to cause pandemics because there are more nonimmune hosts in the population.

The clinical manifestations of H1N1 influenza seemed to be similar to prior influenza outbreaks; however, there were more severe cases and higher mortality in previously healthy young people than in typical influenza epidemics. Testing for H1N1 most commonly involves antigen-based PCR methods with variable sensitivities and specificities. Treatment for severe cases consists either of oral oseltamivir or inhaled zanamivir. Although there have been reports of oseltamivir resistance outside the United States, this currently remains the drug of choice. Of note, the circulating H1N1 strains identified in 2009 were mostly resistant to the older adamantanes (amantadine, rimantadine).

Chikungunya

Another vector-borne disease transmitted primary by *Aedes* spp. mosquitoes, chikungunya was first described in Tanzania in 1953. It often occurs in epidemic outbreaks rather than steady endemic patterns and is most commonly seen in tropical Africa and Asia. More recently, outbreak ranges have expanded slightly, occurring in Italy and Madagascar. In 2006 there were an unprecedented 37 cases diagnosed in the United States; however, all of these were determined to be imported. The clinical hallmark of chikungunya fever is the presence of intense arthralgias and occasionally frank arthritis after a febrile illness with rash and conjunctivitis. Whereas the clinical illness of malaise and fever may last days to weeks, the joint symptoms may last months to years. Other than the possibility of persistent and nagging arthralgias, severity is typically mild, and fatality is rare. Treatment of chikungunya is generally supportive, as there are no specific antivirals available.

Severe Acute Respiratory Syndrome (SARS) From Coronavirus

From 2002–2004, an epidemic of severe pneumonia due to a previously unrecognized coronavirus (SARS-CoV) caused considerable international concern due to its highly infectious nature and high mortality rate. Epidemiologic studies led to identification of palm civets as the main reservoir of transmission to humans from contact in the marketplace. Further studies suggested that horseshoe bats were the likely natural reservoir. The epidemic, which originated in China, eventually spread to 29 countries with an overall mortality rate of 9.6%, which included numerous health care workers. Clinical features included a mean incubation period of 4.6 days with a presentation of severe pneumonia with a high rate of respiratory failure. Additional clinical manifestations included watery diarrhea and hepatitis. Common laboratory features included lymphopenia, neutropenia, and disseminated intravascular coagulation. The cornerstone of treatment was supportive care. Although many subjects received ribavirin, there was no proven role for it or any antiviral agents during the outbreak. Despite the impressive nature of this epidemic, it subsided rapidly and there has not been evidence of ongoing SARS-CoV transmission. This epidemic highlighted an agent with high transmissibility, morbidity, and mortality, yet only a transient global impact.

Bacteria

Drug-Resistant Bacteria

Community-Acquired Methicillin-Resistant Staphylococcus aureus (MRSA)

Methicillin-resistant *S aureus* strains were recognized shortly after the introduction of methicillin in the 1960s and have been a substantive problem in health care settings for several decades. Health-care associated MRSA (HA-MRSA) has well-established risk factors, which include exposure in the health care setting (eg, hospital, nursing facility) and the presence of comorbid medical conditions (eg, malignancy, chronic liver or lung disease, indwelling catheters). In the 1990s, a new strain of community-acquired MRSA (CA-MRSA) appeared that was not associated with these traditional risk factors, as it often was found in otherwise healthy individuals with no health care–related exposure. Furthermore, CA-MRSA carries the *mecA* resistance gene on a Type IV or V chromosomal

cassette in contrast to HA-MRSA, which belongs to Type I through III categories. Community-acquired MRSA is also more likely to contain the Panton-Valentine leukocidin genes, which may encode virulence factors that influence clinical symptoms. These genotypic differences have facilitated epidemiology studies that suggest that CA-MRSA is a distinct MRSA strain that has increased in frequency throughout the United States and is a bona fide emerging pathogen. In addition to genotypic differences, CA-MRSA is less likely to have a multi-drug–resistant susceptibility pattern. Treatment of CA-MRSA follows similar principles to HA-MRSA with the exception that more antibiotic choices are generally available. For an uncomplicated cutaneous abscess, incision and drainage without antibiotics is often sufficient. For deeper or more severe infections, empiric treatment with trimethoprim-sulfamethoxazole, clindamycin, a tetracycline (doxycycline or minocycline), or linezolid are empiric options while awaiting antibiotic susceptibilities. Although linezolid is an effective drug, it is far more expensive than the other choices. Tetracyclines should not be used in children younger than 8. For impetigo and other minor infections, topical mupirocin can be used.

Resistant Gram-Negative Bacteria and Streptococcus pneumoniae

Similar to CA-MRSA, there are other resistant bacteria that have established significant niches. For example, *S pneumoniae* was previously uniformly sensitive to penicillin. Currently, penicillin and ceftriaxone-resistant strains of *S pneumoniae* are now common and circulating in the community. Similarly, a number of gram-negative bacteria, such as *Escherichia coli* and *Klebsiella pneumoniae*, are highly resistant due to a variety of plasmid and chromosomally encoded mechanisms, such as β-lactamases, cephalosporinases, carbapenamases, porins, and efflux pumps. These strains are mostly seen in the nosocomial setting, although community circulation of these strains has also occurred. Although the emergence of these strains is not as extensive or as clearly delineated as CA-MRSA, each of these strains has similarly "emerged" to a prevalence level in the population that substantially impacts human health.

Ehrlichiosis and Anaplasmosis

Ehrlichia chaffeensis (agent of human monocytotropic ehrlichiosis [HME] and *Anaplasma phagocytophilum* (agent of human granulocytotropic anaplasmosis [HGA], formerly human granulocytotropic ehrlichiosis are examples of infections that emerged due to new diagnostic tests. Both infections were initially recognized as infections of the veterinary world until the application of molecular methods to humans with undiagnosed febrile illnesses. They have likely caused human disease for a long time, although the incidence may have increased with the recent resurgence of populations of some animal reservoirs, such as the white-tailed deer. In the early 1990s, *E chaffeensis* and *A phagocytophilum* were identified as human pathogens that are transmitted by ticks. *Ehrlichia chaffeensis* is transmitted by several ticks (*Amblyomma americanum*, *Dermacentor variabilis*, and *Ixodes pacificus*) and is found in the southeastern and south central United States as well as California. *Anaplasma phagocytophilum* is transmitted by *Ixodes scapularis* and is found in the northern United States. Both agents cause a febrile illness with headache, myalgia, and malaise that is often accompanied by thrombocytopenia, leukopenia, and transaminitis. Rash, which is found in 90% of subjects with Rocky Mountain spotted fever (caused by *Rickettsia rickettsii*), is less often found with HME (31%) and rarely with HGA. Diagnosis of these infections can be made by PCR and less commonly with direct microscopy since the latter methods are insensitive (<10% for HME and 25%–75% for HGA). However, due to the potential severity of the illness, empiric treatment should be initiated if clinical suspicion is high while awaiting the diagnostic workup. The drug of choice for treatment of HGA and HME is doxycycline. Due to a lack of reliable alternative drugs, doxycycline is also recommended for children younger than 8 years.

Fungi

Cryptococcus gattii

Cryptococcus gattii (formerly *Cryptococcus neoformans* var *gattii*) and *C neoformans* are yeast that cause pneumonia and central nervous system infections in immunocompetent and immunocompromised hosts. Although *C neoformans* is present in most regions of the world, *C gattii* has a restricted geographical distribution and previously had been identified in tropical and subtropical countries such as Australia, New Zealand, and Papua New Guinea. In the early 2000s, *C gattii* was identified as a cause of meningoencephalitis for the first time on Vancouver Island in British Columbia. From 1999–2007, 218 cases were reported with a case-fatality rate of 8.7%. Subsequent studies identified its presence in the Pacific Northwest, including the states of Washington and Oregon. Similar to many emerging pathogens, the increased numbers of cases may be due to improved diagnostics and surveillance as opposed to the actual emergence of a new infection to a region. However, some molecular evidence suggests that the strain on Vancouver Island is novel. Clonal analysis suggests that it arose from an unusual type of sexual mating that generated a strain that is hypervirulent. This mechanism of emergence suggests that a species endemic to an original location (eg, tropics) can emerge in a new geographic region (Vancouver Island) in a clonal manner. The clinical presentation of *C gattii* is similar to *C neoformans*, although there may be an increased frequency of cryptococcoma in the lungs and central nervous system caused by *C gattii*. Treatment principles are the same for both species and include initial treatment with amphotericin B and 5-fluorocytosine for meningitis followed by consolidation therapy with fluconazole. For uncomplicated pulmonary disease, fluconazole is the cornerstone of treatment. *Cryptococcus* spp., including *gattii*, infect children and treatment principles are similar to those for adults.

Summary

Contrary to myopic claims that public health would conquer infectious diseases in the 20th century, new pathogens have continued to emerge and old ones have reemerged time and time again, making for a challenging future of disease identification and control. The

tools employed by public health include surveillance and response, yet most of the major epidemics identified in the last 20 years began with astute clinical observation at the primary care level. It is thus essential for primary care providers and others caring for children to remain vigilant to the constant and unpredictable nature of emerging infectious diseases. With astute primary care clinicians, attentive scrutiny of new outbreaks and collaboration with regional and national public health laboratories and officials, the medical field will hopefully keep pace with emerging and reemerging pathogens.

CASE RESOLUTION

The patient was hospitalized and underwent an extensive diagnostic workup for infectious causes of fever and rash. A lumbar puncture revealed a mild lymphocytic pleocytosis. He received 2 days of empiric antibiotic therapy, which was discontinued when cultures were negative for 48 hours. The pediatrician notified the local health department, which facilitated laboratory testing performed by the state public health laboratory, and the Centers for Disease Control and Prevention (CDC).

Serologic testing at the state health department was positive for IgM antibodies against dengue virus. This was confirmed on samples sent to the CDC, and in addition, CSF sent to the CDC was positive by reverse-transcriptase PCR for dengue virus serotype 1. The patient recovered uneventfully over the following 2 weeks, but a public health investigation was launched that eventually resulted in the identification of 27 total cases of dengue fever acquired in Key West, FL. Subsequently, an adult serosurvey was conducted indicating recent exposure to dengue in 5.4% of adults.

This outbreak, which occurred in 2009–2010, represented the first reported cases of dengue fever acquired in Florida since 1934. Although dengue is the most common virus transmitted by mosquitoes in the world, no cases had been acquired in the continental United States between 1946 and 1980 and, subsequently, only sporadic cases were known along the Texas-Mexico border. Reported dengue cases have increased 4-fold in Latin America since 1980, and incidence has risen steadily among returning US travelers. Dengue represents a truly reemerging infectious disease and primary clinicians should be aware of its rising incidence.

Internet Resources

www.cdc.gov

www.cdc.gov/dengue

Selected References

Centers for Disease Control and Prevention. Addressing emerging infectious disease threats: a prevention strategy for the United States. Executive summary. *MMWR Recomm Rep.* 1994;43(RR-5):1–18

Centers for Disease Control and Prevention. Diseases and the vaccines that prevent them: measles. http://www.cdc.gov/vaccines/spec-grps/hcp/conv-materials.htm#disvp

Centers for Disease Control and Prevention. Locally acquired dengue—Key West, Florida 2009–2010, *MMWR Morb Mortal Wkly Rep.* 2010;59(19):577–581

Centers for Disease Control and Prevention. Preventing emerging infectious diseases: a strategy for the 21st century. Overview of the updated CDC plan. *MMWR Recomm Rep.* 1998;47(RR-15):1–14

Centers for Disease Control and Prevention. Update: chikungunya fever diagnosed among returning travelers—United States, 2006, *MMWR Morb Mortal Wkly Rep.* 2007;56(12):276–277

Centers for Disease Control and Prevention. Update: mumps outbreak—New York and New Jersey June 2009—January 2010. *MMWR Morb Mortal Wkly Rep.* 2010;59(5):125–129

Datta K, Bartlett KH, Baer R, et al. Spread of *Cryptococcus gattii* into the Pacific Northwest Region of the United States. *Emerg Infect Dis.* 2009;15(8):1185–1191

David MZ, Daum RS. Community-associated methicillin-resistant *Staphylococcus aureus:* epidemiology and clinical consequences of an emerging epidemic. *Clin Microbiol Rev.* 2010;23(3):616–687

Feikin D, Lezotte DC, Hamman RF, Salmon DA, Chen RT, Hoffman RE. Individual and community risks of measles and pertussis associated with personal exemptions to immunization. *JAMA.* 2000;284:3145–3150

Fraser JA, Giles SS, Wenink EC, et al. Same-sex mating and the origin of the Vancouver Island *Cryptococcus gattii* outbreak. *Nature.* 2005;437:1360–1364

Freed GL, Clark SJ, Butchart AT, et al. Parental vaccine safety concerns in 2009. *Pediatrics.* 2010;125(4):654–659

Hagmann S, Neugebauer R, Schwartz E, et al. Illness in children after international travel: analysis from the GeoSentinel Surveillance Network. *Pediatrics.* 2010;125(5): e1072–e1080

Hui DS, Chan PK. Severe acute respiratory syndrome and coronavirus. *Infect Dis Clin North Am.* 2010;24:619–638

Hviid A, Rubin S, Mühlemann K. Mumps. *Lancet.* 2008;371:932–944

Institute of Medicine Immunization Safety Review Committee. *Immunization Safety Review: Vaccines and Autism.* Washington, DC: National Academies Press; 2004. http://www.iom.edu/Reports/2004/Immunization-Safety-Review-Vaccines-and-Autism.aspx

Liu C, Bayer A, Cosgrove SE, et al. Clinical practice guidelines by the Infectious Diseases Society of America for the treatment of methicillin-resistant *Staphylococcus aureus* infections in adults and children. *Clin Infect Dis.* 2011;52:e18–e55

Morens DM, Folkers GK, Fauci AS. The challenge of emerging and re-emerging infectious diseases. *Nature.* 2004;430:242–249

Morse S. Factors in the emergence of infectious diseases. *Emerg Infect Dis.* 2005;1(1):7–15

Perfect JR, Dismukes WE, Dromer F, et al. Clinical practice guidelines for the management of cryptococcal disease: 2010 update by the Infectious Diseases Society of America. *Clin Infect Dis.* 2010;50:291–322

Sabella C. Measles: not just a childhood rash. *Cleve Clin J Med.* 2010;77(3):207–213

Walker DH, Paddock CD, Dumler JS. Emerging and re-emerging tick-transmitted rickettsial and ehrlichial infections. *Med Clin North Am.* 2008;92:1345–1361

CHAPTER 56

Febrile Seizures

Kenneth R. Huff, MD

CASE STUDY

A 12-month-old girl is brought to the emergency department by paramedics because she is having a seizure. She is unresponsive and hypertonic, with arched trunk and extended arms and legs that are jerking rhythmically. Her eyes are open, but her gaze is directed upward. She has bubbles of saliva around her lips as well as circumoral cyanosis. Her vital signs are a respiratory rate of 60 breaths/min, heart rate of 125 beats/min, blood pressure of 130/78 mm Hg, and temperature of 105.8°F (41.0°C). An assessment of her respiratory status discloses that she is moving air in all lung fields, and there is no evidence of upper airway obstruction.

The paramedics inform you that the girl has been convulsing with varying intensity of tone and movements but remaining unresponsive for approximately 6 minutes. Glucometer testing reveals a normal serum glucose. Blood samples for other tests are sent to the laboratory, and urine is collected. An intravenous (IV) line is started, and the girl is given lorazepam by IV push. Within 2 minutes, the movements cease, and her respirations become slow and even. Her physical examination shows no signs of trauma. Her only abnormality other than her unresponsive mental status is an inflamed and bulging right tympanic membrane.

The girl's parents tell you that she has had a mildly stuffy nose for 2 days but has been afebrile and has seemed to be her usual self. While she was playing, she became cranky, and her parents put her in her crib for her nap. Thirty minutes later they heard grunting noises, found her in the midst of a seizure, and called the paramedics. The girl has never had a seizure before. Her father recalls that his mother once told him that he had several "fever seizures" as an infant.

Questions

1. What are the characteristics of simple febrile seizures?
2. What is the appropriate evaluation of children with febrile seizures, whether it is the first one or a recurrence?
3. What is the recurrence risk for febrile seizures and the risk of developing unprovoked seizures following a febrile seizure?
4. What are the treatment options for children with febrile seizures?

Febrile seizures are easily recognized, dramatic, generalized convulsions. These seizures are defined by the presence of a fever or an acute inflammatory illness (often sudden) from a source outside the nervous system; patient age of about 5 years or younger; absence of chronic brain pathology, including developmental delay; and absence of metabolic or structural abnormalities of the brain. Frequently, familial predisposition to similar seizures or a history of similar events in other family members is present. Despite the relatively uniform presentation of the seizure, genetic abnormalities in channels, neurotransmitter receptors, or hippocampal damage may influence prognosis, and individual clinical variables and social factors may play a part in the treatment.

Epidemiology

Febrile seizures occur in children between the ages of 6 months and approximately 5 years but are more common in those who are younger than 3 years. Some studies indicate that as many as 5% of all children experience at least one febrile seizure. The recurrence rate is 30% to 50% in children younger than 1 year, but drops to 25% between 1 and 3 years, and is only 12% after 3 years. Seizures usually occur with the rise in temperature and often so suddenly that the febrile illness is not recognized by the family prior to the seizure. Frequently, the febrile illness is eventually diagnosed as an upper respiratory tract or influenza infection. Febrile seizures are seen often in children who have a first-degree relative who experienced the problem at the same age.

Clinical Presentation

Simple febrile seizures are characterized by a single episode of generalized, symmetrical, tonic posturing and clonic movements of a few minutes' duration that occur suddenly in children whose developmental progress is generally normal. Fever or an acute inflammatory illness is present, although it may not have been recognized before the seizure, and its source is outside the nervous system. A short time after the seizure (after usually 1–2 hours of postictal sleepiness), children become neurologically normal again (Dx Box).

Dx Febrile Seizures

- Sudden unresponsiveness, tonic posturing, and generalized rhythmic jerking
- Fever or acute inflammatory illness source outside nervous system
- Age 6 months to approximately 5 years
- Normal neurodevelopmental history

Recently described generalized epilepsy with febrile seizures plus (GEFS+) is characterized by the association of generalized febrile seizures beyond the age of 6 years and afebrile generalized convulsions, a positive family history of epilepsy with variable phenotypes, and a benign prognosis in most cases. The same families may have simple febrile seizures, febrile seizures beyond the age of 6 years, febrile seizures and absences, atonic or myoclonic seizures, and myoclonic-astatic epilepsy.

Pathophysiology

The susceptibility of young children to febrile seizures may be related to an increased incidence of sudden high fevers in this age group, a developmental genetic factor that may lower the seizure threshold, or both. Animal models indicate that the immature brain has a lower seizure threshold than the adult, and seizures in the immature brain are more likely to occur by a different mechanism than those in the adult. A sudden increase in temperature to a sufficiently high level can provoke seizures regardless of age. Seizures occur more frequently with fever in many seizure-prone patients who have seizures of different etiologies, including genetic epilepsies. Perhaps circulating pyrogens interact with a brain cellular circuitry mechanism or susceptible ion channels, causing hypersynchronous depolarization and a seizure. The multigenerational familial history that is often seen suggests a dominantly expressed genetic transmission.

Both the precise definition of the genetic markers and the mechanisms of generalized seizures in all cases are not yet fully understood. Recent work suggests a possible mechanism. Recently mutations in either γ-aminobutyric acid (GABA) A receptor or sodium channel genes have been found to be associated with febrile seizures and GEFS+ pedigrees. GABA A receptors receive inhibitory transmission and are composed of combinations of 5 subunits. The γ-2 subunit is critical for receptor trafficking, clustering, and synaptic maintenance, and mutations in this subunit have been associated with febrile seizure families. It has also been found that the trafficking of mutant receptors with γ-2 subunit mutations was more highly temperature dependent than mutations of other subunits, and impaired membrane insertion or accelerated receptor endocytosis with brief increases of 37 to 40 degrees occurred. In these families, the febrile seizures may be caused by a fever-induced change in the dynamic membrane state producing reduced numbers of available GABA A receptors.

In other families with GEFS+, it has been found that mutations in the *SCN1A* channel genes have occurred. Mutations in the same gene occur in sequences that encode for the critical "pore" region of the subunit protein that participates in ion selectivity and results in a more severe phenotype with early prolonged resistant seizures, and later severe myoclonic epilepsy of infancy and mental retardation, the Dravet syndrome. The less severe GEFS+ phenotype is correlated with a less functionally critical position of the missense mutation in the *SCN1A* gene.

Differential Diagnosis

When a young child presents with a fever and a seizure, the possibility that the seizure is symptomatic of meningitis, encephalitis, or brain abscess must be considered. Signs of meningeal irritation may not be reliable in children younger than 18 months, and these and other signs of the illness may be obscured in the postictal period. If there is a history of lethargy or persistent vomiting, or the seizure was focal in onset, prolonged, or multiple, or the postictal depression in responsiveness is prolonged, an examination of the cerebrospinal fluid (CSF) should be done. In addition, if the patient is deficient in *Haemophilus influenza* type B or *Streptococcus pneumoniae* immunizations, or the patient has been pretreated with antibiotics, which could mask meningeal signs or symptoms, a CSF examination should be considered. The fever also could be provocative or coincidental to a seizure of different etiology, such as trauma, toxic ingestion, metabolic derangement, degenerative or neurocutaneous disorder, or stroke.

A useful concept for the physician caring for a child with a seizure with fever has been the differentiation of simple febrile seizures from complex febrile seizures (Table 56-1). A question that has prognostic implications is whether children in the appropriate age range have had a true febrile seizure or a seizure with fever, which may be an early fever-provoked episode of a nonfebrile seizure disorder. The factors defining a complex febrile seizure also predict an increased likelihood of later unprovoked nonfebrile seizures. The length of a complex febrile seizure is longer than 15 minutes. Most febrile seizures last fewer than 90 seconds, although a significant number present in status epilepticus. More than one febrile seizure during

Table 56-1. Simple Versus Complex Febrile Seizures		
Feature	*Simple*	*Complex*
Onset of clonic movements	Generalized	Focal
Length	<15 minutes (usually <90 seconds)	>15 minutes
Number of seizures per 24 h febrile illness	1	Recurrent
Neurodevelopmental history	Normal	Abnormal
Parent–sibling history of a febrile seizure	Often positive	Often negative

the same infectious illness or 24-hour period makes these recurrent seizures complex febrile seizures. The history of a focal or partial onset or the presence of postictal focal neurologic signs makes the febrile seizure complex. The presence of an abnormal neurodevelopmental history prior to the febrile seizure or abnormal neurologic examination or brain imaging study before or after the seizure also increases the likelihood of later unprovoked seizures.

Evaluation

History

After the seizure has been controlled and the child has been stabilized, a more detailed history relating to the circumstances of the seizure (the child's state leading up to the seizure; prenatal, birth, and developmental histories; and family seizure history) should be obtained (Questions Box).

Questions

Febrile Seizures

- What were the child's symptoms for the few days before the seizure?
- Where was the child and what was he or she doing immediately before the seizure?
- Were there any pregnancy-related or perinatal complications?
- Has the child's development been normal or similar to that of siblings?
- Have any other family members had seizures of any kind, including during infancy?

Physical Examination

Children should be examined completely after stabilization, noting the possibility that the fever may be coincidental and signs from an unrelated cause inciting the seizure could be present. Physicians should look for bruises, fractures, retinal hemorrhages, or other signs of trauma. The presence of dysmorphic features, enlarged organs, or bony changes should be noted. The skin should be examined for abnormal, pigmented, or textured spots. Lateralized signs of tone or strength should be assessed. An appropriate examination to determine the etiology of the fever should also be performed (see Chapter 54).

Laboratory Tests

If the seizure is prolonged, focal, or multiple; if there is a history of lethargy, stupor, or persistent vomiting before the seizure; or if the patient still appears ill after the postictal period, cultures should be obtained and metabolic and toxicological blood and urine studies sent. A spinal tap for CSF examination for meningitis or encephalitis should be done unless there are signs of increased intracranial pressure or a lateralized neurologic examination, in which case antibiotics should be given and an imaging study obtained prior to the spinal tap.

If the seizure is a simple febrile seizure, an electroencephalogram (EEG) has limited usefulness. The record is often abnormal in a nonspecific way, and not helpful in predicting either future simple febrile seizures or epilepsy. If the patient does not fully recover after the postictal period, the EEG may be useful to help define the nature of the encephalopathy.

Imaging Studies

Computed tomography and magnetic resonance imaging scans have a low yield of abnormal results in children with simple febrile seizures. Children who have had an abnormal neurodevelopmental history or who have had a focal or partial onset to their seizure should have an imaging study to detect a structural lesion that may be the source of the seizure or serve as a nidus for future seizures.

Management

If children are still convulsing on presentation and have been for at least 5 minutes, they should be managed as for status epilepticus (see Chapter 146). The airway must be secure, blood tests drawn and sent to the laboratory, an IV line started, and lorazepam administered in the appropriate dose to stop the seizure.

If children are not in status epilepticus, management decisions are made on a more long-term basis (Box 56-1). Whether to recommend **anticonvulsant prophylaxis** for children who have experienced febrile seizures is controversial. Factors that must be considered include (1) the benign, age-limited nature of the condition; (2) the morbidity of the anticonvulsant treatment; (3) the chance of recurrence of febrile or nonfebrile seizures; (4) the risk of overmedication during an acute recurrence; and (5) the family's reaction and social disruption caused by the seizures. Given the combination of these factors many physicians do not recommend antiepileptic drug prophylaxis for febrile seizures.

Box 56-1. Treatment Options for Febrile Seizures

- Cooling measures during febrile illness (antipyretics or bathing in tepid water)
- Family reassurance and education
- Diazepam, 0.3 mg/kg orally or 5–10 mg rectal gel (Diastat) every 8 h (during febrile illness only)
- Phenobarbital, 3–5 mg/kg orally daily, for prophylaxis
- Valproic acid (divalproex), 30 mg/kg orally divided twice daily, for prophylaxis

---

Daily doses of phenobarbital or valproic acid are effective prophylactic anticonvulsants. The most commonly used regimen is daily phenobarbital, but its potential side effects include hyperactive behavior disorder and depressed cognition and learning. Valproic acid can produce thrombocytopenia and may have the potential of provoking acute liver dysfunction in the patient younger than 2 years who is taking other medications. Fever control measures should be instituted to make the patient more comfortable but have not been found effective as prevention for seizures. Intermittent anticonvulsant therapy with diazepam has the advantage of reducing side effects but relies on recognizing the fever prior to the seizure and mandates greater vigilance for compliance during each fever. Because prolonged febrile seizures tend to recur as repeated prolonged seizures, this group may benefit by having rectal diazepam or intranasal midazolam to administer at home as an abortive drug to stop the seizure earlier in its course while paramedics are being called.

Recommendations for prophylactic anticonvulsant treatment are often individualized. Anticonvulsants are usually not recommended unless the child has presented in status epilepticus, has experienced marked respiratory compromise (perhaps needing ventilatory support) during the seizure, or has had complex febrile seizures. There is no definitive evidence yet that anticonvulsant prophylaxis for simple febrile seizures prevents the development of unprovoked seizures. Children who have had frequently recurring seizures that are extremely disruptive for the family and deleterious to parent–child interactions despite educational efforts by the medical caretakers may also be candidates for prophylactic anticonvulsant treatment.

Prognosis

Febrile seizures are a common age-limited problem. The prognosis for children with simple febrile seizures is generally good; the incidence of seizure episodes later in life is 3 to 6 times higher than in the general population at the same age but is still low: 2% to 3%. Those who have a complex presentation have a higher likelihood of developing a nonfebrile seizure disorder, but this risk is only 6% if 2 of the first 3 factors (Table 56-1) are present or 17% if they are neurodevelopmentally abnormal. Overall, one-third of children with febrile seizures experience a recurrence. The risk of febrile seizure recurrence is most dependent on age: 50% of infants younger than 1 year at the time of their first seizure will have a recurrence, but only 20% of children older than 3 years will have a recurrence. Other factors that have a lesser influence on the recurrence risk include family history of seizures, temperature at the initial seizure, time since the previous seizure, and history of previous recurrences.

Animal models suggest that seizures, even status epilepticus episodes, in the immature brain are less often associated with neuronal death, but that seizures, particularly hyperthermic seizures, can modify brain development by altering the expression of ion channels regulating neuronal excitability, and epileptogenic mechanisms may be more robust than in the adult.

Among patients who had surgery for intractable temporal lobe epilepsy, mesial temporal sclerosis (MTS) was the most frequent pathology, and 30% of these patients had antecedents of prolonged complex febrile seizures compared with 6% in those who did not have MTS. It is possible that MTS is the etiologic consequence of a prolonged seizure when the hippocampus is developmentally vulnerable. Mesial temporal sclerosis is frequently unilateral, however, although focal complex febrile seizures can actually originate in the temporal lobe in some children. An alternative explanation is that some preexisting damage or genetic predisposition may be present in patients with hippocampal sclerosis after prolonged febrile seizures, and the complex febrile seizure is an epiphenomenon.

A small percentage of infants with febrile seizures may develop Dravet syndrome, a phenotype influencing neurocognition as well as later resistant epilepsy, if they carry a particular channel subunit gene mutation.

CASE RESOLUTION

In the case history presented at the beginning of this chapter, the girl had a somewhat prolonged simple febrile seizure, a diagnosis supported by a family history positive for febrile seizures. Her family is educated about treatment options. They become comfortable with a decision to use intermittent therapy with diazepam for her subsequent febrile illnesses, realizing that a fever may not be recognized before the seizure occurs.

Selected References

American Academy of Pediatrics Provisional Committee on Quality Improvement and Subcommittee on Febrile Seizures. Clinical practice guideline: the neurodiagnostic evaluation of the child with a simple febrile seizure. *Pediatrics.* 2011;127:389–394

Baram T, Shinnar S, eds. *Febrile Seizures.* San Diego, CA: Academic Press; 2002

Cendes F. Febrile seizures and mesial temporal sclerosis. *Curr Opin Neurol.* 2004;17:161–164

Jensen F. Pediatric epilepsy models. *Epilepsy Res.* 2006;8:28–31

Kanai K, Hirose S, Oguni H. Effect of localization of missense mutations in SCN1A on epilepsy phenotype severity. *Neurology.* 2004;63:329–334

Kang J, Shen W, Macdonald RL. Why does fever trigger seizures? GABA-A receptor gamma 2 subunit mutations associated with idiopathic generalized epilepsies have temperature-dependent trafficking deficiencies. *J Neurosci.* 2006;26:2590–2597

Korff C, Nordli D. Epilepsy syndromes in infancy. *Pediatr Neurol.* 2006;34:253–263

Nelson KB, Ellenberg JH. *Febrile Seizures.* New York, NY: Raven Press; 1981

CHAPTER 57

Respiratory Distress

David B. Burbulys, MD

CASE STUDY

A 6-month-old boy has been coughing and breathing fast for the past day. This morning he refused feeding and has been irritable. On examination, the infant is fussy. He has a respiratory rate of 60 breaths/min, a pulse of 140 beats/min, and a normal blood pressure and temperature. In addition, he has nasal flaring, intercostal and supraclavicular retractions, and occasional grunting.

Questions

1. What are the causes of respiratory distress in infants and children?
2. What are the signs and symptoms of respiratory distress in infants and children?
3. What are the signs and symptoms of impending respiratory failure in infants and children?
4. What are the critical interventions for infants and children in respiratory distress?

Respiratory distress and respiratory failure may cause significant morbidity and mortality in infants and children. The signs and symptoms of respiratory compromise may be subtle, particularly in small infants. Decompensation may occur rapidly if ventilation or oxygenation is inadequate but may be prevented by prompt recognition and treatment. **Respiratory distress** is defined as increased work of breathing, and it usually precedes respiratory failure. **Respiratory failure** occurs when ventilation or oxygenation is not sufficient to meet the metabolic demands of the tissues. Thus oxygenation of the blood is inadequate or carbon dioxide is not eliminated. This may be caused by diseases of the airway, inadequate gas exchange in the lungs, or poor respiratory effort (Box 57-1). Respiratory failure may lead to cardiopulmonary arrest if not corrected promptly.

Epidemiology

Primary care physicians frequently care for children in respiratory distress in both offices and emergency departments. Respiratory distress continues to be the most common reason for hospital admission. Such admissions usually involve young infants with acute infections such as bronchiolitis or croup. Reactive airways disease (asthma) accounts for respiratory distress–related admission commonly in older children.

Clinical Presentation

Increases in respiratory rate and work of breathing are the most common signs of respiratory disease. Effortless tachypnea may be a sign of respiratory compensation for metabolic acidosis rather than an indication of pulmonary pathology. Similarly, hypoxia that fails to improve with supplemental oxygen may suggest a primary cardiac lesion. Tachycardia is often present, although bradycardia, if present, may be an ominous sign of impending cardiopulmonary failure. Signs of poor oxygenation include alterations in mental status, head bobbing, and change in skin color. Pallor, mottling, and cyanosis are often late signs indicating respiratory failure and shock. Children who are severely hypoxemic may first appear dusky or pale. If children are anemic, cyanosis may not be evident, although the oxygen saturation is low (Box 57-2).

Pathophysiology

The adequacy of respiration depends on effective gas exchange of carbon dioxide and oxygen and the ability to move an adequate volume of gas in and out of the airways. Infants and children generally breathe with minimal effort. In very young children, the **diaphragm** and abdominal musculature are primarily used for ventilation, and the tidal volume is approximately 6 to 8 mL/kg. If the tidal volume is decreased because of obstruction, children compensate by increasing the respiratory rate, thus attempting to maintain adequate **minute ventilation** (minute ventilation = rate × tidal volume). If the minute ventilation is still insufficient for adequate gas exchange, or the

Box 57-1. Causes of Respiratory Distress in Infants and Children

- Infection
- Bronchiolitis
- Pneumonia
- Croup
- Epiglottitis
- Congenital anomalies
- Foreign body aspiration
- Reactive airways disease (asthma)
- Allergic reactions
- Submersion injuries
- Pneumothorax or hemothorax
- Pulmonary contusion
- Smoke inhalation
- Toxin exposure
- Cardiac disease
- Metabolic disease with acidosis
- Neuromuscular disease

Box 57-2. Respiratory Distress

- Increased respiratory rate
- Changes in tidal volume or minute ventilation
- Presence of retractions: intercostal, substernal, diaphragmatic, or supraclavicular
- Nasal flaring
- Decreased or absent breath sounds
- Changes in inspiratory-expiratory ratio
- Production of sounds with respiration (eg, gurgling, stridor, rhonchi, grunting)
- Diaphoresis
- Alterations in mental status
- Poor feeding
- Inability to speak in sentences
- Presence of pale or cyanotic skin
- Presence of central cyanosis

Box 57-3. Comparison of Respiratory Systems in Children and Adults

- The head in children is proportionally larger and has less muscular support.
- The tongue in children is larger in relation to the mouth, is poorly controlled, and can cause airway obstruction.
- The airway diameter is smaller in children and collapses easily. Reductions in size due to secretions or inflammation cause greater resistance to air flow (resistance is proportional to $1/radius^4$).
- The larynx is higher and more anterior in children and the epiglottis is floppy, which makes visualization of the vocal cords more difficult.
- The narrowest part of the airway in children is at the cricoid ring, unlike in adults, where the narrowest point is at the vocal cords.
- The trachea in children is short. In newborns it is 4-cm long, in 18-month-old infants 7-cm long, and in adults 12-cm long.
- The major muscle of respiration in children is the diaphragm. Any interference with diaphragmatic motion in young children impedes respiratory function. Intercostal muscles are immature in children and fatigue easily.
- Children have less pulmonary reserve and higher metabolic demands.
- Normal respiratory rates are higher in children and vary by age.

---

child can no longer sustain the increased work of breathing, then respiratory failure ensues. Respiratory failure may then lead to acidosis, myocardial dysfunction, and shock and may progress to complete cardiopulmonary arrest.

Infants and children are more prone than adults to respiratory distress because of the differences between their respiratory systems (Box 57-3).

Differential Diagnosis

The differential diagnosis of children with respiratory distress can include abnormalities with the pulmonary, cardiovascular, or metabolic systems or be related to a reduction in the central nervous system drive. It is also important to make an initial differentiation between upper and lower airway disease based on the presence or absence of stridor, rhonchi, rales, or wheezes on examination. Many common causes are shown in Box 57-1.

Evaluation

History

A brief history should be taken (Questions Box) while physical examination proceeds and initial treatment is begun.

Questions

Respiratory Distress

- For how long has this problem been occurring? Has a similar problem ever occurred before?
- Did the problem begin while the child was eating or playing?
- Has the child had any recent infections?
- Are any members of the household ill?
- Is the child taking any medications?

Physical Examination

Before a complete assessment can proceed, critical interventions that may change children's clinical status should be made. Children should be placed in a position of comfort and oxygen should be applied. Both **ventilation** and **oxygenation** should be assessed.

Respiratory and heart rates should be determined for a period of at least 30 seconds. In infants, abdominal excursions should be counted and, in older children, chest excursions should be counted. **Respiratory rates** in children are higher than in adults; infants may breathe 40 times per minute, 1-year-olds 25 times per minute, and 10-year-olds 18 times per minute (Table 57-1). These rates vary with age and changes of activity, emotion, and illness. Abnormal respiratory rates are defined as being faster than normal (**tachypnea**), slower than normal (**bradypnea**), or absent (**apnea**). Neonates may exhibit **periodic breathing**, with periods of regular respirations alternating with irregular breathing. This is a normal variant for age. True apnea (cessation of respiration) is accompanied by change in skin color or tone or altered level of consciousness.

The depth of respiration should be noted. Whether breaths are deep, gasping, or shallow should be determined. Rapid, shallow

Table 57-1. Vital Signs by Age

Age	Respiration (breaths/min)	Pulse (beats/min)	Systolic Blood Pressure (mm Hg)
Newborn	30–60	100–160	50–70
1–6 wk	30–60	100–160	70–95
6 mo	25–40	90–120	80–100
1 y	20–40	90–120	80–100
3 y	20–30	80–120	80–110
6 y	12–25	70–110	80–110
10 y	12–20	60–90	90–120

respirations may not provide enough **inspiratory time** for adequate gas exchange. The heart rate may also reflect respiratory compromise. Breath sounds should first be listened to in the axillae and then at the bases and apices. The absence of breath sounds may be an ominous sign. Children's breath sounds are usually well transmitted across the thorax because of the thin chest wall. It is common to hear upper airway noises when auscultating the lungs.

Abnormal sounds are caused by turbulent air passing through a narrowed airway. Resistance to flow through a hollow tube increases exponentially. Thus the smaller the airway, the greater the resistance to flow generated by even small changes in the radius (eg, as with edema, secretions, or foreign bodies). The nature of the sounds produced depends on the location of the narrowing in the airway. **Gurgling, snoring,** and **stridor** come from the upper airway; **rales, rhonchi,** and **wheezing** from the lower airway. If no abnormal sounds are evident and breath sounds are absent or decreased, the upper or lower airways may be totally obstructed. **Grunting** is caused by turbulent air coming in contact with a partially closed glottis. Children who grunt are generating their own partial obstruction of the upper airway and positive end-expiratory pressure to increase oxygenation.

The physician should also observe the effort children expend in breathing. Increased work of breathing occurs when intercostal, subcostal, or supraclavicular **retractions** are present, the **accessory muscles** of respiration are used, breathing is abnormally noisy, or **nasal flaring** is seen. The normal work of breathing consumes 2% to 3% of total oxygen consumption. The increased work of breathing in children with severe respiratory distress can potentially increase total oxygen consumption to 50%. Increased work of breathing can also be demonstrated by feeding difficulties and diaphoresis in young infants.

In addition, the physician should observe the inspiratory-expiratory ratio while assessing the work of breathing. The ratio is approximately 1:1 in most patients. Prolonged expirations are most often seen with reactive airways disease.

Oxygen saturation should be measured by pulse oximetry in all children with respiratory complaints. Levels less than 93% while awake indicate significant hypoxemia.

Laboratory Tests

Although the physical examination is the most important tool for assessing children in respiratory distress, laboratory tests such as complete and differential blood cell counts and blood cultures may help in the diagnosis of infection. It should be remembered that meningitis, sepsis, and metabolic derangement may present with effortless tachypnea not associated with increased work of breathing. Arterial or venous blood gases may be beneficial in this situation but in general should be reserved for patients in impending respiratory failure.

Peak expiratory flow or forced expiratory volume in 1-second determinations (FEV_1) can be helpful in assessing compliant older children with reactive airways disease. Oxygen saturation measurements can also be helpful in these children because reduced levels below 100% often correlate with the severity of disease.

Imaging Studies

Chest radiographs can aid in assessing children in respiratory distress but should not be routinely performed in patients with known reactive airways disease unless children have a fever or are in status asthmaticus. A patient with significant respiratory distress should not be moved from a monitored setting to the radiology suite but rather portable radiographs should be obtained if needed.

Management

All infants or children in respiratory distress should be managed emergently. As stated earlier, in such situations, assessment and intervention often occur simultaneously. All children in respiratory distress should be reassessed frequently. The highest possible oxygen concentration should be delivered. Children who are able to maintain their own airway should never be forced to use an airway adjunct because this may cause increased anxiety and distress. Patients with clear airways can be maintained with simple interventions such as **oxygen** blown by the face or given by mask or nasal prongs. More advanced airway management such as bag-valve-mask ventilation or endotracheal intubation may be necessary for children who need assisted ventilation, airway protection, or hyperventilation.

Position

Children in respiratory distress who are alert and breathing spontaneously should be allowed to choose a **position of comfort.** Small infants who are incapable of positioning themselves are best placed upright with care taken not to flex or extend the neck. Children and their caregivers should be kept together to reduce anxiety.

The proper position for unconscious children is the "sniffing position," with the neck slightly flexed and the head extended to open the airway. This can be facilitated by placing a towel under the occiput of the head or the shoulders. If simple positioning does not relieve an obstruction, then the airway should be opened using the chin lift or jaw thrust. If spinal trauma is a possibility, only the jaw thrust should be used. If this fails, then **airway adjuncts**, such as nasopharyngeal or oropharyngeal airways, can be placed to help prevent the soft tissue of the oropharynx from collapsing against the posterior pharyngeal wall.

Monitoring

All infants and children in respiratory distress should be carefully monitored. Pulse oximetry will assist the clinician in determining the degree of oxygen saturation and, if available, a cardiac and respiratory monitor will provide constant readings of respirations and heart rate. Frequent assessments of the patient are critical to ensure a good outcome.

Oxygen Administration

Oxygen should be delivered by any method tolerated by children. **Nasal prongs** have 2 advantages: They are noninvasive and allow maintenance of a constant gas flow even when talking and eating. The concentration of oxygen delivered is limited, however, and irritation and drying of the mucous membranes may result.

Oxygen masks deliver a higher concentration of humidified oxygen. Disadvantages include obstruction of children's visual field, potential for carbon dioxide retention, and anxiety because the face is covered. Various types of masks are available.

The **simple mask** can deliver 30% to 60% oxygen concentration at flow rates of 6 to 10 L/min. Room air is drawn into the mask through the exhalation ports in the side of the mask.

A **non-rebreathing mask** has valves that allow only oxygen (85%–95%) to flow from the reservoir bag to the patient on inhalation and additional valves on the exhalation ports of the mask that prevent entrapment of room air (Figure 57-1).

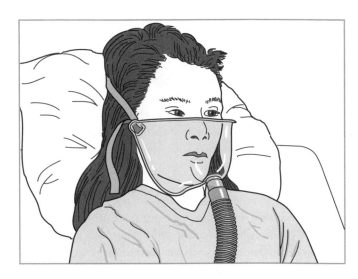

Figure 57-2. Use of a face tent.

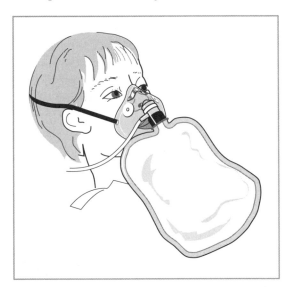

Figure 57-1. A non-rebreathing mask can deliver a high concentration of oxygen to a patient in respiratory distress.

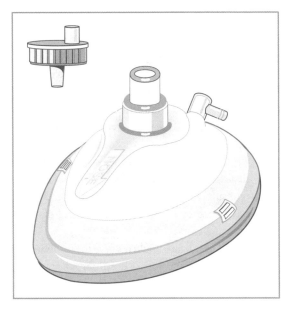

Figure 57-3. A pocket mask with a one-way valve and side oxygen port that can be used for assisted ventilation in the office setting.

The **face tent** is a soft plastic bucket shaped to the chin that is well tolerated by children. The face tent allows up to 40% oxygen to be delivered, and it has the advantage of allowing access to the face and mouth (Figure 57-2).

A **venturi mask** is rarely used in children but has the advantage of precisely titrating the oxygen concentration to be delivered from 24% to 60%.

Children with potential respiratory failure require **assisted ventilation** with **bag-valve-mask** devices or **endotracheal intubation**. Masks of the proper size should be used. The upper edge of the mask should fit snugly over the bridge of the nose without touching the eyes. The lower edge should rest directly on or just above the mandible. An oropharyngeal airway should be inserted in unconscious children to prevent the tongue from obstructing the upper airway. A nasopharyngeal airway may be inserted if the patient has an

intact gag reflex to achieve the same goal. If a bag-valve-mask is not available, assisted ventilation can be given with a **pocket mask** with a one-way valve. Oxygen can be attached to the mask at the side port (Figure 57-3). Endotracheal intubation is indicated in those children who require control of the airway, who need airway protection, or who require hyperventilation.

Prognosis

Respiratory failure and resulting cardiopulmonary arrest are preventable in most infants and children if their condition is carefully assessed and appropriate critical interventions are made. Careful attention to ventilation and oxygenation of patients usually results in a good outcome.

CASE RESOLUTION

The fussy infant discussed in the case history has obvious signs of respiratory distress, including tachypnea, tachycardia, grunting, nasal flaring, and retractions. The differential diagnosis includes foreign body, infection, and reactive airways disease. It is important to place the infant in a position of comfort and provide supplemental oxygen before any diagnostic studies, such as chest radiograph, are performed. Pulse oximetry should be monitored. The clinical status of the infant should be reassessed periodically to prevent further deterioration.

Selected References

Berg MD, Schexnayder SM, Chameides L, et al. Pediatric basic life support: 2010 American Heart Association guidelines for cardiopulmonary resuscitation and emergency cardiovascular care. *Pediatrics.* 2010;126(5):e1345–e1360

Fallot A. Respiratory distress. *Pediatr Ann.* 2005;34:885–891

Kleinman ME, de Caen AR, Chameides L, et al. Pediatric basic and advanced life support: 2010 international consensus on cardiopulmonary resuscitation and emergency cardiovascular care science with treatment recommendations. *Pediatrics.* 2010;126:e1261–e1318

CHAPTER 58

Stridor and Croup

David B. Burbulys, MD

CASE STUDY

A 2-year-old boy has been breathing noisily for 1 day. For the past 3 days he has had a "cold," with a runny nose, fever (temperature: up to 100.4°F [38°C]), and a slight cough. The cough has gradually become worse and now has a barking quality.

On examination, the child is sitting up and has a respiratory rate of 48 breaths/min with marked inspiratory stridor and an occasional barking cough. His other vital signs include a heart rate of 100 beats/min and temperature of 101.2°F (38.4°C). He has intercostal retractions, his breath sounds are slightly decreased bilaterally, and his skin is pale. The remainder of the examination is normal.

Questions
1. What is stridor?
2. What are the common causes of stridor?
3. What is the pathophysiology of viral croup?
4. How are children with stridor managed?

Noisy breathing is a common symptom that often accompanies respiratory infections in children. The presence of **stridor,** a high-pitched crowing sound, often concerns children's caregivers. Some parents try home remedies to alleviate the symptoms, whereas many others immediately seek help in the office or emergency department setting. **Croup** is an inflammation of the larynx, trachea, and upper bronchioles (laryngotracheobronchitis) that causes noisy breathing and stridor. It is one of the most common causes of a seal-like barking cough and stridor in children.

Epidemiology

Croup most commonly affects children between 6 months and 3 years of age, generally in the fall or early winter. Children younger than 1 year make up 26% of cases. The condition is more common in boys than girls; two-thirds of all hospitalized children with croup are boys.

Stridor, which may be indicative of croup, may also be a sign of epiglottitis. The incidence of epiglottitis in children has dramatically decreased since 1988 following the development and widespread use of the vaccine against *Haemophilus influenzae* type b (Hib). Many young children may be incompletely immunized and there are other bacteria that may cause epiglottitis; therefore, epiglottitis should still be considered in toxic-appearing children with rapid onset of symptoms of upper airway obstruction. Prior to Hib immunization, the ratio of cases of epiglottitis to croup was 1:100. Today, epiglottitis in children is exceedingly rare.

Pathophysiology

Stridor

Stridor is generally caused by obstruction of the airway between the nose and the larger bronchi. Obstruction at the level of the nose or pharynx may produce snoring or gurgling sounds. Turbulence of airflow in the laryngeal area or upper trachea causes the high-pitched crowing sound characteristic of stridor. Edema and inflammation at the vocal cords and subglottic areas result in **inspiratory stridor,** whereas obstruction below the cricoid cartilage may lead to both inspiratory and **expiratory stridor.**

Some of the more common causes of stridor are listed in Box 58-1.

The sounds produced at various levels of obstruction can give the primary care provider clues as to the etiology of the problem. The most common cause of stridor that begins shortly after birth is tracheomalacia, a condition secondary to the immaturity of the cartilage of the trachea. Laryngomalacia, which is caused by floppy supraglottic structures, resolves after several months.

The upper airway of infants and children is more susceptible to obstruction as a result of anatomical differences between children and adults. The tongues of children are relatively large and the epiglottis is floppy and shaped somewhat like the Greek letter omega (Ω). The angle between the epiglottis and the glottis is more acute in children, which makes direct visualization of the airway more difficult. Cartilaginous structures are less rigid in infants. During inspiration, negative intraluminal pressure is generated below the level of obstruction, which leads to narrowing of the airway and turbulence of the airflow. This occurs more often in children because the tracheal rings are not well formed. In addition, the smaller size of the airway in children makes resistance to airflow greater when obstruction is present.

Box 58-1. Causes of Stridor	
Congenital Anomalies	**Trauma**
Tracheomalacia	Direct trauma to the upper airway
Laryngomalacia	Post-intubation subglottic stenosis
Choanal atresia	**Neurogenic**
Laryngeal web	Laryngeal paralysis
Laryngocele	Poor pharyngeal muscle tone
Subglottic stenosis	**Caustic or Thermal Injury**
Vascular ring	Lye or caustic ingestion
Macroglossia (Beckwith syndrome)	Hot gas or liquid
Tracheal web or cyst	**Foreign Body**
Inflammatory/Infectious Lesions	Neoplasm
Viral croup	
Epiglottitis	
Abscess (retropharyngeal, peritonsillar, parapharyngeal)	
Tracheitis	
Bronchitis	
Severe tonsillitis	
Angioneurotic edema	
Infectious mononucleosis	
Diphtheria	

The smaller the airway, the greater the resistance to flow (resistance increases exponentially). Alterations in the diameter of the airway are most often caused by edema and inflammation from a variety of conditions, including congenital anomalies, infection, allergic and anaphylactic reactions, cysts, tumors, and trauma. Even small localized areas of airway narrowing in infants and children can lead to respiratory distress because the airway is so small, particularly at the cricoid ring, which is the narrowest portion of the airway in children.

Croup

Croup is most often caused by an infection with **parainfluenza virus** (type I or II). Several other causes include respiratory syncytial virus, influenza virus A or B, adenovirus, rhinovirus, coxsackievirus, measles, and herpes simplex virus. Metapneumovirus and a novel coronavirus, which more commonly cause bronchiolitis, have also been implicated. Particularly severe disease may be associated with influenza A, respiratory syncytial virus, or adenovirus infection. Infection occurs via respiratory droplets spread from other infected individuals.

The virus first attacks the nasopharynx and subsequently spreads to the larynx and upper trachea. The infection causes inflammation and edema of the airway that often involves the vocal cords producing the typical barking cough, hoarseness, and inspiratory stridor. Uncommonly, in severe cases, the lower airways also may be involved, leading to impaired alveolar ventilation and wheezing. In some children, secondary bacterial superinfection may rarely occur with bacterial tracheitis or extension of infection to the lower airway producing pneumonia. Airways of infants are small and particularly susceptible to obstruction because of the narrow subglottic region and the laxity of the cartilaginous structures.

Spasmodic croup, an entirely different disease, is common, frequently occurs at night, and may be recurrent. It is characterized by the sudden onset of hoarseness, barking cough, and stridor. This condition may resolve when children are exposed to humid air. The etiology is unknown but is probably either a reaction to a viral infection or an allergic phenomenon. There may be a family history of recurrent stridor in children with spasmodic croup and it tends to occur in older aged children.

Differential Diagnosis

The differential diagnosis of stridor is presented in Table 58-1.

Evaluation

History

A complete history should be obtained (Questions Box).

Questions

Stridor and Croup

- Did the child have an antecedent respiratory infection?
- Does the child have a fever? If so, how high is the temperature?
- Was the onset of stridor abrupt?
- Is there stridor at rest/sleep or only with agitation?
- Does the child have any ill contacts?
- Does the child have any associated symptoms such as vomiting, diarrhea, or rash?
- Is the child feeding normally?
- Is the child drooling?

Physical Examination

It is important to assess the degree of respiratory distress and to place children in a position of comfort; monitor heart rate, ventilation, and oxygenation; and deliver oxygen (see Chapter 57). The stridorous sounds produced are usually inspiratory but may be inspiratory and expiratory if the disease progresses to the lower airway. The presence of stridor at rest or with sleep should be assessed as well as the severity of retractions with breathing. Breath sounds may be decreased bilaterally, and severe tachypnea, with respiratory rates from 40 breaths/min to 80 breaths/min, may occur. Peripheral or central cyanosis and alterations in mental status associated with severe disease should be noted. Assessment of the croup score may be helpful to direct initial therapy in mild, moderate, or severe cases (Table 58-2).

Laboratory Tests

Investigations, such as a complete blood cell count and cultures, are rarely helpful unless the physician is concerned about secondary bacterial infection. The white blood cell count may be normal or mildly

Table 58-1. Differential Diagnosis of Stridor					
Data	*Viral Croup*	*Spasmodic Croup*	*Bacterial Tracheitis*	*Epiglottitis*	*Foreign Body*
Age	*3–36 mo*	*3–36 mo*	*1–10 y*	*1–8 y*	*All Ages*
Prodrome	Upper respiratory infection symptoms; onset over 2–5 d	None; sudden onset at night	Upper respiratory infection symptoms for days followed by rapid onset fever and respiratory distress	Usually none; rapid onset over several hours	None; sudden onset
Fever	Low grade	None	Low grade initially then higher	Usually above 102.2°F (39°C)	None
Cough	Barking	Barking	Dry initially then barking	None or dry	May or may not be present
Respiratory distress	Present	Present	Absent or mild initially then severe	Present and severe	Usually present
White blood cell count	Normal or slightly elevated	Normal	Normal initially then elevated	Elevated	Normal
Blood culture	No growth	No growth	Growth uncommon	*Haemophilus influenzae*	No growth
Radiograph	Subglottic narrowing; steeple sign	(±) Subglottic narrowing	Subglottic narrowing; steeple sign and ragged trachea	Swollen epiglottis	Air trapping; may show a foreign body

elevated, and the differential count may show a predominance of polymorphonuclear cells. If epiglottitis is being considered, no blood should be drawn until the airway has been visualized and secured.

Imaging Studies

Radiographs of the soft tissues of the upper airway are often helpful. In children with croup, lateral neck films may reveal ballooning of the hypopharynx, a normal epiglottis, and narrowing of the subglottic area (Figure 58-1). The frontal view shows the classic "steeple sign" of the subglottic area where the airway narrows like a church steeple or pencil tip. Radiographic studies should not delay the management of children with suspected epiglottitis nor should children with respiratory compromise be taken from a monitored area for radiographs. Thickening of the epiglottis (thumbprint-shaped) and obliteration of the vallecular space may be seen on lateral neck films in patients with epiglottitis if radiographs are obtained.

Other imaging studies, such as a barium swallow or computed tomography scan of the thorax, are helpful in diagnosing congenital anomalies (eg, vascular ring).

Management

Most children with croup and stridor can be managed as outpatients. Caregivers should be given careful instructions so that they understand the course of the illness, know what to expect, and realize when emergency care is needed. Children with a prolonged or recurrent history of stridor may require consultation with a head and neck specialist. If a specific cause of stridor, such as a foreign body, is identified, appropriate management should be instituted.

Children with croup should be treated with gentleness and should not be upset. They should remain with their caregivers and be allowed to assume a position of comfort. Agitation and crying increase respiratory distress and oxygen demand. Procedures should

Table 58-2. Croup Score[a]				
	0	*1*	*2*	*3*
Stridor	None	Only with agitation	Mild at rest	Severe at rest
Retraction	None	Mild	Moderate	Severe
Air entry	Normal	Mild decrease	Moderate decrease	Marked decrease
Color	Normal	Normal	Normal	Cyanotic
Level of consciousness	Normal	Restless when disturbed	Restless when undisturbed	Lethargic
Disease Category by Score				
Score	*Degree*	*Management*		
≤4	Mild	Consider mist therapy and dexamethasone 0.6 mg/kg orally. Outpatient observation.		
5–6	Mild to moderate	Dexamethasone 0.6 mg/kg orally and consider mist therapy. If child improves after observation, is >6 months, and has a reliable family then outpatient observation.		
7–8	Moderate	Dexamethasone 0.6 mg/kg orally or intramuscularly, consider racemic epinephrine and admission.		
≥9	Severe	Racemic epinephrine, dexamethasone 0.6 mg/kg orally or intramuscularly, oxygen, and admit to intensive care unit.		

[a] Modified from Taussig LM, Castro O, Beaudry PH, Fox WW, Bureau M. Treatment of laryngotracheobronchitis (croup). Use of intermittent positive-pressure breathing and racemic epinephrine. *Am J Dis Child.* 1975;129:790, with permission from the American Medical Association.

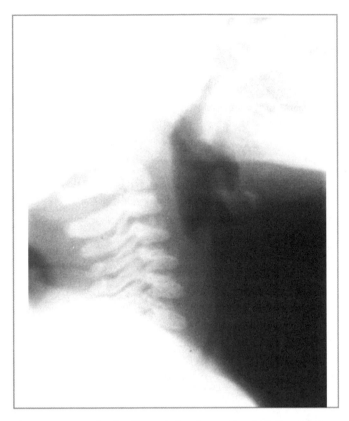

Figure 58-1. Lateral neck radiograph of viral croup. Note the ballooning of the hypo-pharynx and the narrowing in the subglottic area. (Courtesy of Dr J. S. Seidel, Division of General and Emergency Pediatrics, Harbor-UCLA Medical Center.)

be kept to a minimum. The heart rate, respiratory status, and oxygen saturation should be continuously monitored while the patient is being treated and observed. Airway adjuncts that cause increased agitation should not be used.

Cool mist may be provided by blow-by or mask. **Humidified oxygen or air,** which is thought to decrease the viscosity of secretions and reduce the edema of the airway, has been the mainstay of therapy for croup for quite some time. This treatment is currently controversial. Several randomized, controlled trials have questioned this practice demonstrating no benefit of cool humidified mist therapy. Many find it difficult not to continue this treatment practice at this time though. Symptoms of spasmodic croup usually resolve within 6 hours of the onset without treatment but cool, humidified mist is often employed as the sole therapy in this disorder.

Treatment of croup with **corticosteroids** is less controversial. A number of studies have demonstrated that dexamethasone given as a single dose of 0.6 mg/kg is effective in shortening the course and severity of mild, moderate, and severe croup if given in the first 3 days. Several smaller randomized trials have also suggested that half the dose of dexamethasone may be equally effective. It should be given orally but may be given as an intramuscular injection for children who are unable to take oral medication. Use of the tablet preparation ground up in applesauce is recommended because the liquid

preparation does not taste good and is not well tolerated. Recent studies using nebulized budesonide also demonstrate the same efficacy in reducing respiratory distress and lowering of the croup score but at considerably more cost. Continuous or long-term therapy with steroids does not seem to alter the clinical course of the disease or the period of hospitalization and is not recommended. Treatment with antibiotics is not indicated unless infection with bacteria is evident.

Use of **racemic epinephrine** has also been somewhat controversial. Several older studies have shown that there was no difference in the long-term outcome between those children who were treated with epinephrine and those who received a placebo. Other studies have clearly demonstrated an acute effect of the drug when given via nebulizer. This effect lasts a few hours, and repeat respiratory distress after the drug effects have worn off has been reported in the literature. It is therefore prudent that racemic epinephrine only be used on patients who are going to be discharged if they can be observed for 3 to 4 hours after treatment. The anti-inflammatory effects of dexamethasone take several hours for onset, and racemic epinephrine may have more benefit in reducing symptoms during this period.

Hospitalization should be considered for children in severe respiratory distress or with significant stridor at rest who are unable to eat, and those whose parents are unable to cope with the tasks required to manage children at home. It is always indicated for children with a bacterial infection, such as epiglottitis or tracheitis.

About 10% of infants and children with croup may need **controlled ventilation with endotracheal intubation.** The indications for intubation include severe respiratory distress, altered mental status, hypoxia, and hypercapnia. A major complication of endotracheal intubation in children with croup is subglottic stenosis, which develops because the endotracheal tube may traumatize the inflamed airway, leading to permanent damage. Patients should be extubated as soon as possible.

Direct laryngoscopy may be necessary in some children where the etiology of the stridor is not clear. This procedure should be done by a practitioner who is experienced in managing the airway.

Prognosis

Stridor is a serious sign, which is indicative of upper airway obstruction and potential respiratory compromise. Although it has many causes, the prognosis is usually determined by the rapidity of diagnosis and the institution of appropriate therapeutic measures, particularly stabilizing the patient and ensuring patency of the airway. Certain conditions such as croup often resolve spontaneously within a few days, although some children require hospitalization and, rarely, assisted ventilation. Other conditions, such as foreign bodies or tumors, necessitate aggressive intervention to prevent death from airway obstruction.

CASE RESOLUTION

In the case history at the beginning of this chapter, the 2-year-old with the antecedent infection and stridor has the classic signs of croup and a croup score of 6. First, adequate ventilation and oxygenation should be ensured. As soon as the assessment and management of airway, breathing, and circulation are completed, other diagnostic studies and specific therapy, such as dexamethasone or racemic epinephrine, or both, can be considered.

Selected References

Bjornson CL, Johnson DW. Croup-treatment update. *Pediatr Emerg Care.* 2005;21(12):863–870

Cherry JD. Clinical practice. Croup. *N Engl J Med.* 2008;358(4):384–391

Everard ML. Acute bronchiolitis and croup. *Pediatr Clin North Am.* 2009;56(1):119–133

More M, Little P. Humidified air inhalation for treating croup. *Cochrane Database Syst Rev.* 2006;(3):CD002870

Port C. Towards evidence based emergency medicine: best BETs from the Manchester Royal Infirmary. BET4. Dose of dexamethasone in croup. *Emerg Med J.* 2009;26(4):291–292

Sobol SE, ZapataS. Epiglottitis and croup. *Otolaryngol Clin North Am.* 2008;41(3):551–566

CHAPTER 59

Sudden Infant Death Syndrome and Apparent Life-Threatening Events

Lynne M. Smith, MD

CASE STUDY

A 4-month-old male infant is brought to the emergency department (ED) by paramedics after being found blue and not breathing by his mother. He had previously been well except for a mild upper respiratory infection. His mother fed him at 2:00 am, and when she checked on him at 6:00 am she found him blue and lifeless. Although the mother smoked cigarettes during pregnancy, the pregnancy and delivery were otherwise normal. The infant received the appropriate immunizations at 2 months of age.

Questions

1. What factors are associated with sudden infant death syndrome (SIDS)?
2. How are SIDS and apparent life-threatening events (ALTEs) related?
3. How are SIDS and sudden unexplained infant deaths (SUIDs) related?
4. What is the appropriate evaluation of infants who present with an ALTE?
5. What services are available to families who have lost infants to SIDS?
6. What should parents be advised to help prevent SUIDs?

Sudden infant death syndrome, previously referred to as **crib death,** is defined as the sudden, **unexpected death** of an apparently well infant younger than 1 year that is not adequately explained by a comprehensive medical history of the infant and family, a thorough postmortem examination, and a death scene investigation. The syndrome has been known since biblical times; parents were advised not to lie with their children for fear of suffocating them. In the United States, SIDS is the most common cause of death in children younger than 1 year beyond the neonatal period. Research suggests that infants who died of SIDS have **serotonin-mediated dysregulation** of the autonomic nervous system, which increases their vulnerability to exogenous stressors such as prone sleep position and environmental overheating.

Sudden infant death syndrome–like events associated with successful resuscitation were once described as **near-miss SIDS** or **aborted crib death.** The term that is now used is **apparent life-threatening event** and was adopted in 1987 at a National Institute of Health Consensus Development Conference on Infantile Apnea and Home Monitoring. Apparent life-threatening events are characterized by some combination of **apnea, color change, marked change in muscle tone,** and **choking** or **gagging.** Though some have

theorized ALTEs are precursors to SIDS, only approximately 5% to 10% of SIDS victims experienced a previous ALTE. In an attempt to establish the efficacy of home monitoring the **Collaborative Home Infant Monitoring Evaluation (CHIME)** study followed more than 1,000 healthy term infants as well as infants at varying risks for SIDS. The CHIME study found 43% of term infants experienced apnea/bradycardia episodes, indicating these cardiorespiratory events are common in all infants and unlikely to be precursors to SIDS. Further, SIDS usually occurs during infant sleep whereas an estimated 50% of ALTEs occur during wakefulness, which may explain why the Back to Sleep campaign has successfully decreased SIDS but not affected the incidence of ALTEs. Thus SIDS and ALTE should not be considered varying manifestations of a similar disease process.

With the expanded and more thorough home scene investigations, exogenous contributing factors have been increasingly noted in these deaths and are found in the vast majority of what is now referred to as **sudden unexplained infant death.**

Sudden unexplained death in childhood occurs in children older than 12 months. Sudden unexplained death in childhood is rare, with a reported incidence in the United States in 2002 of 1.3

deaths per 100,000 children, compared with 57 deaths per 100,000 live-birth infants under 12 months.

Epidemiology

Sudden unexplained infant death accounts for 2,000 to 3,000 deaths per year in the United States, with an overall incidence of 0.57 per 1,000. These figures were dramatically higher prior to the campaign of the American Academy of Pediatrics (AAP) to place babies in the supine position for sleep. Prior to the institution of the **Back to Sleep** campaign, the annual death rate from SIDS was approximately 5,000 to 8,000 with an incidence of approximately 2 per 1,000. Sudden infant death affects boys more commonly than girls and occurs more often in the winter months. This seasonality may be related to infection with respiratory syncytial virus (RSV). The highest incidence of SIDS occurs at 2 to 3 months of age, with 90% occurring before the age of 6 months.

The frequency of SIDS differs in different populations in both the United States and other countries. Though the incidence of SIDS is decreasing among all groups, SIDS rates in African American and American Indian/Alaska Native children is 2 to 3 times the national average. One factor contributing to the higher SIDS rate is the higher incidence of non-supine sleeping in African American infants. In 2001 the prevalence of prone positioning was 11% for white infants and 21% for African American infants.

Numerous epidemiological, maternal, and infant factors have been associated with SIDS, including **prematurity** and **intrauterine growth restriction** (Box 59-1). Mothers of children with SIDS are frequently young and unwed, smoke cigarettes, and have had fewer doctor visits during the prenatal and postpartum periods. Parental alcohol use is also a risk factor for SIDS. Sudden infant death syndrome rates in one study were 33% higher on New Year's Day, suggesting parents under the influence of alcohol are less able to safely monitor their infants. Despite initial reports and significant research efforts, no clear data have established a causal relationship of ALTEs, apnea, immunizations, or repeated episodes of cyanosis with SIDS.

Box 59-1. Risk Factors for Sudden Infant Death Syndrome

- Male gender
- Maternal youth
- Socioeconomic disadvantage
- Maternal smoking
- Prematurity
- Low birth weight
- Poor prenatal care
- Sleeping in prone or side position
- Soft bedding
- Overheating
- Bed sharing

Clinical Presentation

Victims of SIDS present in **cardiopulmonary arrest,** with a history of previous good health or antecedent upper respiratory infection. They often present in the early morning hours, having succumbed during sleep.

Infants who have experienced an ALTE at home may appear well without any need for medical intervention or resuscitation or may appear in the ED pale, cyanotic, hypotonic, lethargic, and have bradycardia. They often present during the day between the hours of 8:00 am and 8:00 pm, a different time of day than for SIDS victims. If resuscitation is successful en route, infants may look normal and be fully alert.

Pathophysiology and Risk Factors for SIDS

Sudden infant death syndrome is related to the interaction of a number of factors. Sudden infant death syndrome occurs in infants with an underlying vulnerability at a critical time during development when they are exposed to known risk factors such as sleeping in a non-supine position. The AAP recommends only the supine sleep position because side sleeping increases the risk of SIDS 2-fold relative to back sleeping.

Sleeping on a firm crib mattress covered by a fitted sheet is the recommended sleep surface for infants. Soft bedding such as waterbeds, couches, stuffed toys, pillows, quilts, and comforters are to be avoided. Though **bed sharing** has been promoted as enhancing breastfeeding, **accidental suffocation** and sudden infant deaths are associated with this practice. The AAP recommends parents sleep in a separate but proximate sleeping environment from their infant (room sharing but not bed sharing). The importance of a safe sleep environment is underscored by the work of Kemp and colleagues who investigated 119 SIDS cases over a 4-year period following the initiation of the Back to Sleep campaign. Only 8.4% of these SIDS victims were found in a non-prone position, alone in their bed, without any potential obstructions of the external airway by bedding. Overheating can increase the risk of SIDS, so dressing babies in light clothing during sleep and keeping the room temperature at a comfortable level for adults is recommended.

Because approximately 20% of SIDS cases in the United States occur while in the care of someone other than the parent, there is a critical need to educate secondary caregivers and child care centers regarding the need for babies to sleep on their backs. Another group of infants likely to sleep in a non-supine position are infants born weighing less than 1,500 g. These infants are twice as likely to be placed to sleep in the prone position at home than infants weighing 1,500 to 2,500 g. During the first weeks of hospitalization, premature newborns are often placed in a non-supine position because of respiratory complications and gastroesophageal reflux. The children become accustomed to this position, and the parents learn from the hospital staff's modeling to place them in these unsafe positions. The AAP Task Force on SIDS encourages neonatologists and nurses to begin placing premature newborns on their backs "significantly before the infant's anticipated discharge."

One unintended consequence of supine sleep positioning is the increased incidence of **positional plagiocephaly.** To minimize the risk for head deformities and to foster appropriate motor development, parents are encouraged to vary the head position at sleep times, avoid swing and "bouncy" seats that increase pressure on the back of the head, and encourage adult-observed **tummy time** during waking hours starting from birth.

In addition to being exposed to an environment that increases the infant's risk for SIDS, most theories suggest that there is an underlying vulnerability in SIDS victims. The brain stems in infants who died of SIDS have significantly lower concentrations of serotonin and tryptophan hydroxylase, a key biosynthetic enzyme of serotonin; higher **serotonergic neuron** counts; decreased **serotonin 1A receptor** binding; and reduced **serotonin transporter** binding in the medulla. These findings suggest that abnormalities in serotonin synthesis, release, and clearance impair the infant's ability to appropriately regulate arousal and respiratory drive in response to potential life-threatening challenges during sleep.

Numerous other associations with SIDS have been reported including altered polymorphisms of pro-inflammatory cytokines, small mandibular size, disorders of fatty acid oxidation, and cardiac channelopathies including long QT syndrome. The AAP does not currently recommend universal electrocardiogram (ECG) screening at birth to identify potential SIDS victims.

The association between SIDS and **fatal child abuse** has also received attention, though infanticide is estimated to be the cause in less than 5% of suspected SIDS cases. The evaluation of the home environment of SIDS victims, referred to as *death scene investigations,* may reveal factors that contributed to the death of some of these infants. Unsafe sleeping environments (eg, sofas) and parental drug paraphernalia may identify such factors. A complete postmortem examination may reveal prior or recent trauma. The autopsy should include an assessment for long bone fractures as well as intracranial hemorrhage, which establish inflicted trauma as the cause of the sudden death. In some municipalities, child fatality boards review each case of reputed SIDS to determine whether an etiology other than SIDS is present. Infants with parents who have Munchausen syndrome by proxy (MSBP) may present with SIDS or ALTE. Such infants are suffocated by the parents until they become apneic or die. Because distinguishing between SIDS and intentional suffocation is very difficult pathologically, the AAP Committee on Child Abuse and Neglect has cited factors that should heighten the clinician's suspicion for possible child abuse (Box 59-2). The use of in-hospital covert video surveillance has facilitated the recognition of apnea secondary to MSBP.

> **Box 59-2. Circumstances Where the Clinician Should Be Alert About the Possibilities of Child Abuse**
>
> - Previous recurrent cyanosis, apnea, or apparent life-threatening event (ALTE) while in the care of the same person
> - Age at death older than 6 months
> - Previous unexpected or unexplained deaths of one or more siblings
> - Simultaneous or nearly simultaneous deaths of twins
> - Previous death of infants under the care of the same unrelated person
> - Discovery of blood on the infant's nose or mouth in association with ALTE

Differential Diagnosis

The physician is usually not charged with determining the cause of death of the deceased infant; that is the role of the coroner. The major challenge for physicians is to evaluate infants who have experienced an ALTE and determine if any underlying condition caused the episode (Box 59-3). In most cases, no etiology for an ALTE episode is established and the episode represents an isolated event.

> **Box 59-3. Differential Diagnosis of an Apparent Life-Threatening Event**
>
> - Gastroesophageal reflux
> - Lower respiratory tract infection
> - Sepsis
> - Pertussis
> - Respiratory syncytial virus
> - Infantile botulism
> - Seizures
> - Medication misdose or overdose
> - Inborn errors of metabolism
> - Child abuse
> - Intracranial hemorrhage
> - Airway anomalies
> - Aspiration
> - Breath-holding spell
> - Cardiac arrhythmias/anomalies

Sepsis, respiratory infections, seizures, gastroesophageal reflux, inborn errors of metabolism, infantile botulism, cardiac anomalies, and child abuse should all be considered. The circumstances surrounding ALTEs suggest which of these conditions is suspect. A sepsis evaluation is particularly warranted in children who have symptoms such as fever, vomiting, or diarrhea or appear toxic at presentation. Infants with respiratory symptoms such as tachypnea and wheezing may have **RSV** infection, which is associated with apneic episodes, particularly during the first week of illness in infants younger than 3 months who had been premature and experienced apnea of prematurity. Young infants with pertussis do not exhibit the classic cough with whoop and may present with respiratory distress and apnea. Overuse or misuse of over-the-counter cough and cold medication has been associated with drowsiness and seizures, which can present as an ALTE. Infants with abnormal movements or ALTEs when awake may be experiencing seizures. The apnea may represent the seizure or a postictal event. Infantile botulism causes decreased muscle tone and weakness. Apnea may also accompany gastroesophageal reflux. In general, affected infants have a history of eating, regurgitating, and then developing apnea. As previously noted, child abuse, particularly with intracranial hemorrhage or MSBP, may result in apnea or SIDS.

Inborn errors of metabolism are reported in 4% to 8% of cases of ALTE. Inborn errors of metabolism should be considered in infants with other symptoms, such as vomiting or failure to thrive, or in the context of a positive family history. Symptoms may first appear when a previously well infant is metabolically stressed as by an acute infectious illness. Rarely cardiac arrhythmias, most notably long QT interval, are associated with apnea or sudden episodes of bradycardia.

Evaluation

History

The history may provide the clue to the etiology of SIDS or ALTE (Questions Box).

Questions

Sudden Infant Death Syndrome (SIDS) and Apparent Life-Threatening Event (ALTE)

- What were the events leading up to the episode?
- Was the child awake and eating, indicating that gastroesophageal reflux should be considered?
- Was the child awake and did the eyes roll back or the body stiffen or jerk, suggesting that a seizure may have occurred?
- How serious was the event? Did breathing resume spontaneously or did cardiopulmonary resuscitation have to be initiated?
- Have similar events occurred in the past?
- Is the infant basically well? Has the infant been ill recently?
- Has the child had respiratory symptoms such as wheezing or cough?
- Was the child given an over-the-counter cough and cold product?
- Do the siblings have a history of SIDS or ALTE that would suggest the presence of a familial disorder or child abuse?
- Were there any problems with the pregnancy or delivery?
- Is there a history of maternal smoking?
- Does the infant sleep in a supine, prone, or side-down position?

Physical Examination

A complete examination should be conducted. If infants are floppy and have poor color or have required either mouth-to-mouth resuscitation or vigorous stimulation, significant events are likely. Physicians should check for the presence of bruises, retinal hemorrhages, dysmorphic features, growth impairment, and abnormal neurologic or developmental findings, which may suggest an alternative etiology. The presence of tachypnea, retractions, wheezing, or cough is consistent with a respiratory infection such as RSV or pertussis.

Laboratory Tests

In general, the laboratory workup is guided by the findings of the history and physical examination (Box 59-4). A sepsis evaluation, including a complete blood cell count, blood culture, lumbar puncture, and urine culture, is appropriate to rule out sepsis in febrile or toxic-appearing infants. Serum electrolytes, serum ammonia, and glucose are important to check because they may indicate an inborn error of metabolism or other abnormalities (eg, hypoglycemia), which may be associated with apnea with or without the presence of a seizure. Hypotonic infants should be evaluated for infantile botulism by sending a stool specimen for testing. All infants with a history of apnea or ALTE should be admitted to the hospital for

---

Box 59-4. Laboratory Studies to Consider in Evaluating Infants With Apparent Life-Threatening Event

Often Indicated	*Sometimes Indicated*
• Complete blood cell count	• Electroencephalogram
• Blood culture	• Computed tomography scan
• Lumbar puncture	• Barium swallow
• Urine culture	• Electrocardiogram
• Chest radiograph	• Skeletal survey
• Serum electrolytes	
• Blood sugar	
• Serum ammonia	

---

observation, workup, and monitoring. A pilot study has identified a subset of well-appearing, low-risk patients presenting with ALTE episodes that may be safe to discharge home after a thorough evaluation. However, these data need to be validated in a large study that includes children of all ethnicities. In addition, one must be certain that the family is comfortable with this course of action, and know what to do should there be a recurrence.

Imaging Studies

A chest radiograph should be performed to rule out pneumonia if respiratory symptoms are present or sepsis is suspected. If the history and physical examination suggest other etiologies, computed tomography and barium swallow may also be indicated, though the risks of radiation exposure need to be carefully considered.

Diagnostic Studies

An electroencephalogram should be obtained if a seizure disorder is suspected. In-hospital covert video surveillance is a complex procedure that may be undertaken if MSBP is suspected. Multichannel pneumograms detect apnea and bradycardia, but are not able to identify infants at risk for SIDS. They are no longer considered in the routine assessment of infants presenting with ALTE. An ECG may be useful in the rare infant with long QT syndrome.

Management

Infants who have not been fully resuscitated in the field should be resuscitated, stabilized, and admitted. Any identifiable conditions such as sepsis, seizures, and reflux should be appropriately managed. In general, infants who experienced an ALTE but do not have an identifiable precipitating condition are also admitted for monitoring and observation. Recent evidence suggests that infants older than 30 days who have not had multiple ALTEs and have no identifiable medical condition may be safely discharged from the ED. Prior to discharge from the hospital, the parents of infants who experienced an ALTE should receive cardiopulmonary resuscitation training and be advised to eliminate tobacco smoke exposure.

In the past home apnea monitoring was prescribed for newborns at risk for apnea. Based on a plethora of studies, the AAP does not recommend home apnea monitors for the prevention of SIDS. Home apnea monitoring may be indicated for premature infants at risk for repeated episodes of apnea of prematurity on discharge from the hospital. Discontinuation should be considered at approximately 43 weeks' gestation.

Home monitoring may be indicated for individuals who are technology-dependent (home ventilators, tracheostomy) or those with ALTEs if the physician wants to monitor episodes of apnea or respiratory failure. The family of an infant who experienced an ALTE should clearly be informed that a home apnea monitor has not been shown to prevent SIDS and is not indicated for that purpose.

Pacifier use has been associated with a lower incidence of SIDS. The AAP recommends that caregivers consider offering a pacifier at nap time and bedtime throughout the first year of life. The pacifier should not be reinserted once the infant falls asleep or coated in any sweet solution. The pacifier should be cleaned often and replaced regularly. Breastfed infants should have pacifier introduction delayed until 1 month of age to ensure that breastfeeding is well established.

In addition to managing infants with ALTE, physicians must provide care to families whose infants have succumbed to SIDS. In most jurisdictions, cases of SIDS must be reported to the coroner's office. The AAP recommends a prompt death scene investigation; appropriate use of available medical specialists by medical examiners and coroners, including pediatricians; and a postmortem examination within 24 hours of death, including radiographic skeletal surveys and toxicological and metabolic screening. A complete review of the medical records of the victim is essential. It is important for physicians to tell families when they think the cause of death is probable SIDS even before definitive autopsy results are available. A timely information session with parents is recommended when the results of the investigation conclude SIDS or a medical causation for death.

Parents of children who have succumbed to SIDS should be guided through issues such as planning the funeral and ending lactation. For ongoing support they should be referred to groups and agencies to help them deal with the loss of their child. Information about these organizations can be obtained from First Candle (800/221-SIDS; www.firstcandle.org).

Prognosis

Prevention of SIDS has become a focus of public health measures. Improving maternal risk factors involves smoking cessation and access to prenatal care. Parents must be instructed to avoid soft bedding for their infants, not to bed share with their infants, not to place their infants on a sofa for sleep, to avoid overheating, and to place their infants in the supine position in a crib. The prognosis for children who have experienced an ALTE varies and depends on predisposing conditions. Parents can be assured that most ALTEs are isolated events and the risk of a chronic condition, such as seizure disorders, is rare. Abnormal neurodevelopmental conditions are generally associated with a poor prognosis when associated with apnea.

CASE RESOLUTION

The infant presented in the case history succumbed to SIDS. In spite of resuscitative efforts by the paramedics, he could not be revived. The mother is advised of the diagnosis of suspected SIDS and referred to appropriate agencies and support groups. The coroner is notified about the case and the presence of any associated physical findings, such as bruises. The mother is advised that a coroner investigator will visit her to learn more about the circumstances surrounding the sudden death of her infant.

Selected References

American Academy of Pediatrics Committee on Fetus and Newborn. Apnea, sudden infant death syndrome, and home monitoring. *Pediatrics.* 2003;111:914–917

American Academy of Pediatrics Task Force on Infant Sleep Position and Sudden Infant Death Syndrome. The changing concept of sudden infant death syndrome: diagnostic coding shifts, controversies regarding the sleeping environment, and new variables to consider in reducing risk. *Pediatrics.* 2005;116:1245–1255

Blair PS, Mitchell EA, Heckstall-Smith EM, Fleming PJ. Head covering—a major modifiable risk factor for sudden infant death syndrome: a systematic review. *Arch Dis Child.* 2008;93(9):778–783

Claudius I, Keens T. Do all infants with apparent life-threatening events need to be admitted? *Pediatrics.* 2007;119:679–683

Duncan JR, Paterson DS, Hoffman JM, et al. Brainstem serotonergic deficiency in sudden infant death syndrome. *JAMA.* 2010;303(5):430–437

Esani N, Hodgman JE, Ehsani N, Hoppenbrouwers T. Apparent life-threatening events and sudden infant death syndrome: comparison of risk factors. *J Pediatr.* 2008;152:365–370

Farrell PA, Weiner GM, Lemons JA. SIDS, ALTE, apnea, and the use of home monitors. *Pediatr Rev.* 2002;23:3–9

Franco P, Kato I, Richardson HL, Yang JS, Montemitro E, Horne RS. Arousal from sleep mechanisms in infants. *Sleep Med.* 2010;11(7):603–614

Horn MH, Kinnamon DD, Ferraro N, Curley MAQ. Smaller mandibular size in infants with a history of an apparent life-threatening event. *J Pediatr.* 2006;149:499–504

Kemp JS, Unger B, Wilkins D, et al. Unsafe sleep practice and an analysis of bedsharing among infants dying suddenly and unexpectedly: results of a four-year, population-based, death scene investigation study of sudden infant death syndrome and related deaths. *Pediatrics.* 2000;106:e4

Kinney HC, Thach BT. The sudden infant death syndrome. *N Engl J Med.* 2009;361(8):795–805

Phillips DP, Brewer KM, Wadensweiler P. Alcohol as a risk factor for sudden infant death syndrome (SIDS). *Addiction.* 2011;106(3):516–525

Ramanathan R, Corwin MJ, Hunt CE, et al. Cardiorespiratory events recorded on home monitors: comparison of healthy infants with those at increased risk for SIDS. *JAMA.* 2001;285:2199–2207

CHAPTER 60

Syncope

David Atkinson, MD, and Elizabeth A. Edgerton, MD, MPH

CASE STUDY

A 15-year-old boy comes to your office a week before the beginning of the school year complaining of fainting during football practice the previous day. He has been trying out for the varsity football team and they are now in the midst of "hell week," 2-a-day workout drills. He has never fainted before, but has gotten dizzy momentarily after standing up "too fast." His mother contradicts him and says that he fainted about a year ago while having blood drawn. In addition, when he was about 18 months old, he fell off of his parents' bed. He cried, gasped, stopped breathing, became pale, and passed out for about 30 seconds. He was diagnosed with a breath-holding spell. There is no family history of sudden death or seizures.

Prior to the recent event he had been sitting on the team bench when the coach blew his whistle, the boy stood up quickly and became dizzy. He came to on the ground and his coach told him he had passed out for about 10 to 15 seconds. He denies taking any medications or using any illicit drugs. The patient states that he ate his lunch, but did not have anything to drink between the practice sessions. There is no family history of sudden death of seizures. The mother wants to know if it is safe for her son to continue participating in physical activities since she has read about sudden death in high school athletes.

His physical examination is unrevealing and his vital signs are all normal. Electrocardiogram shows normal sinus rhythm with normal voltages and intervals for his age.

Questions

1. What are the causes of syncope?
2. What type of workup is done primarily to evaluate for syncope?
3. When should patients who experience syncope be referred to a subspecialist?
4. Which pediatric subspecialists assist in the evaluation of a patient with syncope?
5. Which patients presenting with syncope are at the greatest risk for sudden death?

Syncope, or **fainting,** is a transient loss of consciousness and is a very common clinical problem in pediatrics, particularly in pubescent and adolescent patients. The most common causes of syncope in pediatrics are benign neurocardiogenic events; however, syncope may rarely be a harbinger of sudden death due to arrhythmia, obstruction of aortic outflow, or other serious cardiovascular events.

There are 3 general categories of syncope: **neurocardiogenic** (also called vasovagal syncope), **cardiac syncope,** and **noncardiac syncope** (Box 60-1). The workup for syncope can easily become expensive and time-consuming, and may provide little information beyond that gleaned by the initial history and physical examination. It is the role of the pediatrician to appropriately direct the evaluation for syncope so that a cost-effective evaluation may occur without missing the patient who may be at risk for a sudden death event.

Epidemiology

Syncope is defined as a temporary, transient loss of consciousness and muscle tone, usually associated with a rapid recovery. It is the result of a decrease in cerebral blood flow that can occur through many different mechanisms. Syncopal events are very common in the pediatric population; up to 50% of college undergraduates have reported experiencing syncope or near syncope, and it accounts for about 1% of all pediatric emergency department visits. Females are more commonly affected than males, and the mean age at presentation is 10 to 12 years. Syncope is uncommon in children younger than 5 years. Many cases of syncope resolve quickly and medical attention is not sought, so the true incidence of syncope is almost certainly underestimated.

Clinical Presentation

The clinical presentation of syncope varies with the etiology. In **vasovagal syncope** there is often a prodrome of symptoms, including lightheadedness, visual disturbances, nausea, and diaphoresis. The patient has usually been standing for a long period or has suddenly gone from the supine or sitting position to standing. Other forms of **neurally mediated syncope** include **hair-grooming syncope,** which occurs mostly in girls while combing, brushing, or blow-drying their hair. Micturition syncope, while more common in the elderly, may occur in all ages of patients. Younger patients tend to be male; predisposing factors may include reduced food intake, fatigue, alcohol ingestion, and recent respiratory infection. The events often occur at night when voiding after awakening from sleep (ie, while standing

Box 60-1. Causes of Syncope
Neurocardiogenic (Vasovagal Syncope)
Cardiac
• Tachyarrhythmias
— Supraventricular tachycardia
— Ventricular tachycardia
• Bradyarrhythmias
— Second or third degree heart block
— Sinus node dysfunction
• Left or right ventricular outflow tract obstruction
— Hypertrophic cardiomyopathy
— Aortic stenosis
• Idiopathic pulmonary hypertension
• Coronary artery disease
— Acquired coronary artery disease
• Kawasaki disease
— Congenital coronary anomaly
• Intramural coronary artery
• Anomalous origin of a coronary artery
• Primary cardiac dysfunction
— Dilated cardiomyopathy
— Non-compaction syndrome
• Secondary cardiac dysfunction
— Viral or idiopathic myocarditis
— Restrictive cardiomyopathy
Noncardiac
• Orthostatic hypotension
• Neurologic (seizures, atypical migraine, dysautonomia)
• Breath-holding spells
• Psychogenic (hysteria, hyperventilation)
• Metabolic abnormality (hypoglycemia, anemia)
• Drug or medication effect

immediately after being recumbent). Recurrences of micturition syncope are rare in young patients. **Breath-holding spells** in toddlers brought on by anger, pain, fear, or frustration may be associated with syncope; this is an infantile form of cardioinhibitory neurally mediated syncope. Infants who suffer syncopal breath-holding spells are more likely to grow up and have neurally mediated syncope (see Chapter 49).

Syncope of cardiac etiology will often lack the prodrome of vasovagal syncope. The main cardiac causes of syncope are arrhythmia and left ventricular outflow obstruction. Patients may complain of palpitations, chest pain, or chest tightness. Cardiac syncope commonly occurs during physical activity and may be accompanied by a complete loss of body tone.

Syncope related to **seizures** generally has a longer recovery time associated with the postictal phase; witnesses may describe the patient as being dazed or "having a blank look on their face" prior to fainting. These episodes may occur whether the patient is recumbent or upright.

Pathophysiology

Autonomic

Autonomic causes of syncope are the most common etiology, accounting for up to 80% of cases of syncope that comes to medical attention. They are also referred to as neurally mediated reflexive syncope, vasovagal syncope, neurocardiogenic syncope and, in toddlers, pallid breath-holding spells. They have in common disturbances in autonomic control of heart rate and blood pressure in response to postural changes, bodily functions, pain, fear, or other strong emotional events. Vasovagal syncopal events usually occur when the patient is upright, resulting in decreased venous return, decreased arterial blood pressure, and decreased left ventricular volume. There is a resultant reflex stimulation of vagal fibers leading to bradycardia, vasodilation, and worsening hypotension (Bezold-Jarisch reflex). There are 3 clinical types of neurally mediated syncope: vasodepressor, which starts and is primarily marked by profound hypotension; cardioinhibitory, marked by severe bradycardia or even brief asystole; and mixed response, which is a mixture of both vasodepressor and cardioinhibitory.

Cardiac

Cardiac causes of syncope are more likely to be associated with sudden death, so it is important to identify and treat these abnormalities. Cardiac mechanisms of syncope are mainly related to arrhythmias or to obstructive lesions. Obstructive lesions lead to decreased ventricular outflow, resulting in decreased cerebral perfusion; arrhythmia may lead to decreased ejection volume, also leading to cerebral hypoperfusion and syncope.

Left-sided obstructive lesions, including aortic stenosis and hypertrophic cardiomyopathy, are the most likely cause of obstructive syncope. Rarely, syncope can be caused by pulmonary stenosis or severe primary pulmonary hypertension, mitral stenosis, atrial myxoma, or cardiac tamponade. Cardiac syncope often occurs during exertion, owing to the inability of the heart to increase cardiac output to meet the demands placed on it by increased physical activity. Increased diastolic pressure caused by an obstructive lesion may also decrease myocardial perfusion leading to cardiac ischemia, dyskinesis, or ventricular arrhythmias, which lead to decreased ventricular output.

Anomalous origin of the coronary arteries, though not an obstructive lesion, may also cause syncope with exercise. The left coronary artery may arise from the pulmonary artery, delivering deoxygenated blood to the left coronary system, or the left coronary artery may arise from the right coronary cusp and course between the aorta and pulmonary arteries. When the patient is in a high cardiac output state, such as during exercise, the left coronary artery may be compressed between the great arteries, leading to ischemia or arrhythmias.

Primary arrhythmias causing syncope are a rare but important cause of syncope. Chest radiograph, echocardiogram, and other imaging modalities will generally be normal, with no evidence of structural heart disease or pulmonary edema. Supraventricular tachycardia may cause syncope or near syncope. In most pediatric patients, the tachycardia is propagated through a concealed pathway, and the resting electrocardiogram (ECG) will be normal if the tachycardia is not occurring while the ECG is being obtained. Supraventricular tachycardia may also be associated with Wolff-Parkinson-White (WPW) syndrome. Wolff-Parkinson-White syndrome is characterized by a short P-R interval followed by an abnormally wide QRS complex with an initial delta wave.

Ventricular tachycardia is rare in children with no underlying structural heart disease, but may be brought on by infection (especially myocarditis or pericarditis), cardiomyopathies, drugs (cocaine, amphetamines), drug interactions (non-sedating antihistamines taken with erythromycin or ketoconazole), and long QT syndrome.

Patients with long QT syndrome have prolonged cardiac repolarization, which will usually manifest on the resting ECG as a prolonged corrected QT interval. The prolongation of the repolarization period of the heart puts patients with long QT syndrome at risk for torsades de pointes, a malignant form of ventricular tachycardia. The genetic forms of long QT syndrome result from mutations in genes that code for ion transport channels or related proteins. Romano-Ward syndrome is an autosomal-dominant form of long QT syndrome that is associated with congenital deafness. Autosomal-recessive long QT syndrome has historically been referred to as Jervell and Lange-Nielsen syndrome. Although the clinical diagnosis of long QT syndrome is based on a QTc that is prolonged for the patient's age, it is estimated that 20% of patients with a gene mutation associated with long QT syndrome will have a normal ECG; therefore, a critical part of the evaluation of the syncopal patient is obtaining a family history of long QT syndrome, sudden death or near sudden death, seizures, or a history of torsade de pointes. Long QT syndrome may also be brought on by electrolyte imbalance, increased intracranial pressure, or medications (Table 60-1).

Noncardiac

Noncardiac causes of syncope include neurologic etiologies (seizures, migraines), metabolic disturbances (hypoglycemia), hyperventilation (panic attacks or self-induced), and hysteria. Low iron stores have been associated with neurally mediated syncope in children and adolescents. Seizures may be difficult to distinguish from vasovagal events because both can have tonic-clonic movements. Unlike vasovagal or cardiac syncope, seizures result in unconsciousness secondary to neurologic dysfunction. Syncope associated with hypoglycemia is due to insufficient substrate being delivered to the brain. Cerebral vasoconstriction secondary to arterial hypocapnia produces syncope with hyperventilation that may be secondary to panic attacks or may be self-induced. Hysterical syncope lacks a true prodrome, and patients usually suffer no injury when they fall. This form of syncope is thought to be related to Munchausen syndrome.

Table 60-1. Drugs Known to Increase the Risk of Ventricular Arrhythmia in Patients With Long QT Syndrome[a]

Drug	Class/Clinical Use
Amiodarone	Antiarrhythmic/abnormal heart rhythm
Arsenic trioxide	Anticancer/leukemia
Bepridil	Anti-anginal/heart pain
Chloroquine	Antimalarial/malaria infection
Chlorpromazine	Antipsychotic/antiemetic/schizophrenia/nausea
Cisapride	Gastrointestinal (GI) stimulant/heartburn
Clarithromycin	Antibiotic/bacterial infection
Disopyramide	Antiarrhythmic/abnormal heart rhythm
Dofetilide	Antiarrhythmic/abnormal heart rhythm
Droperidol	Sedative; antinausea/anesthesia adjunct, nausea
Erythromycin	Antibiotic; GI stimulant/bacterial infection; increase GI motility
Halofantrine	Antimalarial/malaria infection
Haloperidol	Antipsychotic/schizophrenia, agitation
Ibutilide	Antiarrhythmic/abnormal heart rhythm
Levomethadyl	Opiate agonist/pain control, narcotic dependence
Mesoridazine	Antipsychotic/schizophrenia
Methadone	Opiate agonist/pain control, narcotic dependence
Pentamidine	Anti-infective/pneumocystis pneumonia
Pimozide	Antipsychotic/Tourette tics
Procainamide	Antiarrhythmic/abnormal heart rhythm
Quinidine	Antiarrhythmic/abnormal heart rhythm
Sotalol	Antiarrhythmic/abnormal heart rhythm
Sparfloxacin	Antibiotic/bacterial infection
Thioridazine	Antipsychotic/schizophrenia

[a] For a complete list of drugs to avoid in patients with long QT syndrome, visit www.qtdrugs.org.

Differential Diagnosis

The differential diagnosis of syncope is presented in Box 60-1. Events that precede and follow the syncopal event are key in determining the etiology of syncope.

Evaluation

History

A thorough history should be obtained from the family and patient, focusing on the patient's symptoms, the situation surrounding the event, and the family history (Questions Box). A primary goal of the history is to identify any underlying cardiac problems because these patients are at the greatest risk for sudden death.

Syncope

- What was the patient doing when the episode occurred?
- What was the position of the patient?
- Did the patient have any symptoms before the syncopal event?
- Did the patient have any chest pain or palpitations during the event?
- How long did it take for the patient to recover from the syncopal event?
- Were any residual symptoms present after the syncopal event?
- Has the patient recently been ill, dehydrated, or fatigued?
- Does the patient have a history of underlying cardiac disease?
- Is the patient taking any type of medication (prescribed, over the counter, or illicit)?
- Does the patient have a history of breath-holding or pallid spells?
- Is there a family history of sudden death, seizures, deafness, or cardiac abnormalities?

Physical Examination

The patient with syncope needs a thorough physical examination. Vital signs should assess the blood pressure to screen for hypotension and hypovolemia. The cardiac examination should include palpation of the chest for the point of maximal intensity, thrills and lifts, and auscultation to assess the intensity of the heart sounds and to detect the presence of murmurs or other adventitial sounds. Upper- and lower-extremity pulses should be palpated for their presence and quality. The remainder of the examination should focus on identifying any abnormal neurologic findings.

Laboratory Tests

The history and physical examination should guide which laboratory tests are necessary. In general, few tests are needed. Serum glucose shortly after the syncopal event may reveal hypoglycemia. Fasting glucose or glucose tolerance tests are usually normal, and such testing is not indicated. In pubertal females, a pregnancy test should be obtained as well as a hemoglobin level. Iron levels may be low in patients with neurally mediated syncope.

Imaging Studies

Every patient who is being evaluated for syncope requires an ECG. The ECG may reveal WPW or a prolonged QT interval, neither of which can be diagnosed by history and physical examination alone. These studies can also be useful in identifying underlying structural abnormalities such as right ventricular hypertrophy secondary to pulmonary hypertension, left ventricular hypertrophy secondary to hypertrophied cardiomyopathy, or Q waves associated with anomalous origin of the coronary arteries. Patients with findings suggestive of cardiac disease (positive history, physical findings, or an abnormal ECG) require referral to a pediatric cardiologist for further evaluation. The cardiac workup of syncope may include a Holter monitor or an event recorder. The Holter monitor is worn for 24 hours and continuously records the heart rhythm. Because this is a limited window of observation, the Holter monitor will capture arrhythmia less than 20% of the time, even in patients with known arrhythmias. Event recorders are worn for longer periods, often up to several weeks. They can record and retain the cardiac rhythm prior to, during, and following an event. When the patient activates the monitor, the recording is saved for download to the cardiologist. If the monitor is not activated, the event recorder will not save the information but will record over it. Although the event recorder has a higher probability of capturing an arrhythmia if one is present than does a Holter monitor, the tracings are generally lower quality. Exercise stress testing is often used to evaluate the patient's response to exertion and to allow for replication of symptoms in a monitored setting. Electrophysiology studies may be ordered if an arrhythmia is uncovered during the evaluation.

The workup for patients without evidence of cardiac disease (negative family history of cardiac disease or of sudden death and no exertional symptoms such as chest pain) should focus on the noncardiac or autonomic causes of syncope. Patients with prolonged recovery time or persistent neurologic symptoms following an event should be referred to a neurologist and may require an electroencephalogram to rule out seizure disorders.

A tilt test may be used to aid in the diagnosis of vasovagal syncope, although in most cases the history will be sufficient. The patient receiving a tilt test is placed on a table that is then tilted to simulate standing in an upright position, a condition that is commonly associated with vasovagal syncope. Unfortunately, there is great variability in the tilt test, with an incidence of up to 20% of false-positives. Factors that influence the test results include the time of day, whether the patient has fasted, hydration status, and whether the test was augmented with isoproterenol. There are very few false-negative tilt tests, but due to the high number of false-positives, the tilt test should be reserved only for refractory, recurrent, or unexplained syncope.

Management

Management of syncope depends on its cause. Recurrent vasovagal syncope may be treated simply by having the patient increase their fluid intake (including carrying a water bottle in school) and increasing their salt intake. Fludrocortisone, a mineralocorticoid, is the most common medical intervention for vasovagal syncope, although the efficacy is not well established. Other treatments include β-blockers (propranolol or atenolol), vagolytic drugs (disopyramide), or centrally acting drugs (imipramine, fluoxetine). These medications have varied benefits, and results between small controlled trials are not consistent.

Patients with neurologic syncope secondary to seizures should be treated with anticonvulsants. Patients with hyperventilation, hysteria, or hypoglycemia are most amenable to behavioral interventions. Patients with syncope secondary to a cardiac etiology should be referred to a cardiologist for further evaluation and correction of the underlying problem. These types of syncopal episodes may require more aggressive management, such as surgery or cardiac pacing, because they are more likely to result in sudden death.

Prognosis

The prognosis for autonomic and noncardiac syncope is good. Patients with vasovagal syncope will often suffer only a single event, and those with recurrent events can be treated with increased fluid intake or with medication. One subgroup to be aware of is children with pallid breath-holding spells; while most will have resolution of these spells by 5 years of age, up to 17% may continue to have syncope in adulthood. Patients who have syncope with an underlying cardiac etiology are at the greatest risk for sudden death, and it is only through identification and treatment of these structural or rhythm abnormalities that sudden death may be prevented.

CASE RESOLUTION

The adolescent boy in the opening scenario describes symptoms consistent with vasovagal syncope. His family history, physical examination, and ECG do not suggest any underlying cardiac disease. The patient and his family should be informed that certain factors, such as dehydration, fatigue, and hunger, can precipitate syncope. Behavioral changes, such as eating breakfast and drinking plenty of water, should be implemented to prevent or limit recurrence of syncope. The patient should be encouraged to carry a water bottle in school, and a note written to the school to allow him to do so, if necessary. Management with medications is not indicated at this time.

Selected References

Evans WN, Acherman R, Kip K, Restrepo H. Hair-groomin syncope in children. *Clin Pediatr.* 2009;48:834–836

Fischer JWJ, Cho CS. Pediatric syncope: cases from the emergency department. *Emerg Med Clin North Am.* 2010;28:501–516

Goble MM, Benitez C, Baumgardner M, et al. ED management of pediatric syncope: searching for a rationale. *Am J Emerg Med.* 2008;26:66–70

Grubb BP. Neurocardiogenic syncope. *N Engl J Med.* 2005;352:1004–1009

Jarpour IT, Jarpour LK. Low iron storage in children and adolescents with neurally mediated syncope. *J Pediatr.* 2008;153:40–44

Khositseth A, Martinez MW, Driscoll DJ, Ackerman MJ. Syncope in children and adolescents and the congenital long QT syndrome. *Am J Cardiol.* 2003;92:746–749

Klumpf M, Sieverding L, Gass M, Kaulitz R, Ziemer G, Hofbeck M. Anomalous origin of the left coronary artery in young athletes with syncope. *BMJ.* 2006;332:1139–1141

Krongrad E. Syncope and sudden death. In: Emmanouilides GC, ed. *Moss Adams Heart Disease in Infants, Children and Adolescents, Including the Fetus and Young Adult.* 5th ed. Baltimore, MD: Williams & Wilkins; 1995:1604–1619

Massin MM, Malekzadeh-Milani S, Benatar A. Caridac syncope in pediatric patients. *Clin Cardiol.* 2007;30:81–85

Petko C, Bradley DJ, Tristani-Firouzi M, et al. Congenital long QT syndrome in children identified by family screening. *Am J Cardiol.* 2008;101:1756–1758

Piccirillo G, Naso C, Moisè A, et al. Heart rate and blood pressure variability in patients with vasovagal syncope. *Clin Sci.* 2004;107:55–61

Salim MA, DiSessa TG. Effectiveness of fludrocortisone and salt in preventing syncope recurrence in children. *J Am Coll Cardiol.* 2005;45:484–488

Stewart JM. Postural tachycardia syndrome and reflex syncope: Similarities and differences. *J Pediatr.* 2005;154:481–485

Strickberger SA, Benson DW, Biaggioni I, et al. AHA/ACCF scientific statement on the evaluation of syncope: from the American Heart Association Councils on Clinical Cardiology, Cardiovascular Nursing, Cardiovascular Disease in the Young, and Stroke, and the Quality of Care and Outcomes Research Interdisciplinary Working Group; and the American College of Cardiology Foundation: in collaboration with the Heart Rhythm Society: endorsed by the American Autonomic Society. *Circulation.* 2006;113:316–327

Sun BC, Emond JA, Camargo CA. Inconsistent electrocardiographic testing for syncope in United States emergency departments. *Am J Cardiol.* 2004;93:1306–1308

CHAPTER 61

Shock

Kelly D. Young, MD, MS

CASE STUDY

A 7-month-old infant boy is brought in by his parents with a history of vomiting and diarrhea for 2 days. He also has had a low-grade fever and, according to his parents, has become progressively more listless. Vital signs show a heart rate of 200 beats/min, respiratory rate of 30 breaths/min, and blood pressure of 72/35 mm Hg. The infant is lethargic and mottled. Capillary refill time is 3 seconds. His anterior fontanelle is sunken, and his mucous membranes are dry. The abdomen is flat and non-tender and displays hyperactive bowel sounds.

Questions

1. What is shock, and what clinical signs can help in the recognition and assessment of shock?
2. What are the stages of shock?
3. What different types of shock are there, and what are the possible causes for each type?
4. What are the management priorities in treating shock?

Shock is defined as a state of circulatory dysfunction resulting in insufficient delivery of oxygen and other metabolic substrates to the tissues. Shock is not a disease but rather an abnormal physiological state that may result from many disease processes. Early recognition and prompt therapy of shock are critical to avoid permanent end-organ damage or death.

Epidemiology

The most common type of shock in children is hypovolemic shock, and the most common causes are dehydration from gastrointestinal infections that cause vomiting and diarrhea, and hemorrhage from traumatic injury. However, in a case series of 147 pediatric shock patients (excluding trauma patients) from Children's Hospital of Nevada, septic shock was the most common etiology, accounting for 57% of patients. Of the remaining patients, 24% had hypovolemic shock, 14% distributive, and 5% cardiogenic. Shock may be seen in any age group, but it is more difficult to recognize the early stages in young children because early clinical signs of shock in children are subjective and may be attributed to other causes. By the time young children have developed more typical signs, such as thready pulses and hypotension, they are in the late stages of shock.

Clinical Presentation

Early signs of shock include tachycardia; cool, clammy, pale, or mottled skin; and delayed capillary refill time. There may be a history of decreased urine output. In this early stage, perfusion to vital organs such as the brain and heart is maintained by compensatory physiological processes. As the shock state progresses, it becomes uncompensated, resulting in impairment of vital organ perfusion. Signs of uncompensated shock include hypotension; altered mental status

(irritability, lethargy, decreased interactiveness); weak, thready, or absent pulses (although pulses may be bounding in "warm" septic shock); and severely mottled or cyanotic skin (Dx Box). In the Nevada epidemiologic study, young children commonly presented with poor extremity perfusion and poor pulses, while adolescents presented with hypotension. Irreversible shock occurs when multiple organs fail and death occurs.

Dx Shock

Compensated	Uncompensated
• Tachycardia	• Tachycardia or bradycardia
• Normal blood pressure	• Hypotension
• Normal or bounding pulses	• Weak, thready, or absent pulses
• Normal or cool, clammy skin	• Cool, clammy skin
• Pale or mottled skin color	• Severely mottled or cyanotic skin color
• Alert, anxious mental state	• Altered mental state, lethargic
• Mildly delayed capillary refill time	• Delayed capillary refill time
• Decreased urine output	• Decreased or absent urine output

Pathophysiology

Shock occurs when oxygen delivery to tissues is impaired. Adequate oxygen delivery depends on sufficient blood oxygen content and adequate circulatory blood flow (Figure 61-1). The oxygen content in blood depends primarily on the concentration of hemoglobin and the amount of oxygen bound to hemoglobin. In children, oxygen consumption by end organs depends most on oxygen delivery, while in adults it depends on oxygen extraction by the tissues.

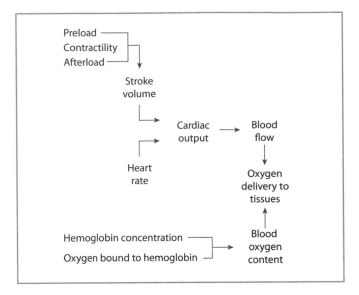

Figure 61-1. Pathophysiology of shock. Factors affecting oxygen delivery to tissue.

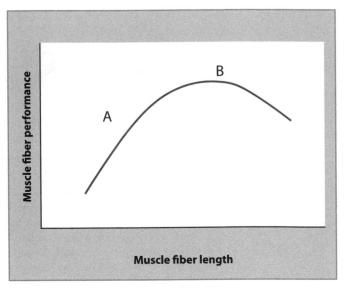

Figure 61-2. Starling curve of cardiac output. A. As muscle fiber length increases, performance increases. B. Muscle fiber reaches its optimal length, after which performance declines.

Blood flow, or cardiac output, is determined by heart rate and stroke volume. Stroke volume depends on preload, contractility, and afterload. Preload refers to the amount of blood entering the heart from the systemic vasculature. Increasing preload, for example, via administration of intravenous (IV) fluid boluses, will increase cardiac output until a point of optimal heart muscle fiber length is reached. The Starling curve demonstrates that increased stretching of a muscle fiber results in improved performance of that muscle fiber (ie, improved stroke volume and cardiac output); but, after the point of optimal stretching is reached, there is decreased performance (Figure 61-2).

Contractility, or inotropy, is the heart's intrinsic ability to contract and pump blood to the body. Afterload refers to the systemic vascular resistance impeding ejection of blood from the ventricles. Optimal cardiac output depends on sufficient preload, unimpaired cardiac contractility, and the ability of the heart to overcome any afterload. During states of decreased cardiac output leading to decreased tissue perfusion, adults compensate primarily by increasing cardiac contractility, whereas children compensate primarily by increasing their heart rate. Irreversible shock in adults is most likely to be due to vasomotor collapse, while in children cardiac failure plays a larger role.

Differential Diagnosis

There are several types of shock depending on the underlying pathophysiology (Table 61-1).

Hypovolemic shock is the most common type seen in children and usually results from dehydration or traumatic hemorrhage. Hypovolemia results in inadequate preload, which leads to impaired cardiac output and impaired perfusion. Other causes of hypovolemic shock include diabetic ketoacidosis (dehydration due to osmotic diuresis) and peritonitis and burns leading to third-spacing of fluids (shifting from intravascular to extravascular sites) with resultant

intravascular hypovolemia. Non-traumatic hemorrhage may occur from entities such as epistaxis, gastrointestinal bleeding, and vessel fistula formation.

Distributive shock is a relative hypovolemia; vasodilation results in inadequate circulating blood volume relative to the vasodilation (ie, the "tank" has been made larger by vasodilation, and now there is insufficient fluid to fill the tank). Causes include anaphylaxis and sepsis, which result in the release of vasoactive mediators that cause

Table 61-1. Types of Shock		
Type of Shock	**Physiological Mechanism**	**Common Causes**
Hypovolemic	Decreased preload	Dehydration Traumatic hemorrhage Non-traumatic hemorrhage Diabetic ketoacidosis Peritonitis Burns
Distributive	Relative hypovolemia due to vasodilation	Sepsis Anaphylaxis Neurogenic Toxin-mediated
Cardiogenic	Decreased contractility	Congestive heart failure from congenital lesions Myocarditis Tachydysrhythmias
Obstructive	Impaired cardiac output to systemic circulation	Pulmonary embolus Pericardial tamponade Tension pneumothorax Ductal-dependent cardiac lesions
Dissociative	Abnormal hemoglobin—inadequate oxygen bound	Carbon monoxide poisoning Methemoglobinemia

vasodilation. Spinal cord injury **(neurogenic shock)** may result in loss of sympathetic nerve–mediated vascular tone and subsequent vasodilation. Finally, certain intoxications such as iron, barbiturates, and tricyclic antidepressants can cause vasodilation and distributive shock.

Cardiogenic shock is an uncommon but important cause of shock in children. Congestive heart failure from a congenital heart lesion, myocarditis, or cardiomyopathy results in impaired cardiac contractility and decreased cardiac output. Tachydysrhythmias, such as supraventricular tachycardia, do not allow sufficient time for the ventricles to fill with blood, resulting in decreased stroke volume.

Rare causes of shock in pediatric patients include obstructive and dissociative types. In **obstructive shock,** there is obstruction to cardiac output to the systemic circulation due to pulmonary embolus, cardiac tamponade, or tension pneumothorax. Closure of the ductus arteriosus in a neonate with a ductal-dependent congenital heart lesion is another cause of insufficient cardiac output and obstructive shock. In **dissociative shock** abnormal hemoglobin such as methemoglobin or carboxyhemoglobin from carbon monoxide poisoning results in decreased oxygen bound to hemoglobin and decreased oxygen delivered to tissues.

Septic shock combines elements of distributive, hypovolemic, and cardiogenic shock. Vasoactive mediators lead to decreased systemic vascular resistance and a relative hypovolemia. Third-spacing of fluid leads to a true intravascular hypovolemia as well. In addition, mediators of sepsis cause impaired cardiac function.

Because shock is a physiological state resulting from a variety of etiologies, and because it is recognized through clinical findings, it is important to interpret individual findings in the context of the patient as a whole. Heart rate may be elevated for many reasons, including fear, anxiety, fever, and other reasons. Capillary refill may appear delayed in the extremities of a child who is cold. Blood pressure may appear artificially low when too large of a cuff is used to measure it. The clinician must consider whether the child's history is consistent with risk for shock, and whether the physical examination taken as a whole supports the diagnosis.

Evaluation

Early recognition and prompt treatment of shock is the goal. A rapid, focused history and physical examination should be performed to identify patients in shock, and then early therapy should be instituted before returning for a more complete evaluation. Recognition of shock depends on history and physical examination alone; therapy should never be withheld while awaiting results of diagnostic tests.

History

A history of vomiting with or without diarrhea, decreased oral intake, and decreased urine output, especially in infants, should alert the clinician to possible hypovolemic shock. Children presenting with major trauma should be evaluated for hemorrhagic shock. A history of fever, lethargy, or irritability, and sometimes a rash, may point toward septic shock. Patients with asplenia, sickle cell disease, or

indwelling catheters and those who are immunocompromised (eg, young infants or children on chemotherapy) are at increased risk for sepsis. Children in cardiogenic shock may have a history of a murmur, poor feeding, sweating with feeds, cyanosis, tachypnea, and dyspnea and, in the older child, palpitations.

Physical Examination

A brief examination to identify shock focuses on mental status, vital signs, pulses, and skin signs. Impaired level of consciousness, such as lethargy or lack of recognition of parents, occurs later in shock. Earlier, children are anxious or fussy but alert. Tachycardia occurs early in shock but must be interpreted in the context of other signs of shock because tachycardia may also result from fever, pain, or simply the child's fear of the examination process. Bradycardia is a late, ominous sign in shock and often results from hypoxemia. Hypotension is also a late sign in shock. It is important to remember that normal values for heart rate and blood pressure vary by age. The lower limit of acceptable systolic blood pressure in a neonate from birth to 1 month is 60 mm Hg; in an infant from 1 month to 1 year is 70 mm Hg. For a child 1 year or older, the lower limit can be estimated using the formula 70 + (2 × age in years) mm Hg; the lower limit is 90 mm Hg for children 10 years or older. Systolic blood pressures lower than these guidelines represent hypotension and late uncompensated shock. Heart rate and blood pressure values requiring immediate attention are shown in Table 61-2.

Table 61-2. Critically Abnormal Heart Rate and Blood Pressure			
Age	**Bradycardia**	**Tachycardia**	**Hypotension**
Neonate 0–28 d	<100 bpm	>180 bpm	<60 mm Hg
Infant 1–12 m	<90 bpm	>160 bpm	<70 mm Hg
Child 1–10 y	<60 bpm	>140 bpm	<70 + (2 x age) mm Hg
Child >10 y	<60 bpm	>120 bpm	<90 mm Hg

Abbreviation: bpm, beats per minute.

Presence and quality of pulses should be checked. Weak, thready, or absent peripheral pulses are indicative of shock. However, in warm septic shock, pulses may be bounding. Skin color, moisture, and temperature give valuable clues to diagnosis. Children in shock may have pale, cyanotic, or mottled skin. Early in shock, however, skin color may be normal. Some infants may also have mottled skin normally. As with tachycardia, isolated signs must be correlated with the bigger clinical picture to diagnose shock. Decreased perfusion in shock leads to cool and clammy skin. This is often best appreciated in the hands and feet initially.

Capillary refill is tested by compressing the capillary bed of a fingertip, palm, or dorsal foot with gentle pressure until it blanches. On release, color should return in 2 seconds or less; a capillary refill time of 3 seconds or more is abnormal and indicative of shock. Children in warm septic shock may display "flash" (ie, shortened) capillary refill time. Capillary refill should be tested with the extremity elevated above the heart so that arterial, not venous, perfusion is tested. Also, cool ambient temperatures can falsely delay capillary refill times.

In hypovolemic shock due to dehydration, look for signs of dehydration such as dry mucous membranes, lack of tears, sunken eyes, sunken anterior fontanelle in infants, and tenting of the skin. The degree of dehydration can often be estimated clinically (see Chapter 66). Patients with hemorrhage, traumatic or non-traumatic, must be examined thoroughly to locate the source of hemorrhage.

Children with congestive heart failure and cardiogenic shock may demonstrate dyspnea on exertion, tachypnea, orthopnea, rales, hepatomegaly, gallop rhythm, and a heart murmur. Jugular venous distention and peripheral edema are appreciated less often in children compared with adults. Other signs may include a cardiac murmur, hepatomegaly, cardiomegaly on chest radiograph, and a differential in pulses or blood pressure between upper and lower extremities.

Ductal-dependent cardiogenic shock should be suspected in the infant in the first few weeks of life presenting with severe cyanosis unresponsive to oxygen therapy and shock. Cardiac tamponade is suspected when there are muffled or decreased heart tones, pulsus paradoxus (decrease in systolic blood pressure >10 mm Hg during inspiration), and distended neck veins. Tension pneumothorax is suspected in patients with deviated trachea (away from the affected side), decreased breath sounds and hyperresonance to percussion on the affected side, and distended neck veins. Pulmonary embolism is rare in pediatric patients, and signs are subtle. It is mainly suspected when there are predisposing factors.

Approximately 20% of children present with the classic adult form of warm septic shock—including increased cardiac output, hypotension, decreased systemic vascular resistance, warm non-mottled skin, bounding pulses, and flash capillary refill. Children are more likely (60%) to present with cold septic shock—including decreased cardiac output; increased systemic vascular resistance; normal blood pressure to hypotension; cool, clammy, or mottled skin; thready pulses; and delayed capillary refill. The remaining 20% of children with septic shock present with both decreased cardiac output and decreased systemic vascular resistance. Petechiae or purpura point toward meningococcemia as the etiology of septic shock. A sunburn-like rash may be seen in toxic shock syndrome due to streptococcus or staphylococcus.

Laboratory Tests

The suspected cause of the shock will determine which laboratory tests are performed. In hypovolemic shock secondary to dehydration, a chemistry panel should be obtained for electrolyte abnormalities and acidosis. Serial hematocrit determinations and a type and crossmatch are important studies in traumatic and non-traumatic hemorrhage, either known or suspected. In septic shock, a complete blood cell count and blood cultures should be obtained, as well as cultures of other potential sources of infection (urine, cerebrospinal fluid, wound, indwelling venous access line, etc). Coagulation studies including panels to evaluate for disseminated intravascular

coagulopathy, and electrolyte studies including calcium and magnesium levels, are frequently abnormal in sepsis. Hypoglycemia is a common finding in any type of shock, and a rapid bedside glucose determination should be performed. Arterial blood gases can demonstrate adequacy of oxygenation and degree of acidosis, and are necessary to diagnose elevated carboxyhemoglobin and methemoglobin levels. Initial lactate levels, particularly for septic shock and trauma patients, may be correlated with overall prognosis, and can be followed serially to chart progress. Troponins may be useful in determining severity of disease and following patients with cardiogenic shock. D-dimer is useful in patients with suspected pulmonary embolism.

Other Studies

Chest radiography, electrocardiogram, and echocardiogram may be obtained in cardiogenic or ductal-dependent obstructive shock to further elucidate the specific etiology. Workup of stabilized trauma patients may include bedside ultrasound, radiographs, or computed tomography scans. Imaging studies contribute to the diagnoses of cardiac tamponade, tension pneumothorax, and pulmonary embolism. Invasive monitoring with arterial lines for systemic arterial blood pressure and central venous lines for central venous pressure or pulmonary artery wedge pressure may be helpful in the ongoing management of shock, particularly fluid-resistant shock.

Management

The first management priority in the treatment of any critically ill child is attention to airway patency and ventilation. If there is significant respiratory compromise, bag-mask ventilation followed by endotracheal intubation is performed. Usually, however, patients in compensated shock do not require immediate attention to airway management. Instead, the immediate priorities are administration of **oxygen** and initiation of **cardiorespiratory monitoring.** Elective, rather than emergent, endotracheal intubation should be considered to reduce metabolic demands caused by increased work of breathing. When intubating patients in shock, induction agents without hemodynamic effects are preferred instead of opiates or benzodiazepines, for example, ketamine and etomidate (although etomidate is not recommended in septic shock due to its effect of cortisol suppression).

Almost concurrently with the above, the next priority is achieving **intravascular access** and, in most cases, administering fluids. Peripheral IV access should be attempted. If this is unsuccessful after 3 attempts or 90 seconds, an intraosseous line may be placed, or IV access may be obtained by placement of a central venous catheter or by cutdown technique. Intraosseous line has been demonstrated to provide much more rapid vascular access compared to central line placement. Umbilical venous lines can sometimes be placed in neonates within the first 1 to 2 weeks of life. More than one intravascular line is usually needed for managing patients in shock.

Decreased preload and hypovolemia (actual or relative) are present in the most common causes of shock. Only cardiogenic shock may not benefit from increasing preload via a fluid bolus. Generally, an **initial fluid bolus of 20 mL/kg isotonic crystalloid fluid,** such as normal saline or lactated Ringer's, should be rapidly infused (this may require manually pushing the fluid using a large syringe). The patient should be assessed for improvement in mentation, vital signs, peripheral pulses, and skin signs after each fluid bolus. **Repeat fluid boluses** of 20 mL/kg to a total of 80 mL/kg or more may be necessary to restore intravascular volume. Colloid fluid (eg, albumin) theoretically has the advantage of staying intravascular longer, but this has not been proved to result in a measurable benefit. Crystalloid fluid is recommended for initial boluses because it is less expensive and more readily available. If a patient with traumatic hemorrhage is still hemodynamically unstable after 2 crystalloid fluid boluses, packed red blood cells at 10 mL/kg may be required. Patients should be reassessed after *each* bolus prior to ordering another bolus. Development of hepatomegaly or rales may indicate fluid overload, and the need to begin other therapies such as vasoactive infusions. This is particularly true for cardiogenic and septic shock.

The mnemonic SHOCKED may be used to recall overall management (Table 61-3). Further management in addition to fluids depends on the specific etiology. Patients in septic shock should receive empiric broad-spectrum antibiotic coverage within the first hour after presentation. A surgeon must assist in identifying the source of hemorrhage and controlling the bleeding in patients with traumatic hemorrhage, and may be required for non-traumatic hemorrhage as well depending on the specific etiology. Blood transfusions may be required. Spinal cord injury is treated with supportive care in consultation with a neurosurgeon. Anaphylactic shock is treated with IV epinephrine, IV diphenhydramine, antihistamine H₂ receptor blockers, glucocorticoids, and nebulized albuterol. Pericardial tamponade is relieved by pericardiocentesis, tension pneumothorax by needle thoracostomy and/or tube thoracostomy, and pulmonary embolus with supportive care and thrombolytics. Carbon monoxide poisoning is treated with 100% oxygen and, if severe, hyperbaric oxygen therapy. Patients with methemoglobinemia appear cyanotic even while receiving 100% oxygen and may be treated with methylene blue. Supraventricular tachycardia should be treated with adenosine if the patient is hemodynamically stable and with synchronized cardioversion if the patient is unstable. Ductal-dependent obstructive shock should be treated with prostaglandin E1 (PGE1) infusion.

Patients with cardiogenic shock require **inotropic agents** to increase cardiac contractility and improve tissue perfusion. Patients in the later stages of other forms of shock (hypovolemic, distributive, septic) may also suffer cardiac dysfunction. In such patients, only after adequate fluid resuscitation has been performed and there are still signs of shock or hypotension should inotropic agents be started. Central venous pressure monitoring may be needed to determine whether fluid resuscitation is adequate. Patients with septic shock may require **vasoactive agents** to reduce or increase systemic vascular resistance.

Dopamine or epinephrine is often the first-line inotropic agent. At low doses (2–5 µg/kg/min), dopamine improves renal blood flow and enhances urine output. At mid-range doses

Table 61-3. SHOCKED Mnemonic for Management	
S	**Sound the alarm:** Obtain help from consultants, intensivists, ancillary personnel. Move the patient to a monitored room, and place on cardiorespiratory monitor, automated blood pressure measurement, and pulse oximetry.
H	**Help hypovolemia:** Get intravascular access and start 20 cc/kg crystalloid fluid bolus. Reassess after each bolus, and continue giving boluses unless hepatomegaly or rales develop. Patients may require 80 cc/kg of fluids or more.
O	**Optimize oxygenation:** Give supplemental oxygen regardless of pulse oximetry values. Consider elective intubation and artificial ventilation to reduce metabolic demands as indicated. Transfusion may be required if hemoglobin is low (<8–10 g/dL).
C	**Constrict and contract:** Use inotropic and vasoconstricting agents as needed for fluid-refractory shock.
K	**Keep in mind underlying causes:** Give or apply therapies specific to the underlying cause.
E	**Electrolytes and glucose normalized:** Measure and normalize electrolytes (especially calcium) and glucose.
D	**Decrease metabolic demand:** Treat hyperthermia and pain to reduce metabolic demand on the patient. Consider elective intubation. Keep patient NPO.

(5–10 µg/kg/min), dopamine exerts primarily a b-adrenergic effect, improving contractility and increasing heart rate. At higher doses (10–20 µg/kg/min), dopamine's a-adrenergic effects cause peripheral vasoconstriction to improve hypotension. **Epinephrine** has predominantly β-adrenergic effects at lower doses (0.05–0.1 µg/kg/min) and α-adrenergic effects at higher doses (up to 1.0 µg/kg/min). Because epinephrine is a strong inotrope, it is recommended for dopamine-resistant cold septic shock. **Norepinephrine** (0.01–1.0 µg/kg/min) has predominantly α-adrenergic vasoconstricting effects, and is therefore preferred for warm septic shock with low systemic vascular resistance and for distributive shock states (anaphylaxis, neurogenic shock, certain toxin-induced shock states). **Dobutamine** (1–20 µg/kg/min) may be the most useful drug for cardiogenic shock because it is selective for β-adrenergic effects, increasing cardiac contractility. However, if hypotension is present, dobutamine-mediated peripheral vasodilation may be detrimental. Dobutamine is typically used in a range of 10 to 20 µg/kg/min. Combinations of inotropic agents may be beneficial to maximize improvements in cardiac contractility and cardiac output without compromising renal perfusion or worsening hypotension. Both dopamine and dobutamine may be less effective in children younger than 6 to 12 months. For this reason, some centers recommend epinephrine as the first-line inotropic agent.

Patients in cardiogenic shock or cold septic shock may also benefit from afterload reduction using systemic vasodilators such as **nitroprusside** (0.5–5 µg/kg/min). If these are used, blood pressure should be continuously monitored, typically in the setting of the intensive care unit. Cold septic shock refractory to epinephrine may also be treated with type III phosphodiesterase inhibitors (**amrinone** 1–20 μg/kg/min, **milrinone** 0.25–1.0 μg/kg/min), which exert inotropic and vasodilator actions. Typically, a pediatric intensive care specialist should be involved in the care of the patient, and central venous pressure monitoring should be begun before vasodilator agents are started.

Neonates with ductal-dependent lesions present with a sudden onset of shock and cyanosis in the second half of the first week of life. Common lesions include hypoplastic left heart syndrome, aortic coarctation, and tricuspid atresia. **Prostaglandin E₁** (0.1 μg/kg/min, titrated to effect), which acts to keep the ductus arteriosus open, should be immediately infused if a ductal-dependent lesion is suspected as the cause of shock. Apnea may result from PGE₁ therapy, and attention to airway management is key.

It used to be common to mix vasoactive infusions using the **rule of 6 and 0.6.** For dopamine, dobutamine, and nitroprusside, mix 6 μg/kg of drug with enough dextrose 5% in water (D5W) to produce a final volume of 100 mL. Infusion at 1 mL/hour provides a dose of 1 μg/kg/min. For epinephrine, norepinephrine, and PGE₁, mix 0.6 μg/kg of drug with enough D5W to produce a final volume of 100 mL. Infusion of 1 mL/hour provides a dose of 0.1 μg/kg/min. However, calculations such as these are error prone, and computerized order forms with automatic error alerts, or "smart" pumps that automatically calculate doses based on the patient's inputted weight, are better choices.

Treatment of patients in shock must include attention to conditions that increase metabolic demand. Acidosis should be assessed and, if severe, treatment with bicarbonate may be considered, although such therapy is controversial. Temperature should be kept neutral with use of antipyretics and cooling measures as needed. Electrolyte abnormalities, particularly hypocalcemia, and hypoglycemia must be assessed and corrected. If a hypothyroid state is suspected, thyroid hormone replacement therapy is important. Blood products may be required for patients with septic shock and disseminated intravascular coagulation. Packed red blood cells, 10 cc/kg at a time, should be given to maintain hemoglobin of at least 10 g/dL. Fresh frozen plasma may be given to correct abnormalities in prothrombin and partial thromboplastin times, but should not be pushed due to its propensity to cause further hypotension. Cryoprecipitate should be reserved for documented hypofibrinogenic states.

An expert panel from the American College of Critical Care Medicine created **clinical practice parameters for the treatment of pediatric septic shock.** Recommended therapy is divided between therapies for the first hour (the "golden hour") and therapies beyond the first hour (often with critical care specialists involved). In the first 15 minutes after recognition of septic shock, practitioners should attend to the airway and establish intravascular access, begin fluid boluses in 20 cc/kg increments, and diagnose and correct any hypoglycemia and hypocalcemia. The goal of therapy is normalization of heart rate, blood pressure, and capillary refill; cardiac index more

than 3.3 and less than 6.0 L/min/m²; and superior vena cava (SVC) oxygen saturation (O₂ sat) 70% or higher. Patients who are responsive to fluid may be observed in the pediatric intensive care unit. Dopamine therapy should be started for those who are still hypotensive after fluid resuscitation. Once dopamine therapy is titrated up to 20 μg/kg/min, epinephrine should be added for dopamine-resistant cold septic shock, while norepinephrine should be added for dopamine-resistant warm septic shock. The updated guidelines emphasize that inotropic therapy should not be withheld because there is no central line, and can be given peripherally if there are no other options. Two studies of patients transferred into a tertiary pediatric medical center showed significantly reduced mortality and morbidity for patients cared for by community practitioners who followed the above guidelines for the first hour of care.

Corticosteroids are controversial in the treatment of sepsis. Guidelines suggest administering "stress doses" of hydrocortisone 2 mg/kg or 50 mg/m² body surface area beyond the first hour of therapy for catecholamine-resistant septic shock when adrenal insufficiency is suspected. Adrenal insufficiency may be suspected in patients with a history of a central nervous system abnormality or pituitary abnormality, a known adrenal gland disorder, recent surgery, history of chronic steroid therapy (eg, for asthma, inflammatory bowel disease, or a rheumatologic condition), and in purpura fulminans. "Shock doses" of hydrocortisone (50 mg/kg) may be given in catecholamine-resistant fulminant septic shock and dopamine-resistant purpura fulminans. It is suggested that a baseline cortisol level be drawn prior to giving corticosteroids.

Following the first hour of therapy, a vasodilator (nitroprusside) or type III phosphodiesterase inhibitor (amrinone or milrinone) along with further volume loading may be helpful in catecholamine-resistant cold septic shock with normal blood pressure and SVC O₂ sat less than 70%. In cases of "cold" septic shock with low blood pressure and SVC O₂ sat less than 70%, continued titration of epinephrine and volume is recommended. For "warm" septic shock, continued titration of norepinephrine and volume is recommended, with the possible addition of vasopressin (0.0003–0.0008 U/kg/min). Vasopressin has not been well studied in children, but shows promise in adults. Finally, for persistent catecholamine-resistant septic shock, consideration may be given to extracorporeal membrane oxygenation. Recombinant activated protein C (drotrecogin alfa) is recommended for some septic adult patients, but not for pediatric patients.

Prevention

Improving outcomes focuses primarily on early recognition and early appropriate therapy of shock. Carcillo et al showed significantly reduced morbidity and mortality in shock patients transferred to a tertiary pediatric medical center if community hospital physicians recognized shock and used pediatric advanced life support (PALS)–recommended interventions early. Appropriate PALS-recommended therapy was defined as more than 20 mL/kg of fluids (except in those with cardiac conditions) and use of inotropes in fluid-refractory shock. Unfortunately, while 37% of the patients transferred during the study period were in shock, as defined by prolonged capillary refill time or hypotension, only 7% were identified as in shock during the referral process. **Early recognition of compensated shock** is a key preventive measure to reduce mortality. In the study, of those in shock only 36% received appropriate PALS-recommended therapy prior to transfer. Community practitioners must concentrate on obtaining vascular access (with an intraosseous needle if necessary), giving fluid boluses early, and starting inotropes (through a peripheral intravenous line if necessary) for fluid-refractory shock within the first hour. **Early therapy,** often before the patient reaches a tertiary care center, is also a key preventive measure. Rapid response teams are increasingly being used in hospitals to institute appropriate medical therapy for inpatients with concerning symptoms or vital signs. At a minimum, community pediatricians should have the ability to obtain intravascular or intraosseous access and administer rapid fluid boluses in their offices.

Prognosis

Children in shock are critically ill and at risk for progression to multi-organ failure and death. Prognosis depends on how early shock is recognized and treated, and on the underlying etiology. Pediatric septic shock carries a 9% mortality rate, which is significantly improved from 60% in the 1980s and 97% in the 1960s, and is also lower than the adult septic shock mortality rate. Mortality rates are even lower (6% in one study) with prompt recognition and adequate treatment.

CASE RESOLUTION

The boy in the case history is in barely compensated (he is not hypotensive) hypovolemic shock due to diarrhea, vomiting, and dehydration. He should receive oxygen and cardiorespiratory monitoring, and intravenous access should be rapidly established. Isotonic fluid boluses of 20 mL/kg should be given with reassessment between each bolus. As much as 80 mL/kg may be needed before improvements in mentation, vital signs, pulses, and skin signs are seen.

Selected References

Brierley J, Carcillo JA, Choong K, et al. Clinical practice parameters for hemodynamic support of pediatric and neonatal shock: 2007 update from the American College of Critical Care Medicine. *Crit Care Med.* 2009;37:666–688

Carcillo JA, Fields AI; American College of Critical Care Medicine Task Force Committee. Clinical practice parameters for hemodynamic support of pediatric and neonatal patients in septic shock. *Crit Care Med.* 2002;30:1365–1378

Carcillo JA, Kuch BA, Yong YH, et al. Mortality and functional morbidity after use of PALS/APLS by community physicians. *Pediatrics.* 2009;124:500–508

Fisher JD, Nelson DG, Beyersdorf H, Satkowiak LJ. Clinical spectrum of shock in the pediatric emergency department. *Pediatr Emerg Care.* 2010;26:622–625

Han YY, Carcillo JA, Dragotta MA, et al. Early reversal of pediatric neonatal septic shock by community physicians is associated with improved outcome. *Pediatrics.* 2003;112:793–799

Kissoon N, Orr RA, Carcillo JA. Updated American College of Critical Care Medicine-Pediatric Advanced Life Support guidelines for management of pediatric and neonatal septic shock. *Pediatr Emerg Care.* 2010;26:867–869

Maar SP. Emergency care in pediatric septic shock. *Pediatr Emerg Care.* 2004;20:617–624

McKiernan CA, Lieberman SA. Circulatory shock in children: an overview. *Pediatr Rev.* 2005;26:451–460

Saladino RA. Management of septic shock in the pediatric emergency department in 2004. *Clin Pediatr Emerg Med.* 2004;5:20–27

Schwarz AJ. Shock. E-medicine. http://emedicine.medscape.com/article/1833578-overview. Accessed December 1, 2010

Silverman AM, Wang VJ. Shock: a common pathway for life-threatening pediatric illnesses and injuries. EB Medicine. http://www.ebmedicine.net/topics.php?paction=showTopic&topic_id=149. Accessed December 1, 2010

CHAPTER 62

Approach to the Traumatized Child

David B. Burbulys, MD

CASE STUDY

A 6-year-old boy is brought to the emergency department after being struck by an automobile while crossing the street. He was found unconscious at the scene. Initial evaluation shows that he has an altered level of consciousness; shallow respirations; ecchymosis across the upper abdomen; and a deformed, swollen left thigh. The pediatric emergency physician is called in to discuss an initial assessment and management plan for the injured child with the trauma surgeon.

Questions

1. What are the most common mechanisms of injury responsible for trauma in children?
2. What are some of the physiological differences between adults and children that make children more susceptible to certain types of injuries?
3. Which areas of the body are most likely to be injured in a typical automobile versus pedestrian collision?
4. What are the components of a primary survey in pediatric trauma patients?
5. What radiographic and laboratory studies should be performed in children with multiple injuries?

Trauma is often referred to as the neglected disease of modern society. Childhood trauma, in particular, is poorly understood and studied. Death from trauma is higher in pediatric patients than in adult patients. Mechanisms of injury may be similar in adults and children, but children have particular anatomical differences and physiological responses to injury. Health care professionals should realize that children have unique anatomical and physiological features compared with adults (Box 62-1). Evaluation and management of traumatized children requires specialized knowledge, training, and equipment. Recognition of such facts, coupled with expertise in the performance of emergency procedures, should improve the outcome of children who sustain major injuries.

Epidemiology

More than 64% of the deaths of children aged 1 to 14 years are caused by traumatic injuries. This number peaks at 8 years of age. Approximately 1.5 million pediatric injuries result in a quarter million to half million hospitalizations, and 15,000 to 25,000 deaths (1.5%) each year. Adolescents are most likely to die in motor vehicle crashes and school-aged children are most likely to die after being struck by automobiles. This figure, unfortunately, may be an underestimation, as most childhood injury fatalities occur in the field prior to arrival at a health care facility. The magnitude of the problem becomes even more evident when morbidity is considered.

Box 62-1. Characteristics of Children That Lead to Increased Susceptibility to Injury

Anatomical Characteristics

- Smaller body size allows for the greater distribution of force with trauma, so multiple system injury is common.
- A prominent occiput, exaggerated head-to-body ratio, weak neck muscles, and higher center of gravity predispose younger children to head injury.
- Cranial bones are thinner and the brain is less myelinated, resulting in more serious head injury.
- Skeletal and ligamentous structures have increased flexibility, which results in greater transmission of force to internal organs.
- Less protective muscle and subcutaneous tissue over internal organs expose them to injury.
- Growth plates are not yet fused, which leads to Salter-type fractures and possible bone growth abnormalities with healing.

Physiological Characteristics

- High body surface area-to-weight ratio predisposes children to hypothermia, which may complicate shock and worsen acidosis and coagulopathy if it is not corrected.
- Hypoxia and respiratory failure are increasingly likely in children.
- Hemorrhagic shock is initially well tolerated by increasing heart rate and peripheral vascular resistance without significant changes in systolic blood pressure.

Between 50,000 and 100,000 children per year become permanently disabled as a result of their injuries. Such disabilities have an enormous impact on society; they result in financial and emotional losses for families and many years of lost productivity for individuals.

Blunt trauma, which is more common than penetrating injury in children, represents about 87% of all childhood injuries. Head injuries, followed by thoracoabdominal injuries, are the leading causes of death in this group. In adolescents, however, penetrating injury (suicide and homicide) accounts for a higher percentage of the total, especially among minority populations in urban areas. Causes of non-penetrating trauma are motor vehicle crashes (>40%), falls (25%–30%), drowning (10%–15%), and burns (5%–10%). Included in the remainder are bicycle-related and automobile versus pedestrian injuries. These numbers vary somewhat by locale. Male children are injured twice as often as female children. Different mechanisms of injury predominate in different age groups; the figures given above refer to overall causes of trauma. Perhaps as much as 25% to 35% of trauma deaths are related to child abuse in some centers.

Clinical Presentation

Children who sustain severe trauma present with multiple organ system injury manifested by shock, respiratory failure, or altered mental status (singly or in combination). Those with mild to moderate injury may present in this way or simply with localized signs and symptoms in the injured area.

Pathophysiology

Patterns of injury are important to identify to develop strategies for injury prevention as well as anticipate injuries during patient management. One common pattern is the triad of injuries that result from an automobile versus pedestrian collision (Waddell triad) (Figure 62-1).

Multisystem injury is the rule rather than the exception in children. Internal injury must always be suspected, even if no evidence suggestive of external trauma is apparent when the mechanism of injury warrants. Because children are anatomically and physiologically different from adults, they are more susceptible to different types of injuries (Box 62-1). The most striking physiological differences between adults and children concern responses to acute blood loss. Children have a tremendous capacity to maintain systolic blood pressure despite 25% to 30% acute blood loss.

Hypovolemic shock secondary to acute blood loss is the most common cause of shock in pediatric trauma patients. In general, hemorrhagic shock is a clinical state where the cardiac output is unable to meet the metabolic demands of the tissues for oxygen and nutrients; it is not defined by any absolute blood pressure value.

Acute blood loss stimulates peripheral and central receptors and results in an increased production of catecholamines and adrenocorticoids. The body responds by increasing peripheral vascular resistance, stroke volume, and heart rate. Children are able to dramatically increase heart rate and peripheral vascular resistance and

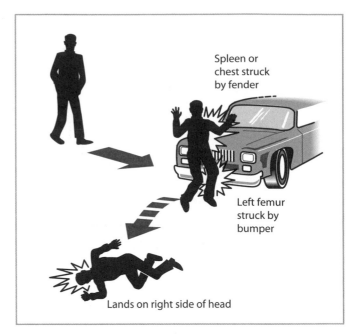

Figure 62-1. Illustration of Waddell triad. Femur, abdominal, and contralateral head injuries (Waddell triad) should be expected to result from automobile versus pedestrian collisions in the United States. A child crossing the street is struck on the left side of the body by an automobile traveling on the right side of the road. The left femur is likely to be injured by the bumper, and the abdomen or chest strikes the grille as the child is lifted into the air and lands on the opposite side of the head, sustaining blunt head trauma. The Waddell triad illustrates the necessity of having a high degree of suspicion for a complex of injuries based on a well-known mechanism.

Labels in figure: Spleen or chest struck by fender; Left femur struck by bumper; Lands on right side of head

they often may exhibit normal blood pressure in the presence of hypovolemic shock. By the time their blood pressure falls, they commonly have lost 20% to 25% of their circulating blood volume. In adults, blood pressure tends to decline after a less significant blood loss and therefore may be recognized sooner (Figure 62-2). Subtle changes in heart rate, blood pressure, pulse pressure, and capillary refill may indicate impending cardiovascular collapse in traumatically injured children and should not be overlooked.

Another obstacle to the recognition of shock in children is the lack of knowledge on the part of many health professionals of age-appropriate vital signs, particularly blood pressure. Table 62-1 gives the normal blood pressure ranges for children of different ages.

Three stages of shock correspond to the progression of volume loss. In the first stage, **compensated shock**, mechanisms for preserving blood pressure are still effective. Decreased capillary refill, diminished pulses, cool extremities, and tachypnea may be apparent, but blood pressure is normal and accompanied by tachycardia. Unrecognized, untreated compensated shock rapidly progresses to **uncompensated shock.** Examination reveals decreased level of consciousness, pallor, reduced urine output, and lower blood pressure with weak, thready pulses and marked tachycardia. With inadequate therapy, uncompensated shock becomes **irreversible shock,** resulting in irreparable organ damage and often unpreventable death. (See Chapter 61 for a more extensive discussion.)

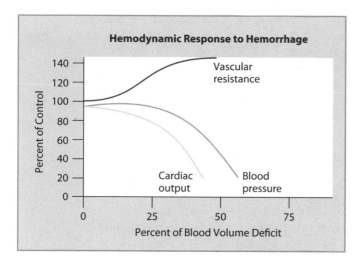

Figure 62-2. Graph showing cardiovascular response to hypovolemia in children. Blood pressure does not begin to decline until the volume deficit is more than 25% because of the compensatory increase in vascular resistance. Cardiac output drops earlier and is manifested clinically as delayed capillary refill; cool, clammy skin; and tachycardia.

Shock has several causes, and it is important to emphasize that, in trauma patients, it should always be initially attributed to hemorrhage. Shock due to obstructive cardiac output causes, such as tension pneumothorax or cardiac tamponade, are much less common. Shock due to spinal cord injury is exceedingly rare. Shock should never be attributed solely to head trauma. The pathways resulting in decreased blood pressure in patients with head trauma are present only at the terminal stages. Therefore, the possibility of blood loss from internal organs should be pursued promptly.

Evaluation and Management

Because of the high potential for serious morbidity and mortality in trauma patients, evaluation and management are performed simultaneously. This care is best handled using an organized, multidisciplinary team approach, with preestablished criteria for activation of the trauma team. History of the event provides important information when implementing these criteria. For example, the entire team responds for all pedestrians struck by an automobile. The types of subspecialists that make up a trauma team are decided by individual institutions.*

Several approaches to the assessment of trauma patients have been developed by professional organizations. The Advanced Trauma Life Support (ATLS) course of the American College of Surgeons and the Basic Trauma Life Support (BTLS) course of the American College of Emergency Physicians (now renamed International Trauma Life Support) are 2 such approaches. Both the ATLS and the BTLS methods stress the importance of a primary evaluation, or primary survey, to identify and treat immediate life-threatening injuries and a more detailed regional examination, or secondary

---

* Most institutions have trauma teams composed of pediatric emergency and critical care specialists, anesthesiologists, trauma surgeons, surgical subspecialists, emergency nurses, respiratory therapists, social workers, and radiograph technicians.

Age	Respiration (breaths/min)	Pulse (beats/min)	Blood Pressure (Systolic)
Newborn	30–60	100–160	50–70
1–6 wk	30–60	100–160	70–95
6 mo	25–40	90–120	80–100
1 y	20–40	90–120	80–100
3 y	20–30	80–120	80–110
6 y	12–25	70–110	80–110
10 y	12–20	60–90	90–120

Table 62-1. Normal Vital Signs for Children of Different Ages

survey, after stabilization to identify and treat all other injuries. In addition, they both adhere to the principles of serial examination and reassessment after each intervention. The primary survey and initial resuscitation efforts must occur simultaneously and within the first several minutes of the evaluation. The secondary survey is meant to enhance the primary survey. Vital signs should be repeated every 5 minutes during the primary survey and every 15 minutes during the secondary survey until the trauma team feels the patient has been adequately stabilized. The reader should understand the rationale for the trauma examination and its parts. (See Selected References for articles that explain the rationale for trauma examination and provide detailed descriptions of evaluation and management techniques.)

Physical Examination

The **primary survey** begins with an assessment of **level of consciousness,** patency of the **airway** (Box 62-2), and quality of **breathing** (Box 62-3). When evaluating injured patients, physicians should always assume that the cervical spine has been injured and should use in-line immobilization to secure it. Basic airway maneuvers for positioning should be performed. The safest method is the jaw thrust to avoid moving the cervical spine (Figure 62-3). The oral cavity should be examined for foreign bodies, blood, or secretions. The most common form of airway obstruction in children is a posteriorly displaced tongue, which is relieved by good airway positioning. Advanced airway maneuvers (bag-valve-mask ventilation

---

Box 62-2. Airway Assessment and Treatment

Assessment
- Airway patency and ability to protect it
- Level of consciousness
- Stridor

Treatment
- Spinal immobilization
- Jaw thrust and suctioning
- 100% oxygen by non-rebreathing mask
- Intubate for Glasgow Coma Scale score <9, no gag reflex

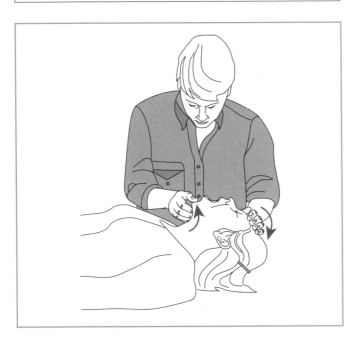

Figure 62-3. Correct method for positioning the head with chin lift or jaw thrust.

or endotracheal tube intubation) are performed during the primary survey if children have apnea, significant respiratory distress, severe head trauma, or an airway that cannot be maintained with basic techniques. All trauma patients are initially given supplemental oxygen by non-rebreathing mask at a concentration of 100% and the adequacy of ventilation is assessed by a general evaluation of the respiratory rate, depth, chest movement and symmetry, and tracheal deviation.

After a patent airway and adequate ventilation have been established, **circulatory status** is assessed. All pediatric trauma patients require placement of the largest bore intravenous catheter obtainable for that patient; these should be placed, if possible, in each antecubital fossa. In life-threatening situations, peripheral vascular access is attempted either 3 times or for 90 seconds, whichever comes first. If peripheral attempts fail, then intraosseous infusion or central venous access should be used. A bolus of 20 mL/kg of an isotonic fluid (normal saline or Ringer's lactate) should be given. This may be repeated,

if necessary, to treat hypovolemic shock. After 60 mL/kg, administration of 10 mL/kg of blood should be considered, and the likelihood of surgical exploration is high. Acutely exsanguinating wounds are treated using direct pressure bandages (Box 62-4).

A brief neurologic assessment to assess patient **disability** is also performed during the primary survey. One rapid assessment technique is the **AVPU** system (**A**, **a**lert; **V**, responds to **v**erbal stimuli; **P**, responds to **p**ainful stimuli; and **U**, **u**nresponsive). Subsequently, a Glasgow Coma Scale score or Children's Coma Scale score should be calculated (Box 62-5).

Once life-threatening conditions are stabilized, more information can be collected. The **secondary survey** involves a complete and thorough head-to-toe examination of the child, fully exposed, to identify additional injuries, while taking great care to maintain normothermia. It also includes a **SAMPLE** history (**s**ymptoms, **a**llergies, **m**edications, **p**ast history/ hospitalizations/surgeries, **l**ast meal, **e**vents preceding trauma). A detailed history of events preceding trauma should ensure that injuries are consistent with the causal mechanism. Health care professionals should be prepared to consider abuse when specific diagnoses do not correlate with either the history given by the caregiver or the developmental ability of the child. Measurement of vital signs should occur as previously described and other devices, such as Foley catheters, nasogastric tubes, and pulse oximetry, should be used at this time. Every time an intervention is performed, repeat assessments that incorporate the elements of the primary survey are made.

Laboratory Tests

Most institutions have a standardized trauma panel (complete blood cell count with differential, electrolytes, blood urea nitrogen, creatinine, glucose, amylase, lipase, prothrombin time, partial thromboplastin time, urine analysis, and blood typing and crossmatching). In addition, drug and alcohol screens may provide important information, particularly in the child with altered mental status. Female children of potential childbearing age should have a point of care pregnancy test performed as well.

Box 62-5. Glasgow Coma Scale Modified for Pediatric Patients

Eye Opening Response

4 Spontaneous

3 To verbal command/shout[a]

2 To pain

1 None

Motor Response

6 Obeys commands/spontaneous[a]

5 Localizes pain

4 Withdraws to pain

3 Decerebrate posturing to pain (flexion)

2 Decorticate posturing to pain (extension)

1 None

Verbal Response

5 Oriented and conversant/appropriate words[a]

4 Confused/inappropriate words[a]

3 Inappropriate words/persistent crying or screaming[a]

2 Incomprehensible sounds/grunts or moans[a]

1 None

Scoring

14–15 Mild

9–13 Moderate

<9 Severe

[a] Younger than 1 year.

Imaging Studies

When major trauma is suspected, radiographs of at least the chest, pelvis/abdomen, and cervical spine should be obtained. This prevents missing injuries in children who may be unconscious or who need lifesaving procedures during resuscitation, which obscure an area of injury from examination. Additional radiographs, for example, of the extremities, may be indicated when other areas of injury are detected on secondary survey. Children are often initially distracted from one injury because of the presence of a more painful one.

More sophisticated imaging techniques, such as computed tomography scans and ultrasound, are a usual part of the evaluation of the seriously injured pediatric trauma patient. The choice of test depends on the experience of the trauma team and the individual characteristics of the patient.

Prognosis

The highest survival rates for seriously injured children have been found among those who are brought to the operating room for treatment within 1 hour of the injury. Definitive care for trauma takes place in the operating room, and initial stabilization takes place in the emergency department. Absolute indications for surgery include hemodynamic instability despite aggressive resuscitation, transfusion of more than 50% of the total blood volume, pneumoperitoneum, intraperitoneal bladder rupture, severe renovascular injury,

gunshot wounds to the abdomen, evisceration, and peritonitis. Other injuries, often in contradistinction to similarly injured adult patients, are frequently treated more conservatively in the intensive care unit after complete consultation with all involved providers.

An organized, preestablished, multidisciplinary approach to care is essential. Studies have shown that the single most important element for any hospital treating injured children is the commitment on the part of the institution and its surgeons. Regional pediatric trauma centers have increased resources for dealing with severely injured patients that include long-term care and rehabilitation. Other non-designated hospitals may do an excellent job in the initial stabilization phase of care. Indications for transfer to a specialty center include inability to provide definitive surgical intervention, inability to provide an appropriate intensive care environment, the presence of multisystem injuries or injuries requiring extensive orthopedic or plastic surgery procedures, or major burns. Health care professionals who treat children should not only become adept at the recognition and initial stabilization of injuries, but should also serve as advocates for injury prevention and coordinated prehospital care services in the community.

CASE RESOLUTION

The 6-year-old boy in the case history sustained multiple trauma from an automobile versus pedestrian collision. He presents with altered level of consciousness; respiratory failure (shallow respirations); potential internal organ injury, which may lead to shock; and probable fracture of the left femur, which may also contribute to the development of shock. These injuries are identified by performance of a primary and secondary survey. Proper management includes stabilization of the cervical spine, airway management, aggressive early shock treatment with fluid replacement, and a vigilant search for additional injuries. Continued reassessment is also an integral part of emergency department stabilization. Due to the presence of multisystem injuries, after initial stabilization, the patient should be transferred to a regional pediatric trauma center for extended care.

Selected References

American College of Surgeons. *Advanced Trauma Life Support (ATLS) Student Manual*. 8th ed. Chicago, IL: American College of Surgeons; 2008

American Heart Association. Pediatric advanced life support: 2010 American Heart Association guidelines for cardiopulmonary resuscitation and emergency cardiovascular care. *Pediatrics*. 2010;126(5):e1361–e1399

Avarello JT, Cantor RM. Pediatric major trauma: an approach to evaluation and management. *Emerg Med Clin North Am*. 2007;25:803–836

Ruddy RM, Fleisher GR. An approach to the injured child. In: Fleisher GR, Ludwig S, eds. *Textbook of Pediatric Emergency Medicine*. 5th ed. Baltimore, MD: Williams & Wilkins; 2005

Swischuk LE. Emergency pediatric imaging: changes over the years (Part I). *Emerg Radiol*. 2005;11:193–198

Ziegler MM, Templeton JM. Major trauma. In: Fleisher GR, Ludwig S, eds. *Textbook of Pediatric Emergency Medicine*. 5th ed. Baltimore, MD: Williams & Wilkins; 2005

CHAPTER 63

Abdominal Trauma

David B. Burbulys, MD

CASE STUDY

An 8-year-old boy who rode a bicycle quickly and unintentionally crashed into a tree is transported to the pediatric emergency department by emergency medical services. On arrival at the trauma center, the paramedics report that the bike handlebars struck the child's stomach, "knocking the wind out of him." The boy complains of dizziness and vomits several times. Initial vital signs show a heart rate of 135 beats/min and a respiratory rate of 24 breaths/min. The abdomen is flat but tender to palpation in the mid-epigastric region and left upper quadrant.

Questions

1. What are the most frequent types of intra-abdominal trauma in children?
2. What are the diagnostic studies used to evaluate abdominal trauma?
3. What are the basic components of the treatment of shock that occurs following abdominal trauma?
4. What is a simple rule for establishing the lower limit of normal blood pressure in children?

Abdominal trauma is the leading preventable cause of fatal injury in trauma patients. Death results when the extent and nature of abdominal injuries are neither appreciated nor appropriately managed, fluid replacement is inadequate, and airway maintenance and surgical intervention are not implemented soon enough. Abdominal trauma is the third leading cause of traumatic death, following head and thoracic injury. Clinicians should be knowledgeable about mechanisms of injury that result in abdominal trauma, the early manifestations of shock, and the methods for aggressive treatment of hemorrhagic shock.

Epidemiology

Twenty-five percent of children who sustain multisystem trauma have significant abdominal injury and 9% die from abdominal-associated trauma. When both head and abdominal injury occur simultaneously, the risk of death is higher than when either occurs alone. Blunt-force mechanisms are responsible for almost 85% of abdominal injuries; the remainder result from penetrating injuries. Examples of blunt-force mechanisms, presented in order of frequency, include motor vehicle crashes (also the most lethal), pedestrian versus automobile collisions, falls, bicycle injuries, sports injuries, and direct blows from both abuse and assault. Injuries to the spleen and liver predominate followed by injuries to the kidney, bowel, and pancreas. In multiple injuries, the incidence of trauma involving pelvic bones and organs (bladder, ureter, iliac vessels) is also high. A straddle injury (eg, fall that occurs when climbing over a fence) can also result in abdominal and pelvic trauma.

Clinical Presentation

Pain, tenderness, ecchymoses, and peritoneal signs tend to be more reliable signs of pathology, whereas distension or the absence of bowel sounds are less consistent as a marker for injury. (See Dx Box for signs and symptoms suggestive of abdominal trauma.) It is particularly important to note that no sign, however, is completely reliable and that acute hemorrhage into the abdomen doesn't lead to irritation initially. Unexplained hypotension or shock mandates further investigation to assess for intra-abdominal hemorrhage.

 Abdominal Trauma

- Pain
- Tenderness
- Distention
- Peritoneal signs (absent or diminished bowel sounds, rebound tenderness)
- Ecchymoses
- Tire tracks
- Seat belt marks
- Urine, stool, or nasogastric aspirate positive for blood
- Unexplained hypotension or other signs of hypovolemic shock

Pathophysiology

Blunt trauma largely involves injury to solid, not hollow, intra-abdominal organs (ie, spleen and liver rather than small bowel) for a variety of reasons. First, the rib cage is flexible in children. Therefore, rib fractures are less likely to occur, reducing the potential for penetration of abdominal organs by broken ribs. Second, children have less well-developed abdominal musculature and less adipose tissue than adults and relatively larger organs. Blunt force is therefore transmitted to the solid organs more easily and more diffusely. Third, because the diaphragm is oriented more horizontally in children than in adults, the liver and spleen lie more anteriorly and caudally within the abdomen.

It is important to emphasize that abdominal injury may lead to excessive blood loss. The pathophysiology of hemorrhagic shock is discussed in detail in chapter 61 and 62. The liver and spleen are highly vascularized organs that bleed profusely when lacerated. Even the accumulation of subcapsular hematomas without rupture may cause a profound drop in hematocrit. Because intra-abdominal organs are not directly visible when a patient is examined, signs and symptoms of injury are not always obvious. Therefore, hemorrhagic shock should always be suspected with abdominal trauma. Likewise, large volumes of blood can accumulate in the pelvis and retroperitoneum, and because of their proximity to the abdomen, they should always be considered as a reservoir for hemorrhage in abdominal as well as pelvic trauma.

Differential Diagnosis

Physicians should be familiar with the most common patterns of abdominal injury, and they should consider the possibility of specific injuries. Any solid abdominal organ can be injured by any mechanism, either blunt or penetrating. The spleen is the most common intra-abdominal organ injured by a blunt force. **Hepatic injuries** are the most common fatal abdominal injuries, although they are less frequent than **splenic injuries.** The right lobe of the liver is injured more frequently than the left lobe.

Injuries to **hollow viscera** such as the stomach and intestines, which represent only about 5% to 15% of injuries from blunt forces, are difficult to diagnose and often present late. Three mechanisms lead to injuries of hollow structures: (1) "crush" between the anterior wall of the abdomen and the vertebral column; (2) deceleration, which causes shearing of the bowel from its mesenteric attachments; and (3) "burst," which occurs when an air-filled or fluid-filled loop of bowel is closed at both ends at the time of impact. Peritonitis may develop in 6 to 48 hours secondary to fecal spillage or devascularization as a consequence of any of these mechanisms. Occasionally, a diagnosis of hollow viscera injury is made incidentally or may be delayed more than 48 hours, highlighting the need for serial examinations. **Duodenal** and **pancreatic** injuries are examples of potentially delayed diagnoses that can have grave consequences. Leakage of bile and enzymes may activate autodigestion of the pancreas and result in sepsis.

Evaluation

Determining which organ or organs may be injured from abdominal trauma is difficult. Children are often uncooperative or unable to assist with the physical examination. Physicians tend to focus on injuries to the extremities, pelvis, face, or chest that are painful and distracting to children and more clinically obvious to the examiner. Initial clinical impressions may be incorrect, causing delay in diagnosis or unnecessary surgical exploration.

History

The history should focus on the mechanism of injury and the physiological response of the child, especially in the pre-hospital setting (eg, initial hypotension, tachycardia, cyanosis) (Questions Box). A poor history concerning the circumstances of the injury may contribute to a delayed diagnosis.

Questions

Abdominal Trauma

- How was the child injured?
- How long ago did the injury occur?
- What parts of the body were injured?
- Has the child received any treatment prior to coming to the hospital, and what was the response?

Physical Examination

An abnormal physical examination may not always be indicative of pathology. Clinicians should avoid relying on physical examination alone as a predictor of abdominal injury. Studies have demonstrated that patients with and without proven injuries often showed no significant differences with respect to physical findings. In particular, children with abusive abdominal trauma often have no cutaneous evidence of bruising, especially immediately after the injury is inflicted (see Chapter 127). Definitive evaluation of the abdomen is therefore mandated with significant mechanism of injury and often includes rapid computed tomography (CT) scan, ultrasound, diagnostic peritoneal lavage, laparoscopy, or laparotomy.

Vital signs should be monitored. In children, the range for normal heart rate, respiratory rate, and blood pressure is age-dependent. A simple rule for calculating the lower limit of normal systolic blood pressure is 70 + (2 x age in years). Physicians should always remember that a drop in blood pressure is a very late sign in the development of shock in children (see chapters 61 and 62).

Serial abdominal examinations increase the likelihood of detecting a previously missed condition. Inspection of the abdomen to look for ecchymoses, distention, tire tracks, penetrations, or paradoxical motion should occur first. Auscultation for bowel sounds follows this inspection, and palpation should come last. Palpation should be done in all 4 quadrants to elicit tenderness, rebound, and guarding. If a hepatic or splenic injury is initially suspected, palpation should be minimized to avoid further hemorrhaging.

Laboratory Tests

Laboratory evaluation should be guided by the history and physical examination. A urinalysis to look for hematuria and check for associated genitourinary injuries is helpful. Elevated serum transaminases, amylase, lipase, and alkaline phosphatase may be indicative of injury, but normal values do not exclude pathology. A comprehensive trauma panel, which usually includes a complete blood cell count and differential, serum electrolytes, blood urea nitrogen, creatinine, glucose, prothrombin time, partial thromboplastin time, urinalysis, and blood type and crossmatch, should be carried out for all patients with serious or multiple injuries (see Chapter 62).

Imaging Studies

Multiple imaging modalities are available to assess the pediatric trauma patient with suspected abdominal injuries. The time to perform an imaging study is after the patient is responding appropriately to resuscitation (ie, fluid therapy). Unstable patients require surgical exploration for definitive treatment of abdominal or pelvic injury.

Computed tomography scanning remains the standard of care for imaging the injured abdomen of a pediatric trauma patient. Computed tomography scans have greater than 97% accuracy in identifying abdominal or retroperitoneal injury, are noninvasive, and most notably provide detailed specific information regarding injuries. The images are also routinely extended to include the pelvis, as necessary. Disadvantages of CT scanning may include the lack of proximity to the trauma suite, which may not be ideal for unstable patients; the length of time it takes to perform the procedure; and the need for an intravenous (IV) contrast, which has inherent risks such as allergic reactions and renal toxicity.

The use of ultrasonography has become very popular, with encouraging results for the identification of abdominal injury, though its use in pediatric trauma patients remains unclear. Ultrasound can rapidly and noninvasively document the presence of intraperitoneal and pelvic fluid (blood). While it is as effective as CT scanning for documenting the **presence of injury** it does not provide as much specific information about the **nature** of the injury. Ultrasound has a few additional advantages: It is relatively inexpensive; does not require contrast or radiation exposure; can be performed in 5 to 10 minutes in the trauma room, thus minimizing the risk to an unstable patient; and can be used many times for serial assessments.

Over the last several decades, diagnostic peritoneal lavage has been a dependable method of detecting intra-abdominal hemorrhage. However, its use may be limited in the pediatric population because many children with blunt trauma to the abdomen are now managed nonoperatively as stated above.

Management

Management of abdominal trauma in children occurs simultaneously with evaluation. The stabilization of children with abdominal trauma, especially in the context of multiple trauma, requires a multidisciplinary team approach that includes surgeons, pediatricians, and emergency physicians. A discussion on the approach to trauma management can be found in Chapter 62.

Hypovolemic shock, if present, is the primary complication of abdominal trauma on which to focus because the leading unrecognized cause of death in affected children is profound blood loss. **Airway problems** and **breathing difficulties** should be addressed initially, followed by **vascular access** and **fluid replacement.** No more than 3 attempts at peripheral vascular access should be made (≤90 seconds) before moving on to more invasive procedures.

The intraosseous route should be used for the next vascular access attempt. The flat, medial portion of the proximal tibia is most commonly used for the procedure, which is performed with an intraosseous, bone marrow, or spinal needle (Figure 63-1). Fluids and medications, delivered into the marrow cavity, then flow into the venous circulation. Intraosseous cannulation is rapid, simple, and may be lifesaving. It is limited by low flow rates (approximately 30 mL/min), which can be augmented either by using pressure on the IV bag or by pushing fluid by hand through a syringe. Complications associated with intraosseous line placement are rare. All physicians who care for pediatric trauma patients should be familiar with this technique.

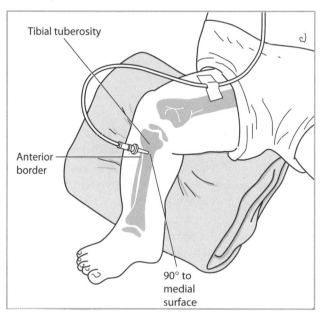

Figure 63-1. **Intraosseous cannulation technique.** (Adapted with permission from American Heart Association. 2005 American Heart Association [AHA] guidelines for cardiopulmonary resuscitation [CPR] and emergency cardiovascular care [ECC] of pediatric and -neonatal patients: pediatric advanced life support. *Pediatrics.* 2006;117:e1005–e1028.)

A variety of central venous access sites, such as femoral, subclavian, and internal jugular, may be used in older children. Upper and lower saphenous vein cutdowns are also possible access sites. The Seldinger technique, with insertion of a large-bore catheter over a guidewire, is often used. A description of these procedures is beyond the scope of this book but may be found in many other publications, including the 2010 American Heart Association (AHA) Guidelines for Cardiopulmonary Resuscitation (CPR) and Emergency Cardiovascular Care (ECC) of Pediatric and Neonatal Patients: Pediatric Advanced Life Support published by the American Heart Association (see Selected References). Intravenous access above the diaphragm is preferred in patients with blunt or penetrating abdominal trauma who have potential disruption of the vena cava or other large veins.

Fluid replacement begins with a 20- to 40-mL/kg bolus of crystalloid solution, either warmed normal saline or Ringer's lactate. If no improvement in circulation occurs, additional 10- to 20-mL/kg boluses may be given, and type-specific blood should be considered. In most scenarios, type-specific blood is given after 60 mL/kg of crystalloid has failed to improve circulatory parameters. Frequent hematocrits or hemoglobins should be determined to monitor ongoing blood loss. Vital signs should be repeated frequently. Serial examinations, which detect the signs and symptoms of shock (Box 63-1), are the most important gauge of hemodynamic recovery and stability. All children require close hospital observation, preferably in a pediatric trauma center and pediatric intensive care unit.

Box 63-1. Signs and Symptoms of Hemorrhagic Shock in Children

- Tachycardia
- Delayed capillary refill (>2 s)
- Cool and mottled skin, pallor
- Respiratory distress
- Anxiety, irritability, decreased responsiveness
- Thirst

Orthostatic fall in blood pressure and supine hypotension (late sign) must be aggressively managed. If hemodynamic stabilization is not achieved after appropriate vascular access and fluid resuscitation, the trauma surgeon will most likely perform an exploratory laparotomy. If children have been stabilized with initial airway and circulatory support, diagnostic procedures such as CT scans can be performed as part of the emergency department evaluation. Once identified, specific organ injury can be managed.

Other specific management concerns for pediatric patients with abdominal injury are early decompression of the stomach with a nasogastric or orogastric tube to prevent respiratory compromise and urinary catheter insertion to decompress the bladder. Before inserting a urinary catheter, the trauma team should evaluate for possible urethral trauma and check for the presence of blood in the urine, which may indicate other genitourinary trauma.

Nonoperative management of minor to moderate liver or spleen injuries is common in children. More severe injuries, including bowel rupture, require surgical intervention.

Prognosis

Morbidity and mortality related to abdominal trauma depend on the specific organ injury and the style of management. More than 40% of patients with major liver injuries die in the prehospital setting. However, a large number of minor liver injuries can be managed nonoperatively. Currently an increasing number of injuries to the spleen and liver are managed with observation in the pediatric intensive care unit. Surgical exploration and repair are performed only if patients become hemodynamically unstable. Reduction in anesthetic-related mortality, post-splenectomy sepsis, and a decrease in other postoperative complications have resulted from this shift in practice style. Without surgical intervention, however, a severe injury such as complete splenic rupture has a 90% to 100% mortality rate.

CASE RESOLUTION

The boy in the case scenario sustained isolated abdominal trauma. Initial presenting signs and symptoms are consistent with internal organ injury, specifically splenic hematoma, pancreatic injury, internal hemorrhage, and compensated shock (eg, tachycardia, tachypnea). The child should undergo initial resuscitation with attention to the airway, breathing, and circulation, especially fluid repletion. Serial hemodynamic measurement and hematocrits, if stable, permit diagnosis of specific injuries by CT scanning. Surgical consultation with expectant observation is the likely management choice. If the child deteriorates, surgical intervention would ensue. Trauma to the small intestine, particularly a duodenal hematoma, must also be suspected because of the mechanism of injury.

Selected References

American College of Surgeons. *Advanced Trauma Life Support (ATLS) Student Manual.* 8th ed. Chicago, IL: American College of Surgeons; 2008

American Heart Association. Pediatric advanced life support: 2010 American Heart Association guidelines for cardiopulmonary resuscitation and emergency cardiovascular care. *Pediatrics.* 2010;126:e1361–e1399

Capraro AJ, Mooney D, Waltzman ML. The use of routine laboratory studies as screening tools in pediatric abdominal trauma. *Pediatr Emerg Care.* 2006;22:480–484

Gaines BA. Intra-abdominal solid organ injury in children: diagnosis and treatment. *J Trauma.* 2009;67(2 suppl):S135–S139

Levy JA, Noble VE. Bedside ultrasound in pediatric emergency medicine. *Pediatrics.* 2008;121:e1404–e1412

Sivit CJ. Imaging children with abdominal trauma. *Am J Roentgenol.* 2009;192:1179–1189

Stylianos S. Outcomes from pediatric solid organ injury: role of standardized care guidelines. *Curr Opin Pediatr.* 2005;17:402–406

Venkatesh KR, McQuay N Jr. Outcomes of management in stable children with intra-abdominal free fluid without solid organ injury after blunt abdominal injury. *J Trauma.* 2007;62:216–220

Wegner S, Colletti JE, Van Wie D. Pediatric blunt abdominal trauma. *Pediatr Clin North Am.* 2006;53:243–256

CHAPTER 64

Head Trauma

Paul Bryan, MD

CASE STUDY

A 2-year-old girl is playing on a window ledge unsupervised. She pushes the screen out and falls onto the concrete sidewalk below, striking her head. A neighbor reports that she is unconscious for 10 minutes. When paramedics arrive, the girl is awake but lethargic. She is transported to the emergency department (ED). Her vital signs are normal. A scalp hematoma is present, and a depressed area of cranial bone is palpated.

Questions

1. What are the priorities in the initial stabilization and management of pediatric head trauma?
2. What is the difference between primary and secondary brain injury?
3. What are the common structural injuries sustained by children with head trauma?
4. What are the various modalities available for treatment of increased intracranial pressure?
5. What are the scoring systems used in the evaluation of mental status in children with head trauma?

Although most childhood head injuries are minor and can be treated on an outpatient basis, it is important for clinicians to become adept at recognizing and managing concussions and more severe forms of head injury. Health care providers can also help lower mortality from head trauma by actively promoting injury prevention to patients and communities.

Epidemiology

Head trauma is one of the most common pediatric injuries and is the leading cause of morbidity and mortality among pediatric trauma patients. Pediatric head trauma accounts for more than 500,000 ED visits; 95,000 hospital admissions; 7,000 deaths; and 29,000 permanent disabilities per year in the United States. The hospital care costs exceed a billion dollars annually. In multiple-injured pediatric patients, 70% of the deaths that occur within 48 hours of hospitalization are the result of trauma to the head. The rates of intracranial injuries in children with only minor head trauma, however, are low with the largest numbers occurring in young children and infants with an incidence of 3% to 6%. Only 0.4% to 1% of children require surgical intervention after minor closed injury.

Falls account for most cases of pediatric head trauma. Other major causes include motor vehicle crashes, vehicle versus pedestrian collisions, bicycle crashes, sports-related injuries, and recreational activities. Non-accidental trauma (ie, child abuse) must be recognized as another important cause of head injury in children, particularly among those younger than 2 years.

Clinical Presentation

Children who have sustained head trauma may present with a history of an antecedent event (eg, fall or collision with another child) or signs and symptoms related to the injury. These include external bruises or lacerations; alterations in the level of consciousness; and neurologic findings, including seizures. Vital signs may be altered; in particular, deep or irregular respirations, hypertension, or bradycardia may be apparent (Dx Box). These changes are indicative of elevated intracranial pressure (ICP).

Pathophysiology

Children have significant anatomical differences from adults that predispose them to head trauma and certain types of intracranial injuries. They have a higher center of gravity, an increased head-to-body ratio, and weaker neck muscles compared with adults. In addition, children have thinner cranial bones and less myelinated brain

Dx | Head Trauma[a]

- Loss of consciousness
- Somnolence
- Pallor
- Emesis/nausea/anorexia
- Irritability
- Lethargy
- Seizure
- Ataxia

- Weakness
- Pain
- Parasthesias
- Amnesia
- Headache
- Visual changes
- Confusion/altered mental status

[a] All of these symptoms may not be present in head trauma.

tissue, predisposing them to intraparenchymal injuries. Whereas adults are more likely to have focal intracranial hematomas, children are more likely to develop diffuse cerebral edema. Cerebral edema can disrupt cerebral blood flow resulting in ischemic injury.

Normally, blood flow to the brain is maintained at a constant rate by a process known as *autoregulation*. With severe brain injury, autoregulation is disrupted and blood flow to the brain is determined by cerebral perfusion pressure (CPP), which is a measure of the mean arterial pressure (MAP) minus ICP [CPP = MAP − ICP]. Cerebral blood flow is therefore compromised when the MAP is too low (ie, hypotension) or the ICP is too high (ie, cerebral edema). Several of the management strategies in severely brain-injured children focus on maintaining MAP and reducing ICP, but control of CPP after head injury can be quite difficult. Children have a greater capacity for recovery than adults, especially infants and very young children, whose open sutures and fontanelles permit expansion of the skull in response to edema and blood.

In head trauma, both primary and secondary brain injury can occur (Figure 64-1). Primary injury is the structural damage that occurs to the cranium and its contents at the time of the injury. Secondary injury is damage to the brain tissue after the initial event. Such damage may result from hypoxia, hypoperfusion, hypercarbia, hyperthermia, and altered glucose or sodium metabolism. The main management strategies for head trauma victims focus on the prevention of secondary brain injury. Primary brain injury can only be prevented through education and safety.

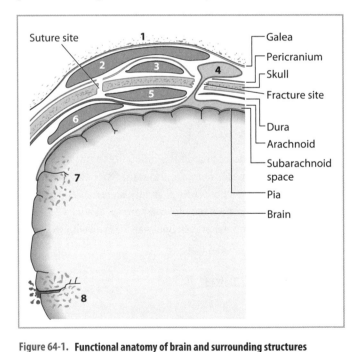

Figure 64-1. Functional anatomy of brain and surrounding structures with sites of pathology. 1. Caput succedaneum. 2. Subgaleal hematoma. 3. Cephalhematoma. 4. Porencephalic cyst or leptomeningeal cyst. 5. Epidural hematoma. 6. Subdural hematoma. 7. Cerebral contusion. 8. Cerebral laceration. (From Tecklenburg FW, Wright MS. Minor head trauma in the pediatric patient. *Pediatr Emerg Care*. 1991;7:40–47, with permission from Wolters Kluwer Health.)

Types of Head Injuries

Even minor head trauma in children can result in fractures to the skull or intracranial injuries. Most skull fractures are simple and linear. Other fracture types are comminuted, diastatic, basilar, and depressed. Comminuted fractures occur when there are multiple skull fragments. Diastatic fractures occur when there is a wide separation at the fracture site. Basilar fractures occur at the base of the skull and often have characteristic findings on physical examination (ie, bilateral periorbital ecchymosis, hemotympanum, postauricular ecchymosis [Battle sign]). Depressed fracture occurs when fragments of the skull are displaced inward, potentially damaging intracranial structures.

Head trauma may result in a **concussion** or mild traumatic brain injury. A concussion is defined as a trauma-induced impairment of neurologic function. This may occur with or without a loss of consciousness (LOC). Neurologic examination is usually normal, but patients may experience somatic symptoms (eg, headache), physical signs (eg, LOC, amnesia), behavioral changes, cognitive impairment, or sleep disturbances. Some of these minor and subtle neurologic sequelae can last for months following the injury (post-concussive syndrome). Most resolve over a relatively short period, typically 7 to 10 days.

A **cerebral contusion** is essentially a bruise of the brain tissue and typically occurs with a more severe injury, such as a high-speed motor vehicle crash. A coup-contrecoup type injury may be produced when the brain strikes the skull on direct impact, bruising one portion of the brain, and then injury occurs to the opposite portion of the brain when rapid deceleration occurs. Clinical manifestations depend on the location of the contusion but often include altered mental status, excessive sleepiness, confusion, and agitation. Small intraparenchymal hemorrhages and swelling of the surrounding tissues are often seen on computed tomography (CT) scan.

Epidural hematomas are collections of blood that accumulate between the skull bone and the tough outer covering of the brain (dura). They are often the result of tears in the middle meningeal artery caused by skull fractures. Classically, patients have initial LOC followed by a lucid interval and then rapid deterioration secondary to brain compression. On CT scan an epidural hematoma appears as a large collection of blood with convex borders next to the skull (Figure 64-2A). Surgical evacuation is required in most cases.

Subdural hematomas accumulate between the dura and the underlying brain tissue. They are associated with both skull fractures and contusions. On CT scan they appear to have crescent-shaped borders (Figure 64-2B). Large subdural hematomas usually require surgical evacuation. In infants and young children, these are often the result of non-accidental trauma.

Diffuse axonal injury occurs when there is extensive damage to the axonal white matter of the brain that results from shearing forces that typically occur with rapid acceleration or deceleration of the brain (Figure 64-2C).

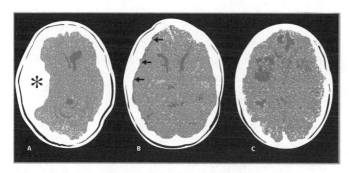

Figure 64-2. A. Epidural hematoma, marked by the asterisk. Note convex borders and midline shift. B. Subdural hematoma. Note crescent shape. C. Diffuse axonal injury. Note ground-glass appearance and tightly compressed ventricles. (Reproduced with permission from Harris JH Jr, Harris WH, Norelline RA. *The Radiology of Emergency Medicine.* **3rd ed. Baltimore, MD: Williams & Wilkins; 1993:15, 16, 17.)**

Evaluation

History

Historical data are obtained during the secondary survey or reassessment phase of evaluation. Prehospital health care providers or witnesses to the injury should be asked about details of the event and the child's status following the event (Questions Box).

Questions

Head Trauma

- What was the mechanism of injury (motor vehicle crash, ejection from motor vehicle, fall, assault)?
- What was the height of the fall?
- What was the type of impact surface?
- What was the shape of the object(s) striking the head?
- What was the child's immediate status after injury?
- What changes in status occurred before arrival at the hospital?
- Did the child lose consciousness? If so, for how long?
- Did the child vomit?
- Did the child have a seizure? If so, when did it occur in relation to the injury and does the child have an underlying seizure disorder?

Physical Examination

Careful attention to the vital signs of children with head injuries is important. The presence of hypertension, bradycardia, and an irregular breathing pattern (**Cushing triad**) all suggest a significant intracranial injury with associated increased ICP.

Secondary survey actions include palpation and inspection of the scalp for soft-tissue swelling, step-offs, lacerations, and fullness of the fontanelle. Facial bones should be tested for stability and deformities. Other clues to possible head trauma include the presence of a septal hematoma, draining blood or fluid from the nose or ears, dental injury, and malocclusion of the mandible. The tympanic membranes should be visualized for the presence of hemotympanum or

cerebrospinal fluid (CSF) otorrhea, which along with postauricular ecchymosis (**Battle sign**), periorbital ecchymosis, or cranial nerve palsies suggest a basilar skull fracture. Funduscopic examination should be performed if possible to look for the presence of papilledema associated with increased ICP or **retinal hemorrhages** that indicate non-accidental trauma.

A comprehensive neurologic examination is the most important part of the secondary survey. This examination should include a mental status assessment, cranial nerve evaluation, presence and quality of deep tendon reflexes, muscle tone, muscle strength, sensation, and cerebellar function. When describing mental status, imprecise terms such as *altered, lethargic,* and *obtunded* should be avoided. Several widely used scoring systems are available for mental status assessment of children who have suffered head trauma that are useful predictors of intracranial injury. A number of scales exist for assessment of the level of consciousness. The most universally accepted and widely used of these scales is the **Glasgow Coma Score** (GCS). It is used routinely in children older than 5 years, but can be modified for younger children. Each scoring system has 3 measured responses (eye opening, verbal, and motor) to a variety of stimuli. Scores should be tabulated when children first present to establish a baseline. They can then be used for reassessment on a regular basis until patients have stabilized or returned to normal mental status. Use of these scores helps promote consistent and accurate communication among health care providers. Tables 64-1 and 64-2 show how to calculate the GCS and modified GCS scores.

Table 64-1. Glasgow Coma Scale	
Elements	*Points*
I. Eye opening	
a. Spontaneous	4
b. To command	3
c. With pain	2
d. No response	1
II. Verbal response[a]	
a. Oriented, converses normally	5
b. Disoriented, confused	4
c. Utters inappropriate words	3
d. Incomprehensible sounds	2
e. No response	1
III. Motor response	
a. Obeys commands	6
b. Localizes pain	5
c. Flexes with pain	4
d. Flexes abnormally with pain	3
e. Extensor response	2
f. None	1
Maximum score	*15*

[a] Assessment of verbal response is modified in children.

Table 64-2. Modified Glasgow Coma Scale for Younger Children	
Elements	**Points**
I. **Eye opening**	
a. Spontaneous	4
b. To command	3
c. With pain	2
d. No response	1
II. **Verbal response**[a]	
a. Coos and babbles	5
b. Irritable cry	4
c. Cries to pain	3
d. Moans to pain	2
e. None	1
III. **Motor response**	
a. Normal spontaneous movement	6
b. Withdraws to touch	5
c. Withdraws to pain	4
d. Abnormal flexion	3
e. Abnormal extension	2
f. None	1
Maximum score	**15**

[a] Assessment of verbal response is modified in children.

The secondary survey should be completed to identify any additional life- or limb-threatening injuries.

Laboratory Testing

All pediatric patients with significant head trauma should have a complete blood cell count and serum electrolytes performed. Bedside glucose should be performed in any child with a head injury with an altered level of consciousness. Toxicological evaluation may be indicated in adolescents who appear to be intoxicated or have an altered level of consciousness. Those infants and children with an intracranial hemorrhage should have screening coagulation studies performed (ie, prothrombin time, activated partial thromboplastin time), as well as a type and screen or crossmatch, should surgery be required.

Imaging Studies

In cases of acute pediatric blunt or penetrating trauma, a non-contrast CT of the head is currently the diagnostic study of choice. It is very sensitive for the detection of acute hemorrhages and skull fractures. It can also provide additional information as to the severity of injury indicating increased ICP, cerebral edema, or pending herniation. Some of the findings on CT that indicate severe brain injury are the shift of midline structures, effacement of the sulci, ventricular enlargement or compression, and loss of the normal gray-white matter differentiation.

Box 64-1. Indications for Computed Tomography Scans in Children With Head Trauma
• Alteration in level of consciousness, with waxing and waning or deteriorating mental status
• Glasgow Coma Score lower than 14
• Focal neurologic deficit(s) on examination
• Examination findings suggestive of a skull fracture
• Posttraumatic seizures
• Persistent vomiting or headache
• Scalp hematoma in a child younger than 2 years
• Prolonged loss of consciousness
• Possibility of penetration of the skull

A list of suggested criteria for obtaining a CT scan for patients with head injuries can be found in Box 64-1. All children classified with moderate to severe head trauma (GCS <14) should have a head CT performed. There is considerable debate about which children who have suffered minor closed head trauma with a normal examination and a GCS of 14 to 15 warrant imaging. There is no pediatric study thus far that has been able to identify a set of clinical criteria to identify all children with radiographic lesions. Vomiting, LOC, and seizures, which can all be seen in intracranial injuries, are relatively poor predictors of radiographic intracranial abnormality in children. The best predictors in children are altered mental status, focal neurologic deficit, and the presence of a skull fracture. Given the small numbers that require actual surgical intervention, some argue that the goal should not necessarily be to identify all of these clinically insignificant lesions but to be selective and thereby minimize unnecessary radiation exposure (see Chapter 15). Others argue that given the lack of reliable clinical criteria, and the possibility of significant intracranial injury in the face of a normal examination, a more liberal use of CT should be employed. The decision to perform a CT scan in these children with minor head trauma currently is based on a variety of factors including historical data, physical findings, age of the child, physician experience, and the psychosocial situation of patients and their families.

With the speed and widespread availability of CT scanners, skull radiographs have relatively little role in the acute evaluation of pediatric head trauma patients. Current CT scans can be performed very quickly, often with the need for no or little sedation. Although sensitive for the detection of skull fractures, plain films do not provide any information about associated intracranial injuries. In addition, several studies have demonstrated that intracranial injuries occur in the absence of a skull fracture, particularly among young pediatric patients. The role of plain films is limited to part of the skeletal survey in suspected cases of non-accidental trauma.

Magnetic resonance imaging (MRI) has little role in the management of the acutely injured head trauma victim. Computed tomography scan is often more sensitive at detecting acute intracranial hemorrhages and is sufficient to guide most immediate patient care issues. Magnetic resonance imaging may be superior to CT for identifying diffuse axonal injury and subtle brain injuries. In general, MRI takes longer to complete, often requires sedation, and the scanners are frequently located away from the ED where the child cannot be monitored appropriately.

One important consideration of any trauma victim is the possibility of a cervical spine injury. Although cervical spine injuries are less common in children, the clinician must maintain a high index of suspicion when presented with a child who has suffered significant head trauma. All children with an altered level of consciousness; significant painful/distracting injuries; an inability to communicate; focal neurologic deficits; or localized pain, swelling, or ecchymosis of the cervical spine require careful evaluation and imaging of the cervical spine.

Management

Assessment and management occur simultaneously when an acutely injured child presents. A primary survey is initially performed with attention to airway, breathing, circulation (ABCs), and cervical spine immobilization. Prompt neurosurgical consultation should be obtained for all children with significant head trauma to assess the need for operative management and ICP monitoring. The primary management goal of significant acute head trauma is the prevention of secondary brain injury by (1) maximizing oxygenation and ventilation, (2) supporting circulation to maximize cerebral perfusion, (3) decreasing elevated ICP, and (4) decreasing cerebral metabolic demands.

Individuals with significant intracranial injuries will often require intubation for airway protection. Those individuals with a GCS of 8 or lower should undergo **rapid sequence intubation** to control the airway. These individuals should be premedicated with etomidate and lidocaine prior to the use of paralytics. Etomidate is a sedative that is cardiovascularly neutral with minimal effect on blood pressure. Most other sedatives can result in hypotension thereby lowering MAP and reducing CPP. Lidocaine is recommended to potentially blunt the transient increase in ICP often associated with orotracheal intubation. In the past, moderate hyperventilation was advocated to reduce ICP. Hyperventilation lowers arterial carbon dioxide partial pressure (Pco_2), leading to cerebral vasoconstriction and decreased cerebral blood flow, lowering ICP. This has been shown to have the unwanted effect of disrupting cerebral metabolism and possibly exacerbating ischemic injury. Currently normoventilation is recommended with the goal of maintaining Pco_2 no lower than 34 mm Hg. Moderate hyperventilation may have a role in the transient management of serious or acute life-threatening elevations in ICP (ie, acute herniation).

Circulation and MAP should be aggressively supported with fluids to prevent hypoperfusion to the brain. Hypovolemia or hypotension should never be assumed to result from head trauma alone. Children should be examined carefully for evidence of additional injury. Central venous pressure monitoring is often necessary to accurately assess volume status. Pressors may be necessary to maintain MAP in euvolemic patients. Morbidity has been shown to significantly increase with subsequent episodes of hypotension that occur.

Elevations in ICP may impede cerebral blood flow and exacerbate ischemic injury. Administration of hypertonic solutions (3% saline), osmotic agents (mannitol), diuretics, and elevation of the head of the bed to 30 degrees to promote venous drainage are all examples of methods used to reduce ICP. Use of mannitol and other diuretics is contraindicated in patients with borderline blood pressures because they can cause hypotension, which can in turn lower MAP, worsening cerebral perfusion. Paralytic agents, sedatives, and analgesics may be needed to prevent agitation, which also leads to increased ICP and increases cerebral metabolic demands. Painful procedures (eg, suctioning) should receive adequate pre-medication with sedatives and analgesics. Intraventricular pressure catheters are often necessary to allow for close monitoring of ICP. In addition, they can be used to drain CSF to help lower elevated ICP.

Hyperthermia and seizure activity should be managed aggressively because these all increase cerebral metabolic demands. Hyperthermia should be managed with antipyretics and active cooling measures. There is conflicting evidence regarding controlled hypothermia in children with severe brain injuries. Future studies will hopefully determine if this is of some benefit as has been shown in certain animal models. Anticonvulsant prophylaxis should also be considered in severely brain-injured children, especially within the first 7 days. It is important to remember that the ability to detect clinical seizure activity is lost if the child is paralyzed.

Serum electrolytes should be followed closely, and any alterations should be minimized. Patients with head injuries should be monitored closely for the development of diabetes insipidus or syndrome of inappropriate secretion of antidiuretic hormone.

Children with large epidural and subdural hematomas will frequently require surgical evacuation. Individuals with depressed skull fractures often require operative management to lift the depressed fragment away from the underlying brain. Children who have suffered significant penetrating head trauma warrant antibiotic and antiepileptic prophylaxis, and may need angiography to assess for vascular injury. They should all have their tetanus status updated if necessary.

Children with minor head injuries (GCS = 14–15) with no LOC or a brief witnessed period of LOC, no focal deficits on neurologic examination, no skull fractures, and without persistent vomiting who demonstrate improvement and normal mental status (GCS = 15) after 4 to 6 hours of observation can be discharged with written instructions if they have adequate transportation back to the hospital, a telephone, and a reliable parent or guardian. Children should be admitted if these criteria cannot be met. Younger children (<2 years of age) are more difficult to assess accurately and consistently and are at higher risk for intracranial injuries. Admission should be strongly considered if their mental status is not completely normal or at baseline. Physicians should be wary of discharging children whose conditions have not improved to baseline following minor injuries or who have persistent emesis, even if their CT scans are normal.

More moderate head injuries (initial GCS = 9–12) necessitate a longer period of evaluation, probably in a monitored setting along with neurosurgical consultation. Severe head injuries (GCS <8) require aggressive stabilization in the ED with the measures described previously and admission to a pediatric intensive care unit.

Children who have suffered a concussion warrant close observation and reevaluation before resuming sporting activities. In the past, grading scales for concussions were devised using severity and duration of symptoms to determine the appropriateness of return to activity. These classification systems have been abandoned, and the decision regarding the resumption of athletic participation should be tailored to the individual. In general, athletes should have complete physical and cognitive rest until they are symptom-free. In addition, they should have a normal neurologic examination, and normal imaging (if performed). Athletes should return to play in a gradual stepwise fashion rather than an abrupt return to full activity and game play. Pediatric and adolescent athletes who have suffered a concussion should never be allowed to return to play the same day of their injury.

Prognosis

Age is the most important prognostic factor in outcome. Younger children tend to do better than older children. It is still difficult to predict the outcome of any individual patient. Scalp lacerations, most skull fractures, and concussions are low-risk injuries. Intracranial hemorrhage, specific skull fractures, head injury secondary to nonaccidental trauma, and trauma accompanied by diffuse cerebral edema are high-risk injuries. If untreated, severe head injury may lead to death from herniation.

Other complications from severe head trauma are posttraumatic seizures, requiring lifelong treatment with anticonvulsants; hydrocephalus, necessitating placement of a ventriculoperitoneal shunt catheter; and persistent vegetative or severely impaired mental states. Penetrating head injuries can result in infections (eg, meningitis, abscess) and vascular injuries (eg, aneurysm, arteriovenous malformations). Sequelae such as post-concussive syndrome may result from less severe head trauma. Some of the characteristics of this syndrome include dizziness, headache, irritability, memory deficits, impaired behavior, and impaired cognitive development. These may persist for months after the head injury and can sometimes be permanent. These children may warrant formal neurobehavioral testing.

Prevention

Despite advancing medical knowledge and excellent critical care available to children with head trauma, little can be done to reduce the severity of primary brain injury once it has occurred. Therefore, pediatric health care providers should make every attempt to educate patients and families about prevention strategies. Some of the most successful prevention strategies involve the required use of restraint devices such as seat belts, and of proper safety gear such as bicycle helmets. Anticipatory guidance and home safety recommendations

provided to parents are also worthwhile. Finally, communities can contribute to injury prevention by providing playground resurfacing, reducing the height of playground equipment, and changing traffic laws. It is only through a combination of these prevention strategies that morbidity and mortality of pediatric head trauma will be truly reduced.

CASE RESOLUTION

The case scenario involves a young child with a significant mechanism of injury; brief LOC; and a depressed, altered mental status. Initial physical findings prompt suspicion of a depressed skull fracture and overlying soft tissue injury. Appropriate diagnostic tools after evaluation of airway, breathing, and circulation are a cranial CT scan followed by admission for observation, monitoring, and serial neurologic examination. Operative repair of the skull fracture may be necessary.

Selected References

American Academy of Pediatrics Committee on Quality Improvement, American Academy of Family Physicians Commission on Clinical Policies and Research. The management of minor closed head injury in children. *Pediatrics.* 1999;104:1407–1415

Atabaki SM, Stiell IG, Bazarian JJ, et al. A clinical decision rule for cranial computed tomography in minor pediatric head trauma. *Arch Pediatr Adolesc Med.* 2008;162:439–445

Bruce DA. Head trauma. In: Fleisher GR, Ludwig S, eds. *Textbook of Pediatric Emergency Medicine.* 5th ed. Baltimore, MD: Williams & Wilkins; 2005

Dunning J, Daly JP, Lomas JP, Lecky F, Batchelor J, Makaway-Jones K. Derivation of the children's head injury algorithm for the prediction of important clinical events decision rule for head injury in children. *Arch Dis Child.* 2006;91:885–891

Goldstein B, Powers KS. Head trauma in children. *Pediatr Rev.* 1994;15:213–219

Halstead ME, Walter KD. Clinical report—sport-related concussion in children and adolescents. *Pediatrics.* 2010;126:597–615

Huh JW, Raghupathi R. New concepts in treatment of pediatric traumatic brain injury. *Anesth Clin.* 2009;27:213–240

Hutchison JS, Ward RE, Jacques L, et al. Hypothermia therapy after traumatic brain injury in children. *N Engl J Med.* 2008;358:2447–2456

Kirkwood MW, Yeates KO, Wilson PE. Pediatric sport-related concussion: a review of the clinical management of an oft-neglected population. *Pediatrics.* 2006;117:1359–1369

Koestler J, Keshavarz R. Penetrating head injury in children: a case report and review of the literature. *J Emerg Med.* 2001;21:145–150

McCrory P, Meeuwisse W, Johnston K, et al. Consensus statement on concussion in sport: the 3rd international conference on concussion in sport held in Zurich, November 2008. *J Athl Train.* 2009;44:434–448

Michaud LJ, Duhaime A, Batshaw ML. Traumatic brain injury in children. *Pediatr Clin North Am.* 1993;40:553–565

Osmond MH, Klassen TP, Wells GA, et al. CATCH: a clinical decision rule for the use of computed tomography in children with minor head injury. *CMAJ.* 2010;182:341–348

Palchak MJ, Holmes JF, Vance CW, et al. A decision rule for identifying children at low risk for brain injuries after blunt head trauma. *Ann Emerg Med.* 2003;42:492–506

Palchak MJ, Holmes JF, Vance CW, et al. Does an isolated history of loss of consciousness or amnesia predict brain injuries in children after blunt head trauma? *Pediatrics.* 2004;113:e507–e513

Rivara FP. Epidemiology and prevention of pediatric traumatic brain injury. *Pediatr Ann.* 1994;23:12–17

Schutzman SA, Barnes P, Duhaime AC, et al. Evaluation and management of children younger than two years old with apparently minor head trauma: proposed guidelines. *Pediatrics.* 2001;107:983–993

Schutzman SA, Greenes DS. Pediatric minor head trauma. *Ann Emerg Med.* 2001;37:65–74

Sun BC, Hoffman JR, Mower WR. Evaluation of a modified prediction instrument to identify significant pediatric intracranial injury after blunt head trauma. *Ann Emerg Med.* 2007;49:325–332

Swaminathan A, Levy P, Legome E. Evaluation and management of moderate to severe pediatric head trauma. *J Emerg Med.* 2009; 37:63–68

Tecklenburg FW, Wright MS. Minor head trauma in the pediatric patient. *Pediatr Emerg Care.* 1991;7:40–47

Zuckerman GB, Conway EE. Accidental head injury. *Pediatr Ann.* 1997;26:621–632

CHAPTER 65

Increased Intracranial Pressure

Kenneth R. Huff, MD

CASE STUDY

A 7-year-old boy has a 2-week history of recurrent vomiting. No fever, abdominal pain, or diarrhea has accompanied the vomiting; the vomiting has no particular relationship to meals; and the boy's appetite has decreased only slightly. The vomiting has gradually increased in frequency and is occurring every night. Yesterday there were 4 episodes. The boy's parents have noticed that their son is generally less active; he spends more time playing on the floor of his room and does not want to ride his bicycle or play with neighborhood friends. Some unsteadiness in the boy's gait has developed in the last few days. His parents attribute this to weakness from the vomiting.

The child's vital signs are normal except for a blood pressure of 130/80 mm Hg. Although the boy is somewhat pale and uncomfortable, he does not appear to be in acute distress. His abdominal examination is unremarkable. His speech is grammatically correct but sparse and hesitant, and he seems inattentive. On lateral and upgaze the boy has coarse nystagmus, and upgaze is somewhat limited.

Some diplopia on left gaze is apparent, with slight failure of left eye abduction. The left eye does not blink as much as the right eye. Fundal examination discloses elevated disks with indistinct margins. No upper extremity weakness is evident. The right foot is slightly weaker than the left, ankle tone is bilaterally increased, and 3 to 4 beats of clonus on the right and bilateral positive Babinski reflexes are present. Some tremor occurs in both arms with finger-to-nose testing. The boy walks with shuffling, small steps; his gait has a slight lurching character; and he veers to the right.

Questions

1. What clinical situations are associated with increased intracranial pressure (ICP)?
2. What is the pathophysiological process leading to ICP?
3. What studies are used to evaluate children with ICP?
4. What measures are used to treat children with ICP?

The signs and symptoms of increased ICP are often a signal of a serious intracranial process that may require surgical or intensive care intervention depending on the underlying cause. Although only a relatively small number of effective medical and surgical treatments for increased ICP are available, greater understanding is accumulating about when to initiate them. It is important to recognize signs and symptoms early and determine the underlying cause; treatment of the cause often resolves the secondarily increased ICP problem, particularly if deployed early in its course. In some cases, however, increased ICP is a potentially life-threatening critical care issue of itself where ongoing management, along with that of the underlying cause, is key for the child's survival.

Epidemiology

Head trauma is a leading cause of increased ICP. Infants may be victims of non-accidental trauma; older children may be stricken pedestrians or bicycle riders, occupants of crashed motor vehicles, or victims of falls or sports injuries; and children of any age may be victims of penetrating trauma such as gunshots. Such trauma is a major source of morbidity in children and requires careful monitoring and management of ICP.

Brain tumors are the most common solid neoplasms in children and frequently lead to increased ICP either by direct mass effect or blockage of cerebrospinal fluid (CSF) flow. Ischemic brain damage resulting from a difficult delivery at birth, a submersion incident, or a major cerebral vessel thrombosis is also a cause of increased ICP. Cytotoxic causes of brain swelling, such as lead intoxication and liver failure in Reye syndrome, are less common etiologies.

Idiopathic intracranial hypertension (also called benign intracranial hypertension or pseudotumor cerebri) may also lead to increased ICP. This condition is associated most frequently with obese adolescent females, but has also been seen with thrombosis of a venous sinus caused by a clotting diathesis or following complicated otitis media or mastoiditis, following the use of high doses of vitamin A or tetracycline, or following withdrawal of steroid therapy.

Clinical Presentation

Children with increased ICP may present with a history of recurrent vomiting, lethargy, and new headaches of increasing frequency or severity (crescendo headaches) or that awaken them from sleep. A prior history of trauma, ischemia, meningitis, or having a CSF shunt, or a concomitant history of intoxication, such as with lead or metabolic aberration (ie, Reye syndrome or diabetic ketoacidosis), may also raise suspicions of increased ICP in the child with compatible examination findings. Neonates with intraventricular hemorrhage or meningomyelocele are prone to hydrocephalus. Children with cyanotic congenital heart disease are prone to abscesses, and children with sickle cell disease can present with strokes or hemorrhages causing increased ICP. In endemic areas of the world, cerebral malaria and intraventricular cysticercosis are frequent causes of increased ICP. Physical findings may include elevated optic disk, failure of upward gaze, hypertonicity of the extremities, and depressed alertness or inattention. Localized findings on neurologic examination may point to a lesion indicative of a space-occupying intracranial mass, which could contribute to increased ICP (Dx Box).

 Increased Intracranial Pressure

- Loss of appetite, nausea, vomiting, headache, or lethargy
- Inattention, decreased arousability
- Papilledema, upward gaze paresis
- Increased tone, positive Babinski reflex
- Focal signs and history compatible with an intracranial mass
- Mass lesion, cerebral edema, or enlarged ventricles in an imaging study
- Elevated cerebrospinal fluid pressure measured manometrically by needle or catheter in the intrathecal or intracranial space

Pathophysiology

The problem of increased ICP can be understood in terms of the Monro-Kellie doctrine, which applies to the rigid cranial compartment and pressure-volume relationships of the contents. This doctrine is conceptually useful even though not always quantitatively predictive because of the variable compliance of the child's skull and dural membranes. Intracranial volume has 3 main components: brain parenchyma, CSF, and blood. Except in the first 2 years of life before most of the cranial sutures are fused, the skull and dura form a relatively rigid compartment; any increase in 1 of the 3 intracranial volume components must occur at the expense of 1 or both of the other 2. Decreased volume leads to increased pressure in a somewhat indirect inverse relationship, however, because of compliance of the skull, sutures, and dura. As compliance decreases, pressure rises more rapidly. Irreversible damage to brain tissue occurs primarily as a result of pressure of the other components overtaking the arterial blood pressure and not allowing adequate tissue perfusion. In younger children, non-fused sutures allow more compliance if volume increases are relatively slow, but this factor is not as

true for acute volume increases. In addition, pressure gradients exist across compartments, sites of CSF flow obstruction, or even around lesions within brain parenchyma, which may lead to focal findings that are more difficult to explain by global ICP or perfusion changes.

Changes in any of the 3 components making up the intracranial volume may result in increased ICP in several ways. First, the brain parenchyma component may be directly increased by mass lesions such as neoplasms, abscesses, or hemorrhages. Edema may increase the brain parenchyma volume. Fluid may accumulate because of vascular leakage due to cytokines, termed vasogenic edema. Brain edema may also result from cytotoxic damage, cell death, and necrosis. Cytotoxic processes include swelling of intact cells, cell rupture producing increased interstitial oncotic pressure from released proteins and ions, and cellular inflammatory and repair processes. Cytotoxic brain edema may be caused by various cellular insults including hypoxemia; ischemia; toxins, including neuronal excitotoxins; and depletion of energy substrates. These cellular insults may in turn be a consequence of a diversity of local or diffuse brain problems including major vessel thrombosis, trauma (eg, local contusion or diffuse axonal injury), anoxia from cardiac arrest, hypertension, encephalitic infection, or metabolic poisoning. Edema with head trauma may be a combination of vasogenic and cytotoxic edema, but also may be related to neurogenic inflammatory release of substance P and calcitonin gene–related peptide.

Second, the pressure of the CSF volume component (ventricles or subarachnoid spaces) may increase in hydrocephalus. Hydrocephalus can result in 2 ways: (1) from a discrepancy in the rate of formation of CSF relative to absorption and (2) from an obstruction between the point of formation in the lateral ventricles and the sites of absorption at the arachnoid granulations in the post-neonatal brain or brain parenchyma itself in the neonatal brain. An obstruction can occur with a congenital malformation; parenchymal or CSF mass such as a cyst or neoplasm; CSF inflammatory cells from meningitis, ventriculitis, or hemorrhage; displaced brain parenchyma; subarachnoid protein or debris; or even overgrowth of dural tissue. The small passageways connecting the ventricular system, the foramen of Monro and the aqueduct of Sylvius; the exits of the ventricular system, the foramen of Magendie and foramen of Luschka; and the cisterns surrounding the brain stem are particularly vulnerable points of obstruction. A third type of brain edema, interstitial edema, is characterized by transependymal transudation of CSF into the adjacent white matter and is generally seen in patients with hydrocephalus.

Third, ICP may rise because the intravascular volume component may increase. One process that leads to this increase is venous outflow obstruction such as occurs with a dural sinus thrombosis. Other processes that raise jugular venous pressure may also increase ICP. In addition, the intracranial arterial vascular volume is affected by carbon dioxide partial pressure. It not only increases with hypercarbia but also decreases with hypocarbia, which allows for central neurogenic or iatrogenic lowering of ICP by hyperventilation.

Because the process is frequently dynamic, it has proven useful to quantitate ICP for management purposes, although values in children are not as well correlated with pathophysiology as in adults. Intracranial pressure is often recorded as cm H_2O while blood pressure is noted as mm Hg, and both types of units are noted here. Normal ICP levels are somewhat lower in the neonatal and infantile period at 2.5 to 6.5 cm H_2O (2–5 mm Hg), but in older children, pressures above 20 cm H_2O (15 mm Hg) are abnormal and may become symptomatic above 26 cm H_2O (20 mm Hg). Although it is possible to have normal mental function up to 52 cm H_2O (40 mm Hg), the ICP becomes clinically significant when the perfusion pressure is compromised, which begins when the ICP is 91 cm H_2O (70 mm Hg) below the mean arterial pressure, and it becomes more dangerous as the ICP approaches 52 to 65 cm H_2O (40–50 mm Hg) below the mean arterial pressure. Decreased perfusion produces swollen, damaged tissue, which further exacerbates the pressure-volume problem in a snowballing fashion.

As ICP increases, brain perfusion pressure may be maintained transiently by a spontaneous increase in mean arterial pressure, a response referred to as Cushing phenomenon. Although the relationship may not be universally reliable, when it is present with other suggestive clinical circumstances, the rise in systemic pressure can be a useful clinical sign of increased ICP. Normally changes in arterial cerebrovascular resistance meet changes in perfusion pressure to maintain constant cerebral blood flow, a process called *autoregulation*. However, this process is frequently compromised after head trauma or asphyxia.

Acute or subacute changes in pressure in an intracranial compartment may produce a pressure gradient that may precipitate a brain herniation syndrome (Figure 65-1). An ominous heralding sign of transtentorial herniation of the uncus of the temporal lobe is loss of the pupillary light reflex caused by entrapment of the third cranial nerve. This herniation often leads to irreversible brain stem damage as well as infarcts and additional secondary edema. Focally increased

posterior fossa pressure may result in a pressure cone downward through the foramen magnum–compressing medullary centers leading to apnea and death. A marginally compensated system could be decompensated by an ill-advised lumbar puncture when the spinal compartment pressure is acutely lowered, increasing the pressure gradient across the foramen magnum.

Differential Diagnosis

Seizures, metabolic derangements, and complicated migraine sometimes have a clinical presentation similar to increased ICP. In children who are only partially responsive, distinguishing an ictal or postictal state from a condition that may be producing increased ICP is sometimes difficult. Findings that suggest a seizure include rhythmic, clonic movements or sudden myoclonic jerks; rapid or variable changes of tone or posturing that are different from decerebrate posturing; abrupt, fluctuating changes of autonomic function (eg, heart rate, blood pressure, pupillary size); saliva production without swallowing; and history of prior seizures. Sometimes, however, only direct electroencephalogram (EEG) monitoring and ICP monitoring are able to distinguish ongoing electrographic "subclinical" seizure activity from increased ICP as the cause of the change in level of responsiveness.

In some cases, diffuse brain dysfunction from a toxic or metabolic etiology mimics increased ICP. Such toxic/metabolic causes include medication toxicity, electrolyte or blood chemistry imbalances, and systemic infections. With toxic/metabolic disorders, inattention is often accompanied by a confusional state with disorientation, incoherence, and sometimes agitation. In contrast, with increased ICP, inattention is frequently accompanied by slowness of thought, perseveration, decreased mental activity, and impaired gait, although these differences are not universal.

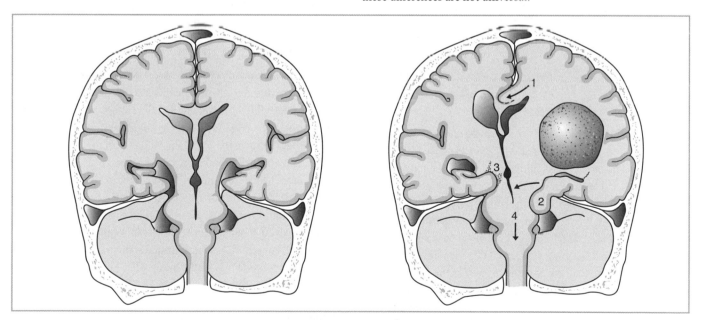

Figure 65-1. Depiction of the anatomy of several potential herniation syndromes caused by intracranial compartment pressure gradients related to a mass (hematoma, neoplasm, or acutely necrotic brain tissue) in a cerebral hemisphere. 1. Transfalcine herniation. 2. Uncal herniation. 3. Contralateral tentorial-midbrain damage. 4. Central herniation and foramen magnum pressure cone. These syndromes often lead to further brain ischemia and additional increases in intracranial pressure. The drawing on the left depicts a normal brain.

The symptoms and signs of complicated migraine sometimes also mimic those of increased ICP. A characteristic prodromal symptom period or the "pounding" nature of the pain may help separate migraine from increased ICP. At the initial headache presentation or when only a short headache history is present, the complicated migraine diagnosis may be one of exclusion, however. If children display focal neurologic signs along with some of the general symptoms of increased ICP, imaging studies to rule out a space-occupying lesion and confirm the safety of a lumbar puncture, and a measurement of normal pressure by lumbar puncture manometry, may need to be performed to support the diagnosis of migraine.

Evaluation

History

A thorough neurologic history should be taken (Questions Box). Headache, nausea and vomiting, drowsiness, personality change, and changes in visual acuity are important historical factors. The headache history may be "crescendo" in frequency or intensity and of only a few days' or weeks' duration. The headache may be worsened by cough, micturition, defecation, or other valsalva-like actions.

Questions

Increased Intracranial Pressure

- How long has the child been vomiting?
- When does the vomiting occur?
- Is the vomiting related to meals?
- Do the headaches awaken the child?
- Has there been a progressive decline in activity level or loss of developmental skills?
- Does the child display weakness or change in gait?
- Does the child have a recent history of trauma or potential ischemic event?

Physical Examination

Vital signs and head circumference should be noted. A careful neurologic examination is warranted whenever increased ICP is suspected. Particular attention should be paid to the components of the mental status and level of responsiveness and alertness of patients. The presence of papilledema and the cranial nerve functions should be assessed. Retinal hemorrhages may raise the suspicion of nonaccidental trauma. Cranial nerve VI is particularly susceptible to increased ICP. Impaired upward gaze and lid retraction may be present. Specific muscle tone and strength as well as the gait characteristics should be evaluated in cooperative children who are able to resist and stand up. Posturing responses and the breathing pattern should be noted in comatose children to help ascertain brain stem localization of the lesion. In such children, findings should be reassessed at frequent intervals to follow a potentially rapid process such

as impending tentorial or brain stem herniation, which would necessitate immediate intervention measures.

Useful quick-assessment instruments for initial, rapid evaluation and subsequent monitoring are the Glasgow Coma Scale (GCS) and Children's (ages ≤4 years) Coma Scale (see Table 64-1 and Table 64-2 in Chapter 64). However, these scales are a useful stratifying "shorthand" description but are not sufficient for every clinical decision related to patients with increased ICP.

In infants, a unique collection of signs—enlarged head circumference; bulging, raised fontanelle; frontal bone bossing with prominent venous distention; "sunset sign" (inability to elevate the eyes and lid retraction from midbrain tectal pressure); hypertonicity; and hyperreflexia—may be secondary to increased ICP from hydrocephalus. Papilledema is not present, perhaps related to greater compliance of the infant skull.

Chronic hydrocephalus may result in optic atrophy, depressed hypothalamic functions, spastic lower limbs, incontinence, and learning problems.

Laboratory Tests

If mental status changes are suggestive of a toxic or metabolic aberration, appropriate laboratory screens should be performed. These may include electrolytes, toxicological screen, liver function tests, and kidney function tests. A CSF examination should be done if signs of meningeal irritation or infection are present without lateralized signs of altered tone or strength. Imaging study evidence of an intercompartmental pressure gradient that could lead to herniation after lumbar puncture would also lead one away from that procedure, but CSF analysis and pressure measurements can also be made from ventricular taps after ventriculostomy. If there are clinical signs of increased ICP and no focal clinical or imaging signs of a mass, then a lumbar puncture can be both diagnostic and therapeutic for idiopathic intracranial hypertension.

Imaging Studies

A computed tomography (CT) or magnetic resonance imaging scan should be performed whenever children's signs or symptoms indicate the possibility of increased ICP. Severe head trauma patients frequently have a dynamic pathophysiology and may benefit from serial CT scanning in the early hours along with their ICP monitoring. Intravenous (IV) contrast should be given if disruption in the blood–brain barrier (eg, infection, inflammation, neoplasia) is suspected and children are not hypersensitive and have adequate kidney function. A magnetic resonance venogram can be obtained if there is a possibility of a venous sinus thrombosis. Computed tomography angiography or traditional intraluminal angiography with the capability of intervention may be the best studies in the case of intracranial hemorrhage of unknown source.

Management

If idiopathic intracranial hypertension is diagnosed, pressure should be monitored periodically with lumbar punctures. Increased

ICP may respond to diuretics such as acetazolamide at high dose (20 mg/kg/d) or furosemide, as well as the removal of CSF during the lumbar puncture. The primary danger in this condition is an expanding blind spot and eventual blindness due to pressure at the optic nerve head. Visual fields should also be monitored, and if medical therapy is not successful, then optic nerve sheath fenestration or lumbar peritoneal shunt placement can be done surgically.

When diagnostic imaging studies reveal an etiology for the increased ICP, if it is a rapidly enlarging surgically accessible lesion such as an epidural hematoma, then management is emergently directed there, and immediate **neurosurgical craniotomy for drainage and hemostasis** may be necessary. Other focal space-occupying lesions seen on scans may not require immediate craniotomy, depending on size, position, and accompanying edema of the lesion as well as the compliance of the surrounding structures and the distortion of normal brain tissue and potential for loss of perfusion; neoplastic lesions may require diagnostic biopsy or excisional biopsy within a few days if surgically accessible. **Mineralocorticoids (dexamethasone 0.25–0.5 mg/kg every 6 hours)** are useful in situations in which the pressure is produced by a component of vasogenic edema, such as that surrounding neoplasms. A histamine H_2 blocker should also be used to help prevent gastric stress ulcer. Hypotonic IV fluids should be avoided, and the patient should be monitored for the syndrome of inappropriate secretion of antidiuretic hormone with serum and urine osmolalities. Hypoglycemia and hyperglycemia should also be avoided. If acute danger of herniation due to a pressure gradient produced by CSF flow blockage is present, then a temporary ventriculostomy may be indicated to relieve the CSF pressure. If an infectious process is present, including focal lesions, abscess, cerebritis, or encephalitis, **antibiotics** and/or **antiviral** agents are indicated after appropriate cultures, serology, and molecular diagnostic tests have been done. Following directed specific treatment of the underlying lesion, increased ICP may eventually resolve spontaneously. If hydrocephalus due to CSF flow obstruction is still present after initial therapy, **ventriculoperitoneal shunting of CSF** may be necessary. Endoscopic third ventriculotomy avoids long-term shunt hardware complications of obstruction and infection, but is less successful in younger children than older ones.

Encephalopathic children whose ICP is markedly elevated or likely to rise rapidly require treatment in an intensive care unit. If there is no mass or other space-occupying lesion or necrotic, traumatized tissue able to be surgically removed, then interventional measures are directed toward preventing eventual loss of perfusion of normal brain tissue. In patients with head injury, a GCS score of 8 or less can be used as a guideline for ICP monitoring. Intracranial pressure can be monitored on an ongoing basis with commonly used neurosurgically placed devices including the fiberoptic microtransducer and intraventricular catheter or ventriculostomy. The former device can measure pressure in brain parenchyma as well as in fluid-filled spaces. An advantage of the latter device is that it also allows for therapeutic CSF drainage to relieve pressure. It carries a slight risk of infection (increasing to a plateau at day 4 of 1%–2% per day) or hemorrhage and may be difficult to place if ventricles are small or shifted. Intracranial pressure monitoring with neurosurgically placed devices and therapy based on the measurements, however, have not been helpful in many cases of ischemic damage, infection, or poisoning because of the totality of brain involvement without normal remaining tissue to which perfusion could be maintained.

Children with a decreased or fluctuating level of responsiveness may require EEG monitoring of cerebral electrical activity. The EEG helps diagnose the abnormal responsiveness as seizure threshold may fluctuate and seizures may occur even in the presence of increased ICP. Anticonvulsant therapy is indicated if evidence of clinical or electrographic seizures is present. In addition, the EEG may be used to monitor barbiturate- or benzodiazepine-induced coma, which may be used for severely increased ICP.

Airway patency and ventilation are important in children with increased ICP because hypoxia and hypercarbia can contribute to vasodilation and increased pressure. Rapid sequence intubation should be performed to minimize elevations of ICP. Ketamine and succinylcholine can increase ICP also. Transmission of elevated intrathoracic pressure to intracranial vessels can be avoided by sedation and decreasing the inspiratory phase of the ventilator. If acute lowering of pressure is necessary, hyperventilation to reduce the intracranial arterial blood volume is most effective, but care must be taken to avoid decreasing brain cell perfusion to the point of producing ischemic damage and exacerbating the problem. It is recommended that carbon dioxide partial pressure be kept at 30 to 35 mm Hg. Elevating the head to about 30 degrees and avoiding flexion or excessive turning of the neck to prevent jugular kinking are also effective in reducing ICP. Because the goal is to ensure perfusion while lowering ICP, maintaining and even elevating systemic mean arterial pressure by appropriate use of fluid therapy and pressor agents are key. Central venous pressure monitoring may also be helpful.

Diuretic agents such as mannitol (osmotherapy) (0.25–1 g/kg bolus) may also be useful in reducing brain volume by removing water, changing the rheologic characteristics of blood, and producing reflex vasoconstriction, but caution is advised. Mannitol, as a chronic infusion, can eventually cross the blood–brain barrier and draw more fluid into the brain. It is most effective where the blood–brain barrier is intact. Hypertonic saline (3%) as a continuous infusion may be an effective alternative. Serum osmolarity greater than 320 mOsm/kg can lead to renal failure. By giving diuretic agents at intervals as a bolus and titrating up to the ICP-lowering dose, such effects can generally be avoided. Sometimes these agents are used to counter ICP plateau waves or increased pressure with endotracheal suctioning or other procedures.

In children with severe refractory increased ICP, especially if secondary to an acute focal process, barbiturates such as pentobarbital or the benzodiazepine midazolam can be given as a continuous IV infusion with appropriate monitoring of brain electrical activity, serum levels, and systemic and brain perfusion pressures

> **Box 65-1. Management Interventions in Increased ICP**
>
> - Maintain serum osmols at 300–320 mOsm.
> - Keep head elevated to 30 degrees.
> - Maintain normal or elevated systemic blood pressure.
> - Control hyperventilation to Pa_{CO_2} at 30–35 mm Hg.
> - Provide supplemental O_2 and PEEP as needed to keep Pa_{O_2} >90 mm Hg and Fi_{O_2} <50%.
> - If ICP progressively rises, pressure waves >20 mm Hg last longer than 5 minutes, or any pressure in first 24 hours is >30 mm Hg, then give mannitol, 250–1,000 mg/kg IV.
> - If mannitol needs repeating in <4 hours or osmolality is >320 mOsm
>   — Give pentobarbital, 5 mg/kg IV, then 2 mg/kg/h IV monitoring to blood level of 25–35 mg/mL, burst-suppression pattern with 10 s between bursts on EEG, and cardiac index >2.7 L/min/m².
>
>   *or*
>
>   — Give midazolam by titrating the dose starting at 0.1 mg/kg/hr IV to the same EEG criteria and limited by the same cardiac index criteria.
>
> If the cerebral lesion is primarily unihemispheric and pressure is rapidly Increasing, hemicraniectomy should be considered
>
> ---
>
> Abbreviations: EEG, electroencephalogram; Fio2, fraction of inspired oxgen; ICP, intracranial pressure; IV, intravenous Paco2, carbon dioxide partial pressure; Pao2, oxygen partial pressure; PEEP, positive end-expiratory pressure.

(Box 65-1). These agents may serve to reduce brain metabolism without impairing vascular autoregulation significantly. Their risk is in reducing cardiac output and with associated infections, particularly pneumonia. Xenon CT measures multiple areas of local blood flow and may be a useful bedside technique to help specify targeted therapies. Decompressive craniotomy or craniectomy in early severe trauma in small series of patients has been associated with up to 50% good outcomes. Hypothermia to 93.2°F (34°C) for head injury and cardiac arrest, and numerous "neuroprotective" agents, have been and continue to be studied as means to slow metabolism and excitotoxic glutamatergic damage and reduce the rate of cytotoxic edema increase and spread in the penumbra surrounding the irreversibly damaged brain tissue.

Prognosis

Children may recover fully from increased ICP if brain perfusion pressure is adequately maintained and the underlying brain lesion generating the increased pressure can be resolved. Ultimately the prognosis depends on the nature of the lesion; its propensity to generate ICP that may be refractory to treatment, leading to irreversible brain tissue damage or death; and its permanence or potential for recurrence.

> **CASE RESOLUTION**
>
> The boy in the case history has focal signs and symptoms referable to the posterior fossa brain stem and cerebellum as well as symptoms of increased ICP. An emergent CT scan shows subacute hydrocephalus due to obstruction of CSF flow produced by a large mass in the cerebellum and brain stem on the left side. He begins taking dexamethasone with some relief of the increased ICP symptoms. Two days later a ventriculostomy is placed along with surgical removal of the mass, which is found to be a medulloblastoma. Because the ICP eventually subsides over the next few days and the CT scans show decreasing ventriculomegally, a ventriculoperitoneal shunt is not required and the ventricular drain is removed. The boy's recovery is otherwise uneventful, and he begins staging evaluation for further malignant brain tumor therapy.

Selected References

American Academy of Pediatrics Committee on Child Abuse and Neglect. Shaken baby syndrome: inflicted cerebral trauma. *Pediatrics.* 1993;92:872–875

Ball A, Clarke C. Idiopathic intracranial hypertension. *Lancet Neurol.* 2006;5:433–442

Del Bigio M. Cellular damage and prevention in childhood hydrocephalus. *Brain Pathol.* 2004;14:317–324

Fishman RA. *Cerebrospinal Fluid in Diseases of the Nervous System.* 2nd ed. Philadelphia, PA: W. B. Saunders; 1992

Garton H, Piatt J. Hydrocephalus. *Pediatr Clin North Am.* 2004;51:305–325

Huff K. Central nervous system failure. In: Osborn L, DeWitt T, First L, Zenel J, eds. *Pediatrics.* Philadelphia, PA: Elsevier; 2005

Kotagal S. Increased intracranial pressure. In: Swaiman K, Ashwal S, Ferriero D, eds. *Pediatric Neurology Principles and Practice.* 4th ed. Philadelphia, PA: Mosby; 2006

Marcoux K. Management of increased intracranial pressure in the critically ill child with an acute neurological injury. *AACN Clin Issues.* 2005;16:212–231

CHAPTER 66

Management of Dehydration in Children: Fluid and Electrolyte Therapy

Sudhir K. Anand, MD

CASE STUDY

A 2-year-old boy presents to your office after 2 days of vomiting and diarrhea. His siblings were both ill a few days ago with similar symptoms. Two weeks ago his weight was 12 kg at a well-child visit. Today his weight is 10.8 kg. He has a pulse of 130 beats/min, respiratory rate of 28 breaths/min, and blood pressure of 85/55. He is alert and responsive but appears tired. He has dry mucous membranes, no tears with crying, and slightly sunken-appearing eyeballs. His capillary refill is 2 seconds. He urinated a small amount about 6 hours ago. Despite his mother's best efforts in your office, the patient has vomited all of the oral rehydration therapy (ORT) given to him. You draw serum electrolytes, blood urea nitrogen (BUN), and creatinine and initiate intravenous (IV) rehydration and give 2 boluses of 240 mL normal saline (NS; 0.9% NaCl solution) each.

Questions

1. How does one assess the magnitude of dehydration in children?
2. What are the different types of dehydration?
3. How does one determine the type and amount of fluid that a dehydrated child requires?
4. How does one assess renal status in a dehydrated child?
5. What is the role of electrolyte and acid-base laboratory studies in the evaluation of the dehydrated child?

Dehydration due to gastrointestinal and other disorders, especially diarrhea, is one of the most common medical problems encountered in children younger than 5 years. During the past 50 years or more, the usual therapy for children who are hospitalized with dehydration has been to administer IV fluids starting with 1 or 2 boluses of NS (0.9% NaCl solution). This is followed by the administration of a sodium solution of variable concentration (usually 0.45% NaCl) mixed with 5% dextrose over next 24 to 48 hours until the child is able to take oral fluids. The exact amount of fluid and electrolytes is calculated using complicated formulas to provide maintenance fluids and correction of remaining deficit (deficit therapy). Holliday, who in the 1950s first recommended the calculation of maintenance therapy, more recently has suggested that dehydration management should focus on rapid restoration of extracellular fluids (ECF deficit) followed by ORT and traditional calculations of fluid deficits should be abandoned. Alternatively, Moritz along with several pediatric nephrologists and intensivists have recommended that we forgo

Na$^+$ calculations in hospitalized children and rely solely on isotonic NS (0.9% NaCl solution) for their management. While this chapter incorporates the above suggestions where appropriate, it continues the traditional approach to maintenance and deficit therapy because an understanding of the pathophysiology of dehydration helps in the management not only of dehydrated children but also of children with other types of fluid and electrolyte disorders.

Epidemiology

Over the past 25 years and associated with the advent of ORT, hospital admissions and mortality due to diarrhea and dehydration have decreased all over the world; nevertheless, diarrhea continues to be one of the leading medical problems in children younger than 5 years. In the United States an estimated 150,000 to 180,000 hospitalizations due to diarrhea occur each year in such children. In addition, diarrhea is responsible for 2 million to 3 million outpatient visits.

Table 66-1. Caloric Method of Determining Maintenance Fluid Requirements in Healthy Children (Holliday-Segar Method)	
Weight	*Maintenance Fluid Requirement for 24 Hours*
3[a]–10 kg	100 mL/kg/d[b] = 4 mL/kg/h
11–20 kg	50 mL/kg/d for each kg above 10 kg + 1,000 mL (fluid requirement for first 10 kg) = 40+2 mL/kg/h for each kg between 11–20 kg
>20 kg	20 mL/kg/d for each kg above 20 kg + 1,500 mL (fluid requirement for first 20 kg) = 60+1 mL/kg/h for each kg >20 kg

[a] Children weighing less than 3 kg may have altered fluid requirements owing to prematurity or other conditions.

[b] During the first 2 to 3 days of life, normal term infants require less fluid (approximately 80 mL/kg) because they mobilize excess extracellular fluid.

Maintenance Fluid and Electrolyte Requirements

The body has a **maintenance fluid requirement** to replace daily normal losses that occur through the kidney, intestines, skin, and respiratory tract. Of the various methods used to determine fluid needs, the most common is the **caloric method,** also called Holliday-Segar method, which is based on the linear relationship between metabolic rate and fluid needs. For every calorie expended in metabolism, a child requires about 1 mL of water. Metabolic rate in children is a function of body surface area. Infants, with higher relative surface areas per unit of body weight, have higher metabolic rates and, therefore, higher fluid requirements per unit weight. As children grow, their relative surface area decreases as does their metabolic rate and fluid requirement per unit weight. Using this relationship, maintenance fluid needs can be calculated for the healthy child using the method outlined in Table 66-1. These calculations of fluid needs are often used to determine the amount of IV fluids provided to a hospitalized child or to calculate the approximate amount of fluid a healthy child requires orally to maintain hydration. However, **these calculations may not be appropriate for critically ill children, some of whom require fluid restriction and others of whom may have increased fluid needs**. Moreover, the caloric method makes no allowance for extra fluid needed for weight gain, growth, activity, or pathophysiological states that increase fluid needs (such as fever). The fluid requirement derived from this method is valid to determine the daily fluid need for an essentially healthy child. Thriving infants normally drink more fluid than this method suggests. On average, growing infants may take 150 to 200 mL/kg/day of milk (breast milk or infant formula) as desired to support the average weight gain of 30 g/day usually observed in the first few months of life.

Replacement of normal daily losses of electrolytes is considered when a child is not able to take an adequate nutritional intake orally (as in the example in Box 66-1, where the child receives nothing orally in preparation for surgery). Electrolyte quantities are usually expressed as milliequivalent (mEq) or millimole (mmol) amount per 100 mL of fluid required. Traditionally, the recommended **sodium**

Box 66-1. Example of Fluid Calculations[a]

Part A

Case: A 22-kg boy is given nothing orally in preparation for an elective abdominal surgery. How much intravenous (IV) fluid per hour should he receive as he awaits the surgery?

- For first 10 kg: 100 mL/kg/d × 10 kg = 1,000 mL
- For next 10 kg (to get to 20 kg): 50 mL/kg/d × 10 kg = 500 mL
- For next 2 kg (to get to 22 kg): 20 mL/kg/d × 2 kg = 40 mL

1,000 mL + 500 mL + 40 mL = 1,540 mL/24 h

IV rate per hour = 64.2 mL/h (with a healthy child, round off to 65 mL/h for ease of administration)

Part B

Question: How much sodium (Na^+) and potassium (K^+) should this patient receive in his IV fluids?

Answer: 3 mEq Na^+/100 mL (1 dL) of fluid = 3 mEq × 15.4 dL = 46.2 mEq Na^+/d in 1,540 mL of water or 30 mEq NaCl/L

2.0 mEq K^+/100 mL (1 dL) of fluid = 2.0 × 15.4 = 30.8 mEq K^+/d in 1,540 mL of water or 20 mEq KCl/L

One possible way to write an IV order for this patient

D5 0.2% NaCl (or 0.25 NS) with 20 mEq KCl/L to run at 65 mL/h.

Abbreviation: D5 = 5% dextrose water.

[a] NS contains 154 mEq NaCl/L and 0.2% NaCl contains 34 mEq NaCl. This solution is a widely available, premade IV solution that provides the approximate daily Na^+ requirement of the patient. Even though the above calculations for sodium concentration are physiologic, at many institutions 0.5 NS in 5% dextrose is used preoperatively to prevent potential post-operative hyponatremia.

(Na^+) requirement for a healthy child is 3 mEq/100 mL fluid required (approximately 0.2% NaCl or 1/4 NS), and the **potassium** (K^+) requirement is 2 to 2.5 mEq/100 mL of fluid (see Box 66-1, part B for sample calculation and IV order). As discussed in more detail below, K^+ should only be given to a patient after ensuring adequate renal function. These estimations of Na^+ and K^+ requirements are meant to replace normal daily losses and would not be adequate in the face of increased electrolyte losses that can occur in a number of pathologic conditions (such as diarrhea). Moreover, there has recently been increasing focus on the risk of hyponatremia and related complications developing in hospitalized ill children (see below for details).

Relatively healthy, well-nourished children receiving IV fluids for a brief period (ie, 1–2 days) while hospitalized do not routinely require supplementation with other electrolytes, such as calcium and magnesium. However, it is important to realize that standard IV fluids containing 5% dextrose, sodium chloride (NaCl), and potassium chloride (KCl) provide only minimal caloric needs and do not adequately support weight gain or provide other necessary nutrients. Children who require prolonged IV therapy because of inadequate gastrointestinal (GI) tract function should receive total parenteral nutrition to better meet their caloric and nutritional needs.

Alterations in Fluid Needs in Illness

A number of conditions alter fluid requirements. Conditions that increase a patient's metabolic rate (eg, fever) will also increase their fluid requirement. A child's metabolic rate is increased 12% for every

1°C temperature elevation above normal. Most otherwise healthy children with free access to fluids will increase their own intake to account for increased needs when febrile. Other less common hypermetabolic states, such as thyrotoxicosis or salicylate poisoning, may have an even more dramatic effect, perhaps increasing metabolic rate by 25% to 50% over maintenance. In these cases and for children who are dependent on others to provide their fluids, clinicians must be aware of the magnitude of increased need and provide supplemental fluids to avoid dehydration.

Other conditions may decrease a child's fluid requirement. In hypometabolic states such as hypothyroidism, metabolic rate and fluid needs are decreased by 10% to 25%. Fluid requirements are decreased by 10% to 25% in high environmental humidity unless the ambient temperature is also high and results in visible sweating. In these situations, a healthy child with normal renal function given extra fluid beyond what is needed can, within limits, effectively excrete any excessive intake. Children with renal failure, however, pose a special challenge for the clinician in the management of fluid and electrolytes. When a child is unable to adequately excrete excessive fluid intake, this fluid can accumulate and lead to complications such as congestive heart failure and pulmonary edema. Without functioning kidneys, only **insensible fluid losses** need to be replaced. Insensible losses occur primarily through the skin and respiratory tract; they account for approximately 40% of maintenance fluid needs. However, fluid needs for patients with renal failure are usually estimated at 30% of the maintenance requirement, with additional fluids provided if needed. This is to avoid giving excessive fluids that may require dialysis for removal.

Fluid requirements may also be decreased under circumstances where **arginine vasopressin** (AVP, also called antidiuretic hormone or ADH) is increased. In addition to hypovolemia or hypertonicity (hyperosmolality), AVP release is also stimulated by pain, nausea, surgery (postoperatively), central nervous system (CNS) infections such as meningitis and encephalitis, severe pneumonia or respirator use, and certain medications (including thiazide diuretics, chemotherapeutic agents, and selective serotonin reuptake inhibitors). Arginine vasopressin release in the absence of hypovolemia or hypertonicity results in hyponatremia, and is referred to as **SIADH** (syndrome of inappropriate antidiuretic hormone secretion). In patients with SIADH, both fluid restriction as well as administration of fluids with a higher Na+ concentration may be indicated.

The most appropriate Na+ concentration of IV fluids for hospitalized children admitted to a pediatric intensive care unit or in postoperative patients is an area of current controversy. Over the past 25 years most such children have been maintained on a solution containing 5% dextrose water in half NS (D5 0.5 NS) or lower Na+ concentrations (D5 0.25 NS). Studies suggest that children, due to the kidney retaining free water in response to excessive AVP, are at risk for hyponatremia, hyponatremic encephalopathy, brain stem herniation, permanent brain damage, or death. Recently, some pediatric nephrologists (see Moritz et al) and intensivists recommended forgoing Na+ calculations in hospitalized very sick children and instead relying solely on isotonic fluids. Others (see Holliday et al

and Friedman) have cautioned that we must make certain that the new recommendations to use isotonic fluids do not result in excessive congestive heart failure or hypernatremia before we abandon previous practices. Regardless of the approach that is taken, close attention to the type and quantity of fluids provided, quantity of body fluid output, weight change, and serial electrolyte assessments are important in the management of all sick children, and fluid and electrolytes must be individualized to prevent serious complications.

Pathophysiology

Dehydration is one of the most common pathophysiological alterations in fluid balance encountered in pediatrics. Although strictly speaking dehydration means deficit of water only, most children with dehydration have lost both water and electrolytes. Dehydration can result from (1) diminished intake, (2) excessive losses through the GI tract (eg, diarrhea or vomiting), (3) excessive losses from the kidney or skin (eg, polyuria due to osmotic diuresis in uncontrolled diabetes), or (4) a combination of these factors.

Children are at increased risk for episodes of dehydration for a number of reasons. Young children have 3 to 4 times the body surface area per unit body weight compared with adults and so have relatively higher fluid needs. It is therefore much easier for children to become dehydrated in the face of the decreased intake or increased losses that often accompany common childhood illnesses. For example, acute gastroenteritis, which is common in young children, often leads to anorexia, recurrent vomiting, and frequent or large-volume stools, with proportionately more severe fluid loss than in older children and adults. In addition, infants and young children are dependent beings who are unable to increase their own fluid intake in response to thirst and must rely on others to provide their fluid needs. If these fluid needs are not met or are underestimated, children can easily become dehydrated.

Dehydration is classified as **isotonic, hypotonic, or hypertonic**. When considering acute dehydration, these terms are often used interchangeably with **isonatremic, hyponatremic,** and **hypernatremic** dehydration, respectively, because it is the Na+ content of the ECF that largely determines serum osmolality in otherwise healthy dehydrated children. In acute **isotonic** or isonatremic dehydration (serum Na+ 135–150 mEq/L), the most common type of dehydration, there is net loss of isotonic fluid containing both Na+ and K+ (Figure 66-1, top). Sodium, the primary ECF cation, is lost not only to the environment but some also shifts to the intracellular fluid (ICF) to balance the loss of K+, because K+ losses from cells are generally not accompanied by intracellular anionic losses in acute dehydration. The Na+ that has shifted into the ICF will return to the ECF compartment with rehydration. There is no net loss of fluid from the ICF in this process; the total water deficit in dehydration comes primarily from the ECF, although some have suggested, in the absence of valid data that two-thirds of the losses come from ECF and one-third from ICF.

There are a variety of mechanisms by which **hyponatremia** (serum Na+ <135 mEq/L) occurs in association with dehydration.

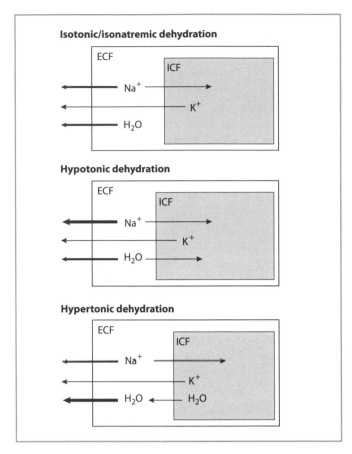

Figure 66-1. Pathophysiology of various types of dehydration.
ECF, extracellular fluid; H₂O, water; ICF, intracellular fluid; K⁺, potassium;
Na⁺, sodium.

In **hyponatremic dehydration**, the ECF volume is compromised to a greater degree than in isotonic dehydration because of osmotic shifts of ECF into the cell, resulting in more severe signs of dehydration (Figure 66-l, middle). Hyponatremic dehydration typically occurs in children with gastroenteritis when there are excessive Na⁺ losses in stool along with a parent giving oral replacement with water or very low Na⁺ beverages such as apple juice or tea. In hyponatremic dehydration, the kidney often excretes a concentrated urine (ie, retains free water) despite hyponatremia because AVP is stimulated by the decreased effective circulating volume. Intravascular volume depletion seems to be a potent stimulus for AVP release, overriding the AVP suppressive effect of hypotonicity/hyponatremia. The result is that serum Na⁺ levels are lowered due to dilution. Hyponatremic dehydration may sometimes also occur due to excessive loss of Na⁺ (relative to body water) in stool (eg, cholera) or in the urine (eg, adrenogenital syndrome, cerebral salt wasting, pseudohypoaldosteronism, and other salt-wasting renal disorders).

Hypertonic or **hypernatremic dehydration** (serum Na⁺ >150 mEq/L) occurs when net loss of water exceeds that of solute loss (Figure 66-1, bottom). It is usually seen in clinical conditions where there is rapid loss of hypotonic fluid in stool, vomit, or urine accompanied by failure of adequate water intake due to anorexia or vomiting. Fever or hyperventilation, if present, may intensify the disproportionate loss of water. Occasionally, hypernatremic dehydration

may be due to excessive solute intake. The urinary excretion of the excess solute obligates loss of large volumes of water, resulting in dehydration. The history may reveal that the child was accidentally fed a high Na⁺ solution due to incorrect mixing of oral rehydration packets or concentrated formula. In hypernatremic dehydration, there is shift of fluid from the ICF to the ECF to attain osmotic balance. As such, the ECF volume is somewhat spared at the expense of the ICF, and signs of dehydration may be delayed. However, fluid loss from the ICF results in intracellular dehydration, the most serious effect of which can occur in the brain. If hypernatremia occurs rapidly, there is not only a decrease in brain size but also a fall in cerebral spinal fluid (CSF) pressure owing to diffusion of water from CSF to the blood. As the brain shrinks, the bridging veins within the skull may stretch and even tear, resulting in subdural hemorrhage or other complications. If the hypernatremic state develops more slowly, the brain cell size may initially shrink minimally but will gradually return to normal size even in the face of continued hypernatremia. The preservation of the brain cell volume despite hypernatremia is thought to be due to the generation of idiogenic osmoles (myoinositol, trimethylamines, taurine, and other amino acids) that prevent water loss and attract water back into the cell and thus maintain cell volume. Rehydration of the patient with hypernatremia must occur slowly and cautiously to avoid brain cell swelling (Figure 66-2). The skin, on clinical examination, in hypernatremic dehydration may sometimes feel "doughy" due to intracellular dehydration. This finding, however, is inconsistent even in the hands of experienced pediatricians and should not substitute for serum Na⁺ measurements to diagnose hypernatremia.

Evaluation

History

In addition to signs and symptoms of the current illness, the history should focus on the cause of dehydration. Parents should be questioned on the type and amount of oral intake; the duration, quality, and frequency of vomiting and/or diarrhea; whether blood is present in the stool; the presence or absence of fever; frequency of urination; and whether a recent pre-illness weight is known for the child (Questions Box). When parents report change in mental status, it is of particular concern because this may occur because of significant electrolyte (eg, Na⁺) disturbance, marked dehydration, or other serious infection or illness. The most accurate way to assess the degree of dehydration is to compare current weight with a recent pre-illness weight, although a prior weight is often unavailable. In acute dehydration, the loss of weight is primarily due to fluid loss. The difference between pre-illness and current weight can be used to determine the degree of the fluid deficit.

Physical Examination

An important goal of the physical examination of the dehydrated child is to assess the degree of dehydration. In the process, vital signs including blood pressure and a current weight should be obtained.

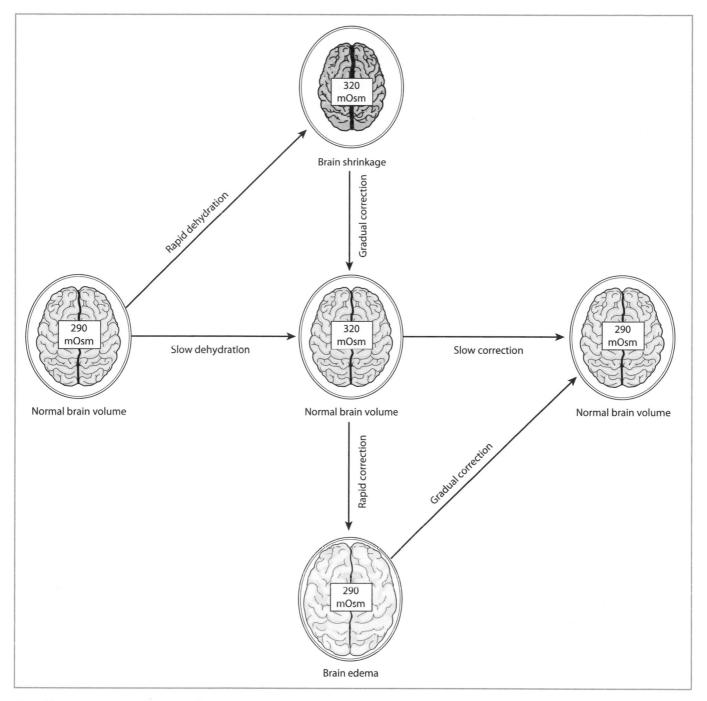

Figure 66-2. **Hypernatremic dehydration. Effects on brain volume of rapid versus slow development of hypernatremia and results of rapid versus slow correction of hypernatremia.**

Questions

Dehydration

- Has the child had vomiting or diarrhea?
- Has the child had fever?
- What has the child been eating or drinking?
- Has the child been urinating? How many wet diapers did the child have?
- How much did the child weigh at the last visit to the physician?
- Is your child's behavior or level of alertness changed from normal?

Specific attention should be focused on the general appearance of the child and in particular whether he or she is ill-appearing, listless, or less reactive. In addition to the usual components of the physical examination, assessing for the following is important: whether the oral mucosal membranes appear tacky or dry, whether tears are present or absent, if tenting of the skin is present (abnormal when tenting remains after the skin is pinched between 2 fingers), and perfusion status of the extremities. In the process, it is important that the clinician recognize whether shock is present because this is a life-threatening condition that requires emergent treatment (see Chapter 61).

	Table 66-2. Clinical Assessment of Magnitude of Dehydration		
Clinical Signs	*Mild Dehydration*	*Moderate Dehydration*	*Severe Dehydration*

Loss of body weight
   Infant/young child
   Older child/adult
	
	5%
	3%
		
		10%
		6%
			
			15%
			9%

Skin turgor	Normal to slightly reduced	Decreased	Markedly decreased (tenting)
Skin color and temperature	Pale or normal	Ashen, cool	Mottled, cool
Dry mucous membranes	±	+	++
Absent tears	±	+	++
Sunken eyeballs	±	+	++
Increased pulse	±	+	++ (may be thready)
Blood pressure	Normal	Normal Postural decrease ±	Reduced (in late shock)
Urine output	Normal or reduced[a]	Oliguria[a]	Oliguria/anuria
Capillary refill time	Slightly prolonged	Prolonged	Prolonged

[a] Usually corrects with restoration of intravascular volume.

Because comparison to an accurate recent pre-illness weight usually is not possible, clinicians must rely on vital signs and clinical signs and symptoms to assess the degree of dehydration (Table 66-2). In infants and young children (<5 years), the estimated fluid loss for mild dehydration is 5% deficit of body water; moderate dehydration, 10%; and severe dehydration, 15%. The corresponding numbers for estimated fluid loss in older children are 3%, 6%, and 9%, respectively. A variety of clinical signs have been proposed to evaluate the degree of dehydration—some more valid and reliable than others. A 2004 systematic review found that assessment of capillary refill was the most useful single sign in detecting 5% or greater dehydration (capillary refill is assessed by placing brief pressure on the distal palmar aspect of a fingertip and assessing the amount of time for the blanched area to refill—normal is considered ≤2 seconds). Two other single signs found to be important in predicting 5% or greater dehydration were abnormal skin turgor (ie, tenting) and respiratory disturbance, in particular hyperpnea (deep, rapid breathing without other signs of respiratory distress) suggestive of acidosis. In general, the more signs that are present the greater the severity of dehydration; however, a combination of delayed capillary refill time, absent tears, dry mucosal membranes, and general ill appearance may be equally as good as capillary refill, tenting, and hyperpnea combined in identifying children who have more than mild dehydration.

Laboratory Studies

Laboratory studies typically are not indicated in children who present with mild dehydration. Dehydrated children who are treated with IV fluids after having failed oral rehydration (at home or in the emergency department) should have initial assessment of their serum electrolytes, BUN, and creatinine. Initial and serial measurements of these laboratory studies should also be performed during rehydration in children with (1) shock, (2) severe dehydration, (3) decreased urine output that does not improve after initial restoration of intravascular volume, or (4) a history and clinical findings inconsistent with straightforward isotonic dehydration or found to have dysnatremia (ie, serum Na+ outside of the normal range [135–150], whether too low or too high). Dehydration in association with dysnatremia can have serious complications, and treatment requires special considerations. Hemolytic uremic syndrome, although uncommon, should be considered in any child with gastroenteritis, particularly with a history of grossly bloody stool, who also has decreased urine output.

Very ill children may require an arterial blood gas measurement to more accurately assess their acid-base status; in others, serum electrolytes are sufficient. The usual acid-base derangement in the moderately dehydrated child is a non-anion gap acidosis (with hyperchloremia) due to bicarbonate losses in the stool. Severely dehydrated children may have an anion gap acidosis due to lactic acid and/or ketone accumulation in the peripheral tissues secondary to the decreased perfusion that accompanies hypovolemia. An interesting exception is seen in infants with pyloric stenosis, who typically manifest a hypokalemic, hypochloremic metabolic alkalosis.

Imaging Studies

Imaging studies such as chest radiograph, abdominal ultrasound, and computed tomography scans are indicated based on the suspected etiology of the dehydration.

Management

The management of the dehydrated child involves consideration of 3 components (1) normal **maintenance** fluid and electrolyte requirement, (2) fluid and electrolyte **deficit** incurred during the present illness, and (3) **ongoing fluid and electrolyte losses.** Most commonly, ongoing losses result from continued vomiting and diarrhea. Losses from diarrhea can be estimated at 10 mL/kg per stool and from vomitus at 5 mL/kg per vomiting episode. Other forms of ongoing losses that occasionally must be considered and replaced include those associated with burns, gastric secretion suctioned via nasogastric tube, hyperventilation, or prolonged fever. The estimation of children's fluid and electrolyte needs and losses are almost always an approximation and require close follow-up, reassessment, and readjustment throughout treatment. At the very least, monitoring during treatment for dehydration requires regular assessment of vital signs, body weight, intake, and output.

Fluid given to dehydrated children may be provided either **enterally** or **parenterally.** Whenever possible, **ORT** using oral rehydration solution (ORS) is preferred for children with mild dehydration and most children with moderate dehydration. Parenteral fluid therapy should be used in children with more severe dehydration, when oral therapy has failed despite an adequate trial (eg, due to intractable vomiting or lethargy), in children in shock or impending shock, or when an anatomical defect such as pyloric stenosis or ileus is suspected.

Parenteral Fluid Therapy

The parenteral management of moderate or severe dehydration can be divided into 2 phases: an initial phase (first 1–2 hours) and the main phase of rehydration. The aim of the initial phase is to restore intravascular volume, thus improving perfusion and renal function and reversing tissue hypoxia, metabolic acidosis, and increased AVP. Regardless of the type of dehydration (isonatremic, hypernatremic, or hyponatremic), NS (0.9% sodium chloride) at 20 mL/kg/hour generally provides the most rapid and effective means to expand the intravascular volume at acute presentation. If shock is present or imminent, the treatment is more aggressive (see Chapter 61). The child should in rapid succession receive 2 to 4 boluses of 20 mL/kg of NS given over 20 to 30 minutes each. After each bolus, the child should be reassessed, and if signs and symptoms of intravascular depletion persist, the next IV bolus of 20 mL/kg of NS should be given over 20 to 30 minutes and the child admitted to the hospital for further careful evaluation, including assessment for other causes of shock such as sepsis. **The rapid restoration of ECF volume with up to 4 boluses of NS is a change in recommendation for the management of dehydrated children when compared with the past** (see Holliday et al and Friedman). However, caution must be used not to give excessive fluids to a child with a compromised heart and thereby induce congestive heart failure. This approach will also decrease AVP/ADH levels and the chances of hyponatremia in subsequent therapy even if 0.45% sodium chloride (1/2 NS) solutions are used instead of NS to correct the remaining deficit and maintenance therapy. All ORT is based on the use of hypotonic fluids generally containing Na$^+$ concentration of 45 to 75 mEq/L.

During the second phase of rehydration, the remaining fluid and electrolyte deficits are replaced based on the magnitude of these losses. These replacements are in addition to the daily maintenance requirements as well as any ongoing losses, as discussed previously, but must take into consideration the NS boluses administered during the initial phase, which may have already restored a substantial portion of the total fluid deficit. Various protocols exist to restore fluid and electrolyte deficits; approaches to treatment of dehydration

at different institutions will vary. Many of the differences in rehydration strategies lie in the composition of treatment fluid and the rate at which it is administered. Some clinicians prefer to administer half of the total fluid needs over the first 8 hours and the remainder over the next 16 hours; others replace the fluid at the same rate over the entire rehydration period. The latter method is presented in the case resolution at the end of the chapter. Usually the fluid deficit is replaced within 24 hours. There are noteworthy exceptions. Treating dehydration associated with **dysnatremia** (ie, abnormally low or high serum Na$^+$) should entail slower return (12 mEq serum Na$^+$ change per 24 hours or 0.5 mEq change per hour) to a normal range and may require 48 to 72 hours for correction.

Sodium replacement in the dehydrated child depends on the type of dehydration. In isotonic dehydration some clinicians elect to replace the entire fluid deficit with NS, others use a saline solution containing 110 mEq Na$^+$/L, and still others use 0.5 NS (77 mEq Na$^+$/L). We recommend NS (154 mEq Na$^+$/L) to replace the fluid deficit (see Case Resolution for example). This amount of sodium is somewhat more than the actual loss of sodium to the environment, which is closer to 110 mEq Na$^+$/L because during isotonic dehydration some Na$^+$, lost from the ECF, is shifted intracelluarly to balance K$^+$ losses and thus will return to the ECF during rehydration. To calculate the ongoing losses, although the content of excreted body fluids can be analyzed for electrolyte content for more exact replacement, the diarrheal stools are commonly replaced with 0.5 NS at 10 mL/kg per stool. (This should be adequate in Na$^+$ content for most cases given diarrhea in rotavirus contains approximately 30 to 40 mEq Na$^+$/L and enterotoxigenic *Escherichia coli*: 50 to 60 mEq/L; however, Na$^+$ stool losses in cholera are 90–120 mEq/L.)

Management of Dehydration With Dysnatremia

In hypernatremic dehydration, the patient is considered to have a relative free water deficit but usually has lost not only body water, but also some Na$^+$. The amount of free water a patient requires to restore their serum Na$^+$ to normal (eg, 145 mEq/L is desired serum Na$^+$) is calculated as follows:

$$\text{[patient's weight in kilograms]} \times \text{[actual serum Na}^+ - 145]$$
$$\times \text{4 mL/kg}$$

For serum Na$^+$ greater than 170 mEq/L, 3 mL/kg of free water is estimated to lower the Na$^+$ to the desired level (and thus the 4 mL/kg in the above equation is changed to 3 mL/kg). The quantity of free water provided by this equation is only part of the patient's total needs. The remainder of their fluid needs include isotonic losses that occurred during the dehydration process, ongoing losses, and maintenance fluids as well. Hypernatremic dehydration is corrected slowly to avoid cerebral edema, which can lead to brain stem herniation and death. In hypernatremia, the various equations used for calculations for phase 2 of therapy, the results for the sodium concentration of the final solution are often less than 30 mEq/L. Many clinicians, however, will initially provide 0.45% NaCl in 5% dextrose (a higher content Na$^+$ fluid than calculated by various equations) to ensure a slow rate of serum Na$^+$ decline and at a later stage decrease the sodium concentration to 0.2 % NaCl. Serial monitoring of electrolytes is important to ensure that the serum Na$^+$ is decreasing at the expected slow rate and not so quickly as to lead to life-threatening brain complications.

Management of **hyponatremic dehydration** also poses challenges. In addition to isotonic losses, additional Na$^+$ loss may have occurred. The amount of additional Na$^+$ (in mEq) to correct the serum Na$^+$ into a normal range (desired Na$^+$ level, eg, 135 mEq/L) has traditionally been calculated by the following equation (where 0.6 represents the body space which is affected by Na$^+$ changes):

$$\text{[patient's weight in kilograms]} \times \text{[135} - \text{actual Na}^+ \text{ level]} \times 0.6$$

This amount of Na$^+$ represents an additional need beyond a patient's isotonic losses, ongoing losses, and maintenance requirements. The use of hypertonic saline (3% containing 513 mEq Na$^+$/L) is generally reserved for children with symptomatic hyponatremia (eg, a child who is seizing). Hypertonic saline is administered as 3.0 mL/kg of 3% saline given by IV over 15 to 30 minutes or until seizures stop. This volume of 3% saline will raise the serum Na$^+$ approximately 2.5 mEq/L and is usually sufficient to correct the serum Na$^+$ to a level where serious signs and symptoms improve. This dose may be repeated once if there is no improvement in the CNS-related symptoms. The remaining hyponatremia is corrected more slowly so as not to exceed 12 mEq/L per 24 hours because too rapid correction of serum Na$^+$, particularly when hyponatremia has been long-standing, can potentially cause pontine demyelination.

Hyponatremia in hospitalized children, as stated earlier (see Maintenance), can result from other factors besides or in addition to Na$^+$ loss. Arginine vasopressin release in response to hypovolemia, hypertonicity, or other stimuli followed by free water retention can lead to dilutional hyponatremia (water intoxication). Hyponatremia in infants given excessively diluted baby formula (WIC [Special Supplemental Nutrition Program for Women, Infants, and Children] syndrome) results from inadequate Na$^+$ intake and free water retention. There have been a number of recent reports of encephalopathy, brain stem herniation, and death occurring in hospitalized children with hyponatremia whose low Na$^+$ level was not appreciated or who received inappropriately low Na$^+$ content IV fluids or excessive volumes of IV fluids (see Moritz et al). The adverse effects of hyponatremia on the CNS seem to be accentuated in the setting of hypoxemia, thus further pointing to the importance of close monitoring of children with electrolyte disturbances. Moreover, with rehydration and provision of Na$^+$, the kidneys excrete relatively more dilute urine that can sometimes lead to rapid and unpredictable increases in serum Na$^+$ levels. As is the case with treatment of hypernatremia, close attention to type and quantity of fluids provided, quantity of body fluid output, weight change, and serial electrolyte assessment is important to prevent serious complications during therapy for low Na$^+$. When faced with such issues, consultation with a pediatric nephrologist or pediatric intensivist experienced in managing alterations in fluid and electrolyte balance is very important.

Potassium Replacement

Potassium deficits are more difficult to determine, and there is no specific method to calculate the exact amount of K$^+$ that a dehydrated child requires. Additionally, as the acidosis that commonly accompanies moderate and severe dehydration corrects, K$^+$ shifts intracellularly. What initially seems to be a normal serum K$^+$ may fall into the hypokalemic zone, potentially resulting in adverse effects on neuromuscular and cardiac function. Frequent reassessment of serum K$^+$ and adjustment of K$^+$ content of the IV fluids may be necessary. In general, once adequate urine output has been established, K$^+$ may be added to the IV fluids to provide 3 to 4 mEq/kg/24 hours. This need can usually be met by adding KCl 20 mEq/L to the IV fluids. Children who have decreased urine output or other indicators of renal impairment should not receive K$^+$ until normal urine output has been restored. Hyperkalemia, a serious and life-threatening condition, may occur if a child is unable to excrete excess K$^+$ via the kidney because of renal impairment.

Oral Rehydration

Oral rehydration therapy refers to specially prepared, balanced preparations of carbohydrates and electrolytes meant for oral consumption. Clinical trials have repeatedly shown that ORT is as efficacious as IV therapy in the treatment of the child with mild or moderate dehydration. Additional advantages of ORT over IV therapy are that it is less expensive and noninvasive, and requires little technology. Oral rehydration therapy has been credited with the dramatic reduction in death associated with diarrhea in the developing world. In 2002 the World Health Organization and UNICEF announced a new ORS with reduced osmolarity (proportionally lower Na$^+$ and glucose concentration) based on a number of clinical studies demonstrating less vomiting, lower stool output, and reduced need for IV fluids relative to the prior formulation.

In the United States, Pedialyte (Ross Laboratories, Abbott) and generic equivalents are the most widely commercially available products. Flavored solutions and ice-pop versions of these solutions are available and often preferred by older children over the unflavored variety. Enfalyte (Mead Johnson) contains rice syrup solids as its carbohydrate source and is only available in unflavored, 6 oz ready-to-use bottles. It is not necessary to change to ORT in a breastfed child who is tolerating breast milk; these children can continue to receive breast milk for rehydration, though they may require shorter, more frequent feedings.

The composition of various ORS is presented in Table 66-3. The cost of commercially available ORS may be prohibitive for some families. Given the simplicity of the ORS packet in the developing world and commercially available ORS in the developed world, these remain the first choice. However, homemade ORT, using the recipes in Box 66-2, can be effective as long as families have, and know how to use, measuring spoons and cups and have a clean source of water. Some solutions, such as fruit juices or chicken broth, do not contain the proper balance of Na$^+$ and carbohydrate to effectively rehydrate a dehydrated patient and should not be used (Table 66-4).

Table 66-3. Composition of Various Oral Rehydration Solution

Solution	Carbohydrate (gm/L)	Sodium (mEq/L)	Potassium (mEq/L)	Base (mmol/L)	Osmolarity (mOsm/L)
Pedialyte	25	45	20	30	250
Enfalyte	30[a]	50	25	34	170
World Health Organization-UNICEF Oral Rehydration Solution	13.5	70	20	30	245

[a] As rice syrup solids.

Table 66-4. Composition of Some Clear Liquids Not Appropriate for Rehydration

Liquid	Carbohydrate (g/L)	Sodium (mEq/L)	Potassium (mEq/L)	Base (mmol/L)	Osmolality
Cola	110	2	0	13	750
Apple juice	120	3	32	0	730
Chicken broth	0	250	8	0	500
Sport beverage	40	20	3	3	330

The amount of ORT fluid needed for rehydration can be calculated much the same way as is done when determining the parenteral fluid requirement for a dehydrated child. However, most children with mild dehydration can be rehydrated relatively quickly and then are likely to request, in response to thirst, the amount of fluid they need. Therefore, a simplified method of determining ORT fluid requirements has been developed (Table 66-5). This quantity of fluid is given over a period of 3 to 4 hours. Children with ongoing losses should have these replaced. For the most part, it is not necessary to calculate the quantity of electrolytes that should be provided because these solutions are designed to adequately replace electrolytes in otherwise healthy children who are dehydrated.

Box 66-2. Recipes for 2 Homemade Oral Rehydration Solutions[a]

Starch-Based Solution
- 1 quart clean water (4 cups, or 32 ounces)
- ½ teaspoon salt
- 1 cup dry baby rice cereal (about 2 ounces in weight)

Sugar-Based Solution
- 1 quart clean water (4 cups, or 32 ounces)
- ½ teaspoon salt
- 6 teaspoons sugar
- One teaspoon of flavored gelatin powder may be added to either recipe to improve palatability.

[a] The proportion of ingredients in these recipes is important. These recipes should only be given to families who have and know how to use measuring spoons and cups. (Courtesy of Kathi Kemper, MD.)

Parents should receive guidance about the volume (converted into common household measures, eg, 5mL = 1 teaspoon and 15 mL = 1 tablespoon of water or ORS) and the frequency and duration of ORT to be given at home. Small volumes of 5 to 15 mL administered with a syringe or teaspoon every 2 to 5 minutes are much more likely to be retained by children who vomit larger volumes. Although this technique is labor intensive, it can be done by the parent and can deliver 150 to 300 mL/hour. As dehydration is corrected, vomiting often decreases and the child is then able to tolerate larger volumes. With ORT the frequency and amount of stooling often increases during the initial period of treatment. Parents should be made aware that the primary purpose of ORT is to rehydrate and not to stop diarrhea, which will gradually decrease spontaneously. "Gut rest" is not appropriate in most cases, and early refeeding with a return to the usual formula or milk and solids, if appropriate, should be prioritized.

Prognosis

Children with mild or moderate dehydration as a consequence of a self-limited childhood illness are likely to recover completely when given timely and appropriate rehydration therapy. It is more difficult to predict the prognosis of children with severe dehydration or significant aberrations in electrolyte balance. If managed appropriately, most of these children also completely recover; however, some, despite closely monitored care, may have permanent sequelae or poor outcomes.

Table 66-5. Treatment With Oral Rehydration Therapy (ORT)

Degree	Dehydration ORT (Given Over 3–4 h)	Replacement of Losses	Dietary Therapy
Mild (5%) (older children = 3%)	50 mL/kg of oral rehydration solution (ORS)	10 mL/kg for each diarrheal stool 5 mL/kg for each vomitus	Return to formula or milk as soon as vomiting resolves. Children who eat solid food can continue their regular diet.
Moderate (10%) (older children = 6%)	100 mL/kg of ORS	10 mL/kg for each diarrheal stool 5 mL/kg for each vomitus	Return to formula or milk as soon as vomiting resolves. Children who eat solid food can continue their regular diet.

CASE RESOLUTION

The opening vignette describes a child who is moderately dehydrated. Based on clinical assessment and weight change since his last clinic visit, he is approximately 10% dehydrated. He does not show evidence of shock. His laboratory studies show an Na$^+$ of 138 mEq/L, K$^+$ of 3.7 mEq/L, chloride of 108 mEq/L, bicarbonate of 14 mEq/L, BUN of 13 mg/dL, and creatinine 0.4 of mg/dL. His renal status is likely to be adequate because he is urinating, and BUN and creatinine are normal for patient age. The child's serum Na$^+$ is 138 mEq/L, which is in the isonatremic range. The serum K$^+$ is 3.7 mEq/L, which is within normal range; however, this may not accurately reflect this patient's total body K$^+$ status. This level may decrease substantially as he is rehydrated and acidosis is corrected, indicating total body K$^+$ depletion. His serum bicarbonate is 14 mEq/L, and his anion gap is 16 [138 − (108 + 14)], which is mildly increased and probably related to ketosis or mild lactic acidosis.

A calculation of this child's fluid and electrolyte needs follows:
His pre-illness weight was 12 kg.

Maintenance
Fluid needs: 1,000 mL for first 10 kg + 100 mL for next 2 kg = 1,100 mL.
Sodium needs: 33 mEq Na$^+$ (3 mEq/100 mL of maintenance fluid requirement)

Deficit
Fluid: 10% of child's weight has been lost during this episode of dehydration = 1,200 mL deficit
Sodium: 185 mEq Na$^+$ (154 mEq/1,000 mL of isotonic losses):
154/1,000 × 1,200 = 185 mEq.

Ongoing Losses
Fluid: Estimate this child's ongoing losses at 10 mL/kg for each stool. He had one loose stool while in the office, so add 120 mL of additional fluid.
Sodium: The Na$^+$ content of diarrhea is variable; however, it is usually replaced with 0.5 NS or about 77 mEq/1,000/mL. We estimate about 9 mEq of Na$^+$ in his one loose stool.
Total fluid needs: 1,100 mL (maintenance) + 1,200 mL (deficit) + 120 mL (ongoing losses) = 2,420 mL/24 hours.

Electrolyte Needs
Sodium: 33 mEq (maintenance) + 185 mEq (deficit) + 9 mEq (ongoing losses) = 227 mEq Na$^+$/24 hours.
Potassium: Estimate his maintenance and replacement needs to be 20 mEq K$^+$/1,000 mL fluid provided.

Treatment
In the initial phase of therapy, provide 40 mL/kg/hour NS for about 2 hours. During this period, his heart rate normalizes and he urinates. The initial parenteral phase provides 480 mL fluid and 74 mEq Na$^+$. This amount of fluid and Na$^+$ is subtracted from the patient's total fluid needs. The remaining amount to be provided is 1,940 mL fluid and 153 mEq Na$^+$, or about 79 mEq Na$^+$/1,000 mL fluid. It is not necessary to prepare a special IV solution; 0.5 NS (77 mEq NaCl/L) with 5% dextrose ordered as **D5 0.5 NS with 20 mEq KCl/L to run at 80 mL/hour** is appropriate. As his GI symptoms improve, IV therapy is discontinued and ORT instituted. The patient tolerates the ORT well and is discharged home.

Selected References

Cheek DB. Changes in total chloride and acid-base balance in gastroenteritis following treatment with large and small loads of sodium chloride. *Pediatrics.* 1956;17:839–847

Denno D. Global child health. *Pediatr Rev.* 2011;32:e25–e38

Fischer TK, Viboud C, Parashar U et al. Hospitalizations and deaths from diarrhea and rotavirus among children <5 years of age in the United states, 1993–2003. *J Infect Dis.* 2007;195:1117–1125

Friedman A. Pediatric hydration therapy: historical review and a new approach. *Kidney Int.* 2005;67:380–388

Holliday MA. The evolution of therapy for dehydration: should deficit therapy be still taught? *Pediatrics.* 1996;98:171–177

Holliday MA, Ray P, Friedman AL. Fluid therapy for children: facts, fashion and questions. *Arch Dis Child.* 2007;92:546–550

Holliday MA, Segar WE. The maintenance need for water in parenteral fluid therapy. *Pediatrics.* 1957;19:823–832

King CK, Glass R, Bresee JS, Duggan C; Centers for Disease Control and Prevention. Managing acute gastroenteritis among children: oral rehydration, maintenance, and nutritional therapy. *MMWR Recomm Rep.* 2003;52:1–16

Moritz ML, Ayus JC. New aspects in the patogenesis, prevention and treatment of hyponatremic encephalopathy in children. *Pediatr Nephrol.* 2010;25:1225–1238

Moritz ML, Ayus JC. Preventing neurological complications from dysnatremias in children. *Pediatr Nephrol.* 2005;20:1687–1700

Rose BD, Post TW. *Clinical Physiology of Acid-Base and Electrolyte Disorders.* New York, NY: McGraw Hill; 2001

Steiner MJ, DeWalt DA, Byerley JS. Is this child dehydrated? *JAMA.* 2004;291:2746–2754

Vernacchio L, Vezina RM, Mitchell AA et al. Diarrhea in American infants and young children in the community setting. *Pediatr Infect Dis J.* 2006;25:2–7

Winters RW, ed. *The Body Fluids in Pediatrics.* Boston, MA: Little Brown; 1973

CHAPTER 67

Acute Kidney Injury

Gangadarshni Chandramohan, MD, MS, and Sudhir K. Anand, MD

CASE STUDY

A 10-month-old girl has a 2-day history of fever, vomiting, and watery diarrhea. The child has previously been healthy. Her diet has consisted of Similac with iron, baby food, and some table food. Since the onset of her illness, she has not been drinking or eating well, and she has thrown up most of what she has eaten. Her mother has tried to give her Pedialyte and apple juice on several occasions but has had limited success. The child has had 8 to 10 watery stools without blood or mucus each day. Her temperature has varied between 98.6°F and 101.8°F (37.0°C and 38.8°C); the mother has given her daughter acetaminophen, which she has vomited. The girl's 4-year-old brother and her parents are doing well and have no vomiting or diarrhea.

The physical examination reveals a severely dehydrated (15%), listless infant. Her weight is 9.4 kg, her height is 74 cm, her temperature is 101.1°F (38.4°C), her heart rate is 168 beats/min, her respiratory rate is 30 breaths/min, and her blood pressure is 72/40 with an appropriately sized cuff. Capillary refill is 2 to 3 seconds. The skin appears dry, but no rash is present. Head and neck, chest, heart, and abdominal examinations are normal. Pending the results of her blood studies, an intravenous (IV) fluid bolus of 180 mL normal saline (20 mL/kg) over 20 to 30 minutes is administered. This is followed by 2 more boluses of 180 mL normal saline each. The girl is catheterized to obtain urine and determine the urine flow rate over the next several hours. A urinalysis is performed.

Questions

1. What are the 3 categories of acute kidney injury (AKI)?
2. What is the etiology of AKI?
3. How would one make an assessment of a patient with AKI?
4. What is the appropriate management for children with AKI?
5. What are the indications for renal replacement therapy?

Acute kidney injury is encountered in both outpatient and hospital inpatient settings and is associated with high morbidity and mortality depending on the primary cause of the insult. There are more than 30 different definitions of AKI in the literature. For the past 50 to 60 years, a sudden decrease in kidney function, signified by the accumulation of nitrogenous waste products (eg, blood urea nitrogen [BUN], creatinine) and often accompanied by a decrease in urine output, has been called acute renal failure. With better understanding of the pathophysiology of acute deterioration in renal function, many nephrologists and intensivists have suggested that the term **acute kidney injury (AKI)** be used instead of acute renal failure (ARF). Acute kidney injury is a more descriptive term that encompasses the full spectrum of renal dysfunction, from early and mild renal injury with only a small elevation in serum creatinine, to severe kidney injury requiring renal replacement therapy (dialysis).

In order to better delineate the progression of AKI as a continuum, in 2004 the Acute Dialysis Quality Initiative work group set forth the "RIFLE" criteria, which is based on serum creatinine level and urine output. The acronym "RIFLE" defines 3 stages of progressively increasing severity of renal injury (*r*isk, *i*njury, and *f*ailure) followed by 2 outcome variables (*l*oss and *e*nd stage renal disease). This criterion was recently modified for the pediatric population (pRIFLE), and the clinical use of it has been shown to improve the outcome in children (Figure 67-1). This classification is in part based on declining urine output; however, in some children, urine output

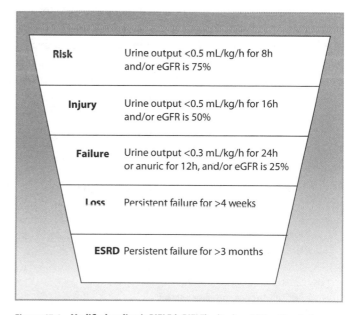

Risk	Urine output <0.5 mL/kg/h for 8h and/or eGFR is 75%
Injury	Urine output <0.5 mL/kg/h for 16h and/or eGFR is 50%
Failure	Urine output <0.3 mL/kg/h for 24h or anuric for 12h, and/or eGFR is 25%
Loss	Persistent failure for >4 weeks
ESRD	Persistent failure for >3 months

Figure 67-1. Modified pediatric RIFLE (pRIFLE) criteria. eGFR, estimated glomerular filatration route; ESRD, end stage renal disease. (Adapted from Bellomo et al.)

may remain normal or even become increased, generally known as nonoliguric renal failure. The pRIFLE criteria, however, are not applicable in newborn infants during the first few days of life because newborns may be physiologically oliguric during the first 24 hours of life and their serum creatinine initially reflects maternal creatinine values.

The pRIFLE classification is intended to emphasize the reversible nature of the renal insult, which is often present in critically ill children admitted in pediatric intensive care units (PICUs). It is anticipated that this precise and universal definition of AKI will probably enable clinicians to rapidly recognize the at-risk individuals and intervene promptly to improve the immediate and long-term outcomes.

Epidemiology

Acute kidney injury occurs in children with a wide variety of medical or surgical conditions and especially in children who are critically ill. The exact incidence of AKI in children is not known, but a late 1990s study from the United Kingdom estimated an incidence of 0.8 per 100,000 children. Acute kidney injury is often observed in patients in PICUs who are septic, have major trauma with severe bleeding, and in the postoperative period following major heart surgery with reported incidence as low as 4.5% and as high as 82% depending on the criteria used for inclusion (see Hsu and Symons in Selected References). Primary renal disease leading to AKI seems to be decreasing in incidence when compared with AKI caused by other systemic illnesses and/or their treatments. The incidence of AKI is about 5% to 10% in neonatal intensive care units and the most common cause in most cases is perinatal hypoxia and hypotension.

Clinical Presentation

Most children with AKI initially present with the clinical findings of the primary condition that ultimately leads to the renal problem. In critically ill children, a small increase in the serum creatinine may be the first indication of AKI. Other findings, such as decreased urine output, edema, and heart failure (following administration of excessive fluids), are specifically related to declining renal function (Dx Box). Additionally, hyperkalemia with cardiac arrhythmia, hyperventilation due to acidosis, and nausea and vomiting due to uremia may occur as renal failure progresses.

Dx **Acute Renal Failure/Kidney Injury**

- Decreased urine output
- Hypertension
- Hematuria
- Edema
- Elevated serum creatinine
- Blood urea nitrogen creatinine ratio <20
- Elevated fractional excretion of sodium

Box 67-1. Etiology of Acute Renal Failure/Kidney Injury in Children

Prerenal Causes
- Decreased plasma volume
- Dehydration
- Hemorrhage
- Third spacing of plasma volume in burns, sepsis, bowel obstruction
- Other causes of renal hypoperfusion
- Shock
- Hypoxia
- Congestive heart failure
- Hepatorenal syndrome
- Bilateral renal artery stenosis
- Cardiac surgery

Postrenal Causes
- Bilateral ureteropelvic or ureterovesical junction obstruction
- Posterior urethral valves
- Trauma to urethra
- Urethral stricture
- Neurogenic bladder
- Ureteropelvic or ureterovesical obstruction of a solitary kidney
- Obstruction due to kidney stone at the bladder neck

Intrinsic Renal Causes
- Vascular: renal artery or vein thrombosis, disseminated intravascular coagulation
- Glomerular: hemolytic uremic syndrome, severe (rapidly progressive) glomerulonephritis from any etiology
- Interstitial: interstitial nephritis due to allergic reaction to drugs (eg, nonsteroidal anti-inflammatory drugs, oxacillin, methicillin), sepsis
- Tubular (acute tubular necrosis [ATN]): sepsis, post-cardiac surgery, ischemia due to prolonged hypoperfusion; all causes listed in prerenal category, if sufficiently prolonged may lead to ATN
- Nephrotoxins: aminoglycoside antibiotics, indomethacin, radiocontrast agents, ethylene glycol, methanol, heavy metals
- Pigments: myoglobinuria, hemoglobinuria
- Uric acid: hyperuricemia, tumor lysis syndrome
- Congenital renal anomalies (especially in newborns and young infants)
- Bilateral cystic dysplastic kidneys, reflux nephropathy, polycystic kidneys, oligomeganephronia

Etiology and Pathophysiology

The causes of AKI are usually grouped into 3 categories: prerenal, intrinsic renal, and postrenal disorders (Box 67-1 and Figure 67-2). Although prerenal failure and acute tubular necrosis (intrinsic renal failure) may actually be on opposite ends of a continuum, rather than separate entities, this classification system still aids in the conceptualization of the underlying problem and formulation of the initial treatment plan. Correspondingly, it is important to note that postrenal failure could also inflict renal damage if intervention is not timely and ultimately can result in intrinsic renal failure.

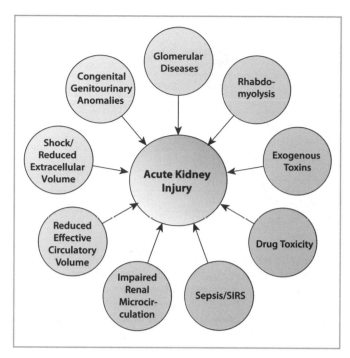

Figure 67-2. Common causes of acute kidney injury in children. SIRS, systemic inflammatory response syndrome.

Prerenal Disorders

Prerenal disorders are the most common cause of AKI in pediatrics and lead to a decrease in total or "effective" circulating blood volume. An absolute decrease in circulating volume can be caused by blood loss from acute hemorrhage secondary to trauma or fluid loss and dehydration secondary to gastroenteritis. Heart failure or redistribution of body fluids (third spacing) can lead to a decrease in effective circulating volume. In each of these situations, the resulting decrease in the glomerular filtration rate (GFR) can be readily reversed by improving renal perfusion in its early stages. If hypoperfusion is prolonged, however, ischemic damage to the kidney occurs and intrinsic renal failure develops (see below).

Postrenal Disorders

Urinary obstruction due to posterior urethral valves or other congenital lesions involving the urinary tract occasionally lead to AKI, especially during infancy. In older children, kidney stones or postoperative complications after pelvic surgeries or trauma could be the cause for postrenal failure.

Intrinsic Disorders

Intrinsic renal failure occurs because of injury to the vascular, glomerular, interstitial, or tubular components of the kidney (see Box 67-1). Intrinsic AKI can result from ischemia, sepsis, or toxins. Acute kidney injury resulting from renal tubular lesions is also called acute tubular necrosis (ATN), although in many patients with ATN, necrosis of tubular cells visible by light microscopy is minimal. Certain histologic changes that characterize ATN include loss of brush border microvilli in tubular cells, detachment of epithelial cells from basement membrane, and cast formation from cellular debris and protein.

Children with prolonged shock due to sepsis, post-cardiac surgery, trauma (hemorrhage), or dehydration often develop ATN if the effective circulating volume is not expanded. This is the most frequent type of intrinsic AKI observed in children. Hemolytic uremic syndrome (HUS) had been the most common cause of AKI in young children in 1970s–1980s, but its incidence has markedly declined in recent years. Nonsteroidal anti-inflammatory drugs are increasingly being recognized as a cause of AKI in children, especially when used in volume-depleted patients. In newborns and young infants, AKI may result from, or be superimposed on, a preexisting congenital renal disorder.

The pathogenesis of ATN in humans is controversial, and no single mechanism completely explains the sequence of events that lead to ATN. Ischemic and toxic ATN results from a complex interplay of hemodynamic, vascular, and tubulointerstitial changes. These include decreased blood flow to glomerular and tubular capillaries, resulting in reduced GFR; injury to cortical and medullary tubules with their cellular debris, leading to tubular obstruction; and "back leak" of solute and water from the lumen to the interstitium with further decrease in GFR. Increased production of endothelin and reduced production of nitrous oxide in the microvascular smooth muscle cells lead to increased vasoconstriction and reduced perfusion, perpetuating the renal injury. Renal tubular cells respond to the injury in many different ways, including no or minimal damage, sublethal injury, apoptosis, or necrosis. In the tubules, at the cellular level, when there is decreased oxygen delivery, there is decreased production of ATP that leads to damage to cell membranes and cell cytoskeletons. The cell damage alters the cell polarity, promotes entry of increased amounts of calcium into the cells, and increases intracellular free radical formation that eventually result in altered cellular function, cellular swelling, and cell apoptosis/necrosis. It is hoped that with better understanding of the pathophysiology of AKI, innovative, improved ways to prevent, diagnose, and treat the disease will be developed.

Differential Diagnosis

The diagnosis of AKI is established by the demonstration of a sudden increase in serum creatinine and/or BUN. Decreased urine output is also helpful. Identification of the clinical disorder that led to AKI is sometimes obvious, but at other times extensive evaluation to discover the etiology of the primary disorder may be necessary. It should also be determined whether children have chronic kidney disease or superimposition of AKI on a preexisting renal condition (Figure 67-2).

Evaluation

This is one of the few settings in which laboratory and radiologic tests are often more helpful diagnostically than history and physical examination.

History

The possibility of developing AKI should be anticipated in all critically ill children. A history of decreasing urine output, hematuria, dysuria, nausea, and vomiting should be sought in all patients. Prenatal and birth history may help to identify causes such as oligomeganephronia in children who were small for gestational age at birth or other complications that would have led to the current condition. The presence of previous genitourinary disorders, delayed growth, and anemia may point to preexisting kidney conditions (Questions Box). Also, family history of renal disorders can help in the differential diagnoses.

Questions

Acute Renal Failure/Kidney Injury

- How frequently is the child passing urine?
- Is the amount of daily urine decreased, increased, or unchanged?
- Does the child have hematuria or dysuria?
- Does the child have nausea or vomiting?
- Has the child had any previous urinary problems?
- (Older children) Does the child have a history of enuresis or nocturia?
- Is the child's physical development normal or delayed?
- Does the child have a history consistent with a primary condition that may have led to the acute renal failure/acute kidney injury?

Physical Examination

An evaluation of physical growth, hypotension or hypertension, arrhythmia, dehydration, or edema should be made. Examination of the flank area for renal enlargement or tenderness and of the bladder for distention is necessary to help determine the etiology of AKI.

Laboratory Tests

The following laboratory tests are recommended in all children with AKI: complete blood cell count, with red blood cell (RBC) morphology and platelet count; serum sodium, potassium, and bicarbonate; BUN; creatinine, uric acid, calcium, and phosphorus; glucose; total protein and albumin serum concentration; urinalysis and urine culture (if indicated); and spot urinary sodium and creatinine concentration and osmolality. If children are not voiding frequently, catheterization of the bladder is advisable temporarily (4–6 hours) to obtain urine for analysis. Residual volume should also be assessed, and the urinary flow rate (especially the response to initial fluid therapy) and presence of an outflow obstruction should be determined. All children with AKI and evidence of hyperkalemia should have an electrocardiogram (ECG).

The diagnosis of AKI can easily be established by laboratory tests and determination of urinary output over a specific time. Oliguria is defined as urine output less than 400 mL/m²/day or less than 1 mL/kg/hour in infants younger than 1 year, less than 0.75 mL/kg/hour in children 2 to 6 years of age, and less than

Table 67-1. Diagnostic Indices in Acute Kidney Injury[a]

Test	Prerenal	Intrinsic Renal
Urinalysis	Normal, occasional granular casts	Renal epithelial cells; pigment casts
Urine osmolality (mOsm/kg H$_2$O)	>600	<400
Urine specific gravity	>1.020	<1.015
Urine sodium (mEq/L)	<15	>40
U-P creatinine	>40	<20
Fractional excretion of sodium (FE$_{Na}$)[b]	<1%	>2%

Abbreviation: U-P creatinine, urine-plasma creatinine ratio (mg/mg).

[a] Values in patients with nonoliguric AKI often overlap and fall between prerenal and renal values. In addition, values in newborn infants differ from those in children beyond 1 year of age.

[b] FE$_{Na}$ = (UNa/UCr) × (PCr/PNa) × 100; UNa = urine sodium (mEq/L)

FENa, fractional excretion of sodium; UCr, urine creatinine (mg/dL); PCr, plasma creatinine (mg/dL); PNa, plasma sodium (mEq/L)

0.5 mL/kg/hour in children older than 6 years. Urinalysis, urine-specific gravity or osmolality, urine-plasma creatinine ratio, urinary sodium concentration, and fractional excretion of sodium help differentiate prerenal from intrinsic AKI (Table 67-1). While a BUN-creatinine ratio of greater than 20:1 suggests prerenal azotemia in adults, this is not necessarily true in infants and young children because they often normally have a BUN-creatinine ratio equal to or greater than 20.

Tubular epithelial cells and brown-pigmented casts are often seen in patients with ATN. Evidence of hematuria or proteinuria signifies glomerular disease, especially glomerulonephritis or HUS. Presence of blood on dipstick but absence of RBCs on sediment examination suggests hemoglobinuria or myoglobinuria as the basis of ATN.

Although urinary indices are helpful in differentiating prerenal from intrinsic AKI, a simple clinical method to distinguish between the 2 can be used. A therapeutic trial of volume expansion with 20 mL/kg of normal saline is administered intravenously over one-half to 1 hour (after the possibilities of congestive heart failure and urinary obstruction are excluded). If oliguria persists at the end of 1 hour, furosemide (2 mg/kg) can be given. If urinary output does not increase following furosemide administration, intrinsic AKI should be suspected and fluid administration should be reduced. Once intrinsic AKI has developed, repeated administration of high-dose furosemide has few benefits and can cause toxicity, especially hearing loss.

Many biomarkers have been investigated for the early diagnosis of AKI in adults and children (see Al-Ismaili et al in Selected References). The hope is that one day biomarkers found in either the serum or urine will allow us to better detect early kidney injury, differentiate among the multiple etiologies, and predict its severity. There are many promising urinary biomarkers, including IL18, KIM-1, NGAL, β$_2$-microglobulin, and osteopontin, which have been recently identified by proteomic analysis and all correlate with AKI to a variable degree. Both NGAL and β_2-microglobulin have been shown to correlate significantly with AKI in children seen in the emergency department with various forms of predisposing conditions. The concept of multiple biomarkers together to determine the changes in the kidneys during the early phase of AKI has been recently entertained, and various investigators are currently studying the value of this tool in clinical practice. Furthermore, more than one genetic polymorphism has identified in adults that are known to be linked to individuals who are susceptible to develop AKI. Perhaps, in the future, this information can help physicians to recognize the at-risk individuals and intervene early to prevent renal injury.

Imaging Studies

Renal ultrasonography is the most useful test for differentiating postrenal from other forms of AKI. Renal ultrasound can detect the presence or absence of kidneys, enlarged kidneys, dilated pelvocalyceal system, a distended bladder, and other congenital anomalies. Other investigative tests, such as voiding cystourethrography, renal scans, angiography, computed tomography, magnetic resonance imaging, or renal biopsy, may occasionally be necessary but are generally not indicated in children with AKI during the initial phase of the workup. Once a glomerular cause is suspected based on laboratory findings or radiologic evaluation, a biopsy will be an appropriate next step. A chest radiograph may also be helpful in detecting cardiac enlargement or pulmonary edema due to fluid overload.

Management

Prerenal azotemia is corrected by reestablishing adequate circulating volume, but unfortunately no current treatment leads to rapid recovery of renal function in humans with established intrinsic AKI. Although low-dose dopamine and furosemide are often used in the initial management of AKI, many studies have shown that these medications do not enhance recovery of renal function. Fenoldapam, a dopamine receptor agonist, has been used in critically ill, hemodynamically unstable patients with AKI to improve renal perfusion with some benefit in selected patients. Certain drugs, such as ATP-magnesium chloride, thyroxine, atrial natriuretic hormone, and insulin-like growth factors (IGF-1) have been used in experimental animals and some human trials without much success. The goal of therapeutic management of intrinsic AKI is maintenance of normal body homeostasis while awaiting spontaneous improvement because proximal tubules can undergo repair and regeneration after damage.

After dehydration is corrected, **daily fluid intake** is limited to replacement of insensible water loss (about 30%–40% of daily recommended fluid intake for age), urinary losses, and fluid losses from non-renal sources (eg, nasogastric drainage). Overhydration should be avoided in patients with AKI because it can cause edema, congestive heart failure, hypertension, hyponatremia, encephalopathy, and seizures.

Patients with complete anuria require no sodium intake. **Sodium** losses should be replaced daily in patients with urinary output, however. Preferably, the amount of sodium required should be determined by measuring daily urinary sodium losses.

Once AKI is suspected, **potassium** intake from all sources should be restricted. Severe hyperkalemia can often be avoided early in the course of the disease with strict adherence to potassium restriction. The level of serum potassium as well as ECG changes should be closely monitored. Patients with mild hyperkalemia may be treated with ion exchange resins; sodium polystyrene sulfonate (Kayexalate) may be given orally every 4 to 6 hours or by retention enema every 1 to 2 hours. Sodium polystyrene sulfonate should be mixed in water and mixtures containing polysorbate avoided because the latter may lead to bowel perforation. Moderate hyperkalemia can be treated with insulin and glucose infusions or β-agonists, which will drive the potassium intracellularly. Calcium gluconate should be given to stabilize the myocardium in patients who have ECG changes of hyperkalemia, such as tall T waves or widened QRS complexes. Dialysis is the most effective treatment for hyperkalemia and may be warranted if serum potassium has been rising slowly over several days or there is evidence of cardiac instability despite conservative treatment. Dialysis is also indicated for other reasons (see below).

Hypocalcemia and hyperphosphatemia are common in AKI, and small alterations in levels of **calcium** and **phosphorus** require no treatment. For serum phosphate greater than 8 mg/dL, phosphate binders such as calcium carbonate or calcium acetate may be used. If serum calcium is less than 8 mg/dL, IV or oral calcium should be given to prevent tetany.

Mild metabolic acidosis is common in AKI and requires no treatment. If blood pH is less than 7.2 or serum bicarbonate is less than 12 mEq/L, sodium **bicarbonate** may be administered.

Adequate nutrition is important in AKI because it prevents excessive tissue breakdown. If renal failure is expected to be short in duration (3–4 days), most calories may be provided as carbohydrates. If AKI is expected to last longer, adequate calories in the form of carbohydrates along with daily protein intake of 1 g/kg should be provided.

Anemia should be identified and corrected if hemoglobin is less than 10g/dL in order to improve the oxygen and nutrient delivery to the tubules to facilitate the regeneration of cells and to establish their function. This can be achieved by maintaining an optimal hemoglobin level either by transfusing packed red cells and by subcutaneous or IV administration of epogen if renal failure is prolonged.

Many children with AKI can be managed by the conservative measures described previously. If renal failure lasts more than a few days or if complications develop, however, **dialysis** should be planned. The usual indications for dialysis include uncontrollable hyperkalemia or acidosis, volume overload with pulmonary edema and/or congestive heart failure unresponsive to diuretic treatment, progressive uremia with BUN greater than 100 mg/dL, or creatinine clearance less than 15 mL/min/1.73 m². In preemies and newborn babies, peritoneal dialysis is usually preferred over hemodialysis to avoid major hemodynamic instability that is often seen with hemodialysis. In critically ill children with overwhelming sepsis or multisystem organ dysfunction, however, early continuous venovenous hemodiafiltration is indicated for more gradual fluid removal, avoiding significant fluctuations in the fluid balance and to optimize nutritional support.

Acute renal failure/AKI can often be prevented by anticipating its possible occurrence in children with high-risk conditions such as dehydration, trauma, sepsis, and shock, or after cardiac surgery. Prompt recognition of prerenal failure and its aggressive management with volume expansion may prevent the development of intrinsic AKI. Nephrotoxic agents such as gentamicin should be avoided in high-risk patients if possible. When these drugs are used, they should be monitored meticulously, with frequent measurement of blood levels.

Prognosis

The duration of oliguria in AKI may be short (1–2 days) or long (a few weeks). Recovery is usually first indicated by an increase in urinary output. Blood urea nitrogen and creatinine may rise during the first few days of diuresis before beginning to return to normal. During diuresis, large quantities of sodium and potassium may be lost in the urine. Serum electrolytes should be closely monitored, and adequate replacements should be made to prevent hyponatremia or hypokalemia.

In children with AKI, outcome largely depends on the primary condition, the severity of damage to other organs, and physician expertise in managing AKI. Nonoliguric AKI is consistently associated with a shorter clinical course and better prognosis than oliguric AKI. Most children with ATN recover completely. However, children with more severe kidney involvement (cortical necrosis) may have residual renal impairment or chronic renal failure, and critically ill children have a 60% mortality rate.

CASE RESOLUTION

In the case scenario, a series of diagnostic studies are performed. The laboratory results are: hemoglobin, 13.8 g/dL; hematocrit, 41%; white blood cell (WBC) count, 12,400/μL; neutrophils, 58%; band forms, 6%; lymphocytes, 32%; monocytes, 3%; and eosinophils, 1%. The platelet count is 277,500/μL. Serum sodium is 136 mEq/L; potassium, 5.1 mEq/L; chloride, 110 mEq/L; bicarbonate, 10 mEq/L; BUN, 84 mg/dL; creatinine, 2.8 mg/dL; and glucose, 68 mg/dL. The specific gravity is 1.015; the specimen shows protein trace, blood, WBC, and nitrite negative; and the sediment has many epithelial cells, 1 to 2 RBCs, and many granular and pigmented casts. Spot urinary sodium is 65 mEq/L, creatinine is 39 mg/dL, and the fractional excretion of sodium is 3.4%.

These results are most consistent with the diagnosis of intrinsic renal failure/AKI because the fractional excretion of sodium is increased. Recovery may take a few days to a few weeks. The patient is admitted to the pediatric step-down unit where fluids are adjusted according to her urine output and electrolytes are monitored frequently.

Selected References

Akcan-Arikan A, Zappitelli M, Loftis LL et al. Modified RIFLE criteria in critically ill children with acute kidney injury. *Kidney Int.* 2007;71:1028–1035

Al-Ismaili Z, Palijan A, Zapitelli M. Biomarkers of acute kidney injury in children: discovery, evaluation, and clinical application. *Pediatr Nephrol.* 2011;26:29–40

Askenazi DJ, Ambalavanan N, Goldstein SL. Acute kidney injury in critically ill newborns: what do we know? What do we need to learn? *Pediatr Nephrol.* 2009;24:265–274

Basu RK, Devarajan P, Wong H, Wheeler DS. An update and review of acute kidney injury in pediatrics. *Pediatr Crit Care Med.* 2011;12(3):339–347

Bellomo R, Ronco C, Kellum JA, Mehta RL, Palevsky P, ADQI Workgroup. Acute renal failure—definition, outcome measures, animal models, fluid therapy and information technology needs: the Second International Consensus Conference of the Acute Dialysis Quality Initiative (ADQI) Group. *Crit Care.* 2004;8:R204–R212

Du Y, Zappitelli M, Mian A, et al. Urinary biomarkers to detect acute kidney injury in the pediatric emergency center. *Pediatr Nephrol.* 2011;26:267–274

Hsu CW, Symons JM. Acute kidney injury: can we improve prognosis? *Pediatr Nephrol.* 2010;25:2401–2412

Lameire N, Biesen WV, Vanholder R. Acute renal failure. *Lancet.* 2005; 365:417–430

Ringer SA. Acute renal failure in the neonate. *NeoReviews.* 2010;11:e243–e251

Schneider J, Robinder K, Grushkin C, Bart R. Serum creatinine as stratified in the RIFLE score for acute kidney injury is associated with mortality and length of stay for children in the pediatric intensive care unit. *Crit Care Med.* 2010;38:933–939

Schrier R, Wang W, Poole B, Mitra A. Acute renal failure: definitions, diagnosis, pathogenesis, and therapy. *Clin Invest.* 2004;5:5–14

CHAPTER 68

Ingestions: Diagnosis and Management

Kelly D. Young, MD, MS

CASE STUDY

A 2-year-old girl is found by her mother with an open bottle of pills and pill fragments in her hands and mouth. She is rushed into the emergency department. She is sleepy but arousable. The vital signs are temperature of 98.8°F (37.1°C), heart rate of 120 beats/min, respiratory rate of 12 breaths/min, and blood pressure of 85/42 mm Hg. Pupils are 2 mm and reactive. Skin color, temperature, and moisture are normal. She has no other medical problems.

Questions

1. What history questions should be asked to help identify the substance ingested?
2. What physical examination findings can give clues to the substance ingested and the seriousness of the ingestion?
3. What other diagnostic tests might be helpful in managing ingestion patients?
4. What are the management priorities?

Ingestions are a common problem faced by pediatric practitioners. Two scenarios frequently encountered are accidental ingestions by preschool-aged children and intentional suicide attempts by adolescents. This chapter discusses the general approach to the child who has ingested a potentially poisonous substance; ingestions of specific substances are beyond the scope of this chapter, as is toxicity occurring by dermal, ophthalmologic, or inhalational routes. However, the general approach to history, physical examination, laboratory tests and diagnostic studies, and management, especially decontamination, is useful for all ingestions.

Epidemiology

Most calls made to poison control centers involve pediatric patients. Poison control center data (2008) show that pediatric patients younger than 20 years accounted for 65% of exposures, and young children aged 0 to 5 years accounted for 52%. For children aged 0 to 12 years, 3% of exposures are intentional, while for adolescent 13- to 19-year-olds 24% are intentional, and for adults 71% are intentional. The most common substances ingested overall are analgesics (including acetaminophen, nonsteroidal anti-inflammatory drugs, and narcotics) and cosmetics/personal care products. The most common fatal ingestion in children is narcotic analgesics (often not their own prescription). Another common fatal poisoning for young children is carbon monoxide poisoning. Fatalities are uncommon overall and are more likely to be seen in intentional ingestions by older children. Poison control center data (2008) revealed 42 pediatric fatalities (0–12 years old) and 74 adolescent fatalities (13–19 years old). Children accounted for 2.6% of total toxicological fatalities for the year, while adolescents accounted for 5.6% and adults for the remainder. Young children tend to ingest either nontoxic substances or small quantities of toxic substances. While 24% of overall children whose caregivers called into poison control centers are managed in a health care facility (as opposed to observed at home), only 10% of children 0 to 5 years old are.

Clinical Presentation

The clinical presentation varies considerably depending on the substance ingested. Some patients may not present with a clear history of a toxic ingestion. The clinician must maintain a high index of suspicion for poisoning as the cause of symptoms such as altered behavior, depressed level of consciousness, cardiac dysrhythmias, vomiting, seizures, and autonomic changes.

Pathophysiology

The pathophysiological picture depends on the substance. Some toxins act on a particular organ system (eg, acetaminophen on the liver, ethanol on the central nervous system), while others act diffusely at the cellular level (eg, cyanide). Generally, drugs are absorbed, distributed within the body, metabolized, then excreted. Drug levels obtained prior to completion of absorption and distribution may not reflect the peak level. Interventions focus on preventing absorption, sometimes on preventing metabolism into a more toxic by-product, and on enhancing excretion. Toxic effects may be delayed or prolonged when an extended-release form of a drug has been ingested, with drugs likely to form concretions (iron, aspirin, theophylline), or when toxicity results from an active metabolite (toxic alcohols, acetaminophen, acetonitrile, dapsone). Pharmacogenetics are increasingly recognized as possibly playing an important role in individual responses to medications and toxins. Genetic variations in enzymatic activity in drug metabolism may result in toxicity through excessively rapid metabolism of a drug to its active metabolite, or through slow metabolism of a drug to its inactive metabolite. For example, a cytochrome P450 CYP2D6 genotype has been linked to rapid metabolism of codeine to active morphine, resulting in toxicity, and even fatality.

Differential Diagnosis

The differential diagnosis of toxic ingestions is broad. If there is a history of ingestion, the differential is narrowed to substances available to the child. If no history of ingestion is given, practitioners should include ingestion in the differential when evaluating symptoms and signs such as altered mental status, altered behavior, metabolic derangements, cardiac dysrhythmias, hypotension and shock states, seizures, respiratory distress or apnea, cyanosis, vomiting, and diarrhea (Symptoms Box). In fact, almost any symptom complex may result from a toxic ingestion.

Symptoms

Suspicious for Poisoning

- Bradycardia or tachycardia
- Hypothermia or hyperthermia
- Respiratory depression or hyperpnea
- Hypotension or hypertension
- Mydriasis or miosis
- Altered mental status or abnormal behavior
- Seizure
- Cardiac dysrhythmias
- Metabolic derangements
- Nausea, vomiting, diarrhea

Evaluation

A detailed history of what and how much the patient ingested is key to the evaluation. Physical examination should focus on identifying symptoms and serious complications. Patients should be monitored and reassessed frequently. Laboratory and other diagnostic studies can be tailored to the specific ingestion.

History

The most important questions address the ingestion (Questions Box): What did the patient ingest? What is the maximum possible amount that was ingested? When did the ingestion occur? What symptoms are occurring? History regarding previous medical conditions is also important to identify increased susceptibility to a particular toxin (eg, seizure disorder with ingestion of a substance that

---

Questions

Poisonings

- What did the child take? (If unknown, what is available to the child?)
- How much did the child take? (If unknown, what is the maximum amount possible?)
- When did the child take it? (If unknown, how long was the child unattended or unobserved?)
- What symptoms have occurred, and when did the symptoms start relative to the time of ingestion?
- What other medical conditions does the child have? What medications does the child take regularly?

---

causes seizures); assess for factors that may have precipitated the ingestion, such as depression; and assess for medications that may interact with or exacerbate the toxic effects of the ingested substance (eg, acetaminophen ingestion in a patient taking a cytochrome P-450 inhibiting medication).

Parents should be encouraged to bring in the container and any remains of the substance ingested. The practitioner should try to obtain the exact formulation because generic and brand name drugs may differ. One must also be aware of possible combination products. Sleuthing methods such as calling or sending a family member to the home to identify the product, calling the pharmacy on a prescription label, or identifying a pill by comparing its picture and imprint to those in a pharmaceuticals reference may be necessary. Internet search engines may be used to search the imprint on a pill, or to identify foreign medications.

Caretakers should be questioned regarding all available drugs or other toxic substances in the household. Sometimes caretakers must be encouraged to mention all substances in the household, even those they don't think the child could possibly have obtained. The practitioner must also ask about medications used by recent visitors (eg, grandparents) and the possibility of an exposure at a recently visited household or location. It is important not to overlook herbal preparations, vitamins, alternative medications, household products (including cleaning and personal care products), gardening products, chemicals used in hobbies or work, and alcohol or drugs of abuse belonging to an adult. Caretakers may initially overlook these as they concentrate only on recalling "medications." It may be helpful to interview siblings or friends of an adolescent suspected of recreational drug use. One must maintain a high index of suspicion for unreported co-ingestants, especially in adolescent suicide attempts.

Although often difficult, it is important to attempt to determine the quantity of drug that was available to the patient and how much is currently missing. One may need to count pills or measure liquid to determine this. For estimating liquids, the approximate volume of a swallow is 0.3 mL/kg. The practitioner should always assume the "worst case" (ie, the patient took all of the drug that is missing). History concerning the amount ingested may be inaccurate, especially when taken from adolescents with intentional ingestion.

Table 68-1. Toxidromes			
Toxidrome	Toxins	Symptoms	Treatment
Narcotic or opiate	Oxycodone, hydrocodone, methadone, fentanyl, heroin, codeine, morphine	Nausea/vomiting, respiratory depression, miosis, altered mental status, or coma	Naloxone, respiratory support
Cholinergic (parasympathomimetic)	Organophosphate and carbamate pesticides	DUMBELLS mnemonic: *d*iarrhea, *u*rination, *m*iosis, *b*ronchorrhea and bronchospasm, *e*mesis, *l*acrimation, *l*ethargy, *s*alivation	Atropine, 2-PAM (pralidoxime)
Anticholinergic	Antihistamines, jimson weed, antipsychotics, some antidepressants, Parkinson's medications	Flushing ("red as a beet"), dry skin and mucous membranes ("dry as a bone"), hyperthermia ("hot as a hare"), delirium ("mad as a hatter"); mydriasis ("blind as a bat"), also tachycardia, urinary retention, ileus/decreased bowel sounds	Supportive care
Sympathomimetic	Cocaine, amphetamines, ephedrine	Mydriasis, anxiety, tachycardia, hypertension, hyperthermia, diaphoresis	Quiet environment, benzodiazepines
Sympatholytic	Clonidine, β-blocker (eg, propranolol)	Bradycardia, hypotension, miosis, may have lethargy	Supportive care, fluids and pressors if needed for hypotension, atropine for symptomatic bradycardia
Tricyclic antidepressant	Imipramine, amitriptyline, many others	Seizures, tachycardia, prolonged QRS complex, altered level of consciousness, cardiac dysrhythmias	Sodium bicarbonate
Salicylate	Aspirin, methyl salicylate, oil of wintergreen	Hyperventilation, nausea/vomiting, tinnitus, hyperthermia, metabolic acidosis	Alkalinization with $NaHCO_3$ (confirm salicylate level)
Serotonin syndrome	Selective serotonin reuptake inhibitors, many other drugs	Altered mental status, neuromuscular rigidity, tremors, or hyperreflexia, autonomic instability: hyperthermia, mydriasis, tachycardia, hyper- or hypotension	Supportive care

The practitioner should try to determine approximately what time the ingestion occurred. Symptoms are usually expected within a defined time range. Recommended observation periods before discharge usually take into account expected symptoms based on the length of time since the ingestion. Timing may also be important in determining what substance was most likely ingested. For example, ingestion of mushrooms that cause a self-limited illness usually causes gastrointestinal (GI) upset within 4 to 6 hours, whereas *Amanita* mushrooms that may ultimately result in hepatic failure typically present with GI upset in 6 to 12 hours.

The practitioner should ask about current symptoms and when they started relative to the time of the ingestion. In a patient without a definite history of ingestion, certain combinations of symptoms may point toward a specific substance or class of substances. Whether the patient is symptomatic and what symptoms are present may guide the workup for an unknown ingestion, determine whether the patient needs to be hospitalized, or dictate therapy.

Physical Examination

If the substance ingested is known, the physical examination should be directed toward identifying expected symptoms of toxicity. A general physical examination should always be performed, however, because co-ingestion of another undisclosed substance must be considered. Particular attention should be paid to all 4 vital signs (temperature, respiratory rate, heart rate, and blood pressure); pupillary size and reaction; breathing (eg, Kussmaul respiration seen in acidosis); mental status; distinctive breath odors; presence or absence of bowel sounds; and skin color, temperature, and moisture. The patient's weight should be measured because toxicity is often estimated based on milligrams of drug ingested per kilogram of body weight. Because symptoms may develop or worsen if peak levels of the toxic substance have not been reached at the time of initial evaluation, continual reassessment and cardiorespiratory monitoring are imperative. A recognizable set of symptoms suggestive of a certain class of medications or toxins is called a toxidrome. If a symptomatic patient is noted to have a typical toxidrome, therapy may be initiated based on the toxidrome without confirmation of the exact substance ingested. Some common toxidromes and their treatments are listed in Table 68-1.

Laboratory Tests (Box 68-1)

Qualitative drug screens (reporting only presence or absence of the drug) of urine or blood are often used when poisoning is part of a broader differential for symptoms such as altered mental status or acute behavioral changes. Such drug screens are rarely helpful acutely in the poisoned patient because results are often not rapidly reported, testing can only be done for a limited number of substances, and false-positives and false-negatives may occur. Given the frequency of narcotic ingestions, it is important to note that synthetic opioids (eg, fentanyl, methadone, oxycodone, and hydrocodone) are not detected by typical hospital immunoassay "tox screens."

Box 68-1. Laboratory Tests and Diagnostic Studies to Consider

- Specific drug levels as indicated
- Qualitative urine or blood "tox screen"
- Acetaminophen level, consider ethanol level and salicylate level
- Serum chemistries, calculated anion gap
- Serum osmolarity, calculated osmolar gap
- Liver function panel, renal function tests
- Rapid bedside glucose test
- Urine pregnancy test
- Pulse oximetry
- Electrocardiogram
- Arterial blood gas with carbon monoxide and methemoglobin levels
- Urinalysis
- Creatinine phosphokinase level
- Chest radiograph
- Abdominal film for radiopaque tablets

However, quantitative drug levels for specific drugs can be helpful to estimate severity of expected symptoms or to rule out ingestion of that drug. Examples include acetaminophen, salicylate, ethanol, methanol, ethylene glycol, iron, theophylline, lithium, anticonvulsants, and levels of carboxyhemoglobin or methemoglobin by blood gas analysis. Such levels should only be measured when suggested by history or physical examination, with the exception of acetaminophen and ethanol. Many experts in toxicology feel that because acetaminophen overdose produces few acute symptoms, may lead to fulminant hepatic failure, and is readily treatable with an antidote, all patients with a history of ingestion should have an acetaminophen level determined. In adolescents and adults, ethanol is a common co-ingestant, and ethanol levels are often routinely measured. Routine salicylate levels are likely to be low yield in the absence of suspicion by history or physical examination, although some practitioners also obtain them.

Serum chemistries and osmolarity may offer clues in ingestion of an unknown substance. The **anion gap** is calculated as [Na] - ([Cl] + [HCO3]) and is normally 8 to 12 mEq/L. An elevated anion gap indicates presence of metabolic acidosis and is seen in ingestions and conditions identified by the **MUDPILES** mnemonic: *m*ethanol, *u*remia, *d*iabetic ketoacidosis, *p*araldehyde and phenformin, *i*ron and isoniazid, *l*actic acidosis, *e*thylene glycol and ethanol, *s*alicylates and solvents (eg, toluene). The **osmolar gap** is the difference between the measured serum osmolarity and the calculated osmolarity (given by the formula 2[Na] + [glucose]/18 + [BUN]/ 2.8). The normal osmolar gap is less than 10 mOsm. An elevated osmolar gap is seen with ingestion of alcohols such as ethanol, methanol, ethylene glycol, and isopropanol.

Depending on one's suspicion for acidosis, hypoxemia, or abnormal hemoglobins (carboxyhemoglobin and methemoglobin), arterial blood gas analysis may be indicated. Because hypoglycemia may be seen with some ingestions and is easily treated, a rapid bedside glucose test should be done on all patients. Urinalysis and creatinine

phosphokinase level tests may be performed to look for signs of rhabdomyolysis if the patient is deemed at risk. All females of child-bearing age should have a urine pregnancy test. Assessment of liver and renal function is often important because many substances are metabolized by these routes.

Diagnostic Studies

Pulse oximetry and cardiorespiratory monitoring should be instituted for all serious ingestions. An electrocardiogram may be indicated if cardiac toxicity is expected. Other studies are tailored to the specific ingestion, such as endoscopy after ingestion of caustic acids or alkalis.

Imaging Studies

Specific imaging studies may be indicated for certain ingestions, such as chest radiography in hydrocarbon ingestion, to look for signs of aspiration. An abdominal film may be helpful in identifying ingestion of radiopaque substances and monitoring the effectiveness of GI decontamination procedures for removing such substances. The mnemonic **CHIPS** can be used for radiopaque medications: *c*hloral hydrate, *h*eavy metals, *i*ron, *p*henothiazines, and *s*low-release (enteric-coated) medications. In practice, abdominal radiography is primarily used in iron ingestion and suspected body-packing with illicit drugs.

Management

Management strategies are specific for the substance ingested. The regional poison control center should be consulted for advice regarding management and length of time to observe asymptomatic patients. A single number, 1-800-222-1222, automatically routes the caller to one of the appropriate 62 regional poison control centers in the nation. In general, the approach to management includes attention to the basic ABCs (airway, breathing, circulation) of resuscitation, decontamination methods, specific antidotes when available and indicated, and meticulous supportive care, often in an intensive care unit.

Decontamination

Decontamination techniques are strategies used to prevent or minimize absorption of the toxic substance and to enhance its elimination. They are a critical part of the management of acutely poisoned patients and should be used whenever a significant ingestion is suspected (Table 68-2).

Syrup of ipecac was commonly recommended in the past for home use to induce vomiting in the event of an accidental ingestion. **Gastric lavage,** in which a large nasogastric tube is placed and the stomach is washed with normal saline, is the hospital counterpart to syrup of ipecac. Both techniques theoretically remove toxic substance from the stomach, thus preventing absorption. However, at best (immediate performance after ingestion), less than a third of gastric contents are removed by these methods. In addition, these techniques may interfere with the use of activated charcoal, usually a more effective therapy. Gastric lavage is technically difficult to

Table 68-2. Summary of Gastric Decontamination Techniques		
Technique	*Dose*	*Contraindications*
Syrup of ipecac	6 months–1 year: 10 mL (use with caution) 1–12 years: 15 mL >12 years: 30 mL Follow with 8 oz water	**Not recommended for routine use** Altered level of consciousness (ALOC) Caustics: acids and alkalis Hydrocarbons Expected ALOC (eg, tricyclic antidepressants)
Gastric lavage	15 mL/kg aliquots normal saline to maximum of 400 mL until lavage fluid is clear (may be several liters)	ALOC with unprotected airway Caustics: acids and alkalis Hydrocarbons Expected ALOC >1 hour since ingestion
Activated charcoal	1–2 g/kg or <6 years: 25–50 g >6 years: 50–100 g	ALOC with unprotected airway Absent bowel sounds or bowel obstruction Substance not bound by charcoal
Cathartics	Magnesium citrate 4 mL/kg 70% sorbitol 1 g/kg	**Not recommended for routine use** Repeated doses can cause dehydration or electrolyte imbalances.
Whole-bowel irrigation	Toddler and preschool age: polyethylene glycol solution 500 mL/h 6–12 y: 1,000 mL/h Adolescent and adult: 1.5–2 L/h Continue until rectal effluent is clear	Bowel obstruction, ileus, perforation, or hemorrhage ALOC with unprotected airway
20% intralipid	1.5 mL/kg initial bolus intravenous, then 0.25 mL/kg/min for 30–60 minutes	For lipophilic drug overdose with severe cardiotoxicity

perform in young children owing to the need to pass a large-bore tube. Gastric lavage also has a high rate of complications, such as aspiration and esophageal trauma. Neither syrup of ipecac nor gastric lavage is recommended for routine use. The American Academy of Pediatrics released a policy statement in 2003 stating that syrup of ipecac should no longer be kept in homes. Syrup of ipecac was administered in less than 0.01% of pediatric ingestions in 2008. The American Academy of Clinical Toxicology (AACT) reserves gastric lavage only for life-threatening ingestions presenting at less than 60 minutes since ingestion, with the caveat that there is no confirmed clinical benefit.

Activated charcoal is the mainstay in decontamination therapy of ingestion. Charcoal binds toxins, and because it is not absorbed in the GI tract, the charcoal-toxin complex passes through and is eliminated. Its efficacy decreases with increasing time since the ingestion, and ideally it should be started within an hour of the ingestion. The optimal dose of charcoal is 10 times the amount of substance ingested. Because the exact amount of toxin ingested is often unknown, activated charcoal is usually dosed at 1 to 2 g/kg. The amount of charcoal given is limited only by what the child is able to tolerate. Only a few substances are not absorbed by activated charcoal. The mnemonic **PHAILS** can be used to remember them: *p*esticides; *h*ydrocarbons and heavy metals; *a*cids, alkalis, and alcohols; *i*ron; *l*ithium; and *s*olvents. The main complication of charcoal administration is aspiration pneumonitis, primarily seen in patients with altered level of consciousness and an unprotected airway. If charcoal is not voluntarily taken by the child, it may be administered via nasogastric

tube. Endotracheal intubation to protect the airway first may be necessary in the patient with altered mental status. It is imperative that nasogastric tube placement in the GI tract (as opposed to the respiratory tract) be confirmed prior to charcoal administration.

Cathartics (most commonly sorbitol) have been used to decrease transit time and improve elimination of the toxin through the GI tract and to counteract activated charcoal-induced constipation. The cathartic is often mixed with the activated charcoal and may serve to improve the palatability of the charcoal. A significant benefit from cathartic use has never been demonstrated, however, and there is a risk of dehydration and electrolyte disturbances, particularly in young children. The AACT recommends *against* use of cathartics. Under no circumstances should repeated doses of cathartics be given.

Multiple-dose charcoal may remove drugs from the bloodstream by promoting diffusion back into the GI tract and subsequent binding to charcoal. It has been called the "GI dialysis." Activated charcoal at the same dose previously used is repeated approximately every 4 hours. Cathartics should *not* be mixed with the charcoal for repeat doses. Multiple-dose charcoal is useful for a small number of drugs, such as phenobarbital, theophylline, carbamazepine, dapsone, and quinine. It should only be used if a potentially life-threatening amount has been ingested. It should not be used for drugs that can cause an ileus (eg, tricyclic antidepressants).

Whole-bowel irrigation involves infusion of a solution usually used for cleansing of the bowel prior to GI surgery (eg, polyethylene glycol). It is especially useful for slow-release medications, for tablets that dissolve slowly and may cause concretions (eg, iron), and in ingestions where charcoal is not likely to be effective (eg, heavy metals). A nasogastric tube is used to infuse the solution at a rate of 500 mL/hour in young children, and 1 to 2 L/hour in older children and adolescents. Clear rectal effluent is the endpoint; a bedpan may be necessary. Whole-bowel irrigation should not be used when there is bowel obstruction, ileus, perforation, or hemorrhage or altered mental status with an unprotected airway.

Hemodialysis may be used for serious ingestions of ethylene glycol, methanol, phenobarbital, lithium, salicylate, or theophylline. **Charcoal hemoperfusion**, in which blood goes through a charcoal cartridge instead of a dialysis machine, is used rarely for severe theophylline poisoning. **Urinary alkalinization** (by administration of sodium bicarbonate) can increase elimination of weak acids by keeping the drug in its ionic state, thus preventing reabsorption in the renal tubule. It is primarily used for significant salicylate, phenobarbital, and isoniazid poisonings.

Intralipid is becoming recognized as a potential treatment for lipophilic drug overdoses, and has been used successfully for treating severe cardiotoxicity from bupivicaine, haloperidol, and verapamil overdoses. It is unclear by what method intralipid works. Although ideal dosing and indications have not been established, one suggested treatment protocol to consider would be: 1.5 mL/kg of 20% intralipid initial bolus, followed by 0.25 mL/kg/min for 30 to 60 minutes. Boluses may be repeated for severe cardiotoxicity and dysrhythmias.

Supportive Care

Attention to the basic ABCs (airway, breathing, circulation) of resuscitation is always the first step in management. **Hypoglycemia** must be assessed and managed as soon as possible. Dextrose 0.5 to 1 g/kg intravenously is given; glucagon may be used if dextrose cannot be given. **Seizures** are generally treatable with benzodiazepines. Glucose and electrolyte levels should be normalized. With isoniazid ingestions, pyridoxine may be helpful. **Shock** requires aggressive fluid resuscitation. Fluid-resistant shock may require vasopressors, most commonly dopamine, epinephrine, or norepinephrine. Resistant shock in a β-blocker ingestion may respond to glucagon, and in a calcium channel blocker ingestion to insulin plus glucose. **Dysrhythmias** should generally be treated by following Pediatric Advanced Life Support (PALS) protocols, although specific ingestions may respond to specific therapies. Sodium bicarbonate is the first-line treatment for dysrhythmias associated with ingestions of antihistamines, class I antiarrhythmics (lidocaine, quinidine, procainamide), cocaine, and tricyclic antidepressants. β-blocker ingestions may respond to atropine and glucagon, while ingestions of calcium channel blockers are managed with calcium. Procainamide, found on PALS algorithms, should be avoided for dysrhythmias due to overdoses of antihistamines, quinidine and other class I antiarrhythmics, digoxin, quinine, and tricyclic antidepressants. Amiodarone, also found on PALS algorithms, should also be avoided in the treatment of antihistamine ingestions. Electrolyte imbalances should be assessed and corrected. **Suicidality** should be assessed, often in conjunction with a mental health professional.

Table 68-3. Antidotes

Toxin	Antidote
Acetaminophen	N-acetylcysteine
Anticoagulants (coumadin-like)	Vitamin K
Anticholinergic	Physostigmine
Benzodiazepine	Flumazenil
β-blocker	Glucagon
Calcium channel blocker	Calcium, insulin + glucose
Carbamate pesticide	Atropine
Carbon monoxide	Oxygen
Cyanide	Cyanide antidote kit
Digoxin	Digibind
Ethylene glycol	Fomepizole, ethanol
Iron	Deferoxamine
Isoniazid	Pyridoxine
Lead	Dimercaprol (BAL), ethylene diamine tetraacetic acid, dimercaptosuccinic acid (DMSA)
Mercury	BAL, DMSA
Methanol	Fomepizole, ethanol
Methemoglobinemia	Methylene blue
Narcotics	Naloxone
Organophosphate pesticide	Atropine, 2-PAM (pralidoxime)
Rattlesnake bite	Crofab (crotalidae polyvalent immune fab [ovine])
Sulfonylurea oral hypoglycemic	Dextrose, octreotide
Tricyclic antidepressant	Sodium bicarbonate

Antidotes

Antidotes or medications that counteract the pathophysiological mechanisms of the toxin are available for only a few ingestions (Table 68-3). Important antidotes are N-acetylcysteine for acetaminophen, naloxone for narcotics, oxygen for carbon monoxide poisoning, bicarbonate for tricyclic antidepressant cardiotoxicity, Digibind for digoxin, and deferoxamine for iron. Antidotes are not without adverse effects themselves and should only be given in cases of symptomatic or potentially symptomatic (acetaminophen) ingestions of significant amounts. The poison control center staff can be very helpful in guiding practitioners in the use of antidotes.

Anticipatory Guidance and Prevention

Most ingestions are nontoxic and require only observation for a few hours. They do, however, provide an excellent opportunity to discuss poisoning prevention with parents and caretakers. Possible toxins, including prescription and over-the-counter medications, cleaning and household products, cosmetics and nail care products, toxic plants, gardening and hobby chemicals, and kitchen items such as alcohol should be kept out of reach of children. Visitors to the household should also be cautioned to keep medications out of reach of children. Substances should never be stored in unmarked containers, particularly in containers that typically hold beverages such as old soda bottles or cups. Medications should not be referred to as "candy" to entice youngsters to take them. Family members and visitors should be asked to store medications out of the child's reach, and to dispose of leftover medications and used transdermal patches safely. Used transdermal patches may still contain up to 75% of the medication dose. Also, chewing on patches, as toddlers may do, releases the medication much faster. Parents should have the universal telephone number for the poison control center and telephone numbers for local emergency departments readily available. Carbon monoxide detectors should be placed near children's bedrooms. Activated charcoal for home use is controversial and not currently recommended, although it is available without prescription from many pharmacies. Parents should not give activated charcoal without speaking to poison control center staff or medical personnel first.

Prognosis

Prognosis depends on the toxicity of the substance ingested. For a few substances, a small amount can be fatal (Box 68-2), whereas for others, even large ingestions are generally benign. Prognosis is generally excellent; fatalities in children are rare. Prognosis is worse for intentional ingestions, often because patients delay or fail to reveal that they attempted overdose.

Box 68-2. Substances Potentially Fatal in 1 to 2 Pills or Teaspoons

- Camphor (found in Vicks VapoRub, Campho-Phenique, Tiger Balm)
- Imidazoline decongestants (found in over-the-counter nasal and eye drops)
- Acetonitrile nail glue remover
- Clonidine (available in transdermal patches also)
- Opiates (available in transdermal patches also)
- Methyl salicylate (oil of wintergreen, Ben-gay)
- Calcium channel blockers
- Toxic alcohols (methanol, ethylene glycol, ethanol, isopropanol)
- Tricyclic antidepressants
- Lomotil (opiate diphenoxylate + atropine)
- Sulfonylurea oral hypoglycemics
- Chloroquine and hydrochloroquine antimalarial agents
- Hydrofluoric acid
- Selenious acid (gun bluing solution)
- Buffered saline solution
- Benzocaine-induced methemoglobinemia

CASE RESOLUTION

Because the respiratory rate of this 2-year-old is slow and there are symptoms of miosis and altered level of consciousness, narcotic ingestion is suspected and naloxone is administered. The child becomes more alert and respiratory rate increases to 24 breaths/min. The father is instructed to retrieve the bottle, and it turns out to be a prescription narcotic analgesic left in the house by a recent visitor. The child is given activated charcoal, observed overnight in the hospital, and discharged on the following day without sequelae.

Selected References

American Academy of Pediatrics Committee on Injury, Violence, and Poison Prevention. Poison treatment in the home. *Pediatrics.* 2003;112:1182–1185

American Association of Poison Control Centers Web site. http://www.aapcc. org/. Accessed November 30, 2010

Bailey B. To decontaminate or not to decontaminate? The balance between potential risks and foreseeable benefits. *Clin Pediatr Emerg Med.* 2008;9:17–23

Barry JD. Diagnosis and management of the poisoned child. *Pediatr Ann.* 2005;34:937–946

Bronstein AC, Spyker DA, Cantilena LR, Green JL, Rumack BH, Giffin SL. 2008 annual report of the American Association of Poison Control Centers' National Poison Data System (NPDS): 26th annual report. *Clin Toxicol.* 2009;47:911–1084

Drugs.com Pill Identifier. http://www.drugs.com/pill_identification.html. Accessed November 30, 2010

Ferreiros N, Dresen S, Hermanns-Clausen M, et al. Fatal and severe codeine intoxication in 3-year-old twins—interpretation of drug and metabolite concentrations. *Int J Legal Med.* 2009;123:387–394

Henry K, Harris CR. Deadly ingestions. *Pediatr Clin North Am.* 2006;53:293–315

McGregor T, Parkar M, Rao S. Evaluaton and management of common childhood poisonings. *Am Fam Physician.* 2009;79:397–403

Smith HS. Opioid metabolism. *Mayo Clin Proc.* 2009;84:613–624

Weinberg G, Picard J, Meek T, Hertz P. LipidRescue resuscitation for cardiac toxicity. http://lipidrescue.squarespace.com/. Accessed November 30, 2010

White ML, Liebelt EL. Update on antidotes for pediatric poisoning. *Pediatr Emerg Care.* 2006;22:740–746

Head, Neck, and Respiratory System

CHAPTER 69

Approach to the Dysmorphic Child

Julie E. Noble, MD

CASE STUDY

A 13-year-old male presents to the office for the first time for an evaluation after moving to the area. Parents note that he has unexplained mental retardation and has had problems with hyperactivity in school. The pregnancy was uncomplicated and the mother, who was a 32-year-old gravida I para I at the time of the child's birth, denies alcohol or drug use or exposure to any teratogens during pregnancy. Delivery was by cesarean section secondary to cephalopelvic disproportion, but Apgar scores were 8 at 1 minute and 9 at 5 minutes. The infant was noted to have macrocephaly and to be large for gestational age. He did well in the newborn period and had no feeding problems. Subsequently, he had no significant medical illnesses, including no seizures, but at 1 year of age was noted to be developmentally delayed. This delay continued, and he has been in special education classes throughout his school career. Family history is negative for any family members with retardation.

On physical examination, the boy is greater than 90th percentile for height and weight. He is mildly prognathic with large ears. He has hyperextensible fingers. A complete examination reveals that his testicles appear large (6 cm) and his sexual maturity rating (Tanner stage) is 3. The rest of the examination is normal.

Questions

1. What history is important to elicit in evaluating a child with dysmorphic features?
2. What are the possible causes of errors in morphogenesis?
3. What clues on physical examination can aid in establishing a specific diagnosis?
4. What laboratory tests can confirm a diagnosis?
5. When is it appropriate to obtain a genetics consultation or refer a patient for genetic counseling?
6. What are the benefits of establishing a specific diagnosis?

Evaluation for structural anomalies is an essential part of all pediatric examinations. Visible errors in morphogenesis give the physician valuable information in evaluating a patient with abnormal symptoms, such as seizures. Additionally, major malformations frequently require treatment, and the presence of one anomaly suggests that others may also exist.

The study of these congenital defects was termed dysmorphology by David Smith in 1966. The anomalies fall into 2 categories: minor and major. Minor malformations are those of "no medical or cosmetic consequence to the patient." An example would be a supernumerary nipple that appears as a hyperpigmented papule along the nipple line. Identification of minor malformations is important because they may indicate the presence of a more generalized pattern of malformation. Major malformations are those that have "an adverse effect on either the function or social acceptability of the individual." A cleft lip and palate are major malformations that have functional as well as cosmetic relevance to the patient's health.

Epidemiology

Structural anomalies are common in the general population. Most are minor. In the first comprehensive analysis of minor structural anomalies, Marden in 1964 identified 7% to 14% of newborn infants with at least one minor anomaly on surface examination. Other studies identify up to 40% of newborns with one anomaly. Three or more minor malformations have predictive value in identifying a major malformation. In newborns, 0.8% have 2 minor malformations, and 11% of these patients will have a major malformation. Three or more minor malformations occur in 0.5% of newborns, and 90% of these will have a major malformation. Data from the National Collaborative Perinatal Program revealed that 44.78% of these anomalies were craniofacial and 45.3% were skin. Males are affected with minor malformations more often than females. Autopsies of dead fetuses reveal an increased incidence of both minor and major malformations. Frequencies of both minor and major malformations vary along racial lines, depending on the specific malformations. For example, postaxial polydactyly is seen in 16 of 10,000 births in the white population and 140 of 10,000 births in the African American population. Hemangiomas are seen in 350 of 10,000 births in whites and only 100 of 10,000 births in African Americans.

Three percent of all pregnancies produce a child with a significant genetic disease or a birth defect. These malformations account for a great proportion of morbidity and mortality in the pediatric population. Of all pediatric hospital admissions, one-third to one-half involve a child with a disease with a genetic component.

Clinical Presentation

With the advent of more prenatal tests and diagnostic modalities (see Chapter 20), the detection of anomalies may first occur in the prenatal period. Routine prenatal screening tests that are abnormal raise the possibility that the infant will have an anomaly. For instance, an elevated maternal α-fetoprotein indicates the possibility of a spinal cord defect. Amniocentesis or chorionic villus biopsy may reveal abnormal chromosomes with associated structural defects. Prenatal ultrasound demonstrates structural defects in utero and a specific fetal ultrasound can further delineate those abnormalities.

Most structural anomalies develop during the first trimester of gestation and, if not detected prenatally, are noted at birth in the delivery room or the newborn nursery. Many major congenital defects are obvious on a thorough physical examination. Some major defects, such as a tracheoesophageal fistula, will not be manifest on surface examination but will be readily apparent as the infant adapts to extra-uterine life and experiences symptoms when feeding begins. Minor anomalies may be overlooked on an infant's initial examination. However, if that infant manifests developmental delay at 6 months of age, the physician may be more inclined to evaluate for minor anomalies that may aid in identifying the cause of the developmental delay.

Sometimes dysmorphic features are not present at birth but become apparent later in life as the child grows and develops. These types of features are associated with dysplasias, defects in cellular metabolism that become manifest after birth. An example is a skeletal dysplasia that becomes more apparent as the bones grow.

Pathophysiology

The pathophysiology of structural defects can be separated into 4 different types of errors in morphogenesis: malformations, deformations, disruptions, and dysplasias (Box 69-1).

Previously, the term **malformation** was used descriptively to denote an anomaly; but it is also used to denote a specific pathogenic mechanism. Malformations are permanent defects in a structure caused by an intrinsic abnormality in the development of that structure. An example of a malformation is an endocardial cushion defect in a patient with Down syndrome. Malformations frequently are caused by chromosomal abnormalities and single-gene disorders that program for abnormal structure.

Deformations occur in an infant when external forces exert a mechanical pressure on the developing fetus. There is no intrinsic defect of the fetus. These deformations from intrauterine forces can

---

Box 69-1. Pathophysiology of Structural Defects
Malformation
Chromosomal abnormality
Single gene disorder
Deformation
Disruption
Vascular compromise
Viral infection
Mechanical—amniotic bands
Teratogens—alcohol, drugs, irradiation
Dysplasia
Metabolic disorder

---

be caused by uterine constraint, an abnormally shaped uterus, or multiparous pregnancy. A flexible clubfoot is a deformation caused by uterine constraint. Deformations can also be caused by extrauterine forces such as plagiocephaly caused by an infant sleeping on his back. **Disruptions** occur when an agent outside a fetus causes cell death and a permanent defect in fetal development. These disruptive events result in tissue destruction. Disruptions can occur during development when there is tissue ischemia secondary to vascular compromise, when a viral infection disrupts development at a critical gestational age, or when a mechanical disruption interferes with normal development. An amniotic band is an example of a mechanical disruptive agent that can cause an amputation of a limb by constricting the extremity during development. Teratogens can also function as disruptive agents by interfering during a critical period in embryogenesis, causing dysgenesis of fetal organs. Alcohol, specific drugs, and irradiation can all be teratogens. Fewer than 30 drugs have been proved to be teratogenic.

Dysplasias, often caused by a single-gene defect, are structural abnormalities that develop from abnormal cellular metabolism and organization. They can occur intrauterine, and be apparent at birth such as a skeletal dysplasia, or extrauterine. Mucopolysaccharidosis is a dysplasia that develops postnatally secondary to the absence of the lysosomal hydrolase of α-L-iduronidase. As a result, mucopolysaccharides accumulate in parenchymal and mesenchymal tissues. As affected children grow, they develop coarse facies, enlarged tongue, misshapen bones, and hepatosplenomegaly among other features.

Differential Diagnosis

In generating an appropriate differential diagnosis for a dysmorphic child, it is essential to identify all minor and major malformations. The differential will vary depending on the specific findings. A thorough history and physical examination will help greatly to establish the list of conditions to consider. If there are multiple anomalies, identifying the most specific and rarest anomaly can direct the practitioner to a narrower list of possible diagnoses. For example, nail hypoplasia, which is seen in fetal hydantoin syndrome, is much rarer than congenital cardiac disease, which is seen in multiple syndromes. A practitioner should be familiar with the prominent features of the more common syndromes but also should have readily available reference texts, such as *Smith's Recognizable Patterns of Human Malformation,* to aid in establishing differential lists as well as finalizing diagnoses. In addition, the Internet has developed into a valuable tool through Web sites such as PubMed or Google, or those specifically developed for the delineation of syndromes and genetic disorders.

In evaluating an infant with congenital anomalies, the practitioner should attempt to separate the findings into 1 of 5 categories: an isolated defect, a developmental field defect, a birth defect association, a sequence pattern, or a dysmorphic syndrome (Box 69-2). The first step is to determine whether the anomaly is **isolated.** If so, does it represent a failure in development in one location, such as a cleft lip? Most isolated anomalies are believed to have a multifactorial inheritance, representing the interaction between multiple genes and unknown external influences. They usually have a recurrence risk of 2% to 5%.

Box 69-2. Categories of Anomalies	
Isolated defect	Sequence pattern
Developmental field defect	Dysmorphic syndrome
Birth defect association	

A **developmental field defect** is a pattern of anomalies that develops in structures that are together during embryologic development. These defects involve one limited region and are secondary to a disruptive event such as vascular compromise. They therefore have a low recurrence risk. An example would be hemifacial microsomia (oculo-auriculo-vertebral defect), where the defects are secondary to disruption in vascular flow to the first and second branchial arches. This disruption results in hypoplasia of the malar, maxillary, and mandibular region on one side with associated microtia and vertebral defects.

Birth defect associations are diagnosed when the combination of anomalies occurs together frequently but the pattern does not fit a known field defect or syndrome. The etiology of association defects is unknown at this time, and the recurrence risk is low. One of the more common associations is the VACTERRL association (*v*ertebral anomalies, *a*nal atresia, *c*ardiac defects, *t*racheoesophageal fistula, *r*adial defects, *r*enal defects, and *l*imb defects). Emerging information in gene research may identify an etiology in the near future.

A **sequence pattern** of anomalies occurs when one malformation leads to multiple dysmorphic features. Potter oligohydramnios sequence results from renal agenesis. The renal malformation causes oligohydramnios with resultant fetal contractures, pulmonary hypoplasia, and a flattened face.

A **syndrome** is a pattern of anomalies that are pathologically related. Chromosomal abnormalities such as Down syndrome (trisomy 21), single-gene disorders, and teratogens fall into this category. Alcohol is the most common teratogen to which fetuses are exposed. Alcohol exposure in utero causes growth failure, developmental delay, microcephaly, a short nose, and small distal phalanges. Children with developmental delay and anomalies have a higher likelihood of having a syndrome and should undergo a chromosome analysis.

Evaluation

History

A complete history is essential (Questions Box). The history begins prenatally with information from the mother on duration of pregnancy, possible teratogen exposure, fetal activity, diagnostic test results, and any complications of pregnancy. The delivery history should include type of delivery, infant presentation, and size at birth, including growth percentiles. Neonatal adaptation and feeding patterns are important parameters to assess. The subsequent medical history should be obtained.

A thorough family history is equally important, and a pedigree should be outlined. Specifically, the family should be questioned for parental age, possible consanguinity, and history of fetal loss or early infant deaths. Family history of birth defects or retardation should be documented.

Questions

The Dysmorphic Child

- How long was the pregnancy?
- Did the mother take any medications, smoke cigarettes, or use alcohol or any illicit drug?
- What was the fetal activity?
- Were there any complications of pregnancy?
- What was the type of delivery and presentation of the baby?
- What was the infant's size at birth?
- How did the infant feed?
- What is the subsequent medical and developmental history?
- Are the parents related?
- What are the parents' ages?
- Is there a history of fetal or infant deaths?
- Is there a history of birth defects in the family?
- Are any family members retarded?

Physical Examination

The physical examination should be extremely thorough with all morphological findings noted. As previously mentioned, the craniofacial area and skin are common sites for anomalies, but all organ systems should be extensively evaluated. Even minor anomalies, such as a supernumerary nipple or clinodactyly, may have significance. Objective measurements should be obtained when possible. Normal grids are available for evaluating inner canthus distance, palpebral fissure length, ear length, etc. Hair whorl patterns and dermatoglyphics should be evaluated. Physical data, including height, weight, and head circumference, should be plotted and the growth percentiles noted. A complete ophthalmologic evaluation may be indicated to detect abnormalities such as cataracts or cherry-red spots.

Laboratory Tests

In assessments of dysmorphic-appearing children, the physical examination is the most important part. Findings on physical examination direct which further studies will be of benefit. Additional studies may give added or confirmatory information regarding a suspected diagnosis. Prenatal screening tests may be used to detect a fetal abnormality, and specific prenatal tests are available to assess a fetus at risk for a given disease. Cytogenetic evaluation is essential in evaluating a child with a suspected syndrome and also in evaluating a child with malformations and developmental delay. Standard chromosomal analysis is the first-line laboratory test but may not detect many small chromosomal or gene defects. More sophisticated testing may be indicated. Small chromosomal aberrations can be detected by FISH (fluorescent in situ hybridization) analysis, in which labeled probes are applied to chromosomal preparations. These probes are specific for given disorders and should be used to confirm a suspected clinical syndrome. Prader-Willi and DiGeorge syndromes may be diagnosed by FISH analysis. FISH probes can now be applied to subtelomeric regions of the chromosome, which are very gene rich. Whole chromosome painting is another technique in which FISH probes are used to paint the entire chromosome, thus identifying the origin of additional chromosomal material or cryptic translocations. Molecular testing is available for many single-gene disorders. Comparative genomic hybridization is a cytogenetic method for analysis of copy number changes in DNA. It is a supplement to karotyping and is the prime genome-wide screening method. This test has revealed genetic etiologies in many previously unidentified patients with abnormalities.

Many dysplasias and some syndromes can be detected by metabolic testing. Serum amino acids and urine organic acids should be ordered if a diagnosis is suspected. Many states are now including an analysis for metabolic disorders in their expanded newborn screening protocols. There is a federal effort to standardize the newborn screening guidelines statewide.

Imaging Studies

Imaging studies are extremely useful in deriving information on internal malformations. Radiographs, including a skeletal survey, may detect skeletal anomalies. Echocardiogram, ultrasound, computed tomography scan, and magnetic resonance imaging (MRI) studies can all be used when appropriate. With the findings of anomalies and global developmental delay in a patient, the American Academy of Neurology recommends routine neuroimaging with an MRI.

Management

When children present with dysmorphic features, they should be evaluated to determine a specific diagnosis. Obtaining a diagnosis is of vital importance to the care of the patient and parental counseling. Knowing the diagnosis can direct subsequent testing for associated abnormalities. Treatment options may also be available for the condition, and a prognosis can be established. Defining the developmental prognosis for children is essential to establish appropriate school planning. If developmental delay is not associated with the diagnosis, such as with cleft lip and palate, the parents should be reassured. Parents also need to know the recurrence risk for themselves and for their children. Occasionally, further testing of the parents may be necessary to determine the accurate recurrence risk. If one of the parents is a translocation carrier, the risk of subsequent children having the abnormality is increased.

Consultation with a geneticist can help the practitioner in establishing the correct diagnosis and provide the practitioner with the latest information regarding evaluation and possible treatment. New information in the field of genetic disease appears daily, and it is difficult for a primary care practitioner to stay abreast. A genetic consultation should also be obtained in most patients with major malformations to confirm the diagnosis and to help counsel parents.

Health supervision strategies have been established for specific disorders. For instance, published guidelines recommend hearing, ophthalmologic, and thyroid screening, among other tests, for patients with Down syndrome. A geneticist can give guidance regarding revised recommendations.

If support groups are available for specific conditions, parents should be referred to these groups. Such groups can be invaluable in helping parents understand as well as adjust to the disorder. They can also advise parents about community and educational resources available for their child's care and help parents advocate for their child's unique needs.

A referral to a genetics counselor can provide parents with education about prenatal testing, recurrence risk, and alternatives for dealing with this recurrence risk. Counseling is extremely useful to help parents understand the inheritance pattern.

Prognosis

As with management, defining an accurate prognosis for each patient depends on recognition of the specific condition. Some conditions, such as trisomy 13, are lethal while other conditions allow for a normal life span.

Malformations are permanent defects that generally have a recurrence risk. They may be correctable with surgery or treatment but frequently leave a residual disability.

Deformations usually resolve with treatment and have no recurrence risk unless the deformation is secondary to a uterine abnormality such as a bicornuate uterus.

A disruption may be treated with surgery or therapy to improve function but, as in malformations, a residual disability frequently remains. When the disruption is due to tissue ischemia or a mechanical agent, there is no recurrence risk. If it is due to a teratogen, the disruption will recur with the same teratogenic exposure.

Dysplasias tend to persist or worsen with time unless a specific treatment is available. Only a limited number of diseases have specific treatments available. Generally, there is a recurrence risk.

CASE RESOLUTION

The child in the case scenario has features that suggest a dysmorphic syndrome. The most specific finding on examination is macro-orchidism. This finding is associated with fragile X syndrome. The patient is referred to a genetic specialist for diagnosis and counseling. Specific DNA-based molecular analysis is performed and is positive for a fragile site on the X chromosome at Xq27.3.

Parents are counseled that this condition has an X-linked inheritance pattern. The child will have a normal life span but may need early intervention services and later a special education program, and may not be capable of independent living as an adult. The primary care physician will be notified of the diagnosis and coordinate further services. Parents are encouraged to attend a parents' support group and consult with experts to learn how their child's full potential may be realized.

Selected References

Aase JM. Dysmorphologic diagnosis for the pediatric practitioner. *Pediatr Clin North Am.* 1992;39:135–156

Friedman JM. A practical approach to dysmorphology. *Pediatr Ann.* 1990;19:95–101

Groupman AL, Batshaw ML. Epigenetics, copy number, variation, and other molecular mechanisms underlying neurodevelopmental disabilities: new insights and diagnostic approaches. *J Dev Behav Pediatr.* 2010;31:582–591

Hunter A. Medical genetics: 2. The diagnostic approach to the child with dysmorphic signs. *Can Med Assoc J.* 2002;167:367–372

Jones KL. *Smith's Recognizable Patterns of Human Malformation.* 6th ed. Philadelphia, PA: W. B. Saunders; 2006

Koren G, Pastuszak A, Ito S. Drugs in pregnancy. *N Engl J Med.* 1998;338:1128–1136

Moeschler J, Shevell M; American Academy of Pediatrics Committee on Genetics. Clinical genetic evaluation of the child with mental retardation or developmental delays. *Pediatrics.* 2006;117:2304–2316

Poot M. A three step workflow procedure for the interpretation of array-based comparative genomic hybridization results in patients with idiopathic mental retardation and congenital anomalies. *Genet Med.* 2010;12:478–485

Shevell M, Ashwal S, Donley D, et al. Practice parameter: evaluation of the child with global developmental delay: report of the Quality Standards Subcommittee of the American Academy of Neurology and The Practice Committee of the Child Neurology Society. *Neurology.* 2003;60:367–380

Toriello V. Role of the dysmorphologic evaluation in the child with developmental delay. *Pediatr Clin North Am.* 2008; 55;1085–1098

Walker W, Johnson C. Mental retardation: overview and diagnosis. *Pediatr Rev.* 2006;27:204–212

CHAPTER 70

Craniofacial Anomalies

Carol D. Berkowitz, MD

CASE STUDY

A 3,500-g boy is born by normal spontaneous vaginal delivery to a 28-year-old gravida III para III mother after an uncomplicated full-term gestation. The Apgar scores are 9 and 10. On physical examination, the infant is well but has an incomplete, left-sided unilateral cleft of the lip and palate.

No other family members have such a deformity, but the mother and father are distantly related. The mother had prenatal care. During the pregnancy she had no illnesses; took vitamins but no other medications; and did not smoke, drink alcohol, or use illicit drugs.

The mother is planning to feed the infant with formula and wonders if she should do anything special. She is also wondering if her son's lip deformity can be repaired before she takes him home from the hospital. Except for the cleft, the physical examination is normal.

Questions

1. What craniofacial anomalies are common in children?
2. What are feeding considerations in infants with cleft lip or palate?
3. What is the appropriate timing of surgery for the more common craniofacial anomalies?
4. What are the major medical problems that children with craniofacial anomalies, particularly clefts of the lip or palate, experience?
5. What is positional plagiocephaly? How is its prevalence related to the Back to Sleep campaign?

Infants may be born with readily apparent craniofacial anomalies such as cleft lip, cleft palate, or microtia, or anomalies may emerge as an infant grows older. The latter includes conditions that may be genetically based but do not manifest until later, such as facial asymmetry (hemifacial microsomia) and premature closure of one or more sutures. Alternatively, these anomalies may be environmentally influenced, such as positional or deformational plagiocephaly. Deformational plagiocephaly is defined as a condition in which the infant's head and sometimes face are misshapen as a result of prenatal and, in recent years, postnatal external molding, which occur on the infant's malleable cranium.

Epidemiology

The overall incidence of cleft lip with or without cleft palate is 1 in 1,000, and that of isolated cleft palate is 1 in 2,500. Cleft lip with or without cleft palate is the fourth most common birth defect. There is racial, ethnic, and geographic variation in the incidence of clefts. For example, the incidence of clefts in parts of the Philippines is 1 in 200. Similarly, cleft lip with or without cleft palate is most common among Native Americans (1 in 230 to 1,000) and least common among African Americans (1 in 1,300 to 5,000). The gender distribution varies with the type of cleft. Isolated clefts of the palate occur twice as frequently in girls, but clefts of the lip with or without clefts of the palate appear twice as often in boys.

The type of cleft, the gender of the child, and whether parents or other siblings are similarly affected influence the risk for recurrence of clefts in subsequent offspring. In general, the risk for recurrence of clefts is 4% to 7% for cleft lip with or without cleft palate and 3% for isolated cleft palate.

Clefts may occur either as isolated findings or as part of syndromes or sequences. In Van der Woude syndrome, clefts of the lip or palate are associated with lip pits. This condition is inherited in an autosomal-dominant manner. There are now more than 200 disorders associated with clefts, although only 10% to 15% of children with clefts fit a syndrome. Pierre Robin sequence includes micrognathia and glossoptosis (retropositioned tongue) and a distinct u-shaped cleft. One theory relates the sequence to failure of the fetal neck to extend normally, leading to compression of the mandible on the chest thereby restricting its growth, causing the tongue to be malpositioned, thus preventing closure of the palate.

True craniosynostosis occurs in about 1 in 2,000 to 3,000 births, and this incidence is the same in all ethnic groups. There is gender variation among the different types of craniosynostosis. Mild deformational plagiocephaly is reported to be present in up to 13% of newborns, 16% of 6-week-olds, and nearly 20% of 4-month-olds. The term plagiocephaly comes from the Greek *plagio,* meaning oblique, twisted, or slanted, and *kephale* for head. First born and male gender increase the risk of deformational plagiocephaly at birth.

Most cases of deformational plagiocephaly resolve over time without specific medical intervention. When infants slept in the prone position, plagiocephaly occurred in 1 in 300. The prevalence of plagiocephaly increased to 1 in 60 following the recommendation for supine sleep position.

Microtia is less common and occurs in 1 in 6,000 to 8,000 births. Other ear malformations, such as auricular dystopia (ear located on the check) or total atresia of the external area, are less common and can be associated with other syndromes.

Clinical Presentation

Most craniofacial anomalies are readily apparent (see Dx Box). Some anomalies, such as cleft lips or microtia, are noted immediately in the delivery room. Other anomalies, such as craniosynostosis, develop over time. Because the onset of craniosynostosis may be gradual, parents may fail to recognize the condition, which usually appears as asymmetry of the face or skull. Deformational plagiocephaly also evolves over time and is more often noted by the clinician rather than the parents.

Children with craniofacial anomalies may also have medical problems that occur secondary to the deformity. Infants with cleft palate may present with failure to thrive because of difficulty feeding. Older infants and children may experience recurrent otitis media, speech impairments, or psychosocial stress. Nasal regurgitation of liquids may occur in children with obvious palatal clefts or more subtle deformities, such as submucous clefts of the soft palate.

Dx Craniofacial Anomalies

- Cleft of the lip or palate
- Small, atretic, or malformed ear
- Asymmetry of the face
- Misshapen skull
- Recurrent otitis media
- Speech impairment

Pathophysiology

Clefts of the lip and palate (Figure 70-1) are believed to develop as a result of an interruption in the merging of the middle and lateral portions of the face during the sixth to seventh week of gestation. The palate normally closes with an anterior to posterior progression. Any interference with this progression (eg, tumor or encephalocele in the roof of the mouth) leads to a cleft. A vascular disruption may also result in ischemia in the involved areas. Although the etiology of clefts is not fully determined, it is felt to be multifactorial. Studies establish a link between clefting and transforming growth factor–α (TGF-α). The locus for TGF-α is on the short arm of 2p13. As with other clinical conditions, genetic predisposition interacts with environmental factors to increase the risk of the emergence of a disorder. Infants with the A2 form of the TGF-α gene are 8 times more

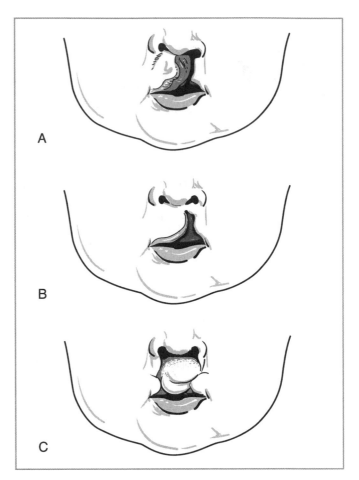

Figure 70-1. Cleft lips. A. Unilateral, complete cleft lip. B. Unilateral, incomplete cleft lip. C. Bilateral, complete cleft lip.

likely to have facial clefts if their mothers smoke. Other environmental teratogens associated with clefts include hydantoin, alcohol, warfarin, trimethadione, thalidomide, aminopterin, and topiramate.

The presence of a cleft palate affects normal oropharyngeal functioning, including sucking and speech. Children may exhibit hypernasal speech, due to the escape of air through the nose, and have articulation problems. Recurrent otitis media seems to be related to dysfunction of the eustachian tube.

Microtia, a small atretic pinna of the ear, results from failure of development of the pinna and portions of the external auditory canal. It is most likely caused by a vascular accident during the 12th week of gestation. Similar anomalies have been created in laboratory animals by ligature of the stapedius artery. Microtia is considered in the spectrum of branchial arch defects.

Craniosynostosis refers to the premature closure of the sutures, which should remain open until 2 to 3 years of age. The newborn skull consists of membranous bones that meet at the suture lines. The newborn skull is therefore moldable, can change during the birthing process, and can expand in response to growth of the brain. Premature closure of the sutures is a pathological process. What initiates this pathologic ossification is unclear. There is some evidence to suggest that skull compression, such as occurs in utero with breech presentation or twins, contributes to the process. When there are other associated anomalies, such as syndactyly, embryologic disturbances in fibrocartilaginous development are suspected. Abnormalities in one region of chromosome 10 are implicated in syndromic synostosis. Genes associated with fibroblast growth factor receptor have been implicated in some genetic syndromes with craniosynostosis. Any or all of the sutures can be affected, and the closure may result in asymmetry of the skull or microcephaly. Single suture synostosis is classified as simple; multiple synostosis is classified as compound. When closure is related to pathology at the suture, the condition is primary. When there is underlying brain pathology, the disorder is secondary. Premature closure of all sutures is often associated with diseases of the central nervous system, with failure of the brain to grow.

Microcephaly may result from premature closure of some or all of the sutures as a primary event or from impairment of the brain and its growth related to some other problem, such as hypoxic encephalopathy or congenital infection. Other disorders involving head size include macrocephaly, where the head circumference is greater than the 97th percentile. There are numerous causes of macrocephaly, including hydrocephalus characterized by enlargement of the ventricular system, and megalencephaly. Megalencephaly may be due to enlargement of the brain from anatomical or metabolic conditions, including the mucopolysaccharidoses. Children who have large heads and are neurologically normal have benign or idiopathic megalencephaly. Measuring parental head size is frequently a clue to the correct diagnosis.

Fusion of individual sutures prevents growth of the skull perpendicular to the suture, and skull expansion proceeds in an axis parallel to that of the suture (Figure 70-2). If the sagittal suture fuses prematurely, the head is long and narrow, a condition referred to as **scaphocephaly** (boat head). This is the most common type of craniosynostosis, occurring in about 54% to 58%. If the coronal sutures fuse too soon, the head is flattened; this condition is called **brachycephaly** and occurs in 18% to 29% of cases of craniosynostosis. The incidence

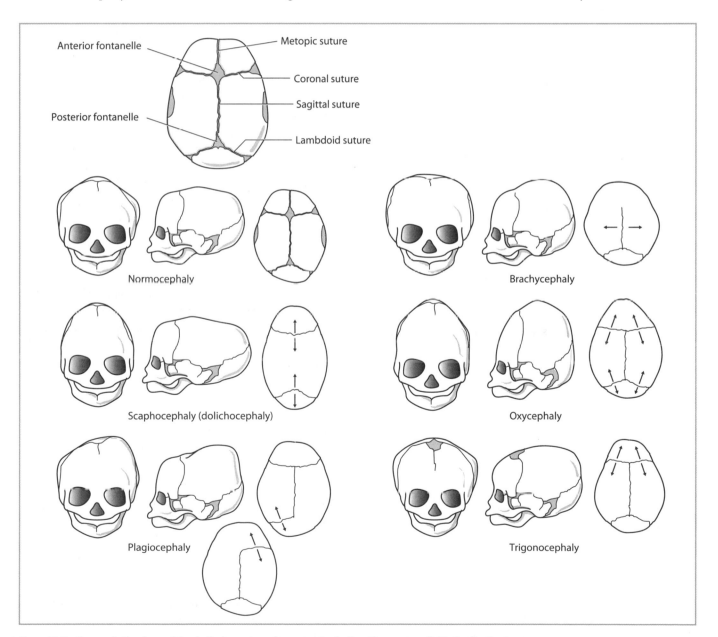

Figure 70-2. Changes in the shape of the skull when sutures fuse prematurely. Growth occurs parallel to the fused suture.

is 1 in 10,000 live births. Unilateral fusion of a coronal suture produces facial asymmetry and a characteristic appearance of the orbit on the affected side called a "harlequin" deformity noted on facial radiograph. Premature closure of the metopic suture results in the triangular-shaped head characteristic of **trigonocephaly,** reported in 4% to 10%. Familial cases have been reported, as well as abnormalities of chromosomes 3, 9, and 11.

Premature closure of the lambdoidal sutures leads to **plagiocephaly** (oblique head) (Figure 70-3). Plagiocephaly may also result from malpositioning in utero or after birth, a condition referred to as non-synostotic, deformational, or positional plagiocephaly. The skull has been likened to a parallelogram in appearance when there is also involvement of the facial structures. Torticollis, often related to injury to the sternocleidomastoid muscle at birth (see Chapter 106) and abnormal positioning after birth, may contribute to plagiocephaly. Plagiocephaly–torticollis sequence occurs in 1 in 300 live births. Malar and contralateral occipital flattening related to preferential positioning by infants are characteristically seen in affected infants. Some affected babies also have hip dislocation or positional clubfoot from in utero constraint (see Chapter 100). Positional plagiocephaly may be seen without torticollis and has been attributed to supine sleeping.

Differential Diagnosis

In general, the differential diagnosis of clefts of the lip and palate presents few problems. However, submucous clefts may be more difficult to diagnose. Children with such clefts may present with recurrent otitis media or hypernasal speech. Physical examination may reveal a bifid uvula and occasionally a notch at the junction of the hard and soft palates.

Determining whether any physical finding represents an isolated anomaly or is part of a genetic syndrome may be challenging. Any associated anomalies (eg, syndactyly or atrial septal defect) suggest the possibility of a genetic problem (Boxes 70-1 and 70-2).

Microtia does not present a diagnostic dilemma. The anomaly usually appears sporadically as an isolated condition although, like a cleft, it may be part of some other syndrome. Microtia is associated with midfacial hypoplasia and antimongoloid slant to the eyes in Treacher Collins syndrome. Microtia may also occur in Goldenhar syndrome, which is characterized by several associated findings, including hemifacial microsomia (one side of the face smaller than the other), epibulbar dermoids, hemivertebrae, microphthalmia, and renal and cardiac anomalies.

Box 70-1. Genetic Syndromes Associated With Clefts	
Ankyloblepharon filiforme adnatum	Optiz
Apert	Oral-facial-digital
Ectrodactyly-ectodermal dysplasia-clefting	Popliteal pterygium
	Stickler
Goldenhar	Treacher Collins
Meckel	Van der Woude

Box 70-2. Anomalies Associated With Cleft Lips and Palates	
Nasal glioma or meningoencephalocele	Sacral agenesis
	Aniridia
Persistent buccopharyngeal membrane	Cleft larynx
	Polydactyly
Congenital neuroblastoma	Anencephaly
Congenital heart disease	Foot deformities
Thoracopagus twins	Oral duplication
Congenital oral teratoma	Spina bifida
Forearm bone aplasia	Aplasia of trochlea
Lateral proboscis	Laryngeal web

Box 70-3. Genetic Disorders With Craniosynostosis	
Apert syndrome	Jackson-Weiss syndrome
Crouzon disease	Pfeiffer syndrome

Craniosynostosis may also be an isolated finding or associated with a condition such as Apert syndrome, in which clefts of the palate are also seen (Box 70-3). A careful neurodevelopmental assessment helps determine whether microcephaly is related to an underlying neurodevelopmental disorder. Plagiocephaly may present a diagnostic dilemma: Is the condition related to unilateral craniosynostosis, torticollis, or supine sleeping? A careful assessment of the neck for masses or mobility helps determine the role of the neck musculature in the cranial flattening and defines the management approach (eg, neck exercises).

Evaluation

Care must be taken to assess children and determine if the anomalies are isolated findings or components of a syndrome. This information is important both in terms of patient care and genetic counseling for parents regarding the likelihood of having future offspring with similar anomalies.

History

A medical, family, and psychosocial history should be obtained (Questions Box). Whether the condition appeared at birth or some time later is particularly significant in lesions affecting the skull, such as craniosynostosis. Maternal use of certain medications, such as diazepam, phenytoin, and isotretinoin (Accutane), and alcohol is associated with an increased incidence of clefts of the lip and palate. Maternal smoking also increases the risk of clefting, especially in a genetically vulnerable population. Maternal smoking and high altitude are associated with an increased occurrence of craniosynostosis.

Physical Examination

Height, weight, and head circumference should be measured and plotted at each visit. Head circumference is especially important in children with craniosynostosis or facial asymmetry. The skull

Questions

Craniofacial Anomalies

- Did the child suffer any injuries at birth?
- Was the child born in an abnormal position?
- What is the child's usual sleeping position?
- Have the findings been present since birth, or did they appear later?
- Has the anomaly led to any changes in the child's health, such as recurrent ear infections or speech difficulties?
- Does the child have any family history of craniofacial anomalies?
- Does the mother have a history of illness during pregnancy?
- Was the mother exposed to any medications, particularly teratogenic agents, during pregnancy?
- Did the mother use alcohol during pregnancy?
- Did the mother smoke during pregnancy?
- Is the child experiencing difficulties in school (eg, teasing)?
- How is the child performing in school?
- Is development progressing normally? What are the child's milestones?
- Is the child's speech understandable?
- Does the child have any trouble with eating or drinking? Are fluids expelled through the child's nose with swallowing?

should be palpated to detect perisutural ridging. Inner canthal distance may reveal hypotelorism, a finding seen in trigonocephaly. The neck should be palpated for masses and the range of neck motion assessed. The growth of children with craniofacial anomalies must be carefully monitored. Problems with adequate weight gain are frequently experienced by infants with clefts.

The physical examination should focus on defining the extent of the anomaly and determining if associated abnormalities are present. Such abnormalities may involve the face or other parts of the body, including the skeleton. The pharynx should be carefully examined for mobility of the palate. While some children with nasal regurgitation have a structural deformity, such as a submucosal cleft, others, including infants with DiGeorge syndrome (22q11 deletion syndrome), have functional impairment with decreased palatal mobility. In children with microtia, the position of the ear should be noted. When the ear is displaced to the cheek, the condition is called *auricular dystopia*. Cardiac murmurs may be noted in children with clefts, and these murmurs should be carefully evaluated.

Children with clefts should be carefully assessed for the presence of otitis media at each visit. Periodic hearing assessments should be carried out in children with clefts or microtia. Speech and development should also be evaluated.

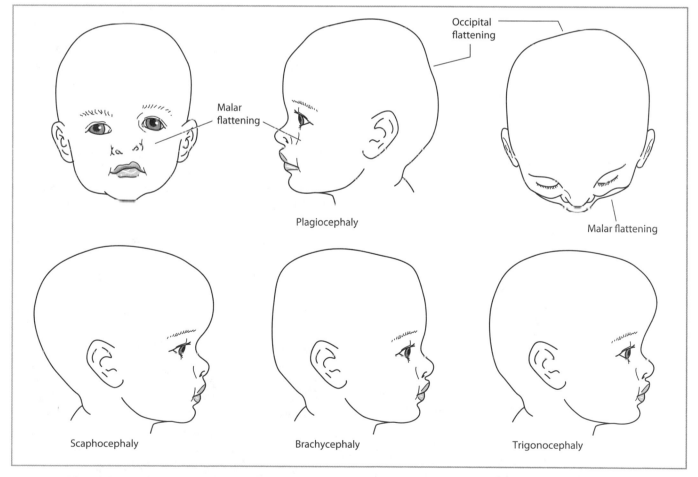

Figure 70-3. **Top row. Classic appearance of an infant with facial asymmetry secondary to plagiocephaly. Bottom row. Classic appearance of infants with craniosynostosis.**

Laboratory Tests

Routine laboratory tests are not indicated in most children with craniofacial anomalies. Chromosomal studies are indicated if a genetic disorder is suspected. Refined studies including FISH (fluorescent in situ hybridization) may be needed to detect certain chromosomal abnormalities (see Chapter 69).

Imaging Studies

Radiographs and imaging studies may be indicated in children with facial asymmetry, microcephaly and macrocephaly, and craniosynostosis. A 3-dimensional computed tomography scan of the skull is particularly helpful in defining which if any sutures are fused. Such studies are helpful in differentiating craniosynostosis and deformational disorders. Renal ultrasound may be indicated in children with microtia or other ear anomalies because of the association between ear and renal anomalies.

Management

The management of children with craniofacial anomalies usually requires the expertise of a multidisciplinary team, including a pediatrician; plastic surgeon; ear, nose, and throat specialist; speech pathologist; social worker; psychologist; orthodontist; and prosthodontist. Primary care physicians who are not part of the team can receive information regarding appropriate patient care and follow-up. It is important for primary care physicians to be familiar with the appropriate nomenclature to be able to communicate with consultants. In brief, clefts of the lip are unilateral or bilateral and complete or incomplete. A complete cleft extends into the nares (see Figure 70-1). Clefts of the palate may involve the entire palate or be confined to the secondary or soft palate.

Routine **well-child care,** including monitoring of growth and administration of immunizations, is most important in the management of children with craniofacial anomalies. Some infants with clefts are slow feeders. Mothers should be told that although breastfeeding can be carried out, it may present unique challenges; however, the compliancy of the breast tissue creates a natural seal for the lip and palate. If difficulties are encountered, consultation with a lactation specialist may be especially helpful. Some formula-fed infants require the use of special adaptive nipples or feeders. A specific cleft palate feeder, which consists of a plastic bottle that allows for compression of the unit during feeding, is available. A soft, premature-type nipple can also be obtained. Long nipples, such as lamb's nipples, which are used to feed infant lambs, are not routinely recommended because they cause infants to gag. Infants who gain weight slowly may need to be given concentrated formulas (see Chapter 129).

Hearing and speech should be monitored. Chronic prophylactic **antibiotics** or the insertion of **pressure equalization tubes** may be needed to manage recurrent otitis media (see Chapter 72). Speech problems require the expertise of a speech pathologist and placement of children in **speech therapy** in either the community or school.

Surgical correction is indicated for many anomalies. Clefts are usually repaired as staged procedures during the first 2 years of life.

Repair of the cleft lip, the first procedure, is traditionally scheduled when infants weigh 10 pounds, are 10 weeks of age, and their hemoglobin is 10 (rule of tens). Appropriate weight gain is therefore critical to ensure timely surgery. If skilled anesthesiologists and nurses are available, cleft lip repair can be carried out within the first 2 weeks of life. Early repair is recommended at some centers. Repair of the cleft palate, the second procedure, is usually undertaken when infants are between 12 and 18 months of age. Better speech develops with earlier palatal repair. Surgical correction of clefts does not alter children's propensity to otitis media. This condition improves as children get older, however. Refinement of the cosmetic results, including rhinoplasty, occurs throughout childhood. Orthodontia is frequently a key component to achieve a cosmetically acceptable result and appropriate occlusion of the dentition for speech and chewing. About 10% to 20% of children will develop velopharyngeal insufficiency following repair of a cleft palate. In these cases, the posterior soft palate fails to make a tight seal with the pharynx. Children may experience nasal regurgitation of food or hypernasal speech. Surgical correction of velopharyngeal insufficiency involves lengthening the shortened palate. Additional surgery may also be required by children who have significant jaw deformities. These may include the placement of bone grafts or maxillary advancement.

Children with isolated unilateral microtia often hear, and surgery is recommended for cosmetic purposes. Surgical correction of microtia is usually initiated when children are 5 years of age, before they start school. At this time the ear has achieved 90% of its growth, and children are spared the potential embarrassment of their deformity in the school setting. Surgical reconstruction can involve the implantation of the child's costal cartilage or a prosthetic device shaped like the pinnae. In either case, several surgical procedures are usually needed. If there are other facial anomalies, more extensive reconstructive surgery is indicated.

Craniosynostosis can be corrected surgically, although the procedure is major and has significant risks. Endoscopic craniosynostosis repair is less invasive and requires shorter operative time and a reduced length of hospital stay. It is the preferred approach in some centers. The age of the infant and the site of the synostosis influence the complexity of the surgical procedure. A controversy about whether neurodevelopmental problems are related to craniosynostosis or whether they represent a preexisting condition has arisen. In developmentally normal children with evidence of closure of all the sutures, surgical repair is believed to be warranted. In other cases, the procedure is thought to be reconstructive because it normalizes the appearance of children with a deformation.

In children with plagiocephaly, where the deformation is believed to be related to torticollis, **passive stretching of the neck** 5 to 6 times a day (with each diaper change) is used to manage the condition. In addition, it is recommended that bright objects such as mobiles be placed over children's cribs to encourage head turning. Changing the crib position, or the position of the infant in the crib, may also encourage movement of the head. Studies have shown that 90% of infants with congenital torticollis improve with manual stretching.

Children who do not improve with stretching, have a deformity related to supine sleeping, or have a deformity that is still present at 6 months of age may be fitted with a specially designed helmet or band referred to as a *dynamic orthotic cranioplasty device* that reshapes the skull. The device is not used prior to 6 months of age and is generally worn for a minimum of 4 months. In an effort to reverse the trend of increasing positional plagiocephaly related to supine sleeping, the American Academy of Pediatrics has recommended that parents rotate their infant's position when they are awake and allow for "tummy time." Tummy time is time when infants are placed prone, sometimes with a rolled receiving blanket under their upper chest. This promotes the development of the neck musculature and head control. Positional plagiocephaly secondary to supine sleeping usually resolves with either repositioning or the use of a helmet and does not require surgical intervention.

Psychological counseling should be available to affected children and their families to help them adjust to the anomalies and the reactions of society. Parents may be referred to community agencies such as the Cleft Palate Foundation (www.cleftline.org) to help them cope with the potential stress related to giving birth to children with this anomaly and to advise them about the medical and surgical interventions that are available. FACES, the National Craniofacial Association (www.faces-cranio.org), is a referral source for parents.

Prognosis

Some anomalies, such as deformational plagiocephaly, resolve spontaneously or with exercise and positioning. Most other anomalies can be surgically corrected, leaving little residual evidence of the deformity. School success and psychological well-being may be more resistant to remediation and are highly dependent on the supportiveness of the family and their emotional resources. Children who grow up in settings where the deformity is thought to be embarrassing have long-term problems with low self-esteem.

CASE RESOLUTION

The infant in the case history has a cleft of the lip and palate. The mother is advised that the infant can be given formula, and she is given a supply of special feeders. She is given the contact information for a parents' support group and meets other parents of children with similar anomalies. During her visit to the local craniofacial team, she views pictures of children who have undergone a repair and feels relieved.

The mother is advised about the timing of surgery and told that the surgery will be scheduled when the infant is approximately 10 weeks old. A follow-up appointment in about 2 weeks is arranged. Weight gain is monitored, and the adjustment between the mother and the infant is assessed.

Selected References

Balasubrahmanyam G, Schere NJ, Martin JA, Michal ML. Cleft lip and palate: keys to successful management. *Contemp Pediatr.* 1998;15:133–153

Connolly JP, Seto ML, Whelan MF, et al. Progressive postnatal craniosynostosis and increased intracranial pressure. *Plast Reconstr Surg.* 2004;113:1313–1323

DaCosta AC, Walters I, Savarirayan R, Anderson VA, Wrennall JA, Meara JG. Intellectual outcomes in children and adolescents with syndromic and nonsyndromic craniosynostosis. *Plast Reconstr Surg.* 2006;118:175–181

Damiano PC, Tyler MC, Romitti PA, et al. Health-related quality of life among pre-adolescent children with oral clefts: the mother's perspective. *Pediatrics.* 2007;120:e283–e290

Denk MJ. Topics in pediatric plastic surgery. *Pediatr Clin North Am.* 1998;45:1479–1506

Graham JM, Gomez M, Halberg A, et al. Management of deformational plagiocephaly: repositioning versus orthotic therapy. *J Pediatr.* 2005;146:258–262

Graham JM, Kreutzman J, Earl D, Halberg A, Samayoa C, Guo X. Deformational brachycephaly in supine-sleeping infants. *J Pediatr.* 2005;146:253–257

Harville EW, Wilcox AJ, Lie RT, Vindenes H, Abyholm F. Cleft lip and palate versus cleft lip: are they distinct defects? *Am J Epidemiol.* 2005;162:448–453

Hunt O, Burden D, Hepper P, Stevenson M, Johnston C. Self-reports of psychosocial functioning among children and young adults with cleft lip and palate. *Cleft Palate Craniofac J.* 2006;43:598–605

Ishimoto S, Karino S, Takegoshi H, Kaga K, Yamasoba T. Hearing levels in patients with microtia: correlation with temporal bone malformation. *Laryngoscope.* 2007;117:416–465

Kane AA, Mitchell LE, Craven KP, Marsh JL. Observations on a recent increase in plagiocephaly without synostosis. *Pediatrics.* 1996;97:877–885

Keating RF. Craniosynostosis: diagnosis and management in the new millennium. *Pediatr Ann.* 1997;26:600–612

Liptak GS, Serletti JM. Pediatric approach to craniosynostosis. *Pediatr Rev.* 1998;19:352–358

Meng T, Shi B, Zheng Q, Wang y, Li S. Clinical and epidemiologic studies of non-syndromic cleft lip and palate in China: analysis of 4268 cases. *Ann Plast Surg.* 2006;57:264–269

Purugganan OH, Adam HM. Abnormalities in head size. *Pediatr Rev.* 2006;27:473–476

Rohan AJ, Golombek SG, Rosenthal AD. Infants with misshapen skulls: when to worry. *Contemp Pediatr.* 1999;16:47–70

Samanich J, Adam HM. Cleft palate. *Pediatr Rev.* 2009;30:230–232

Schuster M, Maier A, Haderlein T, et al. Evaluation of speech intelligibility for children with cleft lip and palate by means of automatic speech recognition. *Int J Pediatr Otorhinolaryngol.* 2006;70:1741–1747

Shaw GM, Carmichael SL, Kaidarova Z, Harris JA. Epidemiologic characteristics of anotia and microtia in California, 1989–1997. *Birth Defects Res A Clin Mol Teratol.* 2004;70:472–475

van Vlimmeren LA, van der Graaf Y, Boere-Boonekamp MM, L'Hoir MP, Helders PJM, Engelbert RHH. Risk factors for deformational plagiocephaly at birth and at 7 weeks of age: a prospective cohort study. *Pediatrics.* 2007;119:e408–e418

CHAPTER 71

Common Oral Lesions

Charlotte W. Lewis, MD, MPH

CASE STUDY

A 7-year-old girl is brought to the office for evaluation of a swelling on the inside of her lower lip of 4 to 6 weeks' duration. Her mother reports that it increases and decreases in size. The girl says that the swelling is not painful, and she cannot remember hurting her lower lip. On examination, a raised, bluish, non-tender, 1 x 1 cm swelling is apparent along the mucosa of the lower lip.

Questions

1. What is the differential diagnosis of lip masses?
2. What laboratory or radiographic tests are useful in the evaluation of oral lesions?
3. What management strategies are used to treat cyst-like oral lesions?
4. When should children with oral lesions be referred to subspecialists?

Primary care physicians are often required to evaluate lesions in the oral cavity. Knowledge of common congenital, developmental, infectious, traumatic, and neoplastic conditions that affect the mouth and its structures can help physicians to recognize and manage these lesions appropriately. Although many oral lesions are benign or represent normal variants, others may require specific medical or surgical treatment. Some oral lesions offer clues to underlying syndromic diagnoses, indicate more serious systemic disease, or occur as side effects of certain medications.

Epidemiology

Oral pathology is common and covers a broad range of lesions. Benign oral lesions such as gingival cysts occur in about 75% of newborns. Approximately 20% of the population has at least a small **torus palatinus,** a benign boney overgrowth of the palate that usually begins in childhood. **Ankyloglossia,** commonly referred to as tongue-tie, affects approximately 5% of newborns. **Fissured tongue** affects approximately 2% of the population. Fissured tongue may be associated with **benign migratory glossitis** (geographic tongue), which occurs in approximately 1% to 2% of children. **Tobacco-associated keratosis** occurs at the site of habitual placement of snuff or chewing tobacco and is estimated to affect more than 300,000 US children. **Leukoplakia,** a premalignant condition associated with smokeless tobacco, occurs in approximately half of users. Although the resulting oral cancer is often diagnosed in the sixth or seventh decade of life, the habit of oral tobacco use typically starts in childhood—typically between 9 to 16 years of age. The popularity of oral forms of snuff and chewing tobacco has rapidly increased in North America, especially among white adolescent males; approximately 10% of male high school students use smokeless tobacco, with quite a bit of variation by state.

Aphthous ulcers (commonly known as canker sores) are one of the most common oral lesions seen in developed countries, with typical onset early in childhood. Approximately 20% to 25% of the US population experiences recurrent aphthous ulcers (RAU). Oral lesions resulting from infections are also common. Approximately 35% of newborns and young infants will develop **oral candidiasis,** commonly known as thrush. Oral **herpes** lesions are also common and are due to herpes simplex virus (HSV) group, usually type 1 (HSV-1). By young adulthood, more than half of US individuals will be seropositive for HSV-1. Approximately 20% to 40% of the population has experienced oral herpes at least one time.

Chronic ("ordinary") gingivitis usually has its onset in older children and will ultimately affect as many as 90% of adults.

Clinical Presentation

Oral lesions may come to the clinician's attention in any number of ways. Some may be obvious at birth, most notably a **congenital epulis,** which while benign in histology typically presents as a mass protruding from an infant's oral cavity and potentially interfering with breathing or eating. Oral lesions may be an incidental finding on physical examination. For example, in examining a newborn, the pediatrician may notice small (approximately 2–3 mm) yellow-white papules along the palatal midline and can then reassure the family that these are Epstein pearls, common lesions of no clinical significance. Most oral vascular malformations (1 of the 3 vessel types usually predominate: arterial, venous, or lymphatic) are present at birth, become more noticeable over time, and rarely regress. Microcystic lymphatic malformations often affect the tongue and surrounding soft tissue, can be friable, may interfere with eating and speaking, and can lead to overgrowth of adjacent bones. When these lesions become infected they rapidly enlarge and can result in potential airway compromise.

Either the clinician or parent may be the first to notice thrush. The incidence of oral candidiasis peaks around the fourth week of life; thrush is uncommon in infants older than 6 to 9 months. Thrush can occur, however, at any age in predisposed patients (ie, immunosuppressed or deficient) and can affect the esophagus as well as the oropharynx. *Candida albicans* in combination with contact irritation has been implicated in **angular cheilitis,** which appear as crusty or scaling erythematous fissures at the corners of the mouth. Other benign oral lesions, such as benign migratory glossitis, are brought to the clinician's attention because parents are concerned that they represent pathology; however, reassurance is appropriate.

Concerns for ankyloglossia may arise when newborns have difficulty breastfeeding or as a cause of speech problems in older children although these connections are controversial. Nevertheless, it can be difficult for children to use their tongue to clean food debris from around their teeth when the lingual frenulum is short. The maxillary labial frenulum can appear quite prominent in young children. It is common for parents to inquire whether this is contributing to what appears to be abnormal spacing between the upper central incisors (midline **diastema**). However, the prominent frenulum may be more a result of a diastema rather than a cause of it.

Clinicians may be the first to note swollen, friable, erythematous gingiva along with plaque buildup on and between the teeth representing the initial presentation of chronic gingivitis. Chronic gingivitis is the first stage of periodontal disease. Onset is typically in peripubertal children. Although young children experience gingivostomatitis from other causes, they do not usually harbor *Actinobacillus actinomycetemcomitans* or *Porphyromonas gingivalis,* and thus do not commonly experience chronic gingivitis or periodontal disease. Thickening of the mucosa, usually in the labial vestibule, offers clues to smokeless tobacco use. The severity of tobacco-related oral lesions demonstrates a dose-response relationship with the amount, frequency, and duration of smokeless tobacco exposure. Tobacco-associated keratosis is a predictable lesion that manifests as an area of thickening at the site of habitual placement of snuff or chewing tobacco. Chronic exposure to smokeless tobacco can lead to the development of opaque-white to yellow-brown lesions with a wrinkled appearance, known as leukoplakia and considered to be a premalignant condition.

Other oral lesions may present in conjunction with systemic symptoms. **Primary herpetic gingivostomatitis** typically occurs in infants and young children with the initial HSV-1 infection and is characterized by multiple oral vesicular or ulcerative lesions, fever, malaise, cervical lymphadenopathy, and decreased oral intake. Reactivation of prior HSV-1 infection often affects the vermillion border of the lip, which is known as herpes labialis. Oral lesions may also indicate underlying serious systemic illness such as Crohn disease, systemic lupus erythematosus, or acute myelogenous leukemia. Some genetic syndromes are first detected because of oral lesions. For example, lip pits or mounds in conjunction with cleft lip/cleft palate are virtually pathognomonic of van der Woude syndrome, an autosomal-dominant cause of orofacial clefting. Hyperpigmented lesions (brown or dark blue, similar to freckles) on the lips or buccal mucosa may provide a clue toward the diagnosis of Peutz-Jeghers syndrome, an autosomal-dominant condition of multiple intestinal hamartomas. Patients with Peutz-Jeghers syndrome may experience recurrent abdominal pain, intestinal obstruction, or bleeding, and have a 15-fold increased risk of intestinal cancer.

Pathophysiology

Neonatal and Other Developmental Lesions

Gingival cysts in the neonate include Epstein pearls, Bohn nodules, and dental lamina cysts and are due to entrapment of tissues during embryologic development. Congenital epulis of the newborn is a rare, gingival tumor of unclear etiology that occurs more commonly in the maxilla than the mandible, with a marked female predilection (8:1), and may occur as a single or multiple tumors. The etiology of fissured tongue and geographic tongue are unknown. Fissured tongue tends to cluster in families, suggesting a genetic etiology, and can also be seen in Down syndrome. Benign migratory glossitis results from the loss of the tiny finger-like projections, called papillae, on the tongue's surface, giving the tongue a map-like appearance. The inciting factors responsible for oral vascular malformations are not well understood.

Traumatic

Some of the most common oral lesions noted on physical examination result from minor accidental self-bites to the lip or buccal mucosa. Most of these resolve quickly, but recurrent trauma may lead to **pyogenic granuloma** or **fibroma** formation. A **mucocele** results from traumatic rupture of a minor salivary gland with subsequent cyst formation.

Infectious

Although an infectious etiology to aphthous ulcers has been proposed, their true etiology remains unclear. Oral herpes lesions are usually due to infection with HSV-1. **Herpangina** results from coxsackievirus A infection. *C albicans* causes oral candidiasis. Thrush occurs when normal host immunity is immature (as in neonates) or suppressed (eg, during steroid treatment) or when normal flora is disrupted (eg, while on antibiotics). Infants may be colonized with *C albicans* during birth. Other sources of transmission to neonates include colonized skin (particularly around the breasts for breast-fed infants) and/or improperly cleaned bottle nipples.

Chronic gingivitis occurs after build-up of bacterial plaque on the teeth, adjacent gingiva, and pockets between teeth and gums. Bacteria within plaque (most common species involved are gram-negative anaerobic bacteria *(A actinomycetemcomitans* and *P gingivalis)* release toxins that cause an inflammatory response.

Other

Drug-induced gingival hyperplasia can occur in patients taking corticosteroids, phenytoin (most common cause in children), cyclosporine-A, and nifedipine. It results from fibrous tissue overgrowth but is exacerbated by poor oral hygiene and presence of plaque in much the same way as ordinary gingivitis is.

Differential Diagnosis

Age at onset, location and characteristics of the lesion, and accompanying signs and symptoms often help to narrow the differential diagnosis. The appearance of 1- to 3-mm cysts in the mouth of a neonate brings to mind (1) **Epstein pearls,** which are the most common and are usually present along the palatal midline; (2) **dental lamina cysts,** which are usually located bilaterally along the crest of the dental ridge about where the first molars usually will erupt; or (3) **Bohn nodules,** which are found on the buccal and lingual aspects of the ridge, away from the midline. A protuberant mass from the anterior maxillary ridge of a newborn should suggest a congenital epulis; however, examination by a pathologist after resection is important to confirm the diagnosis. A mucocele is a painless, clear or bluish, fluid-filled cyst that results from damage to the salivary duct leading to extravasation of mucus from the gland into the surrounding soft tissue.

White plaques involving the buccal, lingual, and palatal mucosa bring to mind oral candidiasis. Thrush can sometimes be confused with milk remaining in the child's mouth after feeding. Scraping the lesion to determine if the white substance is readily removed (as milk is) helps to differentiate this from oral candidiasis, where the white plaques do not easily scrape off, and after scraping, the base of the thrush lesion may be erythematous or bleed. Thrush involving the tongue may also be confused with the erythematous denuded areas of the tongue seen in benign migratory glossitis. In fissured tongue, grooves that vary in depth are noted along the dorsal and lateral aspects of the tongue.

Common oral ulcers include aphthous ulcers, herpes gingivostomatitis, or herpangina. Oral herpes may be characterized by multiple vesicular lesions, which after rupture appear as ulcers, involving the lips, skin around the mouth, tongue, and mucosal membranes, typically in the anterior portion of the mouth. The initial infection may occur between 1 to 3 years of age. Aphthous ulcers also involve the anterior mouth, typically along the wet vermillion, but they usually first appear at a somewhat older age (ie, in the preschool years or later) and with fewer lesions than oral herpes. Herpangina may present similarly to herpes but it more typically involves the posterior pharynx and the palate. Similar lesions on the hands and/or foot, as in hand-foot-and-mouth disease, may lend support to coxsackievirus A as the etiology.

Trauma to the salivary duct may result in a mucocele. In contrast, a pyogenic granuloma is an erythematous, non-painful, smooth or lobulated mass that often bleeds easily when touched, while a fibroma is a moderately firm, smooth-surfaced, pink, sessile or pedunculated nodule, usually noted on the buccal mucosa in the occlusal plane.

Erythematous and friable gums often indicate the presence of chronic gingivitis. Typically plaque is seen on and between the teeth. In contrast to plaque-associated chronic gingivitis, which is usually painless, **acute necrotizing ulcerative gingivitis** is characterized by painful, edematous, bleeding gums with ulcers, necrosis, and pseudomembrane formation in affected areas. When this spreads to the oropharynx, it is referred to as **Vincent angina** (trench mouth), which can progress rapidly and interfere with speech and swallowing, and obstruct the airway.

Evaluation

History

The history is very important in evaluating oral lesions and determining the need for further treatment or referral. Key factors to include in the history are age at onset, duration, inciting factors, other medical problems, medications, use of tobacco, family history, ill contacts, and associated or systemic symptoms such as fever (Questions Box).

Questions

Common Oral Lesions

- How long has the child had the lesion?
- Is the lesion painful?
- Did the child recently injure the affected area?
- Has the child had any fever?
- Is the child eating as usual?
- Does the child have any other lesions?
- Is the child currently taking any medications? Has the child recently taken any medications?

Physical Examination

Physical examination of the oral structures should start with the lip (both the dry and wet vermillion) and surrounding skin (the "white lip"). The examination should then turn to the mucosa, gingiva, teeth, and palate; superior, lateral, and posterior aspect of the tongue; sublingual structures; frena; and posterior pharynx. The clinician should note the number, size, location, and characteristics of the lesions because this information can be helpful in narrowing the differential diagnosis. Whether fever is present should be determined. The rest of the body should be examined with specific attention to the presence of other lesions, rashes, or arthritis.

Laboratory Tests

In otherwise healthy children who present with oral ulcerative lesions, supportive care is typically implemented without pursuing a definitive etiology. When there is need for specific diagnosis, HSV can be diagnosed via polymerase chain reaction techniques, immunofluorescence, or culture. Tzanck smears are no longer commonly performed to diagnose HSV because they require special skills and are not specific to HSV, and more specific tests are available. Likewise, oral candidiasis in an otherwise healthy infant is usually treated without diagnostic tests. However, a potassium hydroxide 10% microscopic slide preparation of scrapings from the lesion should demonstrate the characteristic spherical budding yeasts and pseudohyphae.

An excisional biopsy or resection may be needed to determine histology and diagnosis of an oral lesion.

Laboratory tests, including a complete blood cell count, C-reactive protein, or erythrocyte sedimentation rate, may be helpful in the initial evaluation of the ill-appearing child with oral lesions or when serious infection, systemic illness, or inflammatory conditions are suspected.

Imaging Studies

Imaging studies are not indicated in the evaluation of most oral lesions unless the lesions are related to problems of dentition such as dental abscesses, in which case the radiographs are obtained by the dentist rather than the pediatrician. Computed tomography is usually the best way to initially characterize oral vascular malformations.

Management

Many of the common oral lesions are developmental or normal variants and/or are self-limited, and their management entails observation to ensure the lesions follow their expected course. For example, gingival cysts in newborns typically regress spontaneously. Oral lesions such as torus palatinus or benign migratory glossitis do not require treatment. Although HSV-1 gingivostomatitis is self-limiting, primary infection can cause considerable pain and lead to decreased intake by mouth. Early (within 72 hours) antiviral therapy in the form of acyclovir 5 to 10 mg/kg/dose 5 times per day for 7 to 10 days has been shown to shorten duration of fever, lesions, and odynophagia. Other oral lesions respond well to supportive care. For example, a child with herpangina may benefit from regular ibuprofen or acetaminophen, topical application of a 1:1 mixture of attapulgite (Kaopectate) and diphenhydramine elixir (Benadryl) to form a protective coating over the lesion, avoidance of acidic beverages such as orange juice that may burn on contact with the ulcers, and close attention to fluid intake and signs/symptoms of dehydration. Viscous lidocaine has been associated with systemic absorption and subsequent dysrhythmia or seizure, thus substantial caution is warranted before prescribing. Over-the-counter topical anesthetic agents contain a high content of alcohol and should not be used in children. Amlexanox 5% oral paste or high-dose steroid gel reduces pain, duration, and size of aphthous ulcers and is used in adults with RAU; however, safety of these treatments in children has not been established.

Complicated vascular and lymphatic malformations of the oral cavity require specialty consultation with a team experienced in the care of these lesions. Unlike infantile hemangiomas, vascular malformations do not involute. Treatment of choice for lymphatic malformations is usually surgical resection; however, microcystic lymphatic malformations are difficult to remove and may recur even after resection. Sclerosing therapy and laser treatment are sometimes options. Supportive care includes treatment with antibiotics when the lesion becomes infected and ongoing, aggressive preventive oral hygiene.

Other oral lesions require specific therapy. Thrush is typically treated with nystatin suspension (100,000 units/mL) as 1 mL swabbed to lesions 4 times per day until lesions are resolved. It is important to consider the possibility of an underlying immunodeficiency when thrush occurs outside of infancy or without a reasonable explanation. Angular cheilitis can be treated with nystatin cream or ointment and a low-potency hydrocortisone cream. Some oral lesions are best treated by resection. These would include congenital epulis, mucocele, pyogenic granuloma, and fibroma.

Treatment of gingivitis includes regular rinsing with alcohol-containing phenolic mouth rinse (eg, Listerine) or chlorhexidine gluconate oral preparation, improving oral hygiene (flossing, toothbrushing), and referral for professional dental care. The goals of therapy for gingivitis are to reduce clinical signs of inflammation and gingival bleeding and arrest or reduce the risk of progression of the periodontal disease and maintain dentition. Drug-induced gingival hyperplasia requires similar therapy to ordinary gingivitis. In addition, if the causative medication cannot be discontinued or changed, patients can be referred for surgical removal of excess gingival tissue and fitting of a positive-pressure mouth guard to inhibit further tissue growth. Acute necrotizing ulcerative gingivitis should be treated with penicillin V (or erythromycin for patients allergic to penicillin). Clindamycin can be used in refractory cases.

It is controversial whether treatment of ankyloglossia with frenectomy decreases breastfeeding difficulties, although some small studies suggest there may be a benefit. Consultation with a lactation consultant is often helpful as a first step when questions arise about whether ankyloglossia is contributing to breastfeeding difficulty. Management of oral lesions may require consultation and collaboration with dental, oral surgery, head and neck surgery, or other subspecialty colleagues. If the etiology of a lesion is unclear or if an oral lesion does not follow its expected course, referral is essential to ensure appropriate diagnosis and treatment.

Prognosis

Most oral lesions in children respond to appropriate intervention without residual problems. However, oral lesions can signal the onset of or occur in association with serious systemic conditions. In addition, chronic gingivitis represents the first and only reversible stage of periodontal disease, which is the leading cause of tooth loss in adulthood. Because chronic gingivitis has its onset during childhood, physicians can play an important role in prevention of periodontal disease by promoting oral hygiene early in life. Once periodontal disease extends beyond the gums, it is no longer reversible and gradually destroys the bone and tissue that support the teeth, resulting in halitosis and tooth loss.

CASE RESOLUTION

The child described in the case history at the beginning of this chapter seems to have a mucocele. She should be referred to either an oral or head and neck surgeon for surgical excision of the lesion.

Selected References

American Academy of Pediatric Dentistry Council on Clinical Affairs. Guideline on pediatric oral surgery. *Pediatr Dent*. 2005–2006;27:158–164

Buckmiller LM, Richter GT, Suen, JY. Diagnosis and management of hemangiomas and vascular malformations of the head and neck. *Oral Dis*. 2010;405–418

Ebbert JO, Carr AB, Dale LC. Smokeless tobacco: an emerging addiction. *Med Clin North Am*. 2004;88:1593–1605

Gonsalves WC, Chi AC, Neville BW. Common oral lesions: part I. Superficial mucosal lesions. *Am Fam Physician*. 2007;75:501–507

Gonsalves WC, Chi AC, Neville BW. Common oral lesions: part II. Masses and neoplasia. *Am Fam Physician*. 2007;75:509–512

Scully C. Clinical practice. Aphthous ulceration. *N Engl J Med*. 2006;355:165–172

CHAPTER 72

Otitis Media

Nasser Redjal, MD

CASE STUDY

An 18-month-old male infant is brought to your office with a 2-day history of fever and decreased food intake. He has had symptoms of an upper respiratory infection for the past 4 days but no vomiting or diarrhea. Otherwise he is healthy.

The infant appears tired but not toxic. On physical examination the vital signs are normal except for a temperature of 101°F (38.3°C). The left tympanic membrane (TM) is erythematous and bulging, with yellow pus behind the membrane. The light reflex is splayed, and mobility is decreased. The right TM is gray and mobile, with a sharp light reflex. The neck is supple with shotty anterior cervical adenopathy, and the lungs are clear.

He has a 10- to 15-word vocabulary, and no one smokes in the household.

Questions

1. What are the differences between acute, persistent, and recurrent otitis media (OM)?
2. What factors predispose to the development of ear infections?
3. What are the most common presenting signs and symptoms of an ear infection in infants, older children, and adolescents?
4. How do the treatment considerations differ between acute, persistent, and recurrent ear infections?
5. What are some of the complications of OM?

Otitis media is the second most common reason after well-child care for a visit to the pediatrician and is the most common reason for which antibiotics are prescribed for children. It is estimated that approximately 30 million office visits per year are for the evaluation and treatment of OM and that billions of dollars are spent annually for OM care. Moreover, more than a quarter of all prescriptions written each year for oral antibiotics are for the treatment of middle-ear infections. In addition, many surgical procedures such as **myringotomy** with **tympanostomy tube** placement or adenoidectomy are performed on children for treatment of recurrent disease. Therefore, the primary care physician must have a good understanding of these very common pediatric conditions.

Otitis media can be classified into the following 5 categories: **acute OM (AOM), OM with effusion (OME), recurrent AOM, chronic OME,** and **chronic suppurative OM (CSOM).** It is important to distinguish between each of these entities because their presentation and management differ.

Acute OM (acute suppurative or purulent OM) is the sudden onset of inflammation of the middle ear, which is often accompanied by fever and ear pain (otalgia) (Box 72-1). Otitis media with effusion is the presence of middle-ear fluid after antimicrobial treatment. Resolution of acute inflammatory signs has occurred, with persistence of a more serious, non-purulent effusion. Although the fluid may persist for 2 to 3 months, it resolves within 3 to 4 weeks in 60% of cases. Recurrent OM is defined as frequent episodes of AOM with complete clearing between each episode. A more specific definition is 3 new episodes of AOM requiring antibiotic treatment within a 6-month period, or 4 documented infections in 1 year. This condition affects approximately 20% of children who are "otitis prone"; such children are usually infants who have their first infection at younger than 1 year. Chronic OME (serous OM, secretory OM,

---

Box 72-1. Components of Acute Otitis Media (AOM)[a]

Definition of AOM

A diagnosis of AOM requires

1. A history of acute onset of signs and symptoms
2. The presence of middle-ear effusion (MEE)
3. Signs and symptoms of middle-ear inflammation

Elements of the definition of AOM are all of the following:

1. Recent, usually abrupt, onset of signs and symptoms of middle-ear inflammation and MEE
2. The presence of MEE that is indicated by any of the following:
   a. Bulging of the tympanic membrane
   b. Limited or absent mobility of the tympanic membrane
   c. Air-fluid level behind the tympanic membrane
   d. Otorrhea
3. Signs or symptoms of middle-ear inflammation as indicated by either
   a. Distinct erythema of the tympanic membrane

   or

   b. Distinct otalgia (discomfort clearly referable to the ear[s] that results in interference with or precludes normal activity)

[a] Adapted with permission from American Academy of Pediatrics Subcommittee on Management of Acute Otitis Media. Diagnosis and management of acute otitis media. *Pediatrics.* 2004;113:1451–1465.

non-suppurative OM, mucoid OM, glue ear OM) is a chronic condition characterized by persistence of fluid in the middle ear for 3 months or longer. The TM is retracted or concave with impaired mobility and without signs of acute inflammation. Affected children may be asymptomatic. These children are at greater risk for developing hearing deficits and speech delay. Chronic suppurative OM implies a non-intact TM (perforation or tympanostomy tube present) with 6 or more weeks of middle-ear drainage.

Epidemiology

The overall prevalence of OM is 15% to 20%, with the highest peak in children 6 to 36 months of age. An additional smaller peak occurs at about 4 to 6 years. Otitis media is relatively uncommon in older children and adolescents. The condition is more common in boys than girls.

Several epidemiological risk factors for OM have been identified, including age younger than 2 years; first episode of AOM when younger than 6 months; familial predisposition; siblings in the household; low socioeconomic status; non-breastfed infant; altered host defenses (acquired or congenital immunodeficiencies); environmental factors, such as child care attendance; and the presence of an underlying condition, such as allergic disease of the upper airway, chronic sinusitis, a cleft palate, or other craniofacial anomalies. Children with Down, Goldenhar, and Treacher Collins syndromes and ciliary dysfunction also have an increased risk of OM. Race, bottle feeding, use of pacifier, and exposure to cigarette smoke have not been indentified consistently as risk factors for AOM. As one might expect, the highest rate of OM occurs during the winter months and in early spring, coinciding with peaks in the incidence of upper respiratory infections (URIs).

Worldwide OM leads to an estimated 50,000 deaths per year in children younger than 5 years because of the complications of CSOM. It is estimated to affect 65 million to 33 million people worldwide, 60% of whom suffer significant hearing loss. Chronic suppurative OM is a rare entity in developed countries where most otitis media is AOM or OME.

Etiology

In general 50% to 90% of cases of AOM culture are bacterial, 20% to 50% are viruses and 20% to 30% no growth. Up until the widespread immunization of children with pneumococcal vaccine, the causative microorganisms for AOM were *Streptococcus pneumoniae* (25%–50%), *Haemophilus influenzae* (15%–30% most non-typeable strains), and *Moraxella catarrhalis* (3%–20%). Since vaccine licensure, there has been an overall decrease in the incidence of AOM, especially noted in children who are completely immunized. Group A streptococcus, *Staphylococcus aureus,* alpha-hemolytic *Streptococcus, Pseudomonas aeruginosa,* and anaerobic bacteria are other less common causative organisms. Other uncommon organisms such as *Mycoplasma pneumoniae,* chlamydia, and *Mycobacterium tuberculosis* have also been isolated. Respiratory viruses such as respiratory syncytial virus, adenovirus, rhinovirus, parainfluenza, coronavirus,

and influenza (A and B) also play a role. Respiratory syncytial virus, adenovirus, and coronavirus are associated with a higher rate of AOM, with 50% of children who have URIs caused by these viruses developing AOM compared with only 33% of patients who have URIs caused by rhinovirus, influenza, parainfluenza, or enterovirus. The bacterial pathogens causing AOM in the first 6 weeks after birth are essentially the same as those in older children. However, in a recent study, 10.5% of neonates who had AOM had gram-negative bacilli.

Currently approximately 50% of *H influenzae* and 100% of *M catarrhalis* isolated from the upper respiratory tract are β-lactamase positive and 15% to 50% (average 30%) of *S pneumoniae* are not susceptible to penicillin. The mechanism of penicillin resistance among isolates of *S pneumoniae* is not associated with β-lactamase production but related to an alteration of penicillin-binding proteins. This effect varies widely by geographic location and results in resistance to both penicillins and *cephalosporins.*

Clinical Presentation

Children with AOM often have a history of fever and ear pain. Associated symptoms include URI, cough, vomiting, diarrhea, and nonspecific complaints such as decreased appetite, waking at night, generalized malaise, lethargy, or irritability. Purulent otorrhea with minimal ear pain and hearing loss may also occur. Fever occurs in approximately 30% to 50% of patients. Temperatures exceeding 40°C are uncommon and suggest bacteremia or another complication. Older children may complain of tinnitus, vertigo, and hearing loss. Younger children are not able to express such complaints but may appear ataxic.

Pathophysiology

The most important factor in the pathogenesis of OM is abnormal function of the eustachian tube (Figure 72-1). Eustachian tube dysfunction occurs for 2 main reasons: abnormal patency and obstruction of the tube. Obstruction is either functional (secondary to collapse of the tube), mechanical (from intrinsic or extrinsic causes), or both. Functional obstruction or collapse of the eustachian tube occurs commonly in infants and young children because the tube

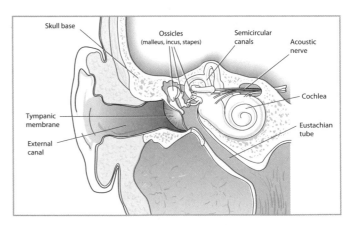

Figure 72-1. Relationship of middle ear to external and inner ears.

is less cartilaginous and therefore less stiff than in adults, as well as more horizontal and shorter. In addition, the tensor veli palatini muscle is less efficient in this age group. Extrinsically, the presence of lymphoid follicles (adenoidal enlargement) or tumors (rare) surrounding the opening of the tube contributes to reflux, aspiration, or insufflation of nasopharyngeal bacteria into the middle ear. Intrinsic mechanical obstruction of the eustachian tube occurs as the result of inflammation secondary to a URI or allergy in patients older than 5 years. In addition, viral infections may occur up to 6 to 12 times per year in children younger than 3 years. Subsequently this causes eustachian tube dysfunction leading to negative middle ear pressure, which occurs in 75% of children who have viral URIs. The presence of a viral URI enhances the ability of bacterial pathogens to adhere and ascend from the nasopharynx to the middle ear via the eustachian tube. In addition, viruses can affect the local host immune response by impairing leukocyte function, exposing receptors for bacteria, and decreasing the effectiveness of the mucociliary escalator (see Figure 72-1).

Hematogenous spread of microorganisms also can lead to infection. Less often, primary mucosal disease of the middle ear from allergies or abnormal cilia contributes to OM.

Differential Diagnosis

The most common cause of otalgia, or ear pain, is AOM. Other causes include mastoiditis, which is almost always accompanied by OM; otitis externa; and referred pain from the oropharynx, teeth, adenoids, or posterior auricular lymph nodes. A foreign body in the canal can produce similar symptoms. In children with ear pain, a search for any of these other conditions must be undertaken if the TM appears completely normal.

Evaluation

History

The history should carefully delineate the symptoms of OM and differentiate from those indicating a more serious condition such as meningitis (Questions Box).

For infants or children with a history of persistent or recurrent OM, it is important to find out when they had their last documented infection and what treatment they received. It is also critical to monitor development, particularly speech.

Physical Examination

To diagnose OM, the TM must be completely visualized and its mobility assessed. Occasionally this may be difficult because of the presence of cerumen or otorrhea. The diagnosis is then made on the basis of the history, and treatment may be initiated without confirmation by physical assessment. In all other cases, the position, color, degree of translucency, and mobility of the TM are evaluated. Classically, in AOM the TM is full, bulging, hyperemic, opaque, and/or has an air fluid level, with limited or no mobility. In addition, the light reflex is usually distorted or absent. In the case of persistent or chronic OM, signs of inflammation are usually absent, and the TM may be retracted, with limited or no mobility.

Associated physical findings with an uncomplicated middle-ear infection may include posterior auricular and cervical adenopathy. Other significant findings on physical examination are pain on movement of the pinna, anterior ear displacement, posterior auricular pain and, rarely, evidence of peripheral facial nerve (cranial nerve VII) paralysis. The presence of these findings suggests other diagnoses such as an associated otitis externa or mastoiditis.

Positioning of infants or young children for examination of the ear is critical for an adequate examination. Several methods have been described, including allowing parents to hold the child in their arms or on their laps or restraining the child on the examination table with or without a papoose board (Figure 72-2). In addition, it may be difficult to visualize the TM in infants because the external auditory canal is slightly angulated. Lateral retraction of the pinna may help correct this problem.

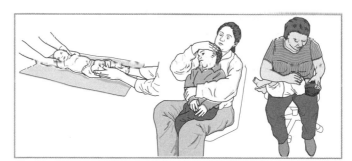

Figure 72-2. Three ways to position the infant or child for examination of the ear.

Laboratory Tests

Although the diagnosis of OM is suspected on the basis of the history and then verified on physical examination, tympanometry may be helpful in distinguishing the normal ear from one with an effusion. In acute cases, audiometry is of limited diagnostic value, but it is helpful in evaluating the effects of a persistent, recurrent, or chronic middle-ear effusion on hearing.

Questions

Otitis Media

- Does the infant or child have fever, ear pain, hearing loss, or otorrhea?
- Is the infant or child inconsolable or lethargic?
- Has the infant or child had a previous ear infection? If so, when?
- Did the child complete the course of prescribed antibiotics?
- How many ear infections has the child had in the past year?
- Is the child taking any medication to prevent recurrent otitis media?
- Does the child attend child care?
- Is the child exposed to passive smoke?
- Is the infant breastfed?
- Does the child seem to hear?
- Is the child's speech development normal?

Tympanocentesis is the most definitive method of verifying the presence of middle-ear fluid and of recovering the organism responsible for the infection. Indications for tympanocentesis or myringotomy are listed in Box 72-2. Nasopharyngeal cultures are not helpful because they do not seem to correlate highly with middle-ear fluid cultures.

Box 72-2. Indications for Tympanocentesis or Myringotomy in Children With Otitis Media (OM)

- OM in patients with severe ear pain, serious illness, or appearance of toxicity
- Onset of OM in children receiving appropriate and adequate antimicrobial therapy
- OM associated with confirmed or potential suppurative complications, such as facial paralysis, mastoiditis, or meningitis
- OM in newborns, sick neonates, or immunodeficient patients, in each of whom an unusual organism may be present
- OM in patients with severe illness who have failed second-line antibiotic management.
- OM in patients with penicillin allergy who have failed first-line agent

---

Prevention

During infancy and early childhood, the incidence of respiratory tract infections and recurrent OM can be reduced by altering child care center attendance patterns.

Immunoprophylaxis with influenza vaccine and pneumococcal conjugate vaccine has proven effective in preventing OM. Avoiding supine bottle-feeding (bottle propping) decreases the incidence of AOM.

Breastfeeding, which provides infants with immunologic protection against URIs, other viral and bacterial infections, and allergies, also has a protective effect. Facial musculature may mature differently in breastfed infants, thus influencing eustachian tube function and reducing the risk of aspiration of fluid into the middle ear. Positioning during breastfeeding also has some protective effect, although immune factors in breast milk may serve as the most important mechanism for the reduced prevalence of OM.

Increased antibiotic resistance has eliminated the utility of routine antibiotic prophylaxis for recurrent AOM as a means of disease prevention.

Management

Current guidelines regarding the treatment of AOM confine the use of antibiotics to young children (<2 years old) or older ones with severe symptoms (Box 72-3). Otherwise, observation without the use of antibacterial agents in a child with uncomplicated AOM is recommended. Antibacterial treatment is deferred in these other children for 48 to 72 hours and management is limited to symptomatic relief. In an era of conjugated pneumococcal vaccine, the likelihood of bacteremia accompanying AOM is remote. Parents may be provided with a prescription to fill without recontacting the physician if the child remains symptomatic. This option is also recommended

---

Box 72-3. Indications for Antibiotics in the Treatment of Otitis Media[a]

Criteria for antibacterial treatment or observation in children with non-severe illness

1. Younger than 6 months: antibacterial treatment
2. 6 months to 2 years: antibacterial treatment with certain diagnosis or severe illness or observation with uncertain diagnosis or non-severe illness
3. 2 years and older: antibacterial treatment with severe or observe with non-severe illness with certain diagnosis; observation for uncertain diagnosis

Obeservation is an appropriate option if
   A. Caregiver is informed and agrees.
   B. Caregiver is able to monitor the child and return should condition worsen.
   C. Systems are in place for ready communication with the clinician, reevaluation, and obtaining medication if necessary.

[a] Adapted with permission from American Academy of Pediatrics Subcommittee on Management of Acute Otitis Media. Diagnosis and management of acute otitis media. *Pediatrics*. 2004;113:1451–1465.

---

to otherwise healthy children 6 months to 2 years of age with non-severe illness at presentation *and* an uncertain diagnosis. Among children 6 to 23 months of age with AOM antibiotic treatment affords a measurable short-term benefit and decreased risk of failure of a watchful waiting strategy. Concern for serious infection among children younger than 6 months influences the decision for immediate antibacterial therapy in this age group. The recommended antibiotic therapy is noted in Table 72-1.

Tympanocentesis is rarely performed nowadays prior to the initiation of antibiotics. Indications for tympanocentesis include severe ear pain (provides relief through decompression) or toxic appearance. Tympanocentesis is occasionally carried out in a child who has been receiving appropriate and adequate antimicrobial therapy but fails to improve; or in the face of confirmed or potential suppurative complications, such as facial paralysis, mastoiditis, or meningitis; or in newborns, sick neonates, or immunodeficient patients, in whom an unusual organism may be present (see Box 72-2).

Adjunctive medications such as topical analgesics and antipyretics are important therapeutic options and should be prescribed for children with significant pain or fever. Antihistamines, decongestants, or steroids play no documented role in the treatment of OME. Most resolving middle-ear effusions seen after AOM in otherwise healthy children do not need to be treated and the "wait-and-watch" approach is recommended.

Failure of antibiotic treatment and chronic effusions warrant a referral to an otolaryngologist for further evaluation for pressure equalization tubes or, if the patient is older than 4 years, a possible adenoidectomy. Other reasons for consultation include evidence of hearing loss; the presence of any anatomical abnormality, such as a defect of the TM (perforations, cholesteatomas) or intranasal problems (deviated septum, polyp); signs and symptoms of an OM but normal physical examination; and a predisposition to chronic recurrent OM (eg, children with a cleft palate or Down syndrome).

Table 72-1. Recommended Antibacterial Agents for Patients Who Have Failed 48 to 72 Hours of Observation or Initial Management With Antibacterial Agents[a]				
1.	*At diagnosis for patients being treated initially with antibacterial agents*			
2.	*Clinically Defined Treatment Failure at 48–72 Hours After Initial Management With Observation Option*		*Clinically Defined Treatment Failure 48–72 Hours After Initial Management With Antibacterial Agents*	
Temperature ≥39°C (102.2°F) and/or Severe Otalgia	*Recommended*	*Alternative for Penicillin Allergy*	*Recommended*	*Alternative for Penicillin Allergy*
No	Amoxicillin, 80–90 mg/kg/d	Non–type I: cefdinir, cefuroxime, cefpodoxime; type I: azithromycin, clarithromycin	Amoxicillin-clavulanate, 90 mg/kg/d of amoxicillin component, with 6.4 mg/kg/d of clavulanate	Non–type I: ceftriaxone, 3 days; type I: clindamycin
Yes	Amoxicillin, clavulanate, 90 mg/kg/d of amoxicillin, with 6.4 mg/kg/d of clavulanate	Ceftriaxone, 1 or 3 days	Ceftriaxone, 3 days	Tympanocentesis, clindamycin

[a] Adapted with permission from American Academy of Pediatrics Subcommittee on Management of Acute Otitis Media. Diagnosis and management of acute otitis media. *Pediatrics.* 2004;113:1451–1465.

Complications

Complications associated with OM are much less common with appropriate antibiotic therapy and follow-up, but occasionally occur. They can be divided into 2 categories: extracranial and intracranial. Extracranial complications include perforation of the TM, conductive and sensorineural hearing loss, cholesteatoma, mastoiditis, facial nerve (cranial nerve VII) paralysis, osteomyelitis of the temporal bone, and Bezold abscess. Intracranial complications are meningitis, extradural as well as subdural abscesses, lateral venous sinus thrombosis, brain abscess, and hydrocephalus.

CASE RESOLUTION

In the case presented at the beginning of the chapter, the child displays the classic signs and symptoms of AOM: fever, upper respiratory infection, decreased appetite, and an abnormal tympanic membrane on physical examination. Because of his age, fever, and the certainty of diagnosis, he should be treated for 10 days with oral amoxicillin. The prognosis is good given his normal speech development.

Selected References

American Academy of Pediatrics. Appropriate use of antimicrobial agents. In: Pickering LK, Baker CJ, Long SS, McMillan JA, eds. *Red Book: 2006 Report of the Committee on Infectious Diseases.* 27th ed. Elk Grove Village, IL: American Academy of Pediatrics; 2006:737–741

American Academy of Pediatrics Subcommittee on Management of Acute Otitis Media. Diagnosis and management of acute otitis media. *Pediatrics.* 2004;113:1451–1465

Apiro DM, Khoon YT, Donald HA, Dziura JD, Baker MD, Shapiro ED. Wait and see prescription for the treatment of AOM. *JAMA.* 2006;296:1235–1241

Arguedas A, Emparanza P, Schwartz RH, et al. A randomized, multicenter, double blind, double dummy trial of single dose azithromycin versus high dose amoxicillin for treatment of uncomplicated acute otitis media. *Pediatr Infect Dis J.* 2005;24:153–161

Berkun Y, Nir-Paz R, Ben Ami A. Acute otitis media in the first two months of life: characteristics and diagnosis difficulties. *Arch Dis Child.* 2008;93:690–694

Brunton S, Pichichero ME. Acute otitis media: influence of the PCV-7 vaccine on changes in the disease and its management. *J Fam Pract.* 2005;54:961–968

Casey JR, Pichichero ME. Changes in frequency and pathogens causing acute otitis media in 1995–2003. *Pediatr Infect Dis J.* 2004;23:824–828

Centers for Disease Control and Prevention. National, state, and urban area vaccination coverage among children aged 19–35 months—United States, 2005. *MMWR Morb Mortal Wkly Rep.* 2006;55:988–993

Coco, A, Vernacchio, L, et al. Management of acute otitis media after publication of the 2004 AAP and AAFP clinical practice guidelines. *Pediatrics.* 2010;125(2):214–220

Damoiseaux RA, van Balen FA, Hoes AW, Vaerheij TJ, de Melker RA. Primary care based randomised, double blind trial of amoxicillin versus placebo for acute otitis media in children aged under 2 years. *BMJ.* 2000;320:350–354

Gould, J, Matz, P. Otitis media. *Pediatr Rev.* 2001;31(3):102–115

Hoberman A, Paradise J, et al. Treatment of acute otitis media in children under 2 years of age. *N Engl J Med.* 2011;364(2):105–115

Ongkasuwan J, Valdez TA, Hulten KG, et al. Pneumococcal mastoiditis in children and the emergence of multidrug-restraint serotype 19A isolates. *Pedatrics.* 2008;122:34

Piglansky L, Leibovitz E, Raiz S, et al. Bacteriologic and clinical efficacy of high dose amoxicillin for therapy of acute otitis media in children. *Pediatr Infect Dis J.* 2003;22:405–413

Rosenfeld RM. Diagnostic certainty for acute otitis media. *Int J Pediatr Otorhinolaryngol.* 2002;64:89–95

Siegel RM, Kiely M, Bien JP, et al. Treatment of otitis media with observation and a safety-net antibiotic prescription. *Pediatrics.* 2003;112:527–531

Wald ER. Acute otitis media: more trouble with the evidence. *Pediatr Infect Dis J.* 2003;22:103–104

Whitney CG, Farley MM, Hadler J, et al. Decline in invasive pneumococcal disease after the introduction of protein-polysaccharide conjugate vaccine. *N Engl J Med.* 2003;348:1737–1746

CHAPTER 73

Hearing Impairments

Julie E. Noble, MD

CASE STUDY

A 15-month-old girl is brought to the office because the parents are concerned that she has not yet begun to speak. The child was the full-term product of an uncomplicated pregnancy. Her 25-year-old mother, who began to receive regular prenatal care during the second month of gestation, had no documented infections during the pregnancy, took no medications, and has denied using illicit drugs or alcohol. The infant was delivered at home by a mid-wife and a newborn hearing screening was never done. The 27-year-old father is reportedly healthy. There is no family history of deafness, mental retardation, or consanguinity.

The girl, who is otherwise healthy, has never been hospitalized, but she has had 3 documented ear infections. She rolled over at 4 to 5 months of age, sat at 7 months, and walked at 13 months. She is able to scribble. The parents report that their daughter smiles appropriately, laughs occasionally, and plays well with other children. As an infant, the girl cooed and babbled, but she now points and grunts to indicate her needs. She does not respond to loud noises by turning her head.

The child's growth parameters, including head circumference, are normal for age. The rest of the physical examination is unremarkable.

Questions

1. When should deafness be suspected in infants or children?
2. What is the relationship between hearing loss and language development?
3. What are the major causes of deafness in children?
4. What neonates are at risk for the development of hearing deficits?
5. What methods are currently available to evaluate hearing in infants and children?
6. What are the important issues to address with families who have infants or children with suspected hearing impairment?

Hearing loss, even in a mild degree, is a significant childhood disability that can compromise speech and language development, academic performance, and psychosocial behavior. It is essential to identify hearing loss as soon as possible to implement early intervention, which has been shown to prevent many adverse consequences. Children may either be born with a hearing deficit, termed *congenital deafness,* or may acquire the condition during childhood, termed *progressive* or *late-onset.* A mild hearing deficit occurs with a 26 to 40 decibel (dB) loss. Severe hearing loss, on the other hand, is defined as 71 to 90 dB, and profound loss is 90 dB or greater. The most important period for speech and language development is from birth to 3 years of age. Reduced hearing acuity in both or even one ear during this time can significantly interfere with this important process (see Chapter 28). Therefore, primary care physicians must have a clear understanding of when to suspect impaired hearing in infancy and early childhood and must be familiar with the identification, evaluation methods, and treatment of hearing loss.

Epidemiology

The prevalence of congenital deafness in children is approximately 0.1%. In other words, 1 in 1,000 children is born severely to profoundly deaf. It has been estimated, however, that 3 to 5 in 1,000 children have mild to moderate hearing loss. The average age at diagnosis of most children who were born deaf was 2 to 3 years of age prior to the initiation of newborn hearing screening. Since its advent, the average age of diagnosis has dropped to 2 to 3 months of age. At this time in the United States, all 50 states have mandated universal newborn hearing screening programs. But as with any screening program, some infants may get missed, especially with at-home births; some infants may be lost to follow-up; and some forms of early-onset hearing loss are not apparent at birth. Therefore, careful assessment of hearing and language development by the pediatrician is essential at each patient encounter.

An estimated 20% to 30% of children who are hearing impaired develop the condition during childhood. Of these, 70% of children with acquired hearing loss are initially identified by the parents rather than physicians. Any concern by the parent that their child might have a hearing problem should be taken seriously by the physician and objective testing performed. Risk factors for acquired hearing loss in childhood include persistent otitis media with effusion, history of head trauma, bacterial meningitis, and the identification of syndromes or neurologic disorders associated with hearing loss.

Graduates of the neonatal intensive care unit have a significant increased risk of bilateral sensorineural hearing loss (1%–3%)

termed auditory neuropathy/dyssynchrony. Associated factors such as prematurity (birth weight <1,500 g), hyperbilirubinemia, prolonged mechanical ventilation, extracorporeal membrane oxygenation treatment, perinatal asphyxia, exposure to ototoxic drugs, and neonatal sepsis increase this risk. Other factors associated with deafness in childhood include meningitis, parental consanguinity, craniofacial malformations, congenital viral infections, exposure to chemotherapy, and a family history of deafness.

Clinical Presentation

Newborns might present to their pediatrician having had an abnormal newborn hearing screening test. The initial newborn screen is mandated by 1 month of age with definite testing by an audiologist for abnormal tests by 3 months of age. Therapy should begin by 6 months. If infants pass hearing testing but have positive risk factors they should have communication skills assessed at every well-child visit and diagnostic audiological assessment by 24 to 30 months of age.

Children with hearing impairments frequently present to physicians with delayed speech. Parents may be concerned that the toddler is indicating his needs by grunting and pointing rather than by using words. Children also may display behavioral problems, such as inattention, temper tantrums, or aggressive play with other children (Dx Box).

Dx Hearing Impairment

- Parental concern or suspicion of hearing loss
- Delayed speech and language development
- Associated risk factors including prematurity, exposure to ototoxic drugs, congenital or acquired central nervous system infections, family history of hearing loss and craniofacial abnormalities
- History of behavioral problems and/or poor school performance
- Abnormal hearing test

Hearing impairment can be more difficult to recognize in infants younger than 6 months because they may have no obvious symptoms of a hearing deficit. They may startle to moderately loud noises and begin to vocalize just as other infants (Figure 73-1). If the history is suggestive of a hearing deficit, audiological testing should be performed.

Pathophysiology

Mechanism of Hearing

Sounds in the form of pressure waves are carried from the environment through the external auditory canal to the tympanic membrane (TM). These waves are then converted to mechanical vibrations by the ossicles, and the mechanical vibrations are then transmitted from the TM to the inner ear, where they are transformed to fluid vibrations. Finally, these fluid vibrations are converted into nerve impulses by nerve endings within the organ of Corti located in the cochlea in

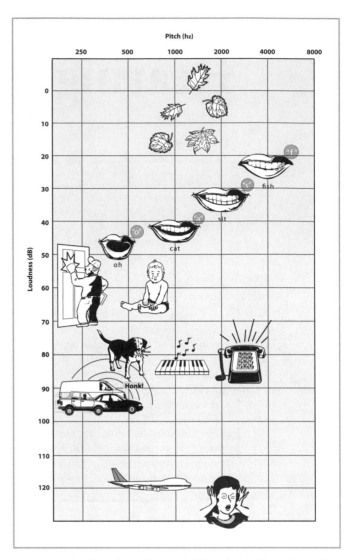

Figure 73-1. Loudness of everyday sounds. (Reproduced with permission from Northern J, Downs M. *Hearing in Children.* **4th ed. Baltimore, MD: Williams & Wilkins; 1991.)**

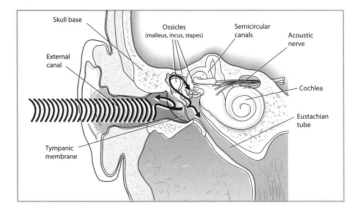

Figure 73-2. Sound waves passing through the external ear into the middle ear.

the inner ear. These impulses are conducted via the auditory nerve to the auditory cortex (Figure 73-2).

Hearing impairments can be classified either according to the part of the auditory system affected or by the cause of the hearing loss.

Types of Hearing Loss

A **conductive hearing loss denotes an abnormality in the outer ear, the TM, or middle-ear ossicles.** Cerumen impaction, otitis externa, serous otitis, recurrent otitis media, TM perforation, and ossicular discontinuity are examples of this type of hearing loss. Middle-ear effusions rarely cause more than a 20- to 30-dB loss.

The cochlea or inner ear or auditory nerve is affected in **sensorineural hearing loss (SNHL).** Congenital infections, anomalies, and genetic disorders lead to this type of loss. The loss of cochlear function is the main cause of permanent childhood hearing loss. A **mixed disorder** has characteristics of both conductive and sensorineural losses. In a **retrocochlear hearing loss,** the auditory nerve, brain stem, or cortex is affected. This includes auditory neuropathy noted in infants following neonatal intensive care unit stays.

Etiology of Hearing Impairment (Box 73-1)

Severe to profound hearing loss has 2 main causes: genetic and acquired environmental. Genetic causes account for approximately 68% of cases. There are more than 500 forms of syndromic hearing loss with associated clinical features. An autosomal-recessive syndrome, Pendred syndrome with thyromegaly is a more common example. Down syndrome and Goldenhar syndrome both have frequently associated hearing impairment. Alport syndrome with progressive SNHL and nephritis is also well recognized. But most cases of genetic hearing loss are non-syndromic and result from a single gene defect encoding connexin, 26(CX26) protein. This recessive disorder with mutations in the *GJB2* gene account for 30% to 50% of all cases in many populations. Genetic malformations of the ear pinnae or ossicles do occur but are the least common cause of hearing loss. Genetic mutations may result in different types of deafness with various presentations and outcomes (ie, hearing loss may be conductive, sensorineural, or mixed, and may be static or progressive with the initial presentation either in infancy or later childhood).

Acquired environmental causes include prenatal, perinatal, or postnatal events and exposures such as congenital infections, bacterial meningitis, hyperbilirubinemia, complications of prematurity, and exposure to ototoxic medications. Cytomegalovirus (CMV) is probably the most frequently unrecognized congenital infection causing deafness. Ten percent of infants with congenital hearing loss are infected with CMV. However, toxoplasmosis, rubella, herpes simplex virus, HIV, and syphilis can also be implicated. Hearing loss associated with bacterial meningitis accounted for as many as 20% of cases, with *Streptococcus pneumoniae* as the prevalent responsible organism. The incidence of both *S pneumoniae* and *Haemophilus influenzae* meningitis have decreased tremendously in young children following the advent of conjugate vaccine, and the prevalence of post-meningitic hearing loss has similarly declined. The role of steroids in the treatment of bacterial meningitis has also contributed to the decrease in sensorineural hearing loss in survivors.

Box 73-1. Major Causes of Childhood Deafness[a]	
Conductive Hearing Loss	*Sensorineural Hearing Loss*
Congenital • Microtia/atresia • Tympanic membrane abnormalities • Ossicular malformations	• Genetic disorders (syndromic, connexin 26, mitochondrial) • In utero infections (cytomegalovirus, measles, mumps, rubella, varicella, syphilis) • Anatomical abnormalities of the cochlea or temporal bone • Exposure to ototoxic drugs during pregnancy (alcohol, isotretinoin, cisplatinum) • Hyperbilirubinemia
Acquired • Infection (acute otitis media, otitis externa, ossicular erosion) • Otitis media with effusion • Foreign body (including cerumen) • Cholesteatoma • Trauma (ossicular disruption, tympanic membrane perforation)	• Infections (bacterial meningitis, measles, mumps, rubella, Lyme disease) • Trauma (physical or acoustic) • Radiation therapy for head and neck tumors • Neurodegenerative or demyelinating disorders (Alport, Cogan syndromes)

[a] Adapted from Gifford KA, Holmes MG, Bernstein HH. Hearing loss in children. *Pediatr Rev.* 2009;30:207–216.

With the recognition and treatment of hyperbilirubinemia in term newborns, this as a cause of hearing loss is now rare in the United States and other developed countries. Prematurity as a cause of hearing loss is, however, not uncommon. Because of associated complications, premature infants have higher rates of severe hearing loss than do full-term infants. Some antibiotics, such as the aminoglycosides, and other medications like furosemide can be irreversibly ototoxic; other drugs may cause only transient effects.

Any head injury causing significant middle-ear trauma may also cause deafness in children. Repeated acoustic trauma from continuous or significant exposure to loud noise can also cause irreversible hearing loss. With children's use of personal listening devices, this cause of hearing loss is increasing.

Differential Diagnosis

In addition to hearing loss, communication disorders should be considered in infants or children with delayed speech and language development. These include problems with speech perception, language comprehension, formulation of language output, and speech production. Unrecognized conditions such as mental retardation or autism can be responsible for some of these disorders. Other etiologies include specific central nervous system deficits as well as impairments of fine motor control of the oropharynx.

Evaluation

Newborn Hearing Screening

In 1994 the Joint Committee on Infant Hearing (JCIH), composed of representatives from several professional organizations, endorsed universal newborn hearing screening. Their goal was the early identification of hearing loss in infants before age 3 months and the implementation of intervention services by 6 months of age. As a result of these recommendations, states have implemented legislation mandating newborn hearing screening and intervention programs. A subsequent position statement was issued in 2000 titled Principles and Guidelines for Early Hearing Detection and Intervention Programs (EHDI). The American Academy of Pediatrics endorsed this statement and promoted newborn hearing screening as well as periodic hearing assessment for every child. The JCIH policy statement was most recently updated in 2007 and includes more specific guidelines for diagnostic audiological evaluation, medical evaluation, and surveillance screening in the medical home. The policy notes that all infants and children regardless of hearing screening results should have ongoing assessment of communication skills beginning at 2 months of age. Any child with evidence of hearing loss in one or both ears should be offered early intervention.

History

Because the primary symptom of deafness is failure to learn to speak at the appropriate age, the most important aspect of the history in children with possible hearing loss is determining whether speech is developing normally. Even deaf infants may begin cooing and babbling in infancy, and these early attempts at verbalization are not useful milestones for assessment of hearing deficits. It helps to ask parents whether they are at all suspicious or concerned about their children's speech or hearing. Guidelines to assess language development are found in Table 73-1 (see Chapter 28). An assessment of risk factors for deafness, such as a positive family history, infection during gestation, history of prematurity, hyperbilirubinemia, neonatal sepsis, and asphyxia, is also important (Questions Box).

Physical Examination

A complete physical examination should be performed on all children. In particular, any dysmorphic facial features that may suggest the presence of a syndrome with an associated hearing deficit should be noted. Other anomalies of the head and neck should be noted as well. Abnormal pigmentary conditions may be important clues. The eyes should be evaluated for heterochromia and hypertelorism findings seen in Waardenburg syndrome, which also includes SNHL. The size and shape of the pinnae and external ear canals should be carefully inspected for abnormalities and patency, respectively. Preauricular pits or tags may be apparent. In addition, the TMs should also be visualized and assessed for the presence of a middle-ear effusion that may influence subsequent audiological tests. Insufflation may be helpful to assess middle-ear effusion. The oropharynx should be examined for a cleft palate or a bifid uvula, which

Table 73-1. Expected Speech-Language-Auditory Milestone[a]		
Age	*Receptive Skills*	*Expressive Skills*
Birth	Turns to source of sound Shows preference for voices Shows interest in faces	Cries
2–4 months		Coos Takes turns cooing
6 months	Responds to name	
9 months	Understands verbal routines (wave bye-bye)	Babbles Points Says ma-ma, da-da
12 months	Follows a verbal command	Uses jargon Says first words
15 months	Points to body parts by name	Learns words slowly
18–24 months	Understands sentences	Learns words quickly Uses 2-word phrases
24–36 months	Answers questions Follows 2-step commands	Phrases 50% intelligible Builds 3- (or more) word sentences Asks "what" questions
36–48 months	Understands much of what is said	Asks "why" questions Sentences 75% intelligible Masters the early acquired speech sounds: m, b, y, n, w, d, p, and h
48–60 months	Understands much of what is said, commensurate with cognitive level	Creates well-formed sentences Tells stories 100% intelligible
6 years		Pronounces most speech sounds correctly; may have difficulty with sh, th as in think, s, z, th as in the, l, r, and the s in treasure
7 years		Pronounces speech sounds correctly, including consonant blends such as sp, tr, bl

[a] Adapted from Feldman HM. Evaluation and management of language and speech disorders in preschool children. *Pediatr Rev.* 2005;26:131–142.

may be associated with a submucous cleft. The manner in which children communicate with parents should be noted, if possible, and the child assessed for response to sound.

Questions

Hearing Impairment

- Does the infant seem to respond to sounds?
- Does the infant attempt to repeat sounds?
- How does the young child indicate his or her desires or needs?
- How are the parents currently communicating with the child?
- Is there any evidence of a congenital infection, structural anomaly of the head and neck, or syndrome?
- Is there a history of prematurity or other prenatal or perinatal problem?
- Have there been any serious bacterial infections such as meningitis?
- Has the child had a history of repeated ear infections or exposure to ototoxic drugs?
- Aside from the hearing problem, is the child developmentally normal?
- Is there a family history of deafness, consanguinity, or multiple miscarriages or stillbirths?

Laboratory Tests

Tympanometry does not measure hearing, but is useful in assessing the presence of middle-ear fluid and the mobility of the TM. Tympanometry can be particularly helpful with uncooperative, crying children in whom assessing the appearance of the TM and insufflation is difficult. Different types of hearing tests for evaluating infants and children for possible hearing deficits are available to general pediatricians (Box 73-2). **Automated auditory brain stem response (ABR)** and **brain stem auditory evoked response (BAER)** are electrophysiological measurements of activity in the auditory nerve and brain stem pathways. Electrodes are placed on the infant or child's head to record brain wave activity while a specific auditory stimulus is presented through earphones to one ear at a time. Auditory thresholds can be estimated. The ABR is used for newborn hearing screening and only takes approximately 10 minutes, whereas the BAER is more comprehensive, requiring up to 90 minutes to perform. **Behavioral observation audiometry** measures a child's response to speech and frequency-specific stimuli presented through speakers in a soundproof room. This method of testing can only assess hearing in the better ear and cannot detect unilateral hearing loss. It is used with children at younger than 6 months' developmental age. **Evoked otoacoustic emissions** can be performed on children of all ages. It measures cochlear function in response to a specific stimulus via a small probe that contains a microphone that is placed in the ear canal. This test can be used for newborn hearing screening in low-risk newborns and also can be performed in approximately 10 minutes. **Conditioned play audiometry** like **conventional audiometric testing** measures auditory thresholds in response to frequency-specific stimuli presented through earphones to one ear at a time. The patient is instructed to perform a particular task, such as put a block in a container versus raise his or her hand, when the stimulus is heard. Children as young as 3 years can be tested by conditioned play audiometry and 4 or 5 years of age via

---

Box 73-2. Tests to Evaluate Hearing

- Automated auditory brain stem response: used for newborn - hearing screening
- Behavioral observation audiometry
- Brain stem auditory evoked response
- Evoked otoacoustic emissions: newer type of newborn hearing screening
- Conditioned play audiometry
- Conventional audiometric testing

---

conventional audiometric testing. These tests should be used in conjunction with evaluations from audiological and otolaryngologic consultations. In the case of high-risk infants, testing should be repeated at least every 6 months until 3 years of age, and at appropriate intervals thereafter depending on the etiology of the suspected hearing loss and the hearing test results.

Diagnostic tests to consider in evaluating the cause of deafness include titers for congenital infections such as CMV, toxoplasmosis, HIV, and rubella and fluorescent treponemal antibody absorption tests for syphilis. In the newborn period, a CMV culture may be helpful. Testing for the *GJB2* gene, the mitochondrial A1555G mutation that predisposes one to ototoxicity from drugs, and the *SLC26A4* gene for Pendred syndrome along with CMV testing would reveal an etiology for 40% of congenital hearing loss and for 60% of late-onset hearing loss. Thyroid function tests are necessary if Pendred syndrome is suspected, especially in school-aged children with goiters. Proteinuria and hematuria should also be ruled out by urine dipstick, especially in boys with a positive family history of deafness and renal failure, findings suggestive of Alport syndrome. An electrocardiogram is recommended to detect conduction defects such as QT prolongation in Jervell and Lange-Nielsen syndrome.

Imaging Studies

Occasionally, a computed tomography or magnetic resonance imaging scan of the temporal bone may be used to view the anatomy of the middle and inner ear, particularly in cases of a suspected cochlear/vestibular malformation or fistula. Necessity for such studies should be determined by the audiologist or otolaryngologist.

Management

Studies have shown that the earlier the hearing deficit is detected and remediation begun in an otherwise normal infant, the greater the likelihood the child will have language development close to that of a hearing infant. Initiation of intervention prior to 6 months of age produces infants who are able to develop language, as well as social and emotional skills appropriate for their age. School performance and communication skills also have been shown to be better in those identified at a younger age. All infants and children identified with a hearing deficit should be referred to an otolaryngologist and audiologist for immediate assessment and recommendation for assistive devices.

Additional assessment includes an ophthalmologic evaluation and referral to a geneticist. Once infants or children are found to have a hearing impairment, careful follow-up is necessary so that any further reduction in hearing is promptly identified. The role of primary care providers thus becomes even more crucial. Coordination of care with speech and language specialists as well as educators that have experience with working with deaf children is essential. Both parents and other family members may initially be devastated by the diagnosis of a hearing impairment, especially if the deficit is severe to profound. They often have multiple questions about children's medical prognosis and educational future. The possibility of further speech and language development may also be a foremost concern in their minds. In addition to providing patients with comprehensive care, all of the parents' questions and concerns must be addressed and anticipated.

Future Audiological Evaluations

In newly diagnosed patients with sensorineural hearing loss, **audiology testing** should be repeated every 3 months in the first year and then every 6 months when children are in preschool. The test should be repeated at least annually after children have begun school. Continued monitoring is essential to detect any progression of the hearing deficit.

Assistive Devices

Although **hearing aids** may not restore normal hearing, all children with conductive as well as sensorineural hearing loss benefit from amplification. Several different types of hearing aids are available for children; these devices should be fitted appropriately and adjusted regularly. In addition, it is also recommended that all patients receive bilateral hearing aids to improve auditory localization and training, particularly in the context of different learning situations.

An **FM system** is an additional assistive listening device that can be used in a classroom. A speaker uses a microphone to transmit to a receiver the child wears to improve reception. **Closed-caption television** (signed or subtitled) is another method of auditory training. In addition, **teletype telephone systems** are available for children who can read.

Cochlear implants may be surgically placed in the cochlea to improve hearing. Implants were first approved by the US Food and Drug Administration in 1990 for use in children. The implant consists of an electrode array that responds to an external microphone and speech processor and produces an electrical discharge within the cochlea. These electrical pulses effectively stimulate the auditory system. The implant can be used in children at 12 months of age or older with profound sensorineural hearing loss. There are ongoing improvements in technology with improving results. Speech, language, and special education resources should also be provided. Most patients with implants show significant improvement in communication skills. Children with cochlear implants are at increased risk for meningitis, therefore pneumococcal vaccine is recommended.

Education and Communication

Much controversy exists regarding the optimal method of communication for deaf children. **Oral communication (lip reading)** and **sign language** each have their advantages as well as disadvantages depending on children's age, the type of deafness, and whether the deficit is congenital or acquired. Whether the children already know a language is also important to consider. The preferred methods seem to vary from region to region; therefore, schools, other institutions, and resource groups often use the most popular communication method in a particular area. In general, some authors recommend that children with minimal hearing loss may do better with lip reading than those with greater hearing loss, who will most likely benefit more from sign language. Early intervention and education programs can be home-based or in a group setting. But it is recommended that the educators be familiar with working with hearing impaired children.

Whether to "mainstream" children with severe hearing loss in a regular classroom with an interpreter or place them in a school for deaf children is another controversial issue. Parents should be encouraged to explore the possibilities of each option and to make a decision based on the individual needs of their children and not current trends. The expertise of an educator who is knowledgeable in this field can also be helpful when making this decision.

Outside Resources and Referrals

As previously mentioned it takes a team to properly evaluate a child with hearing loss. Newly diagnosed children should be evaluated by **otolaryngologists** with pediatric expertise, **audiologists,** pediatric **ophthalmologists,** and medical **geneticists.** Any refractory error should be treated and followed closely because children with severe hearing difficulties are more dependent on vision. A genetics evaluation is important for diagnostic reasons as well as for providing families with information and counseling about the risk of recurrence.

Speech assessment and therapy are an essential part of long-term management as are special education resources. Support groups and referrals to national organizations for hearing impaired individuals can be valuable for parents and families. Resources for financial support should also be explored. Agencies with multidisciplinary teams are particularly important for infants or children with other associated disabilities.

Prognosis

The goals of early recognition and treatment of infants and children with hearing deficits is to minimize the possible long-term sequelae of persistent speech and language problems and to maximize cognitive development. An additional goal is to prevent the development of learning disabilities with subsequent educational failure. The earlier the intervention, the more likely children succeed and maximize their potential. With appropriate treatment the child should be able to lead a normal life.

CASE RESOLUTION

In the opening case, the child has a history classic for a hearing deficit. She does not turn to loud noises, she has not developed any specific words, and she indicates her needs nonverbally. Although there are no obvious historical risk factors for hearing loss, a behavioral audiogram or **BAER** should be performed. The physician's suspicion should be discussed with the family, and a follow-up visit should be arranged to review the hearing test results as soon as possible.

Selected References

American Academy of Pediatrics Task Force on Newborn and Infant Screening. Newborn and infant hearing loss: detection and intervention. *Pediatrics.* 1999;103:527–530

Feldman H. Evaluation and management of language and speech disorders in preschool children. *Pediatr Rev.* 2005;26:131–141

Gifford KA, Holmes MG, Bernstein HH. Hearing loss in children. *Pediatr Rev.* 2009;30:207–216

Harlor A, Bower, C. Clinical report-hearing assessment in infants and children: recommendations beyond neonatal screening. *Pediatrics.* 2009;124:1252–1263

Joint Committee on Infant Hearing. Year 2007 position statement: principles and guidelines for early hearing hearing detection and intervention programs. *Pediatrics.* 2007;120:898–921

Joint Committee on Infant Hearing, American Academy of Audiology, American Academy of Pediatrics, American Speech-Language-Hearing Association, and Directors of Speech and Hearing Programs in State Health and Welfare Agencies. Year 2000 position statement: principle and guidelines for early hearing detection and intervention programs. *Pediatrics.* 2000;106:798–817

Kennedy C, McCann DC, Campbell MJ, et al. Language ability after early detection of permanent childhood hearing impairment. *N Engl J Med.* 2006;354:2131–2141

Kerschner J. Neonatal hearing screening: to do or not to do. *Pediatr Clin North Am.* 2004;51:725–736

Kral A, O'Donoghue G. Profound deafness in childhood. *N Engl J Med.* 2010;363:1438–1450

Lieu JE. Speech-language and educational consequences of unilateral hearing loss in children. *Arch Otolaryngol Head Neck Surg.* 2004;130:524–530

Morton C, Nance W. Newborn hearing screening—a silent revolution. *N Engl J Med.* 2006;354:2151–2164

Papsin B, Gordon K. Cochlear implants for children with severe-to-profound hearing loss. *N Engl J Med.* 2007;357:2380–2387

Smith R, Bale J, White K. Sensorineural hearing loss in children. *Lancet.* 2005;365:879–890

Weichbold V, Nekahm-Heis D, Welzl-Mueller K. Universal newborn hearing screening and postnatal hearing loss. *Pediatrics.* 2006;117:e631–e636

CHAPTER 74

Sore Throat

Stanley H. Inkelis, MD, and Casey Buitenhuys, MD

CASE STUDY

An 8-year-old girl has had a sore throat and fever for 2 days. She also has pain on swallowing, a headache, and a feeling of general malaise but no stridor, drooling, breathing difficulty, or rash. Other than the current illness, the girl is in good health. Although she has had sore throats in the past, she has never had one this severe. One week ago both her mother and father had a sore throat and fever that resolved after 5 days with no medication.

The child has a temperature of 102.2°F (39.0°C). The physical examination is normal except for red tonsils with exudate bilaterally, palatal petechiae, and tender cervical lymphadenopathy.

Questions

1. What are the causes of sore throat in children?
2. What is the appropriate evaluation of children with sore throat? What laboratory tests are necessary?
3. What is the appropriate management for children with sore throat?
4. When should otolaryngologic consultation be obtained?

Sore throat, one of the most common illnesses seen by the primary care physician, is a painful inflammation of the pharynx, tonsils, or surrounding areas. In most cases, children with sore throat have mild symptoms that require little or no treatment. However, sore throat may be the presenting complaint of a severe illness such as epiglottitis or retropharyngeal abscess. Small children are not able to define their complaints very well, which makes a careful history from parents or other caregivers and a good physical examination essential for correct diagnosis. Optimal management of sore throat, especially if group A beta-hemolytic streptococcus (GABHS) is suspected, is still very controversial.

Epidemiology

Sore throat accounts for approximately 7.3 million outpatient physician visits each year and approximately 5% of all pediatric emergency department visits are for pharyngitis. Sore throats are most common in children 5 to 8 years of age, and they continue to occur during later childhood. They are uncommon in children younger than 1 year. Like other respiratory infections, sore throats occur most often in the late fall and winter months. Approximately 11% of all school-aged children receive medical care for pharyngitis. Fifteen percent to 30% or more of cases of pharyngitis in these children are caused by GABHS. The estimated medical and nonmedical costs for GABHS pharyngitis are $205 per visit or approximately $224 to $539 million per year.

The organisms that cause bacterial and viral pharyngitis are present in saliva and nasal secretions and are almost always transmitted by close contact. Spread from child to child in school is the common mode of transmission.

Clinical Presentation

The clinical presentation of sore throat is variable and often depends on etiology (Dx Box and see Differential Diagnosis). Most children with sore throat present with sudden onset of pain and fever. The height of the fever is variable and is typically higher in younger children. In older children, especially if the sore throat is associated

Dx Sore Throat

Viral	Bacterial
• Pain in throat	• Pain in throat, usually sudden onset
• Fever (variable)[a]	• Fever
• Rhinorrhea (common)	• Marked erythema of pharynx, tonsils, or uvula
• Cough (common)	• Headache, nausea, vomiting, abdominal pain
• Erythema of pharynx or tonsils	• Tonsillar and posterior pharyngeal wall exudate
• Follicular, ulcerative, exudative lesions of pharynx or tonsils[a]	• Tender, swollen cervical lymphadenopathy
• Conjunctivitis	• Scarlatiniform rash
	• Absence of rhinorrhea or cough
	• Positive rapid antigen test or throat culture

[a] Dependent on etiology (see Differential Diagnosis).

with a common cold, fever is minimal or absent. The throat or tonsils are red, and the breath may be malodorous. Headache, nausea, vomiting, and abdominal pain may occur, especially if children are febrile. The appetite may be decreased and children may be less active than usual.

In children with the common cold, rhinorrhea and postnasal discharge are present. A pharyngeal and tonsillar exudate is not typical. Although the cervical lymph nodes may be enlarged, they are usually not very tender. In contrast, children with streptococcal pharyngitis typically have high fever, pharyngeal and tonsillar exudate, and tender cervical lymph nodes.

Pathophysiology

Various bacteria and viruses produce sore throat symptoms by causing inflammation in the ring of posterior pharyngeal lymphoid tissue that consists of the tonsils, adenoids, and surrounding lymphoid tissue. This ring of tissue, called Waldeyer ring, drains the oral and pharyngeal cavity and defends against infection of the mouth and throat. Other host defenses that protect against infection include the sneeze, gag, and cough reflexcs; secretory immunoglobulin A; and a rich blood supply.

Viral sore throats may be acquired by inhalation or self-inoculation from the nasal mucosa or conjunctiva. The local respiratory epithelium becomes infected with the virus, and inflammation occurs. In some instances, inflammatory mediators may be responsible for the pain of sore throat. Group A streptococcus and other bacterial organisms directly invade the mucous membranes. Enzymes produced by this organism, streptolysin O and hyaluronidase, aid in the spread of infection.

Differential Diagnosis

Although most children who present with sore throat have common viral or bacterial pharyngitis, other less common disorders such as infectious mononucleosis, acute HIV seroconversion syndrome, epiglottitis, retropharyngeal abscess, or peritonsillar abscess should be considered.

Viral Infection

Viral infection, the most common cause of sore throat in children, is most often associated with an upper respiratory infection caused by a rhinovirus. Cough and rhinorrhea associated with a sore throat suggest this etiology. Influenza virus infections may present with sudden onset of high fever, headache, cough, sore throat, and myalgias.

Adenovirus often leads to exudative pharyngitis, frequently in children younger than 3 years. Pharyngoconjunctival fever, caused by adenovirus 3, is characterized by a high fever (temperature: >102.2°F [39.0°C]) for several days, conjunctivitis, and exudative tonsillitis.

Coxsackievirus and echovirus (enteroviruses) are the usual cause of herpangina. Vesicles and ulcers are generally apparent on the anterior tonsillar pillars and soft palate. They may also be found on the tonsils, pharynx, or posterior buccal mucosa. Children may have a high fever (temperature: >102.2°F [39.0°C]), be irritable, and refuse to eat or drink; dehydration may result. Coxsackievirus A16 and enterovirus 71 cause hand-foot-and-mouth disease, which is characterized by ulcerative oral lesions on the tongue and buccal mucosa and, less frequently, on the palate and anterior tonsillar pillars. Vesicular and papulovesicular lesions are evident on the hands and feet and occasionally on other parts of the body, most commonly the knees and buttocks. Enteroviral infections typically occur in the late spring, summer, and early fall.

Herpes simplex virus (HSV) may lead to pharyngotonsillitis but can be distinguished from most of the enteroviral infections because HSV almost always involves the anterior portion of the mouth and lips and is associated with gingivitis (herpes gingivostomatitis). The lesions often appear as whitish-yellow plaques with an erythematous base and are sometimes ulcerative. This illness is characterized by a high fever (temperature: 102.2°F [39.0°C]) for up to 7 to 10 days and frequent refusal to eat or drink because of the painful lesions. Dehydration may occur.

Epstein-Barr virus (EBV) may cause exudative pharyngotonsillitis either alone or as part of the infectious mononucleosis syndrome that includes fever, malaise, lymphadenopathy, palatal petechiae, and hepatosplenomegaly. Fatigue, malaise, eyelid edema, organomegaly, and a maculopapular rash without the other characteristics of a scarlet fever rash help distinguish between infectious mononucleosis and GABHS infection.

Cytomegalovirus may cause an infectious mononucleosis syndrome similar to EBV but is not as commonly associated with pharyngitis and splenomegaly.

HIV seroconversion syndrome may present with low-grade fevers, myalgias, nonexudative pharyngitis, diffuse adenopathy, anorexia, and weight loss. Usually this constellation of symptoms is attributed to an influenza-like illness. Generally, onset of symptoms is about 1 week after exposure but may be within the first month after exposure.

Bacterial Infection

Group A beta-hemolytic streptococcus is the most common cause of bacterial sore throat in children older than 3 years. The pharynx is typically very red and sometimes edematous, and the tonsils are red, enlarged, and covered with exudate. Occasionally, the uvula is very inflamed as well. Children may also have dysphagia, fever, vomiting, headache, malaise, and abdominal pain. Swollen anterior cervical lymphadenopathy and petechiae on the soft palate and uvula are usually apparent. In addition, the occurrence of a scarlatiniform rash, "strawberry tongue," and Pastia lines (petechiae in the flexor skin creases of joints) indicates scarlet fever, which is diagnostic of group A streptococcal infection (see Chapter 122). Sore throat from GABHS typically occurs in the winter and spring. Rheumatic fever and glomerulonephritis are non-suppurative complications of group A streptococcal infection.

Peritonsillar abscess or cellulitis and cervical lymphadenitis are suppurative complications of GABHS. Children with peritonsillar abscess often experience trismus and drooling and speak with a "hot potato" voice. The abscess in the affected tonsil causes a bulge in the posterior soft palate and pushes the uvula away from the midline to the unaffected side of the pharynx. On palpation, the abscess may feel fluctuant. Peritonsillar cellulitis typically produces a bulge in the soft palate but does not cause deviation of the uvula.

Parapharyngeal and retropharyngeal abscesses that typically occur in children younger than 6 are additional life-threatening complications of GABHS. Sore throat is associated with these conditions, but dysphagia is usually more evident when the child swallows. Children with a retropharyngeal or parapharyngeal abscess are toxic-appearing, also complain of trismus, have a fever, refuse to swallow, drool, have neck pain and rigidity, have dysphonia, or have shortness of breath. A fluctuant mass may be palpated deep to the tonsils. The patient may have pain when the trachea is manipulated in a lateral direction. The neck may be stiff and the patient may resist passive neck movements. Stridor may be present but usually is an ominous sign of impending airway compromise.

Group B, C, and G beta-hemolytic streptococci (non-GABHS) have all been isolated from children with pharyngitis. *Streptococcus pneumoniae* and *Arcanobacterium haemolyticum* infrequently cause pharyngitis in children. The latter organism is associated with a scarlatiniform rash in some patients and is most common in adolescents and young adults. In contrast to scarlet fever, palatal petechiae and strawberry tongue are not present with the pharyngitis caused by this bacterium. Although *Corynebacterium diphtheriae* (diphtheria) rarely causes sore throat in immunized children, this organism should be considered in non-immunized children who have exudative pharyngotonsillitis and a grayish pseudomembrane that bleeds when removal is attempted.

Chlamydia trachomatis may lead to pharyngitis and tonsillitis in adolescents and young adults through sexual transmission. The role of *Chlamydia pneumoniae* as a cause of sore throat in children remains unclear. *Mycoplasma pneumoniae* does not usually produce sore throat in children unless they have lower respiratory tract disease. *Neisseria gonorrhoeae* may lead to sore throat in sexually active adolescents. Its occurrence in prepubertal children is often secondary to sexual abuse. The appearance of the throat is not characteristic, and diagnosis is made by cultures when the degree of suspicion is high. **Tularemia** is a rare cause of exudative pharyngitis in children but should be suspected if contact with wild animals has occurred.

Fusobacterium necrophorum is a gram-negative anaerobe that may cause an exudative pharyngitis, tender adenopathy, and fever. Untreated, it may progress to Lemierre syndrome or septic thrombosis of the internal jugular vein. Direct extension of the bacterial pharyngitis leads to perivenular inflammation and septic thrombosis of the internal jugular vein. Patients may present with fever, severe lateral neck pain, torticollis, and prominent internal and external jugular veins with erythema and induration. Patients may present with additional signs and symptoms if septic emboli propagate, including acute neurologic signs (central nervous system retrograde propagation) and shortness of breath and multilobar pneumonia with or without cavitation (pulmonary propagation). Paradoxical septic emboli may cause other symptoms if a right-to-left cardiac shunt is present.

Other Causes

Candida albicans may be responsible for sore throat in infants and in children who are immunocompromised or taking antibiotics. Children with oral candidiasis usually present with whitish plaques on the labial or buccal mucosa that do not wipe off easily. When the pharynx and tonsils are involved, some discomfort or dysphagia, but usually not significant pain, may occur.

Epiglottitis (supraglottitis) may present as sore throat. Prior to the *Haemophilus influenzae* type B (Hib) conjugate vaccine, epiglottitis typically affected children 2 to 7 years of age who would present with signs of toxicity, stridor, difficulty swallowing, and drooling. In relatively well-appearing children with sore throat but no stridor, neither epiglottitis nor retropharyngeal abscess is a likely cause of sore throat. In the past, epiglottitis was almost always caused by Hib. With the widespread use of the Hib conjugate vaccine, this organism is now rarely the etiology, thus diminishing the prevalence of epiglottitis and making this entity an uncommon cause of sore throat in children. Although rare in adolescents, epiglottitis may present with severe sore throat out of proportion to clinical findings. Other signs and symptoms include dysphagia, odynophagia, a muffled voice, and pain on palpation of the anterior neck around the hyoid bone. *Streptococcus pneumoniae*; *Staphylococcus aureus*; and group A, B, and C beta-hemolytic streptococci are unusual but reported causative agents of epiglottitis.

Children with croup may have sore throat and stridor, but they do not usually appear toxic and do not have difficulty swallowing. Affected children are usually between 6 months and 3 years of age (see Chapter 58).

Trauma from penetrating objects, burns, or exposure to caustic materials may cause sore throat in children. Household smoking may also lead to pharyngeal irritation. In addition, allergic rhinitis with postnasal drip may result in sore throat. Tumor rarely causes sore throat in children but should be considered if a mass is present or pharyngeal inflammation persists. Persistent sore throat may also be a symptom of Kawasaki disease.

Evaluation

History

A thorough history often reveals the etiology of the sore throat (Questions Box). Questions regarding duration, fever, headache, vomiting, pain on swallowing, rash, oral lesions, abdominal pain, and history of contact with other family members or classmates with similar symptoms suggest the most common causes of sore throat (infections with viruses and GABHS). A history of rapid onset of fever, toxicity, difficulty swallowing, drooling, and respiratory distress suggest epiglottitis and retropharyngeal abscess. Voice changes suggest peritonsillar abscess or tonsillar hypertrophy associated with infectious mononucleosis (EBV). Immunization history or history of immigration from a developing country helps assess the risk of diphtheria. Oral sexual activity suggests the possibility of a sexually transmitted infection. A history of allergies, trauma, and environmental smoke may help diagnose other causes of sore throat. Red eye or pinkeye with a rash, persistent fever (>5 days), and sore throat suggest Kawasaki disease. A teenager with at-risk behavior and an influenza-like illness may be presenting with HIV seroconversion syndrome.

Physical Examination

A general physical examination should be performed. It is important to note whether children appear toxic. The skin should be examined for a scarlatiniform, sandpaper-like rash; a vesicular rash involving the hands and feet; or a generalized maculopapular rash. The eyes should be evaluated for conjunctivitis and the nose for rhinorrhea (serous or purulent). The mouth, pharynx, and tonsils should be examined for vesicular lesions, ulcers, and gingivitis. The pharynx should be checked for redness, exudate, vesicles, edema, and foreign bodies. The tonsils and uvula should be examined for these same findings as well as asymmetry, and the neck should be checked for nuchal rigidity. The lymph nodes should be evaluated for enlargement (adenopathy) and inflammation (adenitis). The abdomen should be examined for hepatosplenomegaly.

Laboratory Tests

Although many signs and symptoms may suggest streptococcal pharyngitis, diagnosis can be confirmed only with laboratory tests. The **throat culture** is the gold standard for diagnosis. When done correctly, throat culture has a sensitivity of 90% to 95% in detecting pharyngeal GABHS. Specimens should be obtained from the surfaces of both tonsils and posterior pharynx without touching other parts of the pharynx or the mouth. The main disadvantage of throat culture is that the results are not available for a day or more after the specimen is obtained. Nevertheless, throat culture is the most reliable way to confirm streptococcal infection.

Rapid antigen detection tests (RADTs) are available for on-the-spot diagnosis. False-positive results are uncommon (specificity: ≥95%), but false-negative results for most RADTs occur commonly (sensitivity: 80%–90%). Because a negative test may not exclude a streptococcal infection, it is currently recommended that this result should be confirmed by throat culture. However, newer RADTs using optical immunoassay (OIA) and chemiluminescent DNA probes boast sensitivities of over 99%. Recent data suggest that a negative OIA RADT may not always need routine confirmation with a throat culture, especially if physicians confirm in their practice setting that the newer RADT has a sensitivity comparable to the sensitivity of throat culture. In one study of more than 30,000 patients comparing those managed with throat cultures alone to those managed with a high-sensitivity RADT without throat culture confirmation, it was determined that throat culture confirmation of a high-sensitivity RADT is not necessary to prevent suppurative or non-suppurative complications of group A streptococcal pharyngitis. In addition, it has been suggested in several studies that the recommendation to obtain a backup throat culture in all patients with a negative RADT is not a cost-effective approach. Rapid and sensitive OIA RADTs reduce antibiotic prescription rates by 50% in pediatric emergency care visits related to sore throat. An antistreptolysin-O titer and an anti-DNase-B titer may help confirm a prior streptococcal infection if the throat culture is negative, particularly in children in whom there is a high suspicion of acute rheumatic fever or acute post-streptococcal glomerulonephritis.

Differentiating between viral and bacterial pharyngitis is often difficult, and the rapid streptococcal antigen tests and throat cultures should be reserved for patients who have signs and symptoms common for both illnesses. There are some children whose clinical findings are not consistent with bacterial pharyngitis. For example, afebrile children with a sore throat, runny nose, and cough who have slight pharyngeal erythema almost certainly have viral pharyngitis and do not need further workup. However, children with a constellation of signs and symptoms suggesting bacterial pharyngitis, such as sudden onset of sore throat, fever, headache, swollen and erythematous tonsils, tonsillar or posterior pharyngeal wall exudate, uvulitis, tender and enlarged cervical lymphadenopathy, absence of runny nose or cough, or exposure to an individual with streptococcal pharyngitis may need further testing with RADT or throat culture to confirm group A streptococcal pharyngitis because an accurate diagnosis cannot be made on clinical grounds alone. Approximately 12% of all children are asymptomatic carriers of GABHS in the pharynx. Guidelines for clinical prediction have been evaluated and have suggested different approaches to the need for RADT or throat culture and antibiotic management. The Centor criteria were derived and validated in adult patients and overestimate the likelihood of GABHS pharyngitis in children. A modified McIsaac score predicts better in children but is still neither sensitive nor specific enough to rely on alone. In a meta-analysis of signs and symptoms predicting GABHS, presence of a tonsillar exudate, pharyngeal exudate, or exposure to strep infection in the previous 2 weeks (positive likelihood ratios 3.4, 2.1, and 1.9, respectively) and the absence of tender anterior cervical nodes, tonsillar enlargement, or exudate (negative likelihood ratios of 0.6, 0.63, and 0.74), were most predictive. Guidelines that recommend identifying patients who are likely to have group A streptococcal pharyngitis based on clinical or epidemiological findings and providing antibiotics for only those confirmed by RADT or throat culture decrease the unnecessary overuse of antibiotics.

Viral throat cultures and acute and convalescent titers to determine viral pharyngitis are rarely indicated unless systemic infection occurs (eg, herpes encephalitis). Epstein-Barr virus infection can be determined by specific serologic antibody assays, but nonspecific tests for heterophil antibody (eg, monospot test) are most available and are usually the tests of choice for diagnosing infectious mononucleosis. However, it may be negative in children younger than 4 years or early in the course of the infection. Only 75% of infected children between 2 and 4 years of age, and less than 30% of children younger than 2 years, are identified by this test. The monospot test, a rapid slide test for heterophil antibodies, may remain positive for months after the infection and incorrectly may suggest the diagnosis of infectious mononucleosis in children who do not have this disorder. A complete blood cell count with more than 50% to 60% lymphocytes or more than 10% atypical lymphocytes is suggestive of mononucleosis. When these tests are inconclusive, the specific serologic antibody tests for EBV infection are helpful in establishing the diagnosis. Cytomegalovirus-specific antibody tests should be considered in the patient with a mononucleosis syndrome and negative laboratory tests for EBV. Culture or fluorescent antibody evaluation of the pseudo-membrane may be used to diagnose diphtheria. Culture or presence of serum agglutinins confirms tularemia. Thayer-Martin culture plates should be used to diagnose suspected gonorrheal sore throat. HIV antibody tests are of little use in the evaluation of acute seroconversion syndrome as antibody titers take 4 to 6 weeks to become detectable. If acute seroconversion is suspected, quantitative RNA polymerase chain reaction should be undertaken.

Imaging Studies

If epiglottitis or retropharyngeal abscess is suspected but is not clinically apparent, a lateral neck radiograph may be obtained. The radiograph should be performed with a physician in attendance that is capable of performing endotracheal intubation in case the child has respiratory difficulties (see Chapter 58). Computed tomography of the neck is indicated in the stable patient with suspected deep parapharyngeal or retropharyngeal infection. Emergency bedside ultrasound is an effective and sensitive tool for differentiating between peritonsillar cellulitis and a peritonsillar abscess.

Management

The management of children with sore throat is based on the etiology of the condition. The early recognition of potentially serious conditions based on history and physical examination is essential to providing optimal care. **Otolaryngological consultation** should be obtained in children with peritonsillar abscess, retropharyngeal abscess, parapharyngeal abscess, epiglottitis, significant pharyngeal trauma, or pharyngeal tumor. Recurrent tonsillitis, especially in children who miss school, may be a reason for referral to an otolaryngologist.

Outpatient Treatment

For most children with sore throat, the physician must differentiate between viral and streptococcal pharyngitis. Viral sore throat can be managed symptomatically. Treatment of pain and discomfort with **analgesics such as acetaminophen or ibuprofen to relieve pain and maintaining hydration** are the mainstays of therapy for young children with viral or bacterial sore throat. Gargling with warm water and sucking on hard candy may provide additional symptomatic relief for older children. The use of steroids for reducing pain for pharyngitis is controversial. A recent systematic review demonstrated a relatively small reduction in time to significant pain relief of 4.5 hours and a negligible reduction in pain in 24 hours when a single dose of dexamethasone (0.6 mg/kg, maximum 10 mg) is given. The decision to administer steroids should be made on a case-by-case basis.

The pain from lesions of herpes stomatitis sometimes responds to acetaminophen or ibuprofen. For those children with persistent pain, acetaminophen with codeine or hydrocodone may be helpful. **Anesthetics** such as lidocaine may also decrease the pain. A convenient way of delivering lidocaine is in a mixture (1 part each) of lidocaine, diphenhydramine (Benadryl), and a liquid antacid. This mixture (called "magic mouth wash" by some) may be inserted into each side of the mouth, gargled, or placed on a gloved finger and applied directly on the oral lesions of the tongue and labial and buccal mucosa. It is best used about 15 to 30 minutes before feeding or drinking, especially in children who refuse to drink. Lidocaine should be used cautiously because it can suppress the gag reflex. The dose should never exceed 3 mg/kg/dose. Too much lidocaine may result in seizures. Parents should also be given instruction on how to monitor fluid intake and of the signs of dehydration

In children without clear-cut evidence of streptococcal pharyngitis, a positive rapid streptococcal antigen test helps direct antibiotic treatment. A negative test in the presence of positive symptoms should be accompanied by a throat culture. However, the OIA rapid test may preclude the need for culture confirmation. Patients can await the results of culture before beginning antibiotic therapy. **Antibiotics** without confirmation from rapid streptococcal tests or cultures are indicated in children who appear toxic, who have scarlet fever or peritonsillar cellulitis/abscess, or who have a history of rheumatic fever. Most evidence suggests that early treatment results in more rapid clinical improvement, although this is controversial. Rheumatic fever can be prevented if treatment is started within 9 days of sore throat symptom development. Glomerulonephritis probably is not affected by antibiotic therapy.

Evidence suggests that children with streptococcal pharyngitis should be treated with antibiotics to relieve symptoms; shorten the course of their illness; and prevent disease dissemination, suppurative complications, and rheumatic fever. Penicillin is the antibiotic of choice. It may be administered orally as penicillin V (phenoxymethyl penicillin) in a dose of 250 mg 2 to 3 times a day for 10 days for children and 500 mg 2 to 3 times a day for adolescents and adults. Most patients will feel better after 2 to 3 days, but it is important to stress to parents that their children need to complete the full 10-day course. Amoxicillin, which tastes better, given once a day (50mg/kg, maximum 1,000 mg) for 10 days is as effective as penicillin V given 2 to 3 times a day for 10 days, making compliance more likely. (See Table 74-1 for dosages.) "Magic mouthwash" can also be prepared without lidocaine, especially for younger children.

If the risk of noncompliance is high or if the risk of complication is great (eg, children have a history of rheumatic fever), the penicillin should be administered intramuscularly. Intramuscular penicillin has 2 disadvantages: (1) pain associated with the injection and (2) increased incidence of a potentially more severe allergic reaction. The dose of benzathine penicillin for children weighing less than 27 kg (60 lb) is 600,000 U. The dose for larger children and adults is 1.2 million U. Bicillin CR, which contains 900,000 U of benzathine penicillin and 300,000 U of procaine penicillin, is a satisfactory alternative form of delivering penicillin intramuscularly in children and may be preferable because it causes less pain and less severe local reaction. This preparation has not been determined to be effective in heavier patients (adolescents and adults) and therefore the benzathine preparation noted previously is recommended. The injection of benzathine penicillin is less painful if it is given after it reaches room temperature. (See Table 74-1 for dosage information.) Macrolides such as azithromycin or clarithromycin may be substituted in children who are allergic to penicillin. They are preferred to erythromycin because they are associated with fewer gastrointestinal side effects. Azithromycin has the added advantage of once-a-day dosing and a shortened course of therapy of only 5 days. A first-generation oral cephalosporin is also an acceptable alternative, but should not be used in children with an immediate or Type I hypersensitivity to penicillin. Clindamycin may also be used for penicillin allergic patients; however, the liquid preparation is not palatable and compliance may be poor. Tetracyclines; sulfonamides, including trimethoprim-sulfamethoxazole; and fluoroquinolones are not recommended for the treatment of streptococcal pharyngitis.

If children continue to be symptomatic and have a persistently positive throat culture after completing a course of therapy, they may be re-treated with the same antibiotic, given another oral antibiotic (as noted previously and in Table 74-1), or given an intramuscular dose of penicillin, especially if compliance is in question.

Approximately 12% of children are asymptomatic carriers of group A streptococci. In general, these children do well, and eradication of the bacteria is not necessary. Cultures after treatment are generally not recommended, except for children with recurring or persistent symptoms or those with a previous history of rheumatic fever. In selected cases of children whose throat cultures remain positive, eradication of the pharyngeal carriage should be strongly considered. These indications are as follows: if there is an outbreak of

Table 74-1. Antibiotics Used in the Management of Sore Throat in Children	
Drug **(for Streptococcal Pharyngitis)**	**Dosage**
Penicillin V	250 mg x 2–3/d for children and 500 mg x 2–3/d for adolescents orally for 10 days
Amoxicillin	50 mg/kg once a day orally for 10 days (maximum 1,000 mg)
Azithromycin	12 mg/kg/d, once a day orally for 5 days (maximum 500 mg)
Clarithromycin	15 mg/kg/d every 12 hours orally for 10 days
Cephalexin	25–50 mg/kg/d every 12 hours orally for 10 days (maximum 500 mg every 12 hours)
Benzathine penicillin	600,000 U (<27 kg or 60 lb); 1.2 million U (>27 kg or 60 lb) as single intramuscular injection
Bicillin CR	900,000 U benzathine penicillin and 300,000 U procaine penicillin for children as single intramuscular injection
Rifampin	10 mg/kg/dose orally every 12 hours for 4 days (given last 4 days of treatment with penicillin V or benzathine penicillin for chronic streptococcal carriers)
Clindamycin	20 mg/kg/d in 3 divided doses (maximum 1.8 g/d) orally for 10 days (for chronic streptococcal carriers or suspected *Fusobacterium necrophorum*)
Drug **(for Gonococcal Pharyngitis)**	**Dosage**
Ceftriaxone **Plus**	125 mg intramuscularly in a single dose if <45 kg, 250 mg intramuscularly if in a single dose if >45 kg
Azithromycin **or**	20 mg/kg (maximum 1 g) orally in a single dose
Erythromycin **or (if ≥9 y)**	50 mg/kg/d (maximum 2 g/d) orally every 6 hours for 14 days
Doxycycline	100 mg orally 2 times a day for 7 days

acute rheumatic fever or post-streptococcal glomerulonephritis, if there is an outbreak of group A streptococcal pharyngitis in a closed or semiclosed community, if there is a family history of rheumatic fever, or if repeated episodes of documented symptomatic group A streptococcal pharyngitis recur within a family over several weeks despite appropriate therapy. If cultures remain positive, these children may be treated with benzathine penicillin and oral rifampin for 4 days in an attempt to eradicate the organism. (See Table 74-1 for dosages.) Clindamycin is reportedly more effective in eradication of the organism from symptom-free carriers. (See Table 74-1 for dosages.)

Mycoplasma pneumoniae pharyngitis is usually associated with a generalized infection. Because it is often a self-limited illness, it does not require antibiotic therapy unless symptoms persist. Treatment with any of the macrolide antibiotics may be helpful. However, clarithromycin and azithromycin have fewer side effects and are likely to produce better compliance. Macrolides are also the drugs of choice for children with *Arcanobacterium haemolyticum* pharyngitis.

Diphtheria, seen almost exclusively in less advantaged countries, is a life-threatening infection that requires prompt diagnosis and treatment. Penicillin G or erythromycin must be given to kill *C diphtheriae* and, in addition, equine antitoxin must be administered to neutralize the exotoxin. Tularemia pharyngitis is unusual, but if suspected is treated with gentamicin.

For gonococcal pharyngitis caused by *N gonorrhoeae*, intramuscular ceftriaxone is the drug of choice. (See Table 74-1 for dosages.) Additional antibiotic coverage for associated *C trachomatis* infection should be administered. Oral azithromycin or doxycycline should also be given to children 9 years of age or older. (See Table 74-1 for dosages.) Azithromycin or erythromycin may be used for younger children. Children should be examined and cultured for sexually transmitted infections in other sites and should have a serological test for syphilis at the first visit and have a repeat test 6 to 8 weeks later. They should also be evaluated for concurrent hepatitis B and HIV infection. Sexual abuse should be considered in all cases of gonococcal pharyngitis, particularly in prepubertal children (see Chapters 97 and 128).

Patients with Lemierre syndrome should be admitted and started on intravenous (IV) antibiotics covering polymicrobial organisms, including anaerobic organisms. If simple *Fusobacterium necrophorum* pharyngitis is suspected, antibiotics covering anaerobes are indicated, such as clindamycin.

Children with croup usually respond to steroids. Oral nystatin can be used in children with oral candidiasis. Adolescents with uncomplicated peritonsillar abscess may be managed as outpatients in selected cases with needle aspiration and oral antibiotics.

Inpatient Treatment

Children with sore throat should be admitted to the hospital if they have airway obstruction or need IV hydration or antibiotics. Children with retropharyngeal abscess and epiglottitis require IV antibiotics and should be managed in consultation with an otolaryngologist. Preadolescent children or adolescents with complicated peritonsillar abscess also require IV antibiotics. Surgical intervention is indicated if the abscess is fluctuant, the child is toxic or has severe trismus or airway compromise, or if there is no resolution within 24 hours. Needle aspiration may be acceptable in selected cases. Intravenous hydration is occasionally needed for patients with severe herpes stomatitis who will not drink because of pain and who become dehydrated.

The role of tonsillectomy or adenotonsillectomy for children with recurrent sore throat is still controversial. However, The American Academy of Otolaryngology–Head and Neck Surgery convened a panel of clinicians from various disciplines to develop evidence-based guidelines to identify children who are most likely to benefit from tonsillectomy. These guidelines, containing content based on previous work done by Paradise about children with recurrent sore throats, have been recently published. Most children with sore throat improve on their own, and recommendations are therefore for watchful waiting if there are less than 7 documented sore throat episodes in the past year, less than 5 per year over the past 2 years, and less than 3 per year over the past 3 years. Parental report does not qualify as documentation. If the number of documented sore throats meets or exceeds these numbers, and there are associated findings (temperature of >38.3°C, cervical lymphadenopathy, tonsillar exudate or a positive test for GABHS), the clinician may recommend tonsillectomy. Consultation with an otolaryngologist and a period of watchful waiting should be considered. If the child with recurrent sore throat does not meet these criteria, the child should be assessed for other factors that may favor tonsillectomy over observation. These may include but are not limited to multiple antibiotic allergy/intolerance, PFAPA syndrome (periodic fever, aphthous stomatitis, pharyngitis, and adenitis) or a history of peritonsillar abscess. Although these guidelines are evidence based and the recommendations are better defined than previously, each case should be individualized. As with all clinical decisions, there is a role for shared decision-making with the child's caregiver and primary care physician regarding the need for tonsillectomy.

Education

Both patients and families should receive general education about sore throats. Medication for pain with drugs such as acetaminophen or ibuprofen is useful, especially if children are having difficulty swallowing. Gargling with warm salt water or sucking on hard candy may soothe the pain of sore throat. Children with bacterial pharyngitis may return to school after 24 hours of antibiotic therapy and the disappearance of fever. The practitioner should recommend that symptomatic family members see a physician. Parents should call or return to the physician if their children have respiratory or swallowing difficulties, drooling, severe pain, or fever (temperature: >101.0°F [38.3°C]) for more than 48 hours after the initiation of appropriate antibiotics.

Prognosis

The prognosis for children with viral sore throat is excellent because of its self-limited nature. The outlook for children with streptococcal sore throat is also excellent. If the infection is not diagnosed and treated appropriately, however, suppurative (eg, peritonsillar abscess) and non-suppurative complications (eg, rheumatic fever, acute glomerulonephritis) may occur. With early diagnosis and prompt treatment, the prognosis for unusual, life-threatening causes of sore throat is also very good. In addition, research in the development of a polyvalent synthetic oligosaccharide vaccine to decrease the suppurative and non-suppurative complications of GABHS is underway.

CASE RESOLUTION

In the case presented, the child has palatal petechiae and tonsillar exudate, which are signs and symptoms consistent with streptococcal pharyngitis. A streptococcal rapid antigen detection test is performed, and is positive. The child is treated with oral penicillin. Neither of her parents have sore throat symptoms.

Selected References

American Academy of Pediatrics. Group A streptococcal infections. In: Pickering LK, Baker CJ, Kimberlin DW, Long SS, eds. *Red Book: 2009 Report of the Committee on Infectious Diseases.* 28th ed. Elk Grove Village, IL: American Academy of Pediatrics; 2009:616–628

Ayanruoh S, Waseem M, Quee F, et al. Impact of a rapid streptococcal test on antibiotic use in a pediatric emergency department. *Pediatr Emerg Care.* 2009;25:748–750

Baltimore RS. Re-evaluation of antibiotic treatment of streptococcal pharyngitis. *Curr Opin Pediatr.* 2010;22:77–82

Bisno AL, Gerber MA, Gwaltney JM Jr, Kaplan EL, Schwartz RH. Practice guidelines for the diagnosis and management of group A streptococcal pharyngitis. *Clin Infect Dis.* 2002;35(2):113–125

Bulloch B, Kabani A, Tenenbein M. Oral dexamethasone for the treatment of pain in children with acute pharyngitis: a randomized, double-blind, placebo-controlled trial. *Ann Emerg Med.* 2003;41:601–608

Cherry JD. Pharyngitis (pharyngitis, tonsillitis, tonsillopharyngitis, and nasopharyngitis). In: Feigen RD, Cherry JD, Demler-Harrison GJ, Kaplan SL, eds. *Textbook of Pediatric Infectious Diseases.* 6th ed. Philadelphia, PA: Saunders; 2009:161–170

Clegg HW, Ryan AG, Dallas SD, et al. Treatment of streptococcal pharyngitis with once-daily compared with twice-daily amoxicillin. *Pediatr Infect Dis J.* 2006;25:761–767

Edmonson MB, Farwell KR. Relationship between the clinical likelihood of group A streptococcal pharyngitis and the sensitivity of a rapid antigen-detection test in a pediatric practice. *Pediatrics.* 2005;115:280–285

Fleisher GR. Sore throat. In: Fleisher GR, Ludwig S, eds. *Textbook of Pediatric Emergency Medicine.* 6th ed. Philadelphia, PA: Lippincott; 2010:579–583

Gerber MA. Diagnosis and treatment of pharyngitis in children. *Pediatr Clin North Am.* 2005;52:729–747

Gerber MA, Baltimore RS, Eaton CB, et al. Prevention of rheumatic fever and diagnosis and treatment of acute streptococcal pharyngitis: a scientific statement from the American Heart Association Rheumatic Fever, Endocarditis, and Kawasaki Disease Committee of the Council on Cardiovascular Disease in the Young, the Interdisciplinary Council on Functional Genomics and Translational Biology, and the Interdisciplinary Council on Quality of Care and Outcomes Research. *Circulation.* 2009;119:1541–1551

Gieseker KE, Roe MH, MacKenzie T, et al. Evaluating the American Academy of Pediatrics diagnostic standard for *Streptococcus pyogenes* pharyngitis: backup culture versus repeat rapid antigen testing. *Pediatrics.* 2003;111:666–670

Jaggi P, Shulman ST. Group A streptococcal infections. *Pediatr Rev.* 2006;27:99–105

Joachim L, Campos D Jr, Smeesters PR. Pragmatic scoring system for pharyngitis in low-resource settings. *Pediatrics.* 2010;126:e608–e614

Linder JA, Bates DW, Lee GM, et al. Antibiotic treatment of children with sore throat. *JAMA.* 2005;294:2315–2322

Linder JA, Chan JC, Bates DW. Evaluation and treatment of pharyngitis in primary care practice. The difference between guidelines is largely academic. *Arch Intern Med.* 2006;166:1374–1379

Martin JM, Green M, Barbadora KA, et al. Group A streptococci among school-aged children: clinical characteristics and the carrier state. *Pediatrics.* 2004;114:1212–1219

McIsaac WJ, Kellner JD, Aufricht P, et al. Empirical validation of guidelines for the management of pharyngitis in children and adults. *JAMA.* 2004;291:1587–1595

Millar KR, Johnson DW, Drummond D, Kellner JD. Suspected peritonsillar abscess in children. *Pediatr Emerg Care.* 2007;23:431–438

Paradise JL, Bluestone CD, Colborn K, et al. Tonsillectomy and adenotonsillectomy for recurrent throat infection in moderately affected children. *Pediatrics.* 2002;110:7–15

Park SY, Gerber MA, Tanz RR, et al. Clinicians' management of children and adolescents with acute pharyngitis. *Pediatrics.* 2006;117:1871–1878

Pfoh E, Wessels MR, Goldmann D, et al. Burden and cost of group A streptococcal pharyngitis. *Pediatrics.* 2008;121:229–234

Rafei K, Lichenstein R. Airway infectious disease emergencies. *Pediatr Clin North Am.* 2006;53:215–242

Ramirez-Schrempp D, Dorfman DH, Baker WE, et al. Ultrasound soft tissue applications in the pediatric emergency department: to drain or not to drain? *Pediatr Emerg Care.* 2009;1:44–48

Shaikh N, Leonard E, Martin JM. Prevalence of streptococcal pharyngitis and streptococcal carriage in children: a meta-analysis. *Pediatrics.* 2010;126:e557–e564

Van Howe RS, Kusnier LP II. Diagnosis and management of pharyngitis in a pediatric population based on cost-effectiveness and projected health outcomes. *Pediatrics.* 2006;117:609–619

Webb KH. Does culture confirmation of high-sensitivity rapid streptococcal tests make sense? A medical decision analysis. *Pediatrics.* 1998;101:e2

Webb KH, Needham CA, Kurtz SB. Use of a high-sensitivity rapid strep test without culture confirmation of negative results. *J Fam Pract.* 2000;49:34–38

Wing A, Villa-Roel C, Yeh B, et al. Effectiveness of corticosteroid treatment in acute pharyngitis: a systematic review of the literature. *Acad Emerg Med.* 2010;17:476–483

CHAPTER 75

Nosebleeds

Stanley H. Inkelis, MD, and Katherine E. Remick, MD

CASE STUDY

A 3-year-old boy is brought to the office one winter day. He has had 4 nosebleeds in the past week as well as a cold with a runny nose and cough, which began the day before the first nosebleed. The nosebleeds occurred either at night or during sleep and stopped spontaneously or with gentle pressure. Other than the cold and nosebleeds, the boy is in good health. He is active, with bruises over both tibias but none elsewhere. The many cuts and scrapes he has had in the past resulted in minimal bleeding. His family has no history of a bleeding disorder or easy bruisability.

The child's physical examination is entirely normal except for a small amount of blood in the left anterior naris.

Questions

1. What are the common causes of nosebleeds in children?
2. What systemic diseases are associated with nosebleeds?
3. How should nosebleeds be evaluated in children?
4. How should minor and severe nosebleeds be managed in children?

Nosebleed, or epistaxis, occurs commonly in children, especially in those between the ages of 2 and 10 years. In most cases, nosebleeds are secondary to local trauma and can be cared for by primary care physicians. In rare instances, however, a nosebleed may be difficult to control or may be a manifestation of a serious systemic illness. Referral to an otolaryngologist or a hematologist/oncologist is usually not required except in these situations, and hospitalization is generally unnecessary. Parents and children, who are often frightened by nosebleeds, frequently overestimate the amount of blood lost. Understanding and reassurance are important in allaying anxiety.

Epidemiology

Thirty percent of children have one nosebleed by the time they are 5 years of age. In children between the ages of 6 and 10, the frequency increases to 56%. Nosebleeds are rare in infancy and infrequent after puberty. They occur much more frequently in the late fall and winter months, when upper respiratory infections (URIs) are common, environmental humidity is relatively low, and the use of heating systems results in dryness. Nosebleeds are also more common in children who live in dry climates, especially if they have a URI or allergic rhinitis.

Clinical Presentation

Most children with nosebleeds have a history of bleeding at home and have minimal or no bleeding at the time of presentation (Dx Box). With anterior nosebleeds, blood exits almost entirely from the anterior portion of the nose. With posterior nosebleeds, most of the bleeding occurs into the nasopharynx and mouth, although some blood exits through the nose as well. Posterior nosebleeds are heavier and more difficult to control, and children may present in a hemodynamically unstable condition.

 Nosebleeds

- Blood in anterior nares, nasopharynx, or mouth
- History of any of the following:
  — Frequent digital manipulation (nose picking)
  — Upper respiratory infection (recent)
  — Allergic rhinitis
  — Dry climate
  — Foreign body in nose
  — Trauma to nose
  — Prolonged or difficult-to-stop bleeding or easy bruisability
- Physical examination consistent with any of the following:
  — Rhinorrhea
  — Dry, cracked nasal mucosa
  — Foreign body in nose
  — Trauma to nose
  — Multiple bruises

Children with bleeding disorders may have recurrent nosebleeds and a history of prolonged bleeding, easy bruisability, or multiple bruises in unlikely locations. In unusual situations, children with gastrointestinal or respiratory tract bleeding may present with blood exiting through the nose. Alternatively, some children with nosebleeds may present with hematemesis, hemoptysis, melena, or anemia. In these cases a nasal source should be considered.

Pathophysiology

Nosebleeds may be either anterior or posterior in origin. Most nosebleeds in children (>90%) are anterior and are more easily controlled than posterior nosebleeds. The anterior portion of the nasal septum, about 0.5 cm from the tip of the nose, known as Kiesselbach plexus located in Little's area, is the most common part of the nose involved in anterior nosebleeds. This area is supplied by the anterior and posterior ethmoidal arteries, the sphenopalatine artery, and the septal branches of the superior labial artery (Figure 75-1). The mucosa covering the area is thin and friable, and the small vessels supplying the nasal mucous membrane have little structural support. Congestion of the vessels caused by conditions such as a URI or drying of the mucosa from low environmental humidity makes this area susceptible to bleeding.

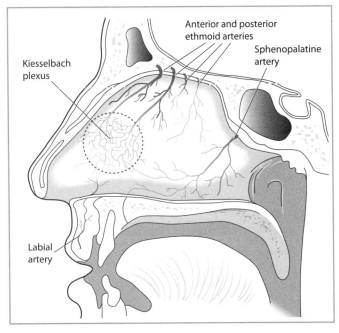

Figure 75-1. Vascular supply of nasal septum. Note the confluence of vessels that forms the Kiesselbach plexus.

Posterior nosebleeds are unusual in children. If bleeding is vigorous, poorly controlled with anterior nasal packing, or involving both nares, a posterior source is likely to be identified. Posterior nosebleeds generally arise from the turbinate or nasal wall. Significant bleeding, usually from a branch of the sphenopalatine artery, may occur. Because of the posterior location, children often present with symptoms other than frank epistaxis (eg, hematemesis, hemoptysis, melena, or anemia).

Differential Diagnosis

Trauma from nose picking and **inflammation** of the nasal mucosa from a URI are by far the most common causes of nosebleeds in children. Repetitive, habitual nose picking results in the formation of friable granulation tissue that bleeds when congested blood vessels are traumatized (epistaxis digitorum). As the nasal mucosa dries, it may lead to crust formation and cracking. Bleeding may occur

spontaneously, but more often it results from forceful nose blowing and sneezing that increases venous pressure in the more vascularized nasal septum. Nosebleeds occur more commonly in children who have nasal colonization with *Staphylococcus aureus*. It is postulated that *S aureus* replaces existing flora and leads to inflammation and new vessel formation.

Other viral respiratory infections, such as infectious mononucleosis and influenza, may also predispose children to nosebleeds because of their local inflammatory effect. Nosebleeds in children with these infections are more common in areas of low environmental humidity. Many children with no URI-like symptoms also suffer from nosebleeds in such environments, usually in winter, when inhaling dry, hot air from heating systems causes desiccation of the nasal mucosa (rhinitis sicca). **Allergic rhinitis** with inflammation and subsequent drying may also lead to nosebleeds. Children with allergic rhinitis who take decongestants or use topical nasal decongestants or topical nasal steroid sprays may be more likely to suffer from nosebleeds. In addition, the dispenser tip of these sprays may traumatize the already dry and friable mucosa causing the nose to bleed.

Foreign bodies may cause direct trauma or pressure necrosis to the vessels of the nasal mucosa. **External trauma** can cause either tears to the nasal mucosa or nasal fractures. If bleeding from mucosal vessels occurs but the mucosa remains intact, a septal hematoma may develop. Abscess formation or septal perforation may occur if the septal hematoma is not drained. **Non-accidental** trauma should be considered in the young child (younger than 2) with a nosebleed.

Although nosebleeds are usually benign conditions, they may be the first sign of serious illness. Persistent or recurrent nosebleeds with no obvious cause should raise the suspicion of **bleeding disorders.** Thrombocytopenia is the most common coagulation defect causing nosebleeds. Idiopathic thrombocytopenic purpura is the most frequent thrombocytopenic disorder associated with nosebleeds. Leukemia, aplastic anemia, and HIV infection must be strongly considered and ruled out in children with nosebleeds and thrombocytopenia. Platelet aggregation disorders may also be a cause of recurrent nosebleeds.

The most commonly inherited bleeding disorder associated with nosebleeds is von Willebrand disease, an autosomal-dominant bleeding disorder characterized by varying degrees of factor VIII deficiency and platelet dysfunction (decreased platelet adhesiveness). Hemophilia (factor VIII, IX, or XI) deficiency, factor VII deficiency, Glanzmann thrombasthenia, and Bernard-Soulier syndrome are other inherited bleeding disorders that may lead to nosebleeds. Hepatic disease, severe vitamin K deficiency, or malabsorption syndrome is associated with an acquired coagulopathy, which may present with nosebleed. Valproic acid administration has been associated with acquired von Willebrand disease and nosebleeds.

Nosebleeds may be a manifestation of **blood vessel disorders,** either hereditary or acquired. Osler-Weber-Rendu syndrome (hereditary hemorrhagic telangiectasia) is an inherited autosomal-dominant disease with multiple mucosal telangiectasias, especially in the nose. Because telangiectasias are deficient in muscular and connective tissue, these telangiectasias may rupture spontaneously and bleed profusely. An association between migraine headaches and recurrent nosebleeds has also been reported.

Neoplasms, particularly malignancies, are uncommon causes of nosebleeds in children. Nasal polyps are usually present in association with cystic fibrosis or allergies. Capillary, cavernous, and mixed hemangiomas may occur in the nose. Juvenile nasopharyngeal angiofibroma occurs almost exclusively in adolescent males who present with nasal obstruction and bleeding. Rhabdomyosarcomas, lymphomas, and squamous cell carcinomas of the nose, sinuses, or nasopharynx are rare causes of nosebleeds.

Drugs such as aspirin and nonsteroidal anti-inflammatory drugs, which interfere with platelet function, and warfarin and heparin, which inhibit clotting factors, increase the risk of nasal hemorrhage with minor trauma, infection, or inflammation. Accidental ingestion of these medications should be suspected if they are available. Cocaine or heroin snorting may cause nasal septal perforation and nosebleeds.

Hypertension is rarely associated with nosebleeds in children. Wegener granulomatosis and lethal midline granuloma are rare idiopathic inflammatory diseases in children that lead to nasal tissue destruction and bleeding. Nosebleeds during menstruation, known as vicarious menstruation, may be secondary to hormonal changes causing vascular congestion of the nasal mucosa.

Evaluation

History

A thorough history often reveals the etiology of the nosebleed (Questions Box). Information concerning the side of the nose from which the bleeding occurred, the amount of bleeding, the measures used to stop the bleeding, and the time required to stop the bleeding may be helpful to quickly assess the severity of the nosebleed.

Physical Examination

A general physical examination should be performed. In children with significant blood loss, particular attention should be directed toward the mental status and vital signs to determine hemodynamic stability. If vital signs are normal, these children should also be evaluated for orthostatic changes. If the blood pressure is elevated, it should be reassessed at a time when the anxiety related to the nosebleed has dissipated.

In addition, the skin and mucous membranes should be checked carefully for petechiae, purpura, and ecchymoses, which are signs of easy bruisability. The abdomen should be examined for hepatosplenomegaly, and the child should be evaluated for lymphadenopathy. Telangiectasias in the oropharynx or mucous membranes suggest Osler-Weber-Rendu syndrome. The oropharynx and nasopharynx should be examined for masses and blood dripping downward from a posterior bleed. The nose should then be inspected for the site of bleeding, with special attention directed toward Kiesselbach plexus

---

Questions

Nosebleeds

- Does the child pick his or her nose?
- Has the child suffered any trauma recently?
- Is there suspicion of non-accidental trauma?
- Has the child recently had an upper respiratory infection?
- Has the child recently had any systemic viral or bacterial illness?
- Does the child have any allergies?
- Is the child exposed to dry conditions (eg, dry climate, dry heat, dehumidified air)?
- Has the child put or tried to put foreign objects in his or her nose?
- Is there a history of easy bruisability or prolonged, difficult-to-stop bleeding in the child or family?
- Does the child or anyone in the family use any aspirin, aspirin-containing medications, nonsteroidal anti-inflammatory drugs, or warfarin?
- Which side of the nose was bleeding?
- How extensive was the bleeding?
- Did the child spit out or swallow blood? Was there blood in the mouth?
- What measures were used to stop the bleeding? How long did it take to stop the bleeding?
- Was this the first nosebleed? If the nosebleeds are recurrent, how often do they occur and how long do they last?

---

in the anterior septum. In children younger than 2 with nosebleeds, suspicion of non-accidental trauma should be considered, especially if nosebleeds are recurrent, the event is not witnessed, or the story given by the caretaker changes.

Diagnostic Studies

Laboratory tests are rarely indicated in most children with nosebleeds. A hematocrit/hemoglobin should be obtained if the nosebleeds are severe or recur frequently. Blood for type and crossmatch should be sent in children who have signs or symptoms of hypovolemia (increased pulse; cool, clammy skin; increased capillary refill; decreased blood pressure; etc) or a marked drop in hematocrit. If the history or physical examination suggests that a coagulopathy may be present, a complete blood cell count with platelet count, prothrombin time, and partial thromboplastin time should be obtained and screening for vonWillebrand disease considered if the other laboratory tests are negative.

Radiographs and other imaging studies are rarely necessary in children with nosebleeds.

Management

Children who present to primary care physicians with a history of a nosebleed or nosebleeds that have resolved spontaneously or with application of pressure to the nose need no further treatment in the office or emergency department setting, provided that the history and physical examination are consistent with a benign cause of the nosebleed. These children or their parents should be instructed to apply **petroleum jelly** or an antibiotic ointment inside the septal portion of the involved naris twice a day for 3 to 5 days with a cotton-tipped swab or with the little finger. Often the child's little finger is used because it is nonthreatening and it "knows where to go." Further nose picking should be discouraged, and fingernails should be trimmed to minimize trauma. In addition, a bedside **humidifier** helps to moisturize the air, especially in dry climates or during the winter when forced hot-air heat is used. Children whose nares moisten from rhinorrhea and then dry and crack also benefit from humidified air. Buffered saline nasal spray may also be helpful in humidifying the nose. Those children who are prone to recurrent nosebleeds in whom serious causes have been ruled out may benefit from regular use of some of the mentioned measures when they have URIs or allergic manifestations, or are in a dry season or environment. In addition, for children with *S aureus* nasal colonization, eradication should be considered.

Children or parents should be given advice about how to care for nosebleeds at home. These instructions can also be given to parents who seek advice over the telephone about how to stop children's nosebleeds. Practitioners should reassure parents and children that most nosebleeds are easily controlled. Children should sit upright and lean forward slightly while **direct pressure** is applied to the nose. External compression of the nares between 2 fingers for 5 to 10 minutes should be sufficient. Pressure applied to the anterior and mid-portion of the nose rather than at the base is more effective in stopping the bleeding because most nosebleeds occur in these parts of the nose.

Children who are actively bleeding through the nose when seen by primary care physicians should be positioned sitting upright and leaning forward slightly, and they should be given a basin and facial tissue. Direct pressure should be applied by a nurse or physician to the anterior and mid-portion of the nose while following universal precautions. A cotton dental roll may be placed under the upper lip to compress the labial artery in older children in whom concern about displacement and possible aspiration of the cotton is minimal. If the bleeding continues after external compression, children should be instructed to blow their noses to remove as much clot as possible. Fresh blood should be removed with suction. Cotton pledgets moistened with a few drops of a topical **vasoconstrictor,** such as 0.05% oxymetazoline (Afrin), 0.25% phenylephrine (Neo-Synephrine) or epinephrine (1:1,000) mixed with 4% lidocaine for local anesthesia, or topical thrombin, should be inserted into the side of the nose involved. Pressure should then be applied for an additional 10 minutes.

If the bleeding persists, **cauterization** of the bleeding site with a silver nitrate stick is indicated. If not already applied, topical anesthesia with 2% to 4% lidocaine should be applied before cauterization. Continued bleeding is slowed by first cauterizing a small ring around the bleeding point to interrupt flow from surrounding vessels and then rolling the tip of the applicator onto the bleeding site for 5 to 10 seconds. Cauterization is often difficult in children, and consultation with an otolaryngologist is advisable. Cauterization should not be performed in children with a bleeding diathesis. In addition, cauterizing both sides of the nasal septum can result in septal ischemia and possible necrosis and ultimately septal perforation.

If the bleeding continues, or as a modality to attempt prior to cauterization, an absorbable **nasal sponge** made from oxidized cellulose (Oxicel, Surgicel) or gelatin (Gelfoam) may be directly applied to the bleeding site to form an artificial clot. Alternatively, a **nasal tampon** (Merocel), made from a dehydrated material that expands when it becomes moist, may be inserted to tamponade the area of bleeding. Applying antibiotic ointment, preferably mupirocin, to the tampon allows for easier insertion and removal as well as potentially preventing *Staphylococcus aureus* infection that may lead to toxic shock syndrome. Avitene, a microfibrillar collagen material, provides for platelet aggregation and clot formation when applied to the bleeding site. Continued uncontrolled bleeding requires anterior **nasal packing** with antibiotic-impregnated, preferably mupirocin, 1-inch petrolatum gauze strips, which should remain in place for approximately 2 to 3 days. Prophylactic **antibiotics** should be started because sinusitis is a complication of anterior nasal packing. Antibiotics providing coverage for staphylococcal organisms, in particular methicillin-resistant *S aureus*, and sinusitis should be strongly considered.

Posterior nosebleeds, which are more difficult to control, should be suspected if (1) the measures described previously are ineffective, (2) bleeding is vigorous and the cause cannot be identified, or (3) most of the bleeding is into the nasopharynx and mouth. A posterior nasal pack can be created using rolled gauze or a nasal tampon. Alternatively, a Foley catheter or an Epistat inflatable nasal balloon catheter may be used to control posterior nosebleeds. Posterior packs should never be used without the presence of a concurrent anterior nasal pack. Thus, double-balloon catheters are now available (eg, Gottschalk Nasostat, Xomed Epistat) such that 2 separate packing mechanisms can be avoided. Posterior packing can result in significant discomfort for the patient and appropriate analgesia should be provided. However, significant pain with balloon inflation should not occur and overinflation may result in ischemia if the balloon is not slightly deflated. Posterior packing should be left in place for 2 to 3 days and antibiotics initiated to prevent sinusitis. In addition, posterior packing can result in hypoventilation and hypoxia. Therefore, all patients with posterior packing should be admitted and placed on a cardiorespiratory monitor. This also allows for monitoring of potential complications, namely aspiration due to accidental dislodgement; septal ischemia secondary to packing; and development of hypotension, bradycardia, or apnea secondary to a pronounced nasal-vagal response.

The need for **otolaryngological consultation** depends on the experience of the individual physician and the availability of consultation. Prompt consultation, if available, should be obtained for children with severe nosebleeds who need volume replacement; with nosebleeds that do not stop or recur after the mentioned measures have been taken; children who may need anterior or posterior nasal packing; and with recurrent, difficult-to-stop nosebleeds. Surgical consultation should be sought in patients with suspected nasal fractures prior to the placement of nasal packing. In some cases, obtaining consultation before cauterization with silver nitrate is advisable, particularly in those patients with known bleeding disorders. Children with septal hematomas, tumors, polyps, telangiectasias, and intractable bleeding should be referred to an otolaryngologist for further care and possible surgical intervention. Children with a documented or suspected bleeding disorder should be referred to a hematologist. Selective angiographic embolization by an interventional radiologist may be indicated for patients with persistent, intractable nosebleeds. Endonasal laser surgery may be indicated in patients with recurrent nosebleeds from abnormal vascular malformations such as Osler-Weber-Rendu syndrome.

Children with severe nosebleeds should have an intravenous line started early; blood sent for type and crossmatch; and fluids replaced, depending on the amount of blood loss and physical evidence of hypovolemia. In children who are frightened or in whom certain procedures (eg, cauterization of bleeding site, drainage of septal hematoma) are performed, procedural sedation should be strongly considered. Intravenous pain medication should be used in children who need anterior or posterior packing. If procedures that cause undue pain or discomfort are necessary, general anesthesia in an operating room setting may be indicated.

Hospitalization is rarely necessary for children with nosebleeds. However, children who are hemodynamically unstable on presentation usually require inpatient treatment. As mentioned previously, children who need placement of a posterior nasal pack should be admitted to the hospital for close airway observation. Hospitalization may be necessary for children with difficult-to-stop bleeds who need an anterior nasal pack or who have a bleeding disorder or underlying chronic illness such as leukemia, aplastic anemia, or HIV infection.

Prognosis

The prognosis for nosebleeds in children is excellent. Almost all nosebleeds are easily controlled with a minimal amount of home care or medical management. Surgery is rarely indicated. Complications associated with significant nosebleeds include hypovolemia from blood loss, and sinusitis and toxic shock syndrome from anterior or posterior nasal packs. Even for rare causes of nosebleeds, the prognosis is very good with prompt diagnosis and treatment.

CASE RESOLUTION

In the case presented, the boy has experienced several nosebleeds of short duration associated with an upper respiratory infection and winter dryness. His history and physical examination are unremarkable for a bleeding disorder or chronic illness. The small amount of blood in his nose is consistent with an anterior nosebleed originating from Kiesselbach plexus with inflammation and drying of the nasal mucosa. Laboratory tests are not indicated. The parents should be instructed to apply petroleum jelly to the septal portion of the left side of the child's nose twice a day for 3 to 5 days and to humidify the child's bedroom. They should also be reassured that their child has a common condition that he will outgrow.

Selected References

Bernius M, Perlin D. Pediatric ear, nose and throat emergencies. *Pediatr Clin North Am.* 2006;53:195–214

Briskin, KB. Epistaxis. In: Baren JM, Rothrock SG, Brennan JA, Brown L, eds. *Pediatric Emergency Medicine.* Philadelphia, PA: Saunders; 2008:402–404

Gifford TO, Orlandi RR. Epistaxis. *Otolaryngol Clin N Am.* 2008;41:525–536

Manning SC, Culbertson MC Jr. Epistaxis. In: Bluestone CD, Stool SE, Alper CM, et al, eds. *Pediatric Otolaryngology.* 4th ed. Philadelphia, PA: Saunders; 2003:925–931

McIntosh N, Mok JY, Magerison A. Epidemiology of oronasal hemorrhage in the first 2 years of life: implications for child protection. *Pediatrics.* 2007;120:1074–1078

Nadel F, Henretig FM. Epistaxis. In: Fleischer GR, Ludwig S, eds. *Textbook of Pediatric Emergency Medicine.* 6th ed. Philadelphia, PA: Lippincott Williams and Wilkins; 2010:236–239

Patel PB, Kost SI. Management of epistaxis. In: King C, Henretig FM, eds. *Textbook of Pediatric Emergency Procedures.* 2nd ed. Philadelphia, PA: Lippincott Williams and Wilkins; 2008:603–614

Riviello RJ, Brown NA. Otolaryngologic procedures. In: Roberts JR, Hedges JR, eds. *Clinical Procedures in Emergency Medicine.* 5th ed. Philadelphia, PA: Saunders Elsevier, 2010:1178–1216

Sandoval C, Dong S, Visintainer P, et al. Clinical and laboratory features of 178 children with recurrent epistaxis. *J Pediatr Hematol Oncol.* 2002;24:47–49

Whymark AD, Crampsey DP, Fraser L, et al. Childhood epistaxis and nasal colonization with *Staphylococcus aureus. Otolaryngol Head Neck Surg.* 2008;138:307–310

CHAPTER 76

Strabismus

Teresa Rosales, MD

CASE STUDY

The mother of an 8-month-old infant complains that every time her son looks to either side his eyes seem crossed. Otherwise, he is growing and developing normally. A symmetrical pupillary light reflex, bilateral red reflex, and normal extraocular eye movements in all directions are noted on physical examination of the eyes.

Questions

1. What is strabismus?
2. What conditions make infants' eyes appear crossed? What is the differential diagnosis?
3. What tests are used in the office evaluation of children suspected of having strabismus?
4. Which infants with crossed eyes require referral for further evaluation and treatment?

Strabismus refers to any abnormality in ocular alignment, whether the eyes go in or out or one eye is higher than the other. It is one of the most common eye problems observed in infants and children. The pediatrician plays an important role in the early detection and prompt referral of children with suspected ocular alignment abnormalities.

Epidemiology

Strabismus affects approximately 3% of the population, and the condition is seen most commonly in children younger than 6 years. About 50% of all affected children have a positive family history of strabismus, although the exact genetic mode of inheritance is unclear. Up to 75% of normal infants have transient intermittent strabismus during the first 3 months of life.

Clinical Presentation

Children with ocular misalignment have an asymmetrical corneal light reflex test. Eye movement is noted with cover testing. Children with paralytic strabismus may present with torticollis or head tilting in an effort to avoid diplopia (Dx Box).

Dx
Strabismus

- Head tilt
- Double vision (diplopia)
- Squint
- Asymmetrical corneal light reflex
- Eye movement with cover testing

Pathophysiology

Normal binocular vision is the result of the fusion of images from both eyes working synchronously across the visual field. Six extraocular muscles control all eye movements. Orthophoria is proper alignment of the eyes, and strabismus results from an imbalance in muscle movements.

Strabismus

The classification of strabismus is complex. Based on etiology, it may be considered non-paralytic (comitant) or paralytic (non-comitant). Strabismus may also be classified as congenital or acquired, intermittent or constant, and alternating or unilateral. In **non-paralytic strabismus,** the extraocular muscles and the nerves that control them are normal. The degree of deviation is constant or nearly constant in all directions of gaze. Non-paralytic strabismus is the most common type of strabismus seen in children, and congenital or infantile esotropia is usually of this kind. Ocular or visual defects such as cataracts or high refractive errors occasionally cause non-paralytic strabismus.

In **paralytic strabismus,** paralysis or paresis of one or more of the extraocular muscles produces a muscle imbalance. The deviation is asymmetrical, and characteristically the degree of deviation is worse when gazing in the direction of the affected muscle. Paralytic strabismus may be congenital or acquired. **Congenital paralytic strabismus** may result from birth trauma, muscle anomalies, abnormal development of the cranial nerve nuclei, or congenital infections affecting the eyes. Congenital strabismus may be seen in association with neurodevelopmental disorders such as cerebral palsy. **Acquired paralytic strabismus** due to extraocular muscle palsies usually indicates the presence of a serious underlying condition, such as an intracranial tumor, a demyelinating or neurodegenerative disease, myasthenia gravis, a progressive myopathy, or a central nervous system (CNS) infection. Children may present with a complaint of double vision or a compensatory torticollis (head tilt) to avoid double vision (diplopia).

Intermittent (latent) misalignment of the eyes is referred to as a **phoria.** Under normal conditions, the fusional mechanisms of the CNS maintain eye alignment. Eye deviation is appreciated only under certain conditions, such as illness, fatigue, stress, or when fusion is interrupted by occluding one eye (eg, during cover testing). Some degree of phoria may be found in almost all individuals and it is usually asymptomatic. Larger degrees of phoria may give rise to troublesome symptoms such as headaches, transient diplopia, or asthenopia (eye strain).

Constant misalignment of the eyes is referred to as **heterotropia.** This condition occurs because normal fusional mechanisms are unable to control eye deviation; children are unable to use both eyes together to fixate on an object. In alternating heterotropias, both eyes appear to deviate equally, and vision generally develops normally in each eye because children have no preference for fixation. If strabismus affects only one eye, the other eye is always used for fixation, and there is a danger of developing amblyopia or loss of vision in the deviating eye.

Convergent deviation, a turning in or crossing of the eyes, is called an esodeviation (eg, esotropia or esophoria). Divergent deviation, a turning out of the eyes, is an exodeviation. Hypertropia is used for upward vertical deviations. Esodeviations are the most common type of ocular misalignment, accounting for 50% to 75% of all cases of strabismus. Vertical deviations represent less than 5% of all cases of strabismus.

Amblyopia

Amblyopia is a potential complication if strabismus is not corrected in a timely manner. It refers to poor vision in one eye or, rarely, both despite correction of any refractive errors. If children have no significant refractive error and the visual acuity of one eye is worse than the other, they have amblyopia. To be considered amblyopia, visual acuity, as measured by reading an eye chart, should differ by at least 2 lines (eg, 20/20 in one eye and 20/40 in the other). It is the leading cause of preventable visual loss in children.

Amblyopia may be classified into 3 major categories. **Deprivational amblyopia** generally results when a unilateral lesion or developmental defect in one of the structures of the eye or its visual pathways obstructs vision. Causes of deprivational amblyopia include congenital cataract, ptosis, corneal opacity, retinal detachment, retinoblastoma, colobomas, optic nerve defects (eg, optic nerve hypoplasia), or orbital tumors. These conditions cause a lack of formation of a retinal image or a blurred retinal image, usually in one eye. **Refractive amblyopia** refers to a blurring of the retinal image due to large or asymmetrical refractive errors. Amblyopia is usually considered a unilateral abnormality, but may be bilateral in cases of large refractive errors (usually astigmatism or hyperopia). In **strabismic amblyopia,** the immature or developing brain suppresses images from the deviating eye to prevent diplopia. Strabismic

amblyopia is most commonly associated with strabismus that develops in children who are younger than 4 years. If the condition leading to the amblyopia is not corrected while the brain's visual pathways are still malleable (eg, before approximately 6–7 years of age), children may have some degree of permanent visual loss.

Differential Diagnosis

The differential diagnosis of strabismus may be divided into 3 categories: transient neonatal strabismus, congenital or infantile strabismus, and acquired strabismus. True strabismus must be differentiated from the illusion of deviation created by facial asymmetry or anatomical variations (ie, pseudostrabismus).

Transient Neonatal Strabismus

Eye alignment in normal infants during the first 2 to 3 months of life may vary from normal to intermittent esotropia or exotropia. These deviations are believed to result from CNS immaturity and resolve spontaneously in most children by 4 months of age. If such deviations are constant or persist beyond this age, children should be referred to an ophthalmologist for further evaluation.

Congenital or Infantile Strabismus

This type of strabismus is defined as a deviation that occurs during the first 6 months of life. Because the deviation may not always be present at birth, the term *infantile* may be more accurate. The differential diagnosis of infantile strabismus is presented in Box 76-1. **Pseudoesotropia** is an illusion or apparent deviation and not a true deviation. In many infants, the broad, flat nasal bridge and prominent epicanthal folds may obscure a portion of the sclera near the nose and create the appearance of esotropia (Figure 76-1). This illusion resolves as children mature. Symmetrical corneal light reflexes or normal cover tests differentiate pseudoesotropia from true esotropia.

Esotropia is one of the more common types of childhood strabismus. The constant deviation of infantile esotropia is usually readily apparent because of the large angle of deviation. Affected children usually have good bilateral vision because of the alternation of fixation from one eye to the other. Cross-fixation, in which children look to the left with the adducted right eye and to the right with the adducted left eye, may be evident because of the large angle of deviation. Rarely, esotropia may be due to palsy of the sixth cranial nerve either in isolation or in association with other cranial nerve palsies (Möbius syndrome).

Infantile exotropia is less common than esotropia. Like esotropia, exotropia develops within the first 6 months of life and is characterized by a large angle of deviation. Other causes of infantile exotropia include congenital third nerve palsy (paralytic strabismus) and abnormalities of the bones of the orbit (eg, Crouzon disease).

Acquired Strabismus

Acquired strabismus may result from a variety of causes (Box 76-1). Accommodative esotropia and intermittent exotropia are the 2 most common types of acquired strabismus. **Accommodative**

Box 76-1. Differential Diagnosis of Strabismus

Congenital or Infantile Strabismus

Esodeviations

Infantile esotropia

Pseudoesotropia

Möbius syndrome

Congenital sixth nerve palsy

Duane syndrome

Exodeviations

Congenital exotropia

Congenital third nerve palsy

Abnormalities of the bony orbit (Crouzon disease)

Both esodeviations and exodeviations

Duane syndrome (esotropia more common than exotropia)

Acquired Strabismus

Esodeviations

Accommodative esotropia

Benign sixth cranial nerve palsy

Exodeviations

Intermittent exotropia

Overcorrection after surgery for esotropia

Both Esodeviations and Exodeviations

Poor vision

Orbital trauma causing entrapment of extraocular muscles

Intracranial tumors or tumors involving the orbit (eg, retinoblastoma)

Myasthenia gravis

Central nervous system (CNS) infection (eg, meningitis)

CNS tumor

Orbital cellulitis

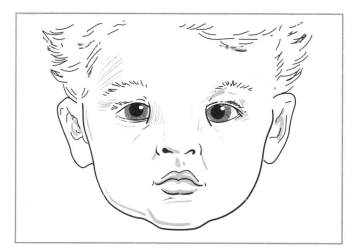

Figure 76-1. Child with pseudoesotropia. Note the wide nasal bridge and prominent epicanthal folds.

esotropia typically develops in children between 2 to 4 years of age but may appear as early as 6 months or as late as 8 years. Children with hyperopia use accommodation (attempts to focus) to see clearly. The accommodative reflex is closely linked to convergence; when accommodation occurs, so does convergence. If children have severe hyperopia (farsightedness), the amount of convergence that occurs with accommodation may be severe and lead to the development of esotropia. Such esotropia is usually intermittent initially and only gradually becomes constant. The deviating eye frequently becomes amblyopic.

Intermittent exotropia, the most common form of exodeviation seen in children, develops between birth and 4 years of age. Although it begins as an intermittent condition in which children's eyes appear to deviate outward, especially when they are tired, ill, or fixating at a distance, the exotropia can become constant with time. Children may also close one eye in bright sunlight, presumably in an effort to prevent diplopia.

Evaluation

History

The evaluation of infants or children suspected of having strabismus should begin with a thorough family history because strabismus often runs in families (Questions Box). Parental description of the ocular deviation is useful because misalignments, especially intermittent deviations that may only become manifest when children are tired, may not always be evident during the office visit. A history of head or orbital trauma may help in the evaluation of acquired strabismus.

Questions

Strabismus

- Does the child have a family history of strabismus?
- Does the child constantly tilt the head toward one side?
- Does the child squint?
- Has the child complained of blurred or double vision?
- Does the child close one eye in bright sunlight?
- Has the child had any recent trauma to the eyes or head?

Physical Examination

On physical examination, the presence of any dysmorphic features and structural abnormalities of the face or neck (eg, torticollis) should be noted. Children with paralytic strabismus (eg, fourth nerve palsy or superior oblique palsy) may compensate for their paretic lesion by tilting their head to avoid diplopia. It is important that visual screening of children begin during the neonatal period. Newborn screening should emphasize the presence of a bilateral red reflex. An abnormal red reflex or a white reflex may indicate the presence of a cataract or retinoblastoma. These require immediate referral to an ophthalmologist. Evaluation for ocular alignment should begin at the 4-month health maintenance visit. Intermittent misalignment of the eyes is often seen in normal infants who are younger than 4 months. However, constant misalignment requires immediate attention at any age.

Vision Testing

Testing visual acuity is essential in the evaluation of children with suspected strabismus. Such testing may be performed as early as 3 years of age if children are cooperative. Charts with symbols, figures, or letters can be used. The traditional Snellen eye chart with letters can generally be used in children who are 4 years of age. Decreased vision in one eye may be indicative of ocular abnormalities, including ocular deviations.

The 2 basic tests for strabismus that can be easily performed in the office are the corneal light reflex test, or Hirschberg test, and the cover test. The pediatrician should be comfortable performing both tests.

The **corneal light reflex test** is the simplest and quickest test for the evaluation of strabismus. In this test, a penlight is projected simultaneously onto the corneas of both eyes as the child looks straight ahead. The examiner compares the placement of the corneal light reflex in each eye with respect to the center of the pupil. If the eyes are straight, the reflection appears symmetrically in the center of both pupils or on the same point on each cornea. If the light reflex appears off center in one eye compared with the other, an ocular deviation or heterotropia is present. Nasal deviation of the light reflex on the cornea indicates exotropia on that side, temporal deviation signifies esotropia, and inferior deviation indicates hypertropia.

Unlike the corneal light reflex test, which may be performed even in uncooperative children, the **cover tests** require a child's cooperation and ability to fixate on a specified object. These tests are used to detect heterophorias. Two types of cover tests, alternate cover and cover-uncover, are used. Only the alternate cover test detects both heterophorias and heterotropias. This test may be preferred by the primary care physician as a screening tool. The cover-uncover test detects only manifest deviations or heterotropias. In the alternate cover test, one eye and then the other is covered as the child fixates on an object at a distance. If neither eye moves as the cover is moved rapidly between the eyes, the eyes are in alignment or orthophoric. With heterotropia, the deviating eye moves when the fixating eye is occluded; in heterophoria, the deviating eye moves when it is uncovered (Figure 76-2).

The alternate cover test may be illustrated with the following example. A child presents with constant esotropia of the left eye. When the right or fixating eye is occluded, the left eye is forced to fixate so that the child can see, and the left eye moves outward as the right eye is occluded. In the case of a child with an esophoria or latent deviation of the left eye, the eye deviates inward when it is occluded because it is not being forced to fixate. As the occluder is moved from the left eye to the right, the left eye moves outward and returns to a position of fixation.

The alternate cover test may be more difficult to interpret in children with bilateral or alternating strabismus who use both eyes in turn for fixation. It is not necessary for the pediatrician to identify exactly what type of strabismus is present; abnormal movement should be noted and children should be referred for further evaluation. An ophthalmologist is able to perform a more detailed examination.

Management

The goals of management are the attainment of the best possible vision in each eye, straight eyes cosmetically, and fusion. The sooner deviations are corrected, the better the child's chances for equal bilateral vision. Treatment includes correction of any underlying

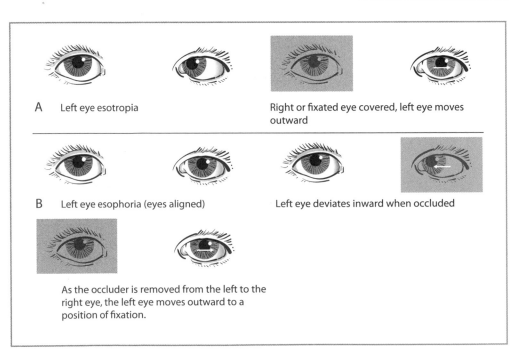

A Left eye esotropia

Right or fixated eye covered, left eye moves outward

B Left eye esophoria (eyes aligned)

Left eye deviates inward when occluded

As the occluder is removed from the left to the right eye, the left eye moves outward to a position of fixation.

Figure 76-2. Alternate cover test in the detection of strabismus. Normally, both eyes appear to be aligned and centrally fixed. A. Detection of esotropia. The right eye is fixating and a left esotropia is present. When the right or fixating eye is covered, the left eye moves outward (away from the nose). B. Detection of esophoria. The eyes are aligned with a left esophoria. When the left eye is covered, it deviates inward. As the occluder is moved from the left eye to the right eye, the left eye moves outward to a position of fixation.

refractive error with **corrective lenses.** Such lenses, which remedy the refractive error and minimize the need for accommodation, are used to treat accommodative esotropia. Glasses are also used in anisometropic amblyopia in which one eye has a significantly different refractive error than the other.

Children who do not see equally well from both eyes may be at risk for amblyopia if they preferentially fixate with only one eye. If detected, amblyopia should be corrected with occlusion therapy of the fixating "good" eye. **Occlusion therapy** forces children to use the amblyopic eye. This treatment is best accomplished by constantly patching the eye with better vision during waking hours, or penalization with dilating drops in the better seeing eye. Children require repeat evaluations and close monitoring during this therapy.

If nonsurgical methods fail to align the eyes, surgical correction may be necessary. **Surgery** may be used to achieve the best possible ocular alignment and is usually required for treatment of infantile esotropia. It is generally performed in children between 6 months and 1 year of age, while the visual system is still pliable enough to allow for development of postsurgical binocular vision. Surgery also may be needed in children with intermittent exotropia if the frequency of the deviation is increasing.

Prognosis

Certain conditions, such as pseudoesotropia or infrequent intermittent exotropia, may resolve as children mature. Others, such as infantile esotropia, require early detection and treatment to achieve the best binocular vision. Amblyopia and permanent vision loss may result if correction of strabismus is delayed.

CASE RESOLUTION

The infant in the case history has pseudoesotropia. Although the boy's eyes appear to deviate, the corneal light reflex and cover tests are normal. Physical examination reveals prominent epicanthal folds and a broad, flat nasal bridge.

Selected References

Bacal DA. Don't be lazy about looking for amblyopia. *Contemp Pediatr.* 1998;15:99–107

Campos EC. Why do the eyes cross? A review and discussion of the nature and origin of essential infantile esotropia, microstrabismus, accommodative esotropia and acute comitant esotropia. *J AAPOS.* 2008;12(4):326–331

Catalano JD. Strabismus. *Pediatr Ann.* 1990;19:289–297

Cheng KP, Biglan AW, Hiles DA. Pediatric ophthalmology. In: Zitelli BJ, Davis HW. *Pediatric Physical Diagnosis.* 3rd ed. St Louis, MO: Mosby-Wolfe; 1997:563–601

Crouch ER Jr, Crouch ER. Pediatric vision screening: why? when? what? how? *Contemp Pediatr.* 1991;8(special issue):9–30

Ekdaw NS, Nusz KJ, Diehl NN, Mohney BG. Postoperative outcomes in children with intermittent exotropia from a population-based cohort. *J AAPOS.* 2009;13(1):4–7

Greenberg AE, Mohney BG, Diehl NN, Burke JP. Incidence and types of childhood esotropia: a population-based study. *Ophthalmology.* 2007;114(1):170–174

Greenwald M, Parks M. Treatment of amblyopia. In: *Duane's Clinical Ophthalmology.* Philadelphia, PA: Lippincott Williams & Wilkins; 2002: 1–10

Keech R. Practical management of amblyopia. In: Wright K, ed. *Focal Points: Clinical Modules for Ophthalmologists.* Vol. XVIII, No. 2. San Francisco, CA: American Academy of Ophthalmology; 2000:1–3

Lavrich JB, Nelson LB. Diagnosis and treatment of strabismus disorders. *Pediatr Clin North Am.* 1993;40:737–752

Louwagie CR, Diehl NN, Grenberg AE, Mohney BG. Long term follow-up of congenital esotropia in a population-based cohort. *J AAPOS.* 2009;13(1):8–12

Mitchell P, Parks M. Concomitant exodeviations. In: *Duane's Clinical Ophthalmology.* Philadelphia, PA: Lippincott Williams & Wilkins; 2002: 1–17

Parks M. Alignment. In: *Duane's Clinical Ophthalmology.* Philadelphia, PA: Lippincott Williams & Wilkins; 2002: 1–12

Parks M, Mitchell P, Wheeler M. Concomitant esodeviations. In: *Duane's Clinical Ophthalmology.* Philadelphia, PA: Lippincott Williams & Wilkins; 2002: 1–21

Simon J, ed. *Pediatric Ophthalmology and Strabismus.* San Francisco, CA: American Academy of Ophthalmology; 2006–2007:9–12, 67–118

Spencer RF, Tucker MG, Choi RY, McNeer KW. Botulinum toxin management of childhood intermittent exotropia. *Ophthalmology.* 1997;104:1762–1767

Wallace DK, Chandler DL, Beck RW, et al. Treatment of bilateral refractive amblyopia in children three to less than 10 years of age. *Am J Ophthalmol.* 2007;144:487–496

CHAPTER 77

Infections of the Eye

Teresa Rosales, MD

CASE STUDY

A 10-day-old neonate has a 1-day history of red, watery eyes and nonproductive cough with no fever. The girl is breastfed and continues to eat well. She was the 7-lb, 2-oz (3,238-g) product of a term gestation, born via normal spontaneous vaginal delivery without complications to a 26-year-old woman. The pregnancy was also uncomplicated. No one at home is ill.

On examination, the infant is afebrile with normal vital signs. Examination of the eyes reveals bilateral conjunctival injection with only a mild amount of purulent discharge. Bilateral red reflexes are present. The rest of the physical examination is within normal limits.

Questions

1. What is the differential diagnosis of conjunctivitis both during and following the neonatal period?
2. What laboratory tests, if any, should be performed?
3. When is a chest radiograph indicated in the evaluation of neonates with conjunctivitis?
4. What are management strategies for eye infections?

Infections of the eye and surrounding structures are commonly seen by pediatricians. Such infections range in severity from common problems such as blepharitis and conjunctivitis, which lack serious sequelae, to severe and less common infections such as periorbital and orbital cellulitis. The presenting complaint in many children with eye infections is a red-appearing eye. Familiarity with the common causes of a red eye makes prompt diagnosis and treatment possible.

Epidemiology

Conjunctivitis, which affects children of all ages, is perhaps the most common eye infection of childhood. The incidence of conjunctivitis in the newborn period is estimated to range from 1.6% to 12%. The incidence of chlamydial conjunctivitis is about 8 in 1,000 live births. About two-thirds of acute childhood conjunctivitis has a bacterial etiology, and one-third is viral. *Haemophilus influenzae* and *Streptococcus pneumoniae* are the most common bacterial agents and account for about 40% and 10% of culture-proven cases, respectively. The incidence of *H influenzae* is decreasing with the advent of the *H influenzae* type b vaccine. *Staphylococcus aureus* is isolated from the conjunctivae of children with acute conjunctivitis, but it is found with about the same frequency in the eyes of children without conjunctivitis. Adenovirus is the most common viral isolate. Most cases of acute conjunctivitis in young adults have a viral etiology. Serious eye infections such as periorbital and orbital cellulitis occur far less often.

Clinical Presentation

Red eyes and discharge are the common presenting signs of infections of the eyelids and conjunctivae. Eyelid edema and erythema surrounding the eye characterize periorbital and orbital cellulitis.

Proptosis, abnormal extraocular movement, or loss of visual acuity may signal spread of the infection beyond the orbital septum (orbital cellulitis) (Dx Box).

Pathophysiology

Eye infections may be divided into 2 types: those affecting the structures surrounding the orbit and those involving the orbital contents themselves (Figure 77-1). Although all structures surrounding the eye may potentially become inflamed or infected, the eyelids, nasolacrimal drainage system (dacryocystitis; see Chapter 78), conjunctiva, and cornea are most commonly involved. Orbital cellulitis is defined as an infection of the orbital structures posterior to the orbital septum. The orbital septum, an extension of the periosteum of the bones of the orbit, extends to the margins of both the upper and lower eyelids and provides an anatomical barrier to the spread of most infectious and inflammatory processes. Preseptal, or periorbital, cellulitis is localized to structures superficial to the orbital septum, whereas post-septal, or orbital, cellulitis implies that the disease process involves orbital structures extending beyond the septum.

Differential Diagnosis

Infections of the eye are included in the differential diagnosis of conditions presenting with red eye (Box 77-1). Also included in the differential diagnosis are congenital, inflammatory, traumatic, and systemic processes. Although infection and irritation are by far the most common causes of an acute onset of red eye, other possibilities, especially trauma, glaucoma, or underlying systemic disease, must be considered.

Dx Eye Infections

Eyelid Infections

- Redness
- Itching (blepharitis)
- Burning (blepharitis)
- Scales at the base of the lashes (seborrheic blepharitis)
- Swelling (hordeolum or chalazion)
- Pain (hordeolum)

Conjunctivitis

- Conjunctival injection and edema
- Excessive tearing
- Discharge or crusting
- Itching (allergic conjunctivitis)

Uveitis

- Conjunctival injection
- Pain
- Blurred vision
- Photophobia
- Headache

Periorbital Cellulitis

- Unilateral eyelid edema
- Erythema surrounding the eye
- Pain
- Fever

Orbital Cellulitis

- Eyelid edema
- Proptosis
- Decreased extraocular movements
- Loss of visual acuity
- Fever
- Ill appearance
- Associated sinusitis

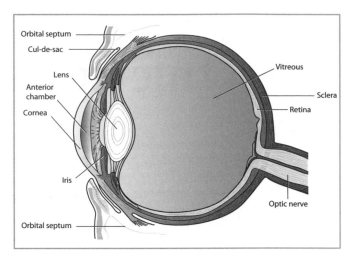

Figure 77-1. The eye and surrounding structures.

pubis, and primary or recurrent herpes simplex virus type 1 infections that may manifest as clusters of vesicles on the eyelids. Acne rosacea may rarely occur in childhood and can present very similarly to chronic blepharitis.

The glands of the eyelid can also be infected. *Staphylococcus aureus* is the most common organism. A **hordeolum,** or common stye, results from an infection of the meibomian glands located along

Box 77-1. Differential Diagnosis of Red Eye
Congenital Anomalies
• Nasolacrimal duct obstruction
• Congenital glaucoma
Infection
• Keratitis
• Conjunctivitis
• Dacryocystitis
• Corneal ulcer
• Periorbital and orbital cellulitis
Inflammation
• Blepharitis
• Hordeolum
• Chalazion
Trauma
• Corneal abrasion
• Foreign body
• Blunt trauma: hyphema
• Perforating injuries
• Exposure to chemicals or other noxious substances
Systemic Illnesses
• Kawasaki disease
• Varicella
• Measles
• Lyme disease
• Stevens-Johnson syndrome
• Ataxia-telangiectasia
• Juvenile rheumatoid arthritis

Eyelid Infections

Common conditions affecting the eyelid and its related structures are blepharitis, hordeolum, and chalazion.

Blepharitis is an inflammation of the lid margins. This condition, which is often bilateral, may be chronic or recurrent. The 2 most common causes of blepharitis are staphylococcal infection and seborrheic dermatitis. Children with staphylococcal blepharitis often present with scales at the base of the lashes, ulceration of the lid margin, and loss of lashes. The infection may spread to the conjunctiva or cornea, producing conjunctivitis or keratitis. In contrast, seborrheic blepharitis is characterized by greasy, yellow scales attached to the base of the lashes. In addition, associated seborrhea of the scalp or eyebrows may be present. Mixed staphylococcal-seborrheic infections, which occur as staphylococcal superinfection, may complicate seborrheic blepharitis. Less commonly seen forms of blepharitis are parasitic blepharitis, which results from infestation of the lids by the head louse, *Pediculus capitis,* or crab louse, *Pediculus* the lid margins. The glands become obstructed and an abscess can form. Affected children present with a well-circumscribed, painful swelling that may be at the lid margin or may be deeper in the lid tissue. These generally rupture or resolve without complications when treated aggressively with hot compresses.

A chalazion is a hordeolum that has not resolved over weeks to months. It is no longer an infectious process but has become a chronic granulomatous inflammation of the meibomian glands. The resulting firm, non-tender, slow-growing mass within the upper or lower eyelid may be painful if secondary infection is present.

Infections of the Conjunctiva

Conjunctivitis refers to any inflammation of the conjunctiva. The condition may be allergic, chemical, viral, or bacterial in etiology. In addition, it may be a sign of systemic disease such as Kawasaki disease or Stevens-Johnson syndrome.

Acute conjunctivitis, or pinkeye, is common during childhood and can be extremely contagious. The usual signs are conjunctival injection, tearing, discharge, crusting of the lashes, and conjunctival edema (chemosis). Pain and decreased vision are uncommon symptoms and may signal corneal involvement.

In general, it is difficult to distinguish bacterial conjunctivitis from viral conjunctivitis on clinical features alone. Certain clinical characteristics may guide the diagnosis. The average age of children affected with **bacterial conjunctivitis** tends to be younger than the age of those with viral conjunctivitis, which occurs more frequently in adolescents; however, considerable overlap occurs. Children with bacterial conjunctivitis typically present with an acute onset of unilateral or bilateral injection and edema of both the palpebral and bulbar conjunctiva, minimal to copious purulent discharge, and crusting of the eyelashes. Children may have difficulty opening their eyes on awakening in the morning because of the exudate. An association between conjunctivitis and concomitant otitis media has been well described. *Haemophilus influenzae,* which is often resistant to ampicillin, is the pathogen most commonly isolated from affected children.

The diagnosis of **viral conjunctivitis** is considered if signs of viral upper respiratory infection (eg, low-grade fever, cough, rhinorrhea) are evident. Viral infection is associated with conjunctival injection, watery or thin mucoid discharge, and only mild lid edema and erythema. Adenoviral infection is usually bilateral, with significant conjunctival injection and chemosis of the conjunctiva, and is often accompanied by a tender preauricular lymph node. Epidemic keratoconjunctivitis is a highly contagious form of adenoviral conjunctivitis. Affected children often complain of foreign body sensation beneath the lids or photophobia due to corneal involvement. Pharyngeal conjunctival fever, another presentation of adenoviral conjunctivitis, usually manifests as conjunctivitis in association with pharyngitis and fever.

Infants who suffer from **chronic or recurrent conjunctival discharge** may have an obstruction of the nasolacrimal duct, whereas older children with chronic conjunctivitis may have allergic diseases, recurrent blepharitis, or chlamydial infections. Blepharitis is the most common cause of chronic conjunctivitis in older children. *Staphylococcus aureus* is frequently implicated in these infections.

Itching, tearing, and conjunctival edema are the hallmarks of **allergic conjunctivitis,** a noninfectious form of conjunctival inflammation often seen in children with other allergic disorders such as asthma or hay fever. Conjunctival injection tends to be mild, bilateral, and seasonal. The etiology is most often a hypersensitivity to pollens, dust, or animal dander. Vernal conjunctivitis is a bilateral, severe form of allergic conjunctivitis seen primarily during childhood. Most cases occur during the spring and summer. Severe itching and tearing are the most frequent complaints. The palpebral conjunctiva may have a cobblestone appearance due to the accumulation of inflammatory cells, or there may be small, elevated lesions of the bulbar conjunctiva at the corneal limbus. The pathogenesis is unclear, but atopy seems to play a role.

Chlamydial conjunctivitis frequently affects both neonates and adolescents. Inclusion conjunctivitis is an acute infection of the eyes caused by sexually transmitted *Chlamydia trachomatis* (usually serotypes D through K). This condition may be seen in neonates or sexually active adolescents. Trachoma, the most common cause of impaired vision and preventable blindness worldwide, is a chronic conjunctivitis usually caused by *C trachomatis* serotypes A, B, and C. Although this disease is rarely seen in North America, it is endemic among certain populations, especially Native Americans. Inclusion conjunctivitis and endemic trachoma are both characterized initially by conjunctivitis with small lymphoid follicles in the conjunctiva.

Neonatal conjunctivitis, or ophthalmia neonatorum, occurs during the first month of life. The major causes of neonatal conjunctivitis are chemical, chlamydial, and bacterial (in decreasing order of frequency). Ophthalmia neonatorum may be produced by the same bacteria that cause childhood conjunctivitis but also results from organisms such as *C trachomatis* or *Neisseria gonorrhoeae.* Newborns may acquire these latter pathogens following premature rupture of membranes or passage through an infected or colonized birth canal. *Chlamydia trachomatis* is the organism most commonly identified. It has been isolated from 17% to 40% of neonates with conjunctivitis. Infants born to mothers with active cervical chlamydial infection have a 20% to 50% chance of developing chlamydial conjunctivitis. Viruses are uncommon causes of neonatal ocular infections. Herpes simplex virus (HSV) is the primary viral agent involved in neonatal conjunctivitis. The presence of characteristic vesicular skin lesions or corneal dendritic lesions helps in the diagnosis.

The time of onset of symptoms is related to the etiologic agent. Inflammation secondary to the **silver nitrate** drops instilled at birth to prevent gonococcal infection presents as mild conjunctivitis 12 to 24 hours after birth in 10% to 100% of treated newborns. This condition usually resolves spontaneously in 24 to 48 hours. This is more of historic interest because erythromycin ointment 0.5% has replaced silver nitrate in most hospitals. (Silver nitrate was ineffective against *C trachomatis.*) Conjunctivitis due to *N gonorrhoeae* appears 2 to 5 days after birth and is associated with copious purulent discharge. Conjunctivitis due to *C trachomatis* occurs at 5 to 14 days, a result of a longer incubation period. The time of onset and the severity of symptoms of these 2 conditions may overlap, however. The presentation of gonococcal infection may be delayed for 5 days or more because of the partial suppression of the infection by the prophylactic drops instilled at birth. Chlamydial infection can vary in severity from mild erythema of the eyelids to severe inflammation and copious purulent discharge. Chlamydial infection is primarily localized to the palpebral conjunctiva and only rarely affects the cornea. Gonococcal conjunctivitis is considered a medical emergency because the gonococcus can penetrate the cornea, resulting in corneal ulceration and perforation of the globe within 24 hours if untreated.

Concomitant nasopharyngeal chlamydial infection is commonly seen. Spread of the organism from the nasopharynx to the lungs is a sequela of colonization. Ten percent to 20% of infants with conjunctivitis have chlamydial pneumonia. It may occur either simultaneously with the conjunctivitis or up to 4 to 6 weeks later. Affected infants are usually afebrile and present with symptoms of increasing tachypnea and cough.

Anterior uveitis may be confused with conjunctivitis. The uvea consists of the iris, the ciliary body, the retina, and the choroid. Inflammation of the iris or ciliary body may produce conjunctival injection, which may be associated with decreased visual acuity, pain, headache, and photophobia. Systemic conditions associated with uveitis include Kawasaki disease, juvenile rheumatoid arthritis, Lyme disease, tuberculosis, sarcoidosis, toxocara infection, toxoplasmosis, and spondyloarthropathies.

Infections of the Eye and Surrounding Tissues

Preseptal cellulitis and **orbital cellulitis** are 2 serious infections of the eyelids and surrounding structures. Although these infections are not as frequent as those that are limited to the eye, they have serious sequelae. The preseptal space is defined by the skin of the eyelid on one side and the orbital septum on the other. Children with preseptal cellulitis, or **periorbital cellulitis,** usually present with acute onset, unilateral upper and lower eyelid edema, erythema, and pain. The condition is often associated with systemic signs and symptoms such as ill appearance, fever, and leukocytosis. The eye itself usually appears normal. Infection may follow hematogenous seeding of the preseptal space, most often with *H influenzae* type b or *S pneumoniae,* or after traumatic breaks in the skin that usually lead to *S aureus* infection.

Orbital cellulitis is an infection of the contents of the orbit posterior to the orbital septum. Usually an insidious onset of eyelid edema, proptosis, decreased extraocular movements, and loss of visual acuity occur. As with periorbital cellulitis, children are often febrile and ill-appearing. Contiguous spread of infection from adjacent sinusitis (most often ethmoid) is the most common cause. The organisms most often involved are the same as those in acute sinusitis (*S aureus, S pneumoniae,* non-typeable *H influenzae,* and

Staphylococcus pyogenes). Untreated, the infection may progress to orbital abscess formation or progress posteriorly in the orbit to the cavernous sinus and the brain.

Primary herpes simplex infection can affect the skin surrounding the eyes as well as the eye itself. Most of these infections are caused by HSV type 1, although type 2 infections may be seen in newborns. Children with **herpetic infections of the eye** usually present with unilateral skin vesicles and a mild conjunctivitis or keratitis. Herpetic keratoconjunctivitis can recur following fever, exposure to sunlight, or mild trauma. The characteristic corneal lesion of herpes keratitis is the dendritic corneal ulcer, which appears as a tree branch pattern on fluorescein staining of the cornea. Although this lesion may be seen with primary infection, it is more common in recurrent infections. Skin vesicles may not appear with a recurrence, which makes it difficult to distinguish herpetic infection from other causes of conjunctivitis. Steroids may lead to progression of the herpetic infection and permanent corneal scarring as well as cataracts and glaucoma. Empiric topical steroid treatment for presumed viral conjunctivitis should be avoided for this reason. Neonatal herpetic infections of the eye primarily result from HSV-2. Infections may be isolated to the eye or the eye may be infected secondarily due to central nervous system (CNS) or disseminated disease. Proper diagnosis is important because disseminated herpetic disease has a mortality of about 85%, and CNS disease has a mortality of 50%. Isolated herpetic eye disease is actually quite rare in neonates.

Evaluation

History

A careful history taken from the parent or primary caregiver as well as the child can guide the diagnosis (Questions Box). It is important to exclude the possibility of ocular trauma or exposure to noxious chemicals when evaluating children with red, irritated eyes.

Questions

Eye Infections

- How long has the child had symptoms?
- Is the child having any difficulty seeing clearly?
- Is he or she complaining of light sensitivity?
- Has the child had fever, cold symptoms, or purulent nasal discharge (eg, green or yellow)?
- Are the eyes pruritic (itchy) or painful?
- Does the child have difficulty opening the affected eye on awakening in the morning or after naps?
- Have the parents noticed any discharge from the eyes or crusting around the eyelids?
- Is the child complaining of earache or sore throat?
- Does the child have allergies, asthma, or hay fever?
- Has there been any trauma or bug bites?

Physical Examination

A thorough examination of the eyes should be performed. The eyelids, conjunctiva, and cornea should be inspected for evidence of inflammation or foreign bodies. The presence of any discharge or crusting of the eyelids as well as light sensitivity or pain should be noted. Extraocular movements should be checked, and their symmetry should be noted. Visual acuity should be determined, and an ophthalmoscopic examination of the retina should be performed whenever possible. A slit-lamp examination of the eye is indicated if uveitis is suspected. In addition, it is important to perform a thorough head and neck examination, noting the presence of associated sinusitis, otitis media, pharyngitis, or preauricular nodes.

Laboratory Tests

Laboratory assessment is guided by the history and physical examination. Although clinical differentiation between a bacterial and viral etiology is difficult, cultures are usually not required because acute conjunctivitis in children is a self-limited disease. In neonatal conjunctivitis, however, the time of onset of illness and the clinical findings overlap, and Gram stain and cultures are essential. Gonococcal infection is assessed by both Gram stain and culture. Treatment may be initiated on the basis of Gram stain alone because of the serious potential for corneal involvement and subsequent loss of visual acuity.

If HSV is suspected, viral cultures should be obtained. If chlamydial infection is suspected, a nasopharyngeal culture should be sent in addition to conjunctival scraping. Purulent material may be examined for gonococci, but conjunctival scrapings are required for chlamydia because chlamydia is an obligate intracellular organism. Laboratory assessment of periorbital cellulitis includes a complete blood cell count (CBC), blood culture, and a lumbar puncture in young infants or in children with signs of meningeal irritation. The reported prevalence of meningitis is 1% in children with periorbital cellulitis and 10% in children with bacteremia and periorbital cellulitis. As with periorbital cellulitis, laboratory assessment of orbital cellulitis includes a CBC and blood culture.

Imaging Studies

Imaging studies are required infrequently in the assessment of eye infections. A chest radiograph to detect pneumonia should be taken if infants with neonatal conjunctivitis have respiratory symptoms. Characteristic features on chest radiograph include hyperinflation and diffuse or patchy interstitial infiltrates. In orbital cellulitis, a computed tomography scan of the orbit and sinuses may be useful for assessing the degree of involvement.

Management

Most common eye infections either resolve spontaneously or respond readily to **hygiene** and **topical antibiotics.** Treatment of both staphylococcal and seborrheic blepharitis consists of daily lid hygiene (usually at bedtime), including application of a warm compress and removal of the scales and crusts with a moistened, warm washcloth.

The eyelashes and lid margins may also be scrubbed with a washcloth soaked in a 50:50 mixture of baby shampoo and water. When staphylococcal blepharitis is present, an ointment containing an anti-staphylococcal antibiotic agent, such as erythromycin, may be applied to the eyelids after cleansing. Treatment of parasitic blepharitis consists of application of petrolatum ophthalmic ointment (to smother the nits) several times a day for 1 week, followed by removal of the remaining parasites and their ova with tweezers or forceps.

Treatment for hordeola consists of application of hot compresses several times a day. This usually causes the abscess to come to a point and drain. Occasionally, surgical excision and drainage may be required if the abscess does not resolve. Unlike the hordeolum, a chalazion generally requires surgical excision, because spontaneous resolution is uncommon.

Most cases of acute childhood conjunctivitis can be managed successfully by primary care physicians. Acute conjunctivitis in childhood is generally a self-limited disease. However, antibiotic treatment of bacterial conjunctivitis hastens recovery and may help prevent secondary cases by eradicating the bacterial pathogen. It is helpful to determine clinically whether the infection is bacterial and initiate empiric treatment with topical antibiotic preparations. Trimethoprim and polymyxin B sulfate (Polytrim), sodium sulfacetamide (Bleph-10), gentamicin (Garamycin), and tobramycin (Tobrex) are some of the commonly prescribed antibiotics. The newest antibiotic of choice is Vigamox (moxifloxacin). Avoid neomycin-containing products because sensitivity to neomycin occurs frequently. Antibiotic ointments may be easier to instill in infants and young children. Antibiotic drops should be used in older children during the day because the ointments can blur the vision. Ointments may be used at bedtime. Systemic therapy can be considered for concomitant conjunctivitis and otitis media. Good hygiene with special attention to hand washing is important to prevent the spread of the infection to the other eye and to family and friends. Children should not go to school until the discharge and drainage have resolved (even if on antibiotic drops). If symptoms persist for more than 7 to 10 days or if the diagnosis is in question, appropriate cultures should be taken. Complicated cases such as suspected herpetic or gonococcal infection, foreign bodies that cannot be removed easily, loss of visual acuity, presence of significant pain, those involving children with a history of recent penetrating ocular trauma or surgery, and those involving children who use contact lenses should be referred to an ophthalmologist immediately. Contact lens wearers with red eyes are at high risk for corneal ulcers. They should be instructed to leave their lenses out until seen by the ophthalmologist.

Allergic conjunctivitis can be managed with cool compresses. Topical decongestant drops may provide symptomatic relief if treatment is indicated. Vernal conjunctivitis may be treated with topical cromolyn sodium drops or medications designed to relieve redness and itching and stabilize mast cells, such as Patanol (olopatadine) or Acular (ketorolac). Caution should be used when prescribing corticosteroid preparations for the eye because they may lead to progression of an undiagnosed herpetic eye infection. Chronic use of topical steroids can cause cataracts and glaucoma.

Treatment of neonatal conjunctivitis depends on the diagnosis. If **gonococcal infection** is suspected and Gram stain is positive for gram-negative diplococci, immediate parenteral therapy with ceftriaxone should be initiated. **Chlamydial** conjunctivitis should be managed with systemic rather than topical treatment to prevent systemic disease. Oral erythromycin is the drug of choice. Although oral treatment provides adequate local antibiotic levels, topical erythromycin ointment may be used in conjunction with systemic therapy to provide more prompt relief of ophthalmic symptoms. The parents should also be treated.

Empiric parenteral antibiotic therapy (eg, cefuroxime) should be initiated for **periorbital cellulitis.** Repeat evaluations for signs of progression should be performed frequently during the initial 24 to 48 hours. If **orbital cellulitis** is suspected, an ophthalmologist should be consulted, and hospitalization and systemic antibiotics should be instituted. Surgical drainage of the sinuses or of an orbital abscess is sometimes necessary.

Children with suspected **herpetic infection** should be referred to an ophthalmologist. Intravenous acyclovir is often recommended for the treatment of isolated herpetic eye infections in neonates.

Prognosis

Most common eye infections such as blepharitis, hordeolum, and acute childhood conjunctivitis resolve without sequelae. Recurrence is common for hordeola, and periorbital cellulitis may be a potential complication in rare or untreated cases. Unlike acute conjunctivitis, chronic conjunctivitis may not be self-limited. Appropriate diagnosis and management are extremely important to prevent serious sequelae in some children. For example, endemic trachoma may progress to produce conjunctival scarring, pannus formation, and even blindness if not appropriately treated with systemic erythromycin or tetracycline. (In general, systemic tetracycline should not be used in children <8 years to avoid discoloration of the teeth.)

Periorbital cellulitis generally resolves without sequelae if treated promptly with systemic antibiotics. Orbital cellulitis should be considered a true ophthalmologic emergency because the potential for complications is high. The optic nerve may become involved, resulting in loss of vision or spread of the infection into the cranial cavity. This spreading may lead to meningitis, cavernous sinus thrombosis, or brain abscess.

CASE RESOLUTION

The infant presented in the case history has neonatal conjunctivitis. A Gram stain of the purulent discharge should be examined, and cultures should be taken from the eye and nasopharynx. If the Gram stain is negative for gonococci, empiric treatment may begin with oral erythromycin.

Selected References

Gigliotti F. Acute conjunctivitis. *Pediatr Rev.* 1995;16:203–207

King RA. Common ocular signs and symptoms in childhood. *Pediatr Clin North Am.* 1993;40:753–766

Liesegang T, Skuta G, Cantor L. Infectious and allergic ocular diseases. *J Pediatr Ophthalmol Strabismus.* 2006;17:215–238

Mets M, Noffke A. Ocular infections of the external eye and cornea in children. *Focal Points.* 2002;2:1–14

McKinley S, Yen M, Miller A, et al. Microbiology of pediatric orbital cellulitis. *Am J Ophthalmol.* 2007;144:497–501

Nageswaran S, Woods DR, Benjamin DK, Givner LB, Shetty AK. Orbital cellulitis in children. *Pediatr Infect Dis J.* 2006;25(8):695–699

O'Hara MA. Ophthalmia neonatorum. *Pediatr Clin North Am.* 1993;40:715–725

Ohnsman CM. Exclusion of students with conjunctivitis from school: policies of state departments of health. *J Pediatr Ophthalmol Strabismus.* 2007;44(2):101–105

Patel PB, Diaz MC, Bennett JE, Attia MW. Clinical features of bacterial conjunctivitis in children. *Acad Emerg Med.* 2007;14(1):1–5

Powell KR. Orbital and periorbital cellulitis. *Pediatr Rev.* 1995;16:163–167

Silver LH, Woodside AM, Montgomery DB. Clinical safety of moxifloxacin ophthalmic solution 0.5% (Vigamox) in pediatric and non-pediatric patients with bacterial conjunctivitis. *Surv Ophthalmol.* 2005;50(suppl 1):S55–S63

Wagner RS. Eye infections and abnormalities: issues for the pediatrician. *Contemp Pediatr.* 1997;14:137–153

Wagner RS. The differential diagnosis of the red eye. *Contemp Pediatr.* 1991;8:26–48

Weiss AH. Chronic conjunctivitis in infants and children. *Pediatr Ann.* 1993;22:366–374

CHAPTER 78

Excessive Tearing

Teresa Rosales, MD

CASE STUDY

A 4-week-old infant girl has had a persistent watery discharge from both eyes since birth. Her mother has noticed white, crusty material on her daughter's eyelids for the past few days. The infant's birth and medical history are unremarkable. Examination of the eyes, including bilateral red reflexes and symmetrical extraocular movements, is normal, except that the left eye appears "wetter" than the right.

Questions

1. What is the differential diagnosis of excessive tearing in infancy?
2. How do physical findings such as corneal enlargement and haziness influence the differential diagnosis?
3. How should infants with excessive tearing be managed?
4. When should a child with excessive tearing be referred to an ophthalmologist?

Infants or young children with excessive tearing or epiphora in one or both eyes are a common pediatric ophthalmologic concern. The pediatrician must be capable of differentiating benign causes of this common childhood condition from other more serious illnesses, such as glaucoma, that potentially threaten vision.

NASOLACRIMAL DUCT OBSTRUCTION

Epidemiology

Congenital obstruction of the nasolacrimal duct or dacryostenosis, which occurs in 1% to 6% of newborn infants, is the most common cause of excessive tearing in infancy. Eighty percent will resolve spontaneously by 6 months of age.

Clinical Presentation

Infants with dacryostenosis usually present with a history of a mucoid discharge and crusting along the eyelid margins. The affected eye appears "wetter" than the normal eye, and a small pool of tears may be noted along the lower eyelid. Frequent tearing is reported. Commonly, the patient has repeated episodes of infection with purulent discharge (Dx Box).

Pathophysiology

The lacrimal system (Figure 78-1) produces and drains tears away from the eyes and into the nose. Reflex tearing is usually present shortly after birth but may be delayed for several weeks to months until the lacrimal gland begins to function. Tears drain away from the eyes through the superior and inferior puncta into the superior and inferior canaliculi and finally into the nasolacrimal duct, which drains beneath the inferior turbinate into the nose.

 Dx Excessive Tearing

- Conjunctival edema or injection
- Crusting of the eyelids
- Rhinorrhea
- Photophobia
- Corneal haziness
- Reflux of tears with gentle pressure on medial canthus
- Wetness of eye

Outflow obstruction, most often due to obstruction of the nasolacrimal duct or dacryostenosis, is the most common cause of excessive tearing in infancy. The obstruction is usually bilateral and occurs during fetal development. Most commonly a persistent, thin membrane (Hasner membrane) obstructs the opening of the sac in the nose. The membrane is usually located in the distal or nasal segment of the duct rather than in the proximal portion. The term *dacryocystitis* is used if acute infection or inflammation is associated with the obstruction. If both the canaliculi and the nasolacrimal duct are obstructed, a mucocele over the nasolacrimal sac may be noted at birth. This sac appears as a bluish, firm mass located over the lacrimal sac. Atresia of some portion of the drainage system may also occur, but this is extremely rare.

Differential Diagnosis

Box 78-1 outlines the differential diagnosis of excessive tearing in infancy. Although obstruction of the nasolacrimal duct is the most common cause of excessive tearing in infants, it is important to consider and rule out glaucoma when evaluating infants with this complaint. Infantile glaucoma may be unilateral or bilateral.

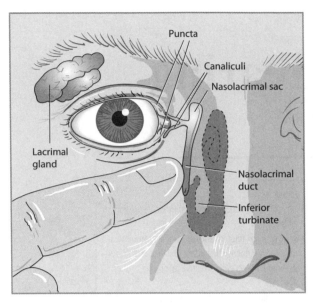

Figure 78-1. The lacrimal system, showing massage of the lacrimal sac.

Box 78-1. Differential Diagnosis of Excessive Tearing in Infants

Increased Production
- Infantile glaucoma
- Allergy
- Conjunctivitis
- Corneal abrasion
- Foreign body under the eyelid

Outflow Obstruction
- Nasolacrimal duct obstruction (dacryostenosis)
- Anomalies of the lacrimal drainage system
- Mucocele of the lacrimal sac
- Atresia of the lacrimal punctum or canaliculus
- Nasal congestion
- Craniofacial anomalies involving the midface

Acute onset of excessive tearing in older children is usually due to ocular irritation. Any irritation of the conjunctiva, cornea, or eyelids may produce tearing. Conjunctivitis and corneal abrasion, usually secondary to a retained foreign body or herpes simplex keratoconjunctivitis, are the 2 most common causes. Eye infections are discussed in Chapter 77.

Evaluation

History

Evaluation of excessive tearing should begin with a thorough history. The nature of any discharge (eg, watery, mucoid, or purulent) should be noted. Parents or other caregivers should be questioned about the appearance of the child's eyes (Questions Box). The excessive mucoid discharge in the medial canthal region and on the eyelashes is noticeable to the family, as is the increased tearing. Crusting

Questions

Excessive Tearing

- How old was the child when the excessive tearing appeared?
- Are one or both eyes affected?
- How does the eye appear? How has its appearance changed?
- Is there a family history of infantile glaucoma?
- Is the child photophobic or light sensitive (eg, closes the eyes in bright sunlight)?
- Has the child had any persistent, watery discharge?
- Does the child have difficulty opening the affected eye on awakening in the morning or after a nap?

along the eyelashes caused by drying of the mucoid material is usually noted when children awaken in the morning or after a nap. Mucopurulent discharge may be noted if an associated acute infection is present (dacryocystitis).

Physical Examination

A careful examination of the eyes in infants includes inspection, evaluation of extraocular movements, and funduscopic examination. Funduscopic examination may be difficult in this age group, but bilateral red reflexes should at least be elicited. Signs of **dacryostenosis,** which usually appear days to weeks after birth, include tearing, mucoid discharge, and crusting of the eyelids. Tearing may be as mild as an increased wetness of the affected eye; this is best evaluated prior to disturbing the child. Visible overflow of tears from the affected eye is not unusual, and is typically seen when the eye is irritated (eg, due to cold or wind). If dacryostenosis is present, there may be associated erythema and edema of the eyelids. Dacryocystitis may also spread to the surrounding tissues, producing a periorbital cellulitis; systemic signs of infection such as fever may be noted. Gentle pressure along the medial canthal region over the lacrimal sac may produce a reflux of tears or mucoid discharge onto the surface of the eye, thus confirming the diagnosis of obstruction.

Laboratory Tests

Routine laboratory assessment is generally not necessary.

Management

Spontaneous resolution of dacryostenosis is common by 6 to 8 months of age. The primary medical treatment of uncomplicated nasolacrimal duct obstruction consists of **local massage** and **cleansing** beginning when the symptoms are noted. Parents are instructed to massage the nasolacrimal duct several times a day by applying firm, downward pressure over the medial canthal region with their finger and then sliding the finger down toward the mouth (Crigler maneuver) (see Figure 78-1). This maneuver attempts to move fluid trapped within the nasolacrimal sac down through the duct in an attempt to break the obstruction with hydrostatic pressure. Parents may be asked to cleanse the eyes with warm water before performing this maneuver. Antibiotic ointments and drops should be prescribed only if the discharge is purulent or associated conjunctivitis is evident.

Controversy exists regarding when probing of the nasolacrimal duct should be performed. Some ophthalmologists prefer probing the duct before children are 6 months of age because prior to this time the procedure may be performed in the office without general anesthesia. Others state that more than 80% of obstructions resolve with conservative medical management by 6 months of age and prefer to delay probing until the age of 9 to 12 months. At this age the procedure needs to be performed under general anesthesia. Deciding when to proceed with the probing depends on the standard of practice within the community, the severity of symptoms, the response to medical management, and the level of parental concern.

Ophthalmologic referral is necessary for affected infants by 6 months of age if the obstruction has not resolved. Referral should be made sooner if symptoms are severe or infections recur.

Prognosis

Most cases of dacryostenosis resolve spontaneously during the first year of life without further sequelae. If tear duct probing is necessary, it is 90% to 95% successful if performed before 13 months of age. The success rate drops to 70% between 13 to 15 months and 50% over 18 months.

CONGENITAL GLAUCOMA

Epidemiology

Congenital or infantile glaucoma, a serious cause of excessive tearing, is quite rare; the incidence is about 1 in 10,000 live births. Although glaucoma may be present at birth, onset during the first few weeks to months of life is more common. Approximately 25% of cases are diagnosed at birth and 80% by 1 year of age. The severity of the disease is worse with earlier onset. Most affected infants are male; the male-female ratio in older infants is 2:1. Infantile glaucoma seems to have a multifactorial inheritance pattern, but most cases are sporadic. In families with one affected child or a parental history of infantile glaucoma, the chance of having a child with glaucoma is about 5%. Although glaucoma may be unilateral or bilateral, most children (75%–90%) who present before 3 months of age have bilateral glaucoma.

Clinical Presentation

In addition to excessive tearing, other clinical signs of infantile glaucoma include blepharospasm (spasmodic blinking of the eyelids), photophobia, corneal enlargement and corneal haziness due to corneal edema, progressive enlargement of the eye (buphthalmos), and cupping and atrophy of the optic nerve (Dx Box).

Pathophysiology

Glaucoma is the most serious and potentially sight-threatening etiology for excessive production of tears. Glaucoma refers to an increase in intraocular pressure that is severe enough to damage the eye and alter vision. In infants and children, glaucoma is usually a result of a developmental abnormality of the iridocorneal angle, interfering with drainage of aqueous humor from the anterior chamber. Young infants differ from adults in that the globe in infants' eyes is distensible; the increased intraocular pressure not only produces corneal enlargement and edema but also expands the globe itself. Breakdown of the corneal epithelium and resultant irritation of the eyes produce reflex tearing and photophobia. Untreated glaucoma may lead to optic nerve damage with resultant loss of visual acuity, decreased visual field, and even blindness. Glaucoma in children younger than 3 years is referred to broadly as infantile glaucoma, and glaucoma that occurs in children between 3 and 20 years of age is called juvenile glaucoma. Infantile glaucoma is further classified as being primary or secondary. Primary glaucoma refers to isolated abnormalities of the iridocorneal angle, whereas secondary glaucoma may be associated with other ocular or systemic diseases. Juvenile glaucoma is a form of open-angle glaucoma.

Differential Diagnosis

Excessive tearing may be due to increased production or to obstruction to outflow (see Box 78-1). Infants with increased production of tears will demonstrate rhinorrhea in association with epiphora, a finding that distinguishes glaucoma from dacryostenosis. Rhinorrhea is not associated with dacryostenosis because the nasolacrimal duct is obstructed and no tears drain out of the nose. Ocular irritation as occurs with conjunctivitis, corneal abrasion, or a foreign body under the eyelid can also produce excessive tearing, especially in older children. Allergies are also associated with excessive tearing due to overproduction.

Disorders associated with outflow obstruction include dacryostenosis, anomalies of the lacrimal drainage system (mucoceles of the lacrimal sac and atresia of the lacrimal punctum or canaliculus), nasal congestion, and craniofacial anomalies involving the midface.

Evaluation

A corneal diameter greater than 12 mm in infants is suggestive of infantile glaucoma. Corneal edema is more common in younger infants (<3 months of age) and may cause the red reflex to appear dull in the affected eye. The optic cup may be enlarged. A cup-to-disk ratio greater than 0.3 or an asymmetry of the ratio between the eyes may indicate glaucoma.

As in adults, loss of visual fields occurs in children with glaucoma. Visual fields are difficult to evaluate in young children because of their inability to cooperate with the examination.

Management

Suspected cases of glaucoma should be referred to an ophthalmologist immediately for further evaluation, including measurement of intraocular pressure. Pressures greater than 20 mm Hg are suggestive of glaucoma (normal pressures are 10–20 mm Hg in infants and young children as well as in adults).

Surgery is the primary treatment. The goal is to normalize intraocular pressure and minimize irreversible corneal and optic nerve damage.

Prognosis

Infantile glaucoma, if left untreated, may progress to blindness. The visual prognosis depends on several factors, including the age at onset of glaucoma (the earlier the onset, the worse the prognosis), the amount of optic nerve damage, and the degree of myopia caused by the enlargement of the eye. In addition, amblyopia, secondary to either deprivation due to corneal opacities or unequal refractive errors, is often seen (see Chapter 76).

CASE RESOLUTION

The infant presented in the case history at the beginning of the chapter has dacryostenosis. She can be managed with medical treatment such as local massage and cleansing at this stage. If her symptoms persist beyond the age of 6 months, consultation with an ophthalmologist is recommended.

Selected References

Beck AD, Lynch MG. Pediatric glaucoma. *Focal Points: Clinical Modules for Ophthalmologists.* Module 5. San Francisco, CA: American Academy of Ophthalmology; 1997;XV:1–14

Becker BB. The treatment of congenital dacryocystocele. *Am J Ophthalmol.* 2006;142:835–838

Guez A, Dureau P. Diagnosis and treatment of tearing in infancy. *Arch Pediatr.* 2009;16(5):496–499

Howard CW. The baby with too many tears: what to do and how to do it. *Int Pediatr.* 1990;5:239–242

Isenberg SJ, Apt L, McCarty J, Cooper LL, Lim L, Del Signore M. Development of tearing in preterm and term neonates. *Arch Ophthalmol.* 1998;116:773–776

Kushner BJ. The management of nasolacrimal duct obstruction in children between 18 months and 4 years old. *J AAPOS.* 1998;2:57–60

Lavrich JB, Nelson LB. Disorders of the lacrimal system apparatus. *Pediatr Clin North Am.* 1993;40:767–776

Olitsky S, Medow N, Rogers G. Diagnosis and treatment of congenital nasolacrimal duct obstruction. *J Pediatr Ophthalmol Strabismus.* 2007;44:80–83

Paysse EA, Coats DK, Bernstein JM, et al. Management and complications of congenital dacryocele with concurrent intranasal mucocele. *J AAPOS.* 2000;4:46–53

Pediatric Eye Disease Investigator Group; Repka MX, Chandler DL, Beck RW, et al. Primary treatment of nasolacrimal duct obstruction with probing in children younger than 4 years. *Ophthalmology.* 2008;115(3):577–584

Robb R. Nasolacrimal duct obstruction in children. *Focal Points: Clinical Modules for Ophthalmologists.* Module 8. San Francisco, CA: American Academy of Ophthalmology; 2004;XXII;1–10

Schnall BM, Christion CJ. Conservative treatment of congenital dacryocele. *J Pediatr Ophthalmol Strabismus.* 1996;33:219–222

Schwartz BA, Manley DR. Disorders of the lacrimal apparatus in infancy and childhood. In: Nelson LB, ed. *Pediatric Ophthalmology.* 4th ed. Philadelphia, PA: W. B. Saunders; 1998:345–352

Stamper RL, Lieberman MF, Drake MV. *Becker-Shaffer's Diagnosis and Therapy of the Glaucomas.* 7th ed. St Louis, MO: Mosby; 1999

Wagner RS. Glaucoma in children. *Pediatr Clin North Am.* 1993;40:855–867

CHAPTER 79

Neck Masses

Stanley H. Inkelis, MD, and Casey Buitenhuys, MD

CASE STUDY

A 2-year-old boy is brought to the office with a 1-day history of an enlarging red, tender "bump" beneath his right mandible. He has a fever (temperature: 101.6°F [38.5°C]) and sores around his nose, upper lip, and cheek. These sores have been present for 3 days and have not responded to an over-the-counter antibiotic ointment. He had an upper respiratory tract infection 1 week ago, which has almost entirely resolved. He is otherwise in good health. The family has no history of tuberculosis or recent travel, and the child has not been playing with cats or other animals.

The physical examination is completely normal except for fever, mild rhinorrhea, honey-crusted lesions on the nares and upper lip, and a 4 × 5-cm, right submandibular neck mass that is erythematous, warm, and tender to palpation.

Questions

1. What are the common causes of neck masses in children?
2. What steps are involved in the evaluation of children with neck masses?
3. What clinical findings suggest that neck masses are neoplasms? When should neck masses be biopsied or removed?
4. What is involved in the treatment of the different types of neck masses in children?
5. When should children with neck masses be referred for further consultation?

Neck masses are any swellings or enlargements of the structures in the area between the inferior mandible and the clavicle. Normal variants, such as the angle of the mandible or tip of the mastoid, may occasionally appear as swellings, and parents sometimes confuse these with neck masses. If the swelling is not a normal structure, a well-directed history and physical examination usually determine the etiology.

Lymphadenopathy from viral or bacterial throat infections is the most common cause of neck masses in children. Therefore, neck masses are common because children frequently have sore throats. Most parents know about swollen lymph glands, and they usually do not seek medical advice unless the glands become very large or do not recede in a few days. Neck masses in children may have many other causes besides lymphadenopathy. Most of these masses may be categorized as inflammatory, neoplastic, traumatic, or congenital in origin. A well-described mnemonic in the adult literature, KITTENS, can summate many of the causes of neck masses in children as well (Table 79-1).

Epidemiology

Most neck masses are benign. Almost 50% of all 2-year-old children and up to 90% of children between 4 and 8 years of age have palpable cervical lymph nodes. Although more than 25% of malignant tumors in children are found in the head and neck region (this is the primary site in only 5%), less than 2% of suspicious head and neck masses are malignant.

The epidemiology of neck masses of infectious origin depends on the infectious agent itself, geographic location of the child, and the child's immediate environment. Neck masses of viral origin may be related to focal infection of the oropharynx or respiratory tract but are often associated with generalized adenopathy. Neck masses of bacterial origin typically occur from normal bacterial flora of the nose, mouth, pharynx, and skin that secondarily spreads to lymph nodes. These organisms are not usually transmitted from person to person. Pathologic flora such as group A streptococcus and *Mycobacterium tuberculosis* that result in neck masses can spread by human-to-human contact, however. Additionally, cat scratch disease is caused by *Bartonella henselae*, a vector-borne pathogen.

Clinical Presentation

Children with neck masses present in a variety of ways depending on the etiology of the mass. Typically a swelling or enlargement in the neck, which parents often notice more than children, is evident. Associated signs and symptoms include fever, upper respiratory tract infection, sore throat, ear pain, pain or tenderness over the mass, changes in skin color over the mass, skin lesions of the head or neck, and dental caries or infections (Dx Box). Malignant tumors are usually slow-growing, firm, fixed, non-tender masses. Congenital neck masses and benign tumors, which have frequently been present since birth or early infancy, are soft, smooth, and cyst-like and may be recurrent. Neck masses associated with trauma are often rapidly evolving and may lead to airway obstruction. Temporal

Table 79-1. KITTENS Mnemonic for Neck Masses		
K	**Congenital/Developmental Anomalies**	• Thyroglossal duct cyst • Branchial cleft cyst • Dermoid cyst • Vascular malformation
I	**Infectious/Inflammatory**	• Lymphadenitis/cervical adenopathy • Viral adenitis (multiple causes) • Bacterial adenitis (multiple causes)
T	**Trauma**	• Hematoma • Pseudoaneurysm • Laryngocele
T	**Toxic**	• Thyroid toxicosis
E	**Endocrine**	• Thyroid neoplasms • Parathyroid neoplasms
N	**Neoplasms**	• Salivary gland • Parapharyngeal space • Lipoma • Lymphoma
S	**Systemic Disease**	• Sarcoidosis • Sjögren syndrome • Kimura disease • Castleman disease

Table 79-2. Rule of Sevens[a]	
Mass duration	*Likely mass etiology*
7 minutes	Trauma
7 days	Inflammation/infection
7 months	Neoplastic
7 years	Congenital

[a] Adapted from Skandalakis LJ, Skandalakis JE, Skandalakis PN, eds. *Surgical Anatomy and Technique.* New York, NY: Springer; 2009.

development of neck masses is a helpful predictor of mass etiology. Skandalakis' rule of seven's may be applied and adapted to pediatric neck masses (Table 79- 2).

Pathophysiology

The pathophysiology of neck masses in children is dependent on etiology. Most neck masses are related to inflammation or infection of lymph nodes. Enlargement of lymph nodes usually results from proliferation of intrinsic lymphocytes or histiocytes already present in the lymph node (eg, lymphadenopathy caused by a viral

Dx Neck Masses

Inflammatory/Infectious
• Swelling or enlargement in the neck
• Fever
• Sore throat, dental infection, skin infection of head or neck
• Pain or tenderness over the mass (usually)

Neoplastic
• Slowly enlarging mass
• Unilateral, discrete
• Firm or rubbery
• Fixed to tissue
• Deep within the fascia
• Non-tender (usually)

Traumatic
• Rapidly enlarging mass
• Hematoma
• Acute airway obstruction

Congenital
• Enlargement in neck (usually present since birth or soon after)
• Soft, smooth, cyst-like
• Non-tender (unless infected)
• Recurrent

infection) or from infiltration of extrinsic cells (eg, lymphadenitis, metastatic tumor). Neck masses from trauma occur from leakage of fluid into the neck, and congenital anatomical abnormalities become apparent because of fluid collection or infection of the defect. The parotid gland may be enlarged from inflammation (eg, blocked salivary gland duct), infection (eg, mumps), or tumor (eg, pleomorphic adenoma), but the swelling primarily involves the face rather than the neck and obscures the angle of the jaw. Other salivary glands may be infected or obstructed and may cause submandibular swelling, erythema, and tenderness.

Differential Diagnosis

Neck masses in children are usually the result of inflammation or infection of lymph nodes, tumors of lymph nodes and other neck structures, trauma, and congenital lesions. The location of the mass is often a clue to its etiology (Figure 79-1).

Lymphadenopathy/Lymphadenitis

Lymphadenopathy is lymph node enlargement or hyperplasia secondary to localized infection or antigenic stimulation proximal to the involved node or nodes. Because lymphoid tissue steadily increases until puberty, palpable lymph nodes, including those in the cervical area, are a common, normal finding in children. Any lymph node in the neck larger than 10 mm qualifies as cervical lymphadenopathy.

The most common cause of cervical lymphadenopathy is a viral infection of the upper respiratory tract. Lymphadenopathy usually begins and resolves with the acute infection. Occasionally the swelling remains for several days or months, however, and children

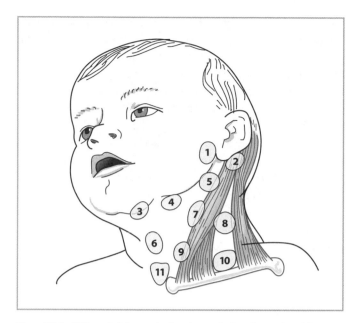

Figure 79-1. Differential diagnosis of neck mass by location. 1. Parotid—cystic hygroma, hemangioma, lymphadenitis, parotitis, Sjögren and Caffey-Silverman syndromes, lymphoma. 2. Postauricular—lymphadenitis, branchial cleft cyst (1st), squamous epithelial cyst. 3. Submental—lymphadenitis, cystic hygroma, thyroglossal duct cyst, dermoid, sialoadenitis. 4. Submandibular—lymphadenitis, cystic hygroma, sialoadenitis, tumor, cystic fibrosis. 5. Jugulodiagastic—lymphadenitis, squamous epithelial cyst, branchial cleft cyst (1st), parotid tumor, normal-transverse process C2, styloid process. 6. Midline neck—lymphadenitis, thyroglossal duct cyst, dermoid, laryngocele, normal hyoid, thyroid. 7. Sternomastoid (anterior)—lymphadenitis, branchial cleft cyst (2nd, 3rd) pilomatrixoma, rare tumors. 8. Spinal accessory—lymphadenitis, lymphoma, metastasis from nasopharynx. 9. Paratracheal—thyroid, parathyroid, esophageal diverticulum. 10. Supraclavicular—cystic hygroma, lipoma, lymphoma, metastasis, normal fat pad, pneumatocele of upper lobe. 11. Suprasternal—thyroid, lipoma, dermoid, thymus, mediastinal mass. (From May M. Neck masses in children: diagnosis and treatment. *Pediatr Ann.* 1976;5:S18–S35, with permission from SLACK Inc.)

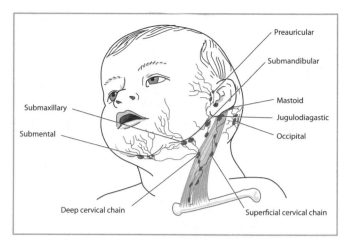

Figure 79-2. The lymphatic drainage and lymph nodes involved in infants and children with cervical lymphadenitis. (Reproduced with permission from Feigin RD, Cherry JD, eds. *Textbook of Pediatric Infectious Diseases.* 5th ed. Philadelphia, PA: Saunders; 2004:186.)

present because of parental concern. Bacterial pharyngitis, usually from infection with group A beta-hemolytic streptococcus (GABHS), is often associated with cervical lymphadenopathy. Cervical as well as generalized lymphadenopathy may be seen in children with systemic illness (eg, Kawasaki disease, sarcoid, HIV). Cat-scratch disease, toxoplasmosis, fungal infection, and mycobacterial and atypical mycobacterial infections may be associated with lymphadenopathy that may later progress to lymphadenitis. Viral illnesses, including Epstein-Barr virus (EBV) (mononucleosis), adenovirus, enterovirus, herpes simplex virus, human herpesvirus 6 (HHV-6), and cytomegalovirus (CMV) commonly cause lymphadenopathy and lymphadenitis.

Lymphadenitis is infection or inflammation of the lymph node that occurs when microorganisms and neutrophils infiltrate the node, leading to necrosis and abscess formation. This condition is usually associated with proximal bacterial infection that drains to the affected nodes by connecting afferent lymphatic channels. Lymphadenitis is often a progression of disease, resulting in enlarged nodes that measure 2 to 6 cm. These nodes, which are typical of

bacterial disease, are often termed hot nodes, and they are erythematous, warm, tender, and sometimes fluctuant. Cold nodes or cold lymphadenitis usually represents subacute or chronic inflammation of lymph nodes typical in illnesses such as cat-scratch disease, mycobacterial infection, or toxoplasmosis. Unlike hot nodes, cold nodes are not warm to the touch and are usually not as tender. They are typically not suppurative and may be difficult to distinguish from nodes that are simply enlarged (Figure 79-2).

Staphylococcus aureus and group A streptococcus are responsible for 50% to 90% of cases of acute unilateral cervical lymphadenitis. These organisms spread from a primary site to the lymph nodes draining those sites. Common primary sites of infection are the throat; teeth and gums; and skin (lesions), particularly on the scalp or ears. Infections at these sites may result from trauma, such as scratches or scabs, or from primary infection, such as impetigo. Anaerobic oral flora constitute a small portion of causes for bacterial cervical adenitis, especially in older children with poor dentition. *Staphylococcus aureus* or group B streptococcus usually causes cervical lymphadenitis in neonates or very young infants. Such staphylococcal infections, which are often nosocomially spread from contact in the newborn nursery, present as discrete masses. Group B streptococcus causes the "cellulitis-adenitis" syndrome, which presents as cervical adenitis associated with a facial cellulitis. *Pseudomonas aeruginosa* is an unusual cause of cervical adenitis in newborns.

Mycobacterial disease must always be considered in children of all ages who present with cervical adenitis particularly involving posterior cervical nodes. The child with *M tuberculosis* cervical adenitis often has multiple nodes, sometimes bilateral, usually non-tender, and usually not erythematous or warm. These children are typically older, commonly reside in an urban setting, have a history of tuberculosis exposure, and often have an abnormal chest radiograph. Intradermal placement of a purified protein derivative (PPD) often produces more than 15 mm of induration in most children with typical mycobacterial infection. A reaction of 5 to 14 mm may be caused by tuberculous or nontuberculous mycobacterial infection. Atypical mycobacterial infection usually occurs in children between 1 and 6 years of age with unilateral rather than bilateral lymph node enlargement and a normal chest radiograph.

Cat-scratch disease should be considered in children who have cats or kittens or who play with them. The infection may result from a cat scratch or from a cat licking a child's broken skin. If the inoculum is near the head and neck area, cervical adenitis develops. Contact with the hand may result in axillary lymphadenitis. Occasionally generalized lymphadenopathy is present. An associated non-painful papule or papules where the cat scratch or lick occurred may be apparent. *Bartonella henselae* has been identified as the organism causing cat-scratch disease.

Toxoplasmosis may be accompanied by adenitis, usually in the posterior cervical area. Nodes are painless and may fluctuate in size, and children are often asymptomatic. Multiple lymph nodes are involved in about one-third to one-half of cases.

Children presenting with recurrent cervical adenitis and recurrent fevers may have PFAPA syndrome characterized by periodic fever, aphthous stomatitis, pharyngitis, and adenitis (cervical). This entity usually occurs in children younger than 5 years and can be aborted with steroids.

Kikuchi disease, or histiocytic necrotizing lymphadenitis, has an Asian and female predilection and is characterized by fever, leukopenia, and cervical lymphadenopathy. The illness is self-limited, and follow-up is recommended because of a possible association with systemic lupus erythematosus.

Less common bacterial, viral, and fungal causes of cervical adenitis are listed in Box 79-1.

Tumors

Compared with other neck masses, **malignant neck tumors** occur rarely; nevertheless, they should be considered in any children with rapidly enlarging or persistent neck masses. Hodgkin disease and non-Hodgkin lymphoma are the most frequent cause of head and neck malignancies in children, accounting for almost 60% of the cases. Rhabdomyosarcomas are the next most frequent head and neck malignancy followed by thyroid tumors, neuroblastoma, and nasopharyngeal carcinomas. Age is an important factor in determining the likelihood of specific tumors. Neuroblastoma and rhabdomyosarcoma are the most common tumor types in children younger than 6 years. Non-Hodgkin lymphoma typically occurs in preadolescence, and Hodgkin disease and thyroid carcinoma are the most common malignancies in adolescents.

Benign neck tumors, with the exception of those mentioned later in the discussion of congenital lesions, are uncommon. They include epidermoid inclusion cysts, lipomas, fibromas, neurofibromas, pilomatrixomas (benign skin neoplasms of hair follicle origin), keloids, goiters, and ranulas (intraoral mucocysts).

Trauma

Trauma to the neck may be associated with bleeding and edema. Large hematomas that affect vital structures are potentially life-threatening. Significant trauma and structural injury usually accompany neck hematomas. In children with mild injuries and neck hematomas, bleeding disorders are a possible cause of the hematoma. Twisting injuries to the neck may lead to muscle spasm of the sternocleidomastoid muscle (torticollis) and an apparent mass that is the contracted muscle. Additonally, intramuscular hematoma and/or bleeding from vaginal delivery may cause torticollis in the neonatal period. The neck is bent toward the side of the affected sternocleidomastoid muscle. Child abuse should also be considered in children who have neck injuries that are not consistent with their histories.

A foreign body in the neck may present as a mass because of the foreign body itself (eg, piece of glass or metal, bullet) or surrounding inflammation. A crepitant neck mass following trauma to the neck or chest suggests subcutaneous emphysema from tracheal injury or a pneumomediastinum. Crepitant neck masses may also be seen secondary to pneumomediastinum in children with obstructive lung diseases such as asthma or cystic fibrosis.

Congenital Lesions

Children with congenital neck lesions can present with a neck mass in early infancy or later in childhood. Some congenital lesions are not discovered until adulthood. The most common of these benign lesions are thyroglossal duct cysts, branchial cleft cysts, lymphatic malformations (cystic hygromas/lymphangiomas), and hemangiomas (Figure 79-3).

Thyroglossal duct cysts are almost always midline in the neck and inferior to the hyoid bone. They usually move upward with

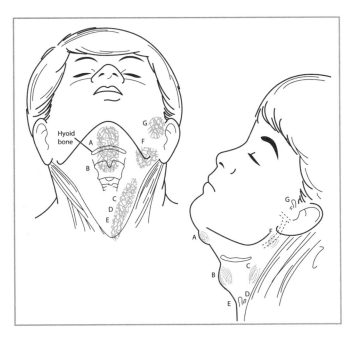

Figure 79-3. Head and neck congenital lesions seen in children in frontal and lateral views. The shaded areas denote the distribution in which a given lesion may be found. A. Dermoid cyst. B. Thyroglossal duct cyst. C. Second branchial cleft appendage. D. Second branchial cleft sinus. E. Second branchial cleft cyst. F. First branchial pouch defect. G. Preauricular sinus or appendage. (Reproduced with permission from Fleisher GR, Ludwig S, eds. *Textbook of Pediatric Emergency Medicine.* 5th ed. Philadelphia, PA: Lippincott Williams & Wilkins; 2006:1594.)

Box 79-1. Differential Diagnosis of Neck Masses		
Cervical Lymphadenopathy/Lymphadenitis	***Tumor***	***Immunologic Disorders***
Bacterial origin	**Malignant**	Local hypersensitivity reaction (sting or bite)
Staphylococcus aureus (methicillin sensitive)	Hodgkin disease	Pseudolymphoma (from phenytoin)
Staphylococcus aureus (methicillin resistant)	Non-Hodgkin lymphoma	Serum sickness
Group A beta-hemolytic streptococcus	Lymphosarcoma	Sarcoidosis
Mycobacterium tuberculosis	Rhabdomyosarcoma	Caffey-Silverman syndrome
Atypical mycobacteria	Neuroblastoma	Kawasaki disease
Cat-scratch disease *(Bartonella henselae)*	Leukemia	Systemic lupus erythematosus
Anaerobes	Langerhans cell histiocytosis	Juvenile rheumatoid arthritis
Gram-negative enteric bacteria	Thyroid tumors	Kikuchi disease (necrotizing lymphadenitis)
Haemophilus influenzae	Nasopharyngeal squamous cell carcinoma	Kimura disease
Plague	Salivary gland carcinoma	
Actinomycosis	**Benign**	**Miscellaneous**
Diphtheria	Epidermoid cyst	Sialadenitis
Tularemia	Lipoma	Parotitis
Brucellosis	Fibroma	Storage disorders
Syphilis	Neurofibroma	Niemann-Pick disease
Group B streptococcus (neonates)	Pilomatrixoma	Gaucher disease
Viral origin	Keloid	Obstructive airway disease (asthma, cystic fibrosis)
Epstein-Barr virus (infectious mononucleosis)	Goiter	
Adenovirus	Osteochondroma	
Cytomegalovirus	Teratoma (may be malignant)	
Herpes simplex virus, types 1 and 2	Ranula	
Enterovirus		
HIV	***Congenital Disorders***	
Measles	**Hemangioma**	
Rubella	Cystic hygroma (lymphangioma)	
Human herpes virus 6	Branchial cleft cyst	
Influenza virus	Thyroglossal duct cyst	
Fungal origin	Laryngocele	
Histoplasmosis	Dermoid cyst	
Coccidioidomycosis	Cervical rib	
Aspergillosis	Sternocleidomastoid tumor	
Candidiasis	**Trauma**	
Sporotrichosis	Hematoma (acute or organized)	
Cryptococcosis	Subcutaneous emphysema	
Parasitic origin	Foreign body	
Toxoplasmosis	Arteriovenous malformation	
Leishmaniasis		

tongue protrusion or swallowing. Most branchial cleft cysts occur anterior to the middle one-third of the sternocleidomastoid muscle. Branchial cleft sinus tracts appear as slit-like openings anterior to the lower third of the sternocleidomastoid muscle and may present as neck masses if they become infected. Thyroglossal duct cysts and branchial cleft cysts may also present for the first time as infected neck masses.

Cystic hygromas are usually large, soft, easily compressible masses found in the posterior triangle behind the sternocleidomastoid muscle in the supraclavicular fossa. They transilluminate well. Two-thirds of cystic hygromas are present at birth, and 80% to 90% are identified before 3 years of age. They are more common on the left side of the neck. Cystic hygromas occasionally become secondarily infected, with findings of erythema, warmth, and tenderness.

Hemangiomas are usually not present at birth but appear in early infancy and may enlarge rapidly. In most cases, they recede spontaneously by 9 years of age. They are usually much smaller than cystic hygromas, do not transilluminate, and may be recognized by their reddish color (capillary or strawberry hemangioma) or by a bluish hue of the overlying skin (cavernous hemangioma).

Small infants who present with torticollis should be examined for a sternocleidomastoid mass ("tumor"), which represents fibrosis and contracture of that sternocleidomastoid muscle so that the head tilts toward the affected side with the chin rotating to the opposite side. Contusion of the sternocleidomastoid muscle from traumatic extraction of the head during delivery with subsequent hemorrhage and healing has been implicated as the cause of the fibrotic mass. However, it is more likely that this mass occurs prior to birth because it contains mature fibrous tissue. In addition, the mass may be present following cesarean section and is associated with hip dysplasia and other congenital lesions, suggesting that the condition is related to abnormal positioning in utero. Venous occlusion of the sternocleidomastoid muscle either in utero or at the time of delivery has also been proposed as a cause.

Evaluation

History

A thorough history is important in establishing the etiology of the neck mass (Questions Box).

Questions

Neck Masses

- How old is the child?
- How long has the neck mass been present?
- What signs and symptoms are associated with the neck mass?
- Has the child been exposed to tuberculosis?
- Has the child ever drunk any unpasteurized cow's milk?
- Has the child been in contact with any cats or kittens? Rabbits? Other animals?
- Has the child traveled to areas where endemic diseases such as histoplasmosis or coccidioidomycosis are prevalent?
- Has the child suffered any trauma recently?
- Does the child have any allergies?
- Does the child have any risk factors for HIV?

Physical Examination

A general physical examination should be performed. The neck mass should be examined for anatomical location, color, size, shape, consistency, tenderness, fluctuance, and mobility. The mass should also be measured. The head, neck, and face should be examined for lesions, most often infections, that drain into neck lymph nodes. Lesions can frequently be found on the scalp, neck, face, ears, mouth, teeth, tongue, gums, and throat. Hairstyles such as tight braids can sometimes provide ports of entry for bacteria. Occasionally, sinus tracts or fistulas may be the entry point of infection. In addition, other lymph node groups should be examined to determine if the lymphadenopathy is local or generalized. Particular attention should be paid to the supraclavicular area because enlarged supraclavicular nodes are more frequently associated with malignant pathology such as Hodgkin disease. The chest should be examined for use of accessory muscles, equality of breath sounds, and wheezing. The abdomen should be examined for hepatosplenomegaly.

Laboratory Tests

Laboratory tests are rarely indicated in children with cervical lymphadenopathy or lymphadenitis of acute onset. Although a rapid streptococcal antigen detection test or throat culture is helpful in children with suspected streptococcal sore throat, it may be unnecessary if antibiotic therapy is empirically prescribed for the lymphadenitis. If the adenitis is fluctuant, aspiration and culture may be helpful in determining the specific bacteriologic diagnosis. Fine-needle aspiration cytology and polymerase chain reaction assays may help differentiate between tuberculous and nontuberculous mycobacterial disease. Superficial cervical nodes or axillary nodes, if enlarged, are appropriate first-line aspiration sites due to their superficial nature. In addition, a PPD test should be applied to all children who present with lymphadenitis.

If the adenitis does not resolve or improve after 2 to 3 days of observation or therapy, laboratory tests directed by the history and physical examination should be considered. A complete blood cell count (CBC) with differential and a monospot or serologic antibody tests for EBV may be helpful in the diagnosis of infectious mononucleosis. If the mass in the neck is a hematoma and a bleeding disorder is suspected, a CBC with platelet count, prothrombin time, and partial thromboplastin time should be obtained. Possible additional tests include an erythrocyte sedimentation rate, C-reactive protein and, if indicated, serologic tests for toxoplasmosis, CMV, HHV-6, coccidioidomycosis, histoplasmosis, tularemia, *B henselae,* and syphilis should be performed. Skin tests for fungi should be considered in those patients coming from endemic areas. These tests should be placed after serologic tests are performed so that false-positive serologic test results are not obtained.

Similar laboratory tests should be considered for children who present for the first time with enlarged or enlarging lymph nodes of long duration or those who do not respond after 2 weeks of antibiotic therapy. The physician may choose to do more of these laboratory tests at the initial evaluation or after a therapeutic trial because the likelihood of viral lymphadenopathy decreases and the possibility of a more unusual etiology increases. HIV testing should also be considered.

Thyroid function tests should be considered in children with a thyroid mass or suspected thyroglossal duct cyst. An ultrasound or a thyroid scan should be considered for the child with a thyroid mass.

Unless cat-scratch disease is very likely, immediate lymph node biopsy is indicated for enlarged supraclavicular nodes or lymph nodes in the lower half of the neck, rapidly progressive and enlarging nodes, fixed nodes, nodes deep within the fascia, or firm or hard nodes. Children who have a persistent fever or weight loss should have a biopsy at 1 week if a diagnosis has not been established. Asymptomatic children without an established diagnosis should have a biopsy at 2 weeks if the node increases in size, at 4 to 6 weeks if the node is not increased in size but is persistent, and at 8 to 12 weeks if the node has not regressed to a normal size. In some cases, the initial biopsy is non-diagnostic but on subsequent biopsy a specific diagnosis may be made. Consequently, children with persistent adenopathy should be followed closely and be biopsied again if indicated. Fine-needle aspiration biopsy in children is controversial, but has some demonstrated benefits. It is being used more often to differentiate between benign and malignant disease and to potentially decrease the need for open biopsy. However, if malignancy is a consideration, consultation with an oncologist is advisable to determine the biopsy method of choice.

Imaging Studies

A chest radiograph should be obtained in all children with suspected tuberculosis or tumor (eg, enlarged supraclavicular nodes) as well as in children with crepitant neck masses or in those children in whom the diagnosis of the adenitis remains uncertain. If a foreign body in the neck is suspected, both anteroposterior and lateral neck radiographs should be obtained.

Almost all neck masses can be evaluated by ultrasonography, computed tomography (CT), or magnetic resonance imaging (MRI). Because there is no ionizing radiation associated with ultrasonography, it is quickly available, is noninvasive, and does not need sedation; it is considered by many to be the initial imaging study of choice, particularly for thyroid masses, thyroglossal duct cysts, branchial cleft cysts, and parotid masses. If malignancy is suspected or the mass cannot be delineated in the field of view, then MRI or CT may be more definitive studies. Ultrasonography with color Doppler is helpful in differentiating cystic from solid masses and determining if the mass is vascular. In addition, demonstration of a normal thyroid gland by ultrasound in patients with a thyroglossal duct cyst confirms a source of thyroid hormone. Consequently, a thyroid scan is not necessary.

Computed tomography and MRI scans provide better definition and extent of the mass. Computed tomography scan with contrast is the preferred method of imaging for deep neck abscesses that present with a neck mass and for enlarged salivary glands. Magnetic resonance imaging provides the best anatomical detail, and it is the preferred imaging study for children with vascular and lymphatic malformations and neoplasms; however, it is not as available as CT and often requires a greater degree of sedation.

Management

Neck masses are rarely acutely life-threatening. If neck masses impinge on the airway, children may experience stridor, hoarseness, drooling, increased

effort of breathing, unequal breath sounds, or evidence of shock. Resuscitation and stabilization should be initiated immediately. The algorithm in Figure 79-4 outlines the management of cervical lymphadenitis.

Children with lymphadenitis who do not appear toxic and have no evidence of sepsis may be treated empirically with **oral antibiotics** that cover *S aureus*, particularly methicillin-resistant *S aureus* (MRSA), and GABHS. Clindamycin or a combination of cephalexin

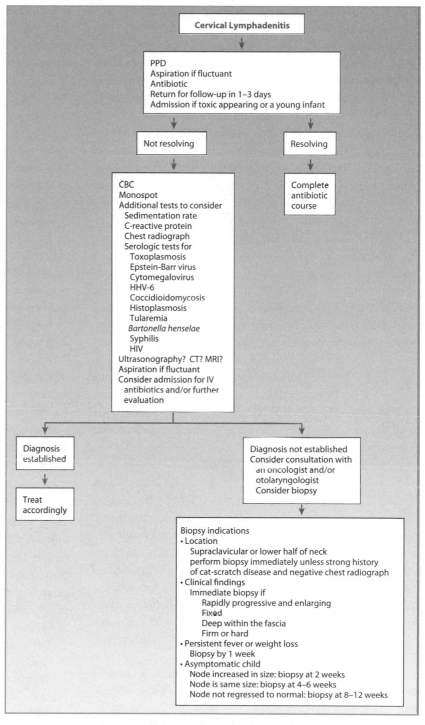

Figure 79-4. Management of cervical lymphadenitis. CBC, complete blood cell count; CT, computed tomography; HHV-6, human herpesvirus 6; HIV, human immunodeficiency virus; IV, intravenous; MRI, magnetic resonance imaging; PPD, purified protein derivative.

(administered until the culture from the lymph node, if available, for group A streptococcus is negative) and trimethoprim-sulfamethoxazole may be used to provide coverage for these organisms. If methicillin-susceptible *S aureus* (MSSA) is cultured and sensitivities are determined, a first-generation cephalosporin such as cephalexin (50 mg/kg/d, dicloxacillin (50 mg/kg/d), or amoxicillin/clavulanic acid (40 mg/kg/d [amoxicillin]) may provide satisfactory coverage. Treatment should be continued for a minimum of 10 days but for no less than 5 days after resolution of acute signs and symptoms. Lack of clinical improvement after 36 to 48 hours suggests that the diagnosis and proposed therapy need to be reevaluated.

Infants and small children, as well as those older children who do not respond to oral antibiotic therapy, may require admission for **intravenous antibiotics** such as clindamycin or vancomycin (especially for a potentially life-threatening infection) until culture results are available. If MSSA is cultured and sensitivities are determined, oxacillin or a cephalosporin may be satisfactory alternatives. Incision and drainage of large, fluctuant nodes that are clearly from bacterial disease should be done in consultation with an otolaryngologist or surgeon to promote resolution of the lymphadenitis. Alternatively, treatment by needle aspiration instead of incision and drainage has been advocated by some physicians. If *M tuberculosis*, atypical mycobacterial infection, or infection with *B henselae* is suspected, incision and drainage should not be done because persistent sinus tracts may result.

Atypical mycobacterial infection is generally unresponsive to treatment with antituberculous medications. **Surgical excision** of all visibly affected nodes, deep as well as superficial, is recommended. However, in cases where surgery is refused or is incomplete or disease is recurrent, macrolide monotherapy (clarithromycin or azithromycin) or a macrolide in combination with ethambutol or rifampin has been helpful in treating nontuberculous adenitis. Tuberculous mycobacterial adenitis usually responds to short-course medical therapy. Antituberculous medication for 6 to 9 months is recommended.

Lymphadenitis from cat-scratch disease usually resolves on its own. Antibiotic therapy is usually not indicated, but if children are severely ill or appear toxic with systemic cat-scratch disease, have hepatic or splenic involvement, are immunocompromised, develop meningoencephalitis, or are admitted for a suppurative adenitis, treatment with oral antibiotics such as azithromycin, rifampin, trimethoprim-sulfamethoxazole, or ciprofloxacin may be beneficial. If there is no improvement, the addition of parenteral gentamicin to the regimen may be considered. **Aspiration** is indicated to relieve symptoms in patients with fluctuant or painful suppurative nodes. Incision and drainage should not be done. Total removal of the node is sometimes necessary to effect a cure.

There is no specific therapy for lymphadenitis caused by *Toxoplasma gondii*. Excision of the affected node may be indicated if the diagnosis is questionable.

If a tumor is suspected, consultation with a pediatric oncologist is recommended. The mass should be biopsied for a definitive diagnosis. If it is malignant, a treatment plan should be generated with the appropriate consultants.

Congenital torticollis from fibrosis of the sternocleidomastoid muscle is best treated with nonoperative intervention. Repetitive passive range-of-motion exercises over several weeks usually result in loosening the tight muscle and increasing the range of motion.

Hemangiomas usually resolve by the time children are 9 years of age, and surgical intervention is rarely indicated. Recent literature has demonstrated a profound benefit with oral propranolol therapy in the management of hemangiomas. Oral propranolol therapy demonstrates a considerable flattening and effacement of both cutaneous and mucous membrane hemangiomas within 24 hours and marked improvement after weeks of propranolol therapy. While studies are still small and underpowered, recent evidence has supported a near 100% efficacy with oral propranolol for the treatment of life-threatening, vital-organ impairing (eg, vision loss), refractory, or disfiguring hemangiomas. Dosing is titrated up to 2mg/kg/day and continued for weeks until resolution of the hemangioma. Patients should be closely monitored for hypoglycemia, bradycardia, hypotension, and congestive heart failure during institution of therapy for adverse effects usually requiring consultation with a cardiologist and a short hospitalization. Corticosteroids, previously the mainline treatment modality for hemangiomas, are now considered an adjunctive treatment with propanolol. Additional therapies include interferon alfa-2a and various cytotoxic medications. Interferon alfa-2a has been associated with transient or permanent neurologic disabilities, so it is important to balance the benefits and risks of this medication.

Surgical excision is usually indicated for cystic hygromas (lymphangiomas), branchial cleft cysts, and thyroglossal duct cysts. A thyroid ultrasound should be performed before removal of a thyroglossal duct cyst to confirm that other thyroid tissue is not present. Endocrinologic consultation is recommended in these cases. Thyroid nodules in children may be cancerous, especially in children who have had irradiation to the head and neck region. Consultation with an endocrinologist and surgeon should be obtained. Goiters in children should be evaluated by an endocrinologist.

Prognosis

The prognosis for children with neck masses is generally excellent but differs depending on the cause. Children with an infectious etiology do very well if diagnosed and treated with appropriate antimicrobials. Mycobacterial lymphadenitis may result in sinus tract formation or disseminated disease. Surgical excision usually cures atypical mycobacterial infection. Cat-scratch disease is usually benign and self-limited. Encephalopathy is a rare complication of this disorder.

The prognosis for benign tumors of the neck is excellent. The outlook for children with malignant neck tumors depends on etiology of the tumor and the spread of the malignancy to other organs. Early diagnosis and treatment are clearly important in improving outcome.

Children with neck masses from trauma usually have had significant injury. The outcome often depends on establishment of an airway, provision of ventilatory support, and management of hemodynamic instability. Availability of surgical support is often essential to a good outcome.

Children with congenital lesions of the neck usually have an excellent prognosis. Some lesions resolve spontaneously, while others require simple surgical excision. Cystic hygromas may require multiple operations for complete removal because of their diffuse nature.

CASE RESOLUTION

In the case presented, the boy has signs and symptoms consistent with submandibular bacterial cervical lymphadenitis. The location of the neck mass in relation to the honey-crusted lesions (non-bullous impetigo) implicates spread of bacteria from the primary site of infection to the lymph nodes. Laboratory tests are unnecessary because the child does not appear septic. Culture of the impetigo may be helpful in determining if the organism causing the infection is MRSA. If the affected lymph node is fluctuant, aspiration of fluid for culture is indicated and incision and drainage should be considered. The child should be treated as an outpatient with an oral antibiotic directed against MRSA and GABHS, such as clindamycin or a combination of cephalexin and trimethoprim-sulfamethoxazole, as well as an analgesic for pain as needed. If MSSA is cultured and sensitivities are determined, cephalexin, amoxicillin-clavulanate acid, or dicloxicillin may be administered. If the child appears toxic, or if there is marked lymph node enlargement, the child should be admitted for intravenous antibiotics. A PPD skin test should be placed. The child should be followed up in 1 to 3 days for clinical improvement depending on the severity of the infection.

Selected References

Acierno SP, Waldhausen JHT. Congenital cervical cysts, sinuses and fistulae. *Otolaryngol Clin North Am.* 2007;40:161–176

Bauer PW, Lusk RP. Neck masses. In: Bluestone CD, Stool SE, Alper CM, et al, eds. *Pediatric Otolaryngology.* 4th ed. Philadelphia, PA: Saunders; 2003:1629–1647

Chadha NK, Forte V. Pediatric head and neck malignancies. *Curr Opin Otolaryngol Head Neck Surg.* 2009;6:471–476

Frieden IJ, Drolet BA. Propranolol for infantile hemangiomas: promise, peril, pathogenesis. *Pediatr Dermatol.* 2009;26(5):642–644

Gross E, Sichel JY. Congenital neck lesions. *Surg Clin N Am.* 86;2006:383–392

Holmes WJM, Mishra A, Gorst C, Liew SH. Propranolol as first-line treatment for rapidly proliferating infantile haemangiomas. *J Plast Reconstr Aesthet Surg.* 2010

Knight PJ, Mulne AF, Vassy LE. When is lymph node biopsy indicated in children with enlarged peripheral nodes? *Pediatrics.* 1982;69:391–396

Lawley LP, Siegfried E, Todd JL. Propanolol treatment for hemangioma of infancy: risks and recommendations. *Pediatr Dermatol.* 2009;26:610–614

Léauté-Labrèze C, Dumas de la Roque E, Hubiche T, et al. Propranolol for severe hemangiomas of infancy. *N Engl J Med.* 2008;358:2649–2651

Malley R. Lymphadenopathy. In: Fleisher GR, Ludwig S, eds. *Textbook of Pediatric Emergency Medicine.* 5th ed. Philadelphia, PA: Lippincott; 2006:421–428

Pasha R. *Otolaryngology: Head and Neck Surgery Clinical Reference Guide.* 2nd edition. San Diego, CA: Plural Publishing, Inc. 2006:79, 207

Pruden CM, McAneney CM. Neck mass. In: Fleisher GR, Ludwig S, eds. *Textbook of Pediatric Emergency Medicine.* 6th ed. Philadelphia, PA: Lippincott Williams and Wilkins; 2010:385–391

Sans V, de la Roque E, Berge J, et al. Propranolol for severe infantile hemangiomas: follow-up report. *Pediatrics.* 2009;124:e423–e431

Skandalakis JE. Neck. In: Skandalakis LJ, Skandalakis JE, Skandalakis PN, eds. *Surgical Anatomy and Technique.* 3rd ed. New York, NY: Springer; 2009:2

CHAPTER 80

Allergic Disease

Nasser Redjal, MD

CASE STUDY

A 3-year-old girl is rushed to the office by her mother after her daughter developed a pruritic rash, facial swelling, and hoarseness shortly after eating a peanut butter sandwich. Previously she has been well except for recurrent nasal congestion every spring that has responded to antihistamines. She has also had an intermittent skin rash that has been treated with topical steroid creams. She has never had an acute reaction before and has no history of asthma. Her father had asthma as a child.

Physical examination reveals a well-developed, 3-year-old girl with marked facial swelling and a **generalized rash** who is in mild respiratory distress. Vital signs, including blood pressure, are normal. Growth parameters are at the 50th percentile. The girl has a diffuse, blotchy,

erythematous rash with central wheals; a hoarse voice; and a mild expiratory wheeze on auscultation of her chest. The remainder of the examination is normal.

Questions

1. What are the various symptoms of allergic disease?
2. What is the appropriate evaluation of children with manifestations of allergic disease?
3. What allergens are common triggers for allergic symptoms?
4. What management is helpful in the treatment of children with manifestations of allergic disease?
5. Can allergic disease be prevented?

Allergic disease, which occurs frequently in the general population, is manifested in many ways. Asthma; atopic dermatitis; allergic rhinitis; allergic conjunctivitis; urticaria; angioedema; anaphylaxis; and food, insect, and drug allergies are all types of allergic diseases. Allergic symptoms result from the production of specific immunoglobulin E (IgE) antibody following exposure to a foreign antigen. The process has 2 steps. The first step is the sensitization or antibody induction stage. The individual develops IgE antibody against an inhaled, ingested, or injected substance. This newly formed IgE antibody adheres to circulating blood basophils or to tissue mast cells. The second step involves reexposure of a sensitized person to the allergen, which then binds to several specific IgE antibodies on the surface of immune cells. The release of inflammatory mediators causes the appearance of the characteristic features of allergic disease, which can range from rhinorrhea to sudden death. Similar non–IgE-mediated symptoms may occur, but these are not true allergic reactions. The reader should refer to Chapter 81 for details concerning asthma and Chapter 121 for a review of atopic dermatitis. This chapter focuses on the remaining manifestations of allergies, including food allergies.

Epidemiology

Allergic disease or some form of allergic symptoms is found in 12% to 20% of the general population. The prevalence of symptoms varies depending on the population being investigated. Factors such as age, genetic background, and place of residence are significant. Allergic rhinitis occurs in 10% of children, as does asthma. Up to 6% of children younger than 3 years develop food allergies. Urticaria occurs at some time in about 10% to 20% of the population.

It is generally accepted that if neither parent is atopic (has the allergic tendency to manufacture IgE on antigen exposure), then the chance that children will develop allergic symptoms is less than 1 in 5. If one parent is atopic, the risk doubles. If both parents are atopic, the chance is greater than 3 in 5.

Clinical Presentation

Children with allergic disease frequently present with persistent, clear rhinorrhea; sneezing; postnasal drip; or injected pruritic conjunctiva. Skin manifestations include dry, scaling, erythematous rashes; wheals; or subcutaneous swelling (Dx Box). A recurrent cough or wheezing on chest examination is further evidence of allergic disease.

Pathophysiology

Allergic rhinitis, like all allergic manifestations, is caused primarily by an antigen-antibody reaction involving IgE. Antigen-specific IgE is produced by the B lymphocytes of allergic patients on exposure to a particular antigen, which attaches to immune cell receptors located on basophils in the circulation and mast cells in the tissue. On reexposure, the antigen reacts with this specific IgE on the mast cells, releasing vasoactive mediators including histamine, leukotrienes, kinins, and prostaglandins. These mediators produce vasodilation and edema, and they also stimulate neural reflexes to produce mucous hypersecretion and sneezing. Eosinophils, and

Dx Allergic Disease

- Chronic, clear rhinorrhea
- Nasal congestion
- Conjunctival tearing and pruritus
- Skin findings of atopic dermatitis or urticaria
- Seasonal variability
- Occurrence of symptoms after exposure to an antigen
- Family history of allergic disease
- Conjunctival injection
- Wheezing
- Chronic cough
- Postnasal drip
- Repetitive sneezing
- Acute onset of symptoms following exposure to possible allergen

other inflammatory cells induced by chemotactic factors, enter the affected organ, releasing mediators, thereby worsening the inflammation and damaging tissues. Secretions and released tissue proteins worsen existing edema. Other immunologic mechanisms can also be involved.

Urticaria, the clinical rash produced by vasodilation and edema of the skin, is the allergic condition that occurs when histamine and other mediators such as prostaglandins and leukotrienes are released from the dermal mast cells. The antigen-specific IgE is located on these mast cells. Otherwise, the pathophysiology is similar to that of allergic rhinitis. Exposure to that antigen causes release of chemical mediators from the mast cells. Other mechanisms, including physical stimuli, can produce urticaria.

Angioedema is the extension of the urticarial process deeper into the dermis of the skin, producing circumscribed swelling. The mucous membranes may be affected. The pathophysiology is the same as for urticaria. A hereditary type of angioedema, which is not allergy related, is caused by the inherited deficiency of the C1 esterase inhibitor.

Anaphylaxis is an acute, systemic allergic reaction resulting from antigen-specific IgE on mast cells and basophils. The pathophysiology is similar to allergic rhinitis, but the reaction occurs in mast cells in many locations simultaneously, and prior sensitization to an allergen is essential. Anaphylactic reactions may be life-threatening. Vasodilation may be so severe that decreased venous return can lead to acute myocardial infarctions and arrhythmias. Reactions can occur in seconds or as late as 1 hour after exposure. Common antigens that precipitate anaphylactic reactions include injections of foreign serum, drugs, foods, and insect venom. Anaphylactoid reactions are clinically indistinguishable from anaphylaxis but are non—IgE-mediated, and include reactions to substances such as intravenous (IV) contrast media, opiates, and deferoxamine. The drug most frequently implicated in anaphylaxis is penicillin. Patients initially experience tightness and intense itching of the skin. Nausea, vomiting, and abdominal pain may ensue. Subsequently, the full spectrum of anaphylaxis appears.

A **food allergy** may produce any of the previously described allergic manifestations, including atopic dermatitis and asthma, as well as vomiting, diarrhea, and failure to thrive. Food intolerance, which has a non-immunologic pathogenesis, should be differentiated from food allergy, which is an IgE-mediated allergic reaction. The localization of the IgE-sensitized mast cells to that specific antigen determines the symptoms produced by the allergy. The antigen enters through the gastrointestinal (GI) mucosal barrier. Intact food proteins may enter the circulation, stimulating the production of antigen-specific IgE.

Major food allergens are usually glycoproteins (Box 80-1), but any food can be sensitizing. Sensitized GI mast cells release mediators, causing vomiting and diarrhea. As a result of the edema and vasodilation of the intestinal wall, the mucosa becomes more permeable to enteric antigens, resulting in more hypersensitivity and inflammation.

Box 80-1. Highly Allergenic Foods		
Egg white	Fish and shellfish	Soy
Cow's milk	Wheat	Corn
Nuts		

Differential Diagnosis

In evaluating children with possible allergic disease, other etiologies for the symptoms should be considered and explored. Allergic rhinitis is most often confused with an upper respiratory infection but may also resemble vasomotor rhinitis, nonallergic rhinitis with eosinophilia syndrome, cerebrospinal fluid rhinorrhea (usually associated with a basilar skull fracture), sinusitis, drug-induced rhinitis, cholinergic rhinitis (skier's/jogger's nose, gustatory rhinitis), or a nasal foreign body. Unlike allergic rhinitis, infectious etiologies of rhinitis result in inflammatory nasal mucosa and possible fever. Foreign bodies elicit a unilateral, purulent, often foul-smelling discharge. Vasomotor rhinitis is usually transient.

Urticaria can resemble insect bites, erythema multiforme, papular urticaria, mastocytosis, or contact dermatitis. Distinct features of urticaria include pruritus, raised erythematous lesions with pale centers and a transient nature, without any epidermal break. It may result from an allergic reaction to drugs, food and food additives, insect bites and stings, inhalant or systemic disease such as endocrine disease, collagen-vascular disease, malignancy, and vasculitis or may occur secondary to an infectious etiology. Parasitic, bacterial, fungal, and viral infections can all cause urticaria. Physical urticaria due to heat, vibration, pressure, ultraviolet light, exercise, or anxiety can also produce the reaction. In addition, a deficiency in factor I in the complement system may cause a genetic form of urticaria.

Anaphylaxis is usually associated with cutaneous, respiratory, cardiovascular, and systemic symptoms, such as skin rash, edema, wheezing, arrythmia, occasionally fever, and shock. A history of an acute exposure is more likely to be seen with anaphylaxis.

Patients with food allergies may present with signs and symptoms of anaphylaxis or their symptoms may resemble those associated with food intolerances, which are nonallergenic. Food intolerances include toxic contamination (eg, scromboids), metabolic disorders (eg, lactose intolerance), and reactions to pharmacologic properties of the ingested food. Associated allergic findings (eg, asthma, atopic dermatitis) may be seen with true allergies. Specific testing of the food or stool, or allergy skin or blood testing, may be necessary to differentiate allergic reactions from food intolerance.

Evaluation: History and Physical Examination

Allergic Rhinitis and Conjunctivitis

Practitioners should determine if children with possible allergic rhinitis have a history of symptoms of sneezing, itching, nasal discharge, and nasal blockage. The eyes, ears, palate, and throat may itch. Children may also have a history of mouth breathing and snoring at night, sleep disturbances and daytime fatigue from nasal obstruction, or signs of complications such as sinusitis, postnasal drip, halitosis, cough, and morning sore throat. Symptoms may be seasonal or associated with a specific stimulus. In addition, systemic symptoms of fatigue, headache, anorexia, and irritability may be present.

The history should also include a search for other manifestations of allergies (eg, wheezing, atopic dermatitis) as well as a family history of atopy. An environmental history of allergen exposure, including pets, is also important to obtain.

The physical examination should be thorough. The skin should be inspected for atopic dermatitis and the lungs for evidence of asthma. The nasal mucosa should be examined with an otoscope. In children with allergic rhinitis, the nasal mucosa is swollen, pale, and sometimes cyanotic with copious clear discharge. Nasal polyps, if present,

should be noted. Although polyps are most often present on an allergic basis, they may occur with cystic fibrosis. A transverse crease across the nose ("allergic creases") can occur from repeatedly using the palm of the hand in an upward thrust on the nares to relieve itching and open the nasal airway ("allergic salute"). Dark circles under the eyes ("allergic shiners") may be present from chronic periorbital edema and venous stasis. Dennie sign (also called Morgan line), a wrinkle just beneath the lower eyelids, is present from early infancy and is associated with atopic dermatitis and allergic rhinitis. Allergic gape or adenoid facies is secondary to chronic mouth breathing during the first several years of life and results in a characteristic pattern of maldevelopment of facial bones, causing a high-arched palate, flat maxilla, and angulated mandible with a recessed chin and dental malocclusion. If affected, the conjunctivae are erythematous with a clear discharge and may have a follicular appearance. The mouth may reveal a high-arched palate from chronic mouth breathing, and hypertrophic lymphoid follicles in the oropharynx often can be seen (Figure 80-1).

Complications of chronic allergic rhinitis may be evident on examination. If children have one of these conditions, such as chronic serous otitis, recurrent otitis media, hearing loss secondary to otitis, sinusitis, nasal polyps, sleep apnea, or dental malocclusion, the possibility of allergic disease as a cause should be explored.

Urticaria and Angioedema

When children present with an acute rash, questions should focus on recent exposures to drugs, dietary changes, new soaps or detergents, and environmental agents. An urticarial rash is acute in onset, extremely pruritic, and typically evanescent. Evidence of infection and a history of chronic disease or any other allergic disease should be explored. The rash should be evaluated carefully. An urticarial rash appears as erythematous lesions of various sizes with pale,

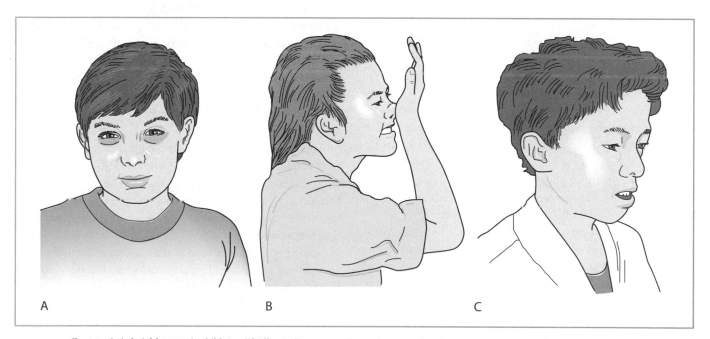

Figure 80-1. Characteristic facial features in children with allergic diseases. A. Allergic shiner. B. Allergic salute. C. Adenoid facies.

papular centers. Lesions may coalesce, the rash blanches on pressure, and the skin is intact.

The physical examination should also assess whether other contributing problems, such as infection, are present.

Anaphylaxis

An acute exposure to a foreign antigen (eg, medication, food, venom) should be elicited in the history of any patient who presents with anaphylaxis.

On physical examination, vital signs indicate hypotension and tachycardia. The skin is erythematous with diffuse edema. Airway edema may produce hoarseness with stridor and wheezing noted on auscultation of the chest. Patients may have severe difficulty breathing. Cardiac examination may reveal arrhythmias.

Food Allergies

An accurate diet diary is essential in diagnosing a food allergy. The timing of symptoms associated with a specific food must be obtained. Personal as well as family history of atopy is important. Allergy skin testing or an allergy blood testing and elimination diet followed by a challenge helps the diagnostic evaluation. The double-blind, placebo-controlled food challenge is the most accurate assessment for diagnosis.

Evaluation

Laboratory Tests

With allergic rhinitis, as with any allergic disease, the diagnosis can usually be made with a thorough history and physical examination. Frequently, therapy can be initiated with no laboratory data.

Screening tests may include a nasal smear for eosinophils. A result of greater than 10% eosinophils is considered confirmatory data for allergic rhinitis. Although serum IgE levels are elevated in 60% of patients with allergic rhinitis and asthma, they are not sensitive or specific and have limited value. A multi-allergen screening test, which gives reliable results when checking for the presence of allergic disease, is currently available.

Skin testing for specific antigens should be performed if desensitization shots or environmental changes are being considered in the management plan. Skin tests are sensitive and accurate. Positive tests indicate the presence of an antigen-specific IgE. Prick tests are used initially. They may be followed by intradermal tests for allergens that are negative on prick testing. Although skin testing may be less reliable in infants because their skin is less reactive, the tests have been performed in children as young as 4 months.

Radioallergosorbent testing (RAST) of sera, which is also available for the laboratory assessment of allergies, provides a semiquantitative measure of the amount of IgE specific for individual allergens. RAST is much more expensive than skin testing and has no advantage unless skin testing cannot be performed, such as in patients with a history of anaphylaxis, poor skin reactivity, current antihistamine use, or dermatographia.

Objective testing with skin tests by the prick method may be helpful in diagnosing food allergies. Negative tests are accurate for excluding food allergies, but positive tests may occur in patients without symptoms related to a particular food. Intradermal skin tests are not indicated. They do not give additional information, and they increase the risk of a serious reaction. RAST of sera may be used for specific foods.

Management

The first line of therapy for all allergic diseases is **avoidance of any precipitants.** For allergic rhinitis, this begins with environmental control, because the most frequent precipitants are inhalant allergens. Reducing exposure to the dust mite, a common allergen, can help control allergic rhinitis. Environmental humidity, which increases the dust mite population, should be decreased. Specifically, parents should be instructed to remove carpets, drapes, and upholstered furniture, which can harbor dust mites, from the house. They should cover mattresses with plastic covers and remove furry pets. Decreasing humidity also helps reduce mold counts, another important allergen, and air-conditioning units with a HEPA filter can lower pollen and mold counts as well. Nonspecific irritants such as smoke should be avoided because they can also precipitate any allergic symptom.

Anaphylaxis is considered a **medical emergency.** The first step in management is to establish an airway. Oxygen therapy should be instituted, and IV access established. Epinephrine is the drug of choice because of its potent vasoconstrictive and myocardial stimulating effects. The dose is 0.01 mL/kg of 1:1,000 aqueous solution, up to 0.5 mL, given subcutaneously. If the blood pressure is decreased, epinephrine may be given intravenously, with normal saline fluid boluses to expand intravascular volume. Intravenous administration of an antihistamine, such as diphenhydramine (5 mg/kg/24 hours) is used as well as a steroid, such as methylprednisolone (2 mg/kg).

The management of urticaria should begin with the **identification of the causal agent** and its elimination. Children who have experienced anaphylaxis should be instructed to avoid future exposure to the precipitating allergen. In addition, they should be instructed to wear a medical alert tag that notifies others of the potential for a severe allergic reaction and carry an epinephrine kit for immediate treatment.

A maintenance diet that does not contain the allergen is the basis for management of food allergies. It is essential that the prescribed diet be nutritionally sound. Families should be instructed by a nutritionist and taught to read food labels appropriately to avoid all exposure to the antigen. They should also be advised about what foods children can consume.

Medications should be used in allergic disease when additional management is indicated by persistent symptoms. Histamine H1 receptor antagonists or **antihistamines** are frequently indicated in the treatment of allergic rhinitis. Diphenhydramine, chlorpheniramine, and brompheniramine have all been useful in relieving symptoms but may be very sedating. The newer antagonists, desloratadine, fexofenadine, cetirizine, and loratadine, do not readily cross the blood-brain barrier and are less sedating. Leukotriene inhibitors, such as montelukast as monotherapy or in combination with an antihistamine, provide effective symptom relief. Oral decongestants have been effective in decreasing nasal congestion. Pseudoephedrine has been used in children. Topical nasal decongestants, which can cause dependence and rebound swelling, should not be used on a long-term basis.

Antihistamines are also used in the symptomatic treatment of urticaria and angioedema. These agents can relieve the rash as well as the itching of the rash. Diphenhydramine (5 mg/kg/d in 4 doses) and hydroxyzine (2 mg/kg/d in 4 doses) are both used. If the urticaria is extensive or severe, epinephrine or Sus-Phrine (epinephrine in oil) may be used subcutaneously. This often provides immediate relief of symptoms and is diagnostic as well as therapeutic.

Cromolyn sodium nasal spray is the next line of treatment for allergic rhinitis in children older than 6 years. A very effective mast cell stabilizer, it suppresses mediator release. Cromolyn spray should be used prophylactically on a regular basis 2 to 4 times per day, one spray per nostril, to prevent symptoms.

Steroids have an anti-inflammatory effect and work well topically for allergic rhinitis. Mometasone, triamcinolone, and flunisolide are available as nasal sprays, and all 3 agents may cause stinging and nasal irritation. Topical antihistamines and mast cell stabilizer, such as azelastine or olapatadine nasal sprays alone or in combination with nasal steroid, are effective. Systemic steroids may also be used for treatment of urticaria, angioedema, and anaphylaxis.

Immunotherapy should be considered for children with allergic rhinitis when avoidance techniques and medications are not controlling symptoms or when there is a history of anaphylaxis, depending on the allergen. This treatment has been effective in relieving symptoms due to dust mites, pollens, animal dander, molds, insect stings, and drug reactions. Immunotherapy involves a series of injections with extracts of allergens specific for individual patients, producing tolerance to particular antigens. The mechanism of action of immunotherapy is related to the development of allergen-specific blocking antibody (IgG), increased allergen-specific suppressor T cells, decreased lymphocyte cytokine response to an allergen, and decreased basophil histamine release in response to an allergen. The results of skin testing dictate which allergens to use. Initially, injections are given weekly. Then they are tapered and given on a maintenance schedule. Although immunotherapy can be performed at any age, the injections are painful and expensive. They necessitate frequent visits. Patients risk an allergic reaction with each injection.

Prevention

The cost of medical care, lost school days and workdays, disability from complications, and actual lives lost from allergic disease take a great toll on the population. Evidence currently suggests that sensitization to foods is more likely to occur in the first 6 to 12 months of life. Avoidance of these allergens at this age may decrease the subsequent development of allergic disease. For children at high risk for the development of allergic disease, which is usually determined by family history, the following steps are recommended:

- Keep the home free of allergens such as dust mites, pollen, etc.
- Keep humidity below 50% in the home to prevent mold and dust mite growth.
- Prevent smoking in the environment.

To reduce the incidence of food allergies, it is recommended that mothers breastfeed infants exclusively for at least the first 6 months of life. When infants are 6 months old, foods can gradually be introduced. Cow's milk, wheat, corn, and citrus should be avoided until after the age of 1 year. Peanuts, eggs, fish, and shellfish should be delayed until 24 months. Postponing the introduction of food allergens may reduce the rate of sensitization in high-risk infants, but this is a controversial issue. Studies have demonstrated that such postponement may only delay the sensitization, though a recent study showed that early food allergen exposure, rather than avoidance, might improve allergic outcome.

Prognosis

The prognosis for children with allergic disease is good when the diagnosis is made correctly. Some patients lose their allergy naturally or following immunotherapy. For others, allergic rhinitis, urticaria, and anaphylactic reactions persist throughout life on exposure to antigens. However, with appropriate management with medication and avoidance of allergens, children with allergic disease can thrive and live a normal life without restrictions on activity. Immunotherapy can be effective in alleviating the allergic response to inhalants in allergic rhinitis and to insect venoms. The chance for resolution of food allergies is very good. Many foods that initially elicit an allergenic reaction can be tolerated after the age of 3 to 4 years; 85% of children with cow's milk, egg, wheat, or soy allergy will experience remission by 5 years, presumably as a result of maturation of the GI mucosa. However, only 20% of young children outgrow peanut allergy.

CASE RESOLUTION

In the case presented at the beginning of the chapter, the girl's symptoms of rash, swelling, and wheezing after exposure to an antigen suggest a systemic allergic reaction with angioedema and asthma. Treatment with epinephrine and antihistamines is clearly indicated. Because of the presence of pulmonary symptoms, admission for observation is warranted. The child and family should be counseled to avoid any foods that contain peanuts in the future. The parents should read all food labels, and carry an epinephrine autoinjector (Epi-pen) at all times for emergency use. The patient should wear a medical alert bracelet indicating peanut allergy. The patient should be referred to an allergist for further evaluation.

Selected References

Barnes ML, Menzies D, Fardon TC, et al. Combined mediator blockade or topical steroid for treating the unified allergic airway. *Allergy.* 2007;62:73–80

Berkowitz RB, McCafferty F, Lutz C, et al. Onset of action of fexofenadine hydrochloride 60 mg/pseudoephedrine hydrochloride 120 mg in subjects aged 12 years with moderate to severe seasonal allergic rhinitis: a pooled analysis of two single-dose, randomized, double-blind, placebo-controlled allergen exposure unit studies. *Clin Ther.* 2006;28:1658–1669

Berger W, Hampel F Jr, Bernstein J, Shah S, Sacks H, Meltzer EO. Impact of azelastine nasal spray on symptoms and quality of life compared with cetirizine oral tablets in patients with seasonal allergic rhinitis. *Ann Allergy Asthma Immunol.* 2006;97:375–381

Bodtger U, Linneberg A. Remission of allergic rhinitis: an 8-year observational study. *J Allergy Clin Immunol.* 2004;114:1384–1388

Burks AW, Sampson H. Food allergies in children. *Curr Probl Pediatr.* 1993;23:230–252

Craig TJ, Ferguson BJ, Krouse JH. Sleep impairment in allergic rhinitis, rhinosinusitis, and nasal polyposis. *Am J Otolarynogol.* 2008;29:209–217

Cutler DL, Banfield C, Affrime MB. Safety of mometasone furoate nasal spray in children with allergic rhinitis as young as 2 years of age: a randomized controlled trial. *Pediatr Asthma Allergy Immunol.* 2006;19:146

Drugs for asthma. *Med Lett Drugs Ther.* 1999;41:5–10

Ellis AK, Day JH. Incidence and characteristics of biphasic anaphylaxis: a prospective evaluation of 103 patients. *Ann Allergy Asthma Immunol.* 2007;98:64–69

Fireman P. Diagnosis of allergic disorders. *Pediatr Rev.* 1995;16:178–183

The Food Allergy and Anaphylaxis Network. www.foodallergy.org. Accessed on November 5, 2007

Joint Task Force on Practice Parameters; American Academy of Allergy, Asthma, and Immunology; American College of Allergy, Asthma, and Immunology; Joint Council on Allergy, Asthma, and Immunology. The diagnosis and management of anaphylaxis: an updated practice parameter. *J Allergy Clin Immunol.* 2005;115:S483

Kim KT, Rabinovitch N, Uryniak T, et al. Effect of budesonide aqueous nasal spray on hypothalamic-pituitary-adrenal axis function in children with allergic rhinitis. *Ann Allergy Asthma Immunol.* 2004;93:61–67

Meltzer EO. Allergic rhinitis: managing the pediatric spectrum. *Allergy Asthma Proc.* 2006;27:2–8

Meltzer EO, Blaiss MS, Derebery MJ, et al. Burden of allergic rhinitis: results from the Pediatric Allergies in America survey. *J Allergy Clin Immunol.* 2009;124:S43–S70

Murphy SJ, Kelly HW. Advances in the management of acute asthma in children. *Pediatr Rev.* 1996;17:227–234

Norman PS. Immunotherapy: 1999–2004. *J Allergy Clin Immunol.* 2004;113:1013–1023

Patel P, Philip G, Yang W, et al. Randomized, double-blind, placebo-controlled study of montelukast for treating perennial allergic rhinitis. *Ann Allergy Asthma Immunol.* 2005;95:551–557

Pitsios, C, Papadopoulos, D, Kompoti, E, et al. Efficacy and safety of mometasone furoate vs nedocromil sodium as prophylactic treatment for moderate/severe seasonal allergic rhinitis. *Ann Allergy Asthma Immunol.* 2006;96:673–678

Platts-Mills TA. Allergen avoidance. *J Allergy Clin Immunol.* 2004;113:388–391

Pratt El, Craig TJ. Assessing outcomes from the sleep disturbances associated with rhinitis. *Curr Opin Allergy Clin Immunol.* 2007;7:249–256

Ramey JT, Bailen E, Lockey RF. Rhinitis medicamentosa. *J Investig Allergol Clin Immunol.* 2006;15:148

Rooklin AR, Gaqchik SM. Allergic rhinitis—it's that time again. *Contemp Pediatr.* 1994;11:19–41

Rudders SA, Banerji A, Vassallo MF, et al. Trends in pediatric emergency department visits for food-induced anaphylaxis. *J Allergy Clin Immunol.* 2010;126:385

Sampson HA, Munoz-Furlong A, Campbell RL, et al. Second symposium on the definition and management of anaphylaxis: summary report—second National Institute of Allergy and Infectious Disease/Food Allergy and Anaphylaxis Network symposium. *J Allergy Clin Immunol.* 2006;117:391

Wallace DV, Dykewicz MS. The diagnosis and management of rhinitis: an updated practice parameter. *J Allergy Clin Immunol.* 2008;122:S1–S84

Wander AA, Bernstein IL, Goodman DL, et al. The diagnosis and management of urticaria: a practice parameter. *Ann Allergy Immunol.* 2005;85:525–544

Wang J, Sampson HA. Food anaphylaxis. *Clin Exp Allergy.* 2007;37:651

Wu CC, Kuo HC, Yu HR, et al. Association of acute urticaria with *Mycoplasma pneunoniae* infection in hospitalized children. *Ann Allergy Asthma Immunol.* 2009;103:134

Zuraw BL, Christiansen SC. Pathogenesis and laboratory diagnosis of hereditary angioedema. *Allergy Asthma Proc.* 2009;30:487–492

CHAPTER 81

Wheezing and Asthma

Nasser Redjal, MD

CASE STUDY

A 7-year-old boy is referred to the office after being seen in the emergency department (ED) for wheezing. He has been treated in the ED for wheezing 4 times in the past month and was once hospitalized for 3 days. The boy's father and paternal grandmother both have asthma.

The child's physical examination is remarkable for end-expiratory wheezing on forced expiration.

Questions

1. What are the most common causes of wheezing in infants and children?
2. What are the causes of reversible bronchospasm?
3. What is the pathophysiology of reversible bronchospasm?
4. How should children with asthma be managed?

Recurrent wheezing is a frequent symptom of obstructive airway disease in children that may be caused by intrinsic or extrinsic compression of the airway, bronchospasm, inflammation, or defective clearance of secretions. Ten percent to 15% of infants wheeze during their first year of life, and as many as 25% of children younger than 5 years present to their clinicians with wheezing during a respiratory illness. Most infants and young children with recurrent wheezing have asthma; however, a wide variety of congenital and acquired conditions can cause narrowing of the extrathoracic or intrathoracic airways, and may present with wheezing. Reactive airways disease is the most common cause of wheezing in childhood. Childhood asthma typically falls into 1 of 3 categories. **Transient wheezers** are infants who wheeze when ill with lower respiratory tract infections but experience no further wheezing after age 3 years. More than 80% of infants with a history of wheezing in their first 12 months fall into this category. **Nonatopic wheezers** are children with somewhat more reactive airways, a history of previous respiratory syncytial virus (RSV) infections, and persistent wheezing beyond 3 years of age, but symptoms may still resolve over time. **Atopic wheezers** are those children who are most likely to develop persistent asthma.

Wheezes can originate from airways of any size, from the large extrathoracic upper airway to the intrathoracic small airways. In addition to narrowing or compression of the airway, wheezing requires sufficient airflow to generate airway oscillation and produce sound. Thus the absence of wheezing in a patient who presents with acute asthma may be an ominous finding, suggesting impending respiratory failure. The audible "musical or squeaking sounds" noted with obstruction are caused by turbulence of the air as it is forced through a narrowed airway. Infants and young children are more prone to wheezing when they have airway obstruction because air forced through smaller airways is more turbulent than air forced through the larger airways of older children and adults. Infection-induced wheezing in children younger than 2 years is associated with RSV, especially in infants with passive exposure to smoke, and with rhinovirus in children older than 2 years. The most common causes of wheezing in infants and children are asthma, bronchiolitis, and pneumonia. Less common causes include congenital structural anomalies, gastroesophageal reflux and aspiration, cardiac failure, cystic fibrosis, foreign bodies, and vocal cord dysfunction (Box 81-1).

The Modified Asthma Predictive Index (API) is a clinical instrument to predict persistence of asthma. Predictive factors include wheezing before 3 years of age and the presence of one major risk factor (parental history of asthma, a personal history of atopic dermatitis, or patient sensitized to aero-allergen) or 2 of 3 minor risk factors (patient sensitized to food, wheezing apart from colds, and/or eosinophilia). The API has a positive predictive value of 76% and a negative predictive value of 95%. More than 80% of infants who have a history of wheezing in the first postnatal years do not wheeze after 3 years of age.

Asthma is a common chronic disorder of the airways characterized by variable and recurring symptoms, airflow obstruction, bronchial hyperresponsiveness, and underlying inflammation. Bronchospasm is reversible either spontaneously or with treatment. In some patients permanent alterations in the airway structure, referred to as **airway remodeling,** develops and is not prevented by, or fully responsive to, currently available treatment. Clinically asthma is characterized by recurrent episodes of cough, chest tightness, dyspnea, prolonged expiration, wheezing, hyperinflation of the chest (air trappings), use of accessory chest muscles (retractions) and, in severe cases, cyanosis.

Epidemiology

Asthma is the most common chronic childhood illness. In 2007 the National Health Interview Survey noted that 9% of children 0 to 17 years of age (6.7 million) had asthma. Asthma is the leading cause

Box 81-1. Causes of Wheezing

Infection
- Bronchiolitis
- Pneumonia
- Bronchitis
- Laryngotracheobronchitis
- Bacterial tracheitis
- Toxocariasis
- Ascariasis

Reactive Airways Disease
- Asthma
- Exercise-induced asthma
- Anaphylaxis
- Nighttime cough asthma
- Toxic exposure (smoke, organophosphate poisoning)
- Allergic aspergillosis

Laryngeal Dysfunction

Congenital Structural Anomalies
- Vascular rings
- Bronchiectasis
- Lung cysts
- Laryngotracheoesophageal cleft
- Tracheobronchomalacia

Defective Secretion Clearance
- Cystic fibrosis
- Immotile cilia syndrome

Tumor
- Mediastinal tumors (lymphoma, teratoma, neuroblastoma, thymoma)

Chronic Aspiration
- Gastroesophageal reflux
- Bulbar palsy
- Tracheoesophageal fistula

Other Causes
- Bronchopulmonary dysplasia
- α_1-Antitrypsin deficiency
- Pulmonary hemosiderosis
- Sarcoidosis

Foreign Body

Cardiac Disease

Immunodeficiency

of ED visits, hospital admissions, and school absenteeism. Over the last several decades, the prevalence of asthma has increased worldwide, an increase that varies from 40% in some areas of the United Kingdom and Australia to 3% in Indonesia, China, and India. Asthma prevalence, mortality, and hospitalization rates are higher in blacks than in whites. One-third of patients initially experience symptoms in the first year of life, and 80% are diagnosed by the time they reach school age. In the United States, asthma is a leading diagnosis for children admitted to children's hospitals. Hospitalization rates have remained relatively stable, with lower rates in some age groups but higher rates in children 0 to 4 years of age. In addition, asthma is a major cause of school absence; 23% of school days missed can be attributed to asthma. The male-female ratio is 2:1 until age 10 and is equal from ages 10 to 14; after puberty, asthma incidence is greater in girls and women.

In recent years, the incidence of more serious disease in younger children and adolescents has increased. Low socioeconomic status is associated with an increase in asthma prevalence, morbidity, and mortality. Inner-city African Americans are most at risk but studies suggest that socioeconomic class and health care disparities only partially account for these differences.

Clinical Presentation

Children with asthma may present with acute symptoms of cough, shortness of breath, prolonged expiration, use of accessory muscles of respiration, wheezing, complaints of chest tightness or congestion, hyperinflation of the chest, cyanosis, exercise intolerance, tachycardia, and abdominal pain.

Wheezing may be audible and detected by the parent or may not be appreciated until the child is examined by a physician. There may be no wheezing in children with severe bronchoconstriction because the flow of air is impeded, but wheezing may appear after bronchodilator treatment, owing to partial opening of the airway.

Some children have cough, which may be nocturnal or recurrent as a predominant symptom. Some pediatric patients have symptoms such as cough or wheezing that are precipitated or exacerbated by exercise (Dx Box).

Dx Asthma
- Recurrent wheezing
- Shortness of breath
- Exercise intolerance
- History of allergies
- History of atopic dermatitis
- Nasal polyps
- History of nighttime cough

Abdominal pain and vomiting also are common in younger children and may be followed by temporary relief of respiratory symptoms. During an acute asthma attack, a low-grade fever, profuse sweating, and fatigue from the hard work of breathing may be apparent.

Pathophysiology

Asthma is a chronic inflammatory disorder of the airways. The immunohistopathologic features of asthma includes alteration and denudation of the airway epithelium, thickening of the basement membrane, fibrotic changes in the sub-basement membrane, bronchial smooth muscle hypertrophy, edema and angiogenesis, mast cell activation, and inflammatory cell infiltration (neutrophils, lymphocytes, eosinophils), which release mediators such as histamine, prostaglandin, leukotriene, major basic proteins, etc. These changes lead to airway hyperresponsiveness, airflow limitation, respiratory symptoms, and disease chronicity. The limitation to the flow of air results from acute bronchoconstriction, airway edema, mucus plug formation, and airway wall remodeling. The unique anatomy and physiology of the lung in infants compared with adults predisposes infants to obstructive airways disease. These anatomical differences include reduced number and size of the pores of Cohn and Lambert canals, causing deficient collateral ventilation and a predisposition to atelectasis distal to obstructed airway. Mucous gland hyperplasia favors increased intraluminal mucus production. Decreased smooth muscle in the peripheral airway results in less support and narrower airways. Decreased number of fatigue-resistant skeletal muscle fibers in the diaphragm, its horizontal insertion to the rib cage (versus oblique in adult), and a highly compliant rib cage increase the work of breathing in children. Decreased static elastic recoil predisposes to early airway closure during tidal breathing, resulting in mismatching of ventilation and perfusion and hypoxemia.

Atopy, the genetic predisposition to the development of immunoglobulin (Ig) E–mediated response to common aeroallergens, is a predisposing factor for developing asthma. There are at least 50 genes that influence susceptibility to asthma and its clinical expression. Sites located on chromosomes 6p, 12q, 5q, 11q, and 16p are known to be associated with allergic diseases and encoding for major histocompatibility complex, IgE, interferon, and cytokine.

Environmental changes such as wind; temperature fluctuations; and increased exposure to allergens or air pollutants, such as tobacco smoke, ozone, sulfur dioxide, and nitrogen dioxide, and particulate matter, such as diesel exhaust and biologic residues (eg, endotoxin), may precipitate clinical attacks. Inhalant allergens, particularly indoors, play an important role. The most important allergens are house dust mite feces (Der p1 and Der p2), cat dander (Feld l), and cockroach saliva (Bla g2, Bla g4, and Bla g5). Other inhalant allergens, such as dog dander, and outdoor fungus (ie, *Alternaria*), and some pollens, also play a role. Infections, particularly respiratory ones, are implicated, influencing not only asthma's exacerbation, but also its inception and persistence. Viral infections, such as RSV, parainfluenza, and rhinovirus, are the most frequent precipitants of asthma exacerbations in infancy. The frequency of lower tract respiratory infection during early childhood with these viruses is a strong independent factor in development of asthma. *Mycoplasma* and *Chlamydia* infections can cause wheezing and persistence of asthma. Emotional stress may also play a role in the exacerbation of asthma.

The physiological changes involved in asthma occur in 2 phases. An immediate response ("early phase") to the offending agent causes edema and bronchial smooth muscle constriction that lead to narrowing of the airway and plugging with secretions. Air is trapped behind the narrowed airways, resulting in altered gas exchange, increased respiratory rate, decreased tidal volume, and increased work of breathing. The late response, which occurs 4 to 12 hours after the initial symptoms, primarily involves infiltration of the airways with inflammatory cells. The end pathway in the disease process is obstruction to airflow. The pathophysiology of asthma is reviewed in Figure 81-1.

Differential Diagnosis

An extensive differential diagnosis is listed in Box 81-1. Most conditions are differentiated from asthma by the presence of associated symptoms or the child's response to bronchodilators.

Evaluation

History

A thorough history including how the child and family are coping with the asthma should be obtained (Questions Box). If acute respiratory distress is present, an abbreviated history focusing on potential precipitating factors and medication use should be obtained first and the more detailed history gotten at a later time.

Physical Examination

Vital signs including pulse oximetry should be obtained. Objective determination of pulmonary function involves measuring the peak expiratory effort. Pulsus paradoxus, the difference between systolic arterial blood pressure during inspiration and expiration, is usually under 10 mm Hg. This difference may be increased during an acute asthma exacerbation, but the measurement is difficult in young children. Breath sounds, work of breathing, the inspiratory-expiratory ratio, use of accessory muscles, presence of retractions, quality of breath sounds (whether decreased), presence of prolonged expiration, and quality of wheezing should be carefully assessed (Table 81-1). Polyphonic wheezing (many different pitches, starting and stopping at varying points in the respiratory cycle) and cough are highly suggestive of asthma. Monophonic wheezing (a single, distinct noise of one pitch and starting and stopping at one discrete time) and cough should always raise suspicion of large airway obstruction caused by foreign body aspiration, vascular ring, or tracheomalacia. The nose and associated nasal passages should be examined for secretions, edema, pallor, and polyps. The skin should be assessed for eczema and other rashes. The chest should be carefully checked for increased anteroposterior diameter of the chest wall, a sign of air trapping. Fingers should be examined for signs of digital clubbing, which suggests a diagnosis other than asthma.

Laboratory Tests

The laboratory assessment of wheezing children is indicated if the diagnosis is unclear or to eliminate disorders that mimic asthma. Pulmonary function tests are noninvasive, objective, and cost-effective in the diagnosis and follow-up of patients with asthma. These tests can be performed in children older than 5 years with appropriate coaching. After the administration of an aerosolized bronchodilator, dynamic tests of airflow increase or return to normal. An improvement in forced expiratory volume in 1 second (FEV_1) greater than

Figure 81-1. Proposed pathways in the pathogenesis of bronchial inflammation and airway hyperresponsiveness. (Reproduced from the National Heart, Lung, and Blood Institute. *National Asthma Education Program Expert Panel Report: Guidelines for Diagnosis and Management of Asthma.* **Bethesda, MD: National Institutes of Health; National Heart, Lung, and Blood Institute; 1991. NIH Publication No. 91-3042.)**

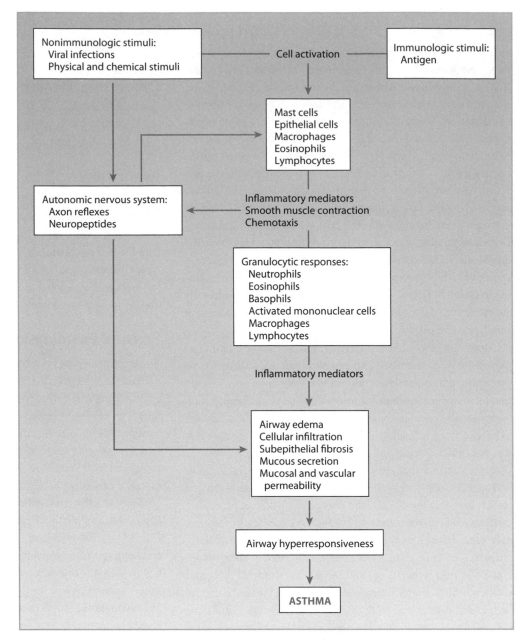

12% is virtually diagnostic, but lack of improvement in FEV$_1$ does not preclude asthma. Exercise tolerance tests using a treadmill or free running followed by pulmonary function tests can be performed; a decrease greater than 12% in FEV$_1$ or 30% in forced expiratory flow is diagnostic of exercise-induced asthma. Peak flow meters, which measure forced peak expiratory flow (PEF), are useful in the office and at home to monitor expiratory flow rate. A decrease in PEF may predict the onset of an exacerbation and suggests the need for early intervention, using additional drug therapy. A complete blood cell count with a differential count may suggest infection or allergies. Peripheral eosinophil counts may be elevated in asthma. Pulse oximetry assesses the degree of oxygen saturation.

Sputum smear, stained with eosin-methylene blue, may show numerous eosinophils and granules from disrupted white blood cells, eosinophils, and epithelial cells. The presence of more than 5% to 10% eosinophils suggests allergic inflammatory disease. Other findings in the sputum include Curschmann spirals, which are threads

of glycoprotein; Creola bodies, which are clusters of epithelial cells; and Charcot-Leyden crystals, which are derived from eosinophils.

Total serum IgE is not as helpful as antigen-specific IgE, and is elevated in 80% of children with allergen-induced asthma. Allergy skin testing or serologic testing, such as radioallergosorbent testing, is indicated to identify potentially important environmental allergens. Allergens may play a significant role in asthma, and 85% of asthma patients have a positive skin test reaction to common aeroallergens. Extensive laboratory testing should be reserved for children with severe disease who may benefit from consultation with an allergy specialist.

Imaging Studies

Children suspected of having asthma rarely require a chest radiograph unless there is concern about other pathology. radiograph findings may range from normal to hyperinflation, increased bronchial

Asthma

Questions

- What symptoms (eg, wheezing, exercise intolerance) does the child experience?
- Does the child experience any nocturnal awakening or cough?
- What time of day and year do the symptoms occur?
- When did the symptoms begin? How old was the child?
- Are the symptoms associated with any particular activity? Does anything seem to trigger the symptoms?
- Are the child's activities limited in any way?
- How often do the asthma attacks occur?
- What is the child's living situation? Are there pets in the home?
- Does anyone smoke in the home?
- Do the asthma attacks cause the child to be absent from school?
- Does the child manage the condition at home with any particular treatments or medications?
- Has the child visited any urgent care and emergency departments for treatment for asthma or related episodes in the past? Has the child had any hospitalizations?
- Does the child have a history of allergies?

marking, and atelectasis, especially during acute exacerbation. Infiltration, pneumothorax, pneumomediastinum, and pneumonia are less common findings.

Management

The long-term goals of asthma therapy are as follows:

- Prevent chronic and disabling symptoms (eg, coughing, sleep disturbances, exercise intolerance, shortness of breath).
- Maintain normal or near-normal pulmonary function.
- Maintain normal activity levels.
- Prevent recurrent exacerbations and minimize the need for ED visits and admission to the hospital.
- Provide drug therapy that is effective with minimal side effects.
- Meet the expectations of the child and the family for the care of asthma.
- Encourage self-management of asthma.

Assessment measures for asthma should include monitoring of the following: signs and symptoms, pulmonary function through peak flow or respirometry, quality of life/functional status, acute disease exacerbations, pharmacologic therapy, and satisfaction of the child and family with their asthma care.

Selecting the appropriate therapy for an asthma patient depends on the age, disease severity, and developmental level of the child; the tolerance for a specific pharmacologic agent; and the routes of administration. The pharmacologic treatment for symptom control and reduction of inflammation is predicated on the severity of the asthma, as categorized, according to National Heart, Lung, and Blood Institute (NHLBI) guidelines. Box 81-2 contains an overview of these medications. Quick-relief medications ("rescue meds") are used for acute exacerbations and the long-term control medications for chronic therapy. Non-pharmacologic measures aim at prevention and serve as an adjunct to drug therapy.

Table 81-1. Parameters Used to Estimate the Severity of Acute Asthma

Sign/Symptom	Mild	Moderate	Severe
Respiratory rate	Normal	Increased	Increased >2 SD
Breath sounds	Normal (some end-expiratory wheezes)	Wheezing in inspiration and expiration	Decreased ± wheezing
Shortness of breath	None (can speak in sentences)	Can speak in phrases	Speaks only single words
Skin color	Normal (pink)	Pale	Pale to cyanotic
Work of breathing	Normal	Moderate retractions; some use of accessory muscles	Severe retractions, nasal flaring, use of accessory muscles
Pulse	Normal	Normal or increased	Increased
Level of consciousness	Normal	Normal	Diminished; may be lethargic or combative
Pulsus paradoxus	<10 mm Hg	10–20 mm Hg	20–40 mm Hg
Oxygen saturation	>95%	90%–95%	<92%
Pulmonary function	80% of predicted	50%–70% of predicted	<50% of predicted

Abbreviation: SD, standard deviation.

Short-term Management

Acute attacks can be managed in the office if the staff is prepared to deal with children in respiratory distress. Otherwise children can be referred to the ED. Equipment and supplies for resuscitation of infants and children must be available in offices that care for children with asthma.

The goal of therapy is to relieve airflow obstruction and prevent respiratory failure. All children with moderate or severe asthma should be placed in a position of comfort and given oxygen by nasal prongs or mask as tolerated. Assessment of work of breathing and the use of pulse oximetry help guide oxygen therapy. Nebulized β_2-agonists such as albuterol are used until symptoms subside. Children may require drug therapy every 20 to 30 minutes. Not only are nebulized β_2-adrenergic agonists more effective than oral medications, they are associated with fewer side effects. Ipratropium bromide used in conjunction with a β-agonist in the urgent care setting has been shown to reduce risk of hospitalization. Systemic corticosteroids, which help reduce the inflammation associated with clinical attacks, are indicated in most moderate and severe cases. Response to therapy is determined by clinical assessment of work of breathing, respiratory rate, objective changes in pulmonary function, and pulse oximetry. Children with incomplete responses to initial therapy may require several hours of treatment or hospitalization.

Long-term Management

The goals of long-term management are shown in Box 81-3.

Continuous and longitudinal primary care of children with asthma can profoundly affect the course of their disease. Primary care practitioners, children, and their families must work together to achieve good control of symptoms. Prevention of exacerbations may be accomplished by removal of offending allergens. Minimization of exposure to known allergens and irritants has been shown to decrease symptoms and exacerbation. The most commonly implicated irritants are tobacco smoke; fumes from gas, oil, and kerosene stoves and wood-burning appliances; and sprays and strong odors. House dust mites are microscopic insects that feed on human scales, require humidity greater than 50%, and are found in stuffed furniture, carpets, and mattresses. House dust mite infestation can be reduced by encasing mattresses, blankets, and pillows in mite-proof covers; removing carpeting; and decreasing humidity to less than 50%.

Allergen immunotherapy may be considered for asthma patients when there is evidence of a clear relationship between symptom and exposure to an allergen, and symptoms are poorly controlled with pharmacologic management (medication ineffective, multiple medications are required, or patient does not accept or tolerate medication). Adherence with appropriate medications and in home peak-flow measurement helps in prevention and control of asthma. Periodic assessment ensures appropriate therapy and compliance with treatment. Practitioners should make sure that families can afford the necessary medications. During routine visits, home monitoring and therapy as well as any diaries and records should be reviewed, children's and families' expectations about the course of the disease should be discussed, and all parties should be allowed to express their concerns regarding the development of a treatment plan. Other factors, such as rhinitis, sinusitis, and gastroesophageal reflux, which may influence the severity of asthma or a child's quality of life, should be assessed and treated appropriately.

Family members and children should be given a written action plan based on patients' personal best peak flow (Figure 81-2) and instructed in the use of peak flow meters to indicate when medical treatment is necessary. Some meters have 3 color zones: a green zone, which indicates good airflow; a yellow zone, which signals the need for treatment; and a red zone, which suggests that a visit to the ED may be indicated.

Pharmacologic Therapy

The 2007 NHLBI guidelines for asthma management are based on age group: children 0 to 4 years of age, children 5 to 11 years of age, children 12 years of age and older (Tables 81-2, 81-3, and 81-4).

Asthma severity is categorized by "impairment" and "risk." Impairment considers the frequency and severity of both daytime and nighttime asthma symptoms, use of short-acting β₂-agonist for other than exercise-associated symptoms, impact on activities, and pulmonary function testing. Risk assesses the frequency of asthma exacerbations requiring the use of oral corticosteroids. The most

---

Box 81-2. Pharmacologic Therapy: An Overview of Medications Used to Treat Asthma

Long-term Control Medications (Controller Class)

Corticosteroids

Most potent and effective anti-inflammatory medication currently available. Inhaled form is used in the long-term control of asthma. Systemic corticosteroids are often used to gain prompt control of the disease when initiating long-term therapy.

Cromolyn Sodium and Nedocromil

Mild anti-inflammatory medication. May be used as monotherapy in mild persistent asthma. Can also be used as preventive treatment prior to exercise or unavoidable exposure to known allergens.

Long-Acting β₂-Agonists

Long-acting bronchodilator used concomitantly with anti-inflammatory medications for long-term control of symptoms, especially nocturnal symptoms. Includes salmeterol and formoterol.

Methylxanthines

Sustained-release theophylline is a mild-to-moderate bronchodilator used principally as adjuvant to inhaled corticosteroids for prevention of nocturnal asthma symptoms. May have mild anti-inflammatory effect.

Leukotriene Modifiers

Montelukast, a leukotriene receptor antagonist, or zileuton, a 5-lipoxygenase inhibitor, may be considered an alternative therapy to low doses of inhaled corticosteroids, or cromolyn or nedocromil, in mild persistent asthma.

Systemic Corticosteroids

- Used for moderate-to-severe exacerbations to speed recovery and prevent recurrence of exacerbations.
- **Omalizimab** (anti-IgE) a recombinant DNA-derived humanized monoclonal antibody of the Fc portion of the IgE antibody, binds to that portion thereby preventing IgE binding to its high-affinity receptor (fcER1) on mast cells and basophils, leads to a decrease in the release of mediators in response to allergen exposure.

Quick-Relief Medications (Reliever Class)

Short-Acting β₂-Agonists

Albuterol and levalbuterol are therapy of choice for relief of acute symptoms and prevention of exercise-induced bronchoconstriction.

Anticholinergics

Ipratropium bromide provides additive benefit to inhaled β₂-agonists in acute exacerbations. May be an alternative bronchodilator for patients who do not tolerate inhaled β₂-agonists.

Box 81-3. Therapeutic Goals for Children With Chronic Asthma

- Maintain a normal, age-appropriate activity level.
- Maintain near-normal pulmonary function.
- Prevent symptoms such as exercise intolerance, chronic cough, and shortness of breath.
- Prevent acute exacerbations of the disease that require acute therapy.
- Minimize adverse effects of the drugs used to treat the disease.
- Promote self-esteem and a sense of well-being.

For: _____   Doctor: _____   Date: _____

Doctor's Phone Number: _____   Hospital/Emergency Department Phone Number: _____

GREEN ZONE

Doing Well

Take these long-term control medicines each day (include an anti-inflammatory).

- No cough, wheeze, chest tightness, or shortness of breath during the day or night
- Can do usual activities

Medicine		How much to take		When to take it
_____	→	_____	→	_____
_____	→	_____	→	_____

And, if a peak flow meter is used,

Peak Flow: more than _____

(80% or more of my best peak flow) _____

My best peak flow is: _____

Before exercise, if prescribed, take: ☐ 2 or ☐ 4 puffs _____
5–60 minutes before exercise

Identify and avoid and control the things that make your asthma worse, like (list here):

_____

_____

YELLOW ZONE

Asthma is Getting Worse →   **First** Add: quick-relief medicine and keep taking your GREEN ZONE medicine

_____ ☐ 2 or ☐ 4 puffs, every 20 minutes for up to 1 hour

(short-acting β_2-agonist) ☐ Nebulizer once

- Cough, wheeze, chest tightness, or shortness of breath, or
- Waking at night due to asthma, or
- Can do some but not all usual activities

– Or –

Peak flow: _____

(50%–79% of my best peak flow)

If applicable, remove yourself from the thing that made your asthma worse.

→ **Second, if your symptoms (and peak flow, if used) return to GREEN ZONE after 1 hour of above treatment:**

☐ Continue monitoring to be sure you stay in the green zone

If your symptoms (and peak flow, if used) do not return to GREEN ZONE after 1 hour of above treatment:

☐ Take: _____ ☐ 2 or ☐ 4 puffs or ☐ Nebulizer
(short-acting β_2-agonist)

☐ Add: _____ mg per day For _____ (3–10 days)
(oral corticosteroid)

☐ Call the doctor _____ ☐ before/☐ within _____ hours after taking oral corticosteroid.

RED ZONE

Medical Alert!

- Very short of breath, or
- Quick-relief medicines have not helped, or
- Cannot do usual activities, or
- Symptoms are same or get worse

After 24 hours in Yellow Zone

– Or –

Peak flow: less than _____

(50% of my best peak flow)

Take this medicine:

☐ _____ ☐ 4 or ☐ 6 puffs or ☐ Nebulizer
(short-acting β_2-agonist)

☐ _____ mg
(oral corticosteroid)

Then call your doctor NOW. Go to the hospital or call an ambulance if:

☐ You are still in the Red Zone after 15 minutes AND

You have not reached your doctor.

DANGER SIGNS

- **Trouble walking and talking due to shortness of breath**
- **Lips or fingernails are blue**
- **Take ☐ 4 or ☐ 6 puffs of your quick- relief medicine AND**
- **Go to the hospital or call for an ambulance** _____

Figure 81-2. Asthma action/medicine plan. (Source: National Heart, Lung, and Blood Institute, National Institutes of Health, US Department of Health and Human Services. NIH Publication No 07-5251, October 2006.)

Table 81-2. Classifying Asthma Severity Ages 0–4 Years[a]

Components of Severity		Classifying of Asthma Severity and Initiating Treatment (0–4 years of age)			
		Intermittent	Persistent		
			Mild	Moderate	Severe
Impairment	Symptoms	≤2 days/week	>2 days/week but not daily	Daily	Throughout the day
	Nighttime awakenings	0	1–2x/month	3–4x/month	>1x/week
	Short-acting β₂-agonist use for symptom control (not prevention of EIB)	≤2 days/week	>2 days/week but not daily	Daily	Several times per day
	Interference with normal activity	None	More limitation	Some limitation	Extremely limited
Risk	Exacerbation requiring oral systemic corticosteroids	0–1/year	≥2 exacerbations in 6 months requiring oral systemic corticosteroids, or ≥4 wheezing episodes/1 year lasting >1 day AND risk factors for persistent asthma		
			Consider severity and interval since last exacerbation. Frequency and severity may fluctuate over time. Exacerbations of any severity may occur in patients in any severity category.		
Recommended Step for Initiating Therapy (See Table 81-5 for treatment steps.)		Step 1: SABA PRN	Step 2: Low-dose ICS	Step 3: Medium-dose ICS and consider short course of OCS	
		In 2–6 weeks, depending on severity, evaluate level of asthma control that is achieved. If no clear benefit is observed in 4–6 weeks, consider adjusting therapy or alternative diagnoses.			

Abbreviations: EIB, exercise-induced bronchoconstriction; ICS, inhaled corticosteroids; OCS, oral corticosteroids; PRN, as needed; SABA, short-acting β₂-agonist.

[a]Adapted from the National Asthma Education and Prevention Program. *Expert Panel Report 3: Guidelines for the Diagnosis and Management of Asthma, 2007.* Bethesda, MD: National Heart, Lung, and Blood Institute; 2007. NIH Publication No. 07-4052.

Table 81-3. Classifying Asthma Severity Ages 5–11 Years[a]

Components of Severity		Classifying of Asthma Severity and Initiating treatment (5–11 years of age)			
		Intermittent	Persistent		
			Mild	Moderate	Severe
Impairment	Symptoms	≤2 days/week	>2 days/week but not daily	Daily	Throughout the day
	Nighttime awakenings	≤2x/month	3-4x/month	>1x/week but not nightly	Often 7x/week
	Short-acting β₂-agonist use for symptom control (not prevention of EIB)	≤2 days/week	>2 days/week but not daily	Daily	Several times per day
	Interference with normal activity	None	More limitation	Some limitation	Extremely limited
	Lung function	Normal FEV_1 between exacerbations FEV_1 >80% predicted FEV_1/FVC >85%	FEV_1 = >80% predicted FEV_1/FVC >80%	FEV_1 = 60%–80% predicted FEV_1/FVC = 75%–80%	FEV_1 <60% predicted FEV_1/FVC <75%
Risk	Exacerbation requiring oral systemic corticosteroids	0–1/year (see note)	≥2/year (see note)		
		Consider severity and interval since last exacerbation. Frequency and severity may fluctuate over time.			
		Relative annual risk of exacerbations may be related to FEV_1.			
Recommended Step for Initiating Therapy (See Table 81-5 for treatment steps.)		Step 1: SABA PRN	Step 2: Low-dose ICS	Step 3: Medium-dose ICS option	Step 3, Medium-dose ICS option or step 4
				Consider short course of OCS.	
		In 2–6 weeks, evaluate level of asthma control that is achieved, and adjusting therapy accordingly.			

Abbreviations: EIB, exercise-induced bronchoconstriction; FEV_1, forced expiratory volume in 1 second; FVC, forced vital capacity; ICS, inhaled corticosteroids; OCS, oral corticosteroids; PRN, as needed; SABA, short-acting β₂-agonist.

[a]Adapted from the National Asthma Education and Prevention Program. *Expert Panel Report 3: Guidelines for the Diagnosis and Management of Asthma, 2007.* Bethesda, MD: National Heart, Lung, and Blood Institute; 2007. NIH Publication No. 07-4052.

Table 81-4. Classifying Asthma Severity ≥12 Years[a]

Component of Severity		Classifying of Asthma Severity and Initiating Treatment (≥12 years of age)			
			Persistent		
		Intermittent	Mild	Moderate	Severe
Impairment	Symptoms	≤2 days/week	>2 days/week but not daily	Daily	Throughout the day
	Nighttime awakenings	≤2x/month	3–4x/month	>1x week, but not nightly	Often 7x/week
	Short-acting β₂-agonist use for symptom control (not prevention of EIB)	≤2 days/week	>2 days/week but not daily and more than 1x on any day	Daily	Several times per day
	Interference with normal activity	None	More limitation	Some limitation	Extremely limited
	Lung function	Normal FEV₁ between exacerbations FEV₁ >80% predicted FEV₁/FVC >85%	FEV₁ = >80% predicted FEV₁/FVC normal	FEV₁ >60, but <80% predicted FEV₁/FVC = reduced 5%	FEV₁ <60% predicted FEV₁/FVC reduced <5%
Risk	Exacerbation requiring oral systemic dorticosteroids	0–1/year	≥2 year		
		Consider severity and interval since last exacerbation. Frequency and severity may fluctuate over time. Exacerbations of any severity may occur in patients in any severity category.			
Recommended Step for Initiating Therapy (See Table 81-5 for treatment steps.)		Step 1: SABA PRN	Step 2: Low-dose ICS	Step 3: Low-dose ICS + LABA	Step 4/5: Medium/ High-dose ICS + LABA
				Consider short course of OCS.	
		In 2-6 weeks, depending on severity, evaluate level of asthma control that is achieved. If no clear benefit is observed in 4–6 weeks, consider adjusting therapy or alternative diagnoses.			

Abbreviations: EIB, exercise-induced bronchoconstriction; FEV₁, forced expiratory volume in 1 second; FVC, forced vital capacity; ICS, inhaled corticosteroids; LABA, long-acting β₂-agonist; OCS, oral corticosteroids; PRN, as needed; SABA, short-acting β₂-agonist.

[a]Adapted from the National Asthma Education and Prevention Program. *Expert Panel Report 3: Guidelines for the Diagnosis and Management of Asthma, 2007*. Bethesda, MD: National Heart, Lung, and Blood Institute; 2007. NIH Publication No. 07-4052.

severe level of symptoms, medication use, and other factors defines the level of severity, which determines the long-term approach to management. Patients with intermittent asthma may respond to short-acting bronchodilator as needed, whereas children with persistent asthma require a controller medication such as inhaled corticosteroids (ICS) to reduce inflammation. The treatment of asthma is based on its severity and control. For **intermittent asthma only** short-acting β₂-agonists are required on an as-needed basis to treat symptoms. Prophylactic use of β₂-agonists, cromolyn, or nedocromil may be used for exercise-induced asthma before the onset of activity. For **mild persistent asthma,** daily anti-inflammatory medications (controllers) are required with low-dose ICS as recommended therapy or alternative monotherapy with cromolyn, nedocromil, or leukotriene modifier agents, such as montelukast. Use short-acting β₂-agonists for acute exacerbations. For **moderate persistent** asthma, medium-dose ICS or low-dose ICS plus a second agent is recommended depending on the age group. Second agents include long-acting β₂-agonists, leukotriene modifiers, and theophylline. For **severe persistent** asthma, usually high-dose ICS plus a second agent is required. Systemic corticosteroids may be required to gain asthma control in moderate to severe persistent asthma patients. In difficult to control patients, especially those experiencing severe exacerbations despite optimal controller therapy, omalizumab has been shown to decrease risk of asthma attacks. Patients of all asthma severities require short-acting β₂-agonists for quick relief of symptoms and prevention of exercise-induced asthma.

Inhaled corticosteroids act topically on lung epithelium, inhibiting cell migration and activation and reducing airway hyperresponsiveness. Inhaled corticosteroids are the most effective anti-inflammatory medication for asthma. Inhaled corticosteroids reduce asthma symptoms, improve lung function, reduce acute exacerbations of asthma, and reduce the risk of death from asthma. Recent data show that ICS are well-tolerated, safe medications at the recommended dosages.

Leukotriene modifiers interfere with the action of leukotrienes, inflammatory mediators released from mast cells, eosinophils, and basophils. Long-acting β₂-agonists provide at least 12 hours of bronchodilation by stimulating β₂ receptors in the airway, which increases the concentration of cyclic adenosine monophosphate, causing relaxation of airway smooth muscle. Long-acting β₂-agonists should never be used alone without concomitant use with ICS in treatment of asthma.

Patients may be started at a higher level of medications at the onset, to establish prompt control, and then step-down reduction should be implemented to reach the minimum medication necessary to maintain control (see Table 81-5).

Table 81-5. Stepwise Approach for Managing Asthma By Age Group[a–d]

Age	Step 1	Step 2	Step 3	Step 4	Step 5	Step 6
0–4 y	SABA PRN	Low-dose ICS alternative: Cromolyn or montelukast	Medium-dose ICS	Medium-dose ICS + either LABA or montelukast	High-dose ICS + either LABA or montelukast	High-dose ICS + OCS + either LABA or montelukast
5–11 y	SABA PRN	Low-dose ICS alternative: Cromolyn, LTRA, or theophylline	Low-dose ICS + either LABA, LTRA, or theophylline OR Medium-dose ICS	Medium-dose ICS + LABA alternative: Medium-dose ICS+ either LTRA OR theophylline	High-dose ICS + LABA alternative: High-dose ICS+either LTRA OR theophylline	High-dose ICS + LABA +OCS alternative: High-dose ICS+either LTRA OR theophylline + OCS
12 y–adult	SABA PRN	Low-dose ICS alternative: Cromolyn, LTRA, or theophylline	Low-dose ICS + LABA OR medium-dose ICS alternative: Low-dose ICS + either LTRA OR theophylline or zileuton	Medium-dose ICS + LABA alternative: Medium-dose ICS + either LTRA OR theophylline or zileuton	High-dose ICS + LABA AND Consider omalizumab for patients who have allergies	High-dose ICS + LABA + OCS AND Consider omalizumab for patients who have allergies

Abbreviations: ICS, inhaled corticosteroid; LABA, long-acting β₂-agonist; LTRA, leukotriene receptor antagonist; OCS, oral corticosteroids; PRN, as needed; SABA, short-acting β₂-agonist.

[a]Adapted from the National Asthma Education and Prevention Program. *Expert Panel Report 3: Guidelines for the Diagnosis and Management of Asthma, 2007*. Bethesda, MD: National Heart, Lung, and Blood Institute; 2007. NIH Publication No. 07-4051.

[b] All patients need quick-relief medication (SABA).

Each Step: Patient education, environmental control, and management of comorbidities.

[c]Steps 2–4 (5 y–adult): Consider subcutaneous allergen immunotherapy for patients who have persistent, allergic asthma.

[d]Steps 5–6 (12 y–adult): Consider omalizumab for patients who have allergies.

Prognosis

Asthma can result in significant morbidity and mortality if children are not managed appropriately. Children without longitudinal primary care generally require expensive therapy in EDs or inpatient settings. A significant number of individuals with asthma have fatal outcomes because of lack of timely and appropriate care. Virtually all of these deaths are preventable.

CASE RESOLUTION

The 7-year-old boy in the case scenario who visits the office for asthma requires not only medication but also education and longitudinal primary care. It is particularly important to assess possible environmental factors (eg, pets), exposure to smoke, and poor compliance with previous recommendations, which have contributed to his recurrent symptoms.

Selected References

Abadolgu O, Mungan D, Pasaoglu G, Celik G, Misirligil Z. Influenza vaccination in patients with asthma: effect on the frequency of upper respiratory tract infections and exacerbations. *J Asthma*. 2004;41:279–283

Akinbami LJ. The state of childhood asthma, United States, 1980–2005. Advance Data from Vital and Health Statistics; No 381. Hyattsville, MD: National Center for Health Statistics; 2006. http://www.cdc.gov/nchs/data/ad/ad381.pdf. Accessed June 2009

Apter AJ, Szefler SJ. Advances in adult and pediatric asthma. *J Allergy Clin Immunol*. 2004;113:407–414

Bacharier LB, Strunk RC, Mauger D, White D, Lemanske RF Jr, Sorkness CA. Asthma severity in children: mismatch between symptoms, medication use, and lung function. *Am J Respir Crit Care Med*. 2004;170:426–432

Bisgaard H, Hermansen MN, Loland L, et al. Intermittent inhaled corticosteroids in infants with episodic wheezing. *N Engl J Med*. 2006;354:1998–2005

Bloom B, Cohen RA. Summary health statistics for U.S. children: National Health Interview Survey, 2007. National Center for Health Statistics. *Vital Health Stat*. 2009;10(239). www.cdc.gov/nchs/nhis.htm. Accessed June 2009

Boushey HA, Sorkness CA, King TS, et al. Daily versus as-needed corticosteroids for mild persistent asthma. *N Engl J Med*. 2005;352:1519–1528

Bousquet J, Wenzel S, Holgate S, Lumry W, Freeman P, Fox H. Predicting response to omalizumab, an anti-IgE antibody, in patients with allergic asthma. *Chest*. 2004;125:1378–1386

Brussee JE, Smit HA, van Strien RT, et al. Allergen exposure in infancy and the development of sensitization, wheeze, and asthma at 4 years. *J Allergy Clin Immunol*. 2005;115:946–952

Bueving HJ, Bernsen RM, de Jongste JC, et al. Influenza vaccination in children with asthma: randomized double-blind placebo-controlled trial. *Am J Respir Crit Care Med*. 2004;169:488–493

Busse W, Corren J, Lanier BQ, et al. Omalizumab, anti IgE recombinant humanized monoclonal antibody for the treatment of severe allergic asthma. *J Allergy Clin Immunol*. 2001;108:184–190

Castro-Rodriguez JA, Holberg CJ, Wright AL, Martinez FD. A clinical index to define risk of asthma in young children with recurrent wheezing. *Am J Respir Crit Care Med.* 2000;162(4 pt 1):1403–1406

Covar RA, Spahn JD, Murphy JR, Szefler SJ; Childhood Asthma Management Program Research Group. Progression of asthma measured by lung function in the childhood asthma management program. *Am J Respir Crit Care Med.* 2004;170:234–241

Eder W, Ege MJ, von Mutius E. The asthma epidemic. *N Engl J Med.* 2006; 355:2226–2235

Friedman H, Wilcox T, Reardon G, Crespi S, Yawn BP. A retrospective study of the use of fluticasone propionate/salmeterol combination as initial asthma controller therapy in a commercially-insured population. *Clin Ther.* 2008;30:1908–1917

Greenstone IR, Ni Chroinin MN, Masse V, et al. Combination of inhaled long-acting beta2-agonists and inhaled steroids versus higher dose of inhaled steroids in children and adults with persistent asthma. *Cochrane Database Syst Rev.* 2005;(4):CD005533

Jenkins CR, Thien FC, Whealtely JR, Reddel HK. Traditional and patient-centred outcomes with three classes of asthma medication. *Eur Respir J.* 2005;26:36–44

Masoli M, Weatherall M, Holt S, Beasley R. Moderate dose inhaled corticosteroids plus salmeterol versus higher doses of inhaled corticosteroids in symptomatic asthma. *Thorax.* 2005;60:730–734

Morgan WJ, Crain EF, Grunchalla RS, et al. Results of a home-based environmental intervention among urban children with asthma. *N Engl J Med.* 2004;351:1068–1080

National Asthma Education and Prevention Program. *Guidelines the Diagnosis and Management of Asthma: Expert Panel Report 3.* Bethesda, MD: National Institutes of Health, National Heart, Lung and Blood Institute; 2007

National Center for Health Statistics. *Reports From the 2005 National Health Interview Survey.* Hyattsville, MD: National Center for Health Statistics, Centers for Disease Control and Prevention; 2005. www.cdc.gov/nchs/about/major/nhis/reports_2005.htm

National Heart, Lung, and Blood Institute. *National Asthma Education and Prevention Program Expert Panel Executive Summary Report: Guidelines for the Diagnosis and Management of Asthma—Update on Selected Topics 2002.* Bethesda, MD: National Institutes of Health; National Heart, Lung, and Blood Institute; 2002. NIH Publication No. 02-5075

Ng D, Salvio F, Hicks G. Anti-leukotriene agents compared to inhaled corticosteroids in the management of recurrent and/or chronic asthma in adults and children. *Cochrane Database Syst Rev.* 2004;(2):CD002314

Pual K, Cover R, Jain N, Gelfand EW, Spahn JD. Do NHLBI lung function criteria apply to children? A cross-sectional evaluation of childhood asthma at national Jewish Medical and Research Center, 1999–2002. *Pediatr Pulmonol.* 2005;39:311–317

Saltpeter SR, Buckley NS, Ormiston TM, Salpeter EE. Meta-analysis: effect of long-acting beta-agonists on severe asthma exacerbations and asthma-related deaths. *Ann Intern Med.* 2006;144:904–912

Sigurs N, Gustafsson PM, Bjarnason R, et al. Severe respiratory syncytial virus bronchiolitis in infancy and asthma and allergy at age 13. *Am J Respir Crit Care Med.* 2005;171:137–141

Verbanck S, Schuermans D, Paiva M, Vincken W. The functional benefit of anti-inflammatory aerosols in the lung periphery. *J Allergy Clin Immunol.* 2006;118:340–346

Wood D, Hill V. Practical management of asthma. *PREP.* 2009;30(10):375–384

Zeiger RS, Hay JW, Contreras R, et al. Asthma costs and utilization in a managed care organization. *J Allergy Clin Immunol.* 2008;121:885–892

CHAPTER 82

Cough

Nasser Redjal, MD

CASE STUDY

A 3-year-old boy presents with a cough that he has had for 4 weeks. In the past he has had coughs with colds, but this cough is persistent and deeper in quality. The cough seemed to develop suddenly when he was playing at a friend's house. It occurs all day and disrupts his sleep at night. The boy has had no nasal congestion, fever, or sore throat. No one at home is coughing, and the boy has not traveled recently. Neither the boy nor his family has a history of allergies or asthma. Over-the-counter cough preparations have not helped relieve his symptoms. On examination, growth parameters are normal. The child has a persistent cough with no respiratory distress. Chest examination reveals a normal respiratory rate, no retractions, and no use of accessory muscles, but diffuse expiratory wheezing is noted in the right lower lobe. The remainder of the examination is normal.

Questions

1. What are common parental concerns regarding cough?
2. What diagnoses in children with persistent cough should be considered?
3. What historical factors and physical findings are important to determine the etiology of cough?
4. What diagnostic workup is appropriate?
5. How should children with chronic cough be managed?

Cough is an essential protective reflex that allows for clearance of secretions and particulates from the airways. Its persistence can be distressing to the patient and often causes parental anxiety due to the concern regarding its etiology and the frequent disruption of sleep. Cough may be acute, subacute, or chronic. Acute cough lasts less than 2 weeks and is often associated with respiratory tract infections in children. Cough lasting 2 to 4 weeks is subacute, and when cough lasts more than 4 weeks, it is persistent or chronic. Parental sensitivity as well as accessibility to medical care influence when in the course of disease children present with this problem.

Epidemiology

Cough is a very common complaint initiating pediatric office visits. In the National Ambulatory Medical Care Survey, 6.7% of pediatric office visits involved children who presented with cough. Typically, preschool children have up to 8 upper respiratory infections with associated cough in a winter season. Persistent cough is also very common, with an estimated prevalence of 5% to 7% in preschoolers and 12% to 15% in older children. Cough is more common among boys than girls up to 11 years of age, and may be less common in developing countries than in affluent countries. Many serious diseases, including cystic fibrosis, congenital heart disease, asthma, and immunodeficiency disorders, may result in cough.

Clinical Presentation

The presentation varies greatly depending on the etiology of the cough. Children may present in severe respiratory distress or have no evidence of respiratory compromise. They may exhibit failure to thrive or appear totally healthy.

Pathophysiology

Coughing is a complicated reflex process that propels excess mucus up the airways at the pressures of up to 300 mm Hg and at flows of up to 5 to 6 L/sec. It is initiated through irritation of one of the multiple cough receptors (Figure 82-1). These receptors are located in the nose, paranasal sinuses, posterior pharynx, larynx, trachea, bronchi, and pleura. They can also be found outside of the respiratory tract in the ear canal, stomach, pericardium, and diaphragm. Stimulation of any of these receptors by an irritant, whether mechanical, chemical, thermal, or inflammatory, can initiate the cough reflex. The proximal airways (larynx and trachea) are more sensitive to mechanical stimulation, and the distal airways more sensitive to chemical stimulation. The lung parenchymal (bronchiolar and alveolar) tissue contains no cough receptors, so pneumonia may not produce a cough. Impulses from stimulated cough receptors traverse afferent nerves (vagus, glossopharyngeal, trigeminal, or phrenic) to a "cough center" in the medulla, which itself is under some control by higher cortical centers. The cough center generates an efferent signal that travels down the vagus, phrenic, and spinal motor nerves to expiratory musculature, thereby producing the cough. The cough center can be voluntarily stimulated or suppressed.

The actual cough experienced by patients may be broken down into 4 phases. First, the glottis opens with an inspiratory gasp. Second, the glottis closes with forceful contraction of the chest wall, diaphragm, and abdominal muscles. Third, the glottis again opens

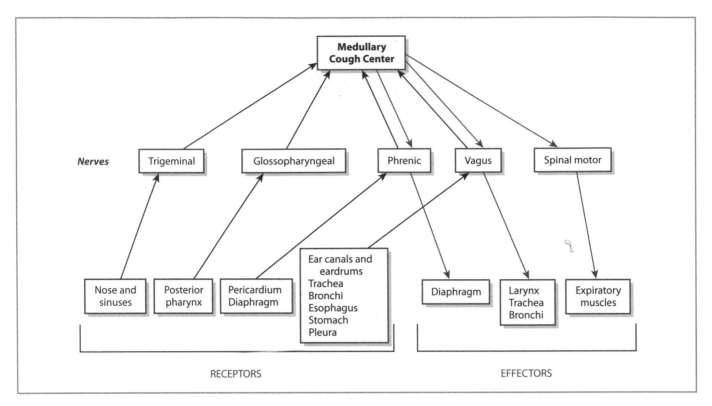

Figure 82-1. The cough reflex.

with release of airway pressure in an expiratory phase. The fourth phase involves relaxation in which the chest wall and abdominal muscles relax. This process expels mucus or irritants from the airways, helping maintain the health of the lungs. Children who do not cough effectively may be at risk for atelectasis, recurrent pneumonia, and chronic airway disease from aspiration and/or retention of secretions.

Differential Diagnosis

The list of differential diagnoses of cough is long (Box 82-1). Narrowing the list of causes can be accomplished by paying attention to several factors (Dx Box).

As with any pediatric symptom, the child's **age** influences the diagnostic possibilities and management of the cough. Congenital anomalies, which are most likely to present in the first few months of life, include tracheoesophageal fistula, laryngeal cleft, vocal cord paralysis, and tracheobronchomalacia. Congenital heart disease

Dx Cough

- Quality: dry, productive, brassy, honking
- Duration: acute, subacute, chronic, recurrent
- Timing: during day, at night, on awakening, with exercise
- Fever or upper respiratory infection associated with infectious origin
- Allergic findings of rhinorrhea, sneezing, wheezing, atopic dermatitis associated with asthma or allergic rhinitis
- Failure to thrive (indicates chronic disease)

can produce a cough from heart failure and pulmonary edema. Congenital mediastinal tumors cause infants to cough if the tumor presses on the bronchial tree. Many children with asthma experience cough and/or wheezing in infancy, often associated with an episode of bronchiolitis.

The **duration of the cough** also suggests its possible cause. Most acute coughs are infectious in origin. Upper respiratory infections can initiate an acute cough through stimulation of the cough receptors in the nose and posterior pharynx. If nasal congestion and cough persist, a diagnosis of allergic rhinitis or sinusitis should be considered. Serous otitis media can also cause a persistent cough and may occur in children with chronic congestion. Children with pneumonia may present with either acute or chronic cough.

The presence of a nighttime cough can be important. Pathologic coughs, including those caused by sinusitis with postnasal drip, gastroesophageal reflux, and asthma, are more likely to occur at night.

The character of the cough is another factor to consider in the differential diagnosis. Certain etiologies are associated with a very specific type of cough. A barking cough is consistent with laryngeal edema and croup. A stridorous cough may be seen with proximal airway disease, such as laryngomalacia or tracheomalacia, laryngotracheobronchitis, or a foreign body. An inspiratory whoop is characteristic of pertussis or parapertussis. Staccato cough in infants can be the result of infection with *Chlamydia trachomatis*. The psychogenic or habitual cough is a strange, honking sound (Canadian goose-like), disappears at night, and is typically at its worst and most disruptive during school classes. Chronic paroxysmal cough triggered by exercise, cold air, sleep, or allergens is often seen in patients with asthma.

Box 82-1. Causes of Cough

Congenital Anomalies • Tracheoesophageal fistula • Laryngeal cleft • Vocal cord paralysis • Mediastinal masses • Pulmonary malformations • Tracheobronchomalacia • Congenital heart disease ***Infections (eg, upper respiratory infection, sinusitis, pneumonia)*** *Viral* • Adenovirus • Influenza • Parainfluenza • Respiratory syncytial virus • Rhinovirus • Human metapneumovirus	*Bacterial* • Pertussis • Pneumococcal • Staphylococcal • Tuberculosis *Fungal* • Coccidioidomycosis *Parasitic infection* • Paragonimiasis • Echinococcosis *Other* • Chlamydial • Mycoplasmosis ***Cardiac Disease*** • Congestive heart failure • Pulmonary hypertension	***Chronic Disease*** • Cystic fibrosis • HIV infection • Immunodeficiency syndrome • Dyskinetic cilia ***Allergic Conditions*** • Allergic rhinitis • Asthma • Serous otitis media ***Mediastinal Tumors*** ***Foreign Body Aspiration*** ***Gastroesophageal Reflux*** ***Environmental Irritants*** ***Psychogenic Cough*** ***Drug-Induced Conditions*** ***Sarcoidosis*** ***Tourette Disorder (tics)***

In contrast, a chronic productive (or "wet") cough suggests a suppurative process, and may require further investigation to exclude bronchiectasis, cystic fibrosis, active infection, immune deficiency, or congenital malformation.

Pneumococcus is the most probable causal agent in acute cough with pneumonia, but when the cough becomes chronic, other infectious agents are more likely. Adenovirus and respiratory syncytial virus, which occur more commonly in infants, and influenza and parainfluenza, which affect children of all ages, are common viral agents that produce chronic cough. *Bordetella pertussis,* mycoplasma, and chlamydia also cause chronic cough. Other infections, such as tuberculosis and coccidioidomycosis, should also be considered in endemic areas or high-risk populations. Chronic infectious coughs, such as those associated with influenza and pertussis, can last up to 6 months. Host factors that may predispose to chronic cough should also be investigated. Children with cystic fibrosis, bronchopulmonary dysplasia, HIV and other immunodeficiency syndromes, and congenital pulmonary malformations may present with chronic, recurrent cough.

The most common triggers of chronic cough are persistent rhinitis and chronic sinusitis followed by gastroesophageal reflux disease and asthma. All of these contribute to the development of an irritable larynx, which causes cough. In fact, cough with no notable wheezing may be the only manifestation of asthma. In infants or neurologically impaired children, chronic cough may indicate gastroesophageal reflux **or** recurrent aspiration. An unexplained persistent cough, primarily in toddlers, may be the result of foreign body aspiration if the initial aspiration was not observed. In some studies a history of choking episodes is absent in approximately 50% and chest radiograph examination produces normal results in approximately 20% to 40% of children who have foreign bodies present on bronchoscopy. The foreign object acts as a chronic airway irritant that stimulates coughing, and it may be the cause of recurrent infections. Other irritants that initiate cough include dust, allergens, wood- and gas-burning stoves, chemicals, and passive or active exposure to smoke from tobacco, marijuana, cocaine, or other substances. Drugs such as β-adrenergic receptor antagonists and angiotensin-converting enzyme inhibitors can also induce a chronic cough, probably by increasing the sensitivity of the cough reflex. Patients previously treated with cytotoxic drugs or thoracic radiation are at risk of interstitial lung disease. Cough along with symptoms of pancreatic insufficiency, recurrent bacterial pneumonia, and/or failure to thrive should raise suspicion of cystic fibrosis. Cough with a history of dyspnea or hemoptysis should trigger a search for organic lung disease. Hemoptysis should also raise concerns of bronchiectasis, cavitary lung disease (tuberculosis or bacterial abscesses), congestive heart failure, hemosiderosis, neoplasm, foreign bodies, vascular lesions, endobronchial lesions, catamenial (ectopic endometrial tissue) bleeding, and clotting disorders.

Evaluation

History

A complete history should be obtained when children present with cough (Questions Box). All symptoms should be noted. Vomiting with cough can indicate phlegm production and the accumulation of mucus in the stomach, with resultant delayed gastric emptying. In some children with a chief complaint of vomiting it is actually the cough that precipitates the vomiting. Post-tussive vomiting is characteristic of pertussis.

Questions

Cough

- How old is the child?
- How long has the child had the cough?
- How frequently does the child cough?
- Does the cough occur at night?
- Does exercise make the cough worse?
- Do any factors such as environmental irritants seem to precipitate the cough?
- Does the child have any related infectious symptoms, including fever and nasal congestion?
- Does the child have any other symptoms?
- Has the child had any previous episodes of coughing or associated symptoms?
- Has the child lost weight recently?
- What is the child's birth history?
- Has the child had any pulmonary injuries?
- What is the child's immunization status?
- Does the child have a history of recent travel?
- Has a family member had similar symptoms?
- Does the family have a history of pulmonary disease or allergies?
- Has the child been treated with any medications for the cough? Have they helped?
- Is the child taking any other medications?

Physical Examination

A complete physical examination should be performed on all children who present with cough. Growth parameters and vital signs should be assessed. Skin should be examined for evidence of cyanosis or atopy. Facial petechiae or subconjunctival hemorrhage indicates particularly forceful coughing. Extremities should be evaluated for fingernail clubbing, which is a sign of chronic pulmonary disease. The nose should be assessed for evidence of congestion. Allergic disease produces pale, edematous mucosa, whereas infection results in more inflammatory mucosa. Tympanic membranes should be examined and mobility tested; halitosis, tonsillar hypertrophy, pharyngeal cobblestoning, and tenderness on the sinus area suggest sinus disease.

The respiratory effort, including the use of accessory muscles, should also be noted. Careful attention should be paid to breath sounds; whether abnormal sounds are in the inspiratory or expiratory phase of respiration should be determined. Stridor is classically an inspiratory sound (see Chapter 58), whereas wheezing is usually an expiratory sound. Chronic cough and wheeze are often noted in combination. Even in the absence of a history of wheeze, clinicians should listen carefully for this finding during the physical examination. Wheezing that is characterized by many different pitches and starting and stopping at varying points in the respiratory cycle is termed *polyphonic* and in association with cough is highly suggestive of asthma. Other causes of polyphonic wheezing include viral bronchiolitis, obliterative bronchiolitis, bronchiectasis, bronchopulmonary dysplasia, congestive heart failure, immunodeficiency, bronchomalacia, and aspiration syndromes.

Monophonic wheezing (a single, distinct, one pitch that starts and stops at one discrete time) and cough should always raise suspicion of large airway obstruction caused by foreign body or by tracheomalacia. Extrinsic airway compression as occurs with vascular rings, lymphadenopathy, and mediastinal tumors is also associated with monophonic wheezing. Tuberculosis should also be considered in a child with a monophonic wheeze, particularly in areas where the disease is prevalent.

Prolongation of the expiratory phase also is associated with wheezing and also indicates airway obstruction. Abnormal breath sounds should be localized if possible. Because the character of the cough can establish the diagnosis, listening to the cough is probably the most important part of the physical examination. A parental description of the cough may be less diagnostic.

Laboratory Tests

After a thorough history and physical examination, laboratory data may not be necessary. Laboratory tests should be ordered when more information is needed to help make a reasonable diagnosis. The laboratory data should be directed at proving or disproving the most likely diagnosis in a specific patient.

If after the history, physical examination, and chest radiograph an infectious etiology for cough is suspected, a complete blood cell count with differential and a purified protein derivative skin test should be ordered. Appropriate cultures should be sent, if possible. Most children swallow their phlegm, so sputum cultures may be difficult to obtain. Gastric aspirates can sometimes yield a reasonable sputum specimen for culture. Nasopharyngeal cultures are useful for diagnosing pertussis and viruses.

If a specific diagnosis is suspected, laboratory tests (Table 82-1) should be directed toward that diagnosis (eg, sweat chloride to rule out cystic fibrosis or quantitative immunoglobulins to rule out immunodeficiency). Allergy skin test or radioallergosorbent testing may be indicated to exclude inhalant allergy.

Imaging Studies

The chest radiograph (anteroposterior and lateral views), the mainstay of the diagnostic evaluation of cough, should be the first test ordered in the evaluation of a chronic cough or if definite findings are evident on physical examination. A lateral decubitus film can provide additional information about pleural fluid or air trapping. Inspiratory and expiratory films can be obtained if a foreign body is suspected. An area of inflation that either fails to deflate on exhalation or remains present in the decubitus position is suggestive of a foreign body. Congenital lobar emphysema and unilateral hyperlucent lung (Swyer-James Macleod) syndrome are rare causes of focal or unilateral hyperinflation. If a nodular pulmonary lesion is found on radiograph, bronchoscopy may be the next step to further define the lesion. Bronchiectasis is a characteristic of cystic fibrosis, immune deficiency, primary ciliary dyskinesia, chronic aspiration, and previous history of severe infection (most commonly adenovirus and pertussis). If sinusitis is suspected, radiographs or a computed tomography scan of the sinuses can be performed. An upper

Table 82-1. Tests to Consider for Evaluation of Chronic Cough	
Allergy	Allergy skin test or blood-specific immunoglobulin E test
Asthma	Pulmonary function test (PFT), bronchial hyperresponsiveness test such as methacholine challenge test, exhaled nitric oxide, trial of asthma treatments
Ciliary dyskinesia	Ciliary function tests
Congenital anomalies	Bronchoscopy, chest radiograph, computed tomography (CT)/magnetic resonance imaging, angiography
Fungal infections	Coccidiomycosis: antibody assay(precipitin, complement fixation) Histoplasmosis: antibody assay (complement fixation, immunoprecipitating) Serum and urine antigen detection
Cystic fibrosis	Sweat chloride test, genetic test
Fibrosing alveolitis, autoimmune disease	PFT and diffusion CT, autoantibodies
Foreign body	Chest radiograph, bronchoscopy
Gastroesophageal reflux	Barium swallow, 24-hour pH recording, and bronchoalveolar lavage (BAL)
Pertussis, chlamydia, or other infectious etiologies	Cultures, serology, polymerase chain reaction testing
Purulent infection	Cultures (sputum, BAL), chest radiograph, CT, microbiology immunology, sweat test
Sinusitis	Imaging of sinuses with radiograph or CT scan
Tuberculosis	Mantoux testing

gastrointestinal series of radiographs or a pH probe study would help to define gastroesophageal reflux if the cough occurs after recurrent episodes of vomiting or at night.

In children with asthma, the chest radiograph may be totally normal. Further diagnostic testing with peak flow measurements or pulmonary function tests in children older than 4 years can be done to demonstrate restriction or obstruction of the airway. The most helpful test to diagnose asthma may be a trial of a bronchodilator (see Chapter 81).

Management

Cough should not be treated until the cause has been identified by a thorough consideration of the differential diagnoses. Therapy should then be directed toward treating that etiology. However, many children do not have any evidence of chronic disease based on a detailed history, physical examination, radiography, and pulmonary function testing. When the initial evaluation outlined previously is unrevealing, cough-variant asthma, post-viral cough, increased cough receptor sensitivity, and functional disorders (including habit cough and tic disorders) should be considered. Empiric courses of therapy for asthma, rhinitis, sinusitis, or gastroesophageal reflux can be considered if suggestive findings exist. The external ear is innervated by the vagus nerve, and removal of irritants from the external auditory canal may reduce the coughing. Airflow obstruction may be apparent at the first visit, and a trial of asthma therapy is warranted, particularly if other signs of allergic disease are present or if the child's cough is precipitated by typical asthma triggers. A cough of an infectious etiology should be treated with the appropriate antibiotics. Expectorants and mucolytic agents in cough syrups have little effect on relieving coughs. Most over-the-counter children's cough medications are marginally effective, provide no greater benefit compared with placebo, and may be associated with adverse or paradoxical reactions.

Prognosis

With thoughtful evaluation, it is usually possible to identify the causes of both acute and chronic cough. Most symptoms resolve with appropriate therapy. If the cough persists with treatment, then alternate diagnoses should be considered.

CASE RESOLUTION

In the case presented at the beginning of this chapter, the child's cough began acutely and developed into a chronic cough. The boy has no history of allergies or symptoms consistent with an infectious process. Physical examination reveals localized wheezing. A chest radiograph is ordered, which reveals hyperinflation of the right lung. His symptoms and presentation are most consistent with foreign body aspiration and he is admitted to the hospital for bronchoscopy.

Selected References

Boat TF. Pulmonary hemorrhage and hemoptysis. In: Chernick V, Boat TF, eds. *Kendig's Disorders of the Respiratory Tract in Children.* 6th ed. Philadelphia, PA: WB Saunders; 1998:623

Bucca CB, Bugiani M, Culla B, et al. Chronic cough and irritable larynx. *J Allergy Clin Immunol.* 2011;127(2):412–419

Carr BC. Efficacy, abuse, and toxicity of over-the-counter cough and cold medicines in the pediatric population. *Curr Opin Pediatr.* 2006;18:184–188

Chang AB. Cough, cough receptors, and asthma in children. *Pediatr Pulmonol.* 1999;28:59–70

Chang AB, Powell CV. Non-specific cough in children: diagnosis and treatment. *Hosp Med.* 1998;59:680–684

Chung KF, Chang AB. Therapy for cough: active agents. *Pulm Pharmacol Ther.* 2002;15:335–338

Chung KF, Pavord ID. Prevalence, pathogenesis, and causes of chronic cough. *Lancet.* 2008;371:1364–1374

de Jongste JC, Shields MD. Cough. 2: chronic cough in children. *Thorax.* 2003;58:998–1003

Eysink PE, Bottema BJ, ter Riet G, Aalberse RC, Stapel SO, Bindels PJ. Coughing in pre-school children in general practice: when are RASTs for inhalation allergy indicated? *Pediatr Allergy Immunol.* 2004;15:394–400

Garrett MH, Hooper MA, Hooper BM, Abramson MJ. Respiratory symptoms in children and indoor exposure to nitrogen dioxide and gas stoves. *Am J Respir Crit Care Med.* 1998;158:891–895

Guilbert TW, Taussig LM. "Doctor, he's been coughing for a month. Is it serious?" *Contemp Pediatr.* 1998;15:155–172

Irwin RS, Baumann MH, Bolser DC, et al. Diagnosis and management of cough executive summary: ACCP evidence-based clinical practice guidelines. *Chest.* 2006;129;1S–23S

Katcher ML. Cold, cough, and allergy medications: uses and abuses. *Pediatr Rev.* 1996;17:12–17

Kelkar P, Weldon D. Approach to the patient with chronic cough. In: Adkinson NF, Bochner BS, et al. *Middleton's Allergy Principle and Practice.* 7th ed. Mayland Heights, MO: Elsevier; 2009:1395–1404

Morice AH, Fontana GA, Belvisi MG, et al. ERS guidelines on the assessment of cough. *Eur Respir J.* 2007;29:1256–1276

Morice AH, Fontana GA, Sovijarvi AR, et al. The diagnosis and management of chronic cough. *Eur Respir J.* 2004;24:481–492

Morice AH, Geppetti P. Cough. 5: the type 1 vanilloid receptor: a sensory receptor for cough. *Thorax.* 2004;59:257–258

Ramanuja, S, Kelkar, P. The approach to pediatric cough. *Ann Allergy Asthma Immunol.* 2010;105(1):3–8

Ramanuja S, Kelkar P. Habit cough. *Ann Allergy Asthma Immunol.* 2009;102:91–95

Santamaria F, Montella S, Camera L, et al. Lung structure abnormalities, but normal lung function in pediatric bronchiesctasis. *Chest.* 2006;130:480–486

Schwartz J. Air pollution and children's health. *Pediatrics.* 2004;113:1037–1043

Stein RT, Holberg CJ, Sherrill D, et al. Influence of parental smoking on respiratory symptoms during the first decade of life: the Tucson Children's Respiratory Study. *Am J Epidemiol.* 1999;149:1030–1037

Tan H, Buyukavci M, Arik A. Tourette's syndrome manifests as chronic persistent cough. *Yonsei Med J.* 2004;45:145–149

Tekdemir I, Aslan A, Elhan A. A clinico-anatomic study of the auricular branch of the vagus nerve and Arnold's ear-cough reflex. *Surg Radiol Anat.* 1998;20:253–257

Hematologic Disorders

CHAPTER 83

Anemia

Wendy Y. Tcheng, MD

CASE STUDY

An 18-month-old girl is brought to the office with a 3-day history of cough, rhinorrhea, low-grade fever, mild scleral icterus and pallor. During her first week of life, the girl had hyperbilirubinemia of unknown etiology that required phototherapy. Her family history is significant for mild anemia in her father; the cause of his condition is unknown. A paternal aunt and grandfather had cholecystectomies while in their 30s.

On physical examination, the girl is tachycardic and tachypneic (no respiratory distress), with scleral icterus and pallor. Her spleen is palpable 3 cm below the midcostal margin. The remainder of her examination is normal.

Questions

1. What hemoglobin/hematocrit values are associated with anemia?
2. What is the appropriate initial evaluation of children with anemia?
3. What emergency situations in children who present with anemia should be recognized by the primary pediatrician?
4. When should a child with anemia be referred to a hematologist?
5. How is the family history relevant in the evaluation of anemia?

Anemia occurs when there is a reduction in hemoglobin concentration or red blood cell (RBC) number, leading to decreased oxygen-carrying capacity of blood. Anemia is defined as a hemoglobin or hematocrit value that is less than 2 SDs below the mean for age and gender. With this statistical definition, 2.5% of the healthy population will be categorized as having anemia. These values vary throughout infancy and childhood as hematopoiesis evolves from fetal to adult type, and it is important to reference normal age and gender-related values when interpreting a hemoglobin or hematocrit result. (See Table 83-1 for normal age-related values.) In addition, there is racial variation with African American children having lower average hemoglobin values when compared to Caucasian children. The cardiopulmonary status should also be considered as children with cyanotic heart disease or chronic respiratory insufficiency typically have hemoglobin values that are higher than the normal range and may be functionally anemic when the hemoglobin value falls even if it is within the lower range of normal.

Epidemiology

Iron deficiency is the most common cause of anemia in childhood, occurring most frequently during late infancy through the first few years of life and again during adolescence. This prevalence pattern corresponds to periods of rapid growth, and when combined with poor dietary intake can predispose to iron deficiency. Other contributing factors to iron deficiency include prematurity, blood loss (most commonly menstrual or gastrointestinal [GI]), and GI conditions associated with decreased iron absorption.

Other epidemiological factors that contribute to anemia are presented in Box 83-1. Anemias that have a genetic etiology, including

Table 83-1. Values (Mean and Lower Limits of Normal) for Hemoglobin, Hematocrit, and Mean Corpuscular Volume Determinations[a]

| Age, y | Hemoglobin (g/dL) | | Hematocrit (%) | | MCV (μ^3) | |
	Mean	Lower Limit	Mean	Lower Limit	Mean	Lower Limit
0.5–1.9	12.5	11.0	37	33	77	70
2–4	12.5	11.0	38	34	79	73
5–7	13.0	11.5	39	35	81	75
8–11	13.5	12.0	40	36	83	76
12–14						
Female	13.5	12.0	41	36	85	78
Male	14.0	12.5	43	37	84	77
15–17						
Female	14.0	12.0	41	36	87	79
Male	15.0	13.0	46	38	86	78
18–49						
Female	14.0	12.0	42	37	90	80
Male	16.0	14.0	47	40	90	80

Abbreviation: MCV, mean corpuscular volume.

[a]From Brugnara C, Oski FA, Nathan DG. Diagnostic approach to the anemic patient. In: Orkin SH, Nathan DG, Ginsburg D, Look AT, Fisher DE, Lux SE eds. *Nathan and Oski's Hematology of Infancy and Childhood.* 7th ed. Philadelphia, PA: Saunders; 2009:456, with permission.

hemoglobinopathies (eg, sickle cell disease, thalassemias), RBC enzyme deficiencies (eg, glucose-6-phosphate dehydrogenase [G6PD], pyruvate kinase), and RBC membrane disorders (eg, hereditary spherocytosis), are commonly diagnosed in childhood. The highest incidence of sickle cell disease, thalassemia, and G6PD deficiency is in individuals of African, Mediterranean, and Southeast Asian descent within the "malaria belt" near the equator, likely reflecting an advantage against malaria. Dietary factors can cause impaired hematopoiesis as in iron, folate, or vitamin B_{12} deficiency. Ingestion of oxidants (eg, fava beans, medications) can trigger hemolysis in G6PD deficiency. Ingestion of toxins such as lead can also result in impaired hematopoiesis. Lead poisoning occurs more commonly in children who live in cities and older housing. In an otherwise healthy child, viral infections can cause a pure red cell aplasia (transient erythroblastopenia of childhood), an autoimmune hemolytic anemia, or an aplastic anemia. Children with congenital hemolytic anemias are at risk for hemolytic and aplastic crises associated with infectious illnesses.

Clinical Presentation

The clinical presentation of anemia depends on the age of the child, the severity and cause of the anemia, and the rapidity of onset (Dx Box). Most often anemia is detected on a routine screen or as part of an evaluation for an acute illness and the child is asymptomatic with no significant physical findings. Children who have developed anemia gradually may be relatively asymptomatic because time has afforded compensatory mechanisms. With severe anemia, easy fatigability and exercise intolerance can develop and pallor, fatigue, headache, dizziness, and irritability may occur. On examination, pallor, tachycardia, tachypnea, edema and, in severe cases, outright congestive heart failure (CHF) may be present. Children with an abrupt drop in hemoglobin due to blood loss or hemolysis will present more acutely with signs of tachycardia, tachypnea, and possible hypotension and shock. If the anemia is due to acute hemolysis, accompanying jaundice, icterus, and dark urine may be seen.

Pathophysiology

Erythrocytes develop from pluripotent stem cells within the bone marrow under the influence of various hematopoietic growth factors. Erythropoietin is the primary growth factor regulating RBC production and is produced primarily in the kidneys. The primary function of the erythrocyte is the delivery of oxygen to tissues for aerobic metabolism. To this end, hemoglobin is the main intracellular protein of the erythrocyte. Hemoglobin consists of 4 polypeptide chains, each containing an active heme group that is capable of binding to an oxygen molecule. A normal erythrocyte has a life span of approximately 120 days and is subsequently removed from circulation as it passes through the reticuloendothelial system. Under steady state conditions, the daily 1% loss of aged erythrocytes is compensated by a normal active erythropoiesis.

Anemia occurs when there is an imbalance between erythrocyte production and destruction. It can arise from conditions leading

---

Box 83-1. Epidemiological Factors Related to Anemia

Genetic
- Autosomal-dominant: hereditary spherocytosis
- Autosomal-recessive: most Embden-Meyerhof pathway enzyme deficiencies (pyruvate kinase deficiency), most hemoglobinopathies (sickle cell disease, β-thalassemia)
- X-linked: glucose-6-phosphate dehydrogenase (G6PD) deficiency

Ethnicity
- Northern European: hereditary spherocytosis, pyruvate kinase deficiency
- Mediterranean (Italian, Greek, North African): β-thalassemia, G6PD deficiency
- African: sickle cell disease, hemoglobin C, hemoglobin D, G6PD deficiency, α-thalassemia trait, hereditary elliptocytosis
- Southeast Asian: α-thalassemia, hemoglobin E, G6PD deficiency

Dietary
Poor dietary intake (iron, folate, or vitamin B_{12} deficiency)
- Iron (excessive cow's milk intake)
- Folate (excessive goat's milk intake)
- Vitamin B_{12} (vegan diet)

Poor gastrointestinal absorption
- Iron, absorbed in duodenum (small bowel disease)
- Folate, absorbed in duodenum and jejunum (small bowel disease)
- Vitamin B_{12}, absorbed in terminal ileum (surgical resection, pernicious anemia, small bowel disease)

Ingestion of oxidants (medications such as sulfa drugs, fava beans in G6PD deficiency)

Toxins (lead)

Socioeconomic
- Living near highways: increased incidence of lead poisoning
- Poverty: associated with pica and lead poisoning

Infectious
- Malaria: heterozygous form of sickle cell disease, thalassemia, G6PD-deficiency confer protection
- Viral infections: transient erythroblastopenia of childhood, autoimmune hemolytic anemias, hemolytic crisis in patients with congenital hemolytic anemias
- Parvovirus: aplastic crisis in patients with hemolytic anemias
- Viral hepatitis: aplastic anemia

Dx   Anemia

- Pallor, fatigue
- Scleral icterus
- Hepatosplenomegaly
- Lymphadenopathy
- Weight loss
- Congestive heart failure

to **decreased production, increased destruction** (ie, hemolysis), or **blood loss.** Deficient production may be due to nutrient deficiency (iron, folate, vitamin B_{12}), bone marrow failure (acquired or inherited), or bone marrow infiltration (eg, malignancy). Increased destruction of erythrocytes can occur as a consequence of disorders intrinsic to the erythrocyte (eg, hemoglobinopathies, enzymopathies, membranopathies) or extrinsic factors (immune or nonimmune etiologies).

Differential Diagnosis

The differential diagnosis of anemia can be determined by considering both the underlying mechanism of anemia (decreased production/increased destruction/blood loss) and the size of the erythrocyte (mean corpuscular volume [MCV]). The differential diagnosis of anemia based on pathophysiology and erythrocyte size can be found in Table 83-2 and Box 83-2. In determining the cause of anemia, the reticulocyte count is the most useful test in ascertaining whether the anemia is due to decreased production or increased destruction. A reduced reticulocyte count indicates decreased marrow production, whereas an elevated reticulocyte count is highly suggestive of hemolysis. Anemia based on erythrocyte size can be classified as microcytic (low MCV), normocytic (normal MCV), or macrocytic (high MCV). Microcytic anemias reflect a defect in hemoglobin synthesis and are most commonly due to iron deficiency, thalassemia, lead poisoning, and chronic disease. Macrocytic anemias reflect a relative decrease in DNA synthesis during erythropoiesis and are usually of nutritional origin (vitamin B_{12} or folate deficiency). The many other causes of anemia commonly fall into the normocytic category and can be further divided based on the reticulocyte count. Etiology and erythrocyte size, the 2 systems for classification of anemia, are not mutually exclusive—simultaneous application of these 2 systems will enable the pediatrician to make a primary diagnosis of anemia and determine its probable causes.

Microcytic Anemias

Iron deficiency is the most frequent cause of microcytic anemia in childhood and occurs as a result of (1) inadequate intake, (2) increased requirements due to growth, (3) blood loss, and (4) malabsorption of iron. As iron deficiency evolves, depletion of iron stores occurs first, then iron-deficient erythropoiesis without anemia and, finally, iron deficiency anemia. The combination of rapid growth and inadequate iron intake is responsible for the common occurrence of iron deficiency anemia in toddlers and adolescents. Most young infants are spared because of adequate iron stores acquired in utero and the ingestion of iron-fortified formulas. Premature infants are the exception as they have lower baseline iron stores (much of the iron stores are acquired by the fetus in the third trimester). As iron stores become depleted during late infancy and cow's milk is introduced into the diet, the ever-growing older infant/toddler becomes at risk for iron deficiency. Excessive cow's milk intake during the first few years of life predisposes to iron deficiency because cow's milk has minimal iron (<1 mg/L). Large intake of cow's milk results in early satiety and prevents adequate intake of other iron-containing

foods. The iron deficiency is often further compounded by trace amounts of GI blood loss due to lack of cytochrome iron and GI mucosal damage or cow's milk allergy enteropathy. Adolescents, particularly menstruating females, are also prone to iron deficiency because of the pubertal growth spurt and suboptimal dietary habits. In young infants and children older than 3 years, dietary iron deficiency is uncommon, and an evaluation for blood loss or malabsorption is warranted. Blood loss can occur as hematochezia or melena (inflammatory bowel disease, diarrhea, Meckel diverticulum, polyp, ulcer), menorrhagia, epistaxis, hematuria (intravascular hemolysis), or rarely as pulmonary bleeding (pulmonary hemosiderosis). Iron is absorbed primarily in the duodenum, and a number of dietary factors (coffee, tea) as well as primary intestinal disorders can impair absorption.

The **thalassemias** are a heterogeneous group of inherited anemias that are characterized by impaired or absent synthesis of either the α or β chains that make up the normal adult hemoglobin tetramer. The **β-thalassemias** are caused by a decrease in the production of β-globin chains. The anemia observed in the severe forms of β-thalassemia occurs as a result of ineffective erythropoiesis. This is due to the instability of the excess α chains, which precipitate and cause oxidative damage to the cell membrane leading to premature destruction of the erythrocyte within the bone marrow. The erythrocytes that do survive in the circulation have a shortened life span because of increased hemolysis. The severe forms (compound heterozygous or homozygous state) are classified as **β-thalassemia intermedia** or **β-thalassemia major** depending on the clinical presentation and degree of anemia. Individuals with β-thalassemia major develop a severe anemia during the first year of life because decreasing levels of fetal hemoglobin ($\alpha_2\gamma_2$) cannot be replaced by normal adult hemoglobin ($\alpha_2\beta_2$). Hemoglobin values fall in the range of 3 to 4 g/dL and regular transfusions are required. Individuals with β-thalassemia intermedia usually present later in life and do not require early intervention with blood transfusions. Hemoglobin values are in the 7 to 8 g/dL range, and individuals may be intermittently transfusion-dependent. Individuals with **β-thalassemia trait** (β-thalassemia minor), the heterozygous form, have a mild microcytic anemia with a hemoglobin that is approximately 2 g/dL below the normal mean for age. Clinically it is an asymptomatic anemia; however, it is of diagnostic relevance in that it must be distinguished from iron deficiency anemia.

The **α-thalassemias** are caused by a decrease in the production of α chains and are generally milder than the β-thalassemias. This reflects the fact that the excess of β chains that occurs in α-thalassemia is more stable, resulting in less membrane damage and intramedullary erythrocyte destruction. In humans, there are 4 α-globin genes. Individuals with a deletion of one α-globin gene are **silent carriers** and are asymptomatic with a normal hemoglobin value and MCV. Individuals with 2-gene deletions have **α-thalassemia trait** and have a very mild microcytic anemia that is asymptomatic. Three α-globin gene deletions causes **hemoglobin H disease,** a moderate chronic hemolytic anemia that may be intermittently transfusion-dependent. This occurs primarily in individuals of Southeast Asian descent.

Table 83-2. Differential Diagnosis of Anemia Based on Pathophysiology[a]

Pathophysiological Mechanism	General Diagnostic Features	Specific Diagnostic Features
Decreased Production of RBCs	**Evidence of decreased production:** ↓ reticulocytes	
Marrow infiltration		
Secondary to tumor infiltration		Pancytopenia due to bone marrow infiltration with leukemia, neuroblastoma, etc
Secondary to infiltration with nonmalignant cells		
Lipidoses		Lipid-filled macrophages
X-linked lymphoproliferative disorder		Hepatosplenomegaly
Decreased production of hematopoietic elements (bone marrow failure)		
Decreased RBC production only		
Constitutional: Diamond-Blackfan syndrome		Multiple physical deformities
Acquired		
Acquired pure red cell aplasia		Associated with thymoma
Transient erythrocytopenia of childhood		Associated with parvovirus infection
Decreased RBC and WBC production		
Constitutional		
Fanconi anemia		Multiple physical deformities
Shwachman syndrome		Pancreatic insufficiency
Decreased production of RBCs, WBCs, and platelets (aplastic anemia)		
Constitutional		
Fanconi anemia		Multiple physical deformities
Shwachman syndrome		Pancreatic insufficiency
Acquired: aplastic anemia		History of hepatitis B, toxin exposure, idiopathic
Dietary deficiency		
Iron deficiency		↓ MCV, ↓ MCH, ↑ RDW, ↓ serum iron, ↓ serum ferritin, excessive milk intake
Folic acid deficiency		↑ MCV, ↑ RDW, megaloblastic marrow, low serum and RBC folate
Vitamin B$_{12}$ deficiency		↑ MCV, ↑ RDW, megaloblastic marrow, low serum B$_{12}$ levels, Schilling test
Vitamin C deficiency		Clinical scurvy
Protein deficiency		Kwashiorkor
Hypothyroidism		Low T4, elevated TSH
Increased Production (Hemolysis)	**Evidence of hemolysis:** ↑ reticulocytes	
Intrinsic RBC defects		
RBC membrane defects (spherocytosis, elliptocytosis)	Hyperbilirubinemia	+ Osmotic fragility, spectrin deficiency (HS)
RBC enzyme defects (G6PD deficiency, pyruvate kinase)	LDH (RBC)	+ Enzyme assays
Hemoglobin defects	MCV may be if reticulocytes high	
1. Qualitative defects (sickle cell anemia, Hb C, Hb E)		Hb electrophoresis
2. Quantitative defects (thalassemia)	MCV 10W with thalassemia	Hb A2 (β-thalassemia), targets cells, basophilic stippling
Extrinsic RBC disorders		
Immune		
Isoimmune hemolytic anemia (eg, ABO, Rh incompatibility)		+ Coombs test
Autoimmune hemolytic anemia		
Idiopathic		+ Coombs test
Secondary: postviral, autoimmune disorders, Evans syndrome		+ ANA
Nonimmune (eg, DIC, HUS)		Concomitant renal disease (HUS)
Blood Loss	**Reticulocytes normal (acute loss),** ↑↓ (chronic)	
Overt (eg, splenic sequestration, gastrointestinal, or nasal bleeding)	↑ Reticulocytes (chronic loss, not iron deficient)	Sickle cell anemia (splenic sequestration)
Occult (eg, bleeding Meckel diverticulum, pulmonary hemosiderosis)	↓ Reticulocytes (chronic loss, iron deficient); may have rapidly falling hematocrit	Pulmonary infiltrates iron deficiency (pulmonary hemosiderosis)

Abbreviations: ANA, antinuclear antibodies; DIC, disseminated intravascular coagulation; G6PD, glucose-6-phosphate dehydrogenase; Hb, hemoglobin; HS, hereditary spherocytosis; HUS, hemolytic uremic syndrome; LDH, lactate dehydrogenase; MCH, mean corpuscular hemoglobin; MCV, mean corpuscular volume; RBC, red blood cell; RDW, red cell distribution width; TSH, thyroid-stimulating hormone; WBC, white blood cell.

[a]Adapted from Lanzkowsky P. *Manual of Pediatric Hematology-Oncology*. New York, NY: Churchill Livingstone; 1989:2–3.

Box 83-2. Differential Diagnosis of Childhood Anemias Based on Red Blood Cell Size

Hypochromic, Microcytic Anemia (Low MCV)
- Iron deficiency anemia
- Thalassemias
- Lead poisoning
- Anemia of inflammation or chronic disease

Normochromic, Normocytic Anemia (Normal MCV)
- High reticulocyte count
  — Intrinsic red cell disorders
- Hemoglobinopathies (hemoglobin SS disease)
- Enzymopathies (G6PD, PK)
- Membranopathies (HS)
  — Extrinsic red cell disorders
- Immune-mediated
- Non-immune (microangiopathic hemolytic anemia [eg, hemolytic uremic syndrome])
- Low reticulocyte count
  — Pure red cell aplasia (Diamond-Blackfan anemia, TEC)
  — Pancytopenia (marrow failure or infiltration)

Macrocytic Anemia (Increased MCV)
- Folate deficiency
- Vitamin B$_{12}$ deficiency
- Diamond-Blackfan anemia
- Myelodysplastic syndromes
- Chemotherapy agents

Abbreviations: G6PD, glucose-6-phosphate dehydrogenase; HS, hereditary spherocytosis; MCV, mean corpuscular volume; PK, pyruvate kinase; SS, 2 sickle β-globin genes; TEC, transient erythroblastopenia of childhood.

Four-gene deletion causes **hydrops fetalis,** an almost universally fatal condition.

Although **lead** inhibits heme synthesis and red cell function on many levels, microcytic anemia is a late finding of lead intoxication. Iron deficiency and lead poisoning often occur together with a complex relationship. In the presence of lead, iron uptake by the erythrocyte is diminished and iron deficiency increases lead retention and toxicity. Intestinal absorption and uptake of lead by red cells is decreased in the presence of iron. In addition, iron deficiency and lead poisoning tend to occur in the same lower socioeconomic population, and both are exacerbated by concomitant nutritional deficiencies.

Anemia of inflammation or chronic disease can be seen in children with chronic infections, generalized inflammatory disorders (rheumatoid arthritis), and some cancers. It is characterized by a decrease in serum iron and iron binding capacity, an increase in ferritin, and the presence of iron in bone marrow macrophages indicating impaired iron mobilization from storage sites. Increased synthesis of hepcidin, an iron regulatory hormone, under the influence of inflammatory cytokines seems to be responsible for the hypoferremia observed in anemia of inflammation. In general, the anemia of inflammation is mild and may be microcytic or normocytic.

Macrocytic Anemias

Both **folate** and **vitamin B$_{12}$ deficiency** cause a macrocytic anemia as a consequence of defective erythroid precursor nuclear maturation and megaloblastic changes in the bone marrow. Folate is absorbed in the duodenum and jejunum and is widely available in meats, green leafy vegetables, and cereals. Because of the ubiquity of folate, dietary deficiency is uncommon; however, infants fed exclusively goat's milk are at risk because of the exceedingly low levels of folate in goat's milk. Individuals with chronic hemolytic anemias may also become folate-deficient because of high bone marrow activity and increased demand.

Vitamin B$_{12}$ is available from animal sources and is actively absorbed in the terminal ileum in association with intrinsic factor. Vitamin B$_{12}$ deficiency can occur in individuals with a strict vegan diet (or in exclusively breastfed infants of women following a strict vegan diet); however, it usually occurs as a consequence of malabsorption. Decreased absorption can occur in the setting of pernicious anemia (decreased intrinsic factor), surgical resection, or GI disease.

Other causes of macrocytic anemias include congenital hypoplastic anemias (eg, Diamond-Blackfan anemia), myelodysplastic syndromes, and chemotherapeutic agents (eg, methotrexate).

Normocytic Anemias

Normocytic anemias can be classified as hemolytic anemias (associated with a reticulocytosis) and hypoplastic anemias (reticulocytopenic). **Hemolytic anemias** can be further divided into disorders that are intrinsic to the RBC or extrinsic to it. Intrinsic RBC disorders include hemoglobinopathies, enzymopathies, and membranopathies.

Sickle cell disease is most common in individuals of African or mixed African and Latino descent. Inheritance of 2 sickle β-globin genes (hemoglobin SS) is the most common form; however, other significant sickle syndromes include hemoglobin SC, Sβ$^+$ thalassemia, and Sβ^0 thalassemia. Hemolytic anemia and painful vaso-occlusive episodes are the hallmarks of sickle cell disease. The anemia is generally well tolerated with hemoglobin values in the 6.5 to 8.5 g/dL range with an associated reticulocytosis (5%–15%). The 2 most common hematologic complications in sickle cell disease are aplastic crises and splenic sequestration—both of which can cause an acute drop in hemoglobin. Aplastic crises are generally the result of infection with parvovirus, which temporarily causes the complete cessation of red cell production. Splenic sequestration occurs most commonly in infants and young children with sickle cell disease, often in association with a viral illness. Large amounts of blood can be quickly trapped in the spleen causing hypovolemia, shock, and massive splenomegaly.

Pyruvate kinase deficiency is the most common red cell enzyme defect causing a chronic congenital hemolytic anemia. The degree of hemolysis is variable, ranging from a mild fully compensated hemolytic process without anemia to a transfusion-dependent anemia. Individuals with severe hemolysis may be chronically jaundiced and may develop the clinical complications of chronic hemolytic states (gall stones, transient aplastic crises in association with infections, folate deficiency and, infrequently, skin ulcers.) The enzymatic activity of G6PD is essential in protecting the red cell proteins from oxidative damage. **Glucose-6-phosphate dehydrogenase deficiency** renders the red cell susceptible to oxidant stress and hemolysis. A number of variants have been defined; however, the most common variants are those associated with acute intermittent hemolytic anemias with exposure to oxidant stresses (fava beans, medications). Variants associated with chronic hemolytic anemias are very rare.

Hereditary spherocytosis is the most common red cell membranopathy and is characterized by the presence of spherical-shaped erythrocytes on the peripheral blood smear. Increased membrane fragility due to defects in proteins of the red cell membrane (spectrin, ankyrin, band 3, protein 4.2) leads to membrane vesiculation and membrane loss and the assumption of a spheroidal shape. Hemolysis occurs as these spherocytes are then trapped within the spleen. Clinically, the degree of hemolysis varies from mild anemia to severe transfusion dependence. The complications of a chronic hemolytic state such as gallstones, aplastic crises, and folate deficiency can also be observed.

Hemolytic anemias that are due to factors extrinsic to the red cell can be further classified as immune-mediated or nonimmune. **Immune-mediated anemias** may be due to alloantibodies that occur in the setting of neonatal Rh or ABO incompatibility or transfusion reactions. Autoantibodies may occur in association with infection, autoimmune disorders, malignancy, or drugs. In children, autoantibodies (warm immunoglobulin G) are often seen in association with a viral illness. **Nonimmune hemolytic anemias** include microangiopathic and macroangiopathic hemolytic anemias due to a myriad of etiologies, including infections, drugs, toxins, burns, and heart valves.

Reticulocytopenic anemias can be congenital or acquired and can occur in isolation or in the setting of pancytopenia. **Diamond-Blackfan anemia** is a ribosomal disorder that causes a congenital pure red cell aplasia that presents early in infancy. The bone marrow typically shows red cell aplasia with a paucity of red cell precursors, and the red cells may be normocytic or macrocytic. Associated congenital anomalies, such as craniofacial anomalies, radial abnormalities, and renal and cardiac defects, are seen in approximately 25% of affected individuals. **Transient erythroblastopenia of childhood** is an acquired reticulocytopenic anemia that typically occurs following a viral illness. The usual age of presentation is between 2 to 3 years in an otherwise healthy child, and complete recovery is the natural course.

Evaluation

History

When evaluating an infant or child with anemia, the age, rapidity of onset of symptoms, MCV, and suspected underlying mechanism of anemia will direct the history (Questions Box). In most instances, it is important to inquire about dietary habits, with particular attention to the type and amount of milk ingested per day (number of bottles/ounces). Ingestion of more than 24 oz of cow's milk should raise

the suspicion for iron deficiency anemia. Medication use, potential toxin ingestion (lead), or a history of pica should be determined as well. In addition, inquiries to potential sources of blood loss (hematochezia, melena, menorrhagia, hematuria, epistaxis, pulmonary) should be addressed. Acute onset of jaundice, icterus, or dark urine is suggestive of hemolysis and should elicit questions regarding possible triggers (fava beans, medications, illnesses). A personal history of neonatal hyperbilirubinemia or a family history of anemia, gallstones, cholecystectomy, or splenectomy is highly suggestive of a congenital hemolytic anemia. Acute onset of hemolysis with a viral illness is consistent with an autoimmune hemolytic anemia. Marrow failure syndromes often present with a prolonged history of increased fatigue and pallor, with occasional history of previous red cell transfusions prior to diagnosis. In acquired marrow failure states such as aplastic anemia, the history is occasionally consistent with antecedent hepatitis, a viral syndrome or, rarely, exposure to toxins such as benzene and toluene-containing compounds, or oral chloramphenicol use (commonly available over the counter in Latin America).

Physical Examination

Most children who present with anemia will have a normal physical examination. Depending on the degree of anemia, pallor, tachycardia, or tachypnea may be present. In severe cases of anemia (hemoglobin <3 g/dL) with chronic onset and moderate anemia (hemoglobin of 3–7 g/dL) with acute onset (blood loss), CHF can occur. Other physical findings are unique to certain red cell disorders. Infants with sickle cell disease may present with dactylitis, a form of painful crisis that manifests as swelling of 1 to 4 digits associated with pain and sometimes fever. Splenomegaly can be seen in sickle cell disease (in younger children prior to autosplenectomy), β-thalassemia major and intermedia, and red cell membrane disorders, most commonly hereditary spherocytosis. In children with severe chronic hemolysis, regardless of etiology, classic facies (often called thalassemic facies) can develop, with frontal bossing and flattened nasal bridge, due to thinning of the facial bones from brisk intramedullary hematopoiesis. Children with Diamond-Blackfan anemia or Fanconi anemia may have physical anomalies, such as thumb or radial abnormalities, short stature, cardiac or renal anomalies, and developmental delay. Aplastic anemia or malignant infiltration of the bone marrow may present with concomitant neutropenia and thrombocytopenia. If neutropenic (absolute neutrophil count <1,000/mL), signs of fever or infection may be present. If thrombocytopenic, bruises; petechiae;

and mucosal bleeding from the mouth, nose, and GI tract may also be present. With malignancy, such as leukemia, lymphadenopathy and hepatosplenomegaly may also be observed.

Laboratory Tests

The complete **blood cell count (CBC)** and peripheral blood smear provide a wealth of information and should be evaluated closely to narrow the differential diagnosis. The first step is to determine if the child is truly anemic by referencing the normal **hemoglobin/hematocrit** values for the child's age and gender. The second step is to evaluate the red cell indices. The **MCV** is a direct measure of red cell size and allows for classification of the anemia as microcytic, normocytic, or macrocytic. The mean corpuscular hemoglobin (**MCH**) is a calculated value that typically parallels the MCV. The **MCH concentration** is a measure of the red cell hydration status and is useful when elevated as this reflects the presence of spherocytes. The red cell volume distribution width reflects the variation in red cell size (usually normal with thalassemia trait and elevated in iron deficiency). The RBC count can be useful because it is typically elevated (>5 million/mL) in a child with thalassemia trait and decreased in iron deficiency anemia. Review of the **white blood cell and platelet count** will provide information as to whether other cell lines are affected. The **peripheral blood smear** provides information regarding RBC morphology characteristic of different red cell disorders (sickle cells, spherocytes, elliptocytes, schistocytes). The presence of polychromasia is suggestive of a hemolytic process. White blood cell morphology can also suggest the etiology of the anemia (hypersegmented neutrophils in folate or vitamin B_{12} deficiency). The **reticulocyte count** provides clues to the underlying mechanism of anemia. An elevated reticulocyte count is consistent with a hemolytic or blood loss picture whereas a reduced or normal reticulocyte count in the face of anemia suggests a production problem. If hemolysis is evident, a **Coombs test (direct antiglobulin test)** should be performed to determine if this is an immune-mediated process.

With the CBC, peripheral blood smear, and reticulocyte count, a focused differential diagnosis can be generated and more specific testing can be performed. Further studies specific for individual hemolytic diseases or particular diseases secondary to marrow failure are summarized in Table 83-2.

Imaging Studies

Few children routinely need imaging studies in the evaluation of their anemia. If performed in children with chronic hemolytic disorders, radiographs may reveal "hair-on-end" appearance of bones due to increased hematopoiesis. Patients who have anemia associated with lead poisoning may have lead deposition, referred to as **lead lines,** in their long bones.

Management

The treatment of anemia varies depending on the etiology. Nutritional anemias require dietary counseling and nutrient supplementation. With **iron deficiency anemia,** oral iron supplementation (3–6 mg/kg/day divided into 2–3 doses) should generate a brisk reticulocytosis within 7 days, and the hemoglobin should increase by 1.0 g/dL/week thereafter. Therapy should be continued for an additional 6 to 8 weeks after the hemoglobin has normalized to replete iron stores. Dietary education is key to ensure that milk intake is reduced and that iron-rich foods are encouraged. Failure to respond to iron therapy is most commonly due to noncompliance; however, alternative diagnoses (thalassemia trait), ongoing blood loss, or malabsorption states should also be considered.

Patients with severe thalassemia syndromes (β-thalassemia major) are transfusion-dependent, often requiring transfusions every 3 to 4 weeks to maintain a hemoglobin level in the 9 to 10.5 g/dL range. With transfusion therapy, progressive iron deposition in tissues occurs leading to cardiac, hepatic, and endocrinologic complications, which can be fatal if not prevented. Iron chelation with deferoxamine or deferasirox has improved survival; however, compliance remains an issue. Bone marrow transplantation has been performed in patients with β-thalassemia major.

Depending on the degree of hemolysis and compensation, individuals with congenital hemolytic anemias may require no transfusions, intermittent transfusions (due to aplastic crises), or regular transfusions. Individuals may require folate supplementation and should be monitored for potential complications such as gallstones and aplastic crises. The more severely affected individuals may benefit from splenectomy. Individuals with G6PD deficiency should be counseled on the avoidance of potential triggers of hemolysis.

Two anemia-related conditions constitute emergencies. Prompt recognition of these conditions is vital if proper treatment is to be initiated. **Splenic sequestration** occurs in infants and young children with sickle cell disease who sequester large volumes of blood within the spleen over a period of hours. This results in a rapidly dropping hemoglobin, clinically resembling anemia due to massive blood loss. The blood pooled in the spleen is not available to the circulation, and affected children are subject to fatal splenic rupture. Treatment involves transfusion or exchange transfusion and early recognition is essential. **Severe autoimmune hemolytic anemia** is the second anemia-related emergency. Children with this disorder can occasionally present with severe Coombs-positive anemia and clinical evidence of rapid hemolysis; their hemoglobin may fall as much as 1 g/dL per hour. These patients generally require hospitalization, transfusion, and treatment with high-dose steroids.

The primary treatment for patients with Diamond-Blackfan anemia is steroids and RBC transfusions. Most patients will respond to steroids (50%–75%) and can be controlled at very low doses. For steroid-refractory patients, alternative immunosuppressive therapy and RBC transfusions are necessary. Bone marrow transplantation has been performed in steroid-refractory patients with Diamond-Blackfan anemia with success.

Prognosis

The prognosis for a child with anemia depends on the underlying cause. Children with anemia due to nutritional deficiencies that are detected and appropriately treated have an excellent prognosis. Children with transient erythroblastopenia of childhood can expect complete recovery. Most immune-mediated anemias are responsive to therapy; however, if associated with an underlying autoimmune disorder, they may have a relapsing course. Children with chronic hemolytic disorders will have varying courses depending on the degree of hemolysis. Early diagnosis and intervention through newborn screening for children with sickle cell disease has significantly reduced early mortality for this disease. Children with β-thalassemia major or severe congenital hemolytic anemias will be transfusion-dependent and will be subject to the complications of iron overload, which can be addressed with chelation therapy. Some children with transfusion-dependent congenital hemolytic anemias may be candidates for splenectomy, with normalization of their hemoglobin values post-splenectomy. The prognosis for children with Diamond-Blackfan anemia depends on their responsiveness to steroid therapy and the need for transfusions. These individuals are also at risk for certain malignancies.

Children with anemia due to chronic inherited or acquired red cell disorders are at risk for complications during the course of their disease and are best served at a center that offers pediatric hematology expertise.

CASE RESOLUTION

The girl described in the case history at the beginning of the chapter has hereditary spherocytosis. Her history is highly suggestive of a hereditary hemolytic disorder, and the combination of spherocytes in the peripheral smear; a negative Coombs test; and a positive, incubated, osmotic fragility test are diagnostic of the condition. At the age of 9 years, she undergoes a splenectomy and has no more hemolytic episodes that require transfusions.

Selected References

American Academy of Pediatrics Committee on Environmental Health. Screening for elevated blood lead levels. *Pediatrics.* 1998;101:1072–1078

Charache S, Lubin B, Reid CD, eds. *Management and Therapy of Sickle Cell Disease.* Bethesda, MD: National Institutes of Health; 1995. NIH Publication No. 96–2117

Cherrick I, Karayalcin G, Lanzkowsky P. Transient erythroblastopenia of childhood. Prospective study of fifty patients. *Am J Pediatr Hematol Oncol.* 1994;16:320

Fixler J, Styles L. Sickle cell disease. *Pediatr Clin North Am.* 2002;49:1193–1210

Gazda HT, Sieff CA. Recent insights into the pathogenesis of Diamond-Blackfan anaemia. *Br J Haematol.* 2006;135:149

Hermiston ML, Mentzer WC. A practical approach to the evaluation of the anemic child. *Pediatr Clin North Am.* 2002;49:877–892

Lo L, Singer ST. Thalassemia: current approach to an old disease. *Pediatr Clin North Am.* 2002;49:1149–1164

McKie VC. Sickle cell anemia in children: practical issues for the pediatrician. *Pediatr Ann.* 1998;27:521–524

Oski, FABrugnara C, Oski FA ,Nathan DG. Diagnostic approach to the anemic patient. In: Orkin SH, Nathan DG, Ginsburg D, Look AT, Fisher DE, Lux SE, eds. *Nathan and Oski's Hematology of Infancy and Childhood.* 7th ed. Philadelphia, PA: Saunders/Elsevier; 2009:455–466

Recommendations to prevent and control iron deficiency in the United States. Centers for Disease Control and Prevention. *MMWR Recomm Rep.* 1998;47:1–29

Robins EB, Blum S. Hematologic reference values for African American children and adolescents. *Am J Hematol.* 2007;82:61

CHAPTER 84

Bleeding Disorders

Wendy Y. Tcheng, MD

CASE STUDY

A 6-year-old girl presents with a several-month history of recurrent epistaxis. Episodes occur every 2 to 3 weeks and last 15 to 20 minutes at a time. Both nares are affected. Her mother also notes that the girl has always bruised easily. On physical examination, several 2- to 3-cm ecchymoses are noted on her lower extremities. Initial laboratory evaluation includes a complete blood cell count, which is normal (platelet count 300,000), a normal partial thromboplastin time of 30 seconds, and a normal prothrombin time of 12.5 seconds, with international normalized ratio (INR) 1:1.

Questions

1. What conditions should be considered when easy bruisability is the chief complaint?
2. What is the appropriate laboratory evaluation for children with clinical signs of bleeding?
3. What management is appropriate for the most common pediatric bleeding disorders?
4. What are the common medical complications that children with bleeding disorders face?
5. When is consultation with a hematologist appropriate in a child with easy bruisability?

When evaluating a child with bruising or bleeding symptoms, the major challenge facing the pediatrician is to ascertain whether the degree of bleeding is appropriate for the hemostatic stress or whether further evaluation for a potential bleeding disorder is warranted. Bruising and bleeding are common childhood complaints and usually follow minor injury or trauma. However, in the child with an underlying hemostatic disorder, non-accidental trauma, or both, the bruising or bleeding may be more extensive than expected. A thorough medical history and physical examination and an understanding of hemostasis will aid in focusing the laboratory evaluation and elucidating the underlying etiology.

Epidemiology

Bleeding disorders can be inherited or acquired. Of the inherited bleeding disorders, von Willebrand disease is the most common, with a reported incidence ranging between 1 in 100 and 1 in 1,000. Von Willebrand disease is autosomally inherited, affecting males and females equally; however, more females are diagnosed because of the inherent hemostatic challenges that females face (menses, childbirth). Hemophilia is the most common severe bleeding disorder affecting about 1 in 5,000 males. Approximately 80% of cases are hemophilia A (factor VIII [FVIII] deficiency) and 20% are hemophilia B (factor IX [FIX] deficiency). Hemophilia is inherited in an X-linked fashion, but a third of newly diagnosed males have no previous family history and represent new mutations. Other inherited coagulation disorders and platelet disorders are rare and are listed in Table 84-1.

Acquired abnormalities of coagulation or platelets are much more common. These can occur in the setting of liver disease, vitamin K deficiency, renal disease, disseminated intravascular coagulation (DIC), infection, medications, malignancy, massive transfusion, post-surgery, and autoimmunity or alloimmunity. Immune thrombocytopenic purpura (ITP) is a common acquired childhood bleeding disorder with an incidence of 4 to 8 per 100,000 children per year. Neonatal alloimmune thrombocytopenia occurs in approximately 1 in 1,800 live births. Common acquired bleeding disorders are also listed in Table 84-1.

Clinical Presentation

Bleeding disorders can present in various ways depending on the etiology. Inherited bleeding disorders will often present during infancy or early childhood; however, mild disorders may go undiagnosed until later in life. In general, disorders of primary hemostasis (ie, von Willebrand disease, platelet disorders, collagen vascular disorders) will present with superficial, immediate, mucocutaneous-type bleeding. Characteristic bleeding symptoms include easy bruising, epistaxis, gum bleeding, menorrhagia, postpartum bleeding, and bleeding with dental extractions or surgeries. Disorders of secondary hemostasis, such as hemophilia A or B, will often present with deep, delayed bleeding, such as hemarthroses or muscular hematomas.

Acquired bleeding disorders typically present with an acute onset and often involve abnormalities of both primary and secondary hemostasis. Acute onset of bleeding symptoms in a toxic or ill-appearing child suggests a systemic process such as sepsis, DIC, malignancy, or hepatic or renal dysfunction. A well-appearing child with acute bleeding symptoms suggests ITP, an acquired inhibitor, or a medication-related cause.

Table 84-1. Inherited Versus Acquired Bleeding Disorders		
Disorder	*Inherited*	*Acquired*

Coagulation	• von Willebrand disease
	• Hemophilia A (FVIII)
	• Hemophilia B (FIX)
	• Hemophilia C (FXI)
	• FII, FV, FVII, FX, or FXIII deficiency
	• Disorders of fibrinogen
	  — Dysfibrinogenemia, hypofibrinogenemia,
	    or afibrinogenemia
	• Disorders of fibrinolysis
	  — α_2-antiplasmin
	• PAI-1 deficiency
		• Vitamin K deficiency
		• Liver disease
		• DIC
		• Massive transfusion syndrome
		• Disorders of fibrinogen (dysfibrinogenemia or hypofibrinogenemia)
		  — Liver disease
		  — Renal disease
		  — Medication
		• Disorders associated with malignancy
		• Coagulation inhibitors

Platelet	• Quantitative
	  — Thrombocytopenia absent radii syndrome
	  — Amegakaryocytic thrombocytopenia
	  — Fanconi anemia
	• Qualitative
	  — Glanzmann thrombasthenia
	  — Storage pool disorders
	  — Release defects
	• Quantitative/qualitative
	  — Bernard-Soulier syndrome
	  — Wiskott-Aldrich syndrome
	  — Gray platelet syndrome
		• Quantitative
		  — Increased destruction
		    ~ Nonimmune-mediated
		      ♦ HUS
		      ♦ TTP
		      ♦ DIC
		    ~ Immune-mediated
		      ♦ ITP
		      ♦ Evan syndrome
		      ♦ NAIT
		      ♦ Medications
		  — Decreased production
		    ~ Aplastic anemia
		    ~ Malignancy infiltrating bone marrow
		    ~ Medications
		• Qualitative
		  — Medication
		  — Liver disease
		  — Uremia
		  — Post-cardiopulmonary bypass surgery

Abbreviations: DIC, disseminated intravascular coagulation; F, factor; HUS, hemolytic uremic syndrome; ITP, immune thrombocytopenic purpura; NAIT, neonatal alloimmune thrombocytopenic purpura; PAI, plasminogen activator inhibitor; TTP, thrombotic thrombocytopenic purpura.

Pathophysiology

Following vascular injury, hemostasis is initiated by exposure of flowing blood to subendothelial collagen and tissue factor. The primary phase of hemostasis leads to the production of a platelet plug. Von Willebrand factor (vWF), a multimeric glycoprotein of varying size, attaches to exposed subendothelial collagen and binds platelets via the platelet glycoprotein IB/IX receptor. Von Willebrand factor also serves as a carrier protein for FVIII, thereby localizing FVIII to areas of endothelial disruption. Once platelets adhere to vWF, they become activated and release their granular contents, produce thromboxane A2, and express the fibrinogen receptor glycoprotein IIb/IIIa (GPIIB/IIIA). The release of thromboxane A2 and other granular contents leads to local vasoconstriction and activation of additional platelets and their respective GPIIB/IIIA receptors, allowing for platelet aggregation. Fibrinogen binds to all of the exposed activated GPIIB/IIIA sites, clumping the platelets together to form a platelet plug. The platelet plug stops local bleeding and provides a phospholipid surface for the coagulation reactions of secondary hemostasis to occur to form a definitive fibrin plug.

Secondary hemostasis is also initiated at the time of endothelial disruption with exposure of tissue factor to circulating blood. Tissue factor binds to FVIIa, and this complex serves as the key initiator of in vivo hemostasis by activating other tissue factor: FVII (TF:FVII) complexes, as well as FIX, and factor X (FX). Once activated (either by FIXa or TF:FVIIa), FXa along with its cofactor, factor Va, activates prothrombin (FII) to thrombin (FIIa). Thrombin cleaves circulating fibrinogen to fibrin monomers that self-polymerize. Factor XIII then stabilizes the fibrin clot by forming cross-links within the clump of fibrin polymers. These coagulation reactions occur on the surface of the platelet plug and, with the generation of cross-linked fibrin, the primary platelet plug is converted into a definitive fibrin plug that prevents further bleeding. An overview of hemostasis is depicted in Figures 84-1 and 84-2. Deficiencies or impairments in any of these elements can lead to inadequate hemostasis and excessive hemorrhage.

The delicate balance of hemostasis and thrombosis is maintained by inhibitors (protein C, protein S, antithrombin, tissue factor pathway inhibitor) at each step of the coagulation cascade. These natural anticoagulants serve to prevent excessive thrombus formation. Fibrinolysis is mediated by plasmin, which cleaves both fibrinogen and fibrin within a thrombus, allowing for restoration of vessel patency following hemostasis. Plasmin is activated by tissue plasminogen activator (tPA) and urokinase. Fibrinolysis is kept in check by plasminogen activator inhibitor (PAI-1), which inactivates tPA, and α_2-antiplasmin, which inactivates plasmin. Any defects in the fibrinolytic system that leads to an increase in fibrinolysis can result in excessive bleeding.

Differential Diagnosis

In developing the differential diagnosis for a child with bleeding symptoms, it is important to obtain a thorough bleeding history and physical examination. The age, bleeding pattern, duration of symptoms, family history, and overall clinical status of the child will help to narrow the spectrum of possibilities.

Child With Chronic History of Mucocutaneous Bleeding

In a child who presents with a history of easy bruising, epistaxis, or menorrhagia, the primary differential diagnosis includes von Willebrand disease, platelet disorders, and collagen vascular disorders (disorders of primary hemostasis). **Von Willebrand disease** is caused by a quantitative or qualitative defect of vWF. Von Willebrand factor plays an important role in both primary hemostasis (mediates platelet adhesion at sites of vascular injury) and secondary hemostasis (stabilizes FVIII in plasma). Von Willebrand disease is autosomally inherited and classified into 3 different types. Type 1 refers to a partial quantitative deficiency of vWF. Type 2 refers to qualitative abnormalities of vWF with a number of subtypes that fall within this classification. Type 3, the most severe form, refers to a complete deficiency of vWF. Type 1 is the most common form, accounting for 70% to 80% of cases. Bleeding symptoms tend to be mild and are characterized by easy bruising, epistaxis, menorrhagia, and prolonged oozing after minor or major surgeries. Only the most severely affected patients (type 3), with very low FVIII levels, will have soft tissue bleeding and hemarthroses similar to an individual with moderate or severe hemophilia.

Qualitative platelet disorders also present with mucocutaneous bleeding, often during infancy. In **Bernard-Soulier syndrome,** the platelets lack a functional glycoprotein IB/IX receptor complex on

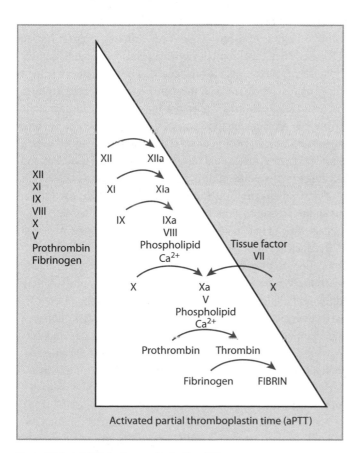

Figure 84-1. Intrinsic pathway reflected by aPTT.

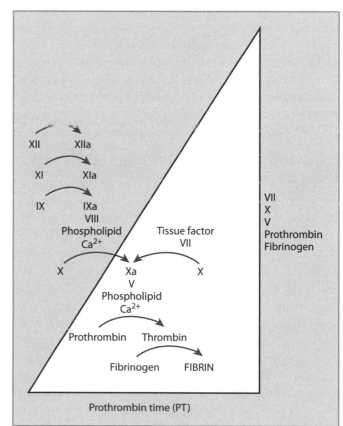

Figure 84-2. Coagulation pathway. Extrinsic pathway reflected by PT.

the platelet surface, resulting in defective platelet adhesion to vWF at sites of vascular injury. It is an autosomal-recessive disorder and is usually seen in consanguineous families. The platelets tend to be large on peripheral smear, and there may be a degree of thrombocytopenia. **Glanzmann thrombasthenia** is characterized by an absence or defect in the platelet membrane GPIIB/IIIA receptor, the main fibrinogen receptor on the platelet surface that allows for platelet aggregation. It is autosomal-recessively inherited and is more common in the presence of consanguinity. Other qualitative platelet disorders such as **storage pool disorders** and **platelet release defects** can also present in a similar manner.

Collagen-vascular disorders, such as Marfan syndrome and Ehlers-Danlos syndrome, can present with bruising and bleeding symptoms. This increased bleeding diathesis is due to an easy disruption of the integrity of the vascular endothelium.

Other rare coagulation disorders to consider in a child with recurrent bleeding symptoms include deficiencies of FXI, FXIII, PAI-1, and α_2-antiplasmin. **Factor XI deficiency,** also known as *hemophilia C,* is a rare bleeding disorder with a high prevalence in the Ashkenazi Jewish population. It differs from the other hemophilias in that it is autosomally inherited and tends to have milder symptoms. Bleeding episodes are typically in response to trauma or surgery, and the deep tissue or intra-articular bleeds characteristic of FVIII or FIX deficiency are not seen. **Factor XIII deficiency** is characterized by delayed or prolonged bleeding because the clots formed are friable owing to the lack of cross-linkage of fibrin monomers by FXIII. It is inherited in an autosomal-dominant pattern, and in the homozygous state usually presents in infancy with umbilical cord bleeding or delayed separation, as well as intracranial hemorrhage. Heterozygotes may present later in life with delayed or prolonged bleeding following trauma or surgery and poor wound healing. **Disorders of fibrinolysis** (deficiency of PAI-1 or α_2-antiplasmin) can also present with prolonged bleeding following trauma.

Child With History of Deep, Delayed Bleeding

Deep tissue and intra-articular bleeding is the hallmark bleeding pattern of **hemophilia.** The differential diagnosis for a child who presents with this type of bleeding is hemophilia A (FVIII deficiency) or B (FIX deficiency), FVII deficiency, and type 3 von Willebrand disease. Clinically, hemophilia is classified according to the factor level with less than 1% factor activity as severe, 1% to 5% as moderate, and greater than 5% as mild. The factor level correlates with the bleeding tendency. Males with severe hemophilia can have "spontaneous" bleeds or bleeding with minimal trauma. Males with moderate or mild hemophilia will bleed with more significant trauma. The bleeding pattern of hemophilia varies as the child grows. Infants may present with a cephalohematoma or intracranial hemorrhage, particularly if the delivery was complicated with the use of forceps or vacuum extraction. Bleeding with circumcision, heel sticks, or blood draws may also occur. As the infant starts crawling, bruises and soft tissue hematomas on the lower extremities become common. As the toddler becomes upright, the first hemarthroses can

occur, typically involving the ankle. The older child has hemarthroses primarily involving the knees and elbows.

Factor VII deficiency is very rare; however, it can present with a bleeding pattern similar to hemophilia A or B. Type 3 von Willebrand disease, which is characterized by an absence of vWF (the carrier protein for FVIII), can have FVIII levels as low as an individual with severe or moderate hemophilia A. In addition to the characteristic mucocutaneous bleeding seen with von Willebrand disease, these individuals can also have deep tissue and intra-articular bleeding.

Well-Appearing Child With Acute Onset of Bleeding Symptoms

An acute onset of bleeding symptoms is consistent with an acquired abnormality of hemostasis. Acute **ITP** is a common acquired bleeding disorder of childhood due to the development of autoantibodies directed against the patient's platelets. These autoantibodies, which cross-react with platelet surface antigens, are thought to develop in response to an infection. Typically, a healthy child (usually between the ages of 2 to 4 years) presents with an abrupt onset of bleeding symptoms, diffuse petechiae and bruising and, occasionally, "wet" bleeding (epistaxis, gum bleeding, gastrointestinal [GI] bleeding). There is often a history of a viral illness or recent immunization. The complete blood cell count (CBC) reveals an isolated thrombocytopenia, and large platelets are seen on peripheral smear reflecting an active marrow with the production of young platelets. In approximately 80% of cases, ITP is an acute, self-limited process resolving within 6 months of diagnosis with or without therapy. Chronic ITP exists when the thrombocytopenia persists beyond 6 months. Although it is not possible to predict at diagnosis whether a patient will go on to have chronic ITP, there are certain presenting features that are associated with a higher risk for chronicity. These include older age at presentation (>10 years), female gender, existing autoimmune disease, and insidious onset of symptoms. In most cases of chronic ITP, the platelet count ranges between 40,000 to 80,000, and bleeding symptoms are minimal.

Acquired coagulation inhibitors are rare in children without an underlying coagulation disorder; however, they can occur in the setting of malignancy, infection, or post-surgery. Acquired FVIII deficiency due to FVIII inhibitor occurs primarily in the adult population, but has been previously reported in children. Acute onset of severe bleeding symptoms is the common presentation. Antiphospholipid antibodies can cause a prolongation of the partial thromboplastin time (PTT) or prothrombin time (PT); however, these antibodies are not associated with bleeding and are typically transient following a viral illness. The exception is if the antiphospholipid antibody is directed against prothrombin, resulting in low levels of prothrombin. In this situation, bleeding may be associated but is usually mild and intervention unnecessary.

Acquired abnormalities of coagulation or platelet function can also occur in association with **medications.** Aspirin and nonsteroidal anti-inflammatory drugs are common medications that affect the function of platelets. Warfarin, a vitamin K antagonist, is commonly used as an anticoagulant. One percent to 3% of patients on therapeutic warfarin can experience bleeding complications. Chronic antibiotic use can result in vitamin K deficiency and a depletion of the vitamin K–dependent factors (II, VII, IX, X).

Ill-Appearing Child With Acute Onset of Bleeding Symptoms

Acute onset of bleeding in an ill-appearing child suggests an acquired systemic process. **Disseminated intravascular coagulation** is a consumptive coagulopathy that can occur secondary to a number of disorders, including sepsis, trauma, or malignancy. Disseminated intravascular coagulation occurs as a result of endothelial disruption and initiation of abnormal coagulation; fibrin deposition; and depletion of multiple clotting factors, inhibitor proteins, and platelets.

Because the liver is the primary site of synthesis for most of the coagulation factors, **liver dysfunction** due to any illness can result in an imbalance in the hemostatic system. In addition, thrombocytopenia may be present with chronic liver disease because of portal hypertension and associated splenomegaly with sequestration. Causes of the depletion of vitamin K–dependent factors, such as obstructive jaundice, malabsorptive states (cystic fibrosis), parenchymal liver disease, and chronic antibiotic use, can also predispose to bleeding.

Renal disease with uremia impairs platelet function and can present with bleeding symptoms as well. A **malignancy** infiltrating the bone marrow, such as leukemia, lymphoma, or neuroblastoma, can cause thrombocytopenia and resultant platelet bleeding. Acquired von Willebrand disease can occur with Wilms tumor and present with mucocutaneous bleeding. **Bone marrow failure syndromes** can also present with thrombocytopenia and associated bleeding.

Infant With Bleeding Symptoms

An infant who presents with bleeding symptoms may have a congenital bleeding disorder or an acquired condition. **Inherited coagulation deficiencies** (VII, VIII, IX, XI, XIII, type 3 von Willebrand disease) and qualitative platelet disorders may present in the newborn period with intracranial hemorrhage or cephalohematoma, bleeding with heel sticks or blood draws, umbilical cord bleeding, and bleeding with circumcision. **Congenital thrombocytopenias** usually present within the first year of life and are associated with other syndromic features. Thrombocytopenia–absent radius (TAR) syndrome is an autosomal-recessive condition, typically recognized in the newborn period, characterized by thrombocytopenia, skeletal anomalies (most commonly radial agenesis), and renal and cardiac abnormalities. Other congenital thrombocytopenias include amegakaryocytic thrombocytopenia, Fanconi anemia, and Wiskott-Aldrich syndrome.

Neonatal alloimmune thrombocytopenia (NAIT) is a rare condition in which an infant inherits platelet antigens from the father that are different from the mother. The mother becomes alloimmunized to the infant's platelet antigens during pregnancy, similar to erythrocyte alloimmunization from Rh incompatibility. The maternal immunoglobulin G alloantibodies cross the placenta and destroy the infant's platelets, resulting in a transient but severe thrombocytopenia in the infant. Antibodies against the human platelet antigen-1a are responsible for 80% of NAIT cases in the Caucasian population. Thrombocytopenia in the infant can last several weeks until the maternal antibody is cleared. Unlike Rh alloimmunization, NAIT can occur in the first pregnancy. The risk of intracranial hemorrhage is significant, with a reported incidence of up to 20% in some series, and can occur in utero. Neonatal thrombocytopenia can also occur as a consequence of **maternal ITP** with maternal transfer of antibody. Bleeding tends to be mild in this setting and intracranial hemorrhage is rare. The thrombocytopenia resolves after several weeks. An acquired thrombocytopenia most often occurs in the setting of an ill infant with sepsis, congenital viral infection (*Toxoplasma*, rubella, cytomegalovirus, HIV), necrotizing enterocolitis, respiratory distress syndrome, asphyxia, or congenital heart disease. Drug-associated thrombocytopenia can also occur in the hospitalized infant.

Vitamin K deficiency in the neonate has 3 different presentations. **Classic hemorrhagic disease of the newborn** presents between days 2 to 7 of life and is due to the immature neonatal liver and impaired clotting factor synthesis, inadequate vitamin K intake, and a sterile neonatal gut. With the advent of vitamin K prophylaxis at birth, this form of vitamin K deficiency is rarely seen. **Early hemorrhagic disease of the newborn** presents in the first 24 hours of life and is due to maternal medications that affect vitamin K metabolism (anticonvulsants). **Late vitamin K deficiency** occurs after the first week of life and is associated with a number of conditions in which vitamin K stores may be low, such as inadequate intake in breastfed infants, impaired absorption in infants with chronic diarrhea, antibiotic use, cystic fibrosis, and other GI disorders. Bleeding symptoms associated with vitamin K deficiency can be quite severe with a significant incidence of GI, deep tissue, and intracranial hemorrhage.

Evaluation

History

A thorough bleeding history and physical examination should enable the pediatrician to determine the likelihood of an underlying bleeding disorder. The pattern of bleeding, the timing of the symptoms (acute vs chronic), the overall health of the child, and the family history are important in helping to determine the underlying etiology. Box 84-1 lists the pertinent questions to ask when obtaining a bleeding history.

Bruises are a common childhood complaint. Normal bruising that occurs in an active child must be differentiated from pathologic bruising owing to a possible bleeding disorder or non-accidental trauma. Bruises over exposed bony prominences such as the anterior tibial region or the knees are common. Bruises of a size inconsistent with the degree of reported trauma, and bruises in nonexposed or unusual areas (back, chest, shoulders, or upper arms) should alert the pediatrician to a possible bleeding disorder or non-accidental trauma. Linear or geometric bruises are concerning for non-accidental trauma. Epistaxis, another common complaint, is most often due to digital trauma or allergic rhinitis. However, epistaxis unrelieved by 15 minutes of appropriately applied pressure or epistaxis requiring packing, cautery, or transfusions is highly suggestive of a bleeding disorder. Menorrhagia, defined as menstrual flow greater than 7 days, and a history of frequently stained clothes or iron deficiency anemia in an adolescent female are concerning. Persistent or recurrent bleeding with dental extractions (beyond the day of the procedure) or with surgeries also merits a closer evaluation. However, if a child has undergone previous dental extractions or surgeries without bleeding complications, an underlying bleeding disorder is unlikely.

Physical Examination

Depending on the underlying bleeding disorder and the time of presentation, the physical examination may be completely normal. If there is active bleeding, physical signs may include petechiae, ecchymoses, mucosal bleeding (nasal, oral, vaginal), hematuria, swollen joints (hemarthrosis), or limited range of motion. Children with bleeding associated with an acquired disorder such as infection, malignancy, autoimmunity, or liver or renal dysfunction may have physical signs specific to the underlying illness. Children with bleeding associated with a genetic disorder may have a normal examination or congenital anomalies associated with a particular syndrome.

Laboratory Tests

The extent of the laboratory evaluation is dependent on the bleeding history and clinical presentation. Initial laboratory studies for a potential bleeding disorder should include a CBC with a peripheral smear, a PT, and an activated PTT (aPTT).

The **CBC** is useful in providing a platelet count to identify suspected thrombocytopenia. In addition, abnormalities in the white blood cell count or red cell indices can provide clues to the underlying process. A microcytic anemia consistent with iron deficiency would suggest chronic blood loss and raise the suspicion for an underlying bleeding disorder. Pancytopenia would suggest an underlying bone marrow failure syndrome or a possible malignancy such as leukemia. Review of the **peripheral smear** can confirm the presence of true thrombocytopenia and allow for an assessment of platelet, white blood cell, and red blood cell morphology.

The **PT** reflects the extrinsic and common pathway and the **aPTT** reflects the intrinsic and common pathway. A prolonged PT or PTT should be followed up with a 1:1 mixing study to determine whether the prolongation is due to a factor deficiency or the presence of an inhibitor. The **bleeding time** is a reflection of primary hemostasis (platelets, vWF, vascular integrity), but is rarely performed in pediatrics because of the unreliability and difficulty of performing this test in children. The **platelet function assay** is a screening test of platelet function, measuring both platelet adhesion and aggregation (primary hemostasis).

A stepwise approach to more specific testing is dictated by the clinical presentation and screening test results and is best performed with the consultation of a pediatric hematologist. When an abnormality of primary hemostasis is suspected, the initial evaluation should focus on von Willebrand disease because it is the most common disorder. A **vWF panel,** which includes vWF antigen, ristocetin cofactor activity (functional measure of vWF), FVIII activity, and a vWF multimer analysis, should be performed. Many factors may transiently increase vWF levels (stress, inflammation, hormones, exercise, oral contraceptives), and normal results are frequently encountered in patients with type 1 von Willebrand disease. Repeat testing is often necessary to make the diagnosis and should be pursued if the suspicion is high. For hemophilia or any other suspected factor deficiency, a specific **coagulation factor assay** must be performed. For patients with suspected qualitative platelet disorder, **platelet aggregation studies** (measuring the degree and pattern of platelet aggregation to various agonists) or **flow cytometry** (measuring the platelet surface GP expression) can be performed. On a case-by-case basis, additional studies such as fibrinogen, d-dimer, fibrin split products, thrombin time, factor inhibitor assay, autoimmune studies, liver function tests, creatinine, or blood urea nitrogen may be indicated. Table 84-2 lists the major screening tests for hemostasis.

Table 84-2. Laboratory Evaluation for Hemostasis

Laboratory Test	Measured Hemostatic Function
CBC	Platelet count
Peripheral blood smear	Platelet morphology
aPTT	Factors I, II, V, VIII, IX, XI, XII (intrinsic and common pathway)
PT	Factors I, II, V, VII, X (extrinsic and common pathway)
aPTT and PT mixing studies	Performed when aPTT/PT is prolonged; patient plasma and normal plasma is mixed 1:1, and then aPTT/PT repeated; if the aPTT/PT corrects, there is a factor deficiency, if not, there is an inhibitor
Bleeding time (not recommended)	Primary hemostasis (platelets, vWF, endothelial integrity)
PFA-100 screen	Primary hemostasis (platelets, vWF)
Thrombin time	Fibrinogen
vWF panel	vWF antigen (amount of vWF) Ristocetin cofactor activity (function of vWF) Factor VIII activity vWF multimer analysis (distribution of multimers)
Coagulation factor assays	Specific factor activity
Platelet aggregation studies	Platelet function; patient platelets are exposed to agonists and the degree of aggregation and pattern of the response is unique for various qualitative platelet disorders

Abbreviations: aPTT, activated partial thromboplastin time; CBC, complete blood cell count; PFA, platelet function assay; PT, prothrombin time; vWF, von Willebrand factor.

Imaging Studies

In general, imaging studies are not indicated. Bone films may be taken of the upper extremities in patients with thrombocytopenia to rule out Fanconi anemia and TAR syndrome.

Management

The management of bleeding disorders is dependent on the underlying abnormality. However, general supportive measures, such as local pressure for bleeding, avoidance of blood draws, and avoidance of medications that affect the function of platelets or hemostasis, can be applied to most clinical scenarios of bleeding.

Treatment of **von Willebrand disease** is dependent on the subtype and the severity of bleeding symptoms. For mild bleeding symptoms, supportive measures alone may be all that is necessary—applying appropriate pressure for epistaxis, ice pack for bruises, and avoidance of antiplatelet medications. For type 1 von Willebrand disease, DDAVP (synthetic vasopressin) can be used and is available as a concentrated nasal spray or intravenously. DDAVP stimulates endothelial release of vWF and can increase levels 2- to 3-fold. For type 3 and most cases of type 2 von Willebrand disease,

replacement therapy with FVIII concentrates that contain vWF is necessary for significant bleeding episodes. Antifibrinolytic agents such as aminocaproic acid are very effective for mucosal bleeding and can be used either alone for mild cases or in conjunction with DDAVP or FVIII concentrates in more severe episodes of bleeding. For females with menorrhagia, a trial of oral contraceptives is reasonable because estrogen can increase vWF levels. This response is variable, however, and if not effective, aminocaproic acid and nasal DDAVP may be necessary

The treatment for most **qualitative platelet disorders** is supportive. Mild bleeding episodes can be treated nonspecifically with antifibrinolytic agents or DDAVP. Platelet transfusions should be reserved for life-threatening bleeds and otherwise avoided because of the risk for developing antibodies.

The management for **acute ITP** consists of family education, supportive measures and, in selected cases, pharmacologic therapies. The use of pharmacologic therapies in acute ITP remains controversial. The natural course of acute ITP is for the platelet count to rise within 1 to 3 weeks of presentation. The impetus to treat is the theoretical prevention of intracranial hemorrhage; however, the incidence of this complication is less than 0.5%, and there are no data to confirm that any of the currently available therapies actually prevent this complication. Pharmacologic intervention will increase the platelet count more rapidly and may prevent a significant bleeding complication. In those at risk, the use of pharmacologic intervention will not reduce the likelihood of developing chronic ITP. The decision to treat must be individualized, taking into consideration the child's age, bleeding symptoms, child's activity level, and parental anxiety level. Treatment options include observation without medical therapy, corticosteroids, intravenous (IV) gammaglobulin, and anti-D immunoglobulin. Anti-D immunoglobulin can only be used in patients who are Rh positive. In all cases, parents should be instructed to avoid the use of aspirin, ibuprofen, and other antiplatelet medications; to avoid intramuscular injections; and to postpone immunizations and allergic desensitization injections that may exacerbate the degree of thrombocytopenia. Physical activity should be limited with specific instruction to avoid activities that may cause head injury. Parents should also be educated to the signs and symptoms of an intracranial hemorrhage and given instructions as to what to do in the event of an emergency. Therapeutic options for **chronic ITP** include observation without therapy, corticosteroids, regular infusions of IV immune globulin (IVIG) or anti-D immunoglobulin (for Rh+ patients), immunosuppressive agents, Rituximab, and laparoscopic splenectomy. Rituximab is a chimeric monoclonal antibody directed against CD20 (found primarily on the surface of B cells) and has been shown to be effective in chronic ITP and other autoimmune conditions. Treatment for acute bleeding in **neonatal alloimmune thrombocytopenia** includes transfusion of maternal platelets and IVIG.

Prevention and early treatment of bleeding episodes, family education, and good well-child care are important in providing comprehensive **hemophilia** care. The current standard of care for patients with severe hemophilia is prophylaxis, the IV administration of factor on a regular schedule (every other day, 3 times a week, or twice a week depending on the type of hemophilia) to prevent bleeding episodes. Prophylaxis is usually initiated during the first few years of life. A subcutaneous central venous catheter is inserted for this purpose and, as the child grows, the parents, and eventually the child, are taught how to administer factor by peripheral infusion. For acute bleeds, prompt treatment is essential to prevent long-term complications. In 30% of patients with hemophilia A and 2% to 3% of patients with hemophilia B, an inhibitor to the respective factor can develop. In the presence of an inhibitor, acute bleeds must be treated with bypassing agents such as prothrombin concentrates or recombinant FVIIa. In the long term, immune tolerance is attempted by exposing the child to high doses of factor on a daily basis in an attempt to eradicate the inhibitor. A number of immune tolerance regimens have been in use with varying success.

Acquired causes of coagulation or platelet abnormalities can be treated supportively or by replacing the deficiency or removing the offending causative agent. Children with **DIC** may be given fresh frozen plasma, cryoprecipitate, and platelets as needed while the underlying etiology of the DIC is treated. In children in whom **vitamin K deficiency** is suspected as the cause of bleeding, one dose of vitamin K should correct the coagulopathy within 12 to 36 hours. Depending on the underlying cause of vitamin K deficiency, regular replacement may be required.

Prognosis

Most patients with inherited bleeding disorders will have an excellent prognosis if the diagnosis is made in a timely fashion and appropriate intervention is initiated.

Patients with **von Willebrand disease** usually have mild bleeding symptoms and, with appropriate education and intervention, the prognosis is excellent. Patients with **hemophilia** will also have an excellent prognosis assuming early diagnosis, family education, prophylaxis, and early treatment of bleeds. With the advent of prophylaxis, the severe hemophilic arthropathy that plagued older generations of males with hemophilia has been largely averted or minimized. In addition, the use of recombinant factor products and highly purified plasma-derived products in the pediatric population has minimized the risk for viral transmission. **Acute ITP** resolves spontaneously by 6 months in 80% of cases, regardless of pharmacologic intervention, and the risk for significant hemorrhage is exceedingly low. For individuals with **chronic ITP,** most cases will also resolve with time, and individuals do not usually have significant bleeding complications.

CASE RESOLUTION

A vWF panel was performed and revealed a vWF antigen of 20%, ristocetin cofactor activity of 30%, FVIII activity of 40%, and a normal multimer analysis. The girl was diagnosed with type 1 von Willebrand disease. A DDAVP challenge was performed in clinic, and she was found to have an excellent response. She was prescribed nasal DDAVP (Stimate) and aminocaproic acid for significant bleeding episodes.

Selected References

Allen GA, Glader B. Approach to the bleeding child. *Pediatr Clin North Am.* 2002;49:1239–1256

Andrew M, Vegh P, Johnston M, et al. Maturation of the hemostatic system during childhood. *Blood.* 1992;80:1998–1905

Astermark J, Petrini P, Tengborn L, et al. Primary prophylaxis in severe haemophilia should be started at an early age but can be individualized. *Br J Haematol.* 1999;105:1109–1113

Cherrick I, Karayalcin G, Lanzkowsky P. Transient erythroblastopenia of childhood. Prospective study of fifty patients. *Am J Pediatr Hematol Oncol.* 1994;16:320

Cines DB, Blanchette VS. Immune thrombocytopenic purpura. *N Engl J Med.* 2002;346:995

Gazda HT, Sieff CA. Recent insights into the pathogenesis of Diamond-Blackfan anaemia. *Br J Haematol.* 2006;135:149

Manco-Johnson MJ, Abshire TC, Shapiro AD, et al. Prophylaxis versus episodic treatment to prevent joint disease in boys with severe hemophilia. *N Engl J Med.* 2007;357(6):535–544

Nichols WL, Hultin MB, James AH, et al. Von Willebrand (VWD): evidence-based diagnosis and management guidelines, the National Heart, Lung, and Blood Institute (NHLBI Expert Panel report (USA). *Haemophilia.* 2008;14(2):171–232

Raipurkar M, Lusher JM. Clinical and laboratory approach to the patient with bleeding. In: Orkin SH, Nathan DG, Ginsburg D, Look AT, Fisher DE, Lux SE, eds. *Nathan and Oski's Hematology of Infancy and Childhood.* 7th ed. Philadelphia, PA: Saunders/Elsevier; 2009:1449–1461

Tarantino MD, Buchanan GR. The pros and cons of drug therapy for immune thrombocytopenic purpura in children. *Hematol Oncol Clin North Am.* 2004; 18:1301

CHAPTER 85

Lymphadenopathy

Wendy Y. Tcheng, MD

CASE STUDY

A 12-year-old girl is brought to the office with swelling of the anterior cervical nodes, which she has had for 2 weeks. Intermittent fever with temperatures as high as 101°F (38.3°C) and decreased appetite have been associated with the condition. On examination, her temperature is 100.4°F (38.0°C), and her other vital signs are normal. Three to 4 non-tender nodes 1 to 2 cm in diameter are present bilaterally. The remainder of the examination is normal.

Questions

1. When is lymphadenopathy of medical concern?
2. What are the clinical features of childhood diseases that present as cervical lymphadenopathy?
3. What are the diagnostic approaches to the evaluation of children with lymphadenopathy?
4. What is an appropriate therapeutic approach to cervical lymphadenopathy in children?

Lymphadenopathy is one of the most common clinical problems encountered in pediatrics. Palpable lymph nodes are a source of anxiety for parents, often prompting a pediatrician visit for evaluation. While most cases are due to a benign, self-limited infectious process, lymphadenopathy may also signal a serious underlying systemic illness. It is important for the pediatrician to make this distinction so that appropriate diagnostic and therapeutic measures can be initiated when necessary.

Epidemiology

Lymphadenopathy occurs frequently in childhood, and even healthy children may have palpable lymph nodes in the anterior cervical, inguinal, and axillary regions. Localized lymphadenopathy is largely due to an infectious etiology, whereas generalized lymphadenopathy occurs with systemic illnesses, such as systemic infections (viral, bacterial, protozoal, fungal), autoimmune disorders, storage disorders, and malignancies.

Clinical Presentation

Lymphadenopathy may be localized or generalized on presentation. **Localized** or **regional** lymphadenopathy refers to enlargement of lymph nodes within contiguous regions, whereas **generalized** lymphadenopathy involves more than 2 noncontiguous lymph node groups (Dx Box). Infection is the most frequent cause of localized lymphadenopathy in children. The anterior cervical lymph node region is the most commonly involved area reflecting the high frequency of upper respiratory infections (URIs). Bilateral cervical lymphadenopathy is often seen with viral and bacterial URIs, and the nodes tend to be soft, mobile, and non-tender. Viruses such as Epstein-Barr virus (EBV) or cytomegalovirus (CMV) can present with prominent posterior cervical lymphadenopathy as well as generalized adenopathy,

---

Dx **Lymphadenopathy**

- Enlarged lymph nodes
- Fever
- Tenderness or warmth over the lymph nodes (lymphadenitis)
- Antecedent infection (eg, pharyngitis, upper respiratory infection, otitis media)
- Pallor
- Weight loss
- Bone pain

---

and occasionally hepatosplenomegaly. Direct bacterial invasion of lymph nodes produces a lymphadenitis, which is typically unilateral, tender, erythematous, and fluctuant. Chronic lymphadenopathy may be due to atypical mycobacterial infections, tuberculosis, cat-scratch disease, EBV, CMV, toxoplasmosis, coccidiomycosis, or HIV. Generalized lymphadenopathy is concerning for an underlying systemic illness (infection, autoimmune process, storage disease, or malignancy). Lymphadenopathy due to malignancy is typically characterized by fixed, firm, non-tender lymph nodes in the setting of other signs and symptoms, such as fever, pallor, night sweats, and weight loss.

Pathophysiology

Lymph nodes are an integral part of the immune system where phagocytic cells filter microorganisms and particulate matter, and antigens are presented provoking a cellular or humorally mediated lymphocyte response. Lymph nodes are distributed in groups throughout the body and drain specific regions (head, neck, axilla, mediastinum, abdomen, extremities) (Table 85-1). Enlargement of a

Table 85-1. Lymph Node Drainage Patterns	
Group	*Drainage Pattern*
Occipital	Posterior scalp
Preauricular	Superficial orbital and periorbital tissue, temporal scalp
Submental/submandibular	Mouth
Cervical	Mouth, pharynx, ear, parotid gland, deep structures of neck (thyroid, larynx, trachea, upper esophagus)
Supraclavicular	Head, neck, arms, lungs, mediastinum, and abdomen
Mediastinal	Lungs, heart, thymus, esophagus
Axillary	Chest wall, breast, upper extremity
Abdominal	Abdominal organs, pelvis, lower extremities
Iliac and inguinal	Lower extremities, genitalia, buttocks, pelvis

lymph node may be due to proliferation of lymphocytes intrinsic to the lymph node (as a physiological immune response or a malignant transformation) or may be due to infiltration by extrinsic inflammatory or metastatic malignant cells.

Differential Diagnosis

The duration and extent of lymphadenopathy (localized vs generalized), the characteristics of the lymph nodes, and the presence of associated symptoms will help to focus the differential diagnosis. A list of the common causes of lymphadenopathy in children is provided in Table 85-2.

Localized lymphadenopathy is most often due to an infectious etiology. Acute bilateral cervical lymphadenopathy is most frequently due to viral URIs (respiratory syncytial virus, adenovirus, influenza virus) or EBV and CMV, which can also cause generalized adenopathy. Bacterial pharyngitis (most commonly *Streptococcus* species) and oral infections/dental abscesses can also present with cervical adenopathy. Unilateral lymphadenitis is most often due to *Staphylococcus aureus,* followed by *Streptococcus pyogenes,* anaerobes, and other species. When the condition appears subacute, cat-scratch disease; tuberculosis (scrofula); atypical mycobacteria; toxoplasmosis; tularemia; and, less commonly, histoplasmosis, brucellosis, and syphilis should be considered. Cervical lymphadenopathy can also occur with Kawasaki disease, along with high fever (5 days), redness/swelling/desquamation of extremities, conjunctivitis, rash, swollen lips/tongue.

Generalized lymphadenopathy may be due to systemic infections (eg, EBV, CMV, HIV, toxoplasmosis), autoimmune disorders (eg, juvenile idiopathic arthritis, systemic lupus erythematosus), storage disorders (eg, Niemann-Pick, Gaucher disease), histiocytic disorders (eg, Langerhans cell histiocytosis, hemophagocytic lymphohistiocytosis), drug reactions (eg, phenytoin), or malignancies. Malignancies include leukemia and lymphoma (Hodgkin and non-Hodgkin lymphoma) as well as solid tumors that can metastasize to lymph nodes (eg, neuroblastoma, rhabdomyosarcoma). With neoplastic infiltration, enlarged nodes are generally non-tender,

firm, rubbery, and immobile. In Hodgkin disease, the nodes enlarge sequentially, with involvement spreading from one chain to the next. Supraclavicular or epitrochlear adenopathy is highly suggestive of malignancy.

A number of head and neck lesions that occur in the pediatric population merit comment because they are often confused with cervical lymphadenopathy. These lesions include cystic hygromas, branchial cleft cysts, thyroglossal duct cysts, and epidermoid cysts. These are congenital malformations that often present as a neck mass in the young child and can easily be mistaken for a lymph node, particularly if infected (see Chapter 79).

Evaluation

History

A thorough history and review of symptoms is essential in determining the underlying etiology of lymphadenopathy in children. Inquiries should be made regarding the duration of the lymphadenopathy, the rate of nodal enlargement, and the occurrence of associated fever and other constitutional symptoms, such as bone pain, weight loss, fever, and night sweats. Recent illnesses or infections, insect or animal bites, and local trauma should be determined. A history of distant travel; recent emigration from countries with endemic tuberculosis (eg, Mexico, Central America, Southeast Asia); recent travel to areas with endemic histoplasmosis (southeastern United States) or coccidioidomycosis (San Joaquin Valley, CA); a detailed history of pet contact (cats/kittens, which can transmit toxoplasmosis and cat-scratch disease); and exposure to ill contacts, particularly individuals known to have tuberculosis, are also important (Questions Box).

Physical Examination

When evaluating a child with lymphadenopathy, the enlarged nodes should be measured and examined at their widest diameter and evaluated for evidence of erythema, tenderness, and warmth, all of which are suggestive of infection. The characteristics of the enlarged lymph node should be noted (eg, soft, firm, rubbery, mobile, matted, tender, discrete). The surrounding skin and soft tissue region that is drained by the involved lymph node should be examined for signs of inflammation or skin breakdown. The extent of the lymphadenopathy should be determined, as well as the presence or absence of hepatosplenomegaly.

Laboratory Tests

In most cases, a thorough history and physical examination can establish the likely diagnosis without any laboratory testing. If studies are deemed necessary, a complete blood cell count, peripheral blood smear, and tests of renal and hepatic function are useful to screen for an underlying systemic illness that may be associated with lymphadenopathy. Lymphocytosis with atypical lymphocytes on peripheral blood smear is consistent with a viral etiology such as EBV or CMV. Leukocytosis with a left shift suggests a bacterial etiology. Cytopenias

Table 85-2. Differential Diagnosis of Lymphadenopathy

Diagnostic Category	Clinical Features	Epidemiological Features	Laboratory Features
Infections			
Viral (EBV, CMV, rubella, HIV)	Usually generalized, not purulent or tender; may have hepatosplenomegaly		EBV/CMV with atypical lymphocytes on peripheral blood smear, viral titers
Mycobacterial (TB, atypical mycobacteria)	Usually localized; often tender, red, flocculent		PPD
Bacterial (staphylococcal and strep-tococcal infections, cat-scratch disease, tularemia, plague, diphtheria)	Usually localized; often tender, red, flocculent		Titers (cat scratch) Gram stain/culture
Protozoal (toxoplasmosis)	Generalized		Titers
Spirochete (syphilis)			Titers
Fungal (histoplasmosis, coccidioidomycosis)	May be generalized	Suspicion should be raised based on regional incidence	Titers
Neoplastic Conditions			
Hodgkin lymphoma	Often associated with "B" symptoms (eg, fever, weight loss, night sweats), pruritus	Common among higher socioeconomic groups, adolescents	ESR (can be >100), LDH, elevated eosinophils, anergy, elevated ferritin
Non-Hodgkin lymphoma	See Hodgkin lymphoma		
Leukemia	Generalized lymphadenopathy, hepatosplenomegaly, petechiae, purpura		Blasts on peripheral blood smear, hyperuricemia, hyperkalemia, hyperphosphatemia, elevated LDH
Solid tumors (eg, rhabdomyosarcoma, neuroblastoma)	Depends on underlying malignancy		
Langerhans cell histiocytosis	Eczema, failure to thrive, bony lesions, diabetes insipidus, proptosis, hepatosplenomegaly all possible		
Sinus histiocytosis with massive lymphadenopathy			
Autoimmune Disorders			
JIA	Generalized lymphadenopathy seen in systemic form (Still) (eg, fever, hepato-splenomegaly, evanescent rash, arthritis)	Equal incidence in males and females	ESR, anemia, negative ANA. and rheumatoid arthritis in Still JRA
Lupus	Arthritis, butterfly facial rash, effusions (lung, joint, cardiac), CNS, nephrotic syndrome	Increased incidence in girls	ESR, positive ANA, anti-ds DNA, ⁻ C3, C4, or CH50, anemia, platelets, proteinuria
Other			
Storage disorders (eg, Niemann-Pick, Gaucher disease)	Generalized lymphadenopathy, hepatosplenomegaly		
Drugs (eg, phenytoin)	Generalized lymphadenopathy		
Sarcoidosis	Bilateral hilar lymphadenopathy, non-caseating granulomas (lung, liver)	In African Americans and those of Irish heritage	Serum angiotensin-1 converting enzyme, serum lysozyme

Abbreviations: ANA, antinuclear antibody; CMV, cytomegalovirus; CNS, central nervous system; EBV, Epstein-Barr virus; ESR, erythrocyte sedimentation rate; HIV, human immunodeficiency virus; JIA, juvenile idiopathic arthritis; LDH, lactate dehydrogenase; PPD, purified protein derivative; TB, tuberculosis.

Lymphadenopathy **Questions**

- How long have the nodes been enlarged?
- Was the child sick before the swelling began?
- Does the child have any symptoms now, such as fever, weight loss, pallor, or anorexia?
- Does the child come in contact with any animals, particularly cats?
- Has the child traveled anywhere?
- Is the child taking any medications?
- Has the child been in contact with anyone who is ill?

or blasts on peripheral blood smear are concerning for leukemia. Uric acid, phosphorus, and lactate dehydrogenase are typically elevated in the setting of leukemia or lymphoma. An erythrocyte sedimentation rate is nonspecific but may be helpful. Depending on the clinical scenario, serum antibody studies for various infections may be warranted (ie, EBV, CMV, HIV, *Bartonella henselae* for cat-scratch disease). In addition, a purified protein derivative (PPD) skin test for tuberculosis or serological tests for fungal disease should be considered. In lupus and juvenile idiopathic arthritis, an antinuclear antibody may be positive and complement levels may be reduced.

If infectious lymphadenitis is suspected, an aspirate for a Gram stain and culture may be helpful, particularly if the infection has been unresponsive to empiric antibiotics. However, if there is *any* concern for malignancy, a fine needle aspiration is *not* the preferred method for diagnosis. An excisional biopsy should be performed so that the entire lymph node can be visualized and adequate samples for testing will be available.

Imaging Studies

A chest radiograph should be performed in any child with significant lymphadenopathy if there is a suspicion of an underlying systemic process. If leukemia or lymphoma is suspected, a chest radiograph is performed to evaluate for an anterior mediastinal mass. Other imaging studies are not routinely performed; however, if the nature of an enlarged lymph node requires further definition, an ultrasound can be done. In the setting of malignancy, additional radiographic studies are performed for staging purposes.

Management

Management is dictated by the underlying cause of lymphadenopathy. Cervical lymphadenopathy associated with URIs will typically resolve without intervention. Bacterial lymphadenitis can be treated with a trial of **antibiotics** with antistaphylococcal and antistreptococcal coverage. Underlying fungal and mycobacterial diseases should be treated with appropriate **antifungal or antibacterial agents,** with the exception of cervical adenopathy due to atypical mycobacteria, which requires **surgical removal.** Malignancies may require **multimodal therapy** with surgery, chemotherapy, and/or radiation, depending on the specific diagnosis and stage (see Chapter 141).

Prognosis

The outcome of lymphadenopathy depends entirely on the underlying etiology. In most cases, the cause is infectious, and the lymphadenopathy is self-limited or resolves with the use of appropriate antibiotics. Lymphadenopathy associated with an underlying systemic illness may have a more chronic or relapsing course depending on the disease.

CASE RESOLUTION

In the case history, the bilateral nature of the swelling and the lack of tenderness of the nodes are very worrisome and suggest a noninfectious etiology. The girl had a throat culture, an intermediate PPD, and a chest radiograph, all of which were negative. A complete blood cell count reveals leukocytosis with 28,000 white blood cells per deciliter (60% lymphocytes), with a normal hemoglobin and platelet count. A heterophil test for infectious mononucleosis is positive. Supportive measures are recommended, and the child makes a complete recovery in 3 weeks.

Selected References

Filston HC. Common lumps and bumps of the head and neck in infants and children. *Pediatr Ann.* 1989;18:180–186

Ginsburg AM. The tuberculosis epidemic: scientific challenges and opportunities. *Public Health Rep.* 1998;113:128–136

Grossman M, Shiramizu B. Evaluation of lymphadenopathy in children. *Curr Opin Pediatr.* 1994;6(1):68–76

Knight PJ, Mulne AF, Vassy LE. When is lymph node biopsy indicated in children with enlarged peripheral nodes? *Pediatrics.* 1982;69:391–396

Knight PJ, Reiner CB. Superficial lumps in children: what, when and why? *Pediatrics.* 1983;72:147–153

Larsson LO, Bentzon MW, Berg Kelly K, et al. Palpable lymph nodes of the neck in Swedish schoolchildren. *Acta Paediatr.* 1994;83(10):1091–1094

Leung AK, Davies HD. Cervical lymphadenitis: etiology, diagnosis, and management. *Curr Infect Dis Rep.* 2009;11(3):183–189

Marcy SM. Infections of lymph nodes of the head and neck. *Pediatr Infect Dis.* 1983;2:397–405

Nield LS, Kamat D. Lymphadenopathy in children: when and how to evaluate. *Clin Pediatr (Phila).* 2004;43(1):25–33

Oguz A, Karadeniz C, Temel EA, Citak EC, Okur FV. Evaluation of peripheral lymphadenopathy in children. *Pediatr Hematol Oncol.* 2006;23(7):549–561

Twist CJ, Link MP. Assessment of lymphadenopathy in children. *Pediatr Clin North Am.* 2002;49(5):1009–1025

Yaris N, Cakir M, Sozen E, Cobanoglu U. Analysis of children with peripheral lymphadenopathy. *Clin Pediatr (Phila).* 2006;45(6):544–549

Zitelli BJ. Evaluating the child with a neck mass. *Contemp Pediatr.* 1990;7:90–112

SECTION VI

Cardiovascular System

CHAPTER 86

Heart Murmurs

Robin Winkler Doroshow, MD, MMS, MEd

CASE STUDY

A 6-year-old girl is brought to the office for a physical examination for school. Her medical history is unremarkable, and her growth and development have been normal. She is asymptomatic. Her physical examination is normal except for a grade II/VI low-pitched vibratory systolic ejection murmur that is loudest at the left lower sternal border, with radiation to the apex and upper sternal border. The murmur increases to III/VI in the supine position.

Questions

1. What is the significance of a heart murmur in asymptomatic children? How reassuring are a negative history and the absence of other physical findings?
2. What workup should be done by primary care physicians?
3. What are the costs of excessive tests and unnecessary consultation? What are the costs of an inadequate workup?
4. When should physicians refer children to specialists for consultation?

Asymptomatic children with heart murmurs are commonly encountered by physicians. A murmur is a finding rather than a medical sign or symptom because it is detected incidentally at an examination conducted for another purpose.

Correct assessment of the significance of a heart murmur is important to ensure appropriate management of children with heart disease. Complications of undiagnosed cardiac disease in children include progressive hemodynamic impairment, endocarditis, and even sudden death.

The misinterpretation of an innocent murmur as organic in nature can also take its toll, primarily as parental anxiety. Unnecessary restriction of activities may result, which can have a negative impact on children's school and social lives as well as self-image. As adults they may be denied health insurance, life insurance, and certain types of employment. In addition, misdiagnosis costs money and uses limited resources, with unnecessary tests and doctor visits, as this "non-disease" is evaluated and followed.

Epidemiology

An estimated 50% of healthy children have heart murmurs. The overall incidence of congenital heart disease (CHD), including symptomatic cases, is just under 1%, and some children with CHD have no murmur. Therefore, about 98 out of 100 murmurs noted during childhood are "innocent" (ie, have no organic basis).

Clinical Presentation

Heart murmurs are usually detected on routine examination for well-child care or on evaluation for an unrelated problem. Innocent murmurs are not associated with signs or symptoms because they are normal findings. Most of the symptoms sometimes associated with

organic murmurs (ie, murmurs of heart disease) are related to the presence of congestive heart failure (CHF) (see Chapter 88) and usually appear during infancy. Some children with murmurs come to medical attention with complaints of exercise intolerance or chest pain. It is necessary to determine whether these problems are actually referable to the heart.

Pathophysiology

A murmur is a sustained sound that can be detected with a stethoscope placed on the chest. This sound is produced by turbulence of blood flow in the heart or great vessels. This turbulence may be due to structural abnormalities (eg, aortic valve stenosis), benign or normal flow patterns (see below), or exaggeration of normal flow patterns (seen in high output states such as fever, exercise, anxiety, or anemia, and sometimes termed *functional*).

Not all significant heart disease in children is heralded by a murmur. Structural heart disease may be silent and be indicated by other findings. For example, transposition of the great arteries results in cyanosis, anomalous pulmonary venous return in pulmonary edema and hypoxia, and anomalous origin of the left coronary artery from the pulmonary artery in CHF. Acquired heart disease, such as Kawasaki disease, myocarditis, or cardiomyopathy, often produces no murmur.

The common innocent murmurs are better recognized than understood. Because they occur in normal, healthy individuals, there are few hemodynamic or anatomical data to correlate with the murmur, and pathophysiology is in some cases conjectural. **Still murmur,** which was once thought to be due to easily appreciated aortic valve flow, is now believed to result from vibration of normal fibrous bands ("false tendons") that cross the left ventricle. This murmur may also be heard in children who have undergone spontaneous closure of a membranous ventricular septal defect, with a small residual aneurysm in the septum. The **pulmonary flow murmur** seems to be caused by normal flow across the pulmonary valve, perhaps made more apparent because of high cardiac output, close proximity to the chest wall, and (in adolescent females) mild anemia. The **venous hum** is attributed to turbulence at the confluence of the innominate veins, which is exacerbated in the upright position by gravity.

The **physiological peripheral pulmonic stenosis (PPPS) murmur** in newborns is produced by turbulence at the origins of the left and right pulmonary arteries. Because less than 10% of the combined ventricular output of the fetus goes to these branches, they are small and arise at a sharp angle from the main pulmonary artery. When postnatal circulation abruptly requires the entire cardiac output to enter these vessels, a relative stenosis is encountered. This physiological stenosis resolves gradually with remodeling of the pulmonary artery tree by 2 to 3 months of age.

Differential Diagnosis

In healthy children, the differential diagnosis of a heart murmur includes innocent murmurs and murmurs resulting from structural lesions, most of which are congenital. The specific features of a particular murmur usually provide most if not all necessary clues to the diagnosis. It is therefore important to develop and maintain auscultatory skills. A good quality stethoscope, with both diaphragm and bell correctly sized for the patient, is essential. Conditions should be optimized: The patient should be kept comfortable and, if necessary, distracted, and extraneous environmental noise should be minimized.

Some features may alert examiners to the organic nature of a murmur. Although very loud murmurs (grades IV–VI; ie, with associated precordial thrill) are usually not innocent, some innocent murmurs may be as loud as grade III, particularly with high cardiac output (eg, fever, anxiety, or anemia). Diastolic murmurs and continuous murmurs, other than the easily recognizable venous hum, are usually pathologic, as are high-pitched and harsh murmurs, which are better heard with the diaphragm of the stethoscope.

The common innocent murmurs of childhood are recognizable on auscultatory examination. **Still murmur,** or the **innocent vibratory murmur,** is a low-pitched, vibratory, or musical murmur that sounds like a groan. Because of its low frequency, the murmur is better heard with the bell. It is loudest at the left lower sternal border but is often distributed widely over the precordium. This murmur is often quite loud, particularly in the supine position, and is extremely common in school-aged children. The characteristics of the murmur are diagnostic, although the absence of other findings is supportive.

The **pulmonary flow murmur,** usually heard in older children, is a short, blowing systolic ejection (ie, crescendo-decrescendo) murmur localized to the left upper sternal border. It may be louder in the supine position.

The **venous hum** is a soft continuous murmur, similar to the sound heard in a seashell. Because of its constancy, it is often

overlooked. This murmur is very commonly heard in preschool and school-aged children. Loudest in the right infraclavicular area, it may also be heard on the left. This murmur is highly variable with head and neck position and compression of the neck veins, which may increase or diminish it. It usually disappears in the supine position.

The **PPPS** murmur is an innocent murmur found in newborns. Best heard at the upper left sternal border, this blowing systolic ejection murmur radiates strikingly over the lung fields into the back and both axillae.

Evaluation

History

The history may be helpful in assessment of the child with a murmur. If a thorough history shows that the child has no symptoms, this suggests the absence of severe heart disease and helps exclude many major or complex defects as well as CHF. The absence of symptoms does not, however, exclude several common defects that may require intervention (Table 86-1).

The most common cardiac symptom reported by children or parents is easy fatigability (Questions Box). This is difficult to quantitate. Determining exercise intolerance on the basis of history is very subjective; it may be due, of course, to noncardiac causes and may be unrelated to the murmur. Easy fatigability during infancy may be reported as slow or poor feeding. Chest pain, a common symptom in adults with heart disease, is rarely cardiac in origin in children. A history of rapid breathing, excessive sweating, and other complaints referable to CHF suggests organic heart disease. Central cyanosis (ie, involving the oral mucosa rather than the perioral area or the fingers) may be reported occasionally by parents of children with cyanotic CHD but is often not recognized.

Physical Examination

The physical examination often gives strong clues to the cardiac diagnosis beyond the murmur itself. Even in children with known CHD, the non-auscultatory portions of the examination are critical in assessing the cardiac status (ie, how the patient is tolerating the defect). **Vital signs,** preferably obtained with the child at rest or sleeping, yield information regarding cardiac status more than

Table 86-1. Common Organic Murmurs in Asymptomatic Children	
Lesion	*Other Clues*
Atrial septal defect	Fixed split S_2
Ventricular septal defect (small to moderate)	Loud heart sounds
Patent ductus arteriosus (small to moderate)	Full or bounding pulses
Pulmonic stenosis	Systolic ejection click (SEC)
Aortic stenosis	SEC; suprasternal thrill
Coarctation of the aorta	Weak or absent femoral pulses

specific diagnosis. Tachypnea and tachycardia are present in CHF. A normal resting respiratory rate (ie, <60 breaths/min in infants) argues strongly against CHF. Blood pressure is normal in most patients with CHD. It may be useful to measure blood pressure in the legs, especially if coarctation of the aorta is suspected because of diminished pulses in the lower extremities.

The **growth pattern** may reflect the presence of any chronic illness, including hemodynamically significant CHD. Affected patients, particularly infants and children with large left-to-right shunts (with or without CHF) gain weight poorly. Height and head circumference are usually normal, although in more severe or prolonged situations height may also be affected.

A complete **cardiac examination** should be performed. Is the chest asymmetrical, a sign of long-standing cardiomegaly? Is the precordial impulse hyperdynamic? Are extra sounds (eg, clicks, rubs, gallops) heard? Is the second sound normal in intensity and in width and motion of splitting (ie, variation with respiration)?

Additional pertinent findings include lethargy, dysmorphic features suggestive of a genetic syndrome, central cyanosis, and clubbing. Hepatomegaly is found in children with CHF. The peripheral pulses should be normal in volume, neither diminished (eg, pedal pulses in coarctation) nor bounding (eg, in patent ductus arteriosus), and equal in all extremities. The temperature and capillary refill of the extremities in children who are not chilled reflect adequacy of the peripheral circulation.

Diagnostic Studies

Routine laboratory studies are not warranted in the evaluation of most murmurs. An **electrocardiogram (ECG)** is indicated when heart disease is known or strongly suspected, but a normal ECG may not rule out significant CHD. A **chest radiograph** may be helpful in this setting, but its potential benefits are usually outweighed by the risks of discomfort and radiation exposure. In the case of some tests, such as **echocardiography**, the manner in which the examination is carried out may vary depending on the suspected diagnosis; direct input from a cardiologist may be necessary to maximize the yield from these studies. Such tests are not suitable for screening purposes and should be obtained only after consultation with a pediatric cardiologist.

Management

If a heart murmur is suspected of being organic in origin because of its features or associated findings, referral to a pediatric cardiologist is indicated. For the young infant (particularly the newborn), prompt referral is essential because of the serious risks inherent in ductus-dependent defects (see Chapter 87), which may present with a simple murmur. In the case of a child who is asymptomatic there is no urgency, but parental and physician anxiety can best be allayed by proceeding to consultation promptly (ie, within weeks). In some cases, a repeat examination may be useful before deciding whether to consult a specialist, particularly if the murmur is initially heard under non-physiological conditions such as fever. Tests are usually best used if selected and ordered by specialists. Not all cardiologists perform all tests on all patients. Management of organic heart disease in infants or children is also best handled by specialists. Treatment may include **medications, interventional catheterization,** or **cardiac surgery.** Communication with the primary care provider, however, is essential to delivery of optimal patient care.

If the murmur is innocent, physicians must complete the following steps:

1. Children and their families must be informed about the presence of the murmur. Even if the murmur is benign, patients have a right to know that it was heard. In addition, they are likely to be examined by other practitioners who will report it, which may lead to the erroneous suspicion of either a new murmur or negligence on the part of the first examiner.

2. The diagnosis must be clearly explained to parents and children (depending on the age). It is essential that they understand that this is a normal finding rather than a minor abnormality. In some cases, notification of teachers or athletic coaches may be appropriate to prevent misunderstanding. Physicians must stress that no further evaluation is needed and no restrictions are indicated. Printed brochures that explain innocent murmurs are available from organizations such as the American Heart Association.

3. The description of the murmur and the diagnosis itself must be documented in the medical record. A murmur that is clearly and unequivocally innocent, with no evidence of heart disease, should not affect the child's access to insurance, participation in sports, etc. Medical documentation also helps protect patients from unnecessary reevaluations in the future.

4. Physicians should proceed no further. No laboratory studies or consultations need be performed. If the evaluation has been completed by a specialist because of suspicion of CHD by the referring physician, no follow-up with the specialist is indicated. The child is referred back to the primary practitioner.

Prognosis

The prognosis for children with heart murmurs depends on the cause of the murmur. Children with an innocent murmur, who by definition have normal hearts, have a normal prognosis—with one exception. If parents mistakenly believe their children to have heart disease, parents may treat the children inappropriately (eg, unnecessary testing, restriction of activities). As a result, children may develop sedentary habits and inferior self-image.

With appropriate medical attention, the prognosis is normal or near normal in most cases of CHD. Children with minor defects not requiring intervention (eg, small ventricular septal defect, mild pulmonic stenosis) need only infrequent cardiology follow-up visits. With the development of refined cardiac surgery and interventional catheterization, even children with the most complex cardiac anomalies now have a good outlook with respect to both daily living and life expectancy.

CASE RESOLUTION

In the case presented, a healthy girl with no history of cardiovascular symptoms has a heart murmur and an otherwise unremarkable physical examination. The murmur is a typical Still (innocent vibratory) murmur, which is identifiable by its low-pitched, vibratory quality. No further evaluation is necessary. The diagnosis is explained, the girl and her parents are reassured, and the murmur and diagnosis are noted in the medical record.

Selected References

Bergman AB, Stamm SJ. The morbidity of cardiac nondisease in school children. *N Engl J Med.* 1967;276:1008–1013

Danford DA, Nasir A, Gumbiner C. Cost assessment of the evaluation of heart murmurs in children. *Pediatrics.* 1993;91:365–368

Gaskin PR, Owens SE, Talner NS, Sanders SP, Li JS. Clinical auscultation skills in pediatric residents. *Pediatrics.* 2000;105:1184–1187

Geggel RL, Horowitz LM, Brown EA, Parsons M, Wang PS, Fulton DR. Parental anxiety associated with referral of a child to a pediatric cardiologist for evaluation of a Still's murmur. *J Pediatr.* 2002;140:747–752

Haney I, Ipp M, Feldman W, McCrindle BW. Accuracy of clinical assessment of heart murmurs by office based (general practice) paediatricians. *Arch Dis Child.* 1999;81:409–412

Hohn AR. Congenital heart disease—the first test. *West J Med.* 1992;156:435–436

Mangione S, Nieman LZ. Cardiac auscultatory skills of internal medicine and family practice trainees. *JAMA.* 1997;278:717–722

Moss AJ. Clues in diagnosing congenital heart disease. *West J Med.* 1992;156:392–398

Newburger JW, Rosenthal A, Williams RG. Noninvasive tests in the initial evaluation of heart murmurs in children. *N Engl J Med.* 1983;308:61–64

Smythe JF, Teixeira OH, Vlad P, Demers PP, Feldman W. Initial evaluation of heart murmurs: are laboratory tests necessary? *Pediatrics.* 1990;86:497–500

Vukanovic-Criley JM, Criley S, Warde CM, et al. Competency in cardiac examination skills in medical students, trainees, physicians, and faculty. *Arch Intern Med.* 2006;166:610–616

CHAPTER 87

Cyanosis in the Newborn

Robin Winkler Doroshow, MD, MMS, MEd

CASE STUDY

A 3,500-g term male infant born to a 29-year-old, gravida II para II, healthy mother by spontaneous vaginal delivery is well until 24 hours of age, when a nurse notes that he is cyanotic. On examination, he appears blue but in no distress. The vital signs are temperature (axillary) 37°C (98.6°F), pulse 130 beats/min, respirations 40 breaths/min, and blood pressure 80/60 mm Hg in the right arm. His general appearance is normal except for the cyanosis. His heart sounds are normal, and no murmur is heard. His liver is not palpable, and the peripheral pulses are normal and equal in all extremities. Capillary refill is normal. Oxygen saturation is 65% by pulse oximetry.

Questions

1. What are the causes of cyanosis in newborns?
2. What is the appropriate evaluation of cyanosis in newborns?
3. How urgent is the assessment? What are the risks and benefits of further evaluation?
4. Which aspects of management should be initiated by a primary physician at a community hospital?
5. Which types of treatment should be undertaken by the consulting pediatric cardiologist at the referral center?

Cyanosis is a bluish appearance of the skin due to the presence of reduced hemoglobin in the tissues. Central cyanosis, which is detected initially in the oral mucosa and nail beds but is generalized when severe, indicates at least 4 to 5 g of reduced hemoglobin per 100 mL blood. Hypoxemia is usually the cause. This condition is frequently present in neonates with pulmonary pathology but is also one of the most common presentations of severe congenital heart disease (CHD).

Because cyanotic CHD in newborns may be life-threatening, it must not go undiagnosed. Most diagnostic studies have minimal risk. Even the risk of cardiac catheterization in this setting is relatively low. Most of the lesions that cause cyanotic CHD can be palliated or corrected, and the prognosis is good.

Epidemiology

Cyanotic CHD occurs in about 2 to 3 of every 1,000 live-born infants. Approximately 80% to 90% of these cases, usually the most severe ones, are detected in the first 30 days of life. However, failure to diagnose major CHD *before newborn discharge* occurs in at least 10% of cases, leading to unnecessary morbidity and mortality. Infants with low pulmonary blood flow or lesions causing poor mixing most often present with obvious cyanosis, although initially they otherwise appear well and comfortable. Those with high pulmonary flow are less blue and often present first with congestive heart failure (CHF) or a murmur, but may be detected earlier using screening pulse oximetry.

Most cyanotic CHD is not diagnosed before birth. The antenatal history, gestational age, birth weight, and delivery room examination are unremarkable. Failure to identify CHD in the setting of a routine obstetric ultrasound study does not rule it out; the sensitivity of such scans in the general population is very low. Congenital heart disease is more likely in some situations that can be anticipated prenatally (Box 87-1). In these settings, increased suspicion may lead to antenatal detection using specialized echocardiography.

Clinical Presentation

Children with cyanotic CHD often present within the first week of life with cyanosis of the oral mucosa. In more severe cases, generalized cyanosis occurs. The abnormal color may be more apparent with effort (eg, feeding, passing stool) or crying. Respiratory distress, heralded by grunting, nasal flaring, and retractions, is minor or absent in many newborn infants with cyanotic CHD. In cases of severe hypoxia, metabolic acidosis leads to poor perfusion and compensatory tachypnea with hyperpnea. Additional findings depend on the nature of the causal lesion (Dx Box). It is important to note that the absence of associated physical findings does not exclude cyanotic CHD.

Box 87-1. Settings With Increased Risk of Congenital Heart Disease

- Genetic syndromes (eg, trisomies, DiGeorge syndrome)
- Certain extracardiac anomalies (eg, omphalocele, forearm anomalies)
- High incidence of congenital heart disease in the family
- Maternal diabetes if poorly controlled during first trimester
- Fetal exposure to cardiac teratogen (eg, lithium, isotretinoin)
- Fetal or neonatal arrhythmia other than premature atrial beats

---

Dx Cyanosis in the Newborn: Possible Associated Findings

- Low oxygen saturation
- No improvement with oxygen
- Heart murmur
- Tachypnea
- Increased perspiration
- Abnormal cardiac silhouette on radiograph
- Abnormal electrocardiogram
- Abnormal echocardiogram

Pathophysiology

Cardiac cyanosis is due to **right-to-left shunting** so that systemic venous blood bypasses the pulmonary circulation and enters the systemic circulation. Two conditions are necessary to produce this type of shunting: a communication, such as a septal defect, for the blood to shunt across and a cause, such as pulmonic stenosis, for the blood to be shunted away from the lungs. The most notable exception is simple transposition of the great arteries (TGA), where the fundamental connections are abnormal, and all systemic venous blood is directed to the systemic arterial circulation. Lesions associated with cyanosis may be divided into 3 groups.

1. The *low pulmonary blood flow (LPBF) group* consists of tetralogy of Fallot, pulmonary atresia with intact ventricular septum, and virtually any combination of defects that includes pulmonary atresia or severe pulmonic stenosis. Pulmonary flow is diminished and may derive entirely from the ductus arteriosus while it remains patent. Aside from obvious cyanosis (and associated oxygen saturation below 80%), infants often appear well.

2. The *high pulmonary blood flow (HPBF) group* includes truncus arteriosus, single ventricle, and combinations of defects that involve mixing of oxygenated and unoxygenated blood and little or no obstruction to pulmonary flow. Although a right-to-left shunt is present, the left-to-right shunt is even greater. Pulmonary venous return is therefore voluminous and contributes disproportionately to systemic output. Cyanosis is less apparent; saturation is greater than 80% and may be as high as 95%. Pulmonary flow increases over the first days and weeks of life as the pulmonary vascular resistance falls, and CHF develops, as in patients with isolated shunt lesions (eg, ventricular septal defect). Some children with HPBF lesions also have obstruction to systemic blood flow (eg, coarctation of the aorta, hypoplastic left heart syndrome) and may depend on the ductus arteriosus to carry some or all of this flow.

3. The *poor mixing group* is limited to TGA and its variants. The right and left circuits are in parallel rather than in series, and survival depends on interchange of oxygenated and unoxygenated blood between them. Most newborns with poor mixing present with marked cyanosis (saturation <80%), like patients in the LPBF group.

Severe hypoxemia (oxygen partial pressure [pO_2] <35 mm Hg for the average newborn) is not compatible with prolonged survival. Infants experience tissue hypoxia, anaerobic glycolysis, and metabolic acidosis. Respiratory compensation may occur at first. Even with a normal pH, however, the presence of metabolic acidosis (large base deficit) indicates life-threatening hypoxia, necessitating immediate intervention, without which death ensues in a matter of hours.

Differential Diagnosis

The major causes of cyanosis are cardiac and respiratory (Box 87-2). Diagnoses in the latter group include problems of the lung, chest, airway, or respiratory drive.

The syndrome of **persistent fetal circulation** is perhaps most often confused with cyanotic CHD. It is also known as **persistent pulmonary hypertension of the newborn.** In this syndrome the heart and great vessels are structurally normal, but high pulmonary vascular resistance, which is often seen in post-term infants with perinatal distress or pulmonary disease, causes blood to shunt away from the lungs at the foramen ovale and ductus arteriosus. Profound cyanosis that is unresponsive to supplemental oxygen may be the only abnormal finding, and echocardiography is required to exclude CHD.

Pulmonary cyanosis may be due to **infection** (eg, group B streptococcal pneumonia); **aspiration** (eg, meconium, tracheoesophageal fistula); **pulmonary hypoplasia** (eg, Potter syndrome, diaphragmatic hernia); **respiratory distress syndrome** (eg, prematurity); or a host of other problems of the lung, chest, or airway. Neurologic depression may produce hypoventilation with resultant hypoxia.

Evaluation

Evaluation of the cyanotic newborn must be expeditious so that management is not delayed. In some cases, therapy may be initiated before the evaluation is complete. All available data, the statistical likelihood of CHD, and the risk-benefit ratio of the treatment must be taken into account.

History

Review of the history may be helpful, particularly in certain situations, such as in children with pulmonary disease (Questions Box). It is important to note that a negative response to any or all of the

Box 87-2. Noncardiac Causes of Neonatal Cyanosis

- Persistent fetal circulation
- Upper airway obstruction (eg, choanal atresia)
- Pulmonary infection (eg, group B streptococcal infection)
- Aspiration (eg, meconium aspiration syndrome, tracheoesophageal fistula)
- Pulmonary hypoplasia (eg, Potter syndrome, diaphragmatic hernia)
- Respiratory distress syndrome (eg, in prematurity)
- Thoracic hypoplasia (eg, thanatophoric dwarfism)
- Hypoventilation (eg, neurologic depression)

Cyanosis in the Newborn

Questions

- Has the infant been in any distress?
- Has the infant had difficulty feeding?
- Was the infant suspected of having a heart problem prior to birth (eg, fetal arrhythmia, abnormal heart on ultrasound)?
- Is the mother diabetic?
- Did the mother take any drugs (prescribed or not) during the pregnancy?
- Was the mother ill during the first trimester?
- Is there a positive family history of congenital heart disease or other birth defects?
- Did any perinatal problems (eg, passage of meconium in utero) occur?

questions does not render cyanotic CHD unlikely; in fact, negative responses are noted in most cases.

Physical Examination

Cyanosis may be the only abnormal physical finding in cardiac patients, but a careful, thorough examination often yields information about the underlying cardiac defect and the overall circulatory status. External anomalies or abnormal phenotypic appearance may indicate a genetic disorder with associated cardiac anomalies. Dyspnea (grunting, nasal flaring, intercostal retractions) is more often seen with lung disease, but tachypnea (rapid respiration) is common with both severe heart disease and pulmonary problems. Tachypnea results from CHF in HPBF lesions, and hyperpnea (deep breathing) from metabolic acidosis in severe hypoxia or impaired perfusion. Poor perfusion is also manifested by abnormal color (a gray or ashen appearance if combined with cyanosis), cool extremities, delayed capillary refill, and diminished pulses.

The peripheral pulses are palpated in all extremities. Abnormalities or discrepancies between extremities must be confirmed by measuring blood pressure. Weak pulses may be found in cardiogenic shock, and bounding pulses may be noted with diastolic runoff lesions such as patent ductus arteriosus or aortic insufficiency. Pulse quality and blood pressure may differ in different extremities if an aortic arch abnormality such as coarctation is present. The abdominal examination may reveal hepatomegaly (in CHF) or abnormal situs (as in asplenia syndrome, usually associated with complex cyanotic CHD).

The cardiac examination may disclose a loud murmur if an obstruction such as pulmonary stenosis is present. The physician should note, however, that atresia, being a total obstruction, produces no murmur. Heart sounds may be loud and the precordium hyperdynamic, particularly in children with HPBF. Splitting of the second sound confirms that 2 patent semilunar valves are present, but this finding is often difficult to appreciate even in normal newborns.

Laboratory Tests

A number of laboratory studies are available (see Chapter 88, Table 88-1). As in CHF, it is initially more important to determine whether patients have heart disease than to obtain a precise, complete diagnosis. In cyanotic CHD, sophisticated studies such as echocardiography, magnetic resonance imaging, and catheterization are usually needed to make a detailed diagnosis.

The suspicion of arterial hypoxemia should be confirmed by **pulse oximetry,** an indirect measurement. It is readily available and noninvasive but has shortcomings. Perfusion must be adequate to obtain a reading. Accuracy is diminished at saturations below 75%, although the presence of profound hypoxia can still be confirmed. Cyanotic CHD cannot be ruled out by pulse oximetry, however, because readings of 100% saturation may reflect pO_2 values that range anywhere between 75 and 250 mm Hg (Figure 87-1). **Arterial blood gases** are more accurate and give important additional information about ventilation and acid-base status. Arterialized capillary gases may suffice if perfusion is adequate.

Oxygenation may differ between the extremities in infants with certain lesions (eg, coarctation). The site of sampling should be noted. If possible, the saturation should be measured at sites both proximal and distal to the ductus arteriosus (ie, from the right arm and either leg).

A **shunt study,** also known as a hyperoxia challenge, may be performed to determine whether a right-to-left cardiac shunt is present, particularly if echocardiography is not readily available. Pure oxygen (fraction of inspired oxygen in gas [FIO_2] = 1.00) is given for 5 to 10 minutes by hood. In patients with LPBF or TGA, increasing the inspired oxygen does not affect the oxygenation of the blood

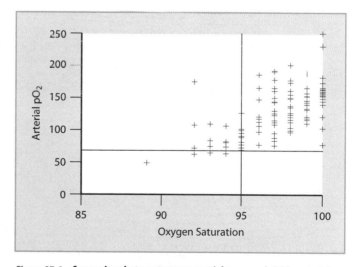

Figure 87-1. Comparison between oxygen partial pressure (pO_2) by arterial blood gas measurement and oxygen saturation by pulse oximetry. (Reproduced with permission from Niehoff J, DelGuercio C, LaMorte W, et al. Efficacy of pulse oximetry and capnometry in postoperative ventilatory weaning. *Crit Care Med.* 1988;16:701.)

because the blood is unable to enter the lungs; this is a positive result. In patients with pulmonary disease or hypoventilation, oxygenation increases strikingly, often to a pO_2 exceeding 200 mm Hg; this negative result rules out cyanotic CHD.

A blunted shunt study, characterized by a rise in pO_2 but rarely to levels above 150 mm Hg, is seen in patients with severe pulmonary disease and in those with HPBF lesions. With such lesions the pulmonary venous blood is high in volume, and the rise in its saturation causes a definite rise in arterial oxygenation. This effect is exaggerated by the further increase in pulmonary flow due to the vasodilating effect of oxygen.

A positive shunt study may be identified with pulse oximetry. It is difficult or impossible, however, to distinguish between a blunted study and a negative one with this tool. The oxyhemoglobin dissociation curve is flattened at the upper end, and the saturation changes very little over a wide range of pO_2 (Figure 87-2). Capillary gases may be equally inaccurate in this range, but directly measured arterial blood gases are highly reliable. In addition, they may reveal hypercapnia, with or without respiratory acidosis, suggesting a pulmonary cause for the hypoxia.

Electrocardiogram (ECG), a fairly inexpensive test, is readily available and noninvasive. However, it does not often help distinguish cyanotic CHD from other causes of cyanosis, particularly for those practitioners who lack experience with neonatal ECGs. The normal range is large in neonates, with much overlap between normal and CHD. Care must also be taken in placing the leads correctly and minimizing artifacts.

Imaging Studies

The **chest radiograph,** a relatively inexpensive and readily available test, is often extremely helpful in differentiating between cardiac and noncardiac disease. Pulmonary disease is often readily apparent on chest radiograph. The radiograph also helps define the cardiac

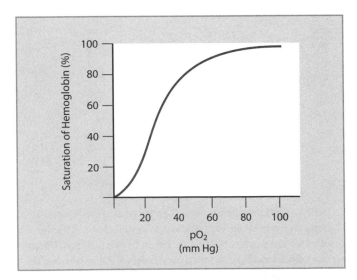

Figure 87-2. Oxyhemoglobin dissociation curve. Note that the position of the curve itself may vary with temperature, pH, oxygen partial pressure (pO₂), and 2,3-diphosphoglycerate.

diagnosis broadly but not precisely. Patients with LPBF lesions have small hearts and diminished pulmonary flow. In contrast, patients with HPBF lesions have large hearts and increased flow, such as is seen in infants with simple left-to-right shunts. With many cyanotic lesions, the cardiac silhouette is abnormal in configuration (eg, boot-shaped heart in tetralogy of Fallot) or position (eg, dextrocardia in patients with heterotaxia syndromes). Transposition of TGA may be more misleading: Pulmonary flow may be increased despite the severe cyanosis, and the heart size may be normal. An apparently normal radiograph does not exclude TGA.

Under optimal conditions, **echocardiography** enables the physician not only to recognize CHD but to identify details of anatomy and physiology. Conversely, a properly performed, complete, negative echocardiogram rules out CHD. The performance of a high-quality study requires the appropriate equipment (with high-resolution imaging), an experienced sonographer, and an experienced cardiologist for interpretation. In the absence of these elements, preliminary echocardiography may be used cautiously as a screening device as part of the initial assessment to confirm heart disease prior to referral to a specialist. Recently, availability of telemedicine for echocardiography has helped to fill this gap in some hospitals and avoid some unnecessary transports. When there is significant suspicion of cyanotic CHD, referral should not be delayed until echocardiography can be performed.

Management

Initial management prior to cardiac consultation (often with transfer to another institution) includes surveillance, assistance, direct medical management, and supportive care.

Close **surveillance,** including transfer to the highest level of neonatal care available, use of a cardiopulmonary monitor and continuous pulse oximetry, frequent monitoring of vital signs, and repeat physical examinations, is begun as soon as cyanotic CHD is identified. Even if the infant is feeding well, it is best to suspend feedings because of the likelihood of invasive procedures or spontaneous deterioration in the near future. An orogastric tube is placed to decompress the stomach, reducing the work of breathing as well as the risk of aspiration. At least one secure intravenous (IV) line should be placed for administration of fluids, glucose, and medications. If umbilical arterial catheterization can be expeditiously established, it will allow close monitoring of arterial blood gases and blood pressure. The latter may be difficult to measure by cuff in the compromised infant.

While undertaking these measures, the physician should make every effort to seek **assistance** from a pediatric cardiologist. A neonatologist may be consulted if a pediatric cardiologist is not immediately available. Much advice may be obtained over the telephone. In addition, plans for immediate consultation or transfer of patients may be discussed in this way.

The need for **supportive care** depends on the case. In the absence of metabolic acidosis or impaired perfusion, no special measures are indicated in this category. In some cases, IV fluid boluses, inotropic agents, and other treatments may be needed as part of the early management. Mechanical ventilation should be used in patients with metabolic acidosis, whether compensated or uncompensated, because of the increased oxygen requirement produced by hyperventilation and the tendency for tiring, leading to superimposed respiratory acidosis.

The temptation to give supplemental oxygen for more than the few minutes necessary to perform a shunt study is great but must be resisted. Oxygen is rarely helpful and may be harmful in this setting. In infants with TGA or LPBF lesions, oxygenation is not affected. In infants with HPBF lesions, oxygenation is usually adequate in room air (saturation >80%), and an increase in FIO_2 may exacerbate the CHF. Patients at greatest risk for deterioration due to administration of oxygen are those with total anomalous pulmonary venous return with obstruction, in whom pulmonary arteriolar vasodilation precipitates severe pulmonary edema and secondary right heart failure. Oxygen may also directly constrict the ductus arteriosus on which the cyanotic newborn may depend.

The possibility of ductal dependency should prompt consideration of administering the ductus dilator, **prostaglandin E_1 (PGE₁)**. The definitive diagnosis of cyanotic CHD need not be made prior to institution of this lifesaving treatment. In infants who remain adequately oxygenated (no acidosis) and perfused, the drug can be prepared but administration deferred pending consultation. The benefits of giving PGE₁ to severely hypoxic infants or infants with compromised perfusion far outweigh the risks, which include apnea and fever. A dramatic improvement is often seen within seconds to minutes, confirming the diagnosis of a ductal-dependent lesion, and enabling the physician to stabilize the patient until more definitive evaluation and intervention can take place.

Prognosis

If untreated, LPBF lesions and TGA are usually fatal during infancy, most often during the neonatal period, because of severe hypoxia. Untreated HPBF lesions may lead to death in infancy from either CHF or complications such as pneumonia. If the systemic blood flow is ductus-dependent (eg, interruption of the aortic arch), death occurs shortly after ductal closure, usually during the first week of life. Delayed diagnosis, even when not fatal, may result in a suboptimal outcome including end-organ injury such as renal dysfunction or neurologic sequelae.

With early recognition and intervention, however, the prognosis for infants with cyanotic CHD is surprisingly good in the absence of a genetic syndrome (eg, trisomy 18) or a major complicating extracardiac malformation (eg, neural tube defect). If diagnosed before the onset of severe circulatory compromise, infants can be stabilized and evaluated promptly, and palliative or corrective procedures can be performed in the operating suite or catheterization laboratory. Most of these patients can survive well into adulthood with a good

quality of life. Infants with lesions in which all 4 chambers are adequate in size (eg, tetralogy of Fallot) have a better lifetime prognosis than those with a hypoplastic chamber (eg, tricuspid atresia). Even infants with abnormalities such as asplenia syndrome or hypoplastic left heart syndrome now have a reasonable outlook with complex reconstructive surgery or heart transplantation.

CASE RESOLUTION

In the case presented at the beginning of the chapter, marked hypoxia is present in the absence of other cardiac findings, such as a heart murmur. The oxygen saturation does not rise after the infant breathes 100% oxygen for 10 minutes. The chest radiograph shows a small, boot-shaped heart and diminished pulmonary blood flow, and the ECG is normal. Transport is arranged. Because of the marked cyanosis, infusion of PGE₁ is begun, and saturation increases to 80%, with the pO_2 rising from 33 to a safer 48 mm Hg. The infant is transferred to a tertiary care center, where consultation is obtained. An echocardiogram is also performed, which demonstrates tetralogy of Fallot with pulmonary atresia. A modified Blalock-Taussig shunt is placed in the newborn period, and complete repair using a pulmonary artery homograft is performed at 1 year of age.

Selected References

Brown KL, Ridout DA, Hoskote A, Verhulst L, Ricci M, Bull C. Delayed diagnosis of congenital heart disease worsens preoperative condition and outcome of surgery in neonates. *Heart.* 2006;92:1298–1302

deWahl Granelli A, Wennergren M, Sandberg K, et al. Impact of pulse oximetry screening on the detection of duct dependent congenital heart disease: a Swedish prospective screening study in 39,821 newborns. *BMJ.* 2009;338:a3037

Freed MD, Heymann MA, Lewis AB, Roehl SL, Kensey RC. Prostaglandin E1 in infants with ductus arteriosus-dependent congenital heart disease. *Circulation.* 1981;64:899–905

Jones RW, Baumer JH, Joseph MC, Shinebourne EA. Arterial oxygen tension and response to oxygen breathing in differential diagnosis of congenital heart disease in infancy. *Arch Dis Child.* 1976;51:667–673

Liske MR, Greeley CS, Law DJ, et al. Report of the Tennessee Task Force on Screening Newborn Infants for Critical Congenital Heart Disease. *Pediatrics.* 2006;118:e1250–e1256

Niehoff J, DelGuercio C, LaMorte W, et al. Efficacy of pulse oximetry and capnometry in postoperative ventilatory weaning. *Crit Care Med.* 1988;16:701–705

Pfammatter JP, Stocker FP. Delayed recognition of haemodynamically relevant congenital heart disease. *Eur J Pediatr.* 2001;160:231–234

Sable CA, Cummings SD, Pearson GD, et al. Impact of telemedicine on the practice of pediatric cardiology of community hospitals. *Pediatrics.* 2002;109:e3

Sasidharan P. An approach to diagnosis and management of cyanosis and tachypnea in term infants. *Pediatr Clin North Am.* 2004;51:999–1021

Victorica BE. Cyanotic newborns. In: Gessner IH, Victorica BE, eds. *Pediatric Cardiology: A Problem Oriented Approach.* Philadelphia, PA: W. B. Saunders; 1993

CHAPTER 88

Congestive Heart Failure

Robin Winkler Doroshow, MD, MMS, MEd

CASE STUDY

A 2-month-old infant is brought to the office by his mother, who complains that her son has been eating poorly and breathing oddly for the past few days. The perinatal history is unremarkable. A heart murmur was noted at the 1-month checkup.

The infant is scrawny and irritable. Physical examination shows that the baby's weight, which was at the 50th percentile at birth, is now at the fifth percentile; his height, which was at the 50th percentile, is now at the 25th percentile. He is afebrile, and his heart rate is 165 beats/min, with respirations 70 breaths/min and shallow but without respiratory distress. The skin is pale and diaphoretic, and the mucous membranes are pink. Examination of the head and neck is normal; no jugular distention is present. The lungs are clear. The precordium is hyperdynamic, and the heart sounds are loud; a prominent systolic murmur is audible at the left lower sternal border. The liver edge is palpable 4 cm below the right costal margin in the right midclavicular line, and the spleen is not palpable. The extremities are thin, with normal pulses and no edema. Capillary refill is slightly delayed.

Questions

1. What are acute and chronic signs of cardiac disease in children?
2. What are the signs of congestive heart failure (CHF) in children? How do these signs in children differ from those in adults?
3. What underlying disorders can cause CHF in young infants?
4. What is the appropriate emergent management for infants with CHF? What are the risks of treatment if the diagnosis is incorrect?

Congestive heart failure is the most common presentation of serious heart disease in infants. Although this condition also occurs in older children, an estimated 90% of cases of CHF in the pediatric population begin in the first year of life. In children CHF is most often caused by structural congenital heart disease (CHD). Compensatory mechanisms are fewer and less successful in small infants. Other causes of CHF are included in Box 88-1.

Epidemiology

The precise incidence of CHF in children is unknown; it is approximately 0.1%. Most cases result from CHD, which occurs in 0.8% of live births. The incidence of CHD varies little with geography, ethnic group, or gender. It is far more common in children with recognizable genetic syndromes (eg, trisomy 21 [Down syndrome], Turner syndrome).

Clinical Presentation

Most commonly, complaints about CHF take the form of concerns about an infant's feeding. Comments are often vague (eg, "my baby is not a good eater") but may be more precise (eg, "he is taking less formula with each feeding," "he is taking longer to nurse"). Parents may also describe rapid breathing, excessive sweating, or decreased activity, but usually only on specific questioning.

Box 88-1. Causes of Congestive Heart Failure in Children

Volume Overload
- Left-to-right shunts (eg, ventricular septal defect)
- Bidirectional shunts (eg, truncus arteriosus)
- Valvular insufficiency (eg, mitral regurgitation)
- Extracardiac conditions (eg, anemia, arteriovenous malformation)

Pressure Overload
- Outflow obstruction (eg, coarctation of the aorta)
- Inflow obstruction (eg, obstructed anomalous pulmonary veins)
- Vascular resistance (eg, hypertension, chronic pulmonary disease)

Myocardial Dysfunction
- Intrinsic conditions (eg, cardiomyopathy, anthracycline toxicity)
- Inflammatory conditions (eg, viral myocarditis, rheumatic fever)
- Coronary insufficiency (eg, anomalous left coronary artery)

Arrhythmias
- Tachyarrhythmia (eg, paroxysmal supraventricular tachycardia)
- Bradyarrhythmia (eg, third-degree atrioventricular block)

Congestive heart failure is also often detected on examination for routine infant checkups or for unrelated complaints. Careful assessment of the physical findings, including vital signs, reveals **tachypnea, tachycardia,** and **hepatomegaly** and frequently signs of underlying structural heart defects, such as a murmur (Dx Box).

Dx Congestive Heart Failure

- Tachycardia
- Tachypnea
- Hepatomegaly
- Sweating
- Decreased feeding
- Irritability
- Easy fatigability

Pathophysiology

High cardiac output may lead to CHF in infants with large left-to-right shunts. Myocardial contractility is relatively normal, and children remain on the "normal" line of the Frank-Starling curve, which relates cardiac output to diastolic volume (also called *preload*) or pressure (Figure 88-1). The shunt requires a very large volume of output, primarily to the pulmonary bed. Although the heart may be able to meet this demand, preload is high, leading to "congestive" signs and symptoms (eg, tachypnea, hepatomegaly). In more severe cases, systemic output may be compromised, resulting in hypotension, renal failure, and metabolic acidosis.

Left-sided failure caused by elevated pulmonary venous pressure produces increased lung water. Initially, this fluid is interstitial, and it does not interfere with gas exchange but does trigger reflex tachypnea. Minute volume is kept normal by decreasing tidal (breath-to-breath) volume, leading to shallow as well as rapid breathing (sometimes called "happy tachypnea" because of the absence of dyspnea). Only when the ability of the pulmonary lymphatics to drain this fluid is overcome by large volume does fluid accumulate in the alveoli; rales and respiratory distress, or dyspnea, then result and gas exchange may be compromised.

Right-sided failure caused by an elevated systemic venous load usually produces more volume than pressure load on this system, possibly as a result of the greater venous compliance in infants compared with adults. The liver becomes very distended and is easily palpated. As long as the liver can absorb the increased venous volume, the portal pressure does not rise, and splenomegaly does not occur. Because the venous pressure rises very little, jugular distention, which is difficult to detect in young infants in any case, is rarely seen, and edema is also rare.

The left and right (systemic and pulmonary) circulations are more interdependent in infants and younger children than they are in older children or adults. As a result, **bilateral heart failure** is much more common than right-sided or left-sided failure alone. Although this means that recognition of CHF may be easier, determination of the underlying condition may be more difficult because the clues are less specific. For example, in an adult with left-sided failure, the differential diagnosis includes mitral, but not tricuspid, valve disease.

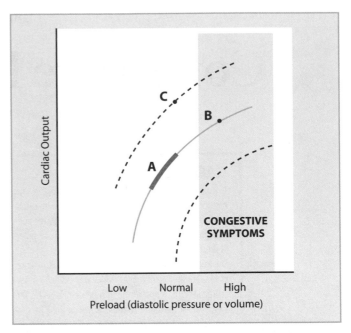

Figure 88-1. Relationship of cardiac output to preload. The solid curve represents normal myocardial contractility, and the dotted curves represent impaired function (shifted downward) and the positive inotropic state (shifted upward). A. Normal range (no heart disease). B. Left-to-right shunt with congestive heart failure (CHF). Note that overall output is high but most of it is shunted. C. Same situation as B but after treatment for CHF. Cardiac output is the same or better, but preload is now out of the range that results in congestive symptoms.

Differential Diagnosis

When tachycardia, tachypnea without dyspnea, and hepatomegaly are present, the diagnosis of CHF is straightforward. Congestive heart failure is most commonly confused with major respiratory infections such as bronchiolitis or pneumonia. Pulmonary infections are frequently associated with dyspnea as well as tachypnea, impaired gas exchange, and other respiratory findings. Rhinorrhea, cough, fever, or wheezing may also be present. Rales may accompany pneumonia but are rare in CHF in infancy or early childhood. Hyperinflation due to lung disease may lead to a false impression of hepatomegaly. In some children, CHD, CHF, and respiratory infections coexist.

Clues to the presence of structural heart disease, such as a murmur or absent femoral pulses, may support the diagnosis of CHF. Severe CHF, with low cardiac output or even shock, has a broader differential diagnosis. In addition to cardiac causes, sepsis, hypovolemia, and disorders associated with inborn errors of metabolism should be considered.

Evaluation

History

The history should include specific questions about feeding and growth (Questions Box). Poor feeding, often a nonspecific complaint in chronically or subacutely ill infants, results from tachypnea and fatigability in infants with heart disease. Growth failure may result from poor feeding and increased cardiopulmonary work. The physician should specifically query parents about possible excessive sweating or rapid breathing in infants, because parents may not volunteer this information (see Chapter 61).

Physical Examination

The diagnosis of CHF is primarily based on clinical findings, and physical examination is essential. The resting respiratory rate must be precisely counted because infants in CHF most often have tachypnea without dyspnea. The liver edge is palpable more than 1 cm below the right costal margin in the midclavicular line, and the degree of enlargement mirrors the severity of the CHF.

In the older child or adolescent, the physical findings are more similar to those of the adult with CHF. Additional findings that may be present in this age group include jugular venous distension, basilar rales, and peripheral pitting edema.

Laboratory Tests

Many laboratory tests can be performed to assess infants' hearts (Table 88-1), including electrocardiogram and echocardiogram. However, some procedures are very costly, and some are invasive and therefore carry risk. The value of most of these tests depends on the expertise of the individuals who perform and interpret them. It is important to remember that although test results and consultation with a pediatric cardiologist may be invaluable in the identification of the underlying lesion, *these procedures are not usually required in order to make a diagnosis of CHF.*

Pressure or volume overload of the ventricles causes them to release a neurohumoral peptide, B-type natriuretic peptide (B-NP), which acts as a natural natriuretic, diuretic, and vasodilator. Studies in adults have demonstrated that blood levels of B-NP are elevated in CHF, and the degree of elevation closely reflects severity of CHF. This test, which may be performed at the bedside, may be used to distinguish between CHF and other similar disorders such as acute pulmonary disease. Because it closely parallels changes in severity of CHF, it may also be used to track response to treatment. Recent studies in children suggest that it may be similarly useful in the pediatric population; B-NP levels may be very effective in distinguishing between cardiac and noncardiac causes of CHF in children (Figure 88-2).

Imaging Studies

Because elucidation of the structure and function of the heart is central to assessment of the underlying cause of CHF in the pediatric population, imaging studies play a key role (see Table 88-1) in evaluation of these patients. Moreover, these tests (particularly

(see Chapter 61).

Questions

Congestive Heart Failure

- How has the infant been feeding? Does he or she get out of breath or appear exhausted?
- Has the infant's growth pattern changed recently?
- Does the infant tire easily? With eating? With playing?
- Does the infant perspire excessively, especially with efforts such as feeding?
- Does the infant breathe rapidly, even at rest?

Table 88-1. Laboratory Tests Used in the Evaluation of Heart Disease in Children	
Test	*Information*
Chest radiograph	Presence and direction of shunt Hints concerning specific diagnosis (and possible pulmonary disease ruled out)
Serum B-type natriuretic peptide	Presence and severity of congestive heart failure
Electrocardiogram (ECG)	Cardiac rhythm and conduction Chamber overload Coronary insufficiency
Ambulatory ECG (24-hour ECG)	Subacute rhythm assessment Correlation of symptoms with rhythm
Oximetry	Presence and degree of hypoxemia
Arterial blood gases	Hypoxemia Acid-base status
Hematocrit	Anemia Polycythemia
Exercise test	Quantitation of exercise tolerance Provocation of symptoms or arrhythmia
Echocardiogram	Specific structural diagnosis and hemodynamics Chamber enlargement and function Presence of pericardial effusion
Cardiac magnetic resonance imaging or computed tomography	Specific structural diagnosis and hemodynamics Chamber enlargement and function
Cardiac catheterization	Specific structural diagnosis and hemodynamics Cardiac electrophysiology
Tilt table test	Autonomic function

echocardiography) may be used as a means of tracking response to treatment.

Chest radiograph, preferably in anteroposterior and lateral projections, may be very useful as a *supportive* study. It may show cardiomegaly, pulmonary venous congestion, and hyperinflation. Cardiomegaly is most commonly due not to myocardial dysfunction,

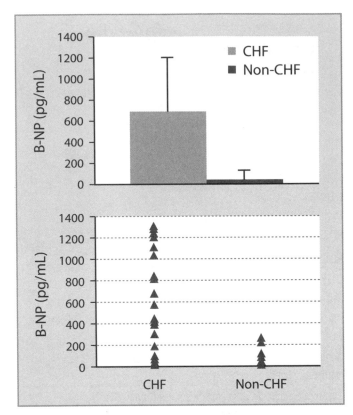

Figure 88-2. Utility of B-type natriuretic peptide (B-NP) in differentiating congestive heart failure (CHF) from lung disease in pediatric patients with respiratory distress. (From Koulouri S, Acherman RJ, Wong PC, Chan LS, Lewis AB. Utility of B-type natriuretic peptide in differentiating congestive heart failure from lung disease in pediatric patients with respiratory distress. *Pediatr Cardiol.* 2004;25:341–346, with permission from Springer Science + Business Media.)

but to volume overload from the shunt. In the absence of cardiac enlargement, the diagnosis of CHF must be seriously questioned. (However, CHF may occur in the absence of cardiomegaly in total anomalous pulmonary venous return with obstruction, which usually presents in the first week of life in association with hypoxia.) Pulmonary venous congestion occurs in left-sided heart failure, but increased pulmonary arterial flow from a left-to-right shunt often obscures the congestion. Hyperinflation resulting from peribronchial edema is also a common finding.

In children with severe CHF, further studies are indicated. **Arterial blood gases** show evidence of metabolic acidosis due to tissue anoxia, with respiratory compensation in early stages and superimposed respiratory acidosis in later stages. A **complete blood cell count** shows leukocytosis due to stress. It may not differentiate between heart disease and sepsis.

Management

All infants and children with CHF should be under the care of a pediatric cardiologist, often in concert with a pediatrician, intensivist, or neonatologist. Prompt referral to a cardiologist will aid not only in management of the CHF, but also in assessment and management of the underlying disorder.

The numerous pharmacologic treatments for pediatric CHF fall into a small number of categories based on mechanism of action (Table 88-2). Preload can be optimized by the administration of diuretics and venodilators, and afterload by the use of arteriolar dilators, some of which also have inotropic effects. Contractility is enhanced by inotropic agents, and antiarrhythmics control tachycardias and bradycardias to optimize heart rate. The most effective control of CHF is attained when more than one mechanism is used.

Inotropes and **diuretics** are used in the initial management of CHF in children. Inotropic support results in a shift to a higher Frank-Starling curve (see Figure 88-1), which allows affected patients to maintain the high volume output necessitated by the underlying CHD at lower diastolic pressures, thus alleviating congestive symptoms. **Digoxin,** a form of digitalis, is the drug of choice in such cases, where cardiac output is not severely impaired, and is therefore often used in outpatients. This agent is readily available, easily absorbed, safe in the therapeutic range, and easy to administer (elixir for oral administration). If digoxin is initially given at the maintenance dose (10 micrograms /kg/d, therapeutic levels are not attained for about a week; therefore, loading is preferable (Table 88-3) but may require hospitalization. Digoxin is well tolerated and rarely causes side effects. Because of the safety and reliability of absorption, blood levels need not be checked unless overdose is suspected (eg, history of over-administration, toxic ingestion, unexplained vomiting, or second- or third-degree heart block). In the neonate, blood levels may be difficult to interpret because of the presence of natural digoxin-like immunoreactive substance in the blood.

Table 88-2. Therapy for Pediatric Congestive Heart Failure	
Category	**Example**
Chronic (Ambulatory)	
Cardiac glycosides	Digoxin
Diuretics	Furosemide, spironolactone
Angiotensin-converting enzyme inhibitors	Enalapril, captopril
Selective β-blockers	Carvedilol, metoprolol
Acute (Inpatient)	
Diuretics	Furosemide, bumetanide
β-agonists	Dobutamine, dopamine
Phosphodiesterase inhibitors	Milrinone, amrinone
Vasodilators	Nitroprusside, oxygen, inhaled nitric oxide
Severe, Refractory	
Mechanical support	Extracorporeal membrane oxygenation, ventricular assist
Cardiac or cardiopulmonary transplantation	
Exogenous B-type natriuretic peptide	Nesiritide

Table 88-3. Digoxin: Total Oral Loading Dose in Children[a]	
Age	*Dose (micrograms/kg)*
Preterm newborns	20–30
Term newborns and infants	25–35
1–5 y	30–40
5–10 y[b]	20–30
10 y to adult[b]	10–15

[a] Intravenous loading dose = 75%–89% of oral dose. Usually given ½, followed 8 hours later by ¼, followed 8 hours later by ¼, followed 12 hours later by initiation of maintenance dose. Assumes normal renal function; the maintenance dose must be adjusted downward for renal failure.

[b] In children older than 5 years, loading dose is more often based on surface area (0.5–1.0 mg/m²).

The elevated diastolic preload of CHF is the result of neurohumorally mediated sodium and water retention. **Diuretics** reverse this phenomenon. **Furosemide,** a potent loop diuretic that is available in an oral suspension and is fairly well absorbed, is the most frequent drug of choice for the outpatient. The starting dose is 1 mg/kg once or twice daily. Initially, furosemide may be given intravenously or intramuscularly rather than orally, which reduces the time to onset of action and is more effective. Such treatment also supports the patient while digoxin loading is in progress. **Spironolactone,** a less potent diuretic, may be used in combination with furosemide for its potassium-sparing effects, and may also reduce the deleterious histopathologic and structural changes known as *myocardial remodeling* that can accompany CHF.

Fluid and sodium restriction, often used in adults with CHF, is difficult to achieve with infants because their diet is predominantly or exclusively liquid. High-calorie diets using concentrated formulas, complex carbohydrate additives, or medium-chain triglyceride oils may reduce the intake of free water and the effort of feeding without compromising caloric intake. Breast milk and most proprietary formulas have a low sodium load. In older infants and children with CHF, salt intake is more easily modified and should be minimized.

Certain pediatric patients with chronic CHF may benefit from the addition of **angiotensin-converting enzyme inhibitors** to their regimen. These arteriolar dilators help control afterload and have been shown to be effective in children with dilated cardiomyopathy and those with large left-to-right shunts, such as ventricular septal defects (VSDs). Recent observations suggest that third-generation β-blockers such as carvedilol may be useful to control chronic CHF in children with dilated cardiomyopathy. Randomized, controlled clinical trials in adults with similar pathology have been very encouraging, despite poor understanding of the mechanism involved; similar trials in children have thus far been disappointing.

Children with acute, severe, or refractory cases of CHF may require additional medications or interventions, necessitating hospitalization, often in an intensive care unit. These therapies include β-**agonists** and **phosphodiesterase inhibitors** for inotropic support and **vasodilators** for afterload reduction, **correction of anemia** (eg, transfusion), **treatment of fever** (eg, antipyretics), and **reduction**

of metabolic demands (eg, ventilatory support, bed rest, sedation). **Diuretics,** usually given intravenously, provide effective control of congestive symptoms. Because of the importance of fluid balance and nutrition in the child hospitalized with CHF, close and accurate monitoring of fluid intake and output, measurement of daily weight, and measurements of serum electrolytes are essential data in the management of CHF.

In a minority of cases, CHF is refractory to all of the above measures. This may be seen in very severe acute myocarditis, longstanding cardiomyopathy of various causes, and during the postoperative period after complex CHD surgery. Additional options include short-term **mechanical support** such as extracorporeal membrane oxygenation and ventricular assist devices. **Exogenous recombinant B-NP** (nesiritide), which has shown some promise in the setting of adult CHF, may be helpful. In some cases, replacement of the ailing heart or heart-lung unit by **transplantation** may be the only remaining alternative.

Ultimately, the best management for CHF is **treatment of the underlying disorder.** In many cases, failure to treat the underlying disorder will result in limited or no success of other treatment modalities. The degree of urgency depends on the nature of the disorder and the severity of the CHF. For example, in neonates with ductus-dependent lesions such as hypoplastic left heart syndrome, maintenance of ductal patency with prostaglandin E_1 is crucial to initial management. In infants with CHF due to supraventricular tachycardia, prompt conversion to normal sinus rhythm is often the only treatment necessary. Congestive heart failure caused by severe anemia responds dramatically to correction of hemoglobin levels, often using exchange transfusion to avoid additional acute volume overload. Cor pulmonale, often seen in children with severe chronic lung disease, is most responsive to measures directed at improving the lung disease and/or decreasing pulmonary vascular resistance, such as supplemental oxygen or inhaled nitric oxide. When CHF is due to structural CHD (the most common situation), surgery or interventional catheterization to palliate the problem (eg, pulmonary artery banding in certain cases with large net left-to-right shunts) or correct the defect (eg, repair of VSD) usually reverses the CHF. Fortunately, it is rarely necessary to "tolerate" prolonged, uncontrolled CHF in children or to treat the condition aggressively at the expense of a major change in lifestyle.

Family counseling, which should begin when CHF is identified, is essential. Several important points should be included, in addition to a general description of both the cardiac defect and CHF. The term *heart failure,* which is commonly thought by laymen to refer to a sudden deterioration of heart function or even cardiac arrest, must be clarified. It is also important to stress that affected infants should be treated as normally as possible, with the exception of administration of medicines and keeping medical appointments. Contrary to popular belief, most infants with cardiac conditions are not fragile. Addressing quality-of-life issues such as parental concern, assuaging guilt, and normalizing existence are key responsibilities of the physician.

Prognosis

In most young infants and children with CHF, the prognosis is excellent. Congestive heart failure responds well to treatment, and the underlying defect can usually be corrected or at least palliated. Without cardiac surgery for CHD, CHF often remits spontaneously over months or years as a result of maturation of compensatory mechanisms, spontaneous improvement in the defect (eg, decrease in the size of a VSD), or increase in pulmonary vascular resistance because of long-standing high pulmonary artery pressure and flow (Eisenmenger syndrome). "Catch-up" growth occurs with remission of CHF, and children have the potential to reach their genetically determined height and weight.

CASE RESOLUTION

The case presented at the beginning of the chapter is typical of an otherwise normal infant with a large VSD who becomes symptomatic with the development of CHF. The baby's growth failure can be attributed to the chronicity of his illness.

The loud murmur and presentation in infancy strongly suggest the existence of underlying structural CHD as the cause of CHF. The time of onset of CHF also suggests a specific mechanism. When the onset is slightly delayed after birth, a lesion with changing postnatal hemodynamics, such as left-to-right shunt, which has increased as pulmonary resistance has fallen, is suggested. (Note that a ductus-dependent defect would have presented more acutely and severely in the first week of life.)

This infant responded fairly well to oral diuretics and digoxin, but continued to grow slowly and tire easily. He underwent surgical repair of this VSD at 5 months of age with an excellent result and no longer has symptoms or requires medication.

Selected References

Bruns LA, Chrisant MK, Lamour JM, et al. Carvedilol as therapy in pediatric heart failure: an initial multicenter experience. *J Pediatr.* 2001;138:505–511

Costello JM, Goodman DM, Green TP. A review of the natriuretic hormone system's diagnostic and therapeutic potential in critically ill children. *Pediatr Crit Care Med.* 2006;7:308–318

Hsu DT, Pearson GD. Heart failure in children: part I: history, etiology, and pathology. *Circ Heart Fail.* 2009;2:63–70

Hsu DT, Pearson GD. Heart failure in children: part II: diagnosis, treatment and future directions. *Circ Heart Fail.* 2009;2:490–498

Koulouri S, Acherman RJ, Wong PC, Chan LS, Lewis AB. Utility of B-type natriuretic peptide in differentiating congestive heart failure from lung disease in pediatric patients with respiratory distress. *Pediatr Cardiol.* 2004;25:341–346

Mahle WT, Cuadrado AR, Kirshbom PM, Kanter KR, Simsic JM. Nesiritide in infants and children with congestive heart failure. *Pediatr Crit Care Med.* 2005;6:543–546

Maisel AS, Krishnaswamy P, Nowak RM, et al. Rapid measurement of B-type natriuretic peptide in the emergency diagnosis of heart failure. *N Engl J Med.* 2002;347:161–167

O'Laughlin MP. Congestive heart failure in children. *Pediatr Clin North Am.* 1999; 46:263–273

Price JF, Thomas AK, Grenier M, et al. B-type natriuretic peptide predicts adverse cardiovascular events in pediatric outpatients with chronic left ventricular systolic dysfunction. *Circulation.* 2006;114:1063–1069

Rosenthal D, Chrisant MR, Edens E, et al. International Society of Heart and Lung Transplantation: practice guidelines for management of heart failure in children. *J Heart Lung Transplant.* 2004;23:1313–1333

Shaddy RE. Optimizing treatment for chronic congestive heart failure in children. *Crit Care Med.* 2001;29(10 suppl):S237–S240

CHAPTER 89

Chest Pain

Robin Winkler Doroshow, MD, MMS, MEd

CASE STUDY

A previously healthy 13-year-old boy comes to the office complaining of recurrent chest pain, occurring approximately once a week over the past 2 months. The pain is stabbing in nature, located over the mid-sternum, not associated with any other symptoms, and occurs randomly, both at rest and with exercise. It lasts for 2 to 3 minutes, is ranked as 4 on a severity scale of 10, and subsides spontaneously. He does not appear very concerned about the pain, but his mother is quite anxious to have it checked out. His teacher has sent him home from school twice because of the pain, and the soccer coach will not let him play until he is cleared by a doctor. His physical examination is unremarkable.

Questions

1. What is the significance of chest pain in an otherwise healthy child?
2. How likely is serious heart disease to be heralded by chest pain?
3. How much testing, and what type, is appropriate in working up chest pain?
4. Which chest pain patients should be referred to a cardiologist? To other specialists?

Chest pain in children is one of the most common reasons for referral to a pediatric cardiologist, second only to heart murmurs. It is, however, one of the least common presenting complaints of cardiac disease. In fact, from an etiologic standpoint, it would be more suitable for this chapter to be located in the section on gastrointestinal disorders, respiratory problems, psychological and psychogenic disorders, or hematology, rather than cardiology.

Why, then, approach it in the cardiology section, along with discussions of heart murmurs, cyanosis, and congestive heart failure? Perhaps the strongest reason is that it is the greatest fear of the patient, parent, and physician that chest pain could herald a serious—even lethal—heart problem in an otherwise healthy youngster. This fear is exacerbated by 2 social phenomena in our culture: the widespread press given to cases of sudden unexpected death in young, apparently healthy athletes (who had not, in fact, experienced chest pain in most cases), and the appropriately high level of concern over the underdiagnosis of ischemic heart disease in the adult population. Public information targeting the adult with chest pain may, unfortunately, be misinterpreted as applying also to the child. It is this apprehension, and the associated medicolegal defensive posture, that can so often drive the patient, and his referring primary care physician, to seek cardiology consultation and testing.

Epidemiology

The epidemiology of pediatric chest pain is not well studied. Published series have looked retrospectively at patients seen in an emergency department (ED), with a rate of about 0.25%; in an outpatient clinic at about 0.3%; or, as mentioned previously, at a high rate in a pediatric cardiology clinic. In the primary care office setting, chest pain is the third most frequent pain complaint, after abdominal pain and headache. The most common age range is 8 to 18 years, peaking between 11 and 13 years of age. There is no gender or racial predilection, although the etiologic distribution may vary by gender.

Cardiac causes of chest pain are very uncommon for 2 reasons. Such pain is either a rare symptom in a common cardiac disorder (eg, aortic stenosis) or caused by a rare condition (eg, anomalous origin of coronary artery [AOCA]).

Clinical Presentation

There is substantial variability in the complaint of chest pain in children (Questions Box). Some youngsters experience a single, protracted, severe episode that brings them to the ED. In that setting, the patient may have other signs or symptoms of an acute medical problem, such as fever, shortness of breath, or hypotension, raising the level of suspicion for a serious organic cause.

More frequently, children report repeated episodes occurring sporadically over a period of months or even years. The pain may be induced or exacerbated by exercise, deep breathing, lying down, or eating. It can begin and end abruptly or gradually. It may be accompanied by other symptoms, which can give major clues to the diagnosis. In cases where the pain occurs on exercise, is this a consistent, predictable experience, or is it unpredictable?

Most (up to 97%) of children seen for chest pain have no serious medical history, and most have an unremarkable physical examination.

Chest Pain

Questions

- What is the pain like? Where is it located? Does it radiate? How severe is it?
- How long has the child been having pain? Did it begin after trauma? How often does the pain occur? How long does it last? Does it start and end suddenly?
- What brings the pain on? Is it related to exercise and, if so, is it consistent?
- Does the child have associated symptoms with the pain, such as syncope, shortness of breath, palpitations, fever, nausea, sour taste, wheezing, or cough?
- Does the child at other times have cardiac symptoms, such as easy fatigability, cyanosis, exertional dyspnea, edema, or syncope?
- Does the child's medical history include potentially pertinent disorders such as asthma, gastroesophageal reflux disease, psychiatric problems, heart disease, or sickle cell disease?
- How much impact is the pain having on the child's life? Is he or she missing school or sports?
- Is there a family history of sudden unexpected death, recurrent syncope, or known genetic syndrome?

Pathophysiology

The pathophysiology varies with the underlying cause of the pain, for which there is a broad differential diagnosis (Box 89-1). It is important for the patient, parent, and physician to understand that thoracic or abdominal pain, and particularly visceral pain, is poorly localized. This makes it difficult to distinguish between, for example, esophagitis and cardiac ischemia; hence, the term "heartburn" for the former. Thus precordial pain may originate from any intrathoracic organ or from the chest wall itself, and the patient cannot identify the source of his discomfort, which in itself is a cause of distress.

Cardiac causes are a heterogeneous category, which can best be viewed as ischemic and non-ischemic in origin (Box 89-2). Ischemic chest pain, or angina, is caused by a drop, often sudden, in the myocardial oxygen supply/demand ratio, causing pain or, in rare cases, sudden death. This may occur because of diseased coronary arteries as in adults, due to accelerated coronary atherosclerosis, which is very rare. It may be seen in progeria, mucopolysaccharidosis, post-transplantation coronary disease, and severe familial hypercholesterolemia. It may occur as a result of previous inflammation (as in Kawasaki disease with coronary aneurysms) leading to coronary artery stenosis. A congenital AOCA from the opposite sinus of Valsalva (Figure 89-1) or from the pulmonary artery may result in ischemia due to compression of the anomalous vessel between the great arteries, obstruction from a slit-like orifice at the origin or, in the case of the pulmonary artery, low pressure and low saturation in the perfusing blood.

The chest pain seen in patients with left ventricular outflow obstruction (aortic valve stenosis and hypertrophic obstructive cardiomyopathy) is likely also due to ischemia. The already diminished

---

Box 89-1. Differential Diagnosis of Chest Pain in Children and Adolescents

Chest Wall
- c   Trauma
- c   Overuse
- c   Inadequate breast support
- c   Chronic cough
- u   Costochondritis
- u   Precordial catch syndrome
- r   Slipping rib syndrome

Gastrointestinal
- c   Gastroesophageal reflux disease
- u   Esophagitis due to repeated vomiting
- r   Esophageal stricture
- r   Foreign body

Pulmonary
- c   Exercise-induced asthma
- c   Pneumonia
- u   Pleurodynia, pleurisy
- r   Pneumothorax/pneumomediastinum
- r   Pulmonary embolism

Psychological
- c   Anxiety disorder
- u   Depression
- u   Conversion reaction
- r   Munchausen syndrome
- r   Bulimia nervosa

Miscellaneous
- c   Idiopathic
- u   Acute chest syndrome (sickle cell disease)
- r   Thoracic tumors
- r   Herpes zoster

Cardiac
See Box 89-2

Abbreviations: c, common cause of chest pain; r, rare cause of chest pain; u, uncommon cause of chest pain.

---

supply/demand ratio due to hypertrophy and hypertension of the left ventricle falls further with strenuous exercise, causing pain and/or arrhythmia.

In abuse of drugs such as cocaine, chest pain may be attributable to arrhythmia, myocardial hypoperfusion, or a combination of the two; this may present as chest pain or overt collapse, in some cases with cardiac arrest.

Although many children with cardiac arrhythmias are asymptomatic or present with palpitations, dizzy spells, or syncope, some do complain of chest pain. In the case of the younger child, this may reflect an inability to express the discomfort of palpitations as other than "hurting." In addition, ischemia does occur in some individuals with tachyarrhythmias, such as paroxysmal supraventricular tachycardia (SVT), due to high myocardial oxygen consumption and

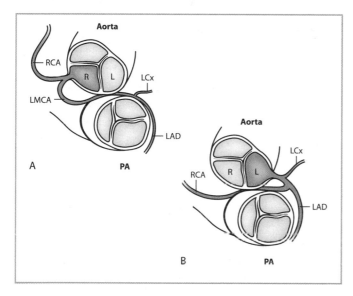

Figure 89-1. Schematic diagram of the 2 forms of anomalous origin of a coronary from the wrong sinus that are associated with myocardial ischemia. A. Anomalous origin of the left main coronary artery (LMA) from the right sinus of Valsalva. B. Anomalous origin of the right coronary artery (RCA) from the left sinus of Valsalva. In each case, the anomalous coronary artery can be seen coursing between the aorta and pulmonary artery (PA). L, left aortic sinus; LAD, left anterior descending; LCx, left circumflex; R, right aortic sinus.

shortened diastole, compromising perfusion. In these patients, ST segment depression may be seen on the electrocardiogram (ECG) during the arrhythmia and may persist for several minutes after the arrhythmia is terminated.

Non-ischemic cardiac causes of chest pain include pericarditis and less commonly myocarditis, aortic dissection, and mitral prolapse. The most common form of inflammatory heart disease is acute viral infection; acute bacterial pericarditis is more severe and associated with greater systemic toxicity. Connective tissue disease, such as lupus erythematosus or juvenile rheumatoid arthritis, is frequently associated with immune-mediated pericarditis, as is the postpericardiotomy syndrome seen shortly after cardiac surgery. In these disorders the pain is due to inflammation of the pericardium and epicardium, directly stimulating the many sensory nerve endings in this area.

Aortic dissection also results in direct stimulation of pain fibers, in this case in the aortic wall. It is very rare in the normal pediatric population but may occur in the setting of Marfan syndrome. Chest pain is also seen in patients with mitral valve prolapse, but it is often difficult to establish a clear causal relationship in this setting. Interestingly, gastroesophageal reflux disease (GERD) can be demonstrated in a high percentage of these patients.

Differential Diagnosis

The differential diagnosis of pediatric chest pain is presented in the Box 89-1, and cardiac causes are listed in Box 89-2. The relative frequencies of these causes vary in reported series, but all report higher frequencies of respiratory, idiopathic, traumatic, and psychogenic etiologies and low frequencies of cardiac etiologies, usually in the range of 1% to 5% in patients with no previous cardiac history. These data must be viewed as approximations because the ultimate etiologic classification of cases in these series is not usually based on a definitive result but rather an attribution by the physician involved. Therefore, cultural factors and individual preferences may lead to higher reported rates of "idiopathic" chest pain in some centers, "chest wall pain" in others, and "anxiety disorder" in still others. Some studies report a higher incidence of cardiac etiologies because they so classify any chest pain patient with a cardiac finding (eg, premature beats, abnormal ECG), regardless of whether it may explain the pain.

Evaluation

The keystones to the evaluation of the child with chest pain are a thorough, methodical history and careful physical examination; indeed, in many cases these will suffice to arrive at a diagnosis and formulate a management plan.

History

The major questions to be addressed are outlined in the Questions Box. Because there are many pertinent details to be included in the **history of present illness,** and they are often provided in a variable sequence, some physicians find it helpful to use a printed format as a guide. Some offer a questionnaire for the patient or parent to complete. Witnesses to the episodes may provide additional helpful information, especially if the patient is not verbally expressive. The witness may estimate a pain score based on observation, which may differ substantially from the score assigned by the patient himself.

Pain that occurs repeatedly over time is less likely due to an organic cause of a serious nature, particularly if it is not reproducible. A severe, protracted episode (eg, lasting hours) is more likely to be organic in origin. The location of the pain has not been a strong predictor of diagnosis in reported series. Its timing and association with other symptoms, however, may provide major clues. Reflux esophagitis may occur after eating, more often when supine or very active, and may be accompanied by a sour taste; it may be relieved by eating or use of an antacid. Associated symptoms that may raise a red flag for a cardiac cause include syncope, palpitations, sweating, and nausea; reproducible pain at a given level of exertion is also more likely anginal. Because pain and accompanying anxiety may cause sinus tachycardia, which can be interpreted by the patient as palpitations, it is important to get a sense of the heart rate experienced by patients with that complaint. The child can be asked to tap his chest or clap his hands as fast as his heart was racing during the palpitations; serious tachyarrhythmias such as supraventricular tachycardia and ventricular tachycardia are usually very rapid.

Recent fever and malaise are often present in pneumonia, pleurisy, or pericarditis. Exercise-induced asthma (EIA), in addition to being related to exertion, is sometimes accompanied by cough and/or wheezing. Shortness of breath is very frequently reported by patients in association with their pain; this may reflect anxiety or sensitivity to movement rather than pulmonary pathology.

In youngsters with psychogenic pain, other symptoms of anxiety or depression may be reported, although not necessarily simultaneously with the chest pain, and a history of recent stressors may be uncovered. These patients may also report other recurrent somatic complaints.

The nature, severity, and abruptness of the pain may also yield diagnostic clues. Exercise-induced asthma is often described as a chest "tightness," is usually gradual in onset, and lasts beyond the exertion itself. The precordial catch syndrome, a poorly understood disorder also known as *Texidor twinge,* is a sudden, sharp, localized pain that is exacerbated by deep breathing, and lasts only seconds or minutes. In contrast, the slipping rib syndrome, in which the cartilaginous tips of the 8th, 9th, and 10th ribs become transiently subluxated, produces pain at the costal margin, is very sensitive to movement, and is often associated with a "popping" or "slipping" sensation in the affected area. Gastroesophageal reflux disease pain is usually described as "burning," and may awaken the patient from sleep. In contrast, the pain of angina is reported as "crushing," and may radiate to the left arm or the neck. The diffuse pain of pericarditis is often ameliorated by sitting forward. Aortic dissection results in an acute, tearing sensation.

A history of recent chest trauma will naturally suggest chest wall injury as the cause, but the fall or sports mishap may be forgotten if the onset of the pain is not temporally associated with the event. Chest wall pain may also result from overuse, as seen in weight lifters, or from inadequate breast support, as seen in female runners. Drug abuse, particularly with cocaine, may be disclosed if the patient is questioned in private. In some cases this may have occurred several days before the onset of pain.

The patient's **medical history,** if positive, may lead the clinician toward the underlying diagnosis. In children with sickle cell disease, acute chest syndrome must be considered early in the assessment. A history of respiratory disease may point to an acute respiratory infection or to EIA. Children with known heart disease, who may experience benign chest pain, are more likely to have a cardiac etiology than their peers, depending on the cardiac diagnosis. Most congenital heart defects, for example, do not cause pain but may raise the level of anxiety in the family and lead to the perception or exaggeration of chest pain. Of greater concern is a history of heart disease that may affect myocardial perfusion, such as Kawasaki disease or cardiac surgery involving the coronary arteries (eg, arterial switch operation for transposition of the great arteries).

The **family history** must not be overlooked. Although most pediatric chest pain is not due to hereditary disorders, some of the more severe causes may be hereditary, such as hypertrophic cardiomyopathy, some arrhythmias, asthma, sickle cell disease, and aortic dissection in Marfan syndrome. It is also noted that in children with nonorganic chest pain, such as psychogenic pain, there is often a history of a close relative having had recent heart surgery or a heart attack, bringing attention to this area during a time of emotional stress.

A complete **review of systems** is essential in the assessment of children with chest pain, due to the wide range of differential diagnoses.

Physical Examination

A careful physical examination is imperative; in children with no history of serious illness, this should be focused on, but not be limited to, the chest. General inspection will immediately aid in distinguishing between the acutely ill child and the otherwise well child with chest pain. Abnormal vital signs, such as fever, tachycardia, or tachypnea, are associated with acute etiologies such as infection or inflammation. The child's pain level should be quantified with the aid of a pain scale. If the patient is dyspneic, pulse oximetry should be measured.

The chest wall should be examined for signs of trauma and for tenderness. Care must be taken with the latter because it is easy to obtain a false-positive examination for costochondritis, for example, because the costochondral junctions have some degree of normal tenderness, as do the female breasts. Asymmetry of tenderness, and a report that the pain produced is similar to that experienced, suggests chest wall injury. In patients with rib injury, the pain can be elicited not only on direct palpation but also indirectly by compression of the thoracic cage from another location. In girls with inadequate breast support, the breast ligaments may be symmetrically tender.

Auscultation of the lungs and heart will, of course, yield useful clues to diagnosis, especially in children with acute inflammatory processes (rales, rub) and in those with left ventricular outflow obstruction, such as aortic stenosis (murmur). It must be remembered, however, that many of the organic causes of chest pain, such as GERD, EIA, intermittent arrhythmias, and AOCA, will have a normal examination if the patient is not experiencing the pain at the time of the visit.

The other portions of the physical examination may also aid in the evaluation of the child with chest pain. Jugular distention, hepatomegaly, and peripheral edema suggest congestive heart failure or pericardial effusion with tamponade. The child's behavior pattern and interaction with his parents may suggest a psychological disorder such as anxiety or depression. Poor dentition and halitosis in an adolescent with weight loss may be a sign of bulimia as a source of esophagitis. Excessive signs of trauma such as multiple ecchymoses may indicate a coagulopathy, and also raise the possibility of non-accidental trauma.

Laboratory Studies

A wide variety of diagnostic studies is available to help in arriving at a diagnosis; it is incumbent on the physician to select those appropriate to the individual patient, guided by the findings of the history and physical examination.

In the patient presenting with **acute chest pain,** often to the ED, there is a greater need for tests because the differential diagnosis more often includes serious, even life-threatening, disorders than in the child with chronic recurrent pain. Reported series show the chest radiograph to have a reasonably high yield of positive findings; a negative radiograph is reassuring in ruling out pathology such as pleural effusion, pneumonia, pneumothorax, pneumomediastinum, and thoracic tumor, but cannot be used to exclude most cardiac etiologies. More detailed imaging such as magnetic resonance imaging may be needed when major chest trauma is reported or aortic dissection suspected. Dyspnea or hypoxemia, particularly in the setting of recent immobilization or in an adolescent female taking oral contraceptives, should lead one to suspect pulmonary embolism, for which a spiral computed tomography or nuclear perfusion scan is indicated.

Although ECG is routinely performed as part of the evaluation for acute chest pain in children, it is rarely helpful in establishing a diagnosis other than arrhythmia, which may be suspected from the history or examination. ST segment changes may reflect pericardial irritation or myocardial ischemia if the ECG is done at the time of the pain. If ongoing myocardial ischemia is suspected, myocardial enzymes (creatine phosphokinase MB fraction, troponin-I) should be measured and a toxicology screen performed. If signs of acute infection such as fever are noted, a complete blood cell count, sedimentation rate or C-reactive protein, and appropriate cultures are indicated. Echocardiography is highly sensitive and specific for pericardial effusion and should be performed early in the evaluation of the patient with chest pain and jugular distention, a friction rub, fever, or ST segment elevation on ECG.

In patients presenting with **chronic recurrent chest pain,** the likelihood of serious pathology is very low. When the examination is normal and the history reassuring, the yield of "screening" tests such as chest radiograph and ECG is extremely poor, and the cost in dollars and anxiety not justifiable. In most cases the history and physical examination are adequate to lead to a focused selection of diagnostic tests, if any are needed. A description of pain suggestive of esophagitis, for example, may lead to endoscopy or upper gastrointestinal series. When EIA is suspected, pulmonary function testing is appropriate, in some cases with an exercise challenge. Strong suspicion of psychogenic causes should prompt further psychological evaluation at the initial encounter, including querying the patient about suicidality; further testing or consultation may be indicated.

The finding of a murmur of left ventricular outflow tract obstruction is an indication for echocardiography, which will confirm the diagnosis and yield further details that will guide management. A history of palpitations or syncope raises the possibility of arrhythmia; an ECG may give clues such as Wolff-Parkinson-White syndrome as a substrate for SVT, but a normal ECG does not rule out arrhythmia if the patient is asymptomatic at the time. Here an ambulatory ECG (Holter) monitor or transtelephonic event detector may enable the clinician to document the rhythm during an episode of pain. Consistent exertional pain merits evaluation for ischemia, using resting ECG and often exercise stress testing. These studies, unfortunately, can be negative between episodes in patients with AOCA. This diagnosis can, however, be identified by echocardiography, but only if the study is deliberately directed toward that diagnosis; therefore, the study should be done in a pediatric echocardiography laboratory, and the sonographer must be aware of the diagnosis in question.

Management

The management of pediatric chest pain depends on the underlying diagnosis or lack thereof. For management of GERD, acute chest syndrome, pneumonia, pericarditis, connective tissue disorders, thoracic tumors, anxiety disorder, pneumothorax, cocaine abuse, and chest wall trauma, as well as other serious disorders discussed under differential diagnosis, the reader is directed to other sources within and beyond this text.

When there is a strong suspicion of cardiac pathology, either on the basis of history and physical examination or on the basis of subsequent testing as described previously, prompt referral to a pediatric cardiologist is indicated. Management may include surgery (eg, for AOCA), antibiotics, anti-inflammatories, pericardiocentesis (eg, for pericarditis), antiarrhythmics, interventional catheterization (eg, balloon angioplasty, radiofrequency ablation), or a combination.

Short-term nonsteroidal anti-inflammatory medication is helpful for chest wall pain due to overuse, trauma, costochondritis, or slipping rib syndrome. In a minority of cases, local injection with anesthetic may be necessary.

Therapeutic trials may be considered in some cases to arrive at a diagnosis. A child with suspected esophagitis may be given an antacid at the time of the pain. If the pain is relieved, further workup and treatment can proceed accordingly. Similarly, a youngster with suspected EIA, particularly if there is a previous history of reactive airways disease, may benefit from a trial of an inhaled bronchodilator at the time of the pain.

In the exceedingly common setting of benign chest pain, such as with minor chest wall trauma, mild somatization, or occasional reflux esophagitis, the most important step in management is reassurance of the patient and family that this is not an indication of a serious disorder. It is essential to clarify how one has arrived at this conclusion, and why further testing is not appropriate.

A frequent observation in this setting is that most families do not require a definitive diagnosis of the cause of the pain. If a serious disorder is excluded—necessary because 50% of patients believe that chest pain means heart disease—all participants are reassured. Follow-up studies have demonstrated that at least 80% of patients in this category do not seek further medical attention for their chest pain or return for follow-up.

Prognosis

The outcome depends on the underlying diagnosis. Most cases of benign chest pain spontaneously resolve, often within a short time of their evaluation. Even in serious and potentially life-threatening causes of chest pain, early diagnosis and intervention will usually lead to an excellent outcome.

CASE RESOLUTION

The patient and his parents are assured that he has no evidence of a serious medical problem. His heart is strong, his lungs clear, and his circulation good. They are told that chest pain in otherwise healthy children may be mysterious but is common, and very rarely a sign of illness. They are told in a gentle but definitive manner that he does not need any more evaluation at this time, but that if the problem does not resolve itself, the child should return for reevaluation.

The boy is delighted to hear that he may return to full sports participation, confirmed in writing to the coach. The parents are very relieved and grateful for the attention and reassurance of the physician.

Selected References

Abdurrahman L, Bockoven JR, Pickoff AS, Ralston MA, Ross JE. Pediatric cardiology update: office-based practice of pediatric cardiology for the primary care provider. *Curr Probl Pediatr Adolesc Health Care.* 2003;33:318–347

Cava JR, Sayger PL. Chest pain in children and adolescents. *Pediatr Clin North Am.* 2004;51:1553–1568

Eslick GD, Selbst, SM, eds. Pediatric chest pain. *Pediatr Clin North Am.* 2010; 57:entire volume

Gumbiner CH. Precordial catch syndrome. *Southern Med J.* 2003;96:38–41

Lipsitz JD, Masia C, Apfel H, et al. Noncardiac chest pain and psychopathology in children and adolescents. *J Psychosom Res.* 2005;59:185–188

Massin MM, Bourguignont A, Coremans C, Comte L, Lepage P, Gerard P. Chest pain in pediatric patients presenting to an emergency department or to a cardiac clinic. *Clin Pediatr (Phila).* 2004;43:231–238

Rowe BH, Dulberg CS, Peterson RG, Vlad P, Li MM. Characteristics of children presenting with chest pain to a pediatric emergency department. *CMAJ.* 1990; 143:388–394

Selbst SM. Chest pain in children. *Pediatrics.* 1985;75:1068–1070

Wiens L, Sabath R, Ewing L, Gowdamarajan R, Portnoy J, Scagliotti D. Chest pain in otherwise healthy children and adolescents is frequently caused by exercise-induced asthma. *Pediatrics.* 1992;90:350–353

Zavaras-Angelidou KA, Weinhouse E, Nelson DB. Review of 180 episodes of chest pain in 134 children. *Pediatr Emerg Care.* 1992;8:189–193

CHAPTER 90

Hypertension

Gangadarshni Chandramohan, MD, MS, and Sudhir K. Anand, MD

CASE STUDY

A 10-year-old girl is seen in the emergency department with a history of severe headache and generalized seizures lasting 2 minutes. Her medical history is remarkable for several episodes of unexplained fever as an infant and an episode of urinary tract infection at age 3 years; no radiologic studies were done. She also has a history of headaches for the past 2 years, which have been treated primarily with acetaminophen. There is no known history of drug ingestion or hypertension in the patient or family members.

The physical examination is remarkable for a pulse of 100 beats/min and a blood pressure of 210/130 mm Hg in the right arm in supine position. Equal pulses are palpable in all 4 extremities. Blood pressure (BP) is 216/134 mm Hg in the right lower extremity. The funduscopic examination reveals evidence of petechial hemorrhages and mild papilledema. Chest examination finds normal breath sounds and an active precordium with the apical impulse shifted to the left; no murmurs are heard. The liver is palpable 1 cm below the right costal margin. The neurologic examination is remarkable for altered sensorium with lethargy;

no focal neurologic deficit is present. A routine urinalysis shows 2+ protein and normal urinary sediment. The hemoglobin is 11.2 g/dL and hematocrit is 33%. Sodium is 139 mEq/L, potassium 3.8 mEq/L, chloride 102 mEq/L, and bicarbonate 22 mEq/L. Blood urea nitrogen is 35 mg/dL and serum creatinine is 1.8 mg/dL. An electrocardiogram shows left ventricular enlargement. Computed tomography scan of the head is normal.

Questions

1. What is the definition of hypertension in children?
2. What are the causes of hypertension in children?
3. What is the appropriate evaluation of hypertension in children?
4. What are the comorbid conditions and long-term complications associated with primary hypertension?
5. What is the appropriate emergency treatment of symptomatic hypertension?
6. What is the long-term management of children with primary hypertension?

Hypertension has become a more common problem among children over the past few decades due to the increased prevalence of obesity, which is associated with primary hypertension. Although the increased prevalence of hypertension in children is predominantly due to increase in primary (essential) hypertension, there is a need with childhood hypertension to identify secondary causes. Secondary causes are proportionately more prevalent among children than adults and, if identified, may be curable, thereby eliminating the need for lifelong medical treatment. Conversely, primary hypertension typically persists into adulthood and is likely to become a major public health concern in the future. With early intervention, however, the long-term adverse consequences of hypertension are preventable. Children who are expected to be at increased risk for end-organ (heart, central nervous system [CNS], kidneys, and eyes) damage as they become adults are those with persistently elevated BP readings, high body mass index, excessive weight gain, and a family history of hypertension.

Normal Blood Pressure and Definition of Hypertension

Both systolic and diastolic BP gradually increase, from the newborn period through adolescence; therefore, age-appropriate norms should be used to classify a given BP reading as normal or hypertensive. For example, a BP reading of 118/76 mm Hg would be regarded as normal for a 16-year-old adolescent, but it would signify stage 2 hypertension in a 2-year-old child, meaning that this child needs urgent medical attention. Blood pressure measurements should be part of routine physical examinations in all children older than 3 years and in all hospitalized children according to the American Academy of Pediatrics (AAP) guidelines. The guidelines also recommend that children who are younger than 3 years who have a history of prematurity, congenital heart disease, recurrent urinary tract infections (UTIs), or chronic systemic illnesses should have their BP measured as a routine part of their well-child care. An appropriately sized BP cuff should be used; the inner cuff width should be approximately 40% of the arm circumference midway between the olecranon and the acromion, and the length should be greater than 80% around the arm circumference at the same point to avoid inaccurately high readings (Dx Box). There are various other factors that should be taken into consideration while measuring BP to minimize errors, which include patient's posture (sitting versus lying down) and level of the arm in relation to level of the heart (elbow to be at the level of the heart) and, if it is the first visit, readings from all 4 extremities to rule out coarctation of the aorta should be performed

Dx Hypertension

- Blood pressure (BP) elevated >95th percentile for age, gender, and height on at least 3 consecutive occasions with the child in a quiet, non-apprehensive state and with BP cuff of appropriate size
- BP checked in both upper and at least one lower extremity
- Fundus examination: vascular changes, exudates, and papilledema
- Abnormal urinalysis

as well. It is also important that the child should remain calm and not be anxious or agitated while the measurement is taken.

Blood pressure values in children are a continuum, with no clear dividing line between normal and high (Tables 90-1 and 90-2). Therefore, the fourth report on high BP in children and adolescents (2004), by using the statistical percentile values, defines hypertension as systolic or diastolic BP of greater than 95th percentile for age, gender, and height on at least 3 occasions (Table 90-3). Furthermore, if the BP readings, either systolic or diastolic, are between the 90th and 95th percentile, it is considered as pre-hypertension. The report further classifies hypertension into 2 categories: (1) stage 1 hypertension, which is when systolic or diastolic BP is persistently between the 95th percentile to 5 mm above the 99th percentiles and (2) stage 2 hypertension, which is when systolic or diastolic BP is persistently more than 5 mm Hg above the 99th percentile. Because this is a statistical definition, 5% of all children (those with BP readings >95th percentile) would be expected to have hypertension. The BP values described in Tables 90-1 and 90-2 were determined from the normal distribution of BP values in healthy children from a study conducted in late 1980s; however, based on more recent data from National Health and Nutrition Survey 2004, the prevalence of hypertension using the BP values described in Tables 90-1 and 90-2 are in fact higher than 5%, suggesting that there is certainly a relative increase in the prevalence of hypertension over the last 2 decades.

Epidemiology

The prevalence of persistent hypertension in children based on the current definition is approximately 3% to 5%; however, it can vary depending on the age, ethnicity, geographic distribution, and type of hypertension. The consensus is that the overall prevalence of primary hypertension has been increasing over the past few decades secondary to increasing prevalence of obesity, cultural factors, and lifestyle changes, which includes increase in stress and sedentary lifestyle. Among those who are obese, the prevalence of hypertension has been reported to be up to 30% from some studies, compared to non-obese children. As in adults, hypertension is more common among African American and Hispanic children compared to Caucasian children. Furthermore, adolescent children and those from urban cities tend to have higher prevalence compared to younger children and to those from rural areas.

Secondary hypertension is more common among infants and young children, whereas primary hypertension is notably more common among adolescents. Children who require hospital admission for their hypertension usually have secondary hypertension, which may have been triggered by an acute event, frequently volume overload. Occasionally the cause of the hypertension is uncertain. In many such children, the acutely increased BP resolves with appropriate medical intervention and most do not require long-term treatment. Data on prevalence of acute hypertension is sparse due to the transient nature of the condition, and there are no major long-term implications.

Clinical Presentation

Mild or stage 1 hypertension in most children is usually asymptomatic. However, children with moderate to severe hypertension can develop headaches, blurring of vision, and sometimes nose bleeds. Acute presentations of hypertension are divided into 3 categories: hypertensive urgencies, hypertensive emergencies, and hypertensive crisis. Occasionally, the terms hypertensive emergency and crisis are used interchangeably to describe the same situation when a patient has very elevated BP. Hypertensive urgency is defined by the sudden development of elevated BP without evidence of severe end-organ damage but can be symptomatic with headache and vomiting. A hypertensive emergency, in comparison, is defined by obvious signs of significant end-organ damage, such as encephalopathy, seizures, papilledema, retinal hemorrhages, or kidney injury, and must be dealt with immediately. Hypertensive crisis is merely a very severe form of hypertension marked by a more than 20% increase in the systolic and/or diastolic BP above the 95th percentile with clinical evidence of malignant hypertension.

Etiology and Pathophysiology

An increase in BP results from an increase in peripheral resistance or cardiac output, or a mixture of the two. The exact cause of hypertension in 90% to 95% of adults is still uncertain; hence, the term essential, primary, or idiopathic hypertension. In the past, hypertension was considered secondary to an underlying disorder in more than 80% of children and fewer than 20% of cases were idiopathic; however, this was true only in children with very severe hypertension. In most obese adolescent children with mild increases in BP, no etiology of hypertension is found and they are classified as having primary or essential hypertension.

Many factors play a role in the development of essential hypertension. Research reveals variable degrees of alteration in cardiac output, extracellular fluid volume, peripheral resistance, renin-angiotensin system, aldosterone, electrolyte balance, catecholamines, sympathetic nervous system, natriuretic hormones, prostaglandins, kinins, antidiuretic hormone, insulin response, endothelins, nitric oxide (endothelium-derived relaxation factors), and others. Whether these abnormalities are primary or secondary and what their exact role is in the pathogenesis of essential hypertension is still uncertain. Barker's hypothesis of epigenetic transmission, a recently promulgated theory, attributes certain disorders, including childhood

Age (Year)	BP Percentile ↓	Systolic BP (mm Hg) ← Percentile of Height →							Diastolic BP (mm Hg) ← Percentile of Height →						
		5th	10th	25th	50th	75th	90th	95th	5th	10th	25th	50th	75th	90th	95th
1	50th	80	81	83	85	87	88	89	34	35	36	37	38	39	39
	90th	94	95	97	99	100	102	103	49	50	51	52	53	53	54
	95th	98	99	101	103	104	106	106	54	54	55	56	57	58	58
	99th	105	106	108	110	112	113	114	61	62	63	64	65	66	66
2	50th	84	85	87	88	90	92	92	39	40	41	42	43	44	44
	90th	97	99	100	102	104	105	106	54	55	56	57	58	58	59
	95th	101	102	104	106	108	109	110	59	59	60	61	62	63	63
	99th	109	110	111	113	115	117	117	66	67	68	69	70	71	71
3	50th	86	87	89	91	93	94	95	44	44	45	46	47	48	48
	90th	100	101	103	105	107	108	109	59	59	60	61	62	63	63
	95th	104	105	107	109	110	112	113	63	63	64	65	66	67	67
	99th	111	112	114	116	118	119	120	71	71	72	73	74	75	75
4	50th	88	89	91	93	95	96	97	47	48	49	50	51	51	52
	90th	102	103	105	107	109	110	111	62	63	64	65	66	66	67
	95th	106	107	109	111	112	114	115	66	67	68	69	70	71	71
	99th	113	114	116	118	120	121	122	74	75	76	77	78	78	79
5	50th	90	91	93	95	96	98	98	50	51	52	53	54	55	55
	90th	104	105	106	108	110	111	112	65	66	67	68	69	69	70
	95th	108	109	110	112	114	115	116	69	70	71	72	73	74	74
	99th	115	116	118	120	121	123	123	77	78	79	80	81	81	82
6	50th	91	92	94	96	98	99	100	53	53	54	55	56	57	57
	90th	105	106	108	110	111	113	113	68	68	69	70	71	72	72
	95th	109	110	112	114	115	117	117	72	72	73	74	75	76	76
	99th	116	117	119	121	123	124	125	80	80	81	82	83	84	84
7	50th	92	94	95	97	99	100	101	55	55	56	57	58	59	59
	90th	106	107	109	111	113	114	115	70	70	71	72	73	74	74
	95th	110	111	113	115	117	118	119	74	74	75	76	77	78	78
	99th	117	118	120	122	124	125	126	82	82	83	84	85	86	86
8	50th	94	95	97	99	100	102	102	56	57	58	59	60	60	61
	90th	107	109	110	112	114	115	116	71	72	72	73	74	75	76
	95th	111	112	114	116	118	119	120	75	76	77	78	79	79	80
	99th	119	120	122	123	125	127	127	83	84	85	86	87	87	88
9	50th	95	96	98	100	102	103	104	57	58	59	60	61	61	62
	90th	109	110	112	114	115	117	118	72	73	74	75	76	76	77
	95th	113	114	116	118	119	121	121	76	77	78	79	80	81	81
	99th	120	121	123	125	127	128	129	84	85	86	87	88	88	89
10	50th	97	98	100	102	103	105	106	58	59	60	61	61	62	63
	90th	111	112	114	115	117	119	119	73	73	74	75	76	77	78
	95th	115	116	117	119	121	122	123	77	78	79	80	81	81	82
	99th	122	123	125	127	128	130	130	85	86	86	88	88	89	90

Table 90-1. Blood Pressure Levels for the 90th and 95th Percentiles of Blood Pressure for Boys Aged 1–17 Years by Percentiles of Height

Table 90-1. Blood Pressure Levels for the 90th and 95th Percentiles of Blood Pressure for Boys Aged 1–17 Years by Percentiles of Height, continued

Age (Year)	BP Percentile ↓	Systolic BP (mm Hg) ← Percentile of Height →							Diastolic BP (mm Hg) ← Percentile of Height →						
		5th	10th	25th	50th	75th	90th	95th	5th	10th	25th	50th	75th	90th	95th
11	50th	99	100	102	104	105	107	107	59	59	60	61	62	63	63
	90th	113	114	115	117	119	120	121	74	74	75	76	77	78	78
	95th	117	118	119	121	123	124	125	78	78	79	80	81	82	82
	99th	124	125	127	129	130	132	132	86	86	87	88	89	90	90
12	50th	101	102	104	106	108	109	110	59	60	61	62	63	63	64
	90th	115	116	118	120	121	123	123	74	75	75	76	77	78	79
	95th	119	120	122	123	125	127	127	78	79	80	81	82	82	83
	99th	126	127	129	131	133	134	135	86	87	88	89	90	90	91
13	50th	104	105	106	108	110	111	112	60	60	61	62	63	64	64
	90th	117	118	120	122	124	125	126	75	75	76	77	78	79	79
	95th	121	122	124	126	128	129	130	79	79	80	81	82	83	83
	99th	128	130	131	133	135	136	137	87	87	88	89	90	91	91
14	50th	106	107	109	111	113	114	115	60	61	62	63	64	65	65
	90th	120	121	123	125	126	128	128	75	76	77	78	79	79	80
	95th	124	125	127	128	130	132	132	80	80	81	82	83	84	84
	99th	131	132	134	136	138	139	140	87	88	89	90	91	92	92
15	50th	109	110	112	113	115	117	117	61	62	63	64	65	66	66
	90th	122	124	125	127	129	130	131	76	77	78	79	80	80	81
	95th	126	127	129	131	133	134	135	81	81	82	83	84	85	85
	99th	134	135	136	138	140	142	142	88	89	90	91	92	93	93
16	50th	111	112	114	116	118	119	120	63	63	64	65	66	67	67
	90th	125	126	128	130	131	133	134	78	78	79	80	81	82	82
	95th	129	130	132	134	135	137	137	82	83	83	84	85	86	87
	99th	136	137	139	141	143	144	145	90	90	91	92	93	94	94
17	50th	114	115	116	118	120	121	122	65	66	66	67	68	69	70
	90th	127	128	130	132	134	135	136	80	80	81	82	83	84	84
	95th	131	132	134	136	138	139	140	84	85	86	87	87	88	89
	99th	139	140	141	143	145	146	147	92	93	93	94	95	96	97

Abbreviation: BP, blood pressure.

*The 90th percentile is 1.28 SD, 95th percentile is 1.645 SD, and the 99th percentile is 2.326 SD over the mean.

hypertension, to altered gene expression from malnutrition or other adverse events during intrauterine life. This hypothesis has been further supported by data demonstrating association between fewer nephrons in children who were born small for gestational age and later development of hypertension.

Other important factors in the development of hypertension include race, heredity, stress response, sleep apnea, obesity, hyperlipidemia, and increased salt intake. Recently obesity has been strongly implicated in the increase in incidence of hypertension in the United States. Mirroring the increase in obesity, average BPs rose by 1.4 to 3.3 mm Hg between 1990 and 2000. Studies showing that weight reduction in obese patients lowers BP strengthen the argument that obesity contributes to hypertension. There also seems to be strong associations between sleep-disordered breathing, sleep apnea, and hypertension.

Recent knowledge from ambulatory BP (ABP) monitoring has contributed significantly to the understanding of hypertension in children by revealing different BP responses under different clinical settings. Ambulatory BP involves using a continuous monitor such as is done when children have a Holter monitor to detect episodic cardiac arrythmias. The device particularly assesses changes in BP during sleep and notes whether an individual has dips ("dipper") or no dips ("non-dipper"). The apparatus is somewhat cumbersome, the study is costly, and sleep may be disturbed by the cuff inflation, thereby influencing the results. In adults, surges of BP in the morning are felt to be predictive of strokes.

Table 90-2. Blood Pressure Levels for the 90th and 95th Percentiles of Blood Pressure for Girls Aged 1–17 Years by Percentiles of Height

Age (Year)	BP Percentile ↓	Systolic BP (mm Hg) ← Percentile of Height →							Diastolic BP (mm Hg) ← Percentile of Height →						
		5th	10th	25th	50th	75th	90th	95th	5th	10th	25th	50th	75th	90th	95th
1	50th	83	84	85	86	88	89	90	38	39	39	40	41	41	42
	90th	97	97	98	100	101	102	103	52	53	53	54	55	55	56
	95th	100	101	102	104	105	106	107	56	57	57	58	59	59	60
	99th	108	108	109	111	112	113	114	64	64	65	65	66	67	67
2	50th	85	85	87	88	89	91	91	43	44	44	45	46	46	47
	90th	98	99	100	101	103	104	105	57	58	58	59	60	61	61
	95th	102	103	104	105	107	108	109	61	62	62	63	64	65	65
	99th	109	110	111	112	114	115	116	69	69	70	70	71	72	72
3	50th	86	87	88	89	91	92	93	47	48	48	49	50	50	51
	90th	100	100	102	103	104	106	106	61	62	62	63	64	64	65
	95th	104	104	105	107	108	109	110	65	66	66	67	68	68	69
	99th	111	111	113	114	115	116	117	73	73	74	74	75	76	76
4	50th	88	88	90	91	92	94	94	50	50	51	52	52	53	54
	90th	101	102	103	104	106	107	108	64	64	65	66	67	67	68
	95th	105	106	107	108	110	111	112	68	68	69	70	71	71	72
	99th	112	113	114	115	117	118	119	76	76	76	77	78	79	79
5	50th	89	90	91	93	94	95	96	52	53	53	54	55	55	56
	90th	103	103	105	106	107	109	109	66	67	67	68	69	69	70
	95th	107	107	108	110	111	112	113	70	71	71	72	73	73	74
	99th	114	114	116	117	118	120	120	78	78	79	79	80	81	81
6	50th	91	92	93	94	96	97	98	54	54	55	56	56	57	58
	90th	104	105	106	108	109	110	111	68	68	69	70	70	71	72
	95th	108	109	110	111	113	114	115	72	72	73	74	74	75	76
	99th	115	116	117	119	120	121	122	80	80	80	81	82	83	83
7	50th	93	93	95	96	97	99	99	55	56	56	57	58	58	59
	90th	106	107	108	109	111	112	113	69	70	70	71	72	72	73
	95th	110	111	112	113	115	116	116	73	74	74	75	76	76	77
	99th	117	118	119	120	122	123	124	81	81	82	82	83	84	84
8	50th	95	95	96	98	99	100	101	57	57	57	58	59	60	60
	90th	108	109	110	111	113	114	114	71	71	71	72	73	74	74
	95th	112	112	114	115	116	118	118	75	75	75	76	77	78	78
	99th	119	120	121	122	123	125	125	82	82	83	83	84	85	86
9	50th	96	97	98	100	101	102	103	58	58	58	59	60	61	61
	90th	110	110	112	113	114	116	116	72	72	72	73	74	75	75
	95th	114	114	115	117	118	119	120	76	76	76	77	78	79	79
	99th	121	121	123	124	125	127	127	83	83	84	84	85	86	87
10	50th	98	99	100	102	103	104	105	59	59	59	60	61	62	62
	90th	112	112	114	115	116	118	118	73	73	73	74	75	76	76
	95th	116	116	117	119	120	121	122	77	77	77	78	79	80	80
	99th	123	123	125	126	127	129	129	84	84	85	86	86	87	88

		Table 90-2. Blood Pressure Levels for the 90th and 95th Percentiles of Blood Pressure for Girls Aged 1–17 Years by Percentiles of Height, continued													

Age (Year)	BP Percentile ↓	Systolic BP (mm Hg) ← Percentile of Height →							Diastolic BP (mm Hg) ← Percentile of Height →						
		5th	10th	25th	50th	75th	90th	95th	5th	10th	25th	50th	75th	90th	95th
11	50th	100	101	102	103	105	106	107	60	60	60	61	62	63	63
	90th	114	114	116	117	118	119	120	74	74	74	75	76	77	77
	95th	118	118	119	121	122	123	124	78	78	78	79	80	81	81
	99th	125	125	126	128	129	130	131	85	85	86	87	87	88	89
12	50th	102	103	104	105	107	108	109	61	61	61	62	63	64	64
	90th	116	116	117	119	120	121	122	75	75	75	76	77	78	78
	95th	119	120	121	123	124	125	126	79	79	79	80	81	82	82
	99th	127	127	128	130	131	132	133	86	86	87	88	88	89	90
13	50th	104	105	106	107	109	110	110	62	62	62	63	64	65	65
	90th	117	118	119	121	122	123	124	76	76	76	77	78	79	79
	95th	121	122	123	124	126	127	128	80	80	80	81	82	83	83
	99th	128	129	130	132	133	134	135	87	87	88	89	89	90	91
14	50th	106	106	107	109	110	111	112	63	63	63	64	65	66	66
	90th	119	120	121	122	124	125	125	77	77	77	78	79	80	80
	95th	123	123	125	126	127	129	129	81	81	81	82	83	84	84
	99th	130	131	132	133	135	136	136	88	88	89	90	90	91	92
15	50th	107	108	109	110	111	113	113	64	64	64	65	66	67	67
	90th	120	121	122	123	125	126	127	78	78	78	79	80	81	81
	95th	124	125	126	127	129	130	131	82	82	82	83	84	85	85
	99th	131	132	133	134	136	137	138	89	89	90	91	91	92	93
16	50th	108	108	110	111	112	114	114	64	64	65	66	66	67	68
	90th	121	122	123	124	126	127	128	78	78	79	80	81	81	82
	95th	125	126	127	128	130	131	132	82	82	83	84	85	85	86
	99th	132	133	134	135	137	138	139	90	90	90	91	92	93	93
17	50th	108	109	110	111	113	114	115	64	65	65	66	67	67	68
	90th	122	122	123	125	126	127	128	78	79	79	80	81	81	82
	95th	125	126	127	129	130	131	132	82	83	83	84	85	85	86
	99th	133	133	134	136	137	138	139	90	90	91	91	92	93	93

Abbreviation: BP, blood pressure.

*The 90th percentile is 1.28 SD, 95th percentile is 1.645 SD, and the 99th percentile is 2.326 SD over the mean.

There are 2 different situations where casual BP measurements in the office setting can significantly differ from ABP or home BP readings: (1) when office BP readings are higher, which is known as white-coat hypertension, and (2) when they are lower, which is called masked hypertension. The prevalence and long-term significance of these 2 types of hypertension is still unclear. White-coat hypertension is usually considered a benign finding. Some studies, however, show significant association between white-coat hypertension and increased left ventricular mass index, but long-term cardiac outcome has not been studied in this population yet. Children with masked hypertension are twice as likely to have a family history of hypertension. If they also have a high pulse rate and body mass index, their risk of developing cardiovascular disorders is increased. It is a significant challenge for pediatricians to diagnose these 2 conditions, particularly masked hypertension, in which BP is increased only when away from the usual office or clinic settings. These findings also raise a question regarding which children need home BP monitoring or ABP monitoring to detect these conditions. In the future, we may better understand white-coat and masked hypertension and whether there are long-term sequelae of these conditions.

Secondary hypertension is more likely in very young children with hypertension, those who meet the criteria for stage 2 hypertension,

Table 90-3. Definitions of Hypertension[a]	
Term	Definition
Normal blood pressure (BP)	Systolic and diastolic BPs <90th percentile for age, gender, and height
Pre-hypertension	Average systolic and/or average diastolic BP between 90th and 95th percentiles for age, gender, and height
	Any BP >120/80 mm Hg regardless of age
Stage 1 hypertension	Average systolic and/or average diastolic BPs ≥95th percentile to 5 mm above 99th percentile for age, gender, and height with measurements obtained on at least 3 occasions
Stage 2 hypertension	Average systolic and/or diastolic BP >5mm above the 99th percentile for age, gender, and height

[a]From the National High Blood Pressure Education Program Working Group on High Blood Pressure in Children and Adolescents. The fourth report on the diagnosis, evaluation, and treatment of high blood pressure in children and adolescents. *Pediatrics.* 2004;114:555–576.

and those with systemic symptoms of hypertension. The etiology of secondary hypertension varies with the age of the patient and with the nature of the hypertension (ie, whether the condition is acute or chronic). Renal abnormalities account for 70% to 80% of secondary hypertension in children. The pathogenesis of the hypertension may be related to either an increase in extracellular fluid volume (eg, acute glomerulonephritis or chronic renal failure), an increase in renin-angiotensin II activity (eg, renal artery stenosis, renin-producing tumor, pheochrmocytoma or reflux nephropathy), or a combination of both mechanisms (eg, a patient with chronic renal failure caused by reflux nephropathy).

Differential Diagnosis

A reasonable effort should be made to identify the cause of hypertension in all young children who are diagnosed with hypertension because only 30% of them are likely to have essential hypertension (see Boxes 90-1 and 90-2). In older children and adolescents with mildly elevated BPs, primary hypertension is the most likely diagnosis, but must remain a diagnosis of exclusion. The cause of hypertension is often obvious from a detailed history, complete examination, and simple laboratory tests. However, extensive evaluation is sometimes necessary to determine the etiology of hypertension, especially in cases of renovascular hypertension.

Evaluation

When a child is identified as having an elevated BP on any occasion, the finding should be verified with at least 2 additional measurements. The physician should also verify that an appropriately sized cuff is being used to take the measurements and that efforts have been made to put the child at ease. Many children develop mild increases of BP (which can extend into the hypertensive range) when they visit a doctor's office because of anxiety or apprehension ("white coat hypertension"). Sometimes 24-hour ABP readings are necessary

Box 90-1. Causes of Acute or Intermittent Increases in Blood Pressure in Children

Renal Causes
- Acute glomerulonephritis
- Hemolytic uremic syndrome
- Henoch-Schönlein purpura nephritis
- Renal trauma
- Renal artery or vein thrombosis
- After renal biopsy
- Acute obstructive uropathy
- Post-genitourinary surgery
- Blood transfusions in patients with renal failure
- After kidney transplant or with transplant rejection

Drug-Induced Causes
- Corticosteroids
- Amphetamine overdose
- Phencyclidine overdose
- Cocaine overdose
- Anabolic steroids
- Oral contraceptives
- Excessive erythropoietin use in patients with end-stage renal disease
- Cyclosporine A and tacrolimus

Central Nervous System Causes
- Increased intracranial pressure (eg, subdural hematoma, meningitis, tumors)
- Encephalitis
- Poliomyelitis
- Guillain-Barré syndrome
- Porphyria
- Familial dysautonomia

Miscellaneous Causes
- Wrong blood pressure cuff size
- Anxiety, apprehension (white coat hypertension)
- Pain
- Fractures
- Orthopedic procedures (especially leg lengthening and those requiring traction)
- Burns
- Leukemia
- Stevens-Johnson syndrome
- Bacterial endocarditis
- Hypernatremia
- Hypercalcemia
- Heavy metal poisoning

to confirm whether hypertension is present. An isolated finding of a mild increase in BP with normal subsequent readings does not indicate hypertension. Once hypertension is confirmed, a detailed history, complete physical examination, and appropriate laboratory evaluation should be performed.

Box 90-2. Causes of Chronic Hypertension in Children

Renal
- Scarred kidney: due to pyelonephritis and/or vesicoureteral reflux nephropathy
- Chronic glomerulonephritis
- Connective tissue disease: systemic lupus erythematosus, Henoch-Schönlein purpura
- Hydronephrosis
- Congenital dysplastic kidneys, multicystic kidney
- Polycystic kidney disease
- Solitary renal cyst
- Tumors: Wilms, pericytoma (renin-producing tumor)

Renal Vascular Lesions
- Renal artery stenosis (fibromuscular dysplasia)
- Renal artery thrombosis (especially in the newborn following umbilical artery catheterization)
- Renal vein thrombosis
- Renal artery lesions with neurofibromatosis, tuberous sclerosis

Other Vascular Lesions
- Coarctation of aorta: thoracic, abdominal
- Polyarteritis nodosa and other vasculitides

Endocrine
- Corticosteroid treatment
- Neuroblastoma or other neural crest tumors
- Pheochromocytoma
- Congenital adrenal hyperplasia with 11β- or 17α-hydroxylase deficiency
- 11β-hydroxysteroid dehydrogenase deficiency
- Liddle syndrome
- Primary hyperaldosteronism
- Dexamethasone-suppressible hyperaldosteronism
- Hyperthyroidism
- Hyperparathyroidism
- Cushing syndrome

Central Nervous System
- Intracranial hemorrhage
- Intracranial mass
- Sleep apnea/disordered breathing

Essential (Primary) Hypertension

As stated earlier ABP monitoring may be indicated in the evaluation of hypertension in select children where BP readings are consistently increased in the physician's office but the history suggests severe anxiety associated with the visit. Ambulatory BP monitoring may also help in identifying masked hypertension or a pre-hypertensive state in children by detecting the usual nocturnal dips in the BP. Because ABP monitoring is expensive, home BP monitoring twice a day in adults has been shown to be as effective as ABP monitoring, and it is currently used by many practitioners. Therefore, home or school BP monitoring should be considered as an alternative by pediatricians who have no access to ABP devices.

History

Information should be obtained about the child's symptoms that may be associated with hypertension, such as headaches and visual difficulties (Questions Box). Inquiry should also be made about the child's history of renal disease, especially previous UTIs, unexplained fevers during infancy and early childhood, edema, hematuria, enuresis or nocturia, duration of gestation, birth weight, and the use of umbilical artery catheterization during the newborn period. Information regarding the child's physical growth; BP recordings during previous physical examinations; eating habits, especially salt intake; use of drugs, especially illicit drugs; and the family's history of hypertension and renal disease should be obtained.

Physical Examination

A thorough examination is essential for determining the etiology of hypertension and the extent of target organ damage caused by hypertension. Poor physical growth or short stature may indicate the presence of an underlying condition, such as Turner syndrome or chronic renal disease with or without renal failure; it may also be the consequence of long-standing severe hypertension alone. Fundus examination is essential to determine if hypertension has been severe and chronic leading to arterial changes, exudate, hemorrhages, and/or papilledema. Tachycardia may signify heart failure or thyrotoxicosis. The child's pulses should be felt in both the upper and lower extremities, and the BP should be measured in all 4 extremities to evaluate for coarctation of the aorta and other vascular lesions. A heart murmur may also be present in patients with coarctation of the aorta. Some patients may present in heart failure secondary to chronic severe hypertension or renal disease with fluid retention. The abdomen should be carefully examined for presence of masses caused by cystic kidneys, Wilms tumor, or neuroblastoma and for tenderness, especially in the costovertebral angle (CVA). Bruits sometimes may be heard over the CVA in patients with renal artery stenosis. Presence of café-au-lait spots or depigmented spots on the skin may signify hypertension secondary to neurofibromatosis or tuberous sclerosis, respectively.

Questions

Hypertension

- Does the child have any symptoms associated with hypertension (eg, headache, dizziness, nosebleed, visual difficulty, or shortness of breath)?
- Have blood pressure readings been taken during previous routine physical examinations?
- Has the child had any hematuria, generalized swelling of the body (edema), enuresis (nocturia), burning urination, previous urinary tract infection, or other kidney problems?
- How much salt does the child take? Does he or she love to put extra salt on most foods and frequently like to eat salty foods?
- How has the child been growing?
- Is there a history of use of illicit drugs or oral contraceptives?
- Is there a family history of hypertension or renal disease?

Laboratory Tests

The extent of laboratory evaluation depends on the clinical findings, the nature of the hypertension (eg, stage 1 or stage 2, acute or chronic), and whether an etiology is apparent or obscure. This can be done in 3 different phases in order to minimize unnecessary cost and discomfort to patient. Box 90-3 outlines suggested laboratory workups for patients with stage 1 or stage 2 hypertension.

Presence of hematuria, heavy proteinuria, pyuria, and/or elevated blood urea nitrogen or plasma creatinine would clearly imply a renal disorder as the cause of hypertension and require an appropriate renal evaluation. A kidney biopsy should be performed to diagnose glomerulonephritis, and radiographic investigations, such as ultrasound and nuclear medicine scans, can help identify scarred kidneys, hydronephrosis, cystic kidneys, or tumors.

The presence of electrolyte abnormalities, such as hypokalemia, hypochloremia, or metabolic alkalosis, would indicate the presence of an increased mineralocorticoid hormone either on a primary basis (primary hyperaldosteronism, adrenogenital syndrome with 11β- or 17α-hydroxylase deficiency, Liddle syndrome, 11β-hydroxysteroid dehydrogenase deficiency, etc) or secondary basis to increased renin activity in renovascular hypertension, renin-producing tumor, or reflux nephropathy; these values would also indicate a need to measure plasma renin activity and urinary or plasma aldosterone levels. Endocrine-based causes of hypertension in children are uncommon, and tests like plasma or urinary fractionated metanephrines and catecholamines, plasma cortisol, thyroid-stimulating hormone, and triiodothyronine are measured on an individual basis depending on the clinical evaluation of the patient to rule out neuroendocrine tumors, Cushing syndrome/disease, or hyperthyroidism, respectively.

Imaging Studies

Although electrocardiograms and chest radiographs are often requested to evaluate the effects of hypertension on the heart, in most instances they are normal until the patient enters the late stages of severe hypertension. Echocardiography is now the recommended primary tool for assessing for the presence of target organ damage and, according to the AAP guidelines, is included as part of the initial evaluation of patients with hypertension. In several studies, left ventricular hypertrophy is present even in children with untreated mild, white-coat or masked hypertension, especially when they are overweight. Newer recommendations also include obtaining sleep studies in overweight patients to evaluate for obstructive sleep apnea, which can contribute to the development of hypertension and left ventricular hypertrophy. Evidence suggests that with appropriate treatment to improve sleep apnea, BP normalizes and end-organ damage is prevented.

If the history, physical examination, and initial investigation do not reveal the etiology of severe hypertension in a young child, renovascular disease should be investigated with a renal Doppler ultrasound, enalapril- or captopril-enhanced iodine-131 mercaptoacetyl triglycine renal scan, renal vein renin measurements, or selective renal arteriography (sometimes magnetic resonance imaging angiography may be used as a substitute) (Box 90-3). However, in a patient with suspected renal artery narrowing, interventional renal angiography is the gold standard that can be done not only for diagnostic evaluation but also for therapeutic purposes if these patients require angioplasty or stent placement during the study.

Management

As previously stated, an effort should be made to identify a remediable cause in all children diagnosed with hypertension so that an appropriate medical or surgical treatment can be offered.

Patients with stage 1 hypertension can be initially managed with non-pharmacologic measures unless the patient is symptomatic or has significant cardiovascular risk factors, such as diabetes or hyperlipidemia, and a strong family history of hypertension, or stroke, or myocardial infarction in young age. These strategies include supportive care, reduction in sodium intake to about 80 to 100 mEq/d, weight reduction if the child is obese, and biofeedback. The 2004 report also recommends treating obstructive sleep apnea if present. If after a 3- to 6-month observation period BP remains persistently elevated, drug treatment should be initiated and a decision should be made whether the child needs a more thorough laboratory evaluation. Drug therapy may begin with a β-blocker (eg, atenolol), a calcium channel blocker (eg, amlodipine or isradipine), an angiotensin converting enzyme (ACE) inhibitor (eg, enalapril), an angiotensin II blocker (eg, losartan), or a diuretic (eg, hydrochlorothiazide).

Box 90-3. Laboratory and Radiologic Evaluation of Hypertension

Phase 1: Initial Evaluation (to identify common causes of hypertension and evaluate for cardiac end-organ damage)

1. Urinalysis (urine culture if indicated)
2. Complete blood cell count, serum electrolytes, blood urea nitrogen, and creatinine; lipid profile for obese patients
3. Urine toxicology screening in adolescent children
4. Echocardiography

Phase II: More Extensive Evaluation (to rule out rare causes of hypertension)

1. Liver profile, calcium, phosphorus, and PTH
2. Plasma renin activity and plasma aldosterone, cortisol, and TSH
3. Plasma fractionated catecholamines and metanephrines
4. 24-hour urine for creatinine, catecholamines, metanephrines, VMA, HVA, and aldosterone (if plasma aldosterone is high)
5. Renal Doppler ultrasonography
6. Enalapril- or captopril-enhanced iodine-131 MAG3 renal scan
7. Renal arteriography (selective if necessary)

Phase III: To Identify Specific Etiologies (studies done mostly by specialists)

1. Diuretic renal scan, DMSA scan, or voiding nuclear cystogram
2. Renal biopsy
3. Specific imaging studies, including nuclear scan to rule out pheochromocytoma or neuroblastoma
4. Other endocrine, neurology, or cardiology studies

Abbreviations: DMSA, 99mTc dimercaptosuccinic acid; MAG3, mercaptoacetyl triglycine; PTH, parathyroid hormone; TSH, thyroid stimulating hormone; VMA, vanillylmandelic acid.

A child can have more than one risk factor that becomes important when instituting a treatment plan. For example, an obese child with a family history of hypertension may also have chronic kidney disease as well as other risk factors contributing to the development of hypertension and/or end-organ damage. Therefore, management should be targeted not only toward aggressive control of BP using medications appropriate for a patient with kidney disease, but also recommendations for weight reduction, dietary modifications, and increased physical activity. If a patient smokes cigarettes, cessation of smoking is essential as well.

Patients with stage 2 hypertension may require combination therapy or the use of additional drugs, such as α-blockers (eg, prazosin), combined α-β–blockers (eg, labetalol), peripheral vasodilators (eg, hydralazine, minoxidil), or centrally acting drugs (eg, clonidine). The use of one or more of these drugs controls the BP in most patients within a satisfactory range and has a limited number of side effects. Patients with renal artery stenosis can be successfully treated with balloon dilatation of the stenosis or placing a stent. If this procedure is unsuccessful or restenosis occurs, surgical correction of the stenosis is usually successful.

Hypertensive emergencies require immediate and rapid intervention with intravenous (IV) medications such as labetalol, nicardipine, or sodium nitroprusside. Hypertensive urgencies may be treated initially with either the above IV medications or oral labetalol or an ACE inhibitor. In both cases, the aim is to lower the BP by about 20% to 25% of the presenting values in the first 8 hours. Over the following days to weeks, BP can gradually be controlled to come within normal values for age.

Prognosis

The long-term outcome of hypertension in children depends on the underlying etiology. In children with severe hypertension, BP control improves growth and overall well-being. The very long-term (40–50 years) prognosis for children with persistent, mild essential hypertension is largely unknown; however, adequate BP control should prolong life and reduce cardiovascular, CNS, renal, and retinal morbidity. In untreated or poorly controlled hypertension the prognosis is poor, especially in combination with obesity and hyperlipidemia, where hypertension is linked with severe cardiovascular morbidity and mortality in adults.

Prevention

While there are no specific predictors for the development of hypertension later in life, it is likely that early childhood health plays a role. Children who are small at birth and undergo rapid catch-up growth seem to have a higher incidence of both obesity and hypertension later in life, while breastfed infants have a slower catch-up rate and subsequently have lower rates of hypertension as adults. As a result, it has been postulated that encouraging breastfeeding may have a protective effect. In addition, limiting intake of sodium and caffeine may reduce rates of hypertension in adolescents. Of course, programs aimed at preventing childhood obesity will likely prevent hypertension as well.

CASE RESOLUTION

Because of the elevated BP and evidence of end-organ dysfunction, the case presented is a clear-cut hypertensive emergency. The history of previous UTI and the laboratory findings of proteinuria and elevated plasma creatinine suggest chronic pyelonephritis with scarred kidneys secondary to vesicoureteral reflux and chronic renal failure. The elevated creatinine also suggests that both kidneys are affected either by the primary process or as a consequence of severe hypertension. After controlling the initial severe increase in BP, a renal Doppler ultrasound is the appropriate test to determine the kidney size, the extent of kidney damage, and possibly the etiology.

Selected References

Collins RT, Alpert BS. Pre-hypertension and hypertension in pediatrics: don't let the statistics hide the pathology. *J Pediatr.* 2009;155:165–169

Constantine E, Linakis J. The assessment and management of hypertensive emergencies and urgencies in children. *Pediatr Emerg Care.* 2005;21:391–396

Flynn J. Hypertension in childhood and adolescence. In: Kaplan NM, ed. *Clinical Hypertension.* 9th ed. Philadelphia, PA: Lippincott, Williams & Wilkins Company; 2006;465–485

Flynn JT. Neonatal hypertension: diagnosis and management. *Pediatr Nephrol.* 2000;14:332–341

Garin EH and Araya CE. Treatment of systemic hypertension in children and adolescents. *Curr Opin Pediatr.* 2009;21:600–604

Harshfield GA, Alpert BS, Pulliam DA, Somes GW, Wilson DK. Ambulatory blood pressure recordings in children and adolescents. *Pediatrics.* 1994;94 (2 pt 1):180–184

Lande MB, Meagher CC, Fisher GS, Belani P, Wang H, Rashid M. Left ventricular mass index in children with hypertension. *J Pediatr.* 2008;153:50–54

National High Blood Pressure Education Program Working Group on High Blood Pressure in Children and Adolescents. The fourth report on the diagnosis, evaluation, and treatment of high blood pressure in children and adolescents. *Pediatrics.* 2004;114:555–576

Sorof JM, Lai D, Turner J, Poffenbarger T, Portman RJ. Overweight, ethnicity, and the prevalence of hypertension in school-aged children. *Pediatrics.* 2004;113:475–482

Genitourinary Disorders

CHAPTER 91

Ambiguous Genitalia

Jennifer K. Yee, MD, and Catherine S. Mao, MD

CASE STUDY

A term infant is being evaluated in the newborn nursery. The mother received prenatal care from the 8th week of gestation, reportedly had no problems during the pregnancy, and took no medications except prenatal vitamins with iron. She specifically denies taking any progesterone-containing drugs. Her previous pregnancy was uneventful, and her 3-year-old son is healthy.

On physical examination, the infant is active and alert, with normal vital signs. Aside from a minimum amount of breast tissue bilaterally, the physical examination is unremarkable, except for the genitalia. The labioscrotal folds are swollen bilaterally with slight hyperpigmentation and mild rugae. No masses are palpable in the labioscrotal folds. The clitoris/phallus is 1.5 cm in length. Labioscrotal fusion is present, with a very small opening at the anterior aspect. The urethra cannot be visualized.

Questions

1. What conditions should be considered in newborns with ambiguous genitalia?
2. What should families of such infants be told regarding the gender of the newborns?
3. What key historical information should be obtained from families of such newborns?
4. What laboratory studies must be obtained to aid in the diagnosis?
5. What psychosocial issues should be addressed with families while infants are in the newborn nursery?

Ambiguous genitalia result from disorders of sex development (DSD) in newborns and are classified according to the chromosomal status and gonads present. This standard classification, using newer nomenclature with previously used nomenclature in parentheses, includes 46XX DSD (female pseudohermaphroditism) and 46XY DSD (male pseudohermaphroditism), ovotesticular DSD (true hermaphroditism), and 46XX testicular DSD or 46XY gonadal dysgenesis (complete or mixed gonadal dysgenesis). Gonadal dysgenesis in 45XO and 46XX individuals do not present with ambiguous genitalia but are also classified as DSD.

A multidisciplinary health care team should be involved in the care of infants with ambiguous genitalia. In addition to the general pediatrician, the nurses, social workers, neonatologists, pediatric endocrinologists, geneticists, and surgeons are all significant members of the team. The role of primary care physicians, however, cannot be underestimated because they are always involved in the initial evaluations of the newborns and often have already established relationships with the families.

Epidemiology

The prevalence of ambiguous genitalia in newborns is approximately 1:3,000 to 1:4,000 live births. 46XX DSD is characterized by female chromosomes (46XX), normal ovaries and müllerian structures, and virilized external genitalia. The most common DSD, 46XX DSD, is most often caused by congenital adrenal hyperplasia (CAH). Neonatal screening studies suggest that the incidence of CAH is 1:5,000 to 1:15,000.

46XY DSD occurs in genetic males (46XY) who have testes but insufficient masculinization of the external genitalia. This disorder most commonly results from androgen insensitivity. Ovotesticular DSD is a rare condition in which both ovarian and testicular tissues are present. Seventy percent to 80% of affected individuals have the 46XX karyotype, and the morphology of the external genitalia varies widely.

The mixed variant of 46XY gonadal dysgenesis is characterized by one testis and an abnormal streak gonad. Reports indicate that this condition is the second most common form of ambiguous genitalia. Affected newborns often have chromosomal mosaicism (45X/46XY).

Clinical Presentation

Variability in the phenotypic as well as clinical presentation of these disorders is considerable (Dx Box). The newborn with ambiguous genitalia may have an enlarged clitoris or small phallus and varying degrees of labioscrotal fusion. Signs of virilization in the female infant might include hyperpigmented labia and the presence of labial rugae. Other findings suggestive of a 46XX DSD are perineal hypospadias or an inguinal hernia. More dramatic presentations, such as severe dehydration and shock in a neonate, are associated with CAH of the salt-wasting form. Females with gonadal dysgenesis often present in adolescence with primary amenorrhea (see Chapter 98). Turner syndrome (45XO) is a common cause of gonadal dysgenesis and may present with additional clinical features, but 46XX pure gonadal dysgenesis is a distinct entity.

Dx Ambiguous Genitalia

- Indeterminate or ambiguous genitalia
- Enlarged clitoris or small phallus
- Hyperpigmented, rugated labia majora that may be fused
- Blind-ending or completely absent vaginal pouch
- Phenotypic male neonate with hypospadias and/or bilateral cryptorchidism
- Phenotypic female neonate with an inguinal hernia or mass

Pathophysiology

In order to appropriately evaluate and interpret laboratory results of neonates with ambiguous genitalia, it is important to understand the physiology of sexual differentiation and how deviations from this process lead to DSD.

Normal Sexual Differentiation

Normally, before embryos are 6 weeks old, undifferentiated bilateral gonads into which germ cells migrate from the yolk sac have developed. Both wolffian and müllerian duct systems are present at this time, making the embryonic gonads of males and females indistinguishable.

If a Y chromosome is present, a testes-determining factor (known as the sex determining region of the Y chromosome, or SRY) induces differentiation of these gonads into testes, thus blocking female development. This process involves the formation of seminiferous tubules that surround the germ cells. Leydig cells begin to produce testosterone, which in turn acts on the wolffian duct to result in the male internal genitalia: vas deferens, epididymis, and seminal vesicles. Concurrently, regression of the müllerian ducts occurs secondary to Sertoli cell production of anti-müllerian hormone (AMH), also called müllerian-inhibiting substance. For normal male external genitalia to form, testosterone must be converted to dihydrotestosterone (DHT) via 5 α-reductase. Dihydrotestosterone then combines with a specific androgen receptor, which allows formation of the phallus and scrotum from the previously undifferentiated external genitalia. The process primarily involves growth and fusion. Later in gestation, the testes migrate into the scrotum.

For the undifferentiated gonads to develop into female organs, the Y chromosome must be absent and 2 intact and normal functioning X chromosomes must be present. Because androgens are not produced and there is no AMH, the wolffian duct degenerates, and the müllerian duct develops into the internal female structures: fallopian tubes, uterus, and upper vagina. Fusion of undifferentiated external genitalia does not occur in the absence of DHT, so folds and swellings become the labia, and the genital tubercle becomes the clitoris. Female differentiation was previously believed to be the default development in the absence of SRY, but recent studies support the existence of female determining factors as well.

Development of Ambiguous Genitalia

Congenital adrenal hyperplasia is the most common cause of virilization of the female and is an autosomal recessively inherited defect. Congenital adrenal hyperplasia is the result of an enzymatic deficiency in the pathway for synthesis of cortisol and aldosterone from cholesterol. The most common of these enzymatic defects is 21α-hydroxylase deficiency. Other less common defects are 11β-hydroxylase deficiency and 3β-hydroxysteroid dehydrogenase deficiency. Lipoid adrenal hyperplasia results from a defect in the steroidogenic acute regulatory protein (StAR) enzyme that transports cholesterol across the mitochondrial membrane for steroid synthesis. A recently identified rare form of CAH is P450 oxidoreductase deficiency, which can be associated with Antley-Bixler syndrome. Prenatally, circulating levels of androgens are abnormally high from the overproduction of precursors in the steroid synthesis pathways. Hence, the external genitalia of the fetus, which are controlled by androgens, are virilized in the female. Internal female organs, however, are normal, because their development is not influenced by androgens. Males may exhibit hyperpigmentation and rugosity, but otherwise have normal external genitalia.

The salt-wasting form of 21α-hydroxylase deficiency is found in approximately two-thirds of patients with classic CAH. As a result of low levels of aldosterone, sodium resorption in the renal tubules is reduced, leading to hyponatremia and hyperkalemia. If this salt-wasting condition goes undiagnosed and untreated, shock and death may result in the first few weeks of life. Newborn screening programs are currently in place in all 50 United States. These programs screen for elevated 17α-hydroxyprogesterone, targeting identification of patients with 21α-hydroxylase deficiency, and are less sensitive for detection of infants with 11β-hydroxylase deficiency and 3β-hydroxysteroid dehydrogenase deficiency.

46XY DSD is secondary to insufficient testosterone production or insensitivity at the cellular level. Androgen insensitivity, the most common cause of this disorder, is the result of either an abnormality or a reduction in the number of androgen receptors. Not all affected individuals present with ambiguous genitalia at birth because the spectrum of sensitivity is broad. If the androgen receptor is completely nonfunctional or absent, the external genitalia are those of a normal female (complete testicular feminization). When there is partial function of the androgen receptor, genital ambiguity does occur. This is an X-linked condition so that only 46XY individuals are affected.

Other causes of 46XY DSD are (1) inadequate testosterone production secondary to low levels of fetal gonadotropins; (2) defects in testosterone synthesis from enzyme deficiencies or disruption of electron transport; (3) failure to convert testosterone to DHT as a result of 5α-reductase deficiency; (4) deficient müllerian duct–inhibiting substance, which can be autosomal recessive or X-linked recessive; and (5) intrauterine loss of both testes secondary to torsion or another prenatal event. The defect in testosterone synthesis resulting in 46XY DSD include congenital adrenal hyperplasia due to deficiencies of StAR, P450scc, 3-β-hydroxysteroid dehydrogenase, 17α-hydroxylase, and P450 oxidoreductase.

Although most causes of ambiguous genitalia are related to chromosomal abnormalities and inherited enzymatic defects, exogenous sources of hormones can affect the differentiation of sexual organs. In most cases, the effect is minimal, and no ambiguity develops. Masculinized female external genitalia can occur, however, depending on the timing and duration of prenatal exposure to androgens or other virilizing drugs. Currently the most commonly used androgens are probably anabolic steroids. An infant may even be exposed prenatally through transdermal passage to the mother from a family member using androgen creams. An adrenal tumor or poorly controlled CAH in the mother will also lead to virilization of the female fetus. Birth control pills do not contain sufficient androgens to cause a problem.

Differential Diagnosis

The differential diagnosis of ambiguous genitalia depends on the classification of the DSD (Table 91-1). Some causes of this condition can be life-threatening and therefore must be recognized immediately (eg, salt-wasting CAH).

Table 91-1. Classification and Causes of Ambiguous Genitalia in the Newborn

Disorder	Causes
46XX DSD	Congenital adrenal hyperplasia
	Maternal androgen ingestion
	Maternal virilizing hormones
	Idiopathic, associated with dysmorphic syndromes
46XY DSD	Biochemical defects in testosterone biosynthesis (enzyme deficiencies)
	Androgen insensitivity (complete or partial receptor defects)
	5α-reductase deficiency
	Persistent müllerian duct syndrome
	Gonadotropic failure
	Dysgenetic testes
	Bilateral vanishing testes syndrome
	Idiopathic, associated with dysmorphic syndromes
Ovotesticular DSD	Chimerism
46XX testicular DSD or 46XY complete gonadal dysgenesis	Chromosomal mosaicism

Abbreviation: DSD, disorders of sex development.

Evaluation

History

The general obstetric history should be reviewed, although it may not be helpful in all cases. Probably the most important source of information on family history can be derived from family pedigrees (Questions Box). The mother of affected infants should be interviewed thoroughly for any clinical findings that might suggest the mother as the source of androgens. Undiagnosed chromosomal disorders, consanguinity, and recurrent medical conditions may be established or inferred from the family background.

Questions

Ambiguous Genitalia

- Did the mother take any medications containing estrogen, progestins, or androgens during the pregnancy? Did she use any other virilizing drugs, such as danazol, during pregnancy?
- Was the mother in contact with anyone using hormonal creams or gels?
- Does the mother have poorly controlled congenital adrenal hyperplasia or an adrenal tumor? Does the mother have any virilizing symptoms that suggest she should undergo an evaluation for the above conditions?
- What is the mother's prior obstetric history?
- Did she have any problems with any previous pregnancies?
- Is there a history of any unexplained neonatal deaths, particularly in male offspring?
- Are her other children growing and developing normally?
- Is there a family history of ambiguous genitalia, including microphallus, hypospadias, and cryptorchidism?
- Is there a family history of sterility, female hirsutism, or amenorrhea?
- Are the parents or other family members consanguineous?

Physical Examination

A complete physical examination of newborns must be performed in the nursery, in addition to a detailed assessment of the genitalia. In particular, the presence of dysmorphic features (eg, microcephaly, low-set ears, micrognathia), which suggests the presence of a chromosomal abnormality, should be appreciated. The areola should be examined for any evidence of hyperpigmentation, and the inguinal area should be palpated for any masses or hernias.

A thorough genital examination should then be performed. The appearance and size of the labioscrotal folds should be noted in terms of pigmentation, presence of rugae, and size. Physicians should keep in mind that normal female labia majora may not completely cover the labia minora, and that the labia may be extremely underdeveloped in premature infants. Practitioners should determine whether any masses are palpable in what appear to be the labia and whether the testes are palpable in what appears to be the scrotum. The size of the phallus/clitoris should be measured; a normal stretched phallus is at least 2.5 cm long, whereas a normal clitoris should not exceed 1 cm in term infants. The labioscrotal folds should then be spread apart to look for a vaginal introitus. The presence of posterior labioscrotal fusion, which may preclude this, confirms the suspicion of indeterminate genitalia. The clitoral index (product of clitoral transverse and sagittal dimensions) and the anogenital distance can be determined by an experienced clinician. Limited data on these measurements in normal children is available in the literature. Finally, the location of a urethral meatus should be noted, because if hypospadias and cryptorchidism occur together, the chance of a DSD disorder is approximately 50%. A rectal examination may help detect the presence of a uterus or prostate but may be difficult.

Laboratory Tests

The most important study to obtain is a karyotype, which can be performed in 24 to 48 hours by many laboratories. Examination of Barr bodies in a buccal smear is not recommended because this test is unreliable. In addition, serum electrolytes should be ordered in the nursery and monitored closely if CAH is suspected. A serum 17α-hydroxyprogesterone level is mandatory in evaluation for CAH. Other intermediate metabolites, such as 11-deoxycortisol, androstenedione, dehydroepiandrosterone sulfate, and sex steroids (eg, testosterone and dihydrotestosterone) can also be measured to evaluate for androgen excess or deficiency. Measurement of 17-ketosteroids and pregnanetriol in the urine may provide supportive data in newborns with ambiguous genitalia, especially in newborns whose gonads are not palpable.

A human chorionic gonadotropin stimulation test may be performed to measure response in testosterone production if ovotesticular DSD is suspected.

Imaging Studies

Pelvic ultrasonography is effective in determining if müllerian structures are present, but this technique is not as useful for locating the gonads. If the gonads are not palpable, magnetic resonance imaging of the pelvis may be considered. Genitography can aid in visualizing the duct structures under fluoroscopy.

Management

An interdisciplinary team consisting of a pediatrician, pediatric endocrinologist, medical geneticist, urologist, social worker, and psychologist or psychiatrist should be involved in the care of infants with ambiguous genitalia. All aspects of treatment can then be addressed in an efficient and comprehensive manner. A consensus statement regarding management of infants with DSD and proposed ethical guidelines for management are available (see Selected References).

Initial Phase: Delivery Room and Newborn Nursery

If the gender of the newborn is uncertain, it should not be assigned in the delivery room. Parents and nursing staff should be notified immediately of the ambiguity, and a unisex name should be assigned such as "Baby Smith" instead of "Baby Boy Smith" or "Baby Girl Smith." Hospital name plates should also reflect a gender neutral status in wording and in color. Physicians should congratulate the parents on the birth of their child, then inform them of the genital ambiguity. Physicians should then reassure parents that they will determine the baby's gender as soon as possible, but that additional tests would be necessary to find out. Parents should be encouraged not to speculate on the gender of the infant in the meantime.

During the initial hours after birth, parents may have difficulty comprehending the condition. An open line of communication must be maintained with the family, however, even while waiting for test results. Parents should be assured that gender assignment will be made as soon as possible and that more information will follow with test results. Gender assignment can potentially be made within 3 to 5 days or even earlier in some institutions because most preliminary laboratory results are reported in 24 to 48 hours. However, some cases may require more extensive workup, such as a trial of testosterone in partial androgen insensitivity, so gender assignment in these infants may take more time. The interval of time to gender assignment, therefore, must be individualized. Necessary radiographic studies should be ordered as soon as possible.

Intermediate Phase: Psychological Issues

Several psychological issues should be addressed at the time of diagnosis. Alleviation of parental anxiety regarding the cause of the condition should be the priority; general questions can also be answered. For example, parents may be unclear about what to tell others about the gender of the infant and find this process very awkward. In addition, parents should be educated about the normal sexual differentiation. Pediatricians must emphasize that during the first 6 to 8 weeks of gestation, sexual organs are undifferentiated. Ambiguous genitalia should be explained as overdevelopment or underdevelopment rather than as freaky or highly unusual. For parental perspective, genital ambiguity can be compared to another type of birth defect, such as a cardiac septal defect.

Primary care physicians must also assess parents' level of sophistication and their cultural and religious beliefs about gender identity and sexuality. The gender preference for newborn infants should be addressed. Were the parents hoping for a boy or girl? Do they feel strongly about one gender? The medical team can also help families establish a plan for newborns regarding what they want to tell the extended family and in what detail they want to disclose the information. After the initial meeting and while awaiting laboratory data, other questions regarding sexual orientation, puberty, fertility, and self-esteem may arise.

Final Phase: Gender Assignment

After the karyotype is confirmed and the type of DSD has been considered, team members should meet with families to discuss gender assignment before discharge from the hospital. Traditionally, gender assignment was based on size of the phallus, potential response to androgen stimulation, and potential for fertility. More recently, additional factors have been recognized as important in gender assignment, including in utero brain exposure to androgens and likely adult gender identity, quality of sexual function with or without surgery, and psychosocial risk for patient and family in the event of gender dysphoria. Parents must be involved in this decision and must agree with the final outcome. Some investigators strongly believe that gender reassignment and genital surgery should be discussed with the patient at a later date rather than assigned during the neonatal period. Such an approach involves consistent counseling for the patient, open discussion among the family, and a primary care physician willing to work diligently with both the patient and the family. Support groups should also be offered regardless of the decision regarding gender reassignment.

Detailed information should be given once again regarding the origin of the condition. The timing and nature of any future hormonal treatment and surgical procedures should be addressed as well. Parents should be urged to move beyond the issue of ambiguous genitalia once a decision regarding gender has been made. They must then deal with activities such as birth announcements and inquiries regarding gender from extended family, siblings, and babysitters. The entire medical team should offer parents encouragement concerning their parenting ability.

Treatment

Hormone replacement therapy is indicated for some newborns with ambiguous genitalia. Cortisol replacement is mandatory in infants with CAH at daily physiological doses of 10 to 20 mg/m²/d. In infants with salt-wasting or classic 21α-hydroxylase deficiency, mineralocorticoid replacement is indicated. Oral fludrocortisone should be administered at doses that suppress plasma renin activity to normal levels without causing hypertension.

Testosterone or estrogen replacement is needed at puberty in disorders in which the gonads failed to develop or were surgically removed. For disorders involving microphallus, injections of testosterone enanthate at regular intervals may be used to increase the length and width of the phallus. Recombinant human growth hormone replacement may also be considered for short stature in mixed gonadal dysgenesis.

Surgical procedures may be necessary in many cases, but can be done later in infancy. Although laparoscopy or laparotomy may be indicated for a gonadal biopsy, this is generally not needed in the neonatal period for gender assignment. A gonadectomy is indicated prophylactically in all phenotypic females with all or part of a Y chromosome because of the potential for malignant conversion of gonadoblastoma. Clitoral reduction and recession, vaginoplasty,

and labioscrotal reduction are usually performed if infants are to be raised as females. For children to be raised as males, orchiopexy, hypospadias repair, and chordee release are often indicated, but these surgical procedures may be difficult. In some specific cases, however, surgical procedures should be delayed until response to medical treatment is evaluated. For example, in CAH, clitoral size may decrease with glucocorticoid replacement.

Psychological support for the patient and family will be necessary during the child's growth and development into adulthood. Issues revolving around gender identity, gender role, and sexual orientation require ongoing discussion with the patient and the parents. Gender dissatisfaction may occur later in life.

Prognosis

The prognosis for most infants with ambiguous genitalia is excellent. Problems arise with undiagnosed CAH, which may lead to shock and death in the neonatal period if unrecognized and untreated. Otherwise, children should be able to live long, healthy lives once their families have come to grips with the diagnosis. Amenorrhea in females and sterility in males or females will need to be addressed during adolescence, at which time psychological services should be provided.

CASE RESOLUTION

In the case described at the beginning of the chapter, the infant has ambiguous genitalia. The parents should be informed immediately of this finding, and all references related to gender should be avoided. A karyotype and 17α-hydroxyprogesterone analyses should be performed immediately. In addition, serial serum electrolytes should be performed starting at 12 to 24 hours of life. The physician should then meet with the family to further discuss DSD and explain the diagnostic workup. General psychological services and information regarding support groups should also be provided.

Selected References

Blizzard RM. Intersex issues: a series of continuing conundrums. *Pediatrics.* 2002;110:616–621

Hughes IA, Fekete-Nihoul C, Thomas B, Cohen-Kettenis PT. Consequences of the ESPE/LWPES guidelines for diagnosis and treatment of disorders of sex development. *Best Pract Res Clin Endocrinol Metab.* 2007;21:351–365

Krone N, Dhir V, Ivison HE, Arlt W. Congenital adrenal hyperplasia and P450 oxidoreductase deficiency. *Clin Endocrinol (Oxf).* 2007;66:162–172

Lee PA, Houk CP, Ahmed SF, Hughes IA. Consensus statement on management of intersex disorders. *Pediatrics.* 2006;118:488–500

Mieszczak J, Houk CP, Lee PA. Assignment of the sex of rearing in the neonate with a disorder of sex development. *Curr Opin Pediatr.* 2009;21(4):541–547 Ogilvy-Stuart AL, Brain CE. Early assessment of ambiguous genitalia. *Arch Dis Child.* 2004;89:401–407

Ottolenghi C, Pelosi E, Tran J, et al. Loss of Wnt4 and Foxl2 leads to female-to-male sex reversal extending to germ cells. *Hum Mol Genet.* 2007;16(23):2795–2804

Sane K, Pescovitz OH. The clitoral index: a determination of clitoral size in normal girls and in girls with abnormal sexual development. *J Pediatr.* 1992;120:264–266

Wiesemann C, Ude-Koeller S, Sinnecker GH, Thyen U. Ethical principles and recommendations for the medical management of differences of sex development (DSD)/intersex in children and adolescents. *Eur J Pediatr.* 2010;169:671–679

Vidal I, Gorduza DB, Haraux E, et al. Surgical options in disorders of sex development (DSD) with ambiguous genitalia. *Best Pract Res Clin Endocrinol Metab.* 2010;24:311–324

Verkauskas G, Jaubert F, Lortat-Jacob S, Malan V, Thibaud E, Nihoul-Fekete C. The long-term follow-up of 33 cases of true hermaphroditism: a 40-year experience with conservative gonadal surgery. *J Urol.* 2007;177:726–731

CHAPTER 92

Inguinal Lumps and Bumps

Julie E. Noble, MD

CASE STUDY

A 2-month-old male infant presents to your office for evaluation of a lump in his right groin for 1-week duration. The lump has been coming and going, and his mother notices that it is larger when he cries. Today, the lump is prominent, and the infant seems fussy. He has been crying more often and vomited once today. His history is remarkable for having been born at 32 weeks' gestation by spontaneous vaginal delivery. Birth weight was 1,500 g, and he did well in the nursery with no respiratory complications. He was sent home at 4 weeks of age and has had no other medical problems. He breastfeeds well and has normal stools.

Physical examination reveals a well-nourished, irritable infant in no acute distress. His vital signs demonstrate mild tachycardia and temperature to 100°F (37.8°C). His abdomen is soft, and the genitourinary examination is significant for a swelling in the right inguinal area that extends into his scrotum. The mass is mildly tender and cannot be reduced. The rest of the examination is normal.

Questions

1. What are the possible causes of inguinal masses?
2. How does age affect the diagnostic possibilities?
3. How do you differentiate between acute and non-acute conditions?
4. What diagnostic modalities can help with the diagnosis?
5. What are the treatment choices for inguinal masses?
6. Are there long-term consequences?

Inguinal masses occur either from disease in normal tissue in the inguinal area or from ectopic tissue, frequently of embryological origin. A child may present with the chief complaint of an inguinal mass, and the mass may vary in position from anywhere along the inguinal canal to the scrotum or labia (Figure 92-1). Along the inguinal canal, a mass might be an enlarged **lymph node,** a **retractile testis,** an **ovary,** or a **synovial cyst.** At the inguinal ring, a mass might also be a testis or an ovary, or an inguinal hernia. In the scrotum, swelling could be due to a **hernia, hydrocele, varicocele, trauma,** or **testicular pathology.** Labial lesions could be secondary to trauma, an **ectopic ovary, mixed gonadal tissue,** an actual testis as in testicular feminization, or a **Bartholin gland cyst.** The differential diagnosis and the subsequent evaluation will vary not only according to the location of the mass and the patient's age but also with the acuity of presentation of the mass.

Epidemiology

Inguinal masses are a fairly frequent complaint in the office setting. The usual cause is an enlarged lymph node, but **hernias and hydroceles** are also common. Surgical repair of hernias and hydroceles are the most common surgical procedures performed in children. The incidence of inguinal hernias has been estimated at 1 to 4 per 100 live births. There is a 60% risk of incarceration in the first 6 months of life. For this reason surgical correction is recommended early. Hernias are present on the right side in 60% of cases, on the left in 30%, and bilateral in 10%. Of affected children, males outnumber females 4:1. Femoral and direct hernias are more common in girls. Certain conditions are associated with a higher incidence of hernias (Box 92-1). The most significant predisposing factor is prematurity, with hernias reported in 30% of infants weighing less than 1,000 g at birth.

The other common acute scrotal lesions—**testicular torsion** and **torsion of the appendix testis**—have an incidence of 1:160 in

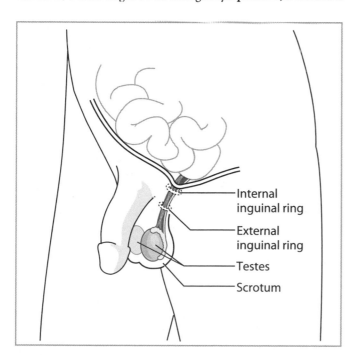

Figure 92-1. The inguinal area.

- Internal inguinal ring
- External inguinal ring
- Testes
- Scrotum

Box 92-1. Conditions Associated With Hernias	
• Abdominal wall defect	• Low birth weight
• Ascites	• Mucopolysaccharidosis
• Connective tissue disease	• Prematurity
• Cystic fibrosis	• Undescended testis
• Family history	• Urologic malformations

males. The peak incidence of testicular torsion occurs in the perinatal period and again at puberty. Torsion of the appendix testis is most likely to occur between ages 7 and 10. **Varicoceles** occur in pubertal and postpubertal males, with a fairly high incidence of up to 15%. **Testicular tumors** are rare in childhood. They occur at an incidence of 0.5 to 2.0 per 100,000 children and account for only 1% of all pediatric solid tumors. But in adolescence, testicular cancer is the most common cause of cancer in young males and may affect as many as 1 in 10,000.

Clinical Presentation

The child with an inguinal mass presents either acutely or non-acutely. In the acute presentation, the swelling occurs rapidly and is associated with pain. There may be systemic symptoms of nausea and vomiting. Inguinal pathology should be suspected in any child with abdominal pain. The involved area may be extremely tender. Non-acute masses appear more slowly. Some may be present from birth. They may come and go, especially with crying or straining. Non-acute masses usually are not tender and are not associated with systemic symptoms (Dx Box).

 Dx **Inguinal Masses**

Acute	Non-acute
• Rapid onset	• Slower onset
• Painful	• Not painful
• Tender	• May fluctuate in size
• Nausea and vomiting	• Cremasteric reflex present
• Fever	
• Overlying skin red	
• Cremasteric reflex absent	

Pathophysiology

Pathophysiological developmental features of an inguinal mass vary depending on the cause of the mass. An enlarged lymph node may result from proliferation of intrinsic lymphocytes or inflammatory infiltrate from infection (lymphadenitis). The etiology of lymphadenopathy is extensive (see Chapter 85). Any of these processes can appear in the inguinal nodes. An enlarged node can also be secondary to metastatic infiltration from another cell line and represent tumor spread.

A hydrocele develops secondary to failure of obliteration of the patent processus vaginalis during embryologic development. During the 27th to 28th weeks of gestation, the testicle, gubernaculum, and processus vaginalis descend from the peritoneum through the inguinal canal into the scrotum. The processus vaginalis begins closing prior to birth and attaches to the testis, forming the tunica vaginalis testis. The closure is complete by 1 to 2 years of age. Failure of closure results in a hydrocele (a peritoneal connection with fluid) or a hernia, with intra-abdominal contents. Either may bulge into the inguinal canal and scrotum. If the hernia cannot be reduced and abdominal contents are at risk for vascular compromise, the hernia is termed *incarcerated*. This condition is a surgical emergency.

Sometimes a parent may misinterpret a normal testicle in the process of descent as an abnormal mass. A delay in the normal descent process of the testis occurs occasionally, and the testicle may not be in the scrotum at the time of birth. Torsion of the testis after it has reached the scrotum can occur in the newborn if the testis twists on the spermatic cord. Similarly, the testicle can also twist in the pubertal period on its own vasculature within the tunica vaginalis. This is frequently secondary to a high attachment of the tunica vaginalis to the spermatic cord, allowing the testis to hang freely, like a bell clapper. Both types of torsion cause vasculature compromise and an ischemic testis.

Likewise, a vestigial remnant called the appendix testis can twist, resulting in vascular compromise of that localized part of the testis.

Pathologically, a traumatic scrotal mass is usually a hematoma, although testicular rupture may occur if the tunica albuginea is torn as a result of trauma. Testicular neoplasms in prepubertal children tend to be germ cell tumors. Yolk sac carcinoma, teratomas, and mixed germ cell tumors with infiltration of their respective cell lines are the usual diseases found.

A varicocele, another scrotal mass, is caused by increased pressure within the venous drainage of the testicle with subsequent dilatation of the veins, producing a mass. Because of the anatomy of the venous drainage, 90% of varicoceles occur on the left side.

Infections of the epididymis or testis can cause an inflammatory infiltrate and swelling. In the female, infection of Bartholin gland in the labia creates an abscess and leads to an acute, painful mass.

Differential Diagnosis

Location, acuity, and patient age aid in establishing the differential diagnosis.

Non-acute masses, which have a slow onset and are not painful, include lymphadenopathy, a retractile testis, hydrocele, hernia, varicocele, tumor, and ectopic ovary.

Acute masses that have a sudden onset and are associated with pain include epididymitis, orchitis, testicular torsion, traumatic hematoma, torsion of the appendix testis, lymphadenitis, and incarcerated hernia (Box 92-2).

Skin changes can mimic an acute scrotal mass. Henoch-Schönlein purpura, a vasculitis of unclear etiology, can develop in the scrotal area. Scrotal edema can also occur acutely.

Testicular torsion occurs most commonly in the newborn period and again at puberty. Incarcerated hernias are seen most often in the

Box 92-2. Differential Diagnosis of Inguinal Masses

Non-acute	*Acute*
• Ectopic ovary	• Bartholin abscess
• Hernia	• Epididymitis
• Hydrocele	• Henoch-Schönlein purpura
• Lymphadenopathy	• Idiopathic scrotal swelling
• Retractile testis	• Incarcerated hernia
• Synovial cyst	• Lymphadenitis
• Testicular tumor	• Orchitis
• Varicocele	• Testicular torsion
• Venous aneurysm	• Torsion of appendix testis
	• Trauma

first 6 months of life. Varicoceles are noted almost always at adolescence and are located in the upper left area of the scrotum. Testicular tumors are also much more common in adolescence.

The gender of the patient will also influence the differential diagnosis of the lesion as well as the workup.

Evaluation

History

A thorough, focused history will help define the differential diagnosis (Questions Box). Inquiring about systemic symptoms should always be included and, if positive, may suggest a more generalized process such as a tumor or systemic infection. Symptoms of dysuria would point to epididymitis or orchitis. A history of trauma or possible sexual abuse should always be sought. Hernias and testicular torsion may have a family history positive for the same condition.

Physical Examination

A complete physical examination should always be performed in assessing any pediatric complaint. Evidence of diffuse adenopathy may be present. With an inguinal mass, a concentrated, thorough examination of the inguinal area and lower extremity is needed. A lower extremity lesion may indicate a reactive adenopathy. If the mass is not apparent on inspection and it comes and goes, ask the

Questions

Inguinal Masses

- How long has the mass been present?
- Is it painful?
- Does it come and go?
- Was there a history of trauma?
- Does the child have dysuria?
- Is there fever or vomiting?
- Are there any other masses?
- Has the child had any lower extremity infections?
- Is there a history of renal disease?
- Is there a history of preterm delivery?
- Is there a positive family history?

parent to point to its location. Observe the skin for evidence of erythema, swelling, or bruising. Gently palpate the inguinal canal to see if you can feel a mass, then assess the scrotal or labial area. If the mass is of acute onset, observe the scrotum and try to localize the tenderness. An incarcerated hernia, testicular torsion, torsion of the appendix testis, epididymitis, and orchitis are extremely tender. If there is torsion of the appendix testis, there may be a classic blue dot at the upper pole of the testis. Try to elicit a cremasteric reflex. If present, it virtually eliminates testicular torsion. If the testis has a horizontal lie, it may indicate a bell clapper type of abnormal fixation. The pain of epididymitis and orchitis is relieved partially when the testis is elevated (Prehn sign). Transilluminating the mass may be helpful. A fluid-filled mass, such as a hydrocele, will definitely transilluminate; incarcerated bowel may also transilluminate.

Any mass should be accurately measured. Evaluating the borders of an inguinal mass is important. A hydrocele does not extend into the inguinal canal; therefore, the top border can be felt below the pubis. A hernia will extend into the inguinal canal, so an upper border will not be apparent. Reduction of any hernia with gentle pressure should be attempted. To detect a hernia that is not readily apparent, causing the infant to cry increases intra-abdominal pressure and may demonstrate the hernia. An older child should be asked to stand and cough while the inguinal canal is palpated. A varicocele, which feels like a bag of worms, is a non-tender mass over the spermatic cord and is readily palpated if the teen is in a standing position.

Laboratory Tests

The laboratory tests should be directed toward the most likely diagnosis as determined by the history and physical examination.

If an infection is suspected, a complete blood cell count (CBC) should be obtained. If the infection is thought to be epididymitis or orchitis, a urinalysis and urine culture, along with gonorrhea and chlamydia cultures, should also be obtained. If lymphadenopathy is suspected, a CBC, mononucleosis test, cat-scratch disease test, and possible biopsy may be necessary. An inguinal mass in a female may be a normal testes, and chromosomal evaluation may be indicated to diagnose a disorder of sexual differentiation (see Chapter 91). If a tumor is suspected, the α-fetoprotein level, which is elevated in 90% of yolk sac tumors, and β-human chorionic gonadotropin should be assayed.

Imaging Studies

Ultrasound can be helpful in defining inguinal masses and is the best test to define scrotal contents. It can be useful in differentiating between a hydrocele or hernia and enlarged lymph nodes where a characteristic central echolucent area can be seen. It gives accurate information in evaluating tumors. Ultrasound can provide information in identifying a mass as ovarian or testicular because the ovary is smaller, more echogenic, and may have follicular cysts. Color Doppler ultrasonography is the test of choice in evaluating the scrotum when symptoms are acute to identify a testicular fracture and also assess blood flow in testicular torsion, but has a longer time frame and may not be practical in the acute setting. Nuclear imaging may be possible, but also has a long time frame. If incarceration of a hernia is suspected, a flat plate radiograph of the abdomen is helpful to detect signs of intestinal obstruction. Computed tomography and magnetic resonance imaging are only moderately effective in evaluations.

Management

Many inguinal masses require surgical treatment. Acute symptoms involving the scrotum present a surgical emergency. There may not be time to perform diagnostic studies. If there is a high probability of a testicular torsion, the scrotum should be surgically explored immediately. Surgery within 6 hours of symptom onset has an excellent rate of a viable testis. If surgery is beyond 6 hours, the possibility of a viable testis is progressively worse. After 48 hours it is unlikely that the testis will be salvaged. If the testis is nonviable, it is removed. Torsion of the appendix testis does not need to be explored if the diagnosis is certain.

Surgical intervention may also be indicated with scrotal trauma, which can cause torsion or testicular rupture. A urological referral is indicated for assessment.

All hernias require surgical repair at some time. Immediate surgery is indicated for an incarcerated hernia that cannot be reduced. If it is reduced, then elective surgical repair can be scheduled. There is controversy regarding the indications for surgery on the contralateral side. An infant younger than 1 year has a 20% chance of developing a hernia on the other side, and most surgeons repair both sides at the same time. Other accepted indications for exploration of the unaffected side include preterm infant, twin gestation, left-sided hernia, increased abdominal pressure, and female gender. Currently some surgeons use laparoscopy at the time of the hernia repair to define a patent processus vaginalis on the opposite side and repair it if patency is found. Hydroceles do not have to be repaired surgically unless they persist beyond 1 year of age. This persistence implies a peritoneal connection and an impending hernia, so repair is indicated. A fracture of the testicle also dictates the need for surgical repair. Varicoceles are removed if there is significant pain, the testicle shows growth retardation, there is bilateral disease, or the teen has a solitary testis. Subinguinal microsurgical varicocelectomy can now be performed preserving lymphatic drainage. All testicular tumors are removed. Additional antitumor therapy is dependent on the stage and cell line of the tumor.

Infectious inguinal masses are treated according to the specific bacteriologic diagnosis.

Prognosis

After surgical treatment for either an inguinal hernia or testicular torsion, the child generally does well. The most significant long-term complication of hernia surgery is subsequent impaired testicular function, and decreased testicular size is noted in up to 27% of cases. Damage to the vas deferens and testicular vessels may impair spermatogenesis and result in a higher incidence of impaired fertility. Surgery for testicular torsion may also be associated with subsequent infertility, particularly if an affected testis is left in place. Two-thirds of affected testicles demonstrate atrophy. If there is loss of a testis, the physician should offer a prosthesis in the future since there can be significant psychological implications.

There may be recurrence of a hernia following repair. A hydrocele may develop following varicocele repair.

CASE RESOLUTION

In the case presented at the beginning of the chapter, the infant's history of prematurity associated with a mass that comes and goes most likely indicates an inguinal hernia. With the additional symptoms of pain, fever, and vomiting and the findings of an inflamed, non-reducible mass on examination, there is a high likelihood that the hernia is incarcerated. The infant is taken to the operating room where this diagnosis is confirmed. The hernia is reduced and repaired, and the intestine is noted to be viable. The contralateral side is explored and found to be normal. The infant makes an uneventful recovery.

Selected References

Adelman WP, Joffe, A. Testicular masses/Cancer. *Pediatr Rev.* 2005;26:335–337

Cavanaugh RM Jr. Screening for genitourinary abnormalities in adolescent males. *Pediatr Rev.* 2009;30:431–437

Gatti JM, Murphy JP. Acute testicular disorders. *Pediatr Rev.* 2008;29:235–241

Haye JH. Inguinal and scrotal disorders. *Surg Clin North Am.* 2006;86:371–381

Katz DA. Evaluation and management of inguinal and umbilical hernias. *Pediatr Ann.* 2001;30:729–789

Leslie J, Cain M. Pediatric urologic emergencies and urgencies. *Pediatr Clin North Am.* 2006;53:513–527

Maclellan DL, Diamond DA. Recent advances in external genitalia. *Pediatr Clin North Am.* 2006;53:449–464

Maisonet L. Inguinal hernia. *Pediatr Rev.* 2003;24:34–35

Mesrobian H, Balcon A, Durkee C. Urologic problems of the neonate. *Pediatr Clin North Am.* 2004;51:1051–1062

Palmer L. Pediatric urologic imaging. *Urol Clin North Am.* 2006; 33;409–423

Sheldon C. The pediatric genitourinary examination: inguinal, urethral and genital diseases. *Pediatr Clin North Am.* 2001;48:1339–1380

CHAPTER 93

Hematuria

Elaine S. Kamil, MD

CASE STUDY

A 5-year-old boy is brought to the office for a school entry examination. He was the full-term product of an uncomplicated pregnancy, labor, and delivery. Although he has had 4 or 5 episodes of otitis media, he has generally been in good health. He has never been hospitalized or experienced any significant trauma. He has no known allergies, has been fully immunized, and is developmentally normal.

In addition, the physical examination is completely normal. The boy's height and weight are at the 75th percentile, and his blood pressure is 100/64 mm Hg. Screening tests for hearing and vision are completely normal. The boy's hematocrit is 42. His urinalysis comes back with a specific gravity of 1.025, pH 6, 2+ blood, and trace protein. Microscopic examination shows 18 to 20 red blood cells (RBCs) per high-power field; 0 to 1 white blood cells per high-power field; and a rare, fine, granular cast.

Questions

1. What disease entities cause hematuria?
2. How should hematuria be evaluated?
3. How does the approach to hematuria differ in children who complain of dark or red urine?
4. What is the appropriate follow-up of children with asymptomatic microscopic hematuria?

Hematuria is a common problem in pediatrics, and primary care physicians should have a clear understanding of its pathophysiology, etiology, evaluation, and therapy. Hematuria can be caused by a serious medical problem, or it may only be an incidental finding with no potential for impairment of patients' health. In general, hematuria is categorized as either gross or microscopic (microhematuria). The etiology and approach to hematuria vary with its severity. Gross hematuria is defined as red or brown urine caused by the presence of RBCs. Microhematuria is defined as 3 or more consecutive urine samples with a positive dipstick and 6 or more RBCs per high-power field in a fresh, spun urine sample.

Epidemiology

The incidence of **gross hematuria** is about 1.3 in 1,000 patient visits (Table 93-1). In one series, the causes in about half of the patients were readily apparent from the intake history or physical examination. The incidence of gross hematuria may increase in the community during an epidemic of a disease, such as acute glomerulonephritis, a condition often associated with gross hematuria. In another series, approximately 30% of children with gross hematuria had glomerular diseases, most commonly immunoglobulin (Ig) A nephropathy. The incidence of kidney stones is increasing in the pediatric population.

Microscopic hematuria is a more common pediatric problem. Prevalence rates for persistent, microscopic hematuria range from 0.5% to 2.0%, but 4% to 5% of school-aged children may have microhematuria on a single voided specimen. The incidence is artificially increased in late summer because at that time children tend to visit pediatricians for school physicals that typically include a screening urinalysis.

Table 93-1. Etiology of Gross Hematuria in an Unselected Pediatric Population[a]	
Causes	*Patients (%)*
Readily Apparent Causes	
Documented urinary tract infection (UTI)	26
Perineal irritation	11
Meatal stenosis with ulcer	7
Trauma	7
Coagulopathy	3
Stones	2
Total	56
Other Causes	
Suspected UTI	23
Recurrent gross hematuria	5
Acute nephritis	4
Ureteropelvic junction obstruction	1
Cystitis cystica	<1
Epididymitis	<1
Tumor	<1
Unknown	9
Total	44

[a]Modified with permission from Ingelfinger JR, Davis AE, Grupe WE. Frequency and etiology of gross hematuria in a general pediatric setting. *Pediatrics.* 1977;59:557–561.

Clinical Presentation

Children with gross hematuria present with the sudden appearance of red or brown urine, which may be associated with flank or urethral pain or with a history of trauma.

Children with microscopic hematuria may have urinary complaints (eg, dysuria). In children who appear well, microhematuria is usually detected on screening dipstick examination.

Pathophysiology

Gross Hematuria

Gross hematuria occurs because of the presence of large numbers of RBCs in the urine. Blood may enter the urine because of rupture of blood vessels following trauma or inflammation in the glomeruli or interstitial regions of the kidney. It may also occur as a result of severe inflammation of the bladder wall.

Causes of gross hematuria are listed in Box 93-1. The presence of casts in the urine suggests the diagnosis of glomerulonephritis. The most common causes of glomerulonephritis in children include acute poststreptococcal glomerulonephritis, anaphylactoid purpura, IgA nephropathy, membranoproliferative glomerulonephritis (MPGN), and systemic lupus erythematosus (SLE).

Box 93-1. Common Causes of Gross Hematuria in Pediatric Patients

Glomerular Causes
- IgA nephropathy
- Acute poststreptococcal GN
- Lupus nephritis
- Membranoproliferative GN
- Anaphylactoid purpura GN
- Alport syndrome
- Thin basement membrane disease
- Rapidly progressive GN
- Vasculitis, ANCA positive
- Anti-glomerular basement membrane disease
- Hemolytic uremic syndrome

Hematologic Causes
- Sickle cell disease or trait or hemoglobin C
- Hemophilia
- Thrombocytopenia
- Thrombosis (renal arterial or venous)

Other
- Hypercalciuria
- Munchausen by proxy

Structural Causes
- Renal trauma
- Tumor
- Obstruction
- Renal stones
- Polycystic kidney disease

Vascular Abnormalities
- Hemangiomas
- Nutcracker syndrome
- Arteriovenous malformations

Infectious Causes
- Bacterial urinary tract infection
- Viral cystitis
- Schistosomiasis
- Tuberculosis

Interstitial Diseases
- Acute interstitial nephritis
- Tubulointerstitial nephritis with uveitis

Abbreviations: ANCA, antineutrophil cytoplasmic autoantibody; GN, glomerulonephritis; IgA, immunoglobulin A.

Common causes of gross hematuria in the absence of RBC casts include urinary tract infection **(UTI), either from bacteria or some viruses; renal trauma; bleeding diathesis** (eg, hemophilia or idiopathic thrombocytopenic purpura); **renal tumors; obstruction of the urinary tract; renal stones; hypercalciuria; or hemolytic uremic syndrome (HUS).** A hemangioma in the urinary tract is an extremely rare cause of gross hematuria. In endemic areas gross hematuria may be caused by schistosomiasis. Another rare cause of gross hematuria is Nutcracker syndrome caused by left-sided renal vein congestion from compression of the renal vein by the superior mesenteric artery. The symptoms are distinctive, intermittent gross hematuria associated with left-sided flank pain that is relieved by lying down.

Microhematuria

Microhematuria occurs when small numbers of RBCs enter the urine via tiny ruptures in the glomerular capillary walls or in the capillaries of the tubular or bladder lining. One study showed that otherwise healthy children with microscopic hematuria had increased erythrocyte deformability, making it easier for the RBCs to slip through the glomerular capillaries. For purposes of discussion, the following causes of microscopic hematuria are considered: infectious, structural, traumatic, glomerular, and interstitial. Separate consideration of the causes of microscopic and gross hematuria is often helpful, although significant overlap exists. The presence of gross hematuria calls for a more rapid, and usually more extensive, evaluation.

Urinary tract infection is one of the most common **infectious causes** of hematuria. Bacterial infections of the bladder or kidney occur much more frequently than viral cystitis. Adenovirus is the most common viral cause of hemorrhagic cystitis and is usually associated with dysuria. Other viral causes include cytomegalovirus, parvovirus 19, and polyomavirus type BK. Vaginitis in girls and prostatitis in teenaged boys may also result in hematuria.

Any type of congenital obstructive uropathy may lead to massive dilatation of the urinary tract, which makes the urinary tract more susceptible to bleeding, even with trivial trauma. **Chronic urinary tract obstruction** in children (eg, posterior urethral valves or congenital ureteropelvic junction obstruction) is often asymptomatic. In the past these conditions were typically diagnosed when children presented with UTIs or with gross hematuria after relatively trivial trauma. Now they are commonly diagnosed after a prenatal ultrasound reveals hydronephrosis. Nevertheless, urinary tract obstruction may be detected during an evaluation for asymptomatic microhematuria.

Any **tumor** of the genitourinary tract may be associated with both gross and microscopic hematuria. Pelvic tumors rarely cause urinary obstruction in children, although such tumors frequently cause obstruction in adults. Children with Wilms tumor, the most common childhood renal tumor, usually present with an abdominal mass, but may experience hematuria.

Congenital renal malformations are quite common. Any of these may be associated with hematuria and include polycystic kidney disease, renal dysplasia, medullary sponge kidney, and simple cysts. Patients with polycystic kidney disease may even have severe, painful hematuria.

Vascular problems may also lead to hematuria. Hemangiomas of the kidney, bladder, or ureter are very rare. Arteriovenous malformations also occur infrequently. Hematuria may be a sign of a renal artery or vein thrombosis, particularly in sick neonates.

Young children are more susceptible to **renal injury,** which may result in hematuria, than older children or adults because their kidneys are relatively less protected by the rib cage. In addition, children may insert foreign objects into the urethra and bladder that cause pain and hematuria. Microhematuria has also been described after extremely vigorous exercise, such as marathon running. Child abuse or Munchausen by proxy should be considered if any suspicions are raised on the basis of the history or physical examination.

Hypercalciuria is another cause of microscopic hematuria. Children with hypercalciuria often have a family history of urinary calculi. Calcium oxalate crystals may be present on the microscopic examination of the urine. A urinary calcium-creatinine ratio is best obtained on a first morning, fasting urine sample. Calcium excretion varies with age. Normal values are listed in Table 93-2.

Table 93-2. Normal Values for Urinary Calcium-Creatinine Ratios[a]

Age	Urine Calcium-Creatinine	24-Hour Urine Calcium
Preterm	≤ 0.82	≤8.9 mg/kg/d[b]
<7 mo	≤0.86	
7–18 mo	≤0.60	
19 mo–6 y	<0.42	
6 y–adult	≤0.22	<4 mg/kg/d

[a]Samples for calcium-creatinine ratio should be obtained on a fasting, first-voided morning specimen. The calcium and creatinine concentrations must be in the same units (eg, milligrams per deciliter) before the ratio is calculated.

[b]For healthy preterm infants taking no medications. Calcium excretion varies with diet and phosphorus intake and it is higher if patients are treated with furosemide, xanthines, or glucocorticoids.

There are 2 types of hypercalciuria: absorptive and renal leak. Children with absorptive hypercalciuria over-absorb calcium from the gastrointestinal tract, probably because of an exquisite sensitivity to vitamin D, and can be treated with a reduced calcium diet. Children with renal leak hypercalciuria have an inherently higher rate of urinary calcium excretion and may require thiazide diuretics to reduce urinary calcium excretion. **Interstitial nephritis,** usually from drug exposure, may also cause hematuria. Generally patients with interstitial nephritis may exhibit other signs of tubular disease such as glucosuria or proteinuria.

Glomerular disease may cause gross or microscopic hematuria. Etiologies include acute or chronic glomerulonephritis, such as acute post-streptococcal glomerulonephritis, MPGN, antineutrophil cytoplasmic antibody–associated vasculitis, IgA nephropathy, SLE, and Alport syndrome. The red cells originating from the glomeruli are dysmorphic, and these patients often have RBC casts when the urine is carefully examined.

Sickle cell disease, sickle cell trait, and hemoglobin C trait have been associated with gross or microscopic hematuria.

Differential Diagnosis

When children complain of gross hematuria or "red" urine, practitioners must first determine if they have hematuria or pigmenturia by using a urine dipstick. If the dipstick is negative for blood, then the dark urine is due to dyes, drugs, or pigments (Table 93-3). If the dipstick is positive for blood, the red color is caused by intact RBCs, hemolyzed RBCs, hemoglobin, or myoglobin; the clarification is based on microscopic examination of fresh, spun urine.

Children whose dipsticks are positive for blood but show no RBCs may have hemoglobinuria or myoglobinuria. Hemoglobinuria may be seen with acute autoimmune hemolytic anemia, drug-induced hemolysis, paroxysmal nocturnal hemoglobinuria, a mismatched blood transfusion, cardiopulmonary bypass, freshwater drowning and, in some cases, HUS. Myoglobinuria is seen in individuals with rhabdomyolysis. Acute rhabdomyolysis can occur after a crush injury or a very prolonged seizure, and in certain susceptible individuals with an inborn error of muscle metabolism. Myoglobinuria may also be seen with the myositis associated with influenza infections. Both free hemoglobin and myoglobin are toxic to the renal epithelial cells, mandating a generous fluid intake and close monitoring.

Table 93-3. Distinguishing Hematuria From Pigmenturia

Problem	Urine Color	Hemastix	Microscopic Appearance
Hematuria	Red, brown, or red-brown	Positive	Red blood cells
Hemoglobinuria	Red, brown, or red-brown	Positive	Negative
Myoglobinuria	Red, brown, or red-brown	Positive	Negative
Porphyrins	Red	Negative	Negative
Exogenous pigments[a]	Red or orange	Negative	Negative

[a]Some common exogenous pigments include phenytoin, beets, rifampin, nitrofurantoin, sulfas, amitriptyline, methyldopa, phenothiazine, and chloroquine.

Evaluation

Gross Hematuria

History

The history is crucial to an accurate, efficient, and cost-effective evaluation of patients with hematuria (Questions Box). The family should be questioned carefully about trauma (to trunk, abdomen, or perineum), recent skin infection or pharyngitis, dysuria, and abdominal or flank pain. Parents should be asked whether their

Hematuria   **Questions**

- Has the child suffered any recent trauma?
- Has the child had fever or dysuria?
- Does the child have any flank or abdominal pain?
- Does the child have any rashes, joint pains, or edema?
- Does the child have a family history of hematuria, kidney disease, kidney stones, or gross hematuria?
- Is there a family history of bleeding disorders or inborn errors of muscle metabolism?

children appear "puffy." A family history of kidney disease, bleeding diathesis, hemolytic anemia, or inborn error of muscle metabolism may be important.

Physical Examination

A complete physical examination is also essential. Blood pressure should be measured accurately. The skin should be examined thoroughly for rashes or petechiae; the abdomen should be checked carefully for renal masses or tenderness; the genitalia should be examined thoroughly for signs of trauma, masses, or rashes (see Chapter 128); and the joints should be checked carefully for signs of arthritis. Fundi should be examined for any hypertensive changes. Children should be assessed for the presence of edema.

A careful cardiac and chest examination is necessary to detect signs of congestive heart failure (CHF), a finding sometimes seen in acute glomerulonephritis.

Laboratory Tests

Recent studies have shown that careful microscopic examination of a urine sample can help determine whether bleeding originates from the upper urinary tract or the lower urinary tract. Red blood cells originating in the glomerulus have a dysmorphic appearance. The first morning urine sample is the most reliable but is not appropriate in some settings, such as after a motor vehicle crash. Sometimes the gross hematuria is so substantial that spinning the urine results in a large pellet of debris that is difficult to examine. In such instances, it is prudent to examine an unspun sample. The presence of RBC casts indicates glomerulonephritis, but the absence of such casts does not rule out this condition.

If the urine shows RBC casts, then the evaluation should include an antistreptolysin-O (ASO) titer, antinuclear antibody (ANA), C3, complete blood cell count (CBC) and differential with platelet count, blood urea nitrogen (BUN) and creatinine, serum albumin, and a random urine for a urinary total protein-creatinine ratio.

If the urine shows only large numbers of RBCs, no RBC casts, and no bacteriuria, a CBC with differential and platelet count, a urine culture, and a prothrombin time (PT) and partial thromboplastin time (PTT) should be obtained. A sickle cell test should be considered as well. Hypercalciuria can be evaluated by collecting a first morning sample for calcium/creatinine ratio, or a more extensive evaluation to assess risk factors for kidney stones should include a 24-hour

urine for a stone risk profile that includes urinary calcium, citrate, uric acid, and oxalate.

Imaging Studies

If the urine has large numbers of RBCs and no bacteriuria, a renal ultrasound should be obtained. With gross hematuria and a history of serious trauma, an abdominal computed tomography scan should be performed. Computed tomography scan is also an excellent modality to detect kidney stones. Children with RBC casts should also have a chest radiograph to evaluate for signs of CHF. Special renal Doppler ultrasound studies are indicated if Nutcracker syndrome is being considered in the differential.

Microhematuria

The evaluation of microscopic hematuria is similar to that of gross hematuria. Figure 93-1 outlines an approach to the evaluation of microscopic hematuria.

History and Physical Examination

Because many conditions may cause either gross or microscopic hematuria, the same historical questions apply to both conditions, and the same careful physical examination is indicated.

Laboratory Tests

Generally, the initial evaluation includes a urine culture and a careful microscopic examination of the urine. If the culture is negative, the hematuria is minimal with no associated proteinuria, and children are otherwise healthy, the urinalysis should be repeated once or twice over the following 2 weeks. Red blood cell casts always signify a glomerular origin. Casts are best preserved in acidic, concentrated urine. Thus the first morning urine is the best sample to examine for casts. Red blood cell morphology should be assessed. Red blood cells originating in the glomerulus are **dysmorphic** and of smaller caliber, whereas those that come from lower downstream appear like normal **biconcave** disks. Although RBC morphology is best appreciated with the use of a polarizing microscope, with experience, dysmorphic RBCs can be recognized using an ordinary microscope. Red blood cells of glomerular origin have a mean cell volume of 50 µL or less. In contrast, RBCs of non-glomerular origin have a mean cell volume of 80 to 90 µL. The presence of a newly described, special form of dysmorphic erythrocyte, the G1 cell, is even more specific for glomerular bleeding. These cells are doughnut shaped and contain one or more blebs on their surfaces. Clotting ability should be determined with a platelet count, PT, and PTT. A sickle cell test should be performed. Renal function should be screened with a BUN and creatinine, and a urine calcium-creatinine ratio should be determined. A C3, ANA, and ASO titer should also be checked. If a urine dipstick shows more than a trace of protein, a urinary protein-creatinine ratio should also be determined. If there is a family history of renal disease, a hearing screen should be ordered. All immediate family members should have their urine checked for blood.

If a bloody urine sample is analyzed with a Coulter counter, characteristic distribution curves are seen for glomerular and nonglomerular hematuria. This test is not readily available, however.

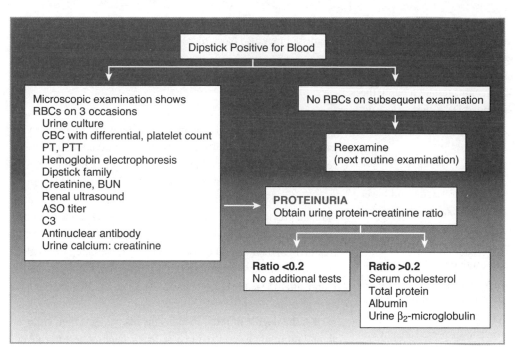

Figure 93-1. Evaluation of asymptomatic, microscopic hematuria. ASO, antistreptolysin-O; BUN, blood urea nitrogen; CBC, complete blood cell count; PT, prothrombin time; PTT, partial thromboplastin time; RBCs, red blood cells.

Imaging Studies

A renal ultrasound should be performed to rule out structural abnormalities and tumors. Chest radiographs should be obtained if acute glomerulonephritis is suspected.

Renal Biopsy

The definitive diagnosis of the etiology of hematuria may require a kidney biopsy. Generally, pediatric nephrologists perform kidney biopsies only in selected instances after ruling out non-glomerular causes for the hematuria. Indications for renal biopsy in a child with hematuria would include an associated abnormal urinary protein excretion, decreased renal function, recurrent macroscopic hematuria, persistently depressed serum complement levels, serologic evidence for SLE, positive ANCA testing, hypertension, or a family history of renal insufficiency of unknown etiology.

Glomerular Diseases Associated With Hematuria

Glomerulonephritis

Both acute and chronic glomerulonephritis are associated with hematuria. The diagnosis of acute poststreptococcal glomerulonephritis requires a "nephritic" urine sediment (RBCs, RBC casts), a low serum complement, and an elevated streptococcal titer (ASO titer, anti-deoxyribonuclease B, or positive streptozyme). It is important to document that the serum complement returns to normal within 3 months because MPGN may present in a similar way. The serum complement is chronically depressed in MPGN.

The most common form of glomerulonephritis in children is **acute poststreptococcal glomerulonephritis.** Many cases are asymptomatic, however, and do not come to the attention of physicians. The resulting hematuria, which may be gross or microscopic, is rarely seen before the age of 2 years. The condition is most commonly diagnosed in preschool-aged and school-aged children, who typically present with gross hematuria, often with some edema and hypertension. The hypertension may be severe, and occasionally children even have hypertensive seizures. The edema results from transient, acute renal failure with salt and fluid retention.

Most children with acute poststreptococcal glomerulonephritis recover completely and have an excellent long-term prognosis. Proteinuria is rarely severe enough to cause nephrotic syndrome, and renal failure is rarely serious enough to require dialysis. If hypertension occurs, the chest radiograph often shows some degree of pulmonary edema, even in the absence of overt clinical signs of CHF. Any hypertension requires treatment. Other infections cause postinfectious glomerulonephritis, but they are less common and less well characterized.

The most common form of chronic glomerulonephritis that affects children is **IgA nephropathy.** On kidney biopsy, patients have mesangial proliferation with mesangial deposits of IgA as the dominant Ig. In the later stages, glomerulosclerosis and interstitial fibrosis are apparent. More than one-third of adults with IgA nephropathy develop end-stage renal disease; the percentage of children who progress to this point is less well known. Gross hematuria in IgA nephropathy is occasionally so severe that patients may pass clots and have flank pain. The presence of persistent proteinuria is considered a poor prognostic sign.

Other forms of primary chronic glomerulonephritis include **MPGN, mesangial proliferative glomerulonephritis,** and **membranous nephropathy,** which is technically not a form of glomerulonephritis because it usually lacks a significant proliferative component. Children with these diseases present with hematuria almost always associated with heavy proteinuria.

Secondary forms of glomerulonephritis include the nephritis of SLE, anaphylactoid purpura, and the nephritis associated with various vasculitides such as Wegener granulomatosis and pauci-immune crescentic glomerulonephritis (ANCA-positive glomerulonephritis). An ANCA panel is indicated in children with glomerulonephritis and decreased renal function. Children with lupus tend to present with multisystem disease but may have only renal manifestations of the disease. Antinuclear antibody is a good screening test for lupus. If the ANA is positive, C3, C4, antidouble-stranded DNA, and a Coombs test should be checked.

Anaphylactoid Purpura

This disease is almost always accompanied by the classical cutaneous vasculitis rash, which is prominent over the lower arms and lower extremities. Abdominal pain may be severe, and affected patients are at risk for the development of intussusception. Children with anaphylactoid purpura have microscopic hematuria, which usually clears, but is occasionally associated with heavy proteinuria and nephrotic syndrome. These children are at risk for developing progressive renal disease. All children with anaphylactoid purpura should have their urine monitored for cessation of hematuria or development of proteinuria. Children with heavy proteinuria and suspected anaphylactoid purpura should have a diagnostic renal biopsy.

Hemolytic Uremic Syndrome

Hemolytic uremic syndrome is a disease characterized by microangiopathic hemolytic anemia, thrombocytopenia, and acute renal failure. It typically follows a prodrome of bloody diarrhea from acute colitis caused by a verotoxin-producing strain of *Escherichia coli* (O157/H7). The verotoxin is believed to be toxic to human endothelial cells. The damaged endothelial cells incite the deposition of fibrin within the glomerular capillaries. These fibrin thrombi lead to the shearing of RBCs and consumption of platelets. Several other organisms, such as pneumococcus and *Shigella,* may precipitate HUS. In atypical cases of HUS, the precipitating event may be an upper respiratory infection. Some cases are familial. Children present with pallor and severe abdominal pain. Urine output may be diminished as a result of renal failure, and in many cases dialysis is required. Hypertension may be severe.

Other Glomerular Diseases

Alport syndrome, thin basement membrane disease (benign familial hematuria), focal segmental glomerulosclerosis (FSGS), and minimal change disease (MCD) are also associated with hematuria. Alport syndrome is a disease of the glomerular basement membrane, where thinning and duplication of the basement membrane occur. The renal involvement eventually leads to end-stage renal disease. Patients or their family members often have nerve deafness or keratoconus. The inheritance of Alport syndrome varies by kindred; it may be either autosomal-dominant, autosomal-recessive, or sex-linked. The sex-linked inheritance is by far the most common mode of inheritance, with female carriers being much less severely affected than the affected males. Thin basement membrane disease also is characterized by thinning of the glomerular basement membrane, but the glomeruli are otherwise normal, and the clinical course is benign. Patients with MCD and FSGS present with nephrotic syndrome but may also have microscopic hematuria.

Management

Gross Hematuria

The management of gross hematuria depends on the underlying cause. Children with a history of trauma should be placed on bed rest pending surgical consultation (see Chapter 63). If the evaluation indicates acute glomerulonephritis and if children are not hypertensive, they can be followed carefully as outpatients with monitoring of blood pressure and renal function with consultation with a pediatric nephrologist. Children with coagulopathies require specific treatment of their bleeding disorders (eg, intravenous gamma globulin for idiopathic thrombocytopenic purpura). If kidney stones are found, after the acute episode has passed, the children should have an evaluation for stone risk factors.

If some degree of renal insufficiency is present, then children should promptly be referred to a pediatric nephrologist to rule out more unusual causes of glomerulonephritis, for consideration of renal biopsy, and for treatment.

Microhematuria

Laboratory tests other than urinalysis may be negative in otherwise healthy children with microscopic hematuria. Some of these children may be recovering from subclinical cases of poststreptococcal glomerulonephritis, which can cause microscopic hematuria for up to 1 year. Others may have early IgA nephropathy and not yet have significant proteinuria, and some may have thin basement membrane disease. As long as children have normal renal function, normal urinary calcium excretion, normal blood pressure, a negative renal ultrasound, no significant proteinuria, and all other tests are normal, it is safe to monitor them every 3 to 6 months until the problem resolves. Healthy children with an otherwise negative workup who show no change in their clinical state for a period of 1 year may subsequently be monitored annually. If hypercalciuria is detected, a low-calcium diet or treatment with thiazide diuretics may be tried. Increased urinary microalbuminuria has been shown to be predictive of glomerular lesions in children with isolated microscopic hematuria.

Prognosis

The prognosis for children with hematuria depends on the underlying cause. Gross hematuria is more often associated with serious renal disease, such as acute glomerulonephritis, HUS, or renal trauma. Even so, most children with gross hematuria have a good prognosis, provided the diagnosis is rapidly discovered and appropriate specific therapy is given. Children with persistent microscopic hematuria who have no family history of the condition, have a negative evaluation, and do not develop hypertension or proteinuria have an excellent long-term prognosis.

CASE RESOLUTION

The boy in the opening scenario shows no worrisome clinical signs, such as hypertension or significant proteinuria. His urine should be rechecked twice more, and if the hematuria persists, his evaluation should follow the algorithm in Figure 93-1.

Selected References

Adams ND, Rowe JC. Nephrocalcinosis. In: Bailie MD, ed. *Clinics in Perinatology.* Philadelphia, PA: W. B. Saunders; 1992:179–195

Assadi FK. Value of urinary excretion of microalbumin in predicting glomerular lesions in children with isolated microscopic hematuria. *Pediatr Nephrol.* 2005;20:1131–1135

Hoppe B, Kemper MJ. Diagnostic examination of the child with urolithiasis and nephrocalcinosis. *Pediatr Nephrol.* 2010;25:403–413

Ingelfinger JR, Davis AE, Grupe WE. Frequency and etiology of gross hematuria in a general pediatric setting. *Pediatrics.* 1977;59:557–561

Kashtan CE. Alport syndrome and thin glomerular basement membrane disease. *J Am Soc Nephrol.* 1998;9:1736–1750

Lettgen B, Wohlmuth A. Validity of G1-cells in the differentiation between glomerular and non-glomerular haematuria in children. *Pediatr Nephrol.* 1995;9:435–437

Meglic A, Kuzman D, Jazbec J. Erythrocyte deformability and microhematuria in children and adolescents. *Pediatr Nephrol.* 2003;18:127–132

Meyers KEC. Evaluation of hematuria in children. *Urol Clin North Am.* 2004; 31:559–573

Pan CG. Evaluation of gross hematuria. *Pediatr Clin North Am.* 2006;53:401–412

Patel HP, Bissler JJ. Hematuria in children. *Pediatr Clin North Am.* 2001;48: 1519–1537

Piqueras AI, White RHR, Raafat F, Moghal N, Milford DV. Renal biopsy diagnosis in children presenting with haematuria. *Pediatr Nephrol.* 1998;12:386–391

Sargent JD, Stukel TA, Kresel J, Klein RZ. Normal values for random urinary calcium to creatinine ratios in infancy. *J Pediatr.* 1993;123:393–397

Savige J, Rana K, Tonna S, et al. Thin basement membrane nephropathy. *Kidney Int.* 2003;64:1169–1178

Tsukahara H, Yoshimoto M, Morikawa K, Okada T, Kuroda M, Sudo M. Urinary erythrocyte volume analysis: a simple method for localizing the site of hematuria in pediatric patients. *J Pediatr.* 1989;115:433–436

Youn T, Trachtman H, Gauthier MB. Clinical spectrum of gross hematuria in pediatric patients. *Clin Pediatr.* 2006;45:135–141

CHAPTER 94

Proteinuria

Elaine S. Kamil, MD

CASE STUDY

A 14-year-old boy is brought to the office for a preparticipation sports physical examination. He has been previously healthy but had one hospital admission at the age of 2 years for treatment of a fractured humerus. He has no acute complaints. The family history is positive for diabetes mellitus in the paternal grandfather and lung cancer in the maternal grandfather. It is negative for renal disease or hypertension. The boy's height and weight are at the 75th percentile for age, and his blood pressure is 110/70 mm Hg.

On physical examination he is a well-developed, well-nourished, athletic teenager. No abnormal findings are present. The complete blood cell count reveals a hemoglobin of 14.8 g/dL, a hematocrit of 48.3%, and a white blood cell (WBC) count of 8,400/mm³ with a normal differential. The urine has a pH of 5, a specific gravity of 1.025, and 3+ protein on dipstick. The rest of the dipstick is negative. Microscopic examination shows 0 to 1 WBC count per high-power field and 0 to 2 hyaline casts per low-power field.

Questions

1. What conditions cause proteinuria?
2. When should children with proteinuria undergo further evaluation?
3. What type of evaluation should be carried out to assess proteinuria?
4. When should children with proteinuria be referred to a pediatric nephrologist?

A small amount of **protein** is normally present in the urine. Urine protein levels increase somewhat under certain conditions, such as vigorous exercise, febrile illnesses, accidental trauma, and congestive heart failure (CHF). Most of the protein in the **glomerular filtrate** is reabsorbed by the tubular cells. Pathologic amounts of protein are present in the urine when the **glomerular leak** of protein is increased, when the **tubules fail to reabsorb** the protein filtered by the glomerulus, or if **inflammation in the renal interstitium** leads to the addition of tubular proteins to the urine.

Urinary protein is initially detected by **urine dipstick,** but this method may be falsely positive in alkaline urine. Dipstick protein is also affected by urine concentration. A dipstick positive for protein of 1+ in concentrated urine may not correlate with an abnormal 24-hour urinary protein excretion, whereas a dipstick of 1+ in very dilute urine may be associated with an abnormal 24-hour urinary protein excretion. Proteinuria may be more accurately determined by performing a timed urine collection or a random sample for chemical determination of the total protein concentration divided by the urinary creatinine concentration (urine TP/Cr).

Epidemiology

The prevalence of **proteinuria** depends on how the condition is defined. In a Texas study, 10 mg/dL of proteinuria was found consistently in the urine of 2% to 3% of children in 3 consecutive urine samples. When 50 mg/dL was used as the cutoff for proteinuria, however, only 0.4% to 0.7% of boys and 0.4% to 2.5% of girls had proteinuria in 2 of 3 consecutive samples. The prevalence of proteinuria increased with age. In Finland, about 11% of school-aged children had at least one episode of proteinuria of 25 mg/dL by dipstick when the urine was tested 4 times. Approximately 2.5% of the children had proteinuria on 2 of 4 occasions.

Clinical Presentation

Proteinuria is a laboratory finding that may present incidentally on a screening urinalysis or be detected during the evaluation of a complaint, such as edema, that may be caused by kidney disease. When proteinuria is detected as an incidental finding in otherwise normal children, the laboratory evaluation of the proteinuria should be delayed until its persistence is confirmed on repeat dipstick, preferably on a first morning urine sample (Dx Box). **Edematous children** with proteinuria most likely have renal lesions or more rarely congestive heart failure. Additional findings on examination could include the presence of hypertension, ascites, pleural effusions, or the rash of systemic lupus erythematosus or anaphylactoid purpura.

Dx Proteinuria

- Presence of dipstick proteinuria (>1+ confirmed on 3 occasions)
- Random urine total protein-creatinine ratio greater than 0.2 or 24-hour urine protein greater than 4 mg/m²/hour
- Orthostatic proteinuria (assessed through separate measurement of afternoon and first morning urine for total protein-creatinine ratios)

Pathophysiology

The glomerular capillaries are adapted to permit the filtration of minimal amounts of plasma proteins, particularly those with a small molecular radius. Approximately 320 mg of albumin and 360 mg of lower molecular weight proteins are filtered by the glomerular capillaries each day. Ninety-five percent of this is reabsorbed by the proximal tubular cells. Normally, children may excrete up to 100 mg/m^2/day of protein. Urinary protein excretion is increased in newborns to about 240 mg/m^2/day and in adolescents to about 300 mg/day. Adults may normally excrete up to 150 mg of protein per day. Only 10% to 15% of this is albumin; the rest of the proteins are other plasma proteins and urinary glycoproteins.

When increased proteinuria results from glomerular disease, higher levels of urinary proteins are primarily due to the enhanced filtration of albumin. Protein excretion may be increased transiently by any condition that raises intraglomerular capillary pressure, such as CHF, strenuous exercise, epinephrine use, fever, or surgery. Children and adults with very early diabetic nephropathy or early end-organ damage from hypertension will show elevated urinary microalbumin/creatinine ratios. Children with diabetes or hypertension should have regular determination of urinary microalbumin/creatinine ratios to detect early, reversible glomerular damage.

Orthostatic proteinuria, which affects some children, is a poorly understood, benign condition. Individuals excrete pathologic amounts of protein in their urine while they are upright, but their urinary protein excretion returns to normal when they are recumbent. This condition seems to be more common in athletic individuals. Orthostatic proteinuria may be due to increased pressure in the renal vasculature while patients are upright. Several investigators have shown partial obstruction of the left renal vein by entrapment between the aorta and the superior mesenteric artery in patients with orthostatic proteinuria while they are standing.

Differential Diagnosis

The proteinuria may be **physiological** (secondary to fever, CHF, **orthostatic, tubular** (as seen in allergic interstitial nephritis), or **glomerular.** Aminoaciduria as a form of tubular proteinuria may occur, as is seen in certain inborn errors of metabolism.

Evaluation

History

It is important to elicit a complete history (Questions Box) in children with proteinuria. When asking about a history of swelling, the practitioner should note that subtle periorbital edema may be present only in the early morning hours. If the proteinuria is detected at a routine screening examination, the conditions under which the urine was obtained should be determined. Children may have been sick with a high fever or have just participated in an athletic event such as a track meet.

Proteinuria — Questions

- Was the mother's pregnancy remarkable in any way? What was the child's birth like?
- Did the child have any neonatal problems that may indicate possible renal damage?
- Is any swelling apparent in areas such as the ankles, the abdomen, or the periorbital region?
- Has the child had any recent illnesses, particularly pharyngitis or impetigo?
- Does the child have a history of joint pains and skin rashes, especially the adolescent patient who may be at greater risk of having a collagen vascular disease?
- Has the child had any previous urinary tract infections, urinary abnormalities, or dark urine?
- Does the child have a history of hypertension or weight loss or gain?
- Is there a family history of renal disease?
- Does the child have diabetes mellitus?

Physical Examination

The physical examination should include a determination of blood pressure and measurement of height and weight. A careful assessment for edema should be made. The skin should be examined for signs of rashes such as that seen in Henoch-Schönlein purpura or healing impetigo. The joints should be inspected for any signs of swelling or joint inflammation. The abdominal examination should include a careful search for ascites or organomegaly.

Laboratory Tests

The extent of the laboratory evaluation depends on the child's general health (eg, the child is ill with another problem), the amount of proteinuria on dipstick, and whether the child has edema. The suggested evaluation is outlined in Figure 94-1. In non-edematous, otherwise healthy children, it is prudent to examine the urine sediment and, if negative, recheck the dipstick in a few days. If proteinuria of 1+ is consistently present and no hematuria is evident, a first-stage evaluation is indicated. If children are ill with a fever or are hospitalized with a serious illness, it is often appropriate to delay the evaluation of the proteinuria until the acute illness is under control, providing no associated hematuria, hypoproteinemia, hypertension, or azotemia is present.

In healthy ambulatory patients with persistent, isolated dipstick proteinuria on 3 occasions, it is important to quantitate the proteinuria (Box 94-1). This may be done simply by ordering a urine protein-creatinine ratio (urine TP/Cr). If the ratio is abnormal (>0.2), children need to be evaluated first for orthostatic proteinuria. Orthostatic proteinuria can be ruled out in several ways. The simplest evaluation involves checking a urine dipstick on a first-voided morning sample and again on an afternoon specimen. This procedure should be repeated on 2 different days. It is critical to be sure that children empty their bladders before going to bed, because urine produced when they are non-recumbent may contain protein

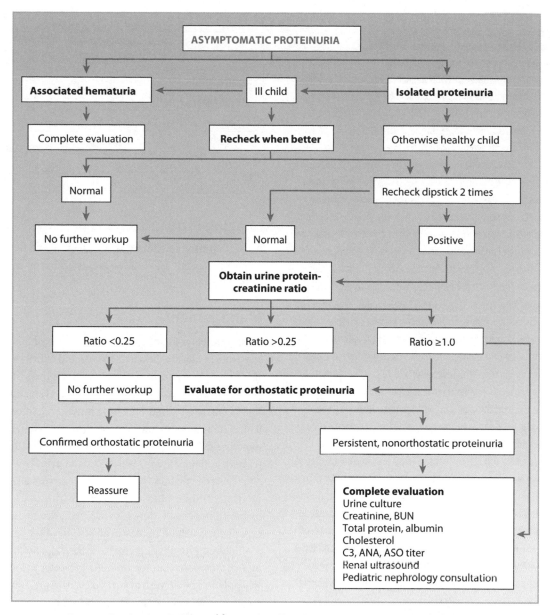

Figure 94-1. **Suggested evaluation of children with asymptomatic proteinuria. ANA, antinuclear antibody; ASO, antistreptolysin-O; BUN, blood urea nitrogen.**

and give an inaccurate result. If the dipstick from the morning urine is negative on a concentrated acid urine, and if the afternoon sample is positive on a concentrated acid urine, the child most likely has orthostatic proteinuria.

A more accurate way of checking for orthostatic proteinuria involves the determination of urine TP/Cr ratios on the first morning and afternoon urine samples. A diagnosis of orthostatic proteinuria can be made if the ratio is normal on the recumbent sample and elevated on the daytime sample. The most accurate way of diagnosing orthostatic proteinuria entails collecting 2 timed urine samples, one during the hours that children are up during the day and the other while they are in bed at night. In most instances of orthostatic proteinuria in children, the total urinary protein excretion is less than 1 g. The urine collected in the recumbent period should contain less than 50 mg/m^2 of protein. If these 2 timed samples meet the criteria

for orthostatic proteinuria, they do not need to be repeated. It is important to remember, however, that even in renal disease proteinuria improves somewhat when patients are recumbent.

If children do not have orthostatic proteinuria, a 24-hour urine protein excretion may be determined. If the collection of a 24-hour urine sample is impractical, the urine protein-creatinine ratio is a reliable alternative. Blood chemistries (eg, blood urea nitrogen [BUN], creatinine) should be obtained to determine renal function. Electrolyte status should be assessed with total carbon dioxide, total protein, albumin, and cholesterol. Serologies should be obtained for antinuclear antibodies, C3, antistreptolysin-O titer, and hepatitis B surface antigen if children come from a population at risk for hepatitis B.

Twenty-four–hour urine protein excretion should be less than 4 mg/m^2/hour. Neonates may excrete as much as 150 mg/m^2/12

Box 94-1. Methods for Assessment of Urinary Protein

Detection of proteinuria by dipstick is only semiquantitative. This examination is affected by urinary pH and concentration and, therefore, more definitive tests are warranted if a patient's urine consistently shows dipstick proteinuria. The sulfosalicylic acid (SSA) turbidity test is also semiquantitative. When SSA is added to an aliquot of urine, it precipitates urinary proteins. The amount of turbidity is graded on a scale of 0 to 4+.

Urinary protein is most accurately quantitated by a chemical determination on a timed urine collection (usually 24 hours). The concentration (measured in milligrams per deciliter) is multiplied by the total urine volume to determine the milligrams of protein excreted in 24 hours. Twenty-four–hour urine samples are difficult to collect in young children. However, several studies have shown that a random urine sample for a protein-creatinine ratio correlates well with the 24-hour urinary protein excretion. The ratio is determined by dividing the urine protein concentration (milligrams per deciliter) by the urine creatinine concentration (milligrams per deciliter). The units must be the same for each component. The urinary protein-creatinine ratio is normally less than 0.2. A ratio of 3.5 or greater in an adult or greater than 1.0 in children indicates nephrotic range proteinuria. A recent study has found that proteinuria in combination with leukocyturia (by dipstick) is likely to indicate more significant noninfectious renal inflammation.

Occasionally it is important to determine whether proteinuria has a tubular or glomerular basis. In these instances, a urinary β_2-microglobulin is helpful. β_2-microglobulin, a very small protein that is freely filtered at the glomerular level, is nearly completely reabsorbed by the proximal tubules. In instances of tubular injury, such as interstitial nephritis, acute tubular necrosis, or nephrotoxic renal injury, urinary β_2-microglobulin is increased. With glomerular proteinuria, urine protein electrophoresis shows a heavy preponderance of albumin. The urine microalbumin-creatinine ratio is an excellent indicator of glomerular proteinuria. It is readily available in most laboratories and will detect minimal but pathologic amounts of glomerular proteinuria such as that seen in early diabetic nephropathy and with early hypertensive glomerular damage.

Table 94-1. Urinary Protein Excretion by Age

Age	24-hour Urine Protein (mg)	Urine Protein-Creatinine
Premature infant	14–60	—
Full-term infant	15–68	—
2–23 mo	17–85	≤0.50
2–4 y	20–121	≤0.2
4–10 y	26–194	≤0.2
10–16 y	29–238	≤0.2

Imaging Studies

A renal ultrasound should be obtained to rule out any structural abnormalities but may not be indicated in the child with simple orthostatic proteinuria.

Management

Most children with normal renal function and normal blood pressure whose evaluation reveals physiological or orthostatic proteinuria should have repeat urinalysis on an annual basis. If the proteinuria worsens or if hematuria develops, a repeat evaluation of renal function is indicated. Children whose initial evaluation reveals persistent, significant proteinuria require careful follow-up to detect and monitor signs of serious renal disease. This follow-up should include repeat blood pressure measurement and urinalysis every 3 months and repeat chemistries (BUN, creatinine, serum albumin) and urine protein-creatinine ratios every 6 months. These children should be managed in consultation with the pediatric nephrologist, whose experience is helpful in reassessing the need for kidney biopsy.

Children with physiological or orthostatic proteinuria who have minimal, persistent proteinuria should be able to follow a full school schedule and be allowed to participate in sports, provided there are no other contraindications. The usual immunization schedule should not be interrupted, and children should follow a regular diet. No increase in dietary protein is necessary to compensate for the minimal amounts of protein lost in the urine. Results of recent studies in nephrotic patients have found that a high-protein diet may actually increase urinary protein losses.

Prognosis

The outlook for children with proteinuria depends entirely on the underlying cause of the proteinuria. Children whose proteinuria is associated with edema or hematuria are more likely to have significant renal disease, such as glomerulonephritis, however, and the prognosis may be less favorable. If the proteinuria is due to a form of chronic glomerulonephritis, children may ultimately develop end-stage renal disease. In individuals with glomerular diseases, persistent proteinuria is a strong risk factor for progressive loss of renal function. If the proteinuria is physiological or orthostatic, however,

hours, however. Table 94-1 gives a summary of normal urinary protein excretion. If children have nephrotic range proteinuria or symptoms consistent with nephrotic syndrome (heavy proteinuria accompanied by hypoalbuminemia and hypercholesterolemia), they require further evaluation for nephrotic syndrome (see Chapter 145). If they do not have nephrotic range proteinuria, abnormal tubular proteinuria should be ruled out. A normal urinary β_2-microglobulin rules out tubular proteinuria. In general, consultation with a pediatric nephrologist is recommended if children have an abnormal 24-hour urinary protein excretion (see Table 94-1). If the proteinuria exceeds 1 g/day or if any other minor signs of renal dysfunction or hematuria are present, a biopsy is warranted. Sometimes, otherwise healthy children with small amounts of isolated proteinuria of less than 750 to 1,000 mg/day are followed by the pediatric nephrologist without a kidney biopsy. However, if this degree of proteinuria persists for 1 year or more, a renal biopsy is warranted.

the long-term prognosis is excellent. The likelihood that these children will develop renal functional impairment is no greater than for the rest of the general population.

CASE RESOLUTION

In the case presented at the beginning of the chapter, odds are that the evaluation of the healthy teenaged boy with isolated proteinuria will reveal that he has orthostatic proteinuria, and his long-term prognosis is good.

Selected References

Abitbol C, Zilleruelo G, Freundlich M, Strauss J. Quantitation of proteinuria with urinary protein/creatinine ratios and random testing with dipsticks in nephrotic children. *J Pediatr.* 1990;116:243–247

Ginsberg JM, Chang BS, Matarese RA, Garella S. Use of single voided urine samples to estimate quantitative proteinuria. *N Engl J Med.* 1983;309:1543–1546

Hogg RJ, Portman RJ, Milliner D, et al. Evaluation and management of proteinuria and nephrotic syndrome in children: recommendations from a pediatric nephrology panel established at the National Kidney Foundation Conference on Proteinuria, Albuminuria, Risk, Assessment, Detection, and Elimination (PARADE). *Pediatrics.* 2000;105:1242–1249

Houser MT, Jahn MF, Kobayashi A. Assessment of urinary protein excretion in the adolescent: effect of body position and exercise. *J Pediatr.* 1986;109:556–561

Koss S, Perl A, Wieder A, et al. Proteinuria and renal disease: prognostic value of urine dipstick testing for leukocytes. *Pediatr Nephrol.* 2006;21:584–587

Pradhan M, Kaplan BS. Proteinuria. In: Kaplan BS, Meyers KEC, eds. *Pediatric Nephrology and Urology: The Requisites in Pediatrics.* Philadelphia, PA: Elsevier; 2005:103–109

Ragazzi M, Milani G, Edefonti A, et al. Left renal vein entrapment: a frequent feature in children with postural proteinuria. *Pediatr Nephrol.* 2008; 23:1837–1839

Reuben DB, Wachtel TJ, Brown PC, Driscoll JL. Transient proteinuria in emergency medical admissions. *N Engl J Med.* 1982;306:1031–1033

Trachtman H, Bergwerk A, Gauthier B. Isolated proteinuria in children. Natural history and indications for renal biopsy. *Clin Pediatr (Phila).* 1994;33:468–472

Vehaskari VM. Mechanism of orthostatic proteinuria. *Pediatr Nephrol.* 1990;4: 328–330

Yoshikawa N, Kitagawa K, Ohta K, Tanaka R, Nakamura H. Asymptomatic constant isolated proteinuria in children. *J Pediatr.* 1991;119:375–379

CHAPTER 95

Urinary Tract Infections

Gangadarshni Chandramohan, MD, MS, and Sudhir K. Anand, MD

CASE STUDY

A 7-month-old girl is brought to the office with a 1-day history of fever (temperature: 103°F [39.4°C]), vomiting, and mild diarrhea. The mother has not noticed any change in urination pattern or any unusual urine odor. The child has been somewhat irritable but fully alert.

Physical examination reveals an active infant. The temperature is 102.6°F (39.2°C), the heart rate is 122 beats/min, the respiratory rate is 30 breaths/min, and the blood pressure is 90/60 mm Hg. The neck is supple. The head, eye, ear, nose, throat, chest, heart, abdominal, and genital examination are all normal. Urinalysis shows specific gravity 1.025, pH 6.0, leukocyte esterase and nitrite both strongly positive, protein trace, and blood trace; the sediment has 15 to 20 white blood cells per high-power field and 2 to 4 red blood cells per high-power field. The Gram stain shows more than 100,000 gram-negative rods, and the urine culture is pending.

Questions

1. What should be the initial approach to children with suspected urinary tract infections (UTIs)?
2. What are the possible diagnoses of children with positive leukocyte esterase or nitrite on urinalysis?
3. What are the indications for hospital admission of children with UTIs?
4. What antibiotics are used in the treatment of UTIs?
5. What is the appropriate diagnostic workup for children with suspected UTIs? When are renal ultrasound, technetium 99m-DMSA renal scan, and voiding cystourethrogram included in the evaluation?
6. If workup reveals vesicoureteral reflux (VUR), how should children be managed over the long term?

Urinary tract infection is one of the most common serious bacterial infections that affect infants and children. Older children with UTI may present with lower urinary tract symptoms such as burning urination, frequency, and urgency with or without flank pain. Infants and newborn babies usually present with nonspecific symptoms, such as fever, vomiting, and diarrhea, or occasionally can develop signs of circulatory failure when complicated by sepsis. In most children UTIs resolve completely with appropriate antibiotic therapy. However, in children with underlying anatomical abnormalities (eg, VUR) or delayed or inadequate antibiotic treatment, UTIs may result in renal scarring that sometimes leads to hypertension or end-stage renal disease.

Urinary tract infection is a nonspecific, generic term implying significant bacteriuria, irrespective of the site of bacterial growth in the urinary tract. In many young children with bacteriuria, clinical findings overlap and precise classification of whether it's an upper or lower tract infection cannot be easily made. We clarify some of the commonly used terms below.

Asymptomatic, covert, and **screening bacteriuria** are synonymous terms usually used when bacteriuria is detected during surveys of healthy children. The term *screening bacteriuria* is more accurate because some affected children may actually have urinary symptoms on close questioning.

Urethritis implies infection of the urethra and is usually seen in the setting of sexually transmitted infections. The usual symptoms are dysuria and urethral discharge.

Cystitis implies infection of the bladder only. Its major feature is voiding symptoms (eg, dysuria, frequency, urgency, enuresis, and foul-smelling urine). Fever, if present, is usually low-grade.

Acute pyelonephritis is a symptomatic infection of renal parenchyma characterized by systemic symptoms such as high fever, chills, flank pain, and vomiting in addition to dysuria.

Recurrent UTI generally refers to reinfection with a new organism (often same species but different strain). According to studies, this condition is common, especially in the first year after initial UTI. If the recurrence occurs within a few months of the initial infection with a negative culture at the time of completing the course of antibiotic and grows the same organism as before, it is considered as persistence of bacteriuria. But, if there was a positive culture after completing the course of antibiotic, and the patient remains symptomatic it would be unresolved bacteriuria. In both of these instances, it could be a result of noncompliance and, therefore, it is essential that the parents become aware of the long-term consequences of an unresolved prolonged course of infection, particularly about the risk of renal scarring and hypertension.

Chronic pyelonephritis is a term that has been used in various ways. Ideally, it should be employed only after renal biopsy specimens reveal renal scarring along with infiltration of plasma cells, monocytes, and macrophages on histology due to chronic repeated infections. Practically, the term often refers to scarred kidneys as demonstrated by nuclear medicine studies and/or reduced kidney function.

Complicated UTI refers to an infection that has an underlying risk factor, such as structural urinary tract defects, functional voiding problems, the presence of stones, or an immunocompromised state.

Epidemiology

Bacteriuria is detected in approximately 1% of girls and 2% of boys during routine screening of healthy newborns and young infants. Approximately 1% of girls continue to have asymptomatic bacteriuria throughout childhood. Bacteriuria in boys older than 1 year is very uncommon. In most affected infants and children, bacteriuria resolves spontaneously with time and does not lead to renal damage. Antibiotic treatment is not indicated unless the child develops a symptomatic infection. Routine screening for bacteriuria in infants and children, however, is not indicated. Symptomatic UTI occurs in approximately 2.5% of children annually and accounts for more than 1 million office visits per year and 14% of pediatric emergency department visits. Among vaccinated febrile infants, UTI is the source of fever in approximately 4% to 8% of patients, even in some of those who have upper respiratory infection symptoms. In early infancy, UTI is about twice as common in boys than in girls and about 5 to 10 times more common in uncircumcised boys than circumcised boys. After the first 6 months of life, the incidence of symptomatic UTI becomes considerably higher in females than males, and the difference between circumcised and uncircumcised males disappears.

Clinical Presentation

Signs and symptoms of UTI in neonates and young infants are usually nonspecific and include fever, irritability, poor weight gain, diarrhea, and vomiting, but many such infants on physical examination do not appear ill. On the other end of clinical spectrum, a few neonates and infants with UTI and bacteremia or sepsis appear quite ill and may also have temperature instability, apnea, bradycardia, cyanosis, anemia, jaundice, and disseminated intravascular coagulation. Older children with symptomatic UTI usually complain of suprapubic, abdominal, or flank pain; dysuria; frequency; urgency; secondary enuresis in a previously toilet trained child; foul-smelling or cloudy urine; and occasionally gross hematuria (Dx Box and Table 95-1).

Pathophysiology

The pathogenesis of UTI involves interaction between various bacterial factors, protective host factors, and environmental factors.

Bacterial Factors

Escherichia coli accounts for 80% to 90% of first-time UTIs. The remainder are caused by other gram-negative enteric bacilli

Dx **Urinary Tract Infection**

Infants
Any unexplained fever
Irritability
Vomiting
Nonspecific symptoms such as apnea, jaundice, or poor feeding
Uncircumcised male infant
History of congenital renal anomalies

Older Children
Abdominal pain
Burning or pain on urination
Urgency
Frequency
Fever
Leukocyturia
Positive nitrite on urinalysis
Positive urine culture

(Proteus, Klebsiella, Enterobacter) and gram-positive cocci (enterococci, *Staphylococcus saprophyticus*). Most organisms that cause UTI originate from the fecal flora. *Staphylococcus saprophyticus* (a coagulase-negative staphylococcus) infections are primarily seen in adolescents with UTI.

Microorganisms that cause UTI usually enter the urinary tract by an ascending route. To initiate colonization and infect the urinary tract, these organisms must first adhere to uroepithelium so they are not swept away during voiding. Bacterial adhesion in *E coli* is mediated by fimbriae, which are fine, hairlike proteins emanating from the bacterial cell wall. One important type of fimbriae, called P-fimbriae, adheres to receptors (Gal-Gal) on the uroepithelium, and some studies have shown that women and children with recurrent UTI have increased numbers of these receptors. P-fimbriae receptors have also been identified in high abundance on the epithelial surface of prepuce in male infants who have recurrent UTIs. In most young children with normal anatomy, acute pyelonephritis is caused by *E coli* with P-fimbriae. In most patients with VUR and scarred kidneys, however, the infection is caused by *E coli* lacking P-fimbriae. Hence, the role of P-fimbriae in the pathogenesis of renal scarring is uncertain. Additionally, many of these bacteria, which are typically extracellular organisms, are able to survive and flourish intracellularly by evading immune defenses and taking advantage of the host cell's nutrients. Other bacterial virulence factors include K and H antigens, colicin, hemolysin, and their ability to acquire iron, but their role in the pathogenesis of UTI is not clearly defined.

Host Factors

There are many unalterable host factors that contribute to the pathogenesis of UTI, including age, sex, genetics, anatomy, and immune response to infection. Preterm babies and neonates carry a higher risk than older children partly related to their immature immune

Table 95-1. Suggested Clinical Approach to Suspected UTI in Children of Different Age Groups

Initial Approach	Follow-up Approach
Infant <2 months old (but >4 weeks) Fever (>39°C)/irritability/lethargy or any other signs and symptoms of infection or dehydration a) Admit the child. b) Perform urine and blood culture (CSF culture is usually indicated). c) Check electrolytes, BUN, and creatinine. d) Start IV antibiotics (broad spectrum). e) Start appropriate IV fluids (even if the child tolerates oral feeds). f) Monitor trend in temperature and urine output closely. g) Obtain renal ultrasound.	If fever does not improve after 48–72 hours—reevaluate. Look for other sources of infection. Check the cultures and sensitivity results. Check the antibiotic dose. Re-culture blood and urine. Obtain renal ultrasound if not already done. Continue IV fluids. If urine and blood cultures are positive, monitor for fever and continue IV antibiotics for 7 days, complete 10–14 days course with PO as outpatient. If urine culture is positive, but blood culture is negative, fever is trending down and the patient is active and tolerating PO, discharge home with oral antibiotics to cover total of 10 days. If both cultures are negative, make a clinical judgment and if the possibility of clinical UTI is strong, treat infant with PO as described above. Renal ultrasound and VCUG (if not already done) to be done as an outpatient as soon as feasible. Repeat urine culture 2 weeks after completing antibiotics.
Children 2 months–2 years old High fever, septic appearing a) Admit. b) Perform urine and blood culture (CSF culture if meningitis suspected). c) Start on broad-spectrum IV antibiotics. d) Start IV fluids. e) Check serum electrolytes, BUN, and creatinine. f) Monitor urine output. Low-grade fever but patient has PO intolerance a) Admit. b) Perform urine culture. c) IV fluids advance to PO as tolerated. Fever, child appearing well a) Treat patient with oral antibiotic for 10 days. b) Encourage fluid intake.	Check urine culture and sensitivity results. If patient continues to have fevers, check antibiotic dose, re-culture urine, request renal ultrasound. Monitor PO intake and determine the need for IV fluid. Renal ultrasound and VCUG to be done as an outpatient as soon as feasible. Repeat urine culture 2 weeks after completing antibiotics.
Children 2 years–12 years a) If PO intolerance, admit. b) IV antibiotics and fluids. c) If tolerating PO well and not appearing septic, treat and do the workup on an outpatient basis.	Check BP. Check electrolytes, BUN, and creatinine. Perform renal ultrasound in all and VCUG in children between 2–5 years of age (particularly in those with hydronephrosis).
Adolescent children a) If PO intolerance, admit, start IV antibiotics and fluids. b) If suspected cystitis or clinically stable pyelonephritis, treat as an out patient with oral antibiotics for 5–7 days.	Check BP. Check electrolytes, BUN and creatinine. Perform renal ultrasound in all cases of pyelonephritis.

Abbreviations: BUN, blood urea nitrogen; CSF, cerebrospinal fluid; IV, Intravenous; PO, oral; UTI, urinary tract infection; VCUG, voiding cystourethrography.

mechanisms. Females seem to be at increased risk because the female urethra is shorter than the male urethra and closer to the anus. As previously stated, the receptors that have the higher affinity to bacterial fimbriae in the uroepithelium of older girls and uncircumcised boys contribute to the gender differences in the prevalence of UTI at different stages of life. In addition, individuals with certain P and Lewis blood groups develop more UTIs than others. Urinary obstruction or other anomalies may contribute to the development of UTIs in about 2% of girls and 5% of boys, especially infants.

Vesicoureteral reflux signifies retrograde passage of urine from the bladder to the ureter. After passage through the bladder wall, the normal ureter tunnels under the bladder mucosa before it opens into the bladder lumen. Under normal circumstances the submucosal segment is compressed when the bladder is filled and during voiding, preventing reflux of urine into the ureter. Most VUR is primary and caused by a congenital abnormality of the ureterovesical junction, with the ureter having a short submucosal segment and more laterally placed openings. Secondary reflux may occur in the presence of normal ureteral anatomy when bladder pressures exceed 40 cm of water, as seen in patients with posterior urethral valves or neurogenic bladders. Vesicoureteral reflux is graded on a scale of I through V, with grade V being the most severe (Figure 95-1).

There are insufficient data on the incidence of VUR in normal infants, but generally the incidence of VUR in normal infants is considered to be less than 2%. In infants with UTI, the incidence of VUR is about 25% to 50%; in school-aged children, about 25% to 30%; and in adolescents, about 10% to 15%. These figures suggest that, with increasing age and maturation of the bladder wall, VUR often spontaneously resolves. The risk of having VUR in those with one of the parents or siblings with VUR is much higher compared to those with no family history of VUR, with reported incidence in 10% to 30% of siblings of index cases. The incidence of UTI is increased in the presence of VUR probably because of incomplete emptying of

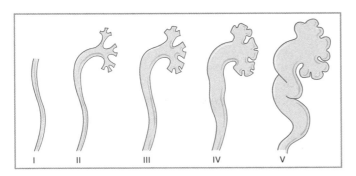

Figure 95-1. Grading of vesicoureteral reflux by vesicoureterogram based on international classification. I. Ureter only. II. Ureter, pelvis, and calyces, but without dilatation. III. Mild or moderate dilatation of ureter and mild or moderate dilatation of renal pelvis, but no or slight blunting of fornices. IV. Moderate dilatation or tortuosity of the ureter with moderate dilatation of renal pelvis and calyces and complete obliteration of the sharp angles of fornices, but maintenance of papillary impressions in most calyces. V. Gross dilatation and tortuosity of ureters, renal pelvis, and calyces; papillary impressions are no longer visible in most calyces.

the bladder; the urine refluxed into the ureters or kidneys returns to the bladder via the abnormally tunneled ureters at the end of voiding. This also provides infected urine direct access to the kidneys, which can lead to pyelonephritis and potential renal scarring.

Intuitively, it would seem that the greater the severity of VUR in children with UTI, the greater the likelihood of renal scarring. Recently, however, it has been clearly recognized that many neonates (especially boys) with antenatal VUR, even in the absence of UTI, have congenital dysplastic renal parenchymal defects, which had been misidentified as infective scars. This suggests that children with VUR can develop scarring even without infections; however, if they develop recurrent infections, it may augment further damage to the kidneys.

Genetic factors: Several gene mutations, candidate genes, and single nucleotide polymorphisms, such as CXCR1, CLR4, tyrosine-related protein 2 and 4, tumor necrosis factor-α and RANTES promoter polymorphisms, have been identified to be associated with high incidence of recurrent UTIs in children in the absence of genitourinary anomalies.

While there are many predisposing host factors that cannot be changed, there are several modifiable behavioral issues that are often associated with UTI in older children. School-aged children with frequent complaints of dysuria or recurrent UTIs who do not have a history of UTI as infants should be questioned for symptoms of dysfunctional voiding. The term *dysfunctional voiding* is often applied in the setting of children (especially girls) who have no neurologic or anatomical abnormalities, but who exhibit abnormal voiding behavior. These girls will often hold their urine for so long that they need to rush to the bathroom only to incompletely empty their bladder, leading to urinary stasis and the potential for infection. Additionally, severe constipation and abnormal stooling patterns are frequently associated with dysfunctional voiding and can also lead to the development of UTI.

Environmental factors: Poor genital hygiene, wiping from back to front, bubble bath use, and wearing of tight nylon panties have often been mentioned in the past as contributing risk factors for UTI; however, the evidence to support these potential risk factors is lacking. Nevertheless, common sense would dictate that fecal contamination of external genitalia and potential colonization be avoided or reduced as much as possible by simple measures such as wiping front to back, avoiding urethral irritation by bubble baths; and wearing loose-fitting cotton underwear in children with UTI.

In the adolescent female, use of spermicidal agents in diaphragms and/or condoms increases the risk of cystitis by altering the normal vaginal flora and enhancing adherence of uropathogenic strains.

Differential Diagnosis

In infants and young children, symptoms of UTI are often nonspecific. Thus a high degree of suspicion for UTI must be maintained. An acute abdomen may rarely be confused with UTI. Some children with dysuria may have chemical irritation from exposure to materials such as bubble baths. Overweight girls may retain urine in their labial folds, which can cause maceration, urethral irritation, or vulvitis. Similarly, some young girls do not sit with their legs spread wide enough on the toilet, which can lead to reflux into the vagina and cause post-void dribbling with subsequent urethral irritation or vulvitis. In these cases, urinalysis and urine culture findings usually help differentiate UTI from vulvitis or urethral irritation. Patients with acute appendicitis may have nonspecific pyuria, which can lead to the misdiagnosis of UTI.

Evaluation

In all infants and young children with fever without an apparent source, urinalysis, urine Gram stain, and urine culture should be obtained to evaluate for UTI.

History

In older children, a history of fever, dysuria, frequency, abdominal pain, and nausea and vomiting is suggestive of UTI. History of previous UTIs, abnormal voiding pattern, and constipation should also be sought. (Also see Table 95-1 and Questions Box).

Physical Examination

The abdomen should be examined for masses and tenderness, the genitalia for local lesions, and the lumbosacral area for anomalies such as deep sacral dimples, lipomas, or tuft of hair that may be suggestive of occult spinal defects that could lead to urinary retention followed by recurrent UTIs. Tenderness is often present in the suprapubic and/or flank regions in children with UTIs. Blood pressure should be measured to evaluate for hypertension secondary to inflammation, scarring, or congenital anomalies of the kidneys. Alternatively, hypotension may be present if the patient is dehydrated or in septic shock.

Questions

Urinary Tract Infection

Neonates and Infants
- Does the urine have unusual odor or color?
- Is the child irritable or not feeding well?
- Is the child urinating like before?
- Is the child a premature or a full-term baby?
- Was the child diagnosed with any previous kidney diseases?
- Is there a family history of urinary tract infections or congenital kidney disorders?

Older Children and Adolescents
- Does it hurt when the child urinates? Does the child scream when urinating?
- Does the child have a good urinary stream? Or does the child dribble?
- Does the child void more frequently?
- Does the urine have an unusual odor?
- Has the child had previous urinary infections?
- If an adolescent, is the teenager sexually active?

Laboratory Tests

The diagnosis of UTI is established by documenting significant bacteria in a urine specimen sent for culture. In young infants the specimen should always be obtained by bladder puncture (suprapubic tap) or catheterization. In infants and children, because of the risk of contamination, a "bag urine" sample is not reliable. In older children with bladder control, a midstream urine collection is satisfactory. The diagnosis of UTI should never be based on the presence or absence of white blood cells alone. Although most older children with symptomatic UTI have pyuria, many neonates and young infants with UTI (25%–50%) may not manifest this finding. Furthermore, leukocyturia may occur in other renal disorders in the absence of UTI. A positive urinary nitrite test is very strongly suggestive of UTI (specificity 95%–100%), but the false-negative rate is nearly 50%.

Most patients with UTI (>85%) have urine bacterial counts greater than 100,000/mL on a voided specimen (ie, significant bacteriuria), although some adult women and teenaged girls with symptomatic recurrent UTI have catheterized or "clean catch" urine colony counts less than 1,000/mL. In general, this has not been observed in young children. Colony counts between 10,000 and 100,000/mL obtained via clean catch are generally unlikely to be significant unless children have symptoms of UTI, associated leukocyturia, and/or cultures that are pure growths of a single organism. Any growth of an organism from a suprapubic tap is considered significant. A colony count of at least 10,000/mL in samples obtained by catheterization is usually necessary to diagnose a UTI. However, in most children with UTIs, urine collected by either of these techniques grows more than 50,000 organisms/mL.

C-reactive protein is usually increased in infants and children with high fever and clinical findings suggestive of acute pyelonephritis. Several other laboratory studies, including erythrocyte sedimentation rate, urinary lactic acid dehydrogenase isoenzymes, urinary concentrating ability, and antibody-coated bacteria, have been used with varying success to differentiate upper (renal) from lower (bladder) UTI in older children and adults. Overall, the reliability of these studies in pediatric patients, especially infants and young children, is not adequate to recommend their routine use. More recently, some studies indicate that with pyelonephritis, increase in procalcitonin level occurs several hours prior to increase in C-reactive protein. This finding may have predictive value in early diagnosis of pyelonephritis and initiating appropriate antibiotic therapy.

Imaging Studies

The last position statement from the American Academy of Pediatrics (AAP) in 1999 states that all girls younger than 2 years and all boys (irrespective of age) should have renal ultrasonography and voiding cystourethrography (VCUG) performed following detection of the first UTI. These 2 studies detect structural renal anomalies and VUR in most patients. In girls, nuclear VCUG instead of contrast VCUG is an acceptable alternative. Renal ultrasound can be performed as soon as feasible after diagnosis. Voiding cystourethrogram may be done once there is clinical evidence that the UTI is resolving, or it may be delayed 4 to 6 weeks depending on the clinical circumstances. Antibiotic prophylaxis, according to the AAP position statement, must be administered until completion of the studies. An excretory computed tomography urogram or intravenous pyelogram is no longer recommended other than under specific circumstances.

Several recent studies (summarized by Feld et al) have demonstrated no or minimal difference in the incidence of repeat UTIs, pyelonephritis, or renal scarring in children who were treated with prophylaxis or no prophylaxis and have questioned the need for routine VCUG in children with their first UTI who have normal renal ultrasound. This controversy is currently unresolved and the AAP has not updated its position statement.

Some authorities recommend a routine technetium 99m-dimercaptosuccinic acid (99mTc-DMSA) renal scan to differentiate upper from lower tract infection. Although the test is positive in 60% to 90% of children with a clinical diagnosis of acute pyelonephritis, the cost, exposure to radiation, and the fact that therapy is usually not altered preclude the routine use of this study. The scan is most helpful in a child where the diagnosis of acute pyelonephritis is in doubt or when used in follow-up to detect development of renal scars, especially in patients with VUR.

Management

All infants younger than 2 months with UTIs should be treated with parenteral **antibiotics,** starting with broad-spectrum antibiotic coverage, such as ceftriaxone, cefotaxime, or ampicillin and gentamicin, pending results of sensitivity studies. Children older than 2 months who appear well and are able to tolerate liquids may receive oral antibiotics on an outpatient basis. Most physicians recommend cephalexin for the first infection until the results of bacterial sensitivity tests are available and treatment is then continued for a total of 10 days. In older children with clear-cut lower tract infection, shorter courses of trimethoprim-sulfamethoxazole are also effective. One should be aware of the local *E coli* resistance patterns because some communities have a high incidence of *E coli* resistance to trimethoprim-sulfamethoxazole. Children who appear toxic and/or are vomiting should be admitted to the hospital and started on parenteral antibiotics until they show clinical improvement, at which time they can be sent home on oral therapy. In most cases there is clinical improvement within 48 hours of initiating treatment and the urine becomes sterile. In high-risk individuals with urinary abnormalities, immunocompromise state or disorders, or sickle cell disease or those who clinically fail to improve within 48 hours a urine culture should be repeated in a timely manner in order to determine whether there is a new infection or the patient has developed resistance to the previous organism. The culture should be repeated again in 2 to 4 weeks after completing the course of antibiotic to determine eradication of the infection. Although recent studies have suggested that prophylactic antibiotics do not necessarily prevent infections or renal scarring and may cause increased risk of resistant infections, most children

with VUR, especially those with grade III or higher, are still placed on low-dose antibiotics (trimethoprim-sulfamethoxazole, cephalexin, or nitrofurantoin) that are continued for 12 to 18 months following treatment for an acute infection. At the end of this period, a radionucleide VCUG is repeated to determine whether reflux has resolved. Development of new renal scars can be best detected by 99mTc-DMSA renal scanning.

Surgery is not necessary in most infants with VUR, including many with severe disease (grades IV and V) because most grade I through III and some grade IV and V reflux in infants disappears with increasing age. In children older than 5 years with grade IV or V reflux, the rate of disappearance with medical treatment is much lower (about 20%–25%). The results of the International Vesicoureteral Reflux Study Group show no difference in the rate of renal scarring between prophylactic medical treatment and surgery. Therefore, surgical reimplantation of the ureter is usually recommended only for those patients who have poor adherence with prophylaxis or breakthrough infections, especially if the upper tract is involved. This latter group seems to have benefited the most from surgery.

An alternate to surgical reimplantation, Deflux is a gel composed of dextranomers and hyaluronic acid that can be injected endoscopically into the ureters. It was approved by the US Food and Drug Administration in September 2001 after having been used extensively throughout Europe with great success. Most pediatric urologists agree that Deflux should be used for persistent grades II through IV, while grade I can be managed expectantly. Severe grade V reflux usually requires surgical reimplantation of the ureter to prevent recurrent infections and scarring of the kidneys.

Prognosis

In most children, UTI is a minor illness with very few long-term or serious consequences. However, UTI commonly reoccurs, especially during the first year following the initial UTI. Repeat urine cultures should be obtained during follow-up assessments in all children with VUR, first at 1- to 2-month intervals and later at 3- to 4-month intervals for at least 1 year or until disappearance of reflux.

The risk factors for the development of renal scars and eventual hypertension and/or renal failure include young age (<1 year), recurrent episodes of acute pyelonephritis, delay in starting effective antibiotic therapy, high-grade reflux, and anatomical or neurogenic obstruction. If repeat infection is prevented in these children, however, development of fresh scars is uncommon, and renal function and growth remain normal. As a group, infants and children younger than 3 years with UTI and high-grade VUR are more likely to develop calyceal clubbing and renal scarring, whereas progressive renal scarring as a result of UTI or reflux after 5 years of age is relatively less common.

CASE RESOLUTION

In the case history, the young girl is hospitalized because of the vomiting. She is started on intravenous ceftriaxone and she improves in 48 hours. Her inpatient renal ultrasound is normal, and she is discharged home with oral antibiotics. Because a radionuclide VCUG is planned in 4 weeks, she is also given a prescription for prophylactic antibiotics to take until the VCUG is completed.

Selected References

American Academy of Pediatrics Committee on Quality Improvement, Subcommittee on Urinary Tract Infection. Practice parameter: the diagnosis, treatment, and evaluation of the initial urinary tract infection in febrile infants and young children. *Pediatrics*. 1999;103:843–852

Chang S, Shortliffe L. Pediatric urinary tract infections. *Pediatr Clin North Am*. 2006;53:379–400

Feld LG, Mattoo TK. Urinary tract infections and vesicoureteral reflux in infants and children. *Pediatr Rev*. 2010;31:451–462

Freedman AL. Urologic Diseases of America project: trends in resource utilization for urinary tract infections in children. *J Urol*. 2005;173:949–954

Hellerstein S. Acute urinary tract infection–evaluation and treatment. *Curr Opin Pediatr*. 2006;18:134–138

Matoo TK. Are prophylactic antibiotics indicated after a urinary tract infection? *Curr Opin Pediatr*. 2009;21:203–206

Schnadower D, Kupperman N, Macias CG, et al. Febrile infants with urinary tract infections at very low risk for adverse events and bacteremia. *Pediatrics*. 2010;126:1074–1083

Shaikh N, Morone N, Bost JE, et al. Prevalance of urinary tract infection in childhood: a meta analysis. *Pediatr Infect Dis J*. 2008;27:302–308

CHAPTER 96

Vaginitis

Monica Sifuentes, MD

CASE STUDY

An 11-year-old girl is brought to your office with vaginal itching for 1 week and a yellow discharge on her panties for the past 4 days. The girl reports no associated abdominal pain, vomiting, or diarrhea. She has no urinary problems and also denies any history of sexual abuse. Although she occasionally bathes with bubble bath, she most often takes showers. Except for the vaginal complaint, she is healthy, and she takes no medications.

The physical examination is notable for a soft, non-tender abdomen with no organomegaly. Bowel sounds are audible in all quadrants. The genitalia are sexual maturity rating (SMR) (Tanner stage) 2. The labia majora and minora and the clitoris all appear normal, and the hymen is annular in shape with a smooth rim. A scant amount of yellow discharge, along with minimal perihymenal injection, is noted at the vaginal introitus. The anal examination is normal, with an intact anal wink.

Questions

1. What are the most common causes for vaginal discharge in prepubescent and adolescent females? How do they differ?
2. What basic historical information must be obtained from all females whose chief complaint is vaginal discharge?
3. What specific methods are used to perform a gynecologic examination in prepubescent and adolescent females?
4. What is the appropriate laboratory evaluation for prepubescent and adolescent females who complain of vaginal discharge? How does this evaluation differ for adolescent females who are sexually active?
5. What are the various treatment options for females with vaginitis?

Vaginal discharge is not an uncommon occurrence in prepubescent and adolescent females. Practitioners are largely responsible for differentiating between a physiological discharge, or leukorrhea, and a pathologic discharge, which occurs, for example, with a bacterial or yeast infection. In cases of an abnormal discharge, the possibility of abuse needs to be considered and investigated appropriately (see Chapter 128). Primary care physicians should become familiar with the various causes of vaginal discharge in both prepubescent and adolescent females. More importantly, they should be comfortable performing gynecologic examinations in these patients so that the appropriate treatment can be initiated.

Vulvovaginitis, which is often used interchangeably with vaginitis or vulvitis, signifies inflammation of the perineal area, often accompanied by vaginal discharge. The discharge may be bloody, malodorous, or purulent, depending on the etiology (Table 96-1).

Epidemiology

Vulvovaginitis is the most common gynecologic complaint in prepubescent girls. Most cases of vulvovaginitis in these girls result from **nonspecific inflammation;** vaginal cultures show normal flora in 33% to 85% of such cases. The incidence of more specific **bacterial causes,** such as group A beta-hemolytic streptococcus (GABHS), has been reported in approximately 14% of patients. However, its occurrence seems to be seasonal, and confirming the diagnosis depends on the use of proper culturing techniques using the appropriate

Table 96-1. Characteristics and Specific Causes of Vaginal Discharge			
Color	Consistency	Amount	Cause
Clear/white	Thin	Variable	Physiological; bacterial vaginosis
White	Cottage cheese like	Moderate	*Candida*
White/yellow	Variable	Variable	Chemical irritation, *Chlamydia trachomatis*
Yellow/green	Thick	Moderate–profuse	*Neisseria gonorrhoeae,* foreign body, *Trichomonas vaginalis*
Bloody	Variable	Variable	*Shigella,* group A streptococcus, foreign body

media. Other bacterial causes include respiratory pathogens such as *Haemophilus influenzae, Neisseria meningitidis, Streptococcus pneumoniae,* and enteric organisms such as *Shigella.* A positive culture for *Chlamydia trachomatis* or *Neisseria gonorrhoeae* can be found in approximately 5% of children who are evaluated for sexual abuse. Higher figures have been reported from selected centers and when data from adolescent victims are included. These organisms are not considered part of the normal flora in prepubescent girls. Vaginal and rectal infections with *C trachomatis* can be acquired perinatally, but usually are not considered perinatally acquired after 2 to 3 years of age.

Parasitic infections may also lead to vaginal symptoms. Twenty percent of females with a rectal infestation of *Enterobius vermicularis*, the organism known as pinworm, have vulvovaginitis. Affected patients often complain of anal pruritus in addition to the vaginal discharge. **Mycotic infections** with organisms such as *Candida albicans* also can cause symptoms in prepubescent girls, although many of these girls have a previous history of oral antibiotic use.

Clinical Presentation

Prepubescent and adolescent females with vulvovaginitis most commonly present with a vaginal discharge, which may be white, purulent (ie, yellow or green), or serosanguineous. Its consistency can range from smooth and thin to thick and cottage cheese–like. The discharge may also be malodorous. In addition, females may complain of associated pruritus, erythema, urinary problems such as dysuria and increased frequency, and abdominal pain (Dx Box). Sexually active adolescent females with vaginitis from a sexually transmitted infection (STI) (eg, gonorrhea) generally have a more profuse, purulent discharge.

| **Dx** | **Vaginitis** |

- Nonphysiological vaginal discharge
- Profuse or malodorous vaginal discharge
- Perineal erythema
- Vaginal pruritus or irritation
- Dysuria

Pathophysiology

Prepubescent girls are at risk for developing vulvovaginitis for both anatomical and physiological reasons. Unlike pubertal adolescents and young women, prepubescent girls have no pubic hair and a smaller labial fat pad to protect the vaginal introitus. The labia minora are small and tend to open when girls are in a squatting position, thereby exposing the vaginal introitus. The relative proximity of the anus to the vagina in young girls also contributes to vaginal contamination with enteric organisms. More importantly, poor hygienic practices (ie, wiping back to front after urination or defecation) can further compound the problem.

In addition, the normal physiology of the vaginal epithelium in prepubescent girls predisposes to vaginitis. The unestrogenized vaginal epithelium is relatively thin, immature, and easily traumatized. In addition, the pH of the vagina is neutral to alkaline, compared with the acidic environment of the vagina in adult females. Local antibody production also may be lacking in the vagina of prepubescent girls.

Differential Diagnosis

A vaginal discharge is normal at 2 distinct times in prepubescent girls: shortly after birth, secondary to the effects of maternal estrogen, and approximately 6 months to 1 year before the onset of menarche, which occurs, in most girls, by SMR (Tanner Stage) 4. Other causes of vaginal discharges in prepubescent and pubescent females are presented in Box 96-1.

Box 96-1. Causes of Vaginal Discharge in Prepubescent and Pubescent Females

Prepubescent Females
- Estrogen withdrawal (neonates)
- Chemical irritation secondary to soaps and detergents
- Mechanical irritation from nylon panties or tight-fitting clothes
- Foreign body in vagina
- Poor hygiene
- Pinworms
- Yeast infection (eg, *Candida*)
- Bacterial infection (eg, group A streptococcus, nonencapsulated *Haemophilus influenzae*, *Shigella* sp, *Salmonella* sp)
- Sexually transmitted infection (eg, gonococcal infection, chlamydial infection, trichomoniasis)
- Congenital abnormality (eg, ectopic ureter [local inflammation])
- Acquired abnormality (eg, labial fusion [pooling of urine in vagina])
- Urethral prolapse
- Systemic illness (eg, scarlet fever, Crohn disease)

Pubescent Females
- Physiological leukorrhea
- Foreign body in vagina (eg, retained tampon or condom)
- Yeast infection (eg, *Candida*)
- Bacterial infection (eg, group A streptococcus, *Staphylococcus aureus*)
- Sexually transmitted infection (eg, gonococcal infection, chlamydial infection, trichomoniasis, bacterial vaginosis)
- Chemical irritation (eg, douches, spermicides, latex [condoms])
- Local trauma (eg, penile studs)

Evaluation

Prepubescent Females

History

A complete history should be obtained in all females with a vaginal discharge (Questions Box). Practitioners should inquire about the appearance of the discharge, its duration, and the relative amount. A profuse, purulent discharge is probably more consistent with one specific etiology (eg, *N gonorrhoeae*) than is a scant, thin discharge that suggests a nonspecific etiology. The existence of urinary problems also should be determined. Pooling of urine in the vagina secondary to labial fusion can lead to vulvovaginitis in addition to a

Vaginitis

Prepubescent Females

- What is the color of the discharge?
- What is the consistency of the discharge?
- How profuse is the discharge?
- Is the discharge malodorous?
- How long has the discharge been present?
- How often does the discharge occur (ie, is it found on the panties daily)?
- Are there any associated problems (eg, dysuria, abdominal pain)?
- What types of laundry soaps or detergents are used?
- Does the child take bubble baths?
- Has the child had any recent illnesses or treatment with oral antibiotics?
- Does the child clean herself after using the toilet, or does she require help?
- In what direction does she tend to wipe after a bowel movement?
- Is there a concern for, or history of, child sexual abuse?

Adolescent Females (all of the above questions plus the following)

- What is the reproductive history (menstrual and sexual)?
- Does the adolescent douche or use scented panty liners?
- Is there a history of sexual assault/abuse?
- If appropriate, is the adolescent using any form of barrier or hormonal contraception? When was the last episode of unprotected intercourse?
- How many sexual partners has the patient had?
- Does the patient or partner have any history of a previous sexually transmitted infection, including hepatitis B or C?

urinary tract infection. Changes in bowel or bladder habits and sudden changes in behavior, such as nightmares or inappropriate stranger anxiety, also should be noted. Such changes in behavior warrant a further inquiry into the possibility of sexual abuse, regardless of the practitioner's index of suspicion. Depending on the information disclosed and the age of the patient, a decision might be made to interview the child and parents independently. Other points to discuss include the type of detergents or soaps used for laundry as well as for bathing, because these may be irritating. Any recent illnesses also should be documented as a possible source of autoinoculation or, if oral antibiotics were required, as a reason for the alteration of the normal vaginal flora. In addition, patients' hygienic practices should be reviewed. Adolescent patients should always be interviewed alone (see Chapter 6). In particular, a reproductive history must be obtained, keeping in mind that puberty and sexual activity both alter vaginal flora.

Physical Examination

Although the genital examination is the priority, a complete physical examination should be performed. This not only allows clinicians to identify other abnormal physical findings, but it also alleviates some of the anxiety often associated with a genital examination. Because most vaginal discharges in prepubescent girls result from nonspecific vulvovaginitis, visualization of the cervix with a speculum is not indicated. Regardless of the gender of the examiner, a chaperone is recommended during the genital examination, particularly in postpubertal patients.

The overall demeanor of young girls at the onset of the genital examination should be noted. Overly compliant, apathetic behavior in children may be a cause for concern regarding abuse, especially in the context of a chronic or recurrent purulent vaginal discharge.

On physical examination, children's SMR must be noted and recorded. In addition, the external genitalia should be examined closely for the presence of any lesions or any evidence of erythema. Chronic changes in labial skin, such as those associated with constant scratching, also should be documented.

Girls should be placed in the modified lithotomy or "frog leg" position, and the labia majora should be gently spread apart to visualize the hymen. The knee-chest position also can be used, depending on the comfort of the practitioner as well as the patient. If the labia cannot be spread apart, the girl may have labial fusion. Perihymenal and periurethral erythema and injection should be noted, in addition to any evidence of edema, trauma, or abnormal masses such as urethral prolapse. Hymenal size and appearance should be carefully evaluated for any evidence of abuse (see Chapter 128). The appearance, consistency, and amount of the vaginal discharge, including the presence or absence of an odor, also should be documented. These findings may vary depending on the characteristics and cause of the discharge. Finally, the anus should be inspected for tone and any evidence of trauma or abnormal lesions such as genital warts. An anal wink is normally elicited. Although not usually indicated, a rectal examination should be performed in an attempt to palpate a foreign body or mass in those patients with a chronic or bloody vaginal discharge.

Laboratory Tests

Laboratory studies are often unnecessary in prepubescent girls with a nonspecific, non-bloody vaginal discharge, diffuse vulvar erythema, and no suspicion or history of sexual abuse. A vaginal culture for isolation of GABHS is indicated in girls with an abrupt onset of a serosanguineous discharge and a history of a systemic illness. The cellophane tape test may be helpful in diagnosing a pinworm infection in girls with associated anal pruritus. A KOH wet mount reveals pseudohyphae if a monilial infection is present, although this diagnosis is often made clinically.

If the discharge is purulent or malodorous or if abuse is suspected, vaginal cultures must be obtained for *N gonorrhoeae* and *C trachomatis*. For suspected cases of sexual abuse or assault, culture remains the gold standard because of the risk of a false-positive result with nonamplified probe tests (direct immunofluorescent smears, enzyme immunoassays) and nucleic acid amplification tests (NAATs). With genital and anal specimens, false-positive results can occur because of cross-reaction with fecal flora. In certain cases, a normal saline wet mount to check for mobile trichomonads may be indicated.

Pubescent Females

History

In adolescent or pubescent females with vaginal discharge, physicians should inquire about a history of sexual activity or assault in addition to other information that relates to their condition (see Questions Box). Questions concerning the possible acquisition of an STI also must be asked in a nonjudgmental confidential manner.

Physical Examination

Virginal adolescents with an uncomplicated history should be examined in a similar fashion as the prepubescent female. The external genitalia should be examined to evaluate the SMR of the patient and the presence of any lesions. Perihymenal or periurethral erythema and hymenal size and appearance should be noted. In the absence of a mucopurulent or bloody discharge, a speculum examination is generally not warranted.

In addition to an overall physical examination, a complete genital examination using a speculum is indicated in the sexually active female. The purpose of the speculum examination is to visualize the cervix, properly obtain vaginal and cervical specimens, and examine the vagina for lesions (eg, condylomata acuminata). A bimanual examination must also be performed to check for cervical motion tenderness as well as adnexal masses or uterine tenderness, which are associated with pelvic inflammatory disease (PID).

Laboratory Tests

Adolescent females who are not sexually active should have a laboratory evaluation similar to that described for prepubescent girls. Sexually active teens, however, warrant a more thorough evaluation to establish the etiology of their symptoms and investigate for cervicitis. In general, because a speculum examination is being performed in these adolescents, a single-swab endocervical sample should be obtained and sent for gonorrhea and chlamydia via NAATs (eg, ligase chain reaction, polymerase chain reaction). Urine also should be sent for *N gonorrhoeae* and *C trachomatis* in those adolescents who refuse a pelvic examination or for screening purposes. Recommendations have changed for teenagers regarding when cervical cancer screening (Pap smear) is indicated (see Chapter 40 for details). A culture or direct fluorescent antibody test for herpes simplex is indicated only if the history of exposure is positive and ulcerative or vesicular lesions are present.

Other causes of vaginal symptoms can be determined by the pH and microscopic analysis of a fresh sample of the vaginal discharge. A normal saline wet mount should be made using a sterile, saline-moistened swab, especially if a nonspecific discharge is present or bacterial vaginosis (BV) is a concern. In addition, motile or static trichomonads may be seen on a wet mount as well as white blood cells. A 10% KOH mount is appropriate in cases of suspected candidiasis. Mixing 10% KOH with the discharge may also produce a "fishy" odor (positive "whiff test"), which is consistent with BV and sometimes a trichomonal infection. In addition, a vaginal pH greater than 4.5 is commonly seen with BV or trichomoniasis, although it is not specific. Commercial kits to evaluate for BV, trichomoniasis, and candida via nucleic acid probes also are available for the office setting where pH paper, KOH, and microscopic analysis of vaginal fluids is not possible. A Gram stain of any purulent material may lead to an early diagnosis of gonococcal cervicitis. Serologies for syphilis should also be obtained in adolescents with suspected (symptomatic) or proven STIs. In addition, these patients should be offered testing for HIV, with appropriate pretest and posttest counseling.

Management

Management of a **nonspecific vaginal discharge** is aimed at relieving the uncomfortable symptoms associated with this type of inflammation. Prepubescent females should be instructed to **discontinue use of all chemical irritants,** including bubble baths, in the genital area. Warm water **sitz baths** should be recommended twice daily for approximately 1 week, or until patients feel better. In addition, females should be instructed in **proper hygiene** (eg, wiping front to back after a bowel movement, appropriate hand washing). The use of cotton or cotton-crotch panties and loose-fitting skirts or pants should be encouraged.

Antifungal medications such as **clotrimazole** (Lotrimin) or **miconazole** (Monistat) cream may be prescribed if a monilial infection is present. Empiric treatment may be warranted in children or adolescents with a previous history of oral antibiotic usage, diabetes mellitus, or other chronic conditions that may alter the normal vaginal flora.

Pinworms are treated with a single oral dose of **mebendazole** (Vermox), 100 mg, or **pyrantel pamoate** (Antiminth), 11 mg/kg/dose (to a maximum of 1 g). Most authorities recommend repeat treatment after 2 weeks to kill worms that may have hatched after the first dose. Bedding and clothing should be laundered.

If a retained foreign body is suspected in prepubescent girls, an examination under general anesthesia may be necessary. Alternatively, practitioners can attempt vaginal irrigation in cooperative children by placing a small feeding tube at the hymenal opening and injecting warm saline. Toilet paper is the most commonly retrieved material in prepubescent girls.

Adolescent females who are not sexually active should be treated as outlined above. If the discharge is believed to be physiological leukorrhea, practitioners should reassure patients and educate them about other issues related to puberty (eg, menarche, body odor). Sexually active adolescents with positive vaginal cultures, NAATs, or highly suspicious vaginal discharges should receive treatment depending on the causal organism (see Chapter 97 for details concerning treatment). Table 96-2 briefly outlines current recommendations.

Any disclosure of molestation by prepubescent or adolescent females must be reported to the appropriate authorities. In addition, abnormal physical findings and positive cultures of STIs in prepubescent females and adolescent females who have never been sexually active must be reported to law enforcement and investigated.

Table 96-2. Treatment Recommendations for Adolescents With Infectious Vaginal Discharge

Organism	Treatment[a]
Neisseria gonorrhoeae	Ceftriaxone, 250 mg intramuscularly, once, or cefixime, 400 mg orally, once
Chlamydia trachomatis[b]	Azithromycin, 1 g orally, once, or doxycycline orally 100 mg twice a day for 1 week
Trichomonas vaginalis	Metronidazole, 2 g orally, once, or tinidazole 2 g orally, once
Bacterial vaginosis	Metronidazole, 500 mg, orally twice a day for 7 days; or clindamycin cream 2%, one applicatorful intravaginally at bedtime for 7 days; or metronidazole gel 0.75%, one applicatorful intravaginally once a day for 5 days
Candida albicans	1% clotrimazole cream 5 g intravaginally for 7–14 days; 2% clotrimazole cream 5 g intravaginally for 3 days; 2% miconazole cream 5 g intravaginally for 7 days; 4% miconazole cream 5 g intravaginally for 3 days; 0.4% terconazole cream 5 g intravaginally for 7 days; 0.8% terconazole cream 5 g intravaginally for 3 days; fluconazole, 150 mg orally once

[a]For a complete list of treatment options, refer to Centers for Disease Control and Prevention, Workowski KA, Berman SM. Sexually transmitted disease treatment guidelines. *MMWR Recomm Rep.* 2010;59:1–110.

[b]May be associated with vaginal discharge becaue it causes cervicitis.

Prognosis

In most prepubescent females, vaginitis resolves spontaneously or after appropriate treatment with no permanent sequelae. In contrast, adolescent females treated for vulvovaginitis or uncomplicated cervicitis from an STI continue to be at risk for the development of PID, HIV, and pregnancy given their high-risk behavior and inconsistent use of barrier contraception (eg, condoms).

CASE RESOLUTION

In the case presented at the beginning of the chapter, the girl and her parents should be assured that the discharge is consistent with a nonspecific process. She should be instructed to take sitz baths for 1 week, discontinue bubble baths and the use of soap in the genital area, and wear loose-fitting clothes with cotton underwear. The girl should be reexamined in 1 to 2 weeks. No laboratory studies are warranted at this time.

Selected References

Braverman PK, Breech L; American Academy of Pediatrics Committee on Adolescence. Gynecologic examination for adolescents in the pediatric office setting. *Pediatrics.* 2010;126:585–590

Burstein GR, Murray PJ. Diagnosis and management of sexually transmitted diseases among adolescents. *Pediatr Rev.* 2003;24:119–127

Centers for Disease Control and Prevention, Workowski KA, Berman SM. Sexually transmitted disease treatment guidelines, 2010. *MMWR Recomm Rep.* 2010;59:1–110

Emans SJ, Laufer MR, Goldstein DP, eds. Vulvovaginal problems in the prepubertal child. In: *Pediatric and Adolescent Gynecology.* 5th ed. Philadelphia, PA: Williams & Wilkins; 2005:83–119

Kokotos R, Adam HM. Vulvovaginitis. *Pediatr Rev.* 2006;27:116–117

Stricker T, Navratil F, Sennhauser FH. Vulvovaginitis in prepubertal girls. *Arch Dis Child.* 2003;88:324–326

Sugar NF, Graham EA. Common gynecologic problems in prepubertal girls. *Pediatr Rev.* 2006;27:213–223

Syed TS, Braverman PK. Vaginitis in adolescents. *Adolesc Med.* 2004;15:235–251

CHAPTER 97

Sexually Transmitted Infections

Monica Sifuentes, MD

CASE STUDY

A 17-year-old male presents with a small red lesion on the tip of his penis. He noticed an area of erythema a few weeks before, but it resolved spontaneously. He reports no fever, myalgias, headache, dysuria, or urethral discharge. He is sexually active and occasionally uses condoms. He did not use a condom during his last sexual encounter 2 weeks ago, however, because his partner uses oral contraception. The adolescent has never been treated for any sexually transmitted infections (STIs) and is otherwise healthy. His partners are exclusively female.

On examination, he is a sexual maturity rating (SMR) (Tanner stage) 4 circumcised male with a 2- to 3-mm vesicle on the glans penis. Minimal erythema is present at the base of the lesion, and there is no urethral discharge. The testicles are descended bilaterally, and no masses are palpable. Bilateral shotty, non-tender, inguinal adenopathy is evident.

Questions

1. What conditions are associated with vesicles in the genital area?
2. What risk factors are associated with the acquisition of STIs during adolescence?
3. What screening tests should be performed in patients with suspected STIs?
4. What recommendations regarding partners of patients with STIs should be given?
5. What issues of confidentiality are important to address with adolescents who desire treatment for STIs?

Most teenagers in the United States have their first sexual experience before they graduate from high school. In the 2009 national Youth Risk Behavior Survey conducted by the Centers for Disease Control and Prevention (CDC), nearly half of all students in high school reported having had sexual intercourse during their lifetime, with 6% of students nationwide reporting sexual intercourse for the first time before age 13 years. More importantly, nearly 16% of boys and 11% of girls in grades 9 to 12 reported having had 4 or more sexual partners during their life. The consequences of sexual activity in adolescents include increased rates of bacterial and viral STIs, unintended pregnancy, and the possible acquisition of long-term infections such as HIV in the 15- to 24-year age group. Without adequate antiretroviral therapy, the average time from acquisition of HIV infection to the development of AIDS is approximately 10 years. Given the complex nature of these consequences, the physician must be skilled in obtaining a complete sexual history in teenaged patients and in diagnosing and treating STIs.

Increasing levels of sexual activity directly affect STI trends in adolescents. Other influential factors include multiple (sequential or concurrent) sexual partners; inconsistent and incorrect use of condoms and other barrier methods; experimentation with drugs, including alcohol, which results in poor judgment concerning sexual activity; poor compliance with antibiotic regimens; and biological factors, such as an earlier age of menarche and the presence of cervical ectopy in adolescent females. The feeling of invulnerability and the associated risk-taking behavior that occurs during adolescence make sexual activity spontaneous rather than premeditated.

As a result, preventive measures are hindered, ignored, or simply unheard of, allowing adolescents to deny the possible consequences of their actions. Other factors influencing STI trends are related to societal norms. Traditionally, educational materials and STI services have not been readily available to adolescents in some areas of the United States, unlike other industrialized countries. Many teens also have difficulty accessing health care in their communities and are concerned about confidentiality when obtaining medical services for sensitive issues. In addition, the depiction of casual sexual relationships in television sitcoms, music videos, and motion pictures may play a major role in glamorizing sex. Advances in technology via Internet access also gives teenagers the opportunity to communicate with peers that were previously unreachable.

Epidemiology

The overall prevalence of STIs in adolescents is difficult to estimate because not all STIs are reportable, and collected data are often influenced by the particular population studied. It has been estimated, however, that nearly 50% of all new STIs diagnosed annually in the United States occur among teenagers and young adults aged 15 to 24 years. *Chlamydia* remains the most common cause of cervicitis and urethritis in adolescents, with age-specific rates highest among girls and young women 15 to 24 years of age and young men 20 to 24 years of age. Additionally, studies have shown that certain adolescent subpopulations are at greater risk for chlamydial infection, such as homeless and incarcerated youth, socioeconomically disadvantaged youth, teenagers attending family planning clinics, and pregnant adolescents. Complications of untreated chlamydial cervicitis occur in 10% to 30% of cases and include pelvic inflammatory disease (PID), ectopic pregnancy, chronic pelvic pain, and infertility. Epididymitis, a result of urethral infection, occurs in 1% to 3% of infected males. Other conditions that are uncommon but may occur in males as a result of an infection with chlamydia include proctitis, prostatitis, and Reiter syndrome.

Teenagers have the highest incidence of **gonorrhea** of any other age group, although the prevalence rates have decreased since 2001. The highest rates of gonorrhea reportedly occur in adolescent females, young men in their early 20s, young adult inner-city minorities, incarcerated youth, men who have sex with men, and prostitutes. A large number of sexual partners, injection drug use, exposure to prostitutes, and casual sexual contacts also contribute to the risk of infection. In 2009 the CDC reported gonorrhea rates to be highest among adolescents and young adults. The incidence of gonorrhea in 15- to 19-year-old women was 568.8 per 100,000. Men aged 15 to 19 years had the second highest rates of gonorrhea (250 per 100,000) compared with men aged 20 to 24 years who had the highest rates of gonorrhea (407.5 per 100,000). Of the more than 1 million cases of PID reported annually in the United States, 20% to 30% are in sexually active adolescents. The risk of developing PID is increased 10-fold in this age group compared with adults for several reasons. Failure to use condoms consistently, new partners within the previous 2 to 3 months, and a history of STIs have been cited as risk factors. Complications of PID, such as tubo-ovarian (TOA) abscess formation, are more likely in adolescents as a result of late presentation, delayed diagnosis, difficulty accessing health care, and noncompliance with prescribed treatment regimens.

Although the rate of primary and secondary **syphilis** declined from 1990 to 2000, the number of cases is now increasing, primarily among men. During 2005 the incidence of syphilis was highest among women in the 20- to 24-year-old age group and among men in their mid-30s. In 2009, however, young men aged 20 to 24 years had the highest rates of syphilis. Studies have shown that people with syphilis, as well as other STIs causing genital ulcers, also are at increased risk for HIV acquisition.

Human papillomavirus (HPV) is the most common STI in the United States, with the highest infection rates among adolescents and young adults. Recent studies report the prevalence in sexually active adolescents to range from 30% to 60% and to decline with age. The prevalence of HPV in adolescents varies widely for 2 reasons: (1) infection with HPV is often latent and generally regresses spontaneously and (2) HPV is not a reportable condition. Behavioral and biological risk factors for HPV infection have been identified and include early age of sexual initiation, multiple sexual partners, partner's number of sexual partners, a lack of consistent condom use, and a history of another STI such as genital herpes, which may facilitate HPV acquisition by compromising mucosal integrity. Cigarette use also increases the risk of infection and HPV-related disease, as does an altered immune system.

Infection with **HSV type 2 (HSV-2)** is underestimated and is the most common cause of genital ulcerative disease in the United States. Reportedly, HSV-2 occurs in approximately 4% of whites and 17% of African Americans by the end of their teenage years.

By 2005 the number of **HIV/AIDS** cases reported in the United States in adolescents aged 13 to 19 years was 6,324; the number of cases in young adults between 20 and 24 years of age was 34,987. As of 2008 there are more than 25,000 adolescents and young adults living with a diagnosis of HIV. Because the time from acute HIV infection to immunosuppression is approximately 10 years for untreated adolescents, estimates of asymptomatic or early HIV infection are often based on reported cases of AIDS in young adults in their 20s. AIDs in adolescents occurs primarily in males and ethnic minorities. Most of these individuals are infected through sexual contact or injection drug use. Teen subpopulations who are at particularly high risk for acquiring HIV are youth who have male-to-male sexual contact; are bisexual, transgendered, and/or homeless or a runaway; injection drug users; incarcerated; mentally ill; in the foster care system; or have been sexually or physically abused.

Clinical Presentation

Adolescents with an STI may go to their physicians with specific complaints related to the genitourinary system, such as painful urination or vaginal discharge. They also may report more generalized complaints, like fever and malaise, especially in cases of primary HSV or HIV (Dx Box: Sexually Transmitted Infections). In addition, some teenagers will use a vague complaint to see their primary care practitioner with the hope that the physician inquires about sexual

---

Sexually Transmitted Infections (STIs)

Males
- Dysuria
- Urethral discharge or pain
- Testicular pain
- Presence of any lesions in the genital area such as ulcers, vesicles, or warts
- Sexual partner who has an STI

Females
- Dysuria
- Abnormal vaginal discharge
- Intermenstrual or irregular bleeding
- Dysmenorrhea
- Dyspareunia
- Postcoital bleeding
- Lower abdominal pain
- Systemic symptoms such as fever, nausea, vomiting, malaise
- Presence of any lesions in the genital area such as ulcers, vesicles, or warts
- Sexual partner who has an STI

activity. It may be only then that they will disclose their true concern if the provider is thorough and appears nonjudgmental.

Pathophysiology

A number of biological factors contribute to the increased prevalence rates of STIs in adolescents, particularly in females. At the onset of puberty, the columnar epithelial cells in the vagina transform to squamous epithelium while columnar cells at the cervix persist (Figure 97-1). With increasing age, the squamocolumnar junction recedes into the endocervix. In adolescent females, however, this junction, referred to as ectopy, is often located at the ectocervix and is relatively exposed, which places these females at particular risk for gonococcal and chlamydial infections. The infectious organisms preferentially attach to cervical columnar cells and infect them. Of note is that the use of oral contraceptives also prolongs this immature histologic state.

The cytologic changes seen in cervical cells of adolescents with HPV infection are also believed to be age-related. The immature cervical metaplastic or columnar cells seem to be more highly vulnerable to infection and neoplastic changes. In addition, exposure to other cofactors (eg, tobacco use, multiple episodes of new HPV infections) is likely to promote the development of squamous intraepithelial neoplasia (SIN) and cervical carcinoma. Not all young women exposed to HPV develop lesions or progress to SIN, however, and most will not remain positive for HPV throughout their lifetime.

The presence of genital ulcers has been shown to facilitate both the transmission and the acquisition of HIV. Such ulcers provide a point of entry past denuded epithelium. In addition, it is hypothesized that many activated lymphocytes and macrophages are located at the base of the ulcer and are therefore susceptible to infection by HIV.

Pelvic inflammatory disease usually develops from an ascending mixed polymicrobial infection, often related to an untreated STI of the cervix and vagina. The infection spreads contiguously upward to the upper genital tract, resulting in inflammation, scarring, and crypt formation in the fallopian tubes. The most common causal organisms, which account for more than half of the cases of PID in most studies, are *Chlamydia trachomatis* and *Neisseria gonorrhoeae*. Other agents include *Escherichia coli*; other enteric flora; and microbes implicated in bacterial vaginosis, such as *Mycoplasma hominis*, *Mycoplasma genitalium*, *Ureaplasma urealyticum*, *Bacteroides* species, and anaerobic cocci. Viruses such as HIV and herpes simplex can facilitate the process of this ascending infection by disrupting normal immunologic barriers to infection, such as altering the vaginal pH and flora and the cervical mucous barrier.

Differential Diagnosis

Most patients with STIs present with 1 of 5 clinical syndromes—urethritis/cervicitis, epididymitis, PID, genital ulcer disease, or genital warts, all of which can be easily diagnosed (Box 97-1). Other conditions that mimic STIs, however, must be considered in certain cases where the adolescent denies sexual activity or where

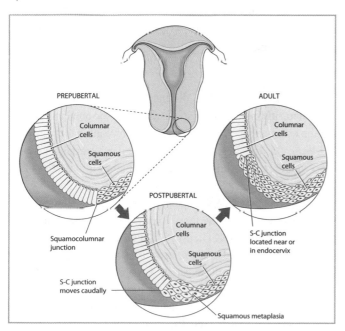

Figure 97-1. Development of the cervical squamocolumnar (S-C) junction, from puberty to adulthood.

Box 97-1. Differential Diagnosis of Sexually Transmitted Infection by Clinical Syndrome

Urethritis
- *Neisseria gonorrhoeae*
- Non-gonococcal disease
  — *Chlamydia trachomatis*
  — *Ureaplasma urealyticum*
  — *Trichomonas vaginalis*
  — Herpes simplex virus
  — Yeasts

Cervicitis
- *C trachomatis*
- *N gonorrhoeae*
- *T vaginalis*
- Herpes simplex virus (especially primary type 2)

Pelvic Inflammatory Disease
- *N gonorrhoeae*
- *C trachomatis*
- Anaerobes
- Gram-negative rods
- Streptococci
- *Mycoplasma hominis*
- *U urealyticum*

Vaginitis
- *T vaginalis*
- *Candida albicans* and other yeast
- *Gardnerella vaginalis*

Genital Ulcers
- *Treponema pallidum* (syphilis)
- Herpes simplex virus, types 1 and 2
- *Haemophilus ducreyi* (chancroid)
- *C trachomatis* (lymphogranuloma venereum)

Genital Warts
- *T pallidum* (condyloma latum)
- Human papillomavirus (condyloma acuminatum)

Proctitis
- *N gonorrhoeae*
- *C trachomatis*
- *T pallidum*
- Herpes simplex virus
- Particular to homosexual youth (in addition to the above)
  — Hepatitis A and B virus
  — *Shigella*
  — *Campylobacter*
  — *Giardia lamblia*
  — *Entamoeba histolytica*

Pharyngitis
- *N gonorrhoeae*
- Herpes simplex virus, types 1 and 2

the disorder does not respond to routine treatment. These disorders include **mucocutaneous ulcers** associated with systemic lupus erythematosus and Behçet disease. Often, systemic disorders such as these can be ruled out historically. **Benign oral lesions** such as aphthous ulcers also can be confused with herpetic ulcers. When evaluating an adolescent female with acute lower abdominal pain, surgical conditions such as **appendicitis, ovarian torsion,** and **ectopic pregnancy** must be ruled out. In the sexually active male with testicular pain, **testicular torsion** must be considered and thoroughly evaluated before a diagnosis of acute epididymitis is made.

Evaluation

In all sexually active adolescents, a complete history, including a sexual history, should be obtained (Questions Box). Because sexual identity and sexual behavior may differ, risk assessment for an STI, particularly HIV, should be based on a review of actual sexual behavior (eg, anal intercourse) rather than on an adolescent's stated sexual orientation. A detailed gynecologic history also should be reviewed with females. The rest of the history should then focus on the particular complaint and any associated symptoms. Sexually active adolescents should have a complete physical examination, including a thorough genital examination. Although diagnostic tests should be determined by the adolescent's risk for a specific STI based on historical and physical findings, one must keep in mind that many adolescent patients are asymptomatic, and screening for common STIs such as chlamydia and gonorrhea should be performed annually on all sexually active teenagers.

Questions

Sexually Transmitted Infections— Questions to Ask the Patient

- Are you currently sexually active?
- At what age did you begin to have sex?
- Do you have sex with men, women, or both?
- How many partners have you had? When was your last contact?
- Have you ever been forced to have sex, or have you ever exchanged sex for food, shelter, money, or drugs?
- Do you or your partner(s) use contraception? What type?
- Do you or your partner(s) use drugs or alcohol?
- Have any of your sexual contacts ever been diagnosed with a sexually transmitted infection?
- Do you have abdominal pain, dysuria, increased urinary frequency, or hesitancy?
- Have you noticed any ulcers, blisters, warts, or other bumps in the genital area? Are the lesions painful?
- For females: Do you have a vaginal discharge or itching? Is sex uncomfortable or painful? Do you have bleeding between periods or after intercourse?
- For males: Do you have a discharge from your penis? Any testicular pain or swelling? Any associated burning or itching?

Urethritis and Epididymitis

History

Because infectious urethritis is more common in young men, all sexually active adolescent males should be asked about the presence of dysuria, urethral discharge, and urethral erythema or pruritis. In females, symptoms such as dysuria may appear more gradually, and dysuria is reported more frequently than other symptoms like meatal edema, erythema, or urethral discharge, which are rarely noticed. General urinary symptoms such as acute urinary frequency or urgency are uncommon with urethritis, especially in males, but all patients should be asked about these symptoms. More often, urethritis is asymptomatic, and the diagnosis is made by routine screening in sexually active adolescents or through known contact with a partner with an STI (eg, *C trachomatis* or *N gonorrhoeae*).

To diagnose acute epididymitis, sexually active males should be asked about testicular pain and swelling. Symptoms associated with urethritis may be present or may have preceded the scrotal symptoms.

Physical Examination

In males, the urethra should be the focus of the genital examination. The presence of a urethral discharge and its consistency (ie, mucoid or purulent) should be noted. Any other urethral or genital lesions also should be assessed. The epididymis, spermatic cord, and testes should be palpated carefully for tenderness and swelling.

In females, a full pelvic examination should be performed after careful examination of the external genitalia for any ulcerative or wart-like lesions. Urethritis is most often caused by *C trachomatis,* but HSV and trichomoniasis can be other causes. The urethra should be inspected for edema, erythema, or any evidence of a discharge prior to speculum insertion. The presence or absence of a vaginal or endocervical discharge also should be noted during the pelvic examination.

Laboratory Tests

A Gram stain of the urethral discharge may confirm the diagnosis of urethritis in males. The specimen should be obtained using a Dacron or cotton swab because calcium alginate inhibits the growth of *Chlamydia*. The presence of gram-negative, intracellular diplococci with the typical "kidney bean" morphology is indicative of an infection with *N gonorrhoeae* (gonococcal urethritis). Five or more polymorphonuclear (PMN) leukocytes per oil immersion field but no organisms indicates the more common type of infection, non-gonococcal urethritis (NGU), usually found in males. In 15% to 40% of cases, NGU is caused by *C trachomatis*. If no PMN leukocytes are seen on Gram stain or if the patient is asymptomatic, assessment for leukocyte esterase with a urine dipstick should be made using the first 10 to 15 mL of a first-voided urine specimen. The sediment also should be examined under the microscope to determine if more than 10 white blood cells per high-power field are present. A routine urine culture is generally not recommended in males and may be of little help in females.

Newer screening tests using urine samples are now available and considered standard of care for detecting gonorrhea and *C trachomatis,* especially in asymptomatic sexually active adolescents. These non-culture tests rely on amplification of DNA (ie, polymerase chain reaction [PCR] and ligase chain reaction) and are highly sensitive and convenient for screening teenagers because the test can be performed on a routine urine specimen. A disadvantage is that these tests are costly and may have a greater potential for false-positive results, making a definitive diagnosis questionable in a judicial setting. In the adolescent population, however, these urine nucleic acid amplification tests (NAATs) are definitely more acceptable than tests requiring a direct urethral swab specimen and can be used to confirm chlamydial or gonococcal urethritis.

Color duplex Doppler ultrasound may be necessary to make an accurate diagnosis of epididymitis, especially if there is any consideration for testicular torsion. If the diagnosis is questionable, a urologic consult should be obtained immediately.

Cervicitis

History

Cervicitis in females is parallel to urethritis in males. Because cervicitis is a local infection, systemic symptoms may not occur, which makes asymptomatic infections, especially with *C trachomatis,* very common. However, a variety of important historical points and associated complaints should be addressed in all sexually active teenagers. Is a vaginal discharge present? If so, does it have an odor? Is the patient experiencing any urinary frequency, urgency, or dysuria? Has she had any non-menstrual vaginal bleeding, including postcoital bleeding? A known exposure to other STIs also must be ascertained. Is the current partner symptomatic or receiving antibiotic treatment? Does the patient or her current or past partners have a history of an STI?

More generalized symptoms, such as moderate lower abdominal pain (either acute or chronic) associated with nausea, vomiting, and fever, may indicate a complication of untreated or undetected cervicitis, such as PID.

Physical Examination

After completing the full physical examination, the physician should focus on the genitourinary examination. The SMR should first be noted, then the presence of any lesions on the external genitalia or inflammation of the perineum. Any urethral erythema or discharge also should be noted. The presence of a vaginal discharge can be assessed more completely when performing the speculum examination, which should be performed in all sexually active adolescent females with vaginal or persistent lower urinary tract complaints.

During the speculum examination, the vaginal mucosa should be inspected, the presence of a vaginal discharge identified, and the appearance of the cervical os should be noted. The physician should determine whether a purulent or mucopurulent exudate is visible in the endocervical canal and should look for any evidence of cervical friability or sustained endocervical bleeding as a swab is gently passed through the cervical os to perform the NAAT and wet mount. Cervical inflammation must be differentiated from normal adolescent ectopy. A presumptive diagnosis of mucopurulent cervicitis is made when there is a discharge from the cervical os, cervical erosion, or friability. A bimanual examination also must be performed to evaluate for cervical motion tenderness (CMT), adnexal masses or fullness, and uterine tenderness.

Laboratory Tests

According to the CDC, NAATs for *N gonorrhoeae* and *C trachomatis* are preferred for the diagnostic evaluation of cervicitis and can be performed on either vaginal, urine, or endocervical specimens. If a pelvic examination is being performed, an endocervical or vaginal swab specimen for NAATs can be collected by direct visualization. A Gram stain of the discharge also can be performed to detect the presence of gram-negative diplococci or PMN leukocytes. The presence of 30 or more PMN leukocytes per oil immersion field is presumptively positive for cervicitis. A wet mount to diagnose associated STIs, such as trichomoniasis, is recommended, especially if the discharge is foul smelling or frothy. Adolescents who are diagnosed with a new STI or engaged in other high-risk behaviors such as unprotected sex, inconsistent condom use, or young men having sex with men also should receive testing for other STIs such as HIV, syphilis, and viral hepatitis.

Pelvic Inflammatory Disease

History

When considering a diagnosis of PID, the history should include a discussion of known risk factors, such as unprotected sexual activity, including the number of sexual partners, especially new partners in the previous 2 months; a previous history of an STI or recent exposure to an STI; the type and consistency of contraceptive use; and the timing of the last menstrual cycle because most women present with PID during the first half of their menstrual cycle. The physician also should ask patients about the presence of symptoms that are often associated with PID: the onset, duration, quality, and location of abdominal pain; urinary symptoms that may indicate concomitant urethritis; intermenstrual bleeding; dysmenorrhea or dyspareunia; abnormal vaginal discharge; right upper quadrant pain; and systemic symptoms such as nausea, vomiting, fever, and malaise. The classic symptoms of PID, which include pelvic or lower abdominal pain, vaginal discharge, fever, and irregular vaginal bleeding, may not be present. More often symptoms are nonspecific or vague, and the practitioner must maintain a high index of suspicion in any sexually active female with pelvic or lower abdominal pain.

Physical Examination

Classic signs of acute PID include fever with lower abdomen pain and tenderness of the cervix, uterus, or adnexa. However, the clinical presentation can vary from vague discomfort to severe disease. A thorough physical examination should be completed before performing the pelvic examination to exclude other common causes of lower abdominal pain. This should include a review of the vital signs, looking for fever or tachycardia. The blood pressure also must be reviewed carefully because hypotension can be seen with a ruptured ectopic pregnancy, which may present with similar symptoms including abdominal pain and vaginal bleeding. The abdomen should be assessed for tenderness and guarding. The location of the pain is particularly relevant because certain acute surgical conditions, such as appendicitis, ovarian torsion, and ectopic pregnancy, are important considerations in the differential diagnosis of PID. In addition, right upper quadrant pain is consistent with perihepatitis, or Fitz-Hugh–Curtis syndrome, which can be seen with a gonorrheal or chlamydial infection. The speculum examination should then be performed, looking for a mucopurulent endocervical exudate or any evidence of cervicitis (cervical friability or erosion). The bimanual examination is the most important part of the physical examination. The cervix should be carefully palpated for any evidence of CMT and the uterus for tenderness or adnexal masses.

Laboratory Tests

The diagnosis of PID is based on clinical findings and a high index of suspicion, after other causes for pelvic or lower abdominal pain have been excluded. Previous CDC criteria for the diagnosis of PID included 3 major components: lower abdominal pain, cervical motion tenderness, and adnexal tenderness. Current recommendations now outline 2 minimal clinical criteria and 5 additional criteria to support the diagnosis (Dx Box: Pelvic Inflammatory Disease). Particularly when evaluating an adolescent for PID, early conservative treatment and maximum sensitivity for clinical findings are paramount to avoid a delayed or missed diagnosis. A NAAT for *N gonorrhoeae* and *C trachomatis* should be sent on the endocervical or vaginal swab specimen obtained during the pelvic examination. If readily available, a Gram stain of any cervical discharge should be performed. The specimen should be examined microscopically for PMN leukocytes as well as gram-negative, intracellular diplococci. The presence of numerous PMN leukocytes per oil immersion field is one of the clinical criteria for making a diagnosis of PID. (See Laboratory Tests section for urethritis and epididymitis.)

Other laboratory studies to obtain include a complete blood cell count with differential and a sedimentation rate or C-reactive protein, although in many cases the laboratory tests are normal. A urine pregnancy test should be performed to exclude the possibility of a concomitant intrauterine or ectopic pregnancy. Additionally, a urinalysis and urine culture should be obtained, as well as a serologic test for syphilis. HIV testing also should be offered to the adolescent female with appropriate verbal pretest counseling. Testing for viral hepatitis is recommended in the patient who has not been immunized against hepatitis B or who has exposure to injection drug use.

 Dx

Pelvic Inflammatory Disease[a]

Pelvic or lower abdominal pain, and one or more of the following minimum criteria on pelvic examination:

- Cervical motion tenderness
- Uterine tenderness
- Adnexal tenderness

Additional Findings

- Oral temperature >38.3°C (101°F)
- Abnormal vaginal or cervical mucopurulent discharge
- Presence of abundant numbers of white blood cells on saline microscopy of vaginal secretions
- Elevated erythrocyte sedimentation rate or C-reactive protein
- Laboratory documentation of cervical infection with *Neisseria gonorrhoeae* or *Chlamydia trachomatis*

Specific Criteria for the Diagnosis

- Inflammatory tubal mass or tubo-ovarian complex seen on magnetic resonance imaging or transvaginal ultrasound, or evidence of pelvic infection (tubal hyperemia) via Doppler
- Histologic evidence of endometritis on endometrial biopsy
- Laparoscopic abnormalities consistent with PID

[a] Centers for Disease Control and Prevention, Workowski A, Berman SM. Sexually transmitted diseases treatment guidelines, 2010. *MMWR Recomm Rep.* 2010;59:64.

Laparoscopy can be performed to make a definitive diagnosis of PID or to obtain direct cultures in cases where the diagnosis is equivocal or the patient is not improving on standard antimicrobial therapy. A gynecologist should be consulted for these challenging cases.

Imaging Studies

A transvaginal ultrasound may help exclude diagnoses such as ectopic pregnancy or ovarian torsion and also can aid in the detection of associated complications of PID, such as TOA. Fluid in the cul-de-sac may be seen on ultrasound; however, it is not specific for the diagnosis of PID.

Genital Ulcers

History

Probably the most important information to obtain from the adolescent with genital ulcers is whether they are painful. A painless chancre on the penis, around the mouth, in the oropharynx, or on the external genitalia in females is consistent with syphilis. If the lesions are painful or are associated with a grouped vesicular eruption, HSV is the likely cause. The presence of systemic symptoms such as fever, chills, headache, or malaise also is important to discern because these symptoms can be seen with a primary infection with HSV or secondary syphilis. Generalized complaints, however, are associated with secondary syphilis only 50% of the time. A history of adenopathy, either localized or generalized, also must be noted, along with dysuria, which may be present in females with HSV. In addition, a history of a viral-like illness accompanied by a rash should be explored further. A diffuse maculopapular rash, especially on the palms and soles, is a classic sign of secondary syphilis. Since a nonspecific rash also can be seen with primary HIV infection, all possible exposures to other STIs should be reviewed with the teenager.

Physical Examination

All adolescents who present with chancres, or ulcers, should receive a complete physical examination. The skin, including the palms and soles, should be examined closely for any dull red to reddish-brown macular or papular lesions. The oropharynx should be carefully checked for chancres or blisters. All lymph nodes should be palpated for pain, enlargement, or induration. Suppurative or fluctuant nodes are often associated with chancroid caused by *Haemophilus ducreyi*. The genital examination should focus on the appearance of the lesions. The following questions should be asked of the patient: Are the lesions ulcerative, clustered, and painful (HSV or chancroid)? Are they associated with grouped vesicles on an erythematous base (HSV)? Is tender inguinal adenopathy present (HSV or chancroid)? Or is there a single, painless, indurated chancre with a clean base and a sharply defined, slightly elevated border (syphilis)? The lymph nodes associated with this syphilitic type chancre are often non-tender but enlarged. Other less common STIs produce genital ulcers that are often painful and deep and may be accompanied by some purulence. Adenopathy can be quite impressive with chancroid and lymphogranuloma venereum (*C trachomatis*).

Laboratory Tests

The necessary diagnostic tests depend on the patient's clinical picture. However, all adolescents who present with an ulcerative lesion should have dark-field microscopy performed for syphilis. Direct fluorescent antibody testing of the lesions is also available and very specific. Non-treponemal serologic tests for syphilis, such as the Venereal Disease Research Laboratory (VDRL) or rapid plasma reagin (RPR) tests, should be done if direct examination is not available or the clinical appearance of the ulcer is nonspecific. In cases of early primary syphilis where the VDRL or RPR may not be reactive initially, the test should be repeated in 1 week. Treponemal tests, such as the fluorescent treponemal antibody absorption test (FTA-ABS), should be used only as confirmatory tests and not for screening purposes.

Viral cell culture and PCR are the preferred HSV tests for persons who seek treatment for genital ulcers or other mucocutaneous lesions. Samples should be obtained from the base of an unroofed vesicle. Herpes simplex virus monoclonal antibody can be performed in older lesions that may be culture-negative and can differentiate between types 1 and 2. Herpes simplex virus serology is generally not helpful. Given the well-described correlation between genital ulcers and HIV, it is recommended that all patients with a diagnosis of syphilis be tested for HIV as well. Conversely, annual syphilis screening is recommended for an adolescent with multiple sexual partners; a history of injection drug use; a history of sex with men, women, or both; or a diagnosed STI.

Genital Warts

History

Risk factors for HPV infection should be assessed in all sexually active adolescents. These include a history of multiple sexual partners, age younger than 25 years, a previous history of STIs, lack of consistent condom use, pregnancy, altered immune response, and tobacco use. Symptoms may include pruritis, pain, or dyspareunia, but often the condition is asymptomatic. Adolescents may inadvertently palpate a lesion on the external genitalia or may note bleeding from larger, traumatized lesions, depending on their location.

Physical Examination

A complete pelvic examination should be performed on all sexually active female adolescents who complain of lower abdominal pain, vaginal discharge or intramenstrual or postcoital vaginal bleeding, or who express concern with "something they felt" in the genital area. Before the speculum is inserted, the external genitalia should be carefully inspected for lesions. Genital warts, or condylomata acuminata, most commonly appear on squamous epithelium as irregular polypoid masses with an irregular, cauliflower-like surface that may coalesce into larger lesions. They are usually located at the posterior introitus, labia minora, and the vestibule in females, and may be found on the cervix and vagina as well. In males, warts are found more commonly on the circumcised penile shaft, glans, or corona, as well as under the foreskin of the uncircumcised penis. They also may appear as flat, flesh-colored papules on the scrotum and anus. Because this is a common location for lesions, the anus should be inspected carefully in both males and females. Intra-anal warts are seen in persons who have receptive anal intercourse, but they can also occur in both men and women who do not have a history of anal sexual contact. Condylomata plana are subclinical lesions that are not grossly visible but are apparent on colposcopy and histology. Condylomata lata are flat, flesh-colored warts that occur in moist areas (anus, scrotum, vulva) and may be associated with other signs of secondary syphilis.

Laboratory Tests

The diagnosis of genital warts is often made by visual inspection and generally does not require confirmation by biopsy. A biopsy may be required in specific instances, such as an uncertain diagnosis; the lesions are not improving or worsen with standard therapy; the lesion is atypical; the patient is immunocompromised; or the warts appear pigmented, indurated, bleeding, or ulcerated. A definitive diagnosis of HPV infection is based on detection of viral nucleic acid or capsid protein. Tests that detect specific types of HPV DNA are available but are not routinely recommended because this information would not alter the clinical management of the condition, except in extraordinary circumstances.

Subclinical HPV infection can be detected using 3% to 5% acetic acid, Schiller iodine, and colposcopy. In the past, suspicious areas of white epithelium or a specific vascular pattern consistent with HPV infection were biopsied. However, this procedure is no longer recommended because prospective studies have shown that many cervical and anogenital lesions, if left untreated in adolescents, resolve spontaneously. For this reason, in 2009 the American College of Obstetrics and Gynecology modified their recommendations regarding screening for cervical cancer in young women to begin at 21 years of age. Of note, the American Cancer Society continues to recommend that young women start cervical screening with Pap tests 3 years after the onset of vaginal intercourse, and no later than age 21 years (see Chapter 40 for details).

NAATs for the detection of gonorrhea or chlamydia can be performed on a urine, endocervical, or vaginal specimen. Additionally, a non-treponemal antibody test for syphilis (RPR or VDRL) is indicated. An HIV antibody test should be offered to all adolescents who are deemed appropriately at risk.

A urinalysis for asymptomatic hematuria is indicated in males with visible condyloma. Its presence would indicate a urethral or meatal lesion.

Management

Although many states differ with regard to the details of health care delivery for adolescents, all 50 states including the District of Columbia allow health care providers to evaluate and treat adolescents for an STI without parental consent, except for unusual circumstances. Routine laboratory screening for common STIs is recommended at least annually in all sexually active adolescents, and as indicated for those who are symptomatic. Positive laboratory results for gonorrhea, chlamydia, syphilis, chancroid, and HIV/AIDS are reportable diseases in every state. Notification of all partners within 60 days of the onset of symptoms or diagnosis of infection or, if greater than 60 days, the last sexual partner is usually anonymous and carried out by local public health officials. Contacts are informed that a partner has been diagnosed with an STI and are instructed to be evaluated and receive treatment.

The complete treatment of the sexual partners of patients diagnosed with an STI is extremely important to prevent reinfection. However, because partners are often asymptomatic and do not seek treatment, and persistent and recurrent infection rates are reported to be particularly high among adolescents, expedited partner therapy (EPT) is now advocated in many states. Expedited partner therapy is the practice of treating the sex partners of persons with STIs without an intervening formal medical evaluation or professional prevention counseling. An extension of EPT, patient-delivered partner therapy, is another practical means for providing patients with medications or prescriptions for their partners. Care must be taken when treating the female partners of men with gonorrhea or chlamydia because of the potential for undiagnosed PID in the female partner. Therefore, as per the CDC guidelines, EPT for female partners should include a review of the symptoms of PID and advice regarding when to seek medical attention in addition to accepting the prescribed medications. Antibiotic recommendations and dosing schedules for the treatment of PID are noted in Box 97-2, as well as in Chapters 96

> ### Box 97-2. Parenteral Regimens for the Treatment of Pelvic Inflammatory Disease
>
> **Parenteral Regimen A**
> Cefotetan, 2 g IV every 12 h
> *or*
> Cefoxitin, 2 g IV every 6 h
> *plus*
> Doxycycline[a], 100 mg PO
> or IV every 12 h
>
> **Parenteral Regimen B**
> Clindamycin 900 mg IV every 8 h
> *plus*
> Gentamicin loading dose IV or IM
> (2 mg/kg body weight), followed by a maintenance dose of 1.5 mg/kg every 8 h (Single daily dosing 3–5 mg/kg may be substituted.)
>
> The above regimens are continued for 24–48 hours after the patient improves clinically. Upon discharge from the hospital, doxycycline is continued orally for a total of 14 days. Clindamycin, 450 mg PO 4 times a day, can be used as an alternative to complete 14 days of treatment.
>
>   When tubo-ovarian abscess is present, clindamycin or metronidazole with doxycycline is recommended rather than doxycycline alone.
>
> ---
> Abbreviations: IM, intramuscularly; IV, intravenously; PO, orally.
> [a]Doxycycline should be administered orally when possible because of the pain associated with intravenous infusion.

(Table 96-2) and 128 (Table 128-1) for other infections. For further details regarding specific conditions and therapies, consult Selected References at the end of the chapter, specifically the CDC 2010 treatment guidelines.

In addition to antimicrobial therapy, management of an adolescent with an STI should include preventive services and counseling regarding risk reduction in a nonjudgmental and developmentally appropriate manner. In addition, the patient's primary language, culture, sexual orientation, and age should be taken into account. Adolescents with a first-time STI as well as those with recurrent STIs should be educated about disease transmission, consequences of delayed treatment, and methods for the prevention of acquiring new and recurrent infections (eg, abstinence, condom use, limiting the number of sexual partners, modifying sexual behaviors, and pre-exposure immunization [Gardasil and Cervarix]). The risk for acquiring other specific STIs, such as HIV, also should be addressed. The physician should spend time with adolescents with recurrent STIs and explore the reasons why preventive methods have failed in the past. Several factors are extremely important to consider, including an untreated partner, poor sexual judgment secondary to substance use or abuse, and noncompliance with previously prescribed treatment regimens.

Except in pregnant women, test-of-cure (repeat testing 3 to 4 weeks after completion of therapy) is not indicated in most routine cases of gonorrhea and chlamydia where the patient has been treated with an appropriate antibiotic regimen. Most post-treatment infections are the result of reinfection rather than treatment failure and occur either because the sex partner did not receive treatment or the initiation of sexual activity with a new infected partner. Because repeat infections can increase the risk of complications such as PID and the rate of reinfection in adolescents is so high, the CDC recommends that patients with gonorrhea and chlamydia be retested 3 months after treatment.

Prognosis

If diagnosed and treated in a timely manner, the prognosis for most STIs is good, especially since the advent of observed single-dose, oral therapies for the most common STIs in adolescents. Sequelae of PID, however, regardless of treatment, include TOA and Fitz-Hugh–Curtis syndrome (perihepatitis). Long-term consequences of PID are chronic abdominal pain, ectopic pregnancy, and infertility. Currently there is no pharmacologic agent to eradicate HSV, HIV, or HPV, although acyclovir, famciclovir, and valacyclovir are useful in treating the signs of primary herpes and reducing the incidence of recurrences. Long-term safety of using valacyclovir or famciclovir for longer than 1 year currently is unknown. The prognosis for HIV is variable, depending on the individual's disease progression at the time of diagnosis and their adherence to antiretroviral therapy. Recurrence of HPV lesions is common since the virus cannot be eradicated completely despite treatment.

CASE RESOLUTION

In the case presented at the beginning of the chapter, a diagnosis of HSV can be made clinically. The adolescent should be counseled with regard to the mode of transmission, the natural history of primary versus recurrent infection, and the role of antiviral agents. A first-void urine sample should be checked for leukocyte esterase or PMN leukocytes and sent for NAATs for the detection of gonorrhea and chlamydia. A serum RPR or VDRL test should be performed as well as a thorough assessment for HIV risk. HIV testing should be offered, allowing the patient time to ask questions or decline testing. The adolescent should be given a return appointment in 1 to 2 weeks to review laboratory results, discuss possible treatment options for recurrent HSV, and explore risk-reduction behavior.

Selected References

American Academy of Pediatrics Committee on Pediatric AIDS, Committee on Adolescence. Adolescents and human immunodeficiency virus infection. *Pediatrics.* 2001;107:188–190

Banikarim C, Chacko MR. Pelvic inflammatory disease in adolescents. *Adolesc Med.* 2004;15:273–285

Burnstein GR, Murray PJ. Diagnosis and management of sexually transmitted disease pathogens among adolescents. *Pediatr Rev.* 2003;24:75–82

Centers for Disease Control and Prevention. *Expedited Partner Treatment in the Management of Sexually Transmitted Diseases.* Atlanta, GA: US Department of Health and Human Services; 2006

Centers for Disease Control and Prevention. Sexually Transmitted Disease Surveillance 2009. Atlanta, GA: US Department of Health and Human Services; 2010

Centers for Disease Control and Prevention, Workowski A, Berman SM. Sexually transmitted diseases treatment guidelines, 2010. *MMWR Recomm Rep.* 2010;59:1–110

Decker MR, Silverman JG, Raj A. Dating violence and sexually transmitted disease/HIV testing and diagnosis among adolescent females. *Pediatrics.* 2005;116:e272–e276

English A. Sexual and reproductive health care for adolescents: legal rights and policy challenges. *Adolesc Med Clin.* 2007;18:571–581

Hogben M, Burstein GR. Expedited partner therapy for adolescents diagnosed with gonorrhea or chlamydia: a review and commentary. *Adolesc Med.* 2006;17:687–695

Kane ML, Rosen DS. Sexually transmitted infections in adolescents: practical issues in the office setting. *Adolesc Med Clin.* 2004;15:409–421

Lehmann C, D'Angelo LJ. Human immunodeficiency virus infection in adolescents. *Adolesc Med.* 2010;21:364–387

Niccolai LM, Hochberg AL, Ethier KA, Lewis JB, Ickovics JR. Burden of recurrent Chlamydia trachomatis infections in young women: further uncovering the "hidden epidemic." *Arch Pediatr Adolesc Med.* 2007;161:246–251

Shafii T, Burnstein GR. An overview of sexually transmitted infections among adolescents. *Adolesc Med Clin.* 2004;15:201–214

Shrier LA. Sexually transmitted disease in adolescents: biologic, cognitive, psychologic, behavioral, and social issues. *Adolesc Med Clin.* 2004;15:215–234

Simpson T, Oh MK. Urethritis and cervicitis in adolescents. *Adolesc Med Clin.* 2004;15:253–271

Trager JDK. Sexually transmitted diseases causing genital lesions in adolescents. *Adolesc Med Clin.* 2004;15:323–352

Wellington MA, Bonnez W. Consultation with the specialist: genital warts. *Pediatr Rev.* 2005;26:467–471

CHAPTER 98

Menstrual Disorders

Monica Sifuentes, MD

CASE STUDY

A 16-year-old female presents with a 9-day history of vaginal bleeding. She has no history of abdominal pain, nausea, vomiting, fever, dysuria, or anorexia, and she reports no dizziness or syncope. Her menses usually last 4 to 5 days and, in general, occur monthly. Her last menstrual period was 3 weeks ago and was normal in duration and flow. Menarche occurred at 14 years of age. She is sexually active, has had 2 partners, and reportedly uses condoms "most of the time." Neither she nor her current partner has ever been diagnosed with or treated for a sexually transmitted infection (STI). She has no family history of blood dyscrasias or cancer, no history of chronic illness, and takes no medications.

On physical examination, she is in no acute distress. Her temperature is 98.4°F (36.9°C). Her heart rate is 100 beats/min, and her blood pressure is 110/60 mm Hg. The physical examination, including a pelvic examination, is unremarkable except for minimal blood noted at the vaginal introitus.

Questions

1. What menstrual disorders commonly affect adolescent females?
2. What factors contribute to the development of menstrual disorders, particularly during adolescence?
3. What relevant history should be obtained in adolescents with menstrual or pelvic complaints?
4. What treatment options are currently available for primary dysmenorrhea?
5. What conditions must be considered in adolescents with abnormal uterine bleeding?
6. How is dysfunctional uterine bleeding managed in adolescent patients?

Gynecologic concerns and complaints are common reasons for adolescent females to visit their primary care physicians. The challenge for practitioners is to differentiate between an organic etiology, functional condition, and psychogenic complaints. When this cannot be readily done or if the physical examination is equivocal, multiple diagnostic procedures may be performed, often with variable results. In addition, many pediatricians are uncomfortable evaluating gynecologic problems in adolescents and performing pelvic examinations, which contributes to this diagnostic dilemma. The purpose of this chapter is to review some of the more common gynecologic conditions affecting the adolescent female and to highlight the significant historical and physical findings associated with each problem. For a discussion of the infectious conditions that cause pelvic pain, see Chapter 97.

Epidemiology

The overall prevalence of menstrual disorders during adolescence is estimated to be 50%, with the most common gynecologic complaint being dysmenorrhea, or painful menstruation. At least 70% to 90% of women have some pain associated with menses regardless of the degree of discomfort. Although most menstruating women report mild to moderate discomfort, severe dysmenorrhea occurs in 10% to 15% of women and has been reported to be responsible for significantly limiting daily activity in these females. Uterine anomalies or pelvic abnormalities such as endometriosis can be found in approximately 10% of adolescents and young women with severe dysmenorrhea.

Prevalence estimates regarding premenstrual syndrome (PMS) are difficult to assess because most studies in adolescents are retrospective and self-reports can be unreliable and misleading. In these studies, between 30% and 75% of older adolescents report significant PMS-type complaints. An estimated 20% to 40% of adult women experience PMS symptoms bothersome enough to impair daily functions, and 5% to 10% have debilitating symptoms. Other menstrual problems in adolescents include abnormal uterine bleeding, vaginal discharge, and amenorrhea.

Several factors contribute to the occurrence of gynecologic problems during adolescence. The average age of menarche in the United States is 12.5 years (range: 9–16 years). Bleeding may be irregular or prolonged initially because 50% to 80% of menstrual cycles are anovulatory and irregular during the first 2 years after menarche. Once ovulatory cycles are established, bleeding problems may resolve, but menstrual symptoms such as pain, headache, and vomiting may predominate. Early sexual activity among adolescents and associated STIs also may contribute to the presence of certain gynecologic conditions in this age group, particularly vaginitis and abnormal uterine bleeding.

Clinical Presentation

Adolescents with menstrual disorders may present in a variety of ways. They may have specific symptoms, such as heavy bleeding, irregular periods, or painful menses, or more general complaints, such as fatigue, dizziness, and syncope (Dx Box). In addition, adolescents or their parents may have questions or concerns about delayed pubertal development and amenorrhea.

 Dx **Menstrual Disorders**

Primary Dysmenorrhea
- Painful menstruation
- Lower abdominal pain associated with menstruation, usually worse on the first few days of bleeding
- Associated back pain
- Pain sometimes accompanied by nausea, vomiting, fatigue, headache, bloating, and diarrhea
- Symptoms began 6 to 12 months after menarche

Dysfunctional Uterine Bleeding
- Prolonged bleeding (>8 days) *or*
- Excessive bleeding (>6 tampons/pads per day) *or*
- Frequent uterine bleeding (≤21 days)
- No demonstrable organic etiology
- Normal laboratory studies, except may have anemia

Primary Amenorrhea
- No spontaneous menstruation in a female of reproductive age
- Absence of menarche by age 16 in a female with normal pubertal development *or*
- Absence of menarche by age 14 in a female with no secondary sexual development *or*
- Absence of menarche within 1 to 2 years of reaching full sexual maturation (sexual maturity rating 5)

Pathophysiology

Puberty and the Normal Menstrual Cycle

Figure 98-1 depicts the menstrual cycle, which typically lasts for 21 to 35 days, with a mean length of approximately 28 days. Normal duration of menses is 4 to 7 days. Blood loss is usually 30 to 40 mL per cycle, and most women do not lose more than 60 mL per cycle. Regular ovulatory cycles usually do not occur until 2 to 3 years after menarche, although 10% to 20% of cycles can remain anovulatory as long as 5 years after menarche.

One-quarter of females begin menstruating when they reach sexual maturity rating (SMR) (Tanner stage) 3 of sexual maturation, but approximately two-thirds do not menstruate until they reach SMR 4 breast and genital development. It is important to note that several other processes occur before the onset of menstruation. Thelarche, or the beginning of breast development, takes place approximately 2 to 3 years before menarche, and growth acceleration usually begins about 1 year before thelarche.

Dysmenorrhea

This condition is often accompanied by other symptoms such as nausea, vomiting, diarrhea, bloating, low back pain, and headaches. It can be classified as either primary or secondary. Primary dysmenorrhea occurs in the absence of any pelvic pathology and is most commonly seen in adolescents once ovulatory cycles are established. Secondary dysmenorrhea refers to painful menses associated with some underlying pelvic pathology, such as pelvic inflammatory disease, endometriosis, ovarian cysts or tumors, or cervical stenosis. A complete list of causes of secondary amenorrhea can be found in Box 98-1. In adolescents, endometriosis is the most common cause of secondary dysmenorrhea.

Numerous studies have shown that cell membrane phospholipids, endometrial prostaglandins, and leukotrienes play a role in the pathogenesis of primary dysmenorrhea. After ovulation, fatty acids build up in the phospholipids of the cell membrane in response to the production of progesterone. Arachidonic acid as well as other omega-7 fatty acids are then released after the onset of progesterone withdrawal before menstruation. A cascade of prostaglandins and leukotrienes is initiated in the uterus during menses, which leads to an inflammatory response. Prostaglandin $F_{2\alpha}$, produced locally by the endometrium from arachidonic acid, is a potent vasoconstrictor and myometrial stimulant that causes uterine contractions, leading to tissue ischemia and pain. Another prostaglandin, $E_{2\alpha}$, causes hypersensitivity of the pain nerve terminals in the uterine myometrium. The cumulative effect of these prostaglandins may cause the pain of primary dysmenorrhea. Hormonal and endocrine factors also may play a role in the etiology of primary dysmenorrhea because ovulatory cycles with estrogen and progesterone are necessary for development of the condition.

Most cases of primary dysmenorrhea begin 6 to 12 months after menarche, and symptoms gradually increase until patients reach their mid-20s. Parity and advancing age are associated with a decrease in symptomatology.

Dysfunctional Uterine Bleeding

Dysfunctional uterine bleeding (DUB) is defined as abnormal or excessive endometrial bleeding in the absence of any pelvic pathology. Menstruation is considered excessive if the cycles are short (<21 days) and the bleeding is prolonged (≥8 days). Although DUB is the most common cause of abnormal or excessive vaginal bleeding in adolescents, it should be considered a diagnosis of exclusion. Other causes of abnormal bleeding should first be investigated by obtaining a thorough history, performing a complete physical examination, and obtaining laboratory studies as indicated.

Dysfunctional uterine bleeding is usually the result of anovulatory, immature menstrual cycles. In adolescents, 50% of menstrual cycles are anovulatory within the first 2 years of menarche. If menarche occurs later in adolescence (ie, at SMR 5), this period of anovulation reportedly lasts even longer. Most cases of DUB in adolescence are thought to result from the delayed maturation of the hypothalamic-pituitary-ovarian axis. Normally, a positive feedback

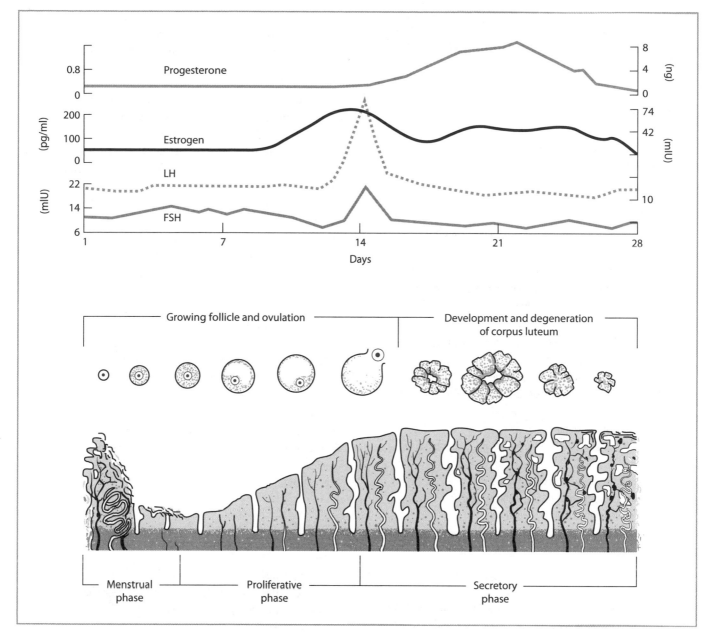

Figure 98-1. The normal ovulatory menstrual cycle. FSH, follicle-stimulating hormone; LH, luteinizing hormone.

mechanism develops with rising estrogen levels, resulting in a surge in luteinizing hormone (LH) and follicle-stimulating hormone (FSH), which triggers ovulation. The progesterone-producing corpus luteum then stimulates development of the secretory endometrium, with subsequent shedding after approximately 14 days if no fertilization occurs (menses). With anovulation, there is no progesterone-producing corpus luteum and, therefore, no development of a secretory endometrium. Thus estrogen remains unopposed, and proliferative endometrium continues to accumulate. Finally, when the tissue can no longer maintain its integrity, it sloughs. In addition, without progesterone, the normal vasospasm that helps limit endometrial bleeding does not occur. Hence, bleeding is prolonged, frequent, and heavy.

Premenstrual Syndrome

Premenstrual syndrome refers to a group of physical, cognitive, affective, and behavioral symptoms that occur prior to menses (during the luteal phase of the menstrual cycle) and resolve within a few days following the onset of menstruation. A variety of mechanisms have been proposed, including an increased sensitivity to the normal cyclic fluctuations in steroid hormones and releasing factors and alterations in neurotransmitters such as endorphins, γ-aminobutyric acid, and serotonin. The exact etiology remains unknown, however, despite multiple studies aimed at pinpointing the cause of this complex condition. Various other hormonal factors have been implicated as possibly having a relationship with PMS, including prolactin,

---

Box 98-1. Differential Diagnosis of Common Menstrual Disorders

Dysmenorrhea
- *Primary*
- *Secondary*
- Endometriosis
- PID
- Uterine myomas, polyps, or adhesions
- Adenomyosis
- Ovarian cysts or tumors
- Presence of an intrauterine device
- Cervical stenosis or strictures
- Congenital malformations (ie, septate uterus, imperforate hymen)

Abnormal Vaginal Bleeding
- Dysfunctional uterine bleeding: anovulation
- Complications of pregnancy: spontaneous/threatened/incomplete abortion, ectopic pregnancy, hydatidiform mole
- Infections of the lower and upper genital tract: PID, cervicitis/vaginitis
- Blood dyscrasias and thrombocytopenia: vWD, ITP, leukemia, platelet defects, leukemia, aplastic anemia
- Endocrine disorders: hypothyroidism and hyperthyroidism, hyperprolactinemia, late-onset 21-hydroxylase deficiency, Cushing or Addison disease, PCOS
- Vaginal anomalies: carcinoma
- Cervical/uterine abnormalities: endometriosis, polyp, hemangioma, sarcoma
- Ovarian abnormalities: ovarian failure, tumors, cysts
- Systemic illness: IBD, malignancy, SLE, diabetes mellitus
- Foreign body: retained condom or tampon, IUD
- Medications: aspirin, anticoagulants, hormonal contraception, androgens
- Trauma or sexual assault

Amenorrhea
- Pregnancy
- Systemic abnormalities: endocrinopathies (hypothyroidism, Cushing syndrome), chronic diseases (IBD, sickle cell disease), poor nutrition (anorexia nervosa), obesity, intense exercise, stress, drugs (opiates, valproate)
- Hypothalamic lesions: tumors, infiltrative lesions (TB, CNS leukemia)
- Pituitary lesions: prolactinoma, drugs causing elevated prolactins (marijuana, cocaine), cranial irradiation
- Ovarian failure: gonadal dysgenesis, autoimmune failure, galactosemia
- Congenital abnormalities of the reproductive tract: imperforate hymen, transverse vaginal septum, absence or abnormality of the uterus, complete androgen insensitivity (46, XY-testicular feminization)
- Androgen excess: PCOS, benign ovarian androgen excess

Abbreviations: CNS, central nervous system; IBD, inflammatory bowel disease; ITP, idiopathic thrombocytopenic purpura; IUD, intrauterine device; PCOS, polycystic ovary syndrome; PID, pelvic inflammatory disease; SLE, systemic lupus erythematosus; TB, tuberculosis; vWD, von Willebrand disease.

---

growth hormone, thyroid hormone, FSH, antidiuretic hormone, insulin, and cortisol. Vitamin deficiencies also have been considered, but have not been documented consistently in the medical literature.

Amenorrhea

Amenorrhea is defined as the lack of spontaneous menstruation in women of reproductive age. Like dysmenorrhea, it can be considered primary or secondary. Traditionally **primary amenorrhea** can be further defined by the following criteria: (1) an absence of menarche by age 16 years in females with otherwise normal pubertal development, (2) an absence of menarche by the age of 14 years in females with no secondary sexual development, and (3) an absence of menarche within 1 to 2 years of reaching SMR 5 pubic hair. Causes of primary amenorrhea range from congenital anatomical anomalies to genetic and endocrine conditions. However, since many of these disorders can be diagnosed and treated earlier than 16 years of age, guidelines have been modified regarding when menstrual conditions should be evaluated (Box 98-2). A detailed discussion of each of these etiologies that cause primary amenorrhea is beyond the scope of this chapter. See Selected References for more information.

Secondary amenorrhea occurs in females who have already established menstruation but have had no periods for 6 months or the equivalent of 3 cycles. The most common cause of secondary amenorrhea is pregnancy, which must be ruled out in all adolescents presenting with this complaint, regardless of their acknowledgment of sexual activity. Other causes include infections, systemic illnesses, significant weight loss, stress, exercise, eating disorders (eg, anorexia nervosa), and certain medications.

Box 98-2. Menstrual Conditions That May Require Evaluation[a]

Menses that
- Have not started within 3 years of thelarche
- Have not started by 13 years of age with no signs of pubertal development
- Have not started by 14 years of age with
  — Signs of hirsutism *or*
  — A history or physical examination suggestive of excessive exercise or eating disorder *or*
  — Concerns about an outflow tract obstruction or anomaly
- Have not started by 15 years of age
- Are regular, occurring monthly, then become markedly irregular
- Occur more frequently than every 21 days or less frequently than every 45 days
- Occur 90 days apart even for one cycle
- Last >7 days
- Require frequent pad/tampon changes (soaking more than 1 every 1–2 hours)

[a]Modified from: American Academy of Pediatrics Committee on Adolescence. Menstruation in girls and adolescents: using the menstrual cycle as a vital sign. *Pediatrics.* 2006;118:2248.

Vaginal Discharge

Vaginal discharge can be normal (physiological). A thin, white discharge, known as leukorrhea, occurs approximately 6 months to 1 year prior to the onset of menarche. A purulent, malodorous, or bloody discharge is considered abnormal, however. Etiologies are varied and may be infectious, inflammatory, or traumatic (see Chapters 96 and 97).

Differential Diagnosis

The differential diagnosis of common menstrual disorders is extensive and can be found in Box 98-1. Other etiologies of pelvic pain include midcycle menstrual disorders (eg, mittelschmerz), urinary tract infections, complications of untreated/inadequately treated PID, and abdominal conditions such as inflammatory bowel disease and irritable bowel syndrome. Psychogenic pain also should be considered as a cause of recurrent pelvic pain and may be secondary to depression, anxiety, previous sexual abuse, or another psychological condition.

Evaluation

History

A thorough history should be obtained in adolescent females with suspected menstrual disorders because many non-gynecologic conditions can affect menses as well. A complete psychosocial assessment also should be performed. The acronym **HEADDSSS** (*h*ome environment, *e*mployment and education, *a*ctivities, *d*iet, *d*rugs, *s*exual activity/sexuality, *s*uicide/depression, *s*afety) serves as a useful tool when interviewing adolescents (see Chapter 6).

Most of the interview should then focus on the gynecologic history (Box 98-3), including pattern of menstrual bleeding, and any associated problems (Questions Box). With primary dysmenorrhea,

---

Box 98-3. Gynecologic History

- Age at menarche
- Date of last menstrual period
- Regularity of menses
- Duration and pattern of bleeding
- Amount of flow (number of pads/tampons used per day and amount of saturation)
- Associated menstrual symptoms such as bloating, headache, lower abdominal pain, and cramping
- Maternal and sibling gynecologic history
- Treatment of menstrual symptoms
- Sexual activity (consensual and nonconsensual)
- Age at debut
- Number of partners and ages
- Date of last sexual encounter
- Protected versus unprotected vaginal intercourse
- Current method of contraception

Questions

Menstrual Disorders

Dysmenorrhea

- What is the pain like?
- Does it always occur with menses?
- When did the pain first begin?
- How frequently does the pain occur?
- How long does the pain last?
- Are any symptoms associated with the pain (eg, nausea, vomiting, diarrhea, headache)?
- Does the adolescent miss a lot of school or work as a result of painful menses?
- Do the painful menses interfere with other activities?
- What does the adolescent do for the pain? Has she tried any medications or complementary or alternative remedies?
- Is there a maternal or sibling history of painful menses?

Abnormal Uterine Bleeding

- Does the adolescent have any symptoms of anemia?
- Is she fatigued, easily tired, dizzy, or short of breath?
- Has she experienced any syncopal episodes?
- Does the adolescent have any history of blood loss in the urine or stool?
- Is there any evidence or a family history of a bleeding disorder (eg, easy bruisability, bleeding from the gums or nares)?
- Does the adolescent have any symptoms of pregnancy (eg, breast tenderness, nausea, fatigue)?
- Is there any known exposure to sexually transmitted infections?
- Is there a marked change in the adolescent's weight? Has the adolescent been on any diets recently?
- Is the adolescent using any medications such as aspirin, oral contraceptives, long-acting progestins, psychotropic medications, or anticoagulants?
- Does the adolescent have a history of a systemic illness such as systemic lupus erythematosus, diabetes mellitus, or renal disease? Does the adolescent have a history of trauma?
- Is the bleeding cyclic in nature?
- Is there breakthrough bleeding throughout the cycle?
- Is there a family history of bleeding disorders, type 2 diabetes mellitus, polycystic ovary syndrome, or thyroid disease?

Amenorrhea

- Has the adolescent ever had a period?
- Has she noticed any other changes associated with puberty (eg, breast development, pubic hair, growth spurt)?
- Does she have any other symptoms such as galactorrhea, weight loss, or hirsutism?
- Has the adolescent experienced significant changes/stressors in her life (eg, parental divorce, new school)?
- How often does the adolescent exercise?
- What is the adolescent's typical diet or are there any dietary restrictions (eg, vegetarian)?

pain that radiates to the anterior thighs or the lower back is not uncommon. The color of the blood may be helpful when assessing abnormal uterine bleeding. Brown or dark blood may be associated with a cervical obstruction or endometriosis, whereas red or pink blood is found with most other conditions. More importantly, the timing of the bleeding is extremely significant. Cyclical bleeding beginning at menarche is more consistent with the presence of a blood dyscrasia. In contrast, breakthrough bleeding throughout the cycle may indicate an infection, endometriosis, or perhaps a polyp. The passing of blood clots on rising in the morning is not uncommon secondary to the vaginal pooling of blood while the patient is supine. Clots throughout the day, however, are not normal and require further investigation.

Physical Examination

A complete physical examination, including an evaluation for stigmata of a systemic illness, must be performed in adolescent females with suspected menstrual disorders. Patients' height and weight should be plotted on the growth chart and compared with previous measurements. Depending on the SMR, physicians can then determine if they have experienced their expected growth spurt. Body mass index (body mass index = weight, kg/[height, m]^2) also should be calculated and compared with previous values, especially in females with amenorrhea. Vital signs, including orthostatic measurements, are a screen for significant blood loss with resultant anemia and are especially important in patients with excessive uterine bleeding. The skin should be inspected for any evidence of androgen excess (eg, hirsutism, acne, acanthosis nigricans), bruising, or petechiae. The thyroid gland should be palpated for masses or any evidence of hypertrophy, and the abdomen and suprapubic area also should be palpated for masses.

In addition, the SMR of the breasts should be noted and compared with pubic hair development, particularly in adolescents with primary amenorrhea. The presence or absence of galactorrhea also should be noted. The external genitalia should then be carefully inspected for clitoral size (normal clitoral glans width 2–4 mm) and patency of the hymen. A bimanual or rectoabdominal examination should be performed in adolescents who are not sexually active to ensure the presence of a normal vagina, uterus, and adnexa. A speculum examination is generally not necessary for the virginal adolescent with suspected DUB or simple primary dysmenorrhea. If the sexually active teen is asymptomatic, screening for STIs, particularly chlamydia and gonorrhea, can be performed noninvasively using a voided urine sample, and the pelvic examination can be deferred. However, in adolescents who are sexually active and have an abnormal vaginal discharge, intercycle menstrual bleeding, history of dyspareunia, or lower abdominal pain, a complete pelvic and bimanual examination is indicated.

Laboratory Tests

The performance of laboratory studies depends on the particular menstrual complaint. No laboratory studies initially are necessary for primary dysmenorrhea because the diagnosis is usually based on

the clinical history and physical examination. The same is true for PMS. For a discussion of the diagnostic evaluation of amenorrhea, refer to Selected References.

In the case of abnormal uterine bleeding, baseline studies must include a hemoglobin or hematocrit. Other initial laboratory studies should include a complete blood cell count to evaluate the red cell indices and platelets, a reticulocyte count, and a urine pregnancy test. Further diagnostic studies depend on the severity of the anemia and findings on history and physical examination. These may include coagulation studies (prothrombin time/partial thromboplastin time), erythrocyte sedimentation rate, and thyroid function tests. Other tests for the evaluation of a blood dyscrasia, such as a von Willebrand panel, should be performed in the patient presenting with severe anemia, especially at menarche. The studies should be performed in consultation with a pediatric hematologist and obtained prior to the administration of any estrogen-containing medications, which may affect the results of certain assays. If the patient is sexually active and a pelvic examination is performed, an endocervical specimen can be obtained for nucleic acid amplification tests (NAATs) for *Chlamydia trachomatis* and *Neisseria gonorrhoeae*. NAATs of the urine to screen for gonorrhea and chlamydia are also available (eg, ligase chain reaction, polymerase chain reaction); however, a speculum examination is still generally indicated for abnormal vaginal bleeding. Follicle-stimulating hormone, LH, prolactin, testosterone, free testosterone, and dehydroepiandrosterone sulfate studies should be performed in patients with a history of chronic anovulation or in whom androgen excess is suspected.

Imaging Studies

A transabdominal or transvaginal pelvic ultrasound or computed tomography scan of the pelvis can be helpful in patients with abnormal uterine bleeding or amenorrhea if a mass is suspected or palpated on physical examination. Complex congenital anomalies, such as a longitudinal vaginal septum with hemi-obstruction, cervical agenesis or stenosis, or a partially obstructing uterine septum, may require magnetic resonance imaging if pelvic ultrasonography is inconclusive. Plain radiographs are not indicated.

Management

With each of these adolescent gynecologic conditions, effective treatment is multifaceted and includes patient and parent education, reassurance regarding the ease with which the condition can be treated, and appropriate medications for those conditions requiring therapy. In general, a **menstrual calendar** or diary initially can be very helpful with most gynecologic conditions to confirm the severity of the bleeding and to assess the pattern of the menstrual cycle.

Dysmenorrhea

General measures in the treatment of dysmenorrhea include education about menstruation, proper nutrition, application of heat (hot water bottle or heating pad), simple exercise, and psychological support. In addition, transcutaneous electrical nerve stimulation has been shown to have some efficacy as a nonpharmacologic therapy for primary dysmenorrhea. It has been reported to work by blocking efferent pain stimuli.

For mild to moderate symptoms of dysmenorrhea, over-the-counter **nonsteroidal anti-inflammatory drugs (NSAIDs),** such as ibuprofen and naproxen sodium, are appropriate for pain management and can also reduce blood loss. Physicians most often suggest that patients use ibuprofen initially because it is safe as well as efficacious when taken in appropriate doses and frequency. The dose is 200 to 400 mg every 4 to 6 hours. Ibuprofen should be taken at the onset of the menstrual cycle and continued for 24 to 72 hours.

For moderate to severe dysmenorrhea in patients who are not sexually active and do not desire birth control, a stronger NSAID, such as naproxen, is the treatment of choice (Table 98-1). The major mechanism of action of NSAIDs is the inhibition of prostaglandin synthesis. Side effects of these drugs, which most commonly relate to the gastrointestinal tract, are nausea, vomiting, and dyspepsia. These reactions can be minimized by taking the medication with food or an antacid. Other adverse reactions include renal effects; skin reactions, such as erythema multiforme and urticaria; and central nervous system effects, including headache and dizziness. Contraindications to NSAID use include peptic ulcer disease, clotting disorders, and renal disease. All NSAIDs should be administered with food and taken for 3 to 4 menstrual cycles before their efficacy is judged.

Low-dose combination oral contraceptives are indicated in adolescents with moderate or severe dysmenorrhea who are sexually active or in patients whose symptoms are not sufficiently relieved by NSAIDs alone and whose own medical or family history does not preclude their use. Oral contraceptives decrease the production of prostaglandins by inhibiting ovulation as well as endometrial growth. Because the symptoms of dysmenorrhea are prevented only after several cycles of oral contraceptive pill (OCP) usage, patients should be told not to expect complete resolution of symptoms during the first month of treatment. Most adolescents who fit the classic clinical presentation of primary dysmenorrhea do not warrant a pelvic examination prior to initiating oral contraceptives. If an adolescent is sexually active, routine STI screening can be performed using urine-based NAATs.

Thirty or 35 µg of ethinyl estradiol-containing oral contraceptives should be used for a minimum of 3 to 4 months. If symptoms do not improve, then an NSAID can be added to the treatment regimen. Oral contraceptives are more than 90% effective in cases of severe dysmenorrhea, and physicians should emphasize this hormonal benefit to both patients and their parents. Although 20 µg of ethinyl estradiol-containing OCP formulations are now available, the literature remains inconclusive regarding their first-line use for primary dysmenorrhea.

If the patient continues to have dysmenorrhea despite the judicious use of NSAIDs and oral contraceptives, a search for other pelvic pathology is warranted and the patient should be referred for possible laparoscopy.

Dysfunctional Uterine Bleeding (Table 98-2)

The management of DUB depends on the severity and frequency of the bleeding and the degree of anemia. The goal of treatment is 4-fold: (1) to control the bleeding, (2) to correct the anemia, (3) to replenish iron stores, and (4) to prevent further episodes of bleeding. Patients with mild or moderate anemia can be treated as outpatients with weekly to monthly follow-up depending on how quickly the bleeding stops. Although monophasic **combination oral contraceptives** are appropriate in the treatment of DUB if the condition is moderate or if birth control is desired, **other hormone regimens,** such

Table 98-1. Nonsteroidal Anti-inflammatory Drugs in the Treatment of Primary Dysmenorrhea

Generic	Trade Name(s)	Dosage
Ibuprofen	Motrin, Advil	200–400 mg every 4–6 h for 24–72 h
Naproxen	Aleve, Naprosyn	440 mg at onset, then 220 mg every 8–12 h 500 mg at onset, then 250 mg every 4–6 h
Naproxen sodium	Anaprox	500 mg at onset, then 275 mg every 6–8 h
Mefenamic acid	Ponstel	500 mg at onset, then 250 mg every 6–8 h

Table 98-2. General Guidelines for the Management of Dysfunctional Uterine Bleeding in Adolescents

	Mild Anemia	Moderate Anemia	Severe Anemia
Hemoglobin (g/dL)	>11	9–11	<9
Management	Reassurance, menstrual calendar, supplemental iron twice daily, COCP 1 pill daily (if sexually active) *Consider NSAID to help reduce blood loss	Initially, 2–3 monophasic COCPs (30–35 µg ethinyl estradiol and potent progestin[a]) every day to control the bleeding with antiemetic, then cycle for minimum of 3 mo; oral iron supplementation *Consider NSAID to help reduce blood loss	Hospitalization if signs of hypovolemia; consider intravenous estrogen until bleeding stops; begin 2–4 monophasic COCPs (50 µg ethinyl estradiol and potent progestin[a]) every day with antiemetic and taper over 21 days, then cycle with monophasic COCPs (30–35 µg ethinyl estradiol) for 3–6 mo; oral iron supplementation
Follow-up	2–3 mo	2–3 wk, then every 2–3 mo	1–2 wk, then every month

Abbreviation: COCP, combination oral contraceptive pill; NSAID, nonsteroidal anti-inflammatory drug.
[a]Potent progestin: norgestrel or levonorgestrel.

as estrogen (alone) or synthetic progestin (alone), also can be used. This is especially important in adolescents who have a medical contraindication or disinterest in combined OCP therapy. **Supplemental oral iron therapy** is also required in all teens who are anemic.

Most adolescent females with severe bleeding and anemia require a more extensive evaluation, and such patients usually are hospitalized for appropriate parenteral therapy and possible blood transfusion. Occasionally, intravenous conjugated estrogens may be required every 4 to 6 hours for the first 24 hours to stop severe acute hemorrhage. Otherwise, in cases of severe anemia, a combination oral contraceptive containing 50 µg or 30 µg of ethinyl estradiol is initiated 3 to 4 times a day; the progesterone component is necessary to stabilize the endometrium. In addition, an antiemetic is often required 1 to 2 hours prior to the OCP during the first few days of therapy. Once bleeding is controlled, the frequency of OCP administration can be tapered, and adolescents can continue a monophasic combined oral contraceptive for a total of 21 days and then switch to a lower-dose combination oral contraceptive for at least 3 cycles. Studies have demonstrated that 20% to 25% of adolescents who require hospitalization for severe anemia within the first year following menarche have an underlying coagulopathy. In cases of DUB where oral contraceptives are used but patients do not desire birth control, oral contraceptives should not be stopped until at least 3 months after the anemia has resolved to ensure restoration of iron stores.

Surgical treatment, such as dilatation and curettage, is rarely indicated in the adolescent patient and is reserved for patients refractory to aggressive medical treatment.

Premenstrual Syndrome

Although various sources have advocated many different treatment regimens for the management of PMS, no definitive studies have been reported, and no single effective treatment has been found. Therapies for mild to moderate symptoms include diet modification for patients who complain predominantly of bloating, promotion of regular aerobic exercise, education regarding menstrual physiology and the relationship of changing hormones to symptoms, stress management, and cognitive-behavior therapy or group therapy. Calcium supplements also can be recommended initially. Although positive outcomes have been reported with vitamin and mineral supplementation as well as with certain herbal preparations, more research is needed to definitively recommend their usage. Of note, some therapies that had been used extensively in the past also have been associated with undesirable outcomes, such as the development of peripheral neuropathy with pyridoxine (B_6) at high doses. Combined OCPs, NSAIDs, and spironolactone may be helpful if physical symptoms predominate. Other medications that may be used when mood symptoms predominate and are significantly impairing function are the selective serotonin reuptake inhibitors such as fluoxetine and/or an anxiolytic, specifically alprazolam.

Vaginitis

See Chapters 96 and 97 for a discussion of the management of vaginal discharge in adolescents.

Prognosis

Most adolescents with common menstrual complaints who receive aggressive, appropriate care are symptom-free after 3 to 4 months of continuous therapy. Complications associated with oral contraceptive use and NSAIDs are rare in this otherwise healthy patient population. Symptoms associated with an immature hypothalamic-pituitary-ovarian axis, such as anovulatory bleeding and DUB, often resolve spontaneously. The prognosis for adolescents with amenorrhea depends in part on the underlying etiology.

CASE RESOLUTION

In the case presented at the beginning of the chapter, more information should be obtained to exclude the numerous other causes of abnormal uterine bleeding in the adolescent before a diagnosis of dysfunctional uterine bleeding can be made. Questions about breast tenderness, galactorrhea, weight loss, fatigue, visual changes, prolonged bleeding, and easy bruisability can be particularly important. If the adolescent has no other complaints, a hemoglobin or hematocrit as well as a complete blood cell count and a pregnancy test should be performed. An endocervical or urine specimen should be sent for NAATs for gonorrhea and chlamydia. Depending on the degree of anemia and the desire for contraception, the adolescent should be placed on twice-daily iron supplementation and oral combined hormonal therapy for at least 3 months.

Selected References

Adams Hillard PJ, Deitch HR. Menstrual disorders in the college age female. *Pediatr Clin North Am.* 2005;52:179–197

American Academy of Pediatrics Committee on Adolescence. Menstruation in girls and adolescents: using the menstrual cycle as a vital sign. *Pediatrics.* 2006;118:2245–2250

American Academy of Pediatrics Committee on Sports Medicine and Fitness. Medical concerns in the female athlete. *Pediatrics.* 2000;106:610–613

Bevan JA, Maloney KW, Hillery CA, Gill JC, Montgomery RR, Scott JP. Bleeding disorders: a common cause of menorrhagia in adolescents. *J Pediatr.* 2001;138:856–861

Bloomfield D. Secondary amenorrhea. *Pediatr Rev.* 2006;27:113–114

Braverman PK. Premenstrual syndrome and premenstrual dysphoric disorder. *J Pediatr Adolesc Gynecol.* 2007;20:3–12

Center for Young Women's Health. http://www.youngwomenshealth.org

Chumlea WC, Schubert CM, Roche AF, et al. Age at menarche and racial comparisons in US girls. *Pediatrics.* 2003;111:110–113

Ellis MH, Beyth Y. Abnormal vaginal bleeding in adolescence as the presenting symptom of a bleeding diathesis. *J Pediatr Adolesc Gynecol.* 1999;12:127–131

Gray SH, Emans SJ. Abnormal vaginal bleeding in adolescents. *Pediatr Rev.* 2007;28:175–182

Harel Z. Dysmenorrhea in adolescents and young adults: etiology and management. *J Pediatr Adolesc Gynecol.* 2006;19:363–371

Hillard PJA. Consultation with the specialist: dysmenorrhea. *Pediatr Rev.* 2006;27:64–71

Kadir RA, Lee CA. Menorrhagia in adolescents. *Pediatr Ann.* 2001;30:541–546

Montgomery RR, Kroner PA. von Willebrand disease: a common pediatric disorder. *Pediatr Ann.* 2001;30:534–540

Rimza ME. Dysfunctional uterine bleeding. *Pediatr Rev.* 2002;23:227–235

Smith YR, Quint EH, Hertzberg RB. Menorrhagia in adolescents requiring hospitalization. *J Pediatr Adolesc Gynecol.* 1998;11:13–15

CHAPTER 99

Disorders of the Breast

Monica Sifuentes, MD

CASE STUDY

A 2-year-old girl is brought to the office for bilateral breast swelling first noticed 3 weeks ago by her mother. The swelling is non-tender and does not appear to be increasing in size. There is no history of galactorrhea. The child is otherwise healthy, takes no medications, and is not using any estrogen-containing creams or other products.

On physical examination, the vital signs are normal, and the child is at the 50th percentile for height and weight. A 1.5-cm firm, non-tender mass is palpated below her left nipple. Below the right nipple, a 1-cm non-tender mass of similar consistency is present. There is no discharge from either nipple and no areolar widening. The abdomen is soft with no masses palpated. The genitalia are those of a normal prepubescent female with no pubic hair and vaginal mucosa that appears red and not estrogenized.

Questions

1. What is premature thelarche, and how can it be differentiated from true precocious puberty?
2. What are the most common causes of breast hypertrophy in the infant?
3. When does pubertal breast development normally occur in females?
4. What are the most common causes of breast masses in adolescent females and how should they be managed?
5. How can transient pubertal gynecomastia be differentiated from pathologic causes of gynecomastia in young males?

Breast disorders can occur in all pediatric age groups. The neonate may present to the pediatrician with bilateral breast hypertrophy and galactorrhea or mastitis. A bewildered parent might bring in a young prepubertal daughter because of early breast development. An anxious adolescent female may notice for the first time that her breasts are asymmetrical, or she may feel a lump beneath the skin. An adolescent male can present with unilateral or bilateral gynecomastia that causes him severe psychological distress. Whatever the underlying cause, breast problems can be disconcerting at any age. Primary care providers should be equipped to differentiate between normal variants of growth and pathologic conditions in infants, children, and adolescents. Although rare, significant disorders can then be diagnosed and treated appropriately.

Epidemiology

Breast problems range from congenital anomalies and benign disorders related to hormonal stimulation to breast masses and tumors. Serious disorders such as breast cancer are practically unheard of in children and adolescents, although inappropriate breast enlargement or gynecomastia as a sign of another neoplastic process is not uncommon.

Benign breast hypertrophy can occur in 60% to 90% of neonates and is seen in both male and female term infants. It may occur unilaterally or bilaterally. Occasionally there is a nipple discharge, particularly in the case of well-intentioned family members who try to "extract the milk," inadvertently promoting the central secretion of prolactin and oxytocin via breast stimulation.

Congenital anomalies of the breast include polythelia, athelia, polymastia, and amastia. Breast deformities such as a tuberous breast anomaly also can be thought of as a congenital anomaly, although it is not manifested until puberty when breast growth normally occurs. Polythelia, or extra nipples, can be found anywhere along the embryonic "milk line" from the axilla to the groin and is seen in 2% of the general population (Figure 99-1). Reportedly, abnormalities of the urologic and cardiovascular systems have been associated with polythelia. Polymastia refers to supernumerary breasts along the milk line and is seen less frequently than polythelia. The usual locations for supernumerary breasts are below the breast on the chest or the upper abdomen. Both polythelia and polymastia may be familial and can occur bilaterally as well as unilaterally.

Amastia (absence of a breast) and athelia (absence of a nipple) are rare occurrences, but their presence often is associated with other anomalies of the chest wall such as pectus excavatum. Amastia also is seen in Poland syndrome (Figure 99-2), which includes absence of the ipsilateral pectoral muscles, various rib deformities and upper limb defects such as syndactyly (webbed fingers), and radial nerve aplasia.

Premature thelarche is isolated unilateral or bilateral breast development in girls between 1 and 4 years of age without other signs of sexual maturation (eg, pubic hair, estrogenized vaginal mucosa, acceleration of linear growth). It has been estimated that 60% of cases occur between 6 months and 2 years of age and that a diagnosis after 4 years of age is uncommon. In contrast, precocious puberty is the appearance of any sign of secondary sexual maturation before age 7

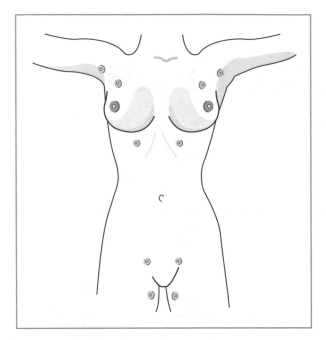

Figure 99-1. Polythelia. Supernumerary nipples along the embryonic mammary ridge (milk line).

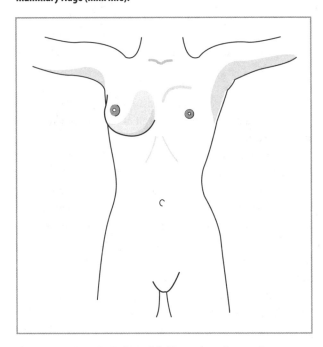

Figure 99-2. Amastia. Unilateral (left) complete absence of breast tissue.

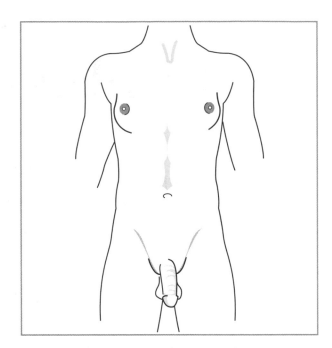

Figure 99-3. Gynecomastia. Breast tissue development in a male.

gynecomastia may be asymmetrical, although concurrent or sequential involvement of both breasts can occur.

In the adolescent female, breast masses are not uncommon; however, clinically significant lesions are rare. Breast cancer per se has an estimated annual incidence of 0.1:100,000 adolescents. In most patient series through age 20, the most common breast tumor is the fibroadenoma, which has been reported in 60% to 95% of biopsied lesions. Two-thirds of these lesions are located in the lateral quadrants of the breast, with most in the upper outer quadrant. Their peak incidence is in late adolescence (17–21 years of age), and they tend to occur more commonly in African American females. In addition, 25% of cases involve multiple fibroadenomas.

Fibrocystic changes are the second most common histologic diagnosis after fibroadenomas. Other breast masses include solitary cysts; abscesses; lipomas; and cystosarcoma phyllodes, a rare, slow-growing, painless breast tumor that is nearly always benign.

Malignancy is reported in less than 1% of excised lesions. There are fewer than 50 cases of primary breast cancer in children and adolescents reported in the literature to date. Rhabdomyosarcoma and fibrosarcomas are among the other rarely reported primary tumors of the breast in adolescents. Metastatic cancer of the breast has been reported in children with primary hepatocellular carcinoma, Hodgkin and non-Hodgkin lymphoma, neuroblastoma, and rhabdomyosarcoma. Of note is the increased lifetime risk for breast cancer in pubertal girls who receive chest wall irradiation, generally administered during treatment for Hodgkin lymphoma.

Normal Breast Development

In the adolescent female, the first sign of puberty is breast development. This begins with the appearance of a breast bud beneath the areola. Under the influence of estrogen, there is an increase in the adipose tissue along with the beginning of ductal and stromal

in Caucasian girls or age 9 in boys. In young females, this involves either breast or pubic hair development, and in males, pubic hair or testicular enlargement.

Gynecomastia commonly occurs in males progressing through puberty and is often called transient or physiological pubertal gynecomastia (Figure 99-3). An estimated 70% of adolescent males are said to be affected, with a peak incidence between ages 13 and 14. This generally corresponds to sexual maturity rating (SMR) (Tanner stage) 2 to 3 genital and pubic hair development in the young male. Like breast development in the pubertal female, transient pubertal growth. Progesterone initiates alveolar budding and lobular growth and contributes to the development of secretory lobules and alveoli. The alveoli are later lined by milk-secreting cells under the influence of prolactin when full maturation occurs during the first pregnancy.

The normal progression of breast growth is divided into 5 stages or SMRs. These descriptions are used to follow normal breast development, which occurs parallel with and generally precedes pubic hair development. It usually takes 2 to 4 years for the completion of breast development although, as in all aspects of puberty, variations do occur. The practitioner should keep in mind that many females will remain in SMR 3 or 4 breast development until pregnancy. Additionally, especially between SMR 2 and 4, significant breast asymmetry can be quite common in the adolescent without indicating a pathologic process. Once both breasts are fully mature and reach SMR 5, adequate catch-up growth usually has occurred.

Clinical Presentation

Infants with breast disorders usually present in the first few weeks of life with bilateral breast enlargement that may be asymmetrical (Dx Box). There may be an associated clear or cloudy nipple discharge. If an infection is present, the overlying skin may be warm and erythematous. Fever or other nonspecific symptoms such as poor feeding and irritability also may be present because mastitis involves the entire breast bud and, although rare, septicemia can occur.

In prepubertal females, benign premature thelarche will present as unilateral or bilateral non-tender subareolar swelling without the appearance of other secondary sexual characteristics. In contrast, girls with precocious puberty may have axillary hair, nipple and areola enlargement and thinning, and pubic hair in addition to early breast development. Adolescent females with a breast problem often will complain of a unilateral breast lump noted incidentally by the teenager. It may be tender, fluctuant, firm, rubbery, or nodular. The adolescent also may complain of painful breasts (mastalgia) that can be cyclic in nature. For most breast masses, the overlying skin is normal, but occasionally skin changes do occur. Rarely, an associated nipple discharge may be present.

Because most breast masses occur in females, gynecomastia is particularly anxiety provoking in young adolescent males. It usually

Dx Breast Disorder

Infants, Prepubescent Children, and Adolescent Males
- Unilateral or bilateral subareolar mass
- Possible associated nipple discharge
- Skin changes such as erythema in infants

Adolescent Females
- Firm, rubbery, freely movable mass
- Possible tenderness
- Breast asymmetry
- Skin changes such as shininess, venous distention, or dimpling (rare)
- Possible associated nipple discharge

appears as a unilateral or bilateral 2- to 3-cm firm mass beneath the areola, which may or may not be tender. There may be irritation of the skin of the nipple from rubbing against the clothing. Galactorrhea rarely accompanies pubertal gynecomastia and may indicate self-stimulation or illicit drug use, including marijuana, heroin, and amphetamines.

Pathophysiology

Neonatal breast hypertrophy seems to be a response to maternal estrogen exposure in utero. Constant stimulation can lead to persistent swelling, galactorrhea, and overt infection (mastitis). Of note, if galactorrhea is present, it should not persist beyond the first few months of life. In general, preterm infants are less responsive to maternal hormones and, therefore, breast hypertrophy occurs less often in this age group. It also may be delayed for weeks.

Central precocious puberty is due to early activation of the hypothalamic-pituitary-gonadal axis and the secretion of gonadotropin-releasing hormone (GnRH)–dependent pituitary gonadotropins in a pulsatile pattern. Although a search for an underlying central nervous system (CNS) or gonadal abnormality may be undertaken, most cases in females are idiopathic. In contrast, less than 10% of males with precocious puberty do not have an identifiable cause, and it has been reported that approximately half of boys with precocious puberty have an identifiable intracranial process. Central nervous system tumors cause precocious puberty by impinging on the neuronal pathways that inhibit the GnRH pulse generator in childhood. Cranial irradiation, received as a part of tumor therapy, also can lead to sexual precocity. Pseudoprecocious puberty is GnRH-independent and is caused by the extrapituitary secretion of gonadotropins or the secretion of gonadal steroids independent of pulsatile GnRH stimulation. (See Muir in Selected References for a complete discussion of precocious puberty.)

Benign premature thelarche is a variation of normal pubertal development with transient elevations in estrogen levels from either functional ovarian cysts or fluctuations in pituitary gonadotropin secretion. Often the breast enlargement occurs without other estrogen effects, such as an increase in uterine size or changes in the appearance of the external genitalia. In general, no linear growth or bone age advancement is associated with this condition.

The cause of fibroadenomas in adolescent females is postulated to be an abnormal sensitivity to estrogen. Observations supporting this hypothesis include the presence of estrogen receptors in the tumor and an increased incidence of this type of tumor during late adolescence. Thus prolonged exposure to estrogen may play a role in its development. Enlargement can occur during pregnancy or toward the end of the menstrual cycle.

The definition of gynecomastia is an increase in the glandular and stromal tissue of the male breast. Transient or physiological gynecomastia is thought to occur from a temporary imbalance of estrogen and androgens during puberty. Alterations in the ratio of these hormones leads to an increase in estrogen relative to testosterone. Certain medications can cause elevations in serum prolactin and lead

<table>
<tr><td colspan="2">

Box 99-1. Causes of Galactorrhea
• Mechanical stimulation of the nipple
• Medications
— Opiates
— Estrogens
— Digitalis
— Butyrophenones (haloperidol)
— Phenothiazines
— Risperidone
— Metoclopramide
— Isoniazid
— Reserpine
— Cimetidine
— Benzodiazepines
— Tricyclic antidepressants
• Illicit drugs
— Marijuana
— Heroin
• Hypothalamic-pituitary disorders

</td></tr>
</table>

Box 99-2. Differential Diagnosis of Precocious Puberty

- Central (true)—gonadotropin-releasing hormone (GnRH)–dependent
- Idiopathic
- Central nervous system
  - Tumor
    - Optic and hypothalamic gliomas (often associated with neurofibromatosis), hypothalamic hamartoma, astrocytoma, ependymoma, craniopharyngioma
  - Lesion
    - Congenital defects, hydrocephalus, cyst in the third ventricle
  - Insult
    - Postinfectious encephalitis or meningitis, static encephalopathy
  - Infection
    - Abscess, tuberculous granulomas of the hypothalamus
  - Head trauma
  - Sequela of cranial radiation
  - Sarcoid granuloma
- Endocrine
  - Hypothyroidism (mechanism unknown)
  - Secondary to GnRH-independent precocious puberty (21-hydroxylase deficiency, McCune-Albright syndrome)
  - Peripheral (pseudo-)—GnRH-independent
  - Adrenal
    - Tumor
    - 21- or 11-hydroxylase deficiency
- Gonadal
  - Tumor
    - McCune-Albright syndrome
    - Familial testotoxicosis
  - Ectopic human chorionic gonadotropin–secreting tumor
  - Exogenous steroids

to gynecomastia and/or galactorrhea (Box 99-1). Some illicit drugs, such as marijuana, contain phytoestrogens that can mimic estrogen or stimulate estrogen receptor sites. Others (eg, spironolactone, cimetidine) interfere with androgen receptors or induce inhibition of enzymes needed in steroid synthesis.

Differential Diagnosis

The differential diagnosis of breast disorders in children and adolescents depends on gender and age at onset. In addition, the presence or absence of other secondary sexual characteristics is helpful to differentiate between a variation of normal pubertal development and a pathologic process.

Infants and Children Younger Than 9 Years

In prepubertal children, the differential diagnosis of isolated early breast development includes exposure to exogenous sources of estrogen such as skin creams, makeup, and medications (oral contraceptives).

For patients with suspected precocious puberty, other etiologies must be considered in addition to exogenous hormones (Box 99-2). Central nervous system tumors, lesions, and insults are among the most common causes. Congenital tumors such as hypothalamic hamartomas are especially important to rule out because they often present before age 3 years. Other CNS tumors to consider are neurofibromas, optic gliomas, astrocytomas, and ependymomas. Specific CNS lesions include cysts in the area of the third ventricle and congenital brain defects. Hydrocephalus, postinfectious encephalitis or meningitis, head trauma, and static cerebral encephalopathy also can lead to sexual precocity. Endocrine disorders include primary

hypothyroidism, estrogen-producing tumors of the ovary or adrenal gland, and ovarian cysts.

Adolescents

The differential diagnosis of breast masses in adolescent females is extensive (Box 99-3). Conditions can be distinguished from one another based on the location of the lesion; its texture, mobility, and size; and how rapidly it is enlarging.

According to some authors, gynecomastia can be classified as type I, II, and III, which is determined by findings on physical examination. Type I is consistent with benign pubertal hypertrophy. The differential diagnosis for types II and III includes physiological gynecomastia (no evidence of an underlying disease process); organic disorders such as hyperthyroiodism, liver disease, and testicular neoplasms; and side effects of medications or drug use (Box 99-4).

Persistent galactorrhea can be caused by several conditions in addition to excessive stimulation of the nipple from sexual activity

Box 99-3. Causes of Breast Masses in the Adolescent Female

- **Fibroadenoma**
- **Breast abscess**
- **Breast cyst**
- Juvenile (giant) fibroadenoma
- Cystosarcoma phyllodes (benign)
- Fat necrosis (secondary to trauma)
- Lipoma
- Hematoma
- Intraductal papilloma
- Adenocarcinoma
- Rhabdomyosarcoma
- Angiosarcoma
- Lymphoma
- Cystosarcoma phyllodes (malignant)

Box 99-4. Causes of Type II Gynecomastia in the Adolescent Male

- Idiopathic
- Tumors
  — Seminomas (40% of germ-cell tumors), Leydig cell tumor, teratoma, feminizing adrenal tumor, hepatoma, bronchogenic sarcoma (ectopic human chorionic gonadotropin production)
- Thyroid dysfunction (hyperthyroidism and hypothyroidism)
- Renal failure and dialysis
- Cirrhosis of the liver
- Klinefelter syndrome (XXY)
- Testicular feminization syndrome (partial androgen insensitivity syndrome)
- Drugs
  — Marijuana, amphetamines, heroin, methadone
  — Alcohol
  — Anabolic steroids
  — Estrogens, testosterone
  — Growth hormone
  — Cimetidine, ranitidine
  — Omeprazole
  — Digitalis
  — Spironolactone
  — Phenytoin
  — Tricyclic antidepressants
  — Risperidone
  — Selective serotonin reuptake inhibitors
  — Isoniazid
  — Ketoconazole
  — HARRT (highly active retroviral treatment)
- Pseudogynecomastia (adipose tissue in obese male)

or jogging without a support bra. Other etiologies include neurologic, hypothalamic, pituitary, and endocrine disorders. Common causes in the adolescent female are prolactin-secreting tumors and hypothyroidism. Drugs that induce galactorrhea in females are the same ones that can cause gynecomastia in males (see Boxes 99-1 and 99-4).

Evaluation

History

In the infant or child, the history should focus on endogenous as well as exogenous sources of estrogen (Questions Box). In addition it is important to ascertain from the parents whether a growth spurt has occurred as well as if other physical features of puberty have appeared. With teenagers, it is important to inquire about drug use as well as systemic illness. All adolescent patients should be interviewed

Questions

Breast Disorder

Prepubertal Children
- At what age was the breast mass first noted?
- Does it seem to be increasing in size?
- Is it tender or erythematous?
- Is there associated discharge from the nipple?
- Has the child been exposed to any estrogen-containing skin creams, medications, or other products?
- In the male patient, is he taking any medications known to cause gynecomastia, such as digoxin, omeprazole, or isoniazid?
- Is the child experiencing any neurologic symptoms such a headaches, ataxia, or visual disturbances?
- Is there a history of head trauma, central nervous system infection, or insult?
- Has the parent noted any other signs of early pubertal development (eg, pubic hair, acne, sudden increase in height)?

Adolescent
- When was the breast mass first noticed, and where is it located?
- Does it seem to be increasing in size?
- Is the lesion tender?
- Is there a history of trauma to the breast?
- Is there any discharge from either nipple?
- In the female, when was the last menstrual period?
- Is there a history of headache or visual disturbances?
- Are there any signs or symptoms of systemic illness, such as weight loss?
- Is there a family history of breast cancer in a first-degree relative, particularly the mother? What was her age at diagnosis?
- Is there a history of chest wall radiation or treatment with chemotherapeutic agents?
- In the male, is he taking any medications that can cause gynecomastia, such as cimetidine?
- Is the adolescent male using anabolic steroids?
- Is the adolescent using any other illicit substances such as marijuana or heroin?
- Is there a family history of gynecomastia or abnormal sexual development?

alone, especially when being asked about illicit substance use (see Chapter 132). The adolescent male may feel particularly embarrassed given the nature of his visit; thus the clinician should be especially patient and supportive during the interview.

Physical Examination

The physical examination includes an assessment of the patient's linear growth, especially in cases of suspected precocious puberty. The height and weight should be plotted on the growth curve and compared with previous measurements. Accelerations in height occur in sexual precocity. Excessive weight gain also should be noted because obesity can stimulate breast enlargement in young females and gynecomastia in males since fatty tissue can be mistaken for breast development if the tissue is not palpated correctly.

The extent of the breast examination depends on the age of the patient. In infants and young children, the breast tissue should be measured and the size recorded so that growth can be monitored over time. Consistency of the tissue and mobility also should be evaluated. Breast growth as a result of neonatal breast hypertrophy and benign premature thelarche is non-tender, firm, and freely mobile. The nipple should be examined for a clear or cloudy discharge by gently compressing each one separately.

In the adolescent female, the breast examination should include visual inspection of the breasts as well as palpation of any lesion and axillary nodes. Ideally this would be performed in the sitting and supine positions, as is done in adult women. Most adolescent females, however, may be uncomfortable with so extensive an examination. The physician must take the time to explain the reasons for the examination to help the patient feel less self-conscious. Male providers always should have a female staff member present to chaperone during the breast examination. In contrast, it is often left to the discretion of the individual female provider as to whether or not to have a chaperone present.

Visual inspection should assess for SMR, appearance of the skin, breast symmetry, and evidence of trauma. Shiny skin or superficial venous distention on one breast would indicate the presence of a large mass. A peau d'orange (orange peel) appearance of the skin or erythema and warmth should be noted as a sign of an infiltrative lesion or infection, respectively.

Palpation of the breast mass can be accomplished with the patient in the supine position using 1 of 3 methods. Using the second, third, and fourth fingers of one hand, the examiner should gently palpate each breast in a pattern of concentric circles, spokes of a wheel, or vertical and horizontal lines. The location of the mass should be noted; a mass beneath the areola might indicate an intraductal lesion, whereas the upper outer quadrant is the classic location for a fibroadenoma. The consistency of the lesion is important. Is it firm, rubbery, and fluctuant, or irregular and lumpy? Is it freely movable or attached to the chest wall? Fibroadenomas tend to be non-tender, firm, discrete, freely movable, and rubbery. A tender, poorly defined mass is consistent with a contusion; a hematoma is more sharply defined with associated skin ecchymoses. Fat necrosis can develop after trauma and is painless, firm, well circumscribed, and

mobile. The size of the mass should be measured and recorded. One must keep in mind that tumor size does not correlate with malignant potential. Finally, each nipple should be gently squeezed to check for a discharge. If present, note whether it is clear, milky, or bloody. A serosanguineous or sanguineous discharge would indicate the presence of an intraductal mass. In addition, a retracted nipple indicates involvement of the areolar area.

In the adolescent male, the breast tissue should be gently palpated in the supine position to distinguish between fatty tissue in the overweight patient and true gynecomastia. Type I gynecomastia presents as a unilateral or bilateral freely mobile subareolar nodule, which is generally up to 3 cm in size. Enlargement beyond the areolar perimeter is consistent with type II; type III resembles SMR 3 breast development in girls. The breast tissue associated with type I and II also is firm and rubbery and may be tender to palpation, whereas type III has a consistency similar to female breast tissue.

The examiner should palpate for axillary lymphadenopathy. Although most clinicians think of its association with breast cancer, it also may be found with infection or necrosis of a benign tumor. In the adolescent male, in addition to palpation of the breast tissue, it is important to evaluate liver size and texture as well as determine the SMR of the genitalia to determine whether pubertal development is consistent with the gynecomastia. The testicles should be palpated carefully for masses and evidence of atrophy (decrease in testicular size). In addition, findings suggestive of hypo- or hyperthyroidism, liver disease, or other stigmata suggestive of a syndrome must be noted.

A detailed neurologic examination should be performed, especially in children with sexual precocity to confirm or detect a CNS disorder.

Laboratory Tests

The laboratory workup for breast disorders is dictated by the findings on history and physical examination. Isolated neonatal breast hyperplasia and premature thelarche require no laboratory studies. Although serum gonadotropin concentrations (luteinizing hormone [LH] and follicle-stimulating hormone [FSH]) and estradiol levels can be obtained in girls with precocious puberty, definitive demonstration of an activated hypothalamic-pituitary axis generally requires the administration of a GnRH stimulation test by the subspecialist. In addition, a morning testosterone level should be ordered in boys. Based on these results, further studies may be indicated, such as a serum human chorionic gonadotropin (hCG) level.

For most breast lesions in adolescent females, no laboratory studies are needed. A fine-needle aspiration (FNA) of the lesion may be performed for those cases that seem to be cystic or if the diagnosis is uncertain. The aspirated fluid should be sent for cytologic analysis if the mass does not completely disappear with this procedure. Sometimes it is necessary to perform another procedure, such as a core needle biopsy, to relieve patient and parental anxiety or to better identify the etiology of the mass. An excision biopsy of the mass allows for more accurate histologic information but is rarely indicated for most lesions.

In the healthy adolescent male with no evidence of systemic illness, no history of medication use or illicit substance abuse, and a normal physical examination including the testicular examination, no further laboratory studies are necessary. If pubertal gynecomastia and other systemic illnesses are ruled out, an endocrine workup is appropriate to elucidate the cause of nonpubertal gynecomastia. This should begin with fasting morning serum levels of hCG, LH, FSH, and serum testosterone and estradiol. DHEAS and liver enzymes also should be obtained. If these laboratory studies are normal, the diagnosis is idiopathic gynecomastia. If they are abnormal, consultation with a pediatric endocrinologist or adolescent medicine specialist should occur.

A pregnancy test and serum prolactin level should be ordered in the adolescent female with galactorrhea, regardless of the menstrual history.

Imaging Studies

Hand and wrist radiographs to determine the child's bone age should be obtained in children with a diagnosis of precocious puberty. In addition, boys should have magnetic resonance imaging (MRI) of the brain to evaluate for a CNS lesion or structural abnormality in the hypothalamus or pituitary gland. Depending on the history, an MRI may be indicated in some girls. Pelvic ultrasound, although rarely necessary, can be performed to rule out the presence of an ovarian tumor or cyst in girls.

Mammograms are not helpful in the pediatric age group, especially in adolescents, and are never indicated in the evaluation of a breast mass. They can be very difficult to interpret because of the dense breast tissue of adolescents. In addition, the risk of breast malignancy is very low. An ultrasound may help distinguish between a cystic lesion and a solid tumor and is noninvasive and not painful. It can also provide more accurate measurement of the size of the lesion and its location prior to the FNA or core needle biopsy.

A testicular ultrasound to search for a tumor is indicated in the adolescent male if the level of hCG or estradiol is elevated, or if a testicular mass is noted on physical examination. Other imaging studies for the evaluation of gynecomastia generally are not useful.

Management

In neonates, mastitis most often is caused by *Staphylococcus aureus* and group B streptococcus. Gram-negative bacilli also have been reported. Parenteral antibiotics should be initiated when the diagnosis is made. Incision and drainage of a breast abscess is rarely indicated and should only be undertaken by an experienced surgeon familiar with the anatomy of the breast to minimize the likelihood of injury to the affected breast bud.

Congenital anomalies such as polythelia and polymastia do not require any treatment. If, however, the patient or parent wants the tissue removed for aesthetic or psychological reasons, it is recommended to do so before puberty. Reconstructive surgery for amastia, as in Poland syndrome, is typically delayed until late adolescence to allow full development of the unaffected breast.

Although no treatment is required for benign premature thelarche, parents need to be reassured that the condition is self-limited. The patient should be reexamined periodically to check for any further progression of puberty, such as persistent breast growth, the appearance of pubic hair, or a growth spurt.

The treatment for central precocious puberty is directed at controlling the secondary sexual development with GnRH agonists. When GnRH is administered continuously, gonadotropin secretion decreases. Currently leuprolide acetate is the only GnRH agonist available for use in the United States. Children should be followed every 1 to 3 months in conjunction with a pediatric endocrinologist to monitor their progression and response to therapy.

Unless otherwise indicated by the type of tumor, children with a CNS lesion as a cause of precocious puberty usually do not require neurosurgical intervention. Therapy should focus on minimizing the degree of growth acceleration and the development of secondary sexual characteristics.

Most breast masses in adolescent females are small, well demarcated, firm or rubbery, and non-tender and can be managed with the "wait and watch" approach. The patient can be followed every 3 to 4 months, preferably allowing a few menstrual cycles to pass between each visit. If there is no change in the lesion or just a small increase in its size, no studies or procedures are indicated because it is most likely a fibroadenoma. As previously noted, an FNA or core needle biopsy may be requested to relieve the anxiety that accompanies the presence of a breast lesion and to confirm the diagnosis. Total excision of the tumor mass and a careful histologic evaluation may be warranted in some cases, but is generally unnecessary in most instances. According to the literature, if findings on physical examination, imaging, and biopsy are consistent with a benign lesion, the diagnosis of a benign mass can be made with 99% accuracy. If this is the case, no further procedures are indicated and the patient can be followed up every 6 months to 1 year. Surgical removal of rapidly enlarging tumors, such as a giant fibroadenoma is important. When the lesion becomes very large, an acceptable cosmetic result is more difficult. Accordingly, the lesion should be removed shortly after the time of diagnosis rather than "waiting and watching."

The primary treatment for transient pubertal gynecomastia, or type I, is reassurance for the adolescent male and his family that the condition is self-limited and should resolve in 1 to 2 years, although some sources state 6 months to 1 year. The teenager should be told explicitly that he is not "becoming a girl." In most cases, he should be reexamined periodically until resolution occurs. Type II gynecomastia may need surgical reduction of the mammary gland, although some studies have shown success with medical therapy. The use of 10 to 20 mg of Tamoxifen orally twice a daily for 3 months has been shown to decrease breast tenderness and pain, followed by a decrease in breast tissue. Plastic surgery intervention may be warranted for cases of persistent breast growth or moderate to severe gynecomastia (SMR 3–4 breasts) in the older adolescent with psychological difficulties related to the condition. Surgical intervention currently involves a combination of ultrasonic liposuction and direct excision of the breast tissue beneath the nipple and areola. The young man may benefit from concurrent psychological counseling as well.

Other underlying causes for gynecomastia should be treated accordingly, and any drugs or medications contributing to the condition should be discontinued, if possible.

Prognosis

The prognosis of a breast disorder in the child or adolescent depends on the particular lesion. In general, most lesions, such as neonatal breast hyperplasia and premature thelarche, are self-limited and resolve on their own. Breast development persists for 3 to 5 years in 50% of cases of premature thelarche, but in one retrospective study, most cases regressed within 6 months to 6 years after the diagnosis. Aside from the short stature that may accompany idiopathic central precocious puberty, these females also tend to have a good prognosis. Fibroadenomas in the adolescent female can recur but typically are benign and have no proven link to the development of breast cancer. Most cases of transient pubertal gynecomastia resolve within 1 to 2 years.

CASE RESOLUTION

The child in the case history has a diagnosis of premature thelarche. She has no known exposure to exogenous sources of estrogen and has isolated breast tissue development with no other signs of pubertal maturation. Her parents should be informed of this diagnosis and reassured that the condition is self-limited and does not indicate that the child is starting puberty. The child should be scheduled for a follow-up visit in 3 to 4 months to remeasure the breast buds and reexamine the genitalia for the appearance of pubic hair as well as to monitor the patient's linear growth.

Selected References

Bock K, Duda VF, Hadji P, et al. Pathologic breast conditions in childhood and adolescence: evaluation by sonographic diagnosis. *J Ultrasound Med.* 2005; 24:1347–1354

De Silva N, Brandt ML. Disorders of the breast in children and adolescents, part 1: disorders of growth and infections of the breast. *J Pediatr Adolesc Gynecol.* 2006;19:345–349

De Silva N, Brandt ML. Disorders of the breast in children and adolescents, part 2: breast masses. *J Pediatr Adolesc Gynecol.* 2006;19:415–418

Diamantopoulos S, Bao Y. Gynecomastia and premature thelarche: a guide for practitioners. *Pediatr Rev* 2007;28:e57–e68

Elger BS, Harding TW. Testing adolescents for a hereditary breast cancer gene (BRCA1). *Arch Pediatr Adolesc Med.* 2000;154:113–119

Greydanus DE, Matytsina L, Gains M. Breast disorders in children and adolescents. *Prim Care.* 2006;33:455–502

Joffe A. Gynecomastia. In: Neinstein LS, ed. *Adolescent Health Care: A Practical Guide.* 5th ed. Baltimore, MD: Lippincott Williams & Wilkins; 2008:180–184

Kronemer KA, Rhee K, Siegel MJ, et al. Gray scale sonography of breast masses in adolescent girls. *J Ultrasound Med.* 2001;20:491–496

Muir A. Precocious puberty. *Pediatr Rev.* 2006;27:373-381

Pacinda SJ, Ramzy I. Fine-needle aspiration of breast masses. A review of its role in diagnosis and management in adolescent patients. *J Adolesc Health.* 1998;23:3–6

Simmons PS. Breast disorders in adolescent females. *Curr Opin Obstet Gynecol.* 2001;13:459–461

Weinstein SP, Conant EF, Orel SG, et al. Spectrum of US findings in pediatric and adolescent patients with palpable breast masses. *Radiographics.* 2000; 20:1613–1621

Orthopedic Disorders

CHAPTER 100

Developmental Dysplasia of the Hip

David P. Zamorano, MD, and Andrew K. Battenberg, BS

CASE STUDY

A 4-month-old girl is seen for her routine health maintenance visit. She is doing well and has no complaints. The results of the entire examination are within normal limits except for limited external rotation and abduction of the left hip, which is approximately 45 degrees, in comparison to that of the right hip, which is almost 90 degrees.

Questions

1. What factors are responsible for normal growth and development of the hip joint?

2. What specific physical maneuvers help in the evaluation of infants with decreased range of motion of the hip?

3. What are the clinical findings of hip dislocation during and after the neonatal period?

4. What are some of the conditions often seen in conjunction with hip dysplasia that may be noted on physical examination?

5. What is the appropriate diagnostic workup of infants with suspected hip dysplasia?

Developmental dysplasia of the hip (DDH) is a common pediatric orthopedic concern that requires a thorough understanding of normal development, pathoanatomy, natural history, and treatment. Developmental dysplasia of the hip defines a range of hip pathology from congenital dysplasia of the hip, partial dislocation of the femoral head, acetabular dysplasia, and complete dislocation of the femoral head from the true acetabulum. Developmental dysplasia of the hip may exist at birth or develop during infancy. In a newborn with true congenital dislocation of the hip, the femoral head dislocates into and out of the acetabulum. In an older child, the femoral head remains dislocated, leading to secondary changes in the head and acetabulum. When DDH is recognized and treated appropriately, children potentially develop completely normally. If the diagnosis is missed or delayed, however, children may suffer significant morbidity, including severe degenerative hip disease.

Epidemiology

Historically, the incidence of DDH is 1 in 1,000 live births. The literature has observed that pediatricians diagnose DDH in 8.6 in 1,000 live births and orthopedic surgeons in 1.5 in 1,000 live births, while the use of ultrasound has resulted in the diagnosis of 25 in 1,000 live births. Hip instability in the neonate is estimated to range from 11.5 to 17 per 1,000 live births. Approximately 50% of these cases resolve by 1 week of age, and 90% resolve by 2 months of age. Approximately 60% of infants affected by DDH are firstborn.

Girls are affected 5 times more frequently than boys. Ethnic variations exist, with incidence highest among the Native American

Navajo, followed by whites and African Americans. Approximately 20% of all DDH occurs in infants born in the breech position. A positive family history of DDH increases the risk by 10%. A female born in the breech position has a 1 in 35 chance of having DDH.

The left hip is involved in 60% of children with DDH, the right hip in 20% of cases, and 20% of cases are bilateral. Developmental dysplasia of the hip has an increased association with lesions of mechanical molding, such as congenital torticollis (approximately 8% of affected children may have DDH), metatarsus adductus (approximately 2%–10% of these children may have DDH), and talipes calcaneovalgus.

Clinical Presentation

The clinical presentation and signs of DDH in children vary with age. In neonates, diagnosis is made primarily by the physical examination (eg, Ortolani and Barlow maneuvers). In older infants, asymmetrical skin folds, limitation of hip abduction, and a positive Galeazzi sign are classic signs of DDH. Physical signs, which become more obvious once children are walking, include waddling gait, limping, and toe-walking (Dx Box).

Pathophysiology

Developmental dysplasia of the hip encompasses a wide variety of conditions ranging from hip instability to dislocation. For normal growth and development of the hip joint to occur, there must be a genetically determined balance of growth of the acetabular and triradiate cartilages and a well-located and centered femoral head. In a normal hip at birth, there is a tight articulation between the femoral head and acetabulum; however, in DDH or dislocation, this tight articulation is lost. Dysplasia refers to (1) a hip that is dislocated but can be relocated, or (2) a hip with a positive Ortolani sign, meaning it can be provoked to dislocate. The term *dislocation* refers to any hip with a negative Ortolani sign, meaning that the hip is not reducible and is associated with secondary adaptive changes such as shortening, decreased abduction, and asymmetrical skin folds.

Dysplasia of the acetabulum is also associated with hip instability. The dysplastic acetabular cavity is shallower with a more vertical inclination angle (Figure 100-1). Although most dislocations occur at or near the time of delivery, this abnormal development of the acetabular cavity helps explain why dislocations can also occur later in infancy. Late hip dislocations are reported in 3% to 8% of affected infants.

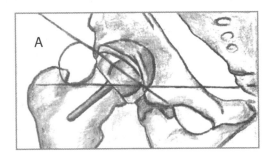

Figure 100-1. **In developmental dysplasia of the hip, inclination angle is increased. Because the acetabulum is more vertical-orientated, the hip articulation is less stable.**

The etiology of DDH is multifactorial, involving genetic and intrauterine environmental factors. The primary **intrauterine environmental factors** are tight maternal abdominal and uterine musculature, breech presentation (causes abnormal hip flexion leading to dislocation of the femoral head), and positioning of the fetal hip against the mother's sacrum. In utero mechanical factors relate to molding and restriction of fetal movement. It is believed that the tight, unstretched maternal abdomen and uterine musculature of primigravidas may restrict fetal movement, thus predisposing firstborn infants to DDH. The increased occurrence of other conditions thought to be secondary to molding (eg, congenital muscular torticollis) with DDH supports this theory of space restriction.

Physiological factors relate to ligamentous laxity. Female infants may be more sensitive to maternal hormones such as estrogen and relaxin, which are present around the time of delivery, resulting in generalized ligamentous laxity, including laxity of the hip capsule. **Environmental factors** that may predispose infants to DDH include swaddling with the legs in extension and adduction, which is still practiced in some societies (eg, Navajos in North America who use cradle boards). Other factors include muscle contractures due to neuromuscular disease, such as cerebral palsy.

Differential Diagnosis

The differential diagnosis of hip dysplasia depends on the age of the child and the presenting complaint. Infants may have a "click" on abduction of the hip that represents the snapping of a ligament rather than the reduction of the dislocated hip into the joint. Infants who have limited abduction may have a neuromuscular disorder such as spastic diplegia, a form of cerebral palsy affecting the lower extremities. Older children who present with gait disturbances such as limp, waddling gait, or toe-walking may have neuromuscular conditions, fractures, or infection (eg, osteomyelitis, septic arthritis).

Evaluation

History

Family history of DDH should be reviewed, and a careful neonatal history should be taken, including presentation (eg, breech versus vertex), type of delivery, history of prenatal problems (eg, oligohydramnios), and presence of congenital torticollis or metatarsus adductus (Questions Box).

Physical Examination

It is important to evaluate the hip joint for instability or dislocation throughout the first year of life or until the child begins to walk. The **Ortolani and Barlow maneuvers** may be used in the neonatal period to evaluate for DDH (Figure 100-2). Both tests are performed with infants in a supine position and the hips and knees flexed to 90 degrees. Infants should be quiet and relaxed because both tests require a cooperative child for adequate results.

The Ortolani Test, also referred to as the *click of entry,* is a diagnostic test used to detect reduction of a dislocated femoral head. To perform, the examiner gently abducts the hip and lifts the femoral head anteriorly. A positive sign is a palpable "clunk," felt when a dislocated femoral head is reduced. This "clunk" differs from the audible hip click, which is due to non-pathologic processes, such as ligamentous snapping. Each leg should be examined separately, not simultaneously.

The Barlow maneuver, also referred to as the *click of exit,* is another diagnostic test; it identifies a dislocatable femoral head in an unstable or dysplastic acetabulum. To perform the maneuver, the hips are adducted and a posterior force is placed along the longitudinal axis of the femur. Subluxations or dislocations are readily palpable. The Ortolani and Barlow tests are rarely used after 6 to 8 weeks of age because the surrounding soft tissues and muscles adapt to the dislocated hip, making it more difficult to reduce.

If the diagnosis of DDH or dislocation is not made shortly after birth, there is a different set of physical findings. There is asymmetry of hip abduction that is secondary to adductor muscle shortening and contracture on the affected side. Limited hip abduction is the most reliable late diagnostic sign.

As the femoral head dislocates posteriorly, the thigh is shortened on the affected side, producing relative limb shortening and asymmetry of the gluteal, thigh, and labial folds. Asymmetrical gluteal folds result from bunching of skin and subcutaneous tissue on the affected side; however, asymmetrical skin folds have not been shown to be reliable signs and assessment for DDH requires further evaluation. **Galeazzi sign** is noted when the femoral head displaces laterally and proximally, causing apparent shortening of the femur on the affected side. On examination, a positive Galeazzi sign may be observed with discrepancy in knee heights noted when infants are supine, the sacrum flat on the examination table, and hips and knees bent (Figure 100-3).

In children of walking age, the physician may notice a limp because of the relative leg length discrepancy. Children may try to disguise the limp by toe-walking. A Trendelenburg test may be positive. Normally, when a child stands on one leg, the hip abductors straighten the pelvis and keep the center of gravity over the femoral head. If the abductors are weak, the weight shifts to the opposite side, causing it to droop. A child with bilateral involvement may display hyperlordosis and a waddling gait.

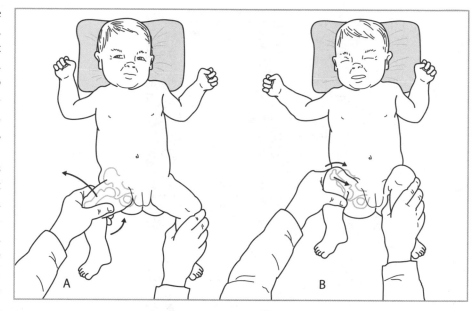

Figure 100-2.   Ortolani and Barlow tests. A. Ortolani (reduction) test. B. Barlow (dislocation) test.

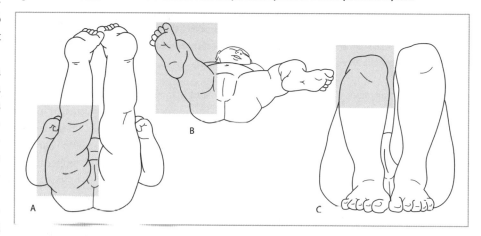

Figure 100-3.   Late signs in the diagnosis of developmental dysplasia of the hip. A. Asymmetry of thigh folds. B. Asymmetry of hip abduction. C. Discrepancy of knee heights.

Imaging Studies

Radiologic and ultrasound evaluations may aid in the diagnosis. Hip sonography helps to confirm the diagnosis and to identify more subtle forms of the disorder. Ultrasonography is the only diagnostic test that allows real-time evaluation and a 3-dimensional view of the neonate's hip. Reliable radiograph changes begin to become evident by 4 to 6 months of age, when the ossific nucleus of the femoral head appears in most infants (Figure 100-4). A flat, shallow acetabulum and delayed ossification of the femoral head are the simplest and most easily recognizable findings.

Management

The need for repeat examinations of the hips during the first year of life cannot be overemphasized. Children suspected of any hip instability or any child with less than 60 degrees of hip abduction should be evaluated with appropriate imaging studies and referred to an orthopedic surgeon for further evaluation. An orthopedic surgeon

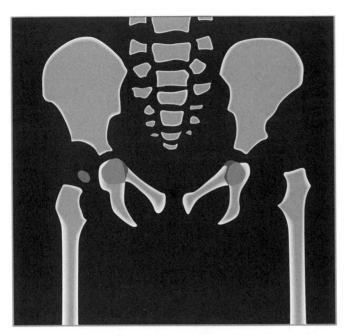

Figure 100-4. **Radiographic findings associated with developmental dysplasia of the hip. The left hip is dislocated. The femur is lateral and proximal, the acetabulum is shallow and flat, and there is delayed ossification of the femoral head, as evidenced by the absence of the ossific nucleus on the left.**

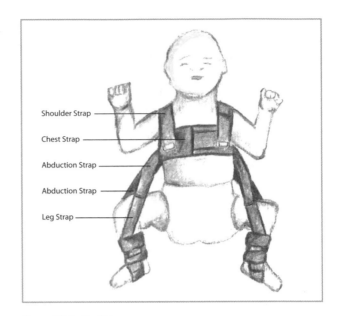

Figure 100-5. Pavlik harness.

can aid the primary care physician in the diagnosis and management of DDH.

The goal of treatment is to return the femoral head to its normal position within the acetabulum and restore normal hip functioning. The common practice of triple diapering should be discouraged because it is unreliable, often delays definitive therapy, and may produce complications, such as avascular necrosis of the femoral head.

The management of DDH is divided into 5 different treatment groups:

1. Newborn to 6 months
2. Infant (6–18 months)
3. Toddler (18–36 months)
4. Child and juvenile (3–8 years)
5. Adolescent to young adult (beyond 8 years)

The **Pavlik harness** is the primary method of treating DDH during infancy. This device has evolved as the clear method of choice for treatment of infants with DDH and has become accepted as the standard of treatment worldwide. The Pavlik harness consists of a chest strap, shoulder straps, and anterior and posterior stirrup straps that maintain the hips in flexion and abduction while restricting extension and adduction (Figure 100-5). When properly used, the harness holds the hips in a flexed and abducted position while allowing infants to move their legs within safe limits of abduction and adduction until stability is achieved. In the newborn with DDH, the harness should be worn for 23 hours daily until the clinical and radiographic examinations are normal. The harness must be worn for a minimum of 3 months by children 3 months and younger, whereas children 4 months or older usually wear the harness for a period of double

their age. A newborn with a diagnosis of true dislocation must wear the harness full time until the dislocatable hip has stabilized in the acetabulum.

The harness should be applied and monitored by an orthopedic surgeon because inappropriate application may lead to adverse outcomes, such as inferior dislocation and, the most serious, avascular necrosis of the femoral head. Parents play a key role in the successful use of the harness and must be educated on the disease process and the proper use of the harness. Overall, the Pavlik harness has an 85% to 95% success rate; however, it loses efficacy as the child ages because of soft tissue contractures that develop in previously untreated individuals.

If this treatment method is ineffective or if the diagnosis is not made until after 6 months of age, **traction** followed by either open or closed **reduction and spica cast immobilization** may be used. Good results are more difficult to obtain with increasing age, especially after children are walking. Operative treatment is required in children older than 18 months to safely reduce the dislocated hip and to surgically re-create normal anatomy. These procedures include (1) **femoral shortening,** (2) **acetabuloplasty** to correct acetabular dysplasia, and (3) **capsulorrhaphy** (suturing the joint capsule).

Prognosis

The prognosis of DDH depends on age at the time of diagnosis and severity of the deformity. The long-term prognosis for satisfactory hip function is good for children when DDH is recognized early and treated appropriately. Generally children with DDH that is diagnosed after the first year of life have a poorer prognosis for satisfactory hip function than those with DDH that is diagnosed during infancy. Left untreated, DDH may result in significant disability, ranging from limp, to pain and stiffness in the hip, to early-onset degenerative joint disease in adult life.

CASE RESOLUTION

The infant presented in the case history has less than 60 degrees of abduction of the left hip, a sign of DDH. An anteroposterior view of the pelvis may be ordered to confirm the diagnosis. Regardless of the radiographic findings, the infant should be referred to an orthopedic surgeon for further evaluation and management. If hip dislocation is confirmed, the initial treatment will involve bracing with the Pavlik harness.

Selected References

Aronsson DD, Goldberg MJ, Kling TF Jr, Roy DR. Developmental dysplasia of the hip. *Pediatrics.* 1994;94:201–208

Ballock RT, Richards BS. Hip dysplasia: early diagnosis makes a difference. *Contemp Pediatr.* 1997;14:108–117

Bialik V, Bialik GM, Blazer S, Sujov P, Wiener F, Berant M. Developmental dysplasia of the hip: a new approach to incidence. *Pediatrics.* 1999;103:93–99

Bond CD, Hennrikus WL, DellaMaggiore ED. Prospective evaluation of newborn soft-tissue hip "clicks" with ultrasound. *J Pediatr Orthop.* 1997;17:199–201

Hensinger RN. Congenital dislocation of the hip: treatment in infancy to walking age. *Orthop Clin North Am.* 1987;18:597–615

Mooney JF, Emans JB. Developmental dislocation of the hip: a clinical overview. *Pediatr Rev.* 1995;16:299–303

Novacheck TF. Developmental dysplasia of the hip. *Pediatr Clin North Am.* 1996; 43:829–848

Theophilopoulos EP, Barrett DJ. Get a grip on the pediatric hip. *Contemp Pediatr.* 1998;15:43–65

Wientroub S, Grill F. Ultrasonography in developmental dysplasia of the hip. *J Bone Joint Surg.* 2000;82:1004–1018

CHAPTER 101

In-toeing and Out-toeing: Rotational Problems of the Lower Extremity

David P. Zamorano, MD, and Andrew K. Battenberg, BS

CASE STUDY

A 3-year-old girl is brought to the office. Her mother is concerned because beginning a few months ago her daughter's feet appeared to "turn in" when she walked. The girl has never walked like this before, and she has no history of trauma, fever, pain, or swelling in the joints. The physical examination is within normal limits except for the in-toeing gait.

Questions

1. How can observation of children's gait help determine the etiology of their in-toeing and out-toeing (rotational problems)?
2. What are the common causes of in-toeing and out-toeing?
3. Does evaluation of in-toeing and out-toeing require any laboratory or radiologic studies?
4. What is the natural history of most rotational problems?

Benign rotational variations of the lower extremities such as in-toeing and out-toeing are seen in many healthy children. Although rotational problems that produce in-toeing and out-toeing may initially be physically alarming, spontaneous resolution occurs in most cases. They are a common cause of parental concern during infancy and childhood; however, they rarely lead to physical limitation. Most of these children can be managed adequately by primary care physicians and do not need orthopedic referral. A thorough understanding of the normal rotational variations that occur in children younger than 10 years of age is essential to proper treatment and patient and parent education. More importantly, a general understanding is imperative to identify more serious underlying structural problems.

Specific terminology used to describe limb positioning is as follows. **Version** is normal variation in limb rotation, whereas **torsion** refers to abnormal conditions (ie, >2 SDs above or below the mean). **Adduction** is movement toward the midline, in contrast to **abduction,** which is movement away from the midline. **Varus angulation** is deviation toward the midline, whereas **valgus angulation** is deviation away from the midline. An **inverted** foot is one turned toward the midline on its long axis. An **everted** foot is one turned away from the midline on its long axis.

Epidemiology

In neonates or young infants, in-toeing is most likely the result of clubfoot (talipes equinovarus), isolated metatarsus adductus, or metatarsus varus. The incidence of clubfoot is 1 in 1,000 live births, with a male to female ratio of 2:1. The condition is bilateral in approximately 50% of cases. The incidence of metatarsus adductus, a much more common problem, is about 1 in 500 live births. It is often bilateral. Internal tibial torsion is the primary cause of in-toeing in the second year of life, and femoral torsion accounts for most cases of this condition during early childhood.

Physiological out-toeing is classically evident in infants who have not yet begun to walk, and is the most common cause of bilateral out-toeing. In older infants and children, however, lateral tibial torsion is believed to be the most common cause of out-toeing.

Clinical Presentation

Children with congenital clubfoot, metatarsus adductus, and metatarsus varus present with in-toeing during infancy. Congenital clubfoot is usually evident at birth. A severe medial, midline, plantar crease is present, and the foot appears C-shaped, with both the heel and forefront turned inward (Figure 101-1). The affected foot is

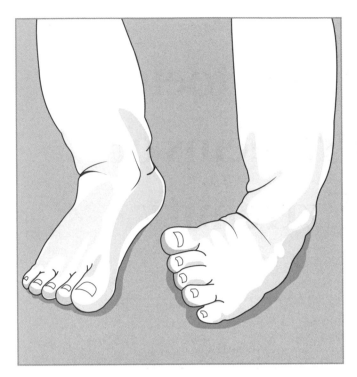

Figure 101-1. Congenital clubfoot.

small, wide, and stiff, and the lower leg appears small due to hypoplasia of the calf muscles. In contrast to clubfoot, only the forefoot turns inward in metatarsus adductus and varus.

Tibial torsion is apparent during the second year of life. In affected children, the feet turn inward during ambulation, but the knees are straight because the deformity is distal to the knee. Medial femoral torsion is evident at 3 to 4 years of age and usually affects girls. Affected children can sit in the "W" position with both legs behind them. As the child walks, both the knees and the feet appear to turn inward because the deformity is proximal to the knee.

Physiological out-toeing is seen in infancy. Classically, parents note that when they hold their child in a standing position, both feet turn outward. Approximately 5 degrees of out-toeing is normal after age 3. Further degrees of out-toeing may be due to lateral tibial torsion.

Pathophysiology

Several factors are involved in the etiology of rotational conditions. Most of these deformations are caused by intrauterine positioning. Genetics are also believed to play a role in the development of rotational problems, as parents may often have the same rotational deformity as their children. Other contributing factors include **bony and neuromuscular abnormalities** in clubfoot and certain sleeping and sitting positions in metatarsus adductus and medial tibial torsion. For example, sleeping in the prone position with the legs internally rotated may worsen internal tibial torsion or metatarsus adductus.

During the early intrauterine period, internal rotation of the lower extremity brings the big toe to the midline. However, during the later intrauterine period, infancy, and childhood, external rotation predominates. Alterations in this normal lateral process are caused by genetic and environmental factors, including intrauterine molding and sleep positions. Conditions influenced by intrauterine position, such as metatarsus adductus and developmental hip dysplasia, are sometimes found in the same children.

Congenital clubfoot is most commonly an isolated birth defect and is considered idiopathic. Two major etiologies have been proposed: (1) a germline defect in the talus results in abnormal bony development leading to plantar flexion, inversion, soft tissue contractures, and hypoplasia of the calf muscles and the bones of the foot and (2) clubfoot represents the final common pathway of disruption anywhere along the neuromuscular unit, including the central nervous system, peripheral nerves, and muscles. Additionally, genetics are believed to play a major role given that 25% of all cases are familial and there is 33% concordance of identical twins. Environmental factors, including intrauterine position and molding, are also thought to contribute.

In-toeing is usually caused by benign conditions such as metatarsus adductus, excessive internal tibial torsion, and excessive femoral torsion. Less frequently, patients have pathologic conditions such as clubfoot, skewfoot, hip disorders, and neuromuscular diseases. Out-toeing is typically caused by external rotation contracture of the hip, external tibial torsion, or external femoral torsion. We will now review the conditions associated with rotational variations in children.

In-toeing

Metatarsus Adductus and Metatarsus Primus Varus

Metatarsus adductus, with or without internal tibial torsion, is the most common cause of in-toeing from birth to 1 year of age. It is a functional deformity in which the forefoot is adducted with respect to the hindfoot with a neutral or slightly valgus heel. It is the most common pediatric foot problem referred to orthopedic surgeons and occurs in 1 in 500 live births and in 1 in 20 siblings of patients with metatarsus adductus. The rate is higher in males, twin births, and preterm babies. Numerous theories exist as to the cause of metatarsus adductus, including in utero positioning, sleeping position of the baby, muscle imbalance, and medial cuneiform abnormality.

Presenting complaints include cosmesis, in-toeing gait, or excessive shoe wear. On physical examination, the foot appears C-shaped with a concave medial border and convex lateral border. The forefoot can be brought into the neutral position either by stroking the lateral border of the foot or by gently straightening it. Metatarsus adductus can be classified into flexible or inflexible based on physical examination. Most cases of flexible metatarsus adductus resolve spontaneously and do not require splinting, bracing, or special shoes. However, patients with rigid metatarsus adductus should undergo early casting; uncommonly, resistant cases may require surgery.

Congenital **metatarsus primus** varus is a bony abnormality characterized by an isolated adducted first metatarsal. Unlike flexible metatarsus adductus, metatarsus varus is a fixed deformity. The foot cannot be brought into the neutral position, and there is a deep vertical skin crease along the medial border of the tarsometatarsal joints. Because it is a more rigid deformity, early casting is recommended and persistent deformity requires surgery.

Skewfoot or Congenital Metatarsus Varus

Skewfoot, also known as *serpentine metatarsus adductus,* is characterized by adducted metatarsals combined with a valgus deformity of the heel and plantar flexion of the talus. It is theorized that improper casting of metatarsus adductus or clubfoot may result in a skewfoot; however, most cases are idiopathic. Patients present with pain or callus formation under the head of the talus and base of the fifth metatarsal. Some feet undergo spontaneous correction, while surgery is indicated for a persistently symptomatic foot.

Dynamic Hallucis Abductus/Searching Toe

Dynamic hallucis abductus/searching toe, also known as *wandering* or *atavistic* toe, can cause in-toeing. Children with a so-called searching toe have a big toe that points medially when they walk. Unlike the other causes of in-toeing, which are structural and present at rest, this condition is a dynamic deformity. Searching toe results from the contraction of the abductors of the big toe during the stance phase of gait, which pulls the toe toward the midline. It usually resolves with age and subsequent development of fine motor coordination.

Clubfoot

Congenital **clubfoot,** a pathologic deformity of the foot, may be identified at birth (Figure 101-1). Clubfoot may be either an isolated deformity or seen in association with other neuromuscular anomalies such as arthrogryposis, myelomeningocele, amniotic band syndrome, cerebral palsy, or poliomyelitis.

The diagnosis of congenital clubfoot is made at birth on the basis of 3 conditions: forefoot varus, heel varus, and ankle equinus. Clubfoot can range in severity from a rigid deformity, in which the forefoot cannot be passively abducted into a neutral position, to nonrigid deformities, in which the forefoot can be gently brought toward the midline. Normal dorsiflexion of the ankle helps distinguish severe forms of metatarsus varus from clubfoot.

Internal Tibial Torsion

Internal tibial torsion is the most common cause of in-toeing from ages 1 to 3 years, is thought to be caused by intrauterine positioning, and is usually first noticed by parents when their child begins to walk. Parents often complain that the child is clumsy and trips frequently. The condition is bilateral in two-thirds of affected children; when unilateral, it more commonly affects the left leg. Observation of gait reveals that the knees point forward but the feet turn inward. Because the knees are straight, the site of the rotational deformity is below this joint. If the feet are normal and no metatarsus adductus or varus is present, the rotational deformity can be isolated to the lower leg. It is important to measure the thigh-foot and transmalleolar axes in the physical examination. Expectant observation is recommended because the natural history of internal tibial torsion strongly favors spontaneous resolution by 4 years of age.

Internal Femoral Torsion

Internal femoral torsion is the most common cause of in-toeing in children presenting at 3 to 6 years of age and is usually bilateral. Children generally present when parents notice worsening in-toeing in a child who has no previous history of in-toeing. Although excessive medial femoral torsion may be present at birth, it is often masked by the external rotatory forces present during infancy. Children with excessive internal femoral torsion characteristically sit with their legs in the "W" position and run with an eggbeater-type motion. No treatment is necessary for most cases of femoral torsion, which usually resolves by 8 years of age.

Out-toeing

Physiological Out-toeing

Out-toeing of infancy, which is most commonly seen in children who are just learning to walk, is caused by intrauterine positioning that leads to external rotatory contractures of the soft tissues surrounding the hip. This condition may be perpetuated in children who sleep in the prone, frog-leg position, which holds the hips in external rotation and prevents normal stretching of the external rotators. Although both feet turn outward when infants stand, the lateral rotation of both hips is normal on examination (Figure 101-2). More serious conditions, such as slipped capital femoral epiphysis, hip dysplasia, or coxa vara, are less common but should be considered.

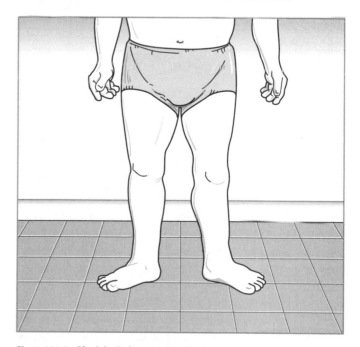

Figure 101-2. Physiological out-toeing of infancy.

External Tibial Torsion

This condition may be suspected in children who are 3 to 5 years of age and present with out-toeing that worsens with time. Increased external tibial torsion is often associated with neuromuscular conditions, such as myelodysplasia and poliomyelitis. Because the tibia normally rotates laterally with development, the condition may become more severe with age. Malalignment between the knee and the direction of gait may produce knee pain.

In-toeing and out-toeing comprise a long list of differential diagnoses; thus, a methodical and meticulous history and physical examination are necessary.

Differential Diagnosis

In-toeing and out-toeing may be classified according to anatomical level and usual age at presentation (Table 101-1). These conditions may be localized to one of 4 areas: toe, foot, tibia, and femur. If in-toeing problems are placed in chronological order by age of presentation, the affected area follows a toe-to-femur sequence.

Table 101-1. Site and Age of Onset of Rotational Problems of the Lower Extremity in Children

Problem	Site of Problem	Age of Onset
In-toeing		
Searching toe	Toe	Infancy
Clubfoot	Foot	Birth
Metatarsus adductus/varus	Foot	Birth/infancy
Medial tibial torsion	Tibia	Toddler stage (12–24 mo)
Medial femoral torsion	Femur	Early childhood (3–5 y)
Out-toeing		
Physiological out-toeing	Hips	Infancy
Lateral tibial torsion	Tibia	Childhood

Evaluation

History

The clinical history must delineate the onset, duration, and progression of any structural problems. The typical natural history of benign rotational conditions shows improvement over time, whereas a more serious condition would have a more progressive deformity. Relevant family and birth history, including gestational age, length of labor, complications, Apgar scores, birth weight, and length of hospital stay, should be noted. These details may heighten suspicion for cerebral palsy or the presence of hereditary disorders, such as vitamin D–resistant rickets, mucopolysaccharidoses, achondroplasia, epiphyseal dysplasia, or metaphyseal dysplasia, that may affect rotational profiles. A thorough developmental history is important because developmental delays may be a sign of underlying neuromuscular or neurologic disorders (Questions Box).

Questions

In-toeing and Out-toeing

- Is there any family history of in-toeing or out-toeing?
- What is the birth history? Was the child a breech presentation?
- At what age did the child begin walking?
- When did the rotational deformity appear? Is it getting better or worse?
- Does the rotational problem produce any disability (eg, tripping or falling a great deal when walking or running)?
- Has any previous treatment been tried?
- In what position does the child sleep? In what position does the child sit?

Physical Examination

Normal variability in the lower extremities of young children must be differentiated from more serious structural problems. A detailed physical examination, including assessment of gait and neurologic and musculoskeletal function, is essential for making the correct diagnosis. The evaluation should determine whether the rotational problem has caused a functional impairment, such as tripping, pain, or footwear difficulties. This evaluation should include examination of the hips for signs of hip dysplasia, which may be associated with metatarsus adductus (see Chapter 100).

Evaluation of postural conditions requires both static and dynamic physical examination. Static examination includes an overall evaluation of the patient and a rotational profile. The child's rotational profile, as described by Staheli, consists of 5 components (Figure 101-3). The 5 components of this profile are internal and external hip rotation, thigh-foot axis, transmalleolar axis, heel-bisector angle, and foot progression angle during gait (Figure 101-4).

Hip rotation in infants averages 40 degrees of internal rotation and 70 degrees of external rotation. By 10 years of age, internal hip rotation averages 50 degrees and external rotation 45 degrees. Internal rotation measuring between 70 and 90 degrees is evidence of femoral torsion.

The **thigh-foot axis** consists of the rotation of the tibia and hindfoot in relation to the longitudinal axis of the thigh and indicates the amount of tibial torsion. In infants, the thigh-foot angle averages 5 degrees internal (range: -30 to +20 degrees). Excessive internal tibial torsion spontaneously resolves by 3 to 4 years of age, and by 8 years of age the thigh-foot axis averages 10 degrees external.

The **transmalleolar axis** also aids in determining the amount of tibial torsion. It is formed by the angle at the intersection of an imaginary line from the lateral to medial malleolus and a second line from the lateral to medial femoral condyles. At gestational age 5 months, the fetus has an average of 20 degrees of internal tibial torsion. During development, the tibia externally rotates to an average final adult position of 23 degrees of external rotation.

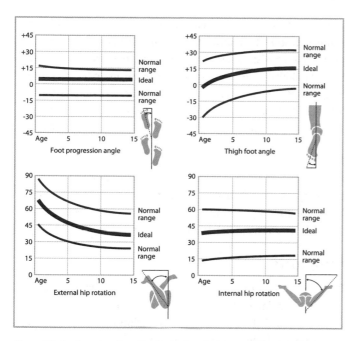

Figure 101-3. Rotational profile. (Reproduced with permission from Wenger DR, Rang M. *The Art and Practice of Children's Orthopedics.* **New York, NY: Raven Press; 1993.)**

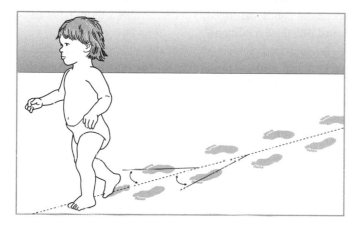

Figure 101-4. Evaluation of foot progression angle.

The **heel-bisector** line examines the foot, and is a line drawn through the midline axis of the hindfoot and forefoot. In a neutral foot, the heel-bisector line passes through the second web space.

Finally, the **foot progression angle during gait** is the angle of the foot relative to an imaginary straight line in the patient's path (see Figure 101-4). Patients who in-toe are assigned a negative value and patient's who out-toe are assigned a positive value. This value represents the sum total effect of the child's structural alignment and dynamic torsion forces resulting from muscle forces.

The examination of infants with clubfoot should include a careful examination of the back for signs of possible spinal dysraphism (eg, skin dimples and hairy patches) and a thorough neurologic examination.

Internal tibial torsion may be diagnosed by having children sit at the end of the examination table with both knees flexed to 90 degrees and palpating the medial and lateral malleoli with the thumb and index finger. Normally, the medial malleolus lies anterior to the lateral malleolus (approximately one fingerbreadth). If the lateral malleolus is on the same plane or anterior to the medial malleolus, internal tibial torsion is indicated.

The diagnosis of tibial torsion can also be made by measuring the thigh-foot angle (Figure 101-5). Measurement of the thigh-foot angle involves having children lie prone on the examination table and observing the relationship of the long axis of the foot compared with the axis of the thigh as viewed from above. The shape of the foot itself can also be assessed with children in this position. Slight internal rotation is normal as children first learn to walk.

Diagnosis of medial femoral torsion can be made by observing children's gaits and measuring hip rotation. For example, when a child with medial femoral torsion ambulates, the knees and feet appear to turn inward. Internal and external hip rotation are evaluated with the child in a prone position, the pelvis flat, and the knees flexed 90 degrees (Figure 101-6). The degrees of normal rotation vary with age (see Figure 101-3). During childhood, internal hip rotation greater than 70 degrees implies medial femoral torsion.

Imaging Studies

Routine imaging studies are not necessary for rotational deformities. Imaging studies may be considered by the orthopedic surgeon in severe deformities when operative correction is being considered. In patients with clubfoot, radiographs are used to assess the relationship and development of the bones and to monitor cast correction.

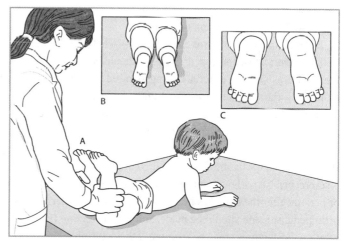

Figure 101-5. Evaluation of the thigh-foot axis. A. Observation with the child in the prone position is best. B. Determination of the thigh-foot axis. C. Assessment of the shape of the foot.

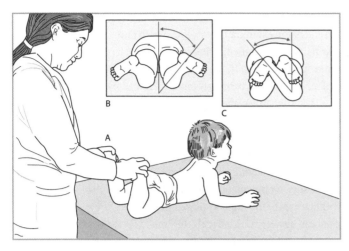

Figure 101-6. Evaluation of hip rotation. A. The child is prone and knees are flexed to 90 degrees. B. Medial rotation is measured. C. Lateral rotation is measured.

Management

In-toeing

Metatarsus adductus generally resolves spontaneously, but stretching exercises for the foot may be advisable, particularly if parents are anxious to "do something." Parents are instructed to manipulate the foot with each diaper change. Because most cases resolve within the first 3 months of life, referral to an orthopedic surgeon should be made if the deformity is still present at 3 to 4 months of age. Cast correction may be required for rigid deformities or deformities that persist beyond 3 to 4 months. Shoe modifications (eg, putting shoes on the wrong foot) should be avoided because they have not been shown to have any long-term benefits.

Because metatarsus varus may progress when children begin walking, referral to an orthopedic surgeon should be made as soon as the condition is detected. Serial casting followed by corrective shoes or inserts is the first line of treatment, and surgery is rarely required. Treatment for medial tibial torsion is rarely required because this problem generally corrects with time when children learn to walk. Night splinting, although still occasionally instituted, has not been shown to affect the natural history of this condition. If the deformity is severe, persists without improvement beyond the age of 18 months, or persists after the child has been walking for 1 year, referral to an orthopedic surgeon should be made. Surgical correction (eg, tibial rotational osteotomy) may be required if the deformity is severe or persists beyond 8 to 10 years of age.

Like other conditions that produce in-toeing, medial femoral torsion generally does not require treatment. Even if it persists into adulthood, it usually produces no disability nor does it increase the risk for degenerative arthritis in the involved joint. Nonoperative treatment is ineffective. Surgical correction may be required if there is a history of repeated falls or severe gait problems. A derotational femoral osteotomy is the only effective method of treatment. It should not be performed until children are at least 8 to 10 years of age.

Clubfoot, unlike other problems, is a pathologic deformity that requires treatment. Treatment, which should begin during the first week of life, consists of serial manipulations of the foot and casting. Several months of casting may be required to attain full correction. Surgery is often required for resistant or recurrent cases. As many as 50% to 75% of patients with clubfoot may eventually require surgery. Surgery is usually delayed until infants are 6 to 12 months of age.

Out-toeing

Physiological out-toeing of infancy is a rotational problem that spontaneously resolves when children learn to walk. Most cases resolve by 18 months of age. Severe lateral tibial torsion may require surgical correction with a tibial rotational osteotomy.

Prognosis

Because the lower extremity rotates laterally with growth, the natural history of internal rotational problems, such as internal tibial torsion and medial femoral torsion, is resolution over time. In contrast, lateral tibial torsion may become worse with time.

The prognosis for most rotational problems is excellent. Parental reassurance and education regarding the natural history of these deformities may decrease anxiety and prevent unnecessary visits to specialists. Functional disability or degenerative arthritis is not associated with these conditions.

Left untreated, clubfoot often leads to considerable pain and disability. The affected foot can be difficult to fit with shoes. Additionally, clubfoot can be unsightly and cause children significant emotional distress.

Selected References

> ### CASE RESOLUTION
>
> The girl described in the case history seems to have medial femoral torsion because she has no history of rotational problems. Her entire leg turns in when she walks. Internal hip rotation greater than 70 degrees confirms the diagnosis. The mother can be reassured that this is a normal, age-related phenomenon that will most likely resolve over time. The child can be reevaluated in 4 to 6 months. Orthopedic referral is not required at this time.

Craig CL, Goldberg MJ. Foot and leg problems. *Pediatr Rev.* 1993;14:395–400

Dobbs MB, Gurnett CA. Update on clubfoot: etiology and treatment. *Clin Orthop Relat Res.* 2009;467(5):1146–1153

Fuchs R, Staheli LT. Splinting and intoeing. *J Pediatr Orthop.* 1996;16:489–491

Hoekelman RA. Foot and leg problems. In: Hoekelman RA, ed. *Primary Pediatric Care.* 3rd ed. St Louis, MO: Mosby-Year Book; 1997:971–979

Hoffinger SA. Evaluation and management of pediatric foot deformities. *Pediatr Clin North Am.* 1996;43:1091–1111

Staheli LT. Lower positional deformity in infants and children: a review. *J Pediatr Orthop.* 1990;10:559–563

Wenger DR, Rang M. *The Art and Practice of Children's Orthopedics.* New York, NY: Raven Press; 1993

CHAPTER 102

Angular Deformities of the Lower Extremity: Bowlegs and Knock-Knees

Carol D. Berkowitz, MD, and Andrew K. Battenberg, BS

CASE STUDY

During the routine health maintenance examination of a 2-year-old child, you observe moderate to severe bilateral bowing of both legs. The child's mother reports that her son began walking at 10 months. She has not noticed problems with his gait and says he does not trip or fall excessively. On examination, the boy's weight is greater than the 95th percentile for age, but otherwise he appears to be a healthy African American child.

Questions

1. What types of angular deformities affect children's lower extremities?
2. How does children's age help determine whether they have physiological or pathologic angular deformities?
3. What clinical measurements can help distinguish physiological from pathologic angular deformities?
4. To what extent are radiographs used in the routine assessment of angular deformities?

With normal growth and development, the angular alignment of children's legs progresses through a series of developmental stages—from relative bowlegs to knock-knees and eventually straight legs. Rotational problems such as in-toeing and out-toeing are deformities in the transverse plane that occur when a bone rotates either internally or externally along its long axis (Figure 102-1). Angular deformities such as bowlegs and knock-knees are deformities in the frontal plane. In bowleg deformity, the legs distal to the knees are angled or tilted toward the midline (tibial varus), whereas they are tilted away from the midline of the body in knock-knee deformity (tibial valgus) (Figure 102-2). Variations in the knee angle that fall outside the normal range (eg, more than ±2 standard deviations of the mean) are referred to as genu varum for bowlegs and genu valgum for knock-knees (Dx Box). Appreciation of the normal developmental sequence in conjunction with a careful history and physical examination can help pediatricians identify pathologic cases of bowlegs and knock-knees and initiate prompt treatment.

Epidemiology

Bowlegs and knock-knees are common in infants and children. While babies are all born bowlegged, parents usually don't appreciate this finding until infants begin to walk. Knock-knees occur less frequently than bowlegs, are seen more often in females, and are

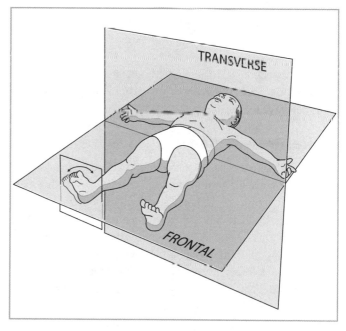

Figure 102-1. Select body reference and rotational planes. Rotational problems are deformities in the transverse plane. Angular deformities are in the frontal plane.

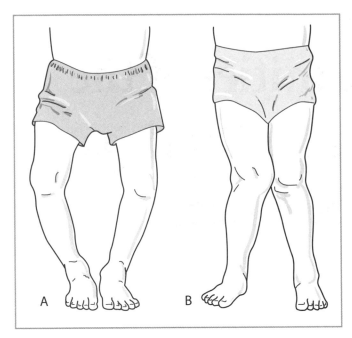

Figure 102-2. Varus and valgus deformities of the lower extremities. A. Bowleg deformity. B. Knock-knee deformity.

Dx Pathologic Bowlegs and Knock-Knees

- Asymmetrical deformity
- Inconsistency with the normal sequence of angular development
- Stature less than the fifth percentile for age
- Severe deformity (>10 cm intermalleolar or intercondylar distance)
- History of rapid progression
- Presence of other musculoskeletal abnormalities

commonly associated with generalized ligamentous laxity. Pathologic cases of bowlegs and knock-knees are uncommon and are defined by the degree of the angulation.

Clinical Presentation

Children with **bowlegs** have a characteristic wide-based stance with increased distance between the knees. They may walk with a waddling gait. In-toeing may be noted as a result of associated internal tibial torsion. Evaluation is required for pathologic bowlegs when the intercondylar distance (distance between the knees) is more than 10 cm with the child lying supine with the medial malleoli touching.

Severe **knock-knees** may produce an awkward gait with the knees rubbing. Children may walk with both feet apart in an effort to avoid knee-to-knee contact. They may need to place one knee behind the other to stand with both feet together. Evaluation for pathologic knock-knees is warranted when the intermalleolar distance (distance between the ankles) is more than 10 cm with the child lying supine with the knees touching.

Pathophysiology

The normal variation in the angular alignment of the lower extremities changes with age. During the first 2 years of life, relative bowing of the legs is common. Although physiological bowing of the lower leg may be appreciated at birth, it is most prominent during the second year of life, when it most commonly involves both the tibia and the femur. When associated with internal tibial torsion, the deformity may appear more striking. Physiological knock-knees develop between 3 and 4 years of age. The knock-knee stage resolves somewhere between 5 and 7 years of age, when normal adult alignment develops. A slight knock-knee appearance remains in normal adults. Bowlegs or knock-knees that develop outside of this sequence require further evaluation for pathologic causes.

The **tibiofemoral angle,** the angle between the long axis of the femur and the long axis of the tibia, is used to assess the angular alignment of the leg. At birth the tibiofemoral angle is approximately 15 degrees varus, and it decreases to 0 between the ages of 18 and 24 months. By 3 to 4 years, the angle peaks at about 10 degrees of valgus angulation. Then between 5 and 7 years it decreases to the normal range of about 7 to 9 degrees in girls and 4 to 6 degrees in boys (Figure 102-3).

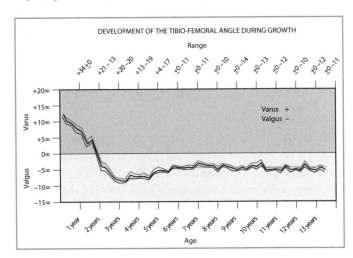

Figure 102-3. Development of the tibiofemoral angle. (Reproduced with permission from Salenius P, Vankka E. The development of the tibiofemoral angle in children. *J Bone Joint Surg.* 1975;57A:259–261.)

Differential Diagnosis

The most common causes of genu varum and genu valgum are presented in Box 102-1. Physiological bowlegs and knock-knees are usually bilateral, and they occur in a sequence that follows the normal developmental pattern. Lateral bowing of the tibia is commonly noted during the first year of life. Bowlegs (involving both the femur and the tibia) are pronounced during the second year, and knock-knees become prominent between 3 and 4 years of age. This is the normal sequence of angular development. Most cases of bowlegs are the result of normal physiological processes, Blount disease (tibia

Box 102-1. Common Causes of Genu Varum and Genu Valgum

Genu Varum

- Physiological bowlegs
- Rickets (vitamin D deficiency [nutritional] or vitamin D resistance [hereditary])
- Blount disease (tibia vara)
- Achondroplasia
- Metaphyseal dysplasia
- Trauma, infection, or tumor of the proximal tibia (resulting in malunion or partial physeal arrest)
- Excessive prenatal fluoride ingestion

Genu Valgum

- Physiological knock-knees
- Rickets (renal osteodystrophy)
- Trauma, infection, or tumor of the distal femur or proximal tibia (resulting in malunion or partial physeal arrest)
- Paralytic conditions (eg, myelodysplasia, polio, cerebral palsy) leading to contracture of the iliotibial band
- Osteogenesis imperfecta
- Rheumatoid arthritis of the knee

vara), and rickets. Common causes of pathologic knock-knees are severe renal rickets and previous fractures of the proximal tibia.

Blount disease, a growth disturbance involving the posterior-medial aspect of the proximal tibia (physis, epiphysis, and metaphysis), is the most common cause of pathologic bowlegs and is due to idiopathic undergrowth of the medial side of the tibia. There are 2 forms of the disease: early-onset (or infantile) and late-onset, which are defined by disease development before or after 4 years of age. The late-onset form is further subdivided into juvenile (4–10 years of age) and adolescent (>10 years of age). At all ages, Blount disease is more common in African Americans.

The infantile form, initially classified by Langenskiöld, is bilateral 80% of the time and is associated with internal tibial torsion. The etiology is believed to involve mechanical stress on the growth plate, thus converting physiological bowlegs to pathologic varus. Affected children are often obese, in the upper growth percentiles, and early walkers, which puts early stress on the growth plate. Blount disease produces a sharp angulation at the proximal tibia, whereas physiological bowlegs lead to a gradual curvature of the legs involving both the femur and the tibia. Six stages of radiograph progression based on the degree of epiphyseal depression and metaphyseal fragmentation at the proximal tibia have been identified (Langenskiöld staging). It may be difficult to distinguish between early stages of Blount disease and physiological bowlegs, though criteria have been established to help predict infantile Blount disease in children presenting with idiopathic bowed legs: (1) a body mass index greater than or equal to 22 and (2) a tibial metaphyseal-diaphyseal angle greater than or equal to 10 degrees. These criteria have been shown to have a sensitivity of 95%, specificity of 100%, positive predictive value of 100%, and negative predictive value of 98%.

The late-onset form of Blount disease is less common than the juvenile form and is usually unilateral. Knee pain, rather than deformity, is the most common presenting sign. It is more common in males than females, and affected children are generally obese but have a normal height. Although the etiology is unclear, it is believed that in predisposed obese adolescents, repetitive trauma due to excess weight leads to decreased growth of the medial tibial physis.

Rickets, a disease of the growing skeleton, is a disorder caused by abnormal calcium and phosphorus metabolism that produces inadequate bone mineralization. Rickets takes several forms, including vitamin D–deficient (nutritional) rickets, vitamin D–resistant (hereditary) rickets (the most common form), and severe renal osteodystrophy. Signs of rickets include short stature, poor muscle tone, joint pain, and angular deformities of the lower extremities. Nutritional rickets may occur in infants who are exclusively breastfed and not supplemented with Vitamin D. The alignment at the time of onset of disease determines the direction of angulation. For example, vitamin D–deficient or vitamin D–resistant rickets generally has an early onset and is more often associated with bowlegs. Children with rickets and bowlegs, unlike those with Blount disease, are late walkers and often have evidence of growth impairment. Renal osteodystrophy, which usually has a later onset, results in a valgus deformity (knock-knees).

Pathologic processes, including trauma (fractures), infections, and tumors, involving the proximal tibia, are additional potential causes of both bowlegs and knock-knees. Overgrowth or malunion following fractures of the proximal tibial metaphysis most commonly results in genu valgum rather than genu varum.

Evaluation

History

A family history; an assessment of the child's growth and nutritional history; and a description of the deformity, its progression over time, impact on function, and prior treatment (Questions Box) should be obtained from the parents or caregivers. A dietary history is also important, particularly whether the infant has been exclusively breastfed because of the risk for vitamin-D deficiency.

Physical Examination

Physical examination begins with a general screening of children's nutritional growth and developmental status. Children's growth parameters (height, weight, head circumference) should be measured and plotted on standard growth curves. The rotational status of the lower limb should be assessed because internal tibial torsion is often associated with bowleg deformity (see Chapter 101). Children should be observed both standing and ambulating to determine the alignment of the legs. The intercondylar and intermalleolar distances can be measured with the child supine to determine the presence of excessive bowlegs or knock-knees (see Clinical Presentation). The intercondylar and intermalleolar distances should be followed every 6 months to monitor the progression of the deformity.

Questions

Pathologic Bowlegs and Knock-Knees

- When was the deformity first noticed?
- Has it changed? If so, how fast?
- Has the problem been treated in any way?
- Does the problem seem to affect how the child walks?
- Has the child had any recent illness or trauma in the affected leg?
- Does anyone else in the family have a similar problem?
- Aside from this condition, is the child growing and developing normally?
- Has the infant been exclusively breastfed?
- Does the child eat a well-balanced diet?
- Does the child have any chronic medical problems such as kidney disease?

Laboratory Tests

Most children with physiological angulation do not require any laboratory studies. A general metabolic screening, including hemoglobin, calcium, phosphorus, vitamin D level, creatinine, and alkaline phosphatase, may be ordered if a systemic or metabolic abnormality is suspected.

Imaging Studies

Radiographs are usually performed in the evaluation of bowlegs or knock-knees if pathology is suspected. True pathology is more likely if the deformity is unilateral, painful, very asymmetrical, or progressing at an accelerated rate. If obtained, radiographs should include the entire lower extremity so that the alignment of the femur and tibia may be assessed. Children should be standing, and a single radiograph of both legs should be taken. Pathologic conditions such as rickets (osteoporosis, metaphyseal fraying, cortical thinning, widening of the growth plates), Blount disease (beaking of the medial metaphysis of the proximal tibia), various bone dysplasias, and forms of dwarfism can usually be ruled out by radiographs. An increased uptake of the proximal medial aspect of the tibia on bone scan may help differentiate early infantile Blount disease from extreme physiological bowlegs.

Management

Angular deformities within normal developmental limits should be managed with continual observation and reassessment. The severity of the deformity should be documented, and children should be followed at 3- to 6-month intervals until the condition resolves. Physicians should **reassure parents** that bowlegs and knock-knees are normal developmental variations that resolve spontaneously with time. Special diets, braces or shoe wedges, arch supports, and bars are generally best avoided; they have not been shown to affect the normal developmental sequence.

Children with physiological varus may be followed clinically until 18 months to 2 years of age. Pathology should be suspected if correction has not begun by this time or if the angulation is progressive. Children with more than 10 degrees of valgus or with an intermalleolar distance greater than 10 cm after 8 to 9 years of age may require further evaluation. Children with suspected cases of pathologic bowlegs and knock-knees require **referral to an orthopedist** for evaluation.

Although treatment of Blount disease in children younger than 3 to 4 years may consist of **bracing** if the deformity is mild and identified early, **surgery** is often necessary. Surgery involves an osteotomy to realign the tibia. Failure to do so may result in damage to the medial aspect of the knee over time. Medical management, such as administration of vitamin D for nutritional rickets, is of primary importance in the treatment of the various forms of rickets. Surgical correction, such as osteotomies to correct varus or valgus deformities, should be reserved until medical management has been maximized because even severe deformities may resolve with conservative management.

Prognosis

Physiological bowlegs and knock-knees spontaneously resolve without further sequelae. Although knock-knees are primarily a cosmetic problem, degenerative arthritis may rarely be a late complication. Surgical correction may be required for adolescents with severe deformity to prevent such late complications.

CASE RESOLUTION

The boy described in the case history should be evaluated for pathologic causes of genu varum, especially Blount disease, for the following reasons: (1) his age is at the upper limit of normal for bowlegs and his deformity is severe, (2) he is African American, (3) he has a history of early walking, and (4) he is obese. A standing radiograph of the lower extremities should be obtained, and the boy should be referred to an orthopedist for further evaluation and management.

Selected References

Bruce RW. Torsional and angular deformities. *Pediatr Clin North Am.* 1996; 43:867–881

Eggert P, Viemann M. Physiologic bowlegs or infantile Blount's disease. Some new aspects on an old problem. *Pediatr Radiol.* 1996;26:349–352

Henderson RC. Tibia vara: a complication of adolescent obesity. *J Pediatr.* 1992;121:482–486

Kling TF. Angular deformities of the lower limbs in children. *Orthop Clin North Am.* 1987;18:513–527

Mankin KP, Zimbler S. Gait and leg alignment: what's normal and what's not. *Contemp Pediatr.* 1997;14:41–70

Sabharwal S. Blount disease. *J Bone Joint Surg Am.* 2009;91:1758–1776

Scherl SV. Common lower extremity problems in children. *Pediatr Rev.* 2004; 25:52–61

Scoles PV. Lower extremity development. In: *Pediatric Orthopedics in Clinical Practice.* 2nd ed. Chicago, IL: Year Book Medical Publishers; 1988:82–121

Scott AC, Kelly CH, Sullivan E. Body mass index as a prognostic factor in development of infantile Blount disease. *J Pediatr Orthop.* 2007;27(8):921–925

Wilkins KE. Bowlegs. *Pediatr Clin North Am.* 1986;33:1429–1438

CHAPTER 103

Orthopedic Injuries and Growing Pains

Sara T. Stewart, MD

CASE STUDY

A 6-year-old boy has a 1-week history of leg pains. He wakes up at night and cries because his legs hurt; yet during the day he is fine, with no pain or movement limitations. He has no history of trauma, fever, or joint swelling. The family history is negative for rheumatic or collagen-vascular disease. The boy's height and weight are at the 50th percentile for age, he is afebrile, and the physical examination is unremarkable.

Questions

1. What is the differential diagnosis of leg pains in school-aged children?
2. What laboratory or radiographic studies are appropriate for children with leg pains?
3. How do musculoskeletal injuries in children differ from those in adults (eg, the type of injury sustained, the location of the injury, etc)?
4. How does one decide the extent of the diagnostic workup in a child with extremity pain?
5. What physiological factors cause musculoskeletal injury patterns to change with age?

Children by nature are active and explorative. They experience cuts, scrapes, minor injuries, and pain routinely. Because primary care physicians are often the first to examine children with injuries, they play an important role in making the preliminary diagnosis and assessment regarding the need for further evaluation and treatment. The more common complaints and injuries seen in the pediatrician's office are discussed in this chapter: growing pains; nursemaids' elbow; and fractures, including growth plate injuries. The evaluation of children with limp is discussed in Chapter 105.

Epidemiology

The term **growing pains** is somewhat misleading because there is no evidence that these pains are associated with growth. The period of middle childhood, when growing pains are diagnosed, is not the period of most rapid growth in the child. *Leg aches* or *idiopathic leg pain* may be better terms, but growing pains is the most widely used term.

The prevalence of growing pains is not well defined, but seems to be between 15% and 30% of all children. They are seen most commonly in children between the ages of 4 and 14 years; the reported age range is infancy to 19 years. Girls are affected more frequently than boys.

Nursemaids' elbow, pulled elbow, or radial head subluxation is the most common joint injury in childhood. It occurs most commonly in children 1 to 4 years of age, with a peak incidence between

2 and 3 years of age. Other ligament and tendon injuries are relatively uncommon in prepubertal children due to the relative strength of these structures in comparison to the growth plate of the adjacent developing bone. Most commonly, fractures involving the growth plate occur before ligamentous injury. When joint dislocations and ligamentous injury occur in children (with the exception of nursemaids' elbow), they are usually due to significant trauma.

Trauma and injury are significant causes of morbidity and mortality in childhood. Injuries are the most common reason for hospitalization in children and adolescents younger than 18 years and are the leading cause of death beyond the first year of life. Musculoskeletal problems account for 15% of all injuries and most commonly occur in the upper extremity. Fractures are perhaps the most common significant form of musculoskeletal injury in children who present to physicians for evaluation and treatment.

Clinical Presentation (Dx Box)

Children with growing pains typically present with a history of intermittent, poorly localized pain in the bilateral lower extremities that occurs at night over a long period. The pain most commonly involves the calves and anterior thighs, never the joints. Symptoms usually resolve over several minutes, and in the morning the child has normal activity.

Nursemaids' elbow is characterized by a sudden onset of elbow pain associated with the traumatic event and subsequent decreased

Dx Growing Pains and Orthopedic Injuries

Growing Pains

- Age between 4 and 14 years
- Normal growth and development
- Intermittent pain or aches in the legs
- Occurrence of symptoms at night
- Pain poorly localized to the anterior thighs, calves, and behind the knees; absence of joint involvement
- Absence of limp, disability, or inflammation
- Response to supportive measures such as heat and massage

Nursemaids' Elbow

- Age between 1 and 4 years
- Elbow pain of acute onset
- History of sudden longitudinal traction on an extended and pronated arm
- Forearm held in a position of flexion and pronation
- Lack of spontaneous movement of the elbow

Fractures

- Obvious deformity
- Swelling or tenderness over the fracture site
- Limited range of movement or absence of movement of the affected extremity

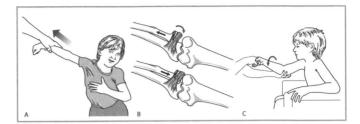

Figure 103-1. Nursemaids' elbow. The sudden traction on the outstretched arm pulls the radius distally, causing a tear in the annular ligament at its attachment to the radius. A portion of the ligament becomes trapped within the joint as the traction is released and the arm recoils. A. Mechanism of injury. B. Pathology. C. Method of reduction (hyperpronation).

between the radius and the capitellum. This injury is seen primarily in young children because the attachment of the ligament to the bone becomes thicker with age and growth.

Because of anatomical and physiological differences (eg, presence of cartilaginous growth plate as well as thicker periosteum and greater plasticity of the skeleton), fracture patterns seen in children often differ from those in adults. Additionally, fractures may influence long-term growth and development of the affected limb in a growing child.

Fractures are classified based on anatomical location, type of fracture, and degree of angulation or displacement. Fracture location may be described as diaphyseal, metaphyseal, or epiphyseal/growth plate depending on the portion of the bone involved (Figures 103-2 and 103-3). Fractures may be either open or closed. In closed fractures, the skin over the fracture site is intact, whereas in open fractures, the skin is broken. When 2 bone fragments are displaced relative to each other, the direction and degree of displacement are based on the distal fragment.

use of the arm. At the time of presentation for medical care, a child with nursemaids' elbow typically appears well, aside from a refusal to use the affected arm. The child typically holds the arm close to the body with the elbow in slight flexion and the forearm pronated. There is usually no gross deformity, swelling, or overlying skin trauma, and the child typically refuses to supinate the forearm during examination. There may also be point tenderness laterally over the radial head.

An underlying **fracture** is strongly indicated by obvious deformity or lack of spontaneous movement in the extremity in question. Localized swelling, tenderness, and limited range of movement may all be signs of a fracture.

Pathophysiology

Growing pains are recurrent aches or pains localized most commonly to the muscles of the legs and occasionally to the muscles of the arms of children. The pain is located deep within the extremity and not in the joints. The etiology is unclear. Emotional and psychological stress, a low pain threshold, bone fatigue, and myalgias secondary to exercise or physical activity have all been implicated as possible contributory factors.

Nursemaids' elbow is a subluxation of the radial head caused by a rapid and forceful extension and pronation of the forearm. This mechanism most commonly occurs when a caretaker pulls a child toward himself or herself and the child resists, wanting to go in the other direction. As illustrated in Figure 103-1, the subluxation occurs due to tearing of the annular ligament, with trapping of the ligament

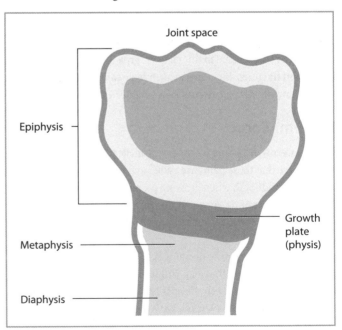

Figure 103-2. Anatomy of a long bone.

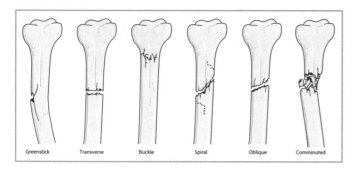

Figure 103-3. **Non-epiphyseal plate fractures.**

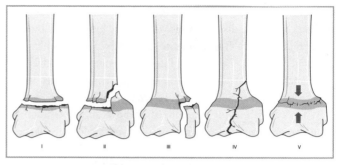

Figure 103-4. **Salter-Harris classification of epiphyseal plate fractures.**

The Salter-Harris classification is used most commonly to classify growth plate injury (Table 103-1, Figure 103-4). Approximately 15% of all fractures in children involve the growth plate. Type I and II fractures are the most common fractures involving the growth plate. Type III and IV fractures involve the epiphysis and are considered to be intra-articular. Type V fractures are uncommon and are due to a crush injury to the growth plate. Initial radiographs in type I and V fractures may appear normal, because bone fragments are not displaced. Due to involvement of the growth plate, there is a risk of growth arrest with any physis injury. The risk is variable, however, depending on the type of injury.

Differential Diagnosis

The diagnosis of **growing pains** is one of exclusion. Leg pain in children has many causes (Box 103-1). If they are limited to vague pains in the legs at night with no associated limp or signs of inflammation, the differential diagnosis may be limited to growing pains, general systemic diseases such as leukemia, benign bone tumors such as osteoid osteoma, and perhaps fibromyalgia. Leukemic infiltration of the bones may cause leg pain before systemic signs such as fever, weight loss, and adenopathy are present. Osteoid osteoma, a benign bone tumor that most commonly occurs in adolescent boys, characteristically causes pain that is worse at night and is usually relieved by anti-inflammatory medications. The pain may be localized in one place, however, unlike with growing pains. Fibromyalgia, which is

Table 103-1. Long Bone Fracture Patterns Seen in Children	
Type	*Description*
Non-Epiphyseal Plate Fractures	
Complete	Both sides of the bone fractured; type depends on direction of fracture line
Transverse	Perpendicular to long axis of the bone
Oblique	At an angle to long axis of the bone
Spiral	Zig-zag course around the bone
Comminuted	Fractures with 3 or more fragments (rare in children)
Buckle or torus	Bone compression causes it to bend or buckle rather than break; occurs at junction of metaphysis and diaphysis
Greenstick	Cortex broken on tension side but intact on compression side
Bowing	Deformation of bone due to bending without fracturing
Classic metaphyseal lesion	Fracture of distal, poorly mineralized metaphysis, perpendicular to long axis of bone; previously termed bucket-handle or chip fracture
Epiphyseal Plate Fractures (Salter-Harris Classification)	
Type I	Horizontal fracture through the physis
Type II	Fracture through the physis, extending into the metaphysis
Type III	Fracture through the epiphysis, extending into the physis
Type IV	Fracture through the epiphysis, physis, and metaphysis
Type V	Crush injury of the physis

Box 103-1. Common Causes of Leg Pain in Children	
Growing Pains (Leg Aches, Idiopathic Leg Pains)	**Collagen-Vascular Disease**
Trauma	• Juvenile rheumatoid arthritis
• Fracture	• Dermatomyositis
• Compartment syndromes	• Fibromyalgia
• Soft tissue injury	• Rheumatic fever
• Muscle strain/sprain	**Other Musculoskeletal Causes**
Infection	• Legg-Calvé-Perthes disease
• Cellulitis	• Slipped capital femoral epiphysis
• Soft tissue abscess	• Osgood-Schlatter disease
• Myositis	• Transient synovitis of the hip
• Osteomyelitis	• Osteochondritis dissecans
• Septic arthritis	• Patellofemoral stress/chondromalacia patellae
Neoplasia	• Generalized ligamentous laxity and joint hypermobility
• Malignant bone tumors (eg, osteogenic sarcoma, Ewing sarcoma)	**Miscellaneous Causes**
• Leukemia	• Sickle cell disease pain crisis
• Metastatic disease (eg, lymphoma, neuroblastoma)	• Psychosomatic conditions
Benign Bone Lesions	
• Osteoid osteoma	
• Bone cysts	
• Histiocytosis X	

probably underdiagnosed in the pediatric population, is a well-recognized cause in adults of chronic, generalized limb pain without a clear, organic source. It is seen more commonly in adolescents than in younger children. This benign, intermittent musculoskeletal pain syndrome is associated with multiple tender "trigger points," stiffness, fatigue, and a non-restorative sleep pattern.

When evaluating for **nursemaids' elbow,** an elbow fracture should be ruled out. Certain fractures and specific features of fractures deserve mention (see Figure 103-3). Fractures that often occur during childhood include clavicular fractures (the most common childhood fracture and most commonly fractured bone from birth trauma) and spiral fractures of the distal tibia—the "toddler's fracture." The toddler's fracture typically occurs in children who have not been walking long, those between 9 months and 3 years of age. It is thought to be due to a rotational force on the lower leg, which could occur as an ambulatory child falls in a twisting motion. Often, when the child presents for medical care the parents are unaware of a history of trauma and the chief complaint is that the child refuses to bear weight on the affected leg. Elbow fractures, including supracondylar humerus, as well as lateral and medial condyle fractures, occur commonly due to a fall directly on the elbow or due to a fall on an outstretched hand. These fractures require careful attention to neurovascular status because of the risk of associated injury to the median or radial nerve, or brachial artery, leading to Volkmann ischemic contracture. A Monteggia fracture is a dislocation of the radial head in association with an ulnar shaft fracture. Long bone fractures in pre-ambulatory children, rib fractures, classic metaphyseal lesions, and the presence of multiple fractures in one child are all concerning for non-accidental trauma and should prompt a more thorough evaluation of possible physical abuse (see Chapter 127).

Because of the relative weakness of the physis compared with the surrounding ligaments, trauma sustained near joints may be more likely to cause a type I Salter-Harris growth plate fracture rather than ligamentous injury (eg, sprain or strain). Therefore, it is important to include this type of fracture in the differential diagnosis of children with point tenderness near the end of a long bone because this injury does require cast immobilization.

Evaluation

Accurate diagnosis of pediatric orthopedic injuries is often challenging because children may be not only poor "historians" but also uncooperative with examinations, especially if they are experiencing pain.

History

A thorough history is essential for the accurate diagnosis of growing pains and orthopedic injuries (Questions Box: Growing Pains and Questions Box: Orthopedic Injuries). A complete history of the events related to the injury, including what happened after the injury was sustained, should be obtained.

Questions

Growing Pains

- When (ie, what time of day) does the pain typically occur?
- How long has the pain been occurring?
- Does the pain resolve and then recur in any predictable manner?
- Where is the pain? Does it change location?
- Does anything make the pain better or worse?
- Is the child sick in any other way?
- Does the pain interfere with the child's activities?
- Does the parent notice any changes such as swelling or redness in the child's legs?

Questions

Orthopedic Injuries

- How did the injury occur?
- How long ago was the injury sustained? When did the symptoms begin?
- Was the incident witnessed by an adult?
- How strong was the injuring force? What direction did it come from?
- What was the position of the affected extremity at the time of the injury?
- Did the child experience any head trauma or loss of consciousness?
- What, if any, first aid was administered at the scene?
- Has the child been able to move the affected extremity since the injury occurred?

Physical Examination

The physical examination of children with suspected **growing pains** should include evaluation for signs of systemic disease such as fever, lymphadenopathy, hepatosplenomegaly, abnormal growth, and generalized weakness or fatigue. Leg length and circumference should be measured. The legs should be palpated and range of motion assessed in the hip, knee, and ankle.

Children with suspected **nursemaids' elbow** should be observed for how they hold the affected arm compared with the unaffected arm. They should be evaluated for limited active motion at the elbow and resistance to attempts at passive movement, especially supination. No swelling should be present, but there may be tenderness over the radial head. The shoulder and wrist should also be well examined.

It is important to undress children with suspected **fractures** and perform a complete physical examination. Simply examining the involved extremity is insufficient. The presence of a deformity, point tenderness, or limitation of motion supports the diagnosis of a fracture. All long bones should be palpated, and the presence of bruises and scars should be noted because these may indicate child abuse. The examination of the involved extremity includes inspection of the overlying skin for swelling, lacerations, or punctures. The degree of active and passive motion and strength compared with the uninvolved side should be noted. In cases of suspected leg injuries, the child's gait should be observed, if possible. Assessment of neurovascular function distal to the injury includes evaluation of capillary refill, peripheral pulses, and motor and sensory function.

Laboratory Tests

A complete blood cell count and erythrocyte sedimentation rate (ESR) may be considered for children with leg pains that do not resolve. Rheumatologic screening tests can be ordered based on abnormalities in these tests (eg, elevated ESR or white blood cell count). Laboratory tests, if obtained, should be normal if a child is diagnosed with growing pains. Routine laboratory studies are not necessary in the evaluation of nursemaids' elbow or fractures. However, because fractures of the femur are often associated with significant blood loss, it is important to monitor the hematocrit in these patients.

Imaging Studies

If leg pains persist and interfere with routine activity, radiographs or a bone scan of the legs may be considered. Radiographic evaluation is not required for children with nursemaids' elbow if presentation is typical and reduction is successful. Radiographs, if taken in such children, are usually completely negative because the dislocation is often corrected during positioning for radiographs. However, radiographs should be obtained in children with suspected fractures. Fractures involving the growth plate, especially type I and V Salter-Harris fractures, may be particularly difficult to diagnose radiographically because the growth plate is primarily cartilaginous and, hence, radiolucent. A bone scan or follow-up radiograph may be used to diagnose suspected fractures when initial radiographs are negative.

Management

Parental education and reassurance regarding the benign nature of **growing pains** are important. The pains themselves usually respond to **supportive measures** such as heat, massage, and analgesia. Stretching exercises for the legs have also been recommended. Referral to an orthopedist should be considered if the pain is severe and persistent and physical examination and laboratory workup fail to reveal a specific diagnosis.

Nursemaids' elbow is one of the few medical conditions that has a dramatic, immediate cure. To treat the elbow, the annular ligament must be reduced back to its anatomical position, and there are 2 common methods of reduction. In both methods the elbow is stabilized with application of pressure laterally over the radial head with the thumb of the medical provider. In the first method, there is rapid, firm hyperpronation of the forearm. In the second, the forearm is firmly supinated then the elbow is flexed. While both methods of reduction have high success rates, several studies suggest superiority of the hyperpronation method. A click may be heard or felt as

the radial head is reduced, and relief of pain is usually immediate for those children treated shortly after the injury. Return of function may require up to 30 minutes, however. If treatment is delayed, such rapid relief of symptoms may not be seen. Following reduction, the parents should be advised that the child may need mild pain medication. Some providers recommend short-term immobilization in a sling or splint to facilitate soft tissue healing. If reduction is unsuccessful, consider the possibility of obtaining radiographs and referring the patient for orthopedic consultation.

Most **fractures** should be referred to an orthopedic surgeon for evaluation and treatment unless the primary care physician is experienced in reducing and casting fractures. Several techniques are used in fracture management. **Closed reduction** is the nonoperative reduction or realignment of fracture fragments. **Open reduction** implies that an incision has been made to expose the fracture and proceed with manipulating the bone fragments into place. Fixation, or stabilization of the fracture with any type of device, may be required following the reduction. This is termed **internal fixation** if the device is under the skin and **external fixation** if the device begins outside of the skin but passes through the skin to bone. Indications for open reduction include failure of closed reduction, need for precise anatomical reduction, and complex multisystem trauma.

Certain fractures are common in pediatrics. Most clavicular fractures do not require reduction and can be treated with immobilization in a sling for 4 to 8 weeks. Elbow fractures (eg, lateral condyle and supracondylar humeral fractures) are at particular risk for neurovascular compromise and often necessitate open reduction to achieve anatomical reduction. Distal forearm fractures are usually managed with closed reduction and casting, but forearm fractures in the middle and proximal thirds of the bone may be harder to reduce in the office setting. Stable metacarpal and phalangeal fractures can be either splinted in an aluminum splint or be taped to an adjacent finger ("buddy taping"). The metacarpophalangeal joints should be maintained in 50 to 90 degrees of flexion, and the interphalangeal joints should be in about 20 degrees of flexion to minimize stiffness. Unstable finger fractures may require open reduction and pin fixation.

Femoral shaft fractures in infants and children can be managed with closed reduction and spica cast placement. As children become older, a fixation device may be required in addition to the closed reduction. Open reduction is necessary on rare occasions. Closed reduction and cast immobilization are usually used in the management of tibial shaft fractures. Short cast immobilization may be required for metatarsal fractures, and buddy taping is used for stable toe fractures.

Because of the potential for infection, open fractures are orthopedic emergencies that require immediate attention and orthopedic consultation. Careful debridement of the wound is required. Antibiotics should be administered, and tetanus immunization may be given based on a review of the immunization history.

Prognosis

Growing pains resolve over time without sequelae. Recurrence of nursemaids' elbow is common, occurring again in up to a third of patients. Therefore, parents should be cautioned regarding pulling children's arms or lifting them by one hand. Fractures in children generally heal faster and remodel (the spontaneous correction of deformity) better than equivalent fractures in adults. Vascular and nerve injuries and growth disturbances are potential complications of fractures and their management. Compartment syndrome, a potentially serious vascular injury, may also develop.

Growth plate injuries require special attention because of the potential for subsequent growth abnormalities of the affected bone. Prognosis of growth plate fractures depends on the type of injury sustained. Salter-Harris type I and II fractures generally have a good prognosis for long-term healing and growth. The severity of the injury and the accuracy of reduction determine the prognosis of type III and IV fractures. Growth arrest is common following type V fractures because the physis itself is injured.

CASE RESOLUTION

The child presented in the opening scenario has the benign condition commonly referred to as growing pains. Management involves parental education and reassurance. Local heat, massage, and analgesia (using ibuprofen) may be recommended.

Selected References

Carson S, Woolridge DP, Colletti J, Kilgore K. Pediatric upper extremity injuries. *Pediatr Clin North Am.* 2006;53:41–67

Hart ES, Albright MB, Rebello GN, Grottkau BE. Broken bones: common pediatric fractures—part I. *Orthop Nurs.* 2006;25:251–256

Hart ES, Luther B, Grottkau BE. Broken bones: common pediatric lower extremity fractures—part III. *Orthop Nurs.* 2006;25:390–407

Kerssemakers SP, Fotiadou AN, de Jonge MC, Karantanas AH, Maas M. Sport injuries in the paediatric and adolescent patient: a growing problem. *Pediatr Radiol.* 2009;39:471–484

Klig JE. Splinting procedures. In: King C, Henretig FM, eds. *Textbook of Pediatric Emergency Procedures.* Philadelphia, PA: Lippincott Williams & Wilkins;2007:919–931

Laine JC, Kaiser SP, Diab M. High-risk pediatric orthopedic pitfalls. *Emerg Med Clin N Am.* 2010;28:85–102

Lowe RM, Hashkes PJ. Growing pains: a noninflammatory pain syndrome of early childhood. *Nat Clin Pract Rheumatol.* 2008;4:542–549

Meckler GD, Spiro DM. Radial head subluxation. *Pediatr Rev.* 2008;29:e42–e43

Tse SML, Laxer RM. Approach to acute limb pain in childhood. *Pediatr Rev.* 2006;27:170–179

CHAPTER 104

Sports-Related Acute Injuries

Monica Sifuentes, MD, and Andrew K. Battenberg, BS

CASE STUDY

A 15-year-old female basketball player complains of 6 months of intermittent pain in her left knee. Occasionally the knee gives out while she is playing ball. The teen denies any associated swelling or erythema over the joint. She is able to walk with no problem and reports no history of direct trauma to the area. She is otherwise healthy.

On physical examination, she is a well-developed, well-nourished teenaged female in no acute distress. The examination is normal except for mild pain to direct palpation of the left patella. No swelling, erythema, or effusion of the knee joint is evident, and the left hip, knee, and ankle have full range of motion. The back is straight.

Questions

1. What are some of the most common orthopedic complaints in adolescent patients, and why do they occur in this age group?
2. What is the pathophysiology of overuse syndromes?
3. What is the purpose of the preparticipation sports physical examination?
4. What conditions disqualify adolescents from participation in competitive sports?
5. What are the current recommendations for the treatment and rehabilitation of acute soft tissue injuries?

Many adolescents with varying degrees of athletic ability participate in sports during their junior high and high school years. Some choose to continue this participation at the college level. Regardless of the ultimate goal, team sports are an important means by which children and adolescents can experience both winning and losing. Individuals learn the importance of group participation and develop interactive skills with other team members. They are exposed to the concept of physical fitness, which can improve body image as well as self-esteem.

Participation in athletics carries significant risks, however. Injuries, inappropriate coaching, and aggressive training sessions are not uncommon occurrences that may have long-term sequelae for young athletes. Primary care practitioners are responsible not only for the evaluation of children prior to their participation in sports but also for the diagnosis, treatment, and prevention of athletic injuries.

Epidemiology

Estimates indicate that as many as 7 million adolescents per year participate in organized sports activities in the United States. Several studies have attempted to quantify the overall injury rate associated with athletic participation. In general, the rate of injury for 13- to 19-year-olds is 7% to 11%. Approximately 20% of those injured sustain a significant injury. For boys, the sport with the highest injury rate in all age groups is football, followed by basketball and soccer. In girls, roller skating and gymnastics accounts for the most injuries. Gender differences between boys and girls have been found in some studies depending on the sport. Overall, boys tend to have more shoulder-related injuries, whereas girls tend to have more knee and ankle injuries and more problems with overuse syndromes. Reports also indicate that the severity of sports-related injuries increases with age.

Preparticipation Physical Evaluation

The goal of the preparticipation physical evaluation (PPE) is the identification of any physical conditions or abnormalities that may predispose young athletes to injury. Examples include a history of concussion with head trauma or an incompletely healed sprain.

The PPE consists of 2 parts: (1) a review of the patient's current health and medical history, including sports injuries and family history relating to participation in strenuous exercise, and (2) a complete physical examination with a focus on the musculoskeletal system. Known as a "2-minute orthopedic examination," the musculoskeletal examination is a detailed assessment of all muscle groups, assessing their strength, tone, and function. Congenital or acquired deformities should also be noted. The American Academy of Pediatrics (AAP) has developed a form specifically for the PPE visit (see Chapter 33).

Disqualification from participation in specific sports is appropriate in certain situations. Competitive sports are classified according to their degree of contact or impact and how strenuous they are. Recommendations differ depending on the adolescent's medical condition and the type of sport the athlete desires to play. For details of these recommendations, see Selected References. Fortunately, many young athletes are healthy and rarely need to be restricted from participation.

Clinical Presentation

Older children and adolescents with sports-related injuries usually present to the practitioner with specific complaints of pain or swelling in a particular joint (Dx Box). In addition, they may complain of nonspecific musculoskeletal pain occurring in certain areas, such as the lower back or shoulder. Other complaints may include a limp, decreased range of motion of an extremity, or an inability to participate in a desired activity without pain.

Dx **Orthopedic Injury**

- Joint pain or swelling
- Tenderness to palpation of the affected joint
- Decreased range of motion of the affected joint or extremity
- May or may not have associated bruising of the skin overlying the injury

Pathophysiology

Adolescents, unlike adults, are particularly susceptible to injury because their bones and joints are not fully mature. Most injuries during adolescence involve the epiphysis, which is the weakest point of the musculoskeletal system. In addition, the presence of congenital anomalies, such as leg length discrepancies or hip rotation abnormalities, puts the young athlete at further risk for injury. Biomechanical and neuromuscular factors, hormonal influences, and anatomical differences have also been proposed reasons for higher rates of some injuries in young female athletes compared to young male athletes. For example, patellofemoral pain syndrome, which presents as knee pain exacerbated by activity, is a very common problem in adolescent females, affecting nearly 1 in 10 of those that are active. Contributing biomechanical factors include tight ileotibial bands, weak gluteal strength, and a relative genu valgum due to wider female hips. This combination leads to valgus stresses at the knee, internal rotation of the femur, and abnormal patellar tracking, which puts the athlete at greater risk for patellofemoral syndrome.

Most orthopedic injuries are the result of either macrotrauma or microtrauma. Sprains are an example of macrotrauma, whereas overuse syndromes can be considered microtrauma. **Macrotrauma** occurs from complete or partial tearing of muscle, ligaments, or tendons and is often associated with acute injuries. In contrast, **microtrauma** is usually produced by chronic repetitive trauma to a particular area, leading to inflammation and ultimately to pain. This most commonly occurs in soft tissues such as the muscle and tendon but can occur in the bone as well.

Definitions

A **sprain** is a stretching injury of a ligament or the connective tissue that attaches bone to bone. A **strain** is a stretching injury of a muscle or its tendon, which is the connective tissue that attaches muscle to bone. **Tendinitis** is an inflammation of the tendon. **Apophysitis** is an inflammation of the apophysis, which is the site of ligament or tendon attachment to growth cartilage (eg, Osgood-Schlatter disease

[apophysitis of the tibial tubercle], Sever disease [calcaneal apophysitis]). A **stress fracture** is an incomplete fracture often occurring in the bones of the legs and feet from repetitive trauma to the area. It is believed that the pain associated with shin splints may be due in part to atypical stress fractures of the distal tibia.

Overuse syndromes occur from repetitive microtrauma to the musculoskeletal system secondary to excessive or biomechanically incorrect activity. They are usually the result of training errors in which athletes are "trying to do too much too fast." Common syndromes in adolescents include Osgood-Schlatter disease, shin splints, and patellofemoral syndrome (chondromalacia patellae).

Grading of Sports Injuries

Sprains can be classified according to the degree of injury and most commonly occur in the knee or ankle. Assigning a grade that describes the injury is useful when considering the prognosis of a particular injury. Consultants also find these grades helpful. Grade I through III is the usual classification used for sprains: Grade I generally refers to stretching of the ligament, Grade II a partial tearing of the ligament, and Grade III a complete tearing of the ligament. Stability of the joint, range of motion, and degree of pain and swelling determine the grade of the sprain. The grading system for **strains,** on the other hand, is based on an assessment of strength. Because strains do not usually cause joint instability, criteria for grading strains are different than for sprains and may be more subjective. A description of these 2 grading systems appears in Table 104-1.

Table 104-1. General Classification of Sprains and Strains					
	Joint	Range of Motion	Weight Bearing	Pain	Swelling
Sprains					
Grade I	Stable	Normal	Normal	+	+
Grade II	Stable	↓	↓	++	++
Grade III	Unstable	↓↓	↓↓	+++	+++
	Strength	Palpable Defect	Pain		
Strains					
Grade I	>4/5	−	+		
Grade II	3/5–4/5	+/−	++		
Grade III	<3/5	+/−	+++		

Differential Diagnosis

The differential diagnosis of orthopedic conditions depends on the anatomical site of the injury or complaint and the mechanism of injury. Box 104-1 lists some of the more common orthopedic conditions by location. Anomalies of skeletal development, such as congenital angular deformities of long bones and soft tissue abnormalities like Ehlers-Danlos syndrome, should be considered as

Box 104-1. Differential Diagnosis Based on the Site of Injury	
Back Injuries • Muscle strain • Spondylolysis • Epiphyseal injury • Herniated disks **Injuries to the Upper Extremity** • Acromioclavicular sprains • Sternoclavicular sprains • Glenohumeral dislocation • Glenohumeral subluxation • Impingement syndrome • Acute elbow injuries • Olecranon bursitis • Lateral epicondylitis • Flexor-pronator tendinitis • Wrist sprains • Scaphoid fractures • Hamate fractures • Finger injuries	**Injuries to the Lower Extremity** • Iliac crest contusion • Iliac apophysitis • Quadriceps contusion • Femoral stress fracture • Medial/lateral ligament sprains • Anterior cruciate ligament sprain • Posterior cruciate ligament sprain • Patellar dislocation/subluxation • Prepatellar bursitis • Patellofemoral stress syndrome • Patellar tendinitis • Osgood-Schlatter disease • Shin splint syndrome • Ankle sprains • Achilles tendinitis • Calcaneal apophysitis • Plantar fasciitis

Questions

Sports-Related Injuries

- What is the acuity of the injury?
- What activity or sport was the patient engaged in at the time of the injury?
- How often has the patient engaged in this sport or particular activity in the past?
- Were there any new additions to the routine this time?
- Did the pain begin after a single injury or after repetitive activity?
- If the injury is related to a repetitive activity, does the pain occur at a specific time during this activity?
- What was the mechanism of injury?
- Is the pain incapacitating?
- Has a similar injury ever occurred in the past?
- How was the injury treated?
- Was there any pain following the previous injury?
- Does the patient feel as if he or she has completely recovered?
- How was this current injury managed acutely?
- Has the patient altered daily activity in any way to compensate for this problem?

possible etiologies for overuse syndromes. Other non-orthopedic conditions, such as collagen-vascular diseases, infections, and tumors, may present with joint or bone symptomatology.

Evaluation

History

The history should focus on the musculoskeletal system and how the injury occurred (Questions Box).

Physical Examination

The physical examination should focus on the musculoskeletal system. If, however, teenagers have not had a physical examination within the past year, a complete physical examination should first be performed to exclude any systemic condition that might manifest itself initially as musculoskeletal pain. This is especially important in adolescents with chronic or systemic complaints, such as intermittent extremity pain, swelling of an affected joint, and fever.

In general, any pain or swelling of an affected joint or muscle should be noted. If there is history of acute trauma, an area of ecchymosis or joint effusion may be seen. The affected joint should be tested for range of motion and joint laxity in order to determine the degree of sprain. Special testing for ligament laxity should be used (Figure 104-1). For the knee, the most common method is the drawer test for anterior and posterior movement of the knee joint. However, the Lachman Test is gaining popularity as it has been shown to be a more sensitive and specific test for anterior cruciate ligament injuries. The patient is examined in a prone position on an examining table and the knee, ligaments, and tibia are assessed.

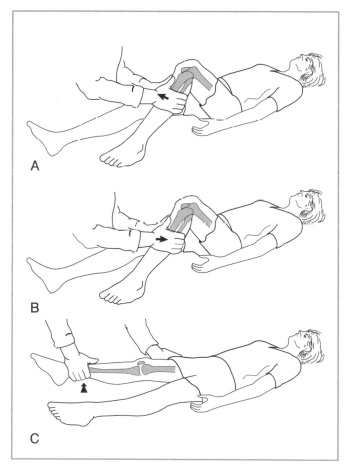

Figure 104-1. Maneuvers used to determine stability of the knee joint. A. Anterior drawer test: Anterior force is applied. B. Posterior drawer test: Posterior force is applied. C. Medial ligament stability: Lateral force is applied.

Muscle spasms and diminished range of motion in an adjacent joint should be noted as these may be signs of a strain injury. Strength of the strained muscle(s) should be assessed, and any pain with palpation or range of motion should be noted. A palpable defect of the muscle suggests complete rupture of the muscle, whereas muscular contusions are associated with localized pain, soft tissue swelling, or hematoma. Pinpoint tenderness over a particular bone may indicate a fracture or, if at the site of a tendon insertion, inflammation. Reviewing the mechanism of injury and the timing of the symptoms is often helpful in differentiating between a fracture and tendinitis.

Laboratory Tests

A complete blood cell count and erythrocyte sedimentation rate may be helpful in adolescents with a history of chronic joint pain or swelling. If the results are abnormal, further workup is indicated to distinguish between a collagen-vascular disease such as systemic lupus erythematosus, an infection such as osteomyelitis or, rarely, an arthritic disorder such as juvenile idiopathic arthritis.

Imaging Studies

A plain radiograph of the involved joint or bone is often the only necessary diagnostic study to perform. Because ankle sprain is such a common occurrence, it is important to understand when a radiograph is needed to rule out fracture: The Ottawa Ankle Rules are guidelines for obtaining radiographs in acute ankle injury, are approximately 100% sensitive, and have been validated for use in children older than 6 years (Box 104-2). Plain radiographs of joints above and below the symptomatic area are also sometimes indicated. One example is the Maisonneuve fracture, a fracture of the proximal fibula near the knee that can occur with serious ankle injury; this fracture can be missed if a knee radiograph is not obtained in addition to ankle views. In general, advanced diagnostic tests such as computerized tomography scanning have limited value in the evaluation of an acute soft tissue injury. Magnetic resonance imaging may be indicated for injuries that do not improve despite adequate treatment and rehabilitation. See Chapter 105 for a discussion of imaging studies used to evaluate a child presenting with limp.

Box 104-2. Ottawa Ankle Rules

- Obtain ankle radiograph if ANY of the following:
  — Bone tenderness at posterior edge or tip of lateral malleolus
  — Bone tenderness at posterior edge or tip of medial malleolus
  — Bone tenderness along distal 6 cm of tibia or fibula
  — Inability to bear weight both immediately after injury AND in emergency department for 4 steps
- Obtain foot radiograph if ANY of the following:
  — Bone tenderness at base of the fifth metatarsal
  — Bone tenderness at navicular bone
  — Inability to bear weight both immediately after injury AND in emergency department for 4 steps

---

Management

With soft tissue injuries, the aim of acute management is to limit the extent of bleeding and inflammation that occur in the first 48 to 72 hours following the injury. The mnemonic **RICE** (rest, ice, compression, elevation) is helpful. Rest should be explained as "relative rest" because the athletes should be allowed to do whatever they want as long as they are pain-free during or within 24 hours of the activity. Ice should be placed in a plastic bag and applied directly to the skin for a continuous 20 minutes. Longer periods of icing are discouraged because this can result in peripheral nerve palsy from cryoinjury. Patients should ice the injury 3 to 4 times a day for the first 48 hours, and then at least once daily until the swelling or pain is gone. Compression is especially important and should be started as quickly as possible. When applying compression bandages, wrapping should begin distal to the injury and should proceed proximally; this prevents trapping of edema and swelling distal to the compression wrap, allowing proper drainage of injured tissue. Elevation of the injured extremity should occur as often as possible. The use of this plan for soft tissue injuries facilitates early healing and allows rehabilitation to proceed more quickly.

Anti-inflammatory or analgesic medications, such as ibuprofen, aspirin, and naproxen, are useful in controlling the symptoms of pain and swelling. For adolescent patients, dosages are similar to those used in adults: aspirin, 650 to 1,000 mg every 6 hours; ibuprofen, 400 to 800 mg every 6 to 8 hours; naproxen, 500 mg twice daily. To minimize gastrointestinal side effects, the medication should be administered with a snack or milk. Ideally, these drugs should be used for 7 to 10 days. Corticosteroids, either oral or parenteral, are not indicated in the management of overuse injuries or acute trauma to the extremities.

After the acute phase, therapy is aimed at rehabilitation and resolution of any edema or hematoma (Box 104-3). Athletes should slowly begin range-of-motion exercises as tolerated. Full tissue healing may take 6 to 8 weeks, but most young athletes do not have to wait that long to return to athletic activity.

Modified activity, depending on the degree of tissue damage, should initially be recommended in athletes who have suffered from overuse syndromes. Complete rest is rarely indicated. Participation in another sport such as swimming or cycling is often preferable to complete immobilization. In addition to the use of anti-inflammatory agents, physical therapy is another important therapeutic modality.

Box 104-3. Principles of Rehabilitation

- Resolution of hematoma
- Resolution of edema
- Regain full range of motion or flexibility
- Regain full muscle strength and endurance
- Regain agility and coordination
- Regain cardiovascular endurance

Cryotherapy, whirlpool, or alternating heat and ice treatments can be helpful. Reconditioning should be continued after 3 to 12 weeks of modified activity, depending on the degree of recovery. This entails gradual strengthening and flexibility training as well as reevaluation of previous modes of training to minimize the risk of reinjury (Box 104-4). Additional aspects to consider are strength imbalances and biomechanics such as those that occur in patellofemoral syndrome. By identifying specific musculoskeletal imbalances, the clinician can suggest stretches and strengthening exercises specific to the patient's deficits.

Box 104-4. Rehabilitation of Musculoskeletal Injuries[a]

Four Phases of Rehabilitation

- Limit additional injury and control pain and swelling (RICE mnemonic).
- Improve strength and flexibility (range of motion) of the injured structures.
- Progressively improve strength, flexibility, proprioception, and endurance training until near-normal function is attained.
- Return to exercise and sports symptom-free.

[a] Modified Hergenroeder AC. Prevention of sports injuries. *Pediatrics.* 1998;101:1057–1063.

Prevention

Injury prevention is an important aspect of sports medicine with which the primary practitioner should be familiar. Because most injuries are the result of "trying to do too much too soon," proper physical **training and conditioning** are essential, no matter how fit the athlete appears. Stretching, warm-up and cool-down exercises, and the type of equipment used for the sport, should be reviewed with the athlete during the sports physical visit. The type of sport to be played should also be reviewed and, if participating in a contact sport, the adolescent should be **matched with other athletes** based on weight and pubertal development rather than age. Some studies suggest that such matching will greatly reduce the risk of injury to the smaller, less mature athlete. Because an old or incompletely healed injury is a significant risk factor for reinjury, all **previous injuries should receive proper treatment and rehabilitation** before the athlete returns to play. **Protective equipment,** especially for collision and contact sports, as well as for those involving a ball or racquet, also should be emphasized to athletes and their parents. In addition, the AAP recommendation of **avoiding strength and weight training** until the athlete reaches sexual maturity rating (Tanner stage) 5 of pubertal development should be endorsed to prevent the risk of serious injury. **Education regarding the hazards of anabolic steroid use and creatine** also may be indicated.

Prognosis

Orthopedic injuries in young athletes and active adolescents have a great capacity for healing if given the opportunity. Early medical intervention to prevent irreversible tissue damage ensures complete recovery in most cases. Long-term sequelae are associated with repeated trauma, incompletely treated cases, and chronic inflammatory changes. Some conditions, however, such as Osgood-Schlatter disease, will resolve even without treatment and do not lead to any permanent damage to the joint.

CASE RESOLUTION

In the case presented at the beginning of the chapter, the teenager has symptoms and physical findings consistent with patellofemoral pain syndrome (traditionally referred to as chondromalacia of the patella). Because plain radiographs are usually not helpful in confirming the diagnosis, none are necessary at this time. Management should include strength training for the quadriceps muscles, activity modification, nonsteroidal anti-inflammatory medication, and ice compresses after activity.

Selected References

American Academy of Pediatrics Council on Sports Medicine and Fitness. Strength training by children and adolescents. *Pediatrics.* 2008;121:835–840

Batra AS, Hohn AR. Palpitations, syncope, and sudden death in children. Who's at risk? *Pediatr Rev.* 2003;24:269–275

Brenner JS; American Academy of Pediatrics Council on Sports Medicine and Fitness. Overuse injuries, overtraining, and burnout in child and adolescent athletes. *Pediatrics.* 2007;119:1242–1245

Carry PM, Kanai S, Miller NH, Polousky JD. Adolescent patellofemoral pain: a review of evidence for the role of lower extremity biomechanics and core instability. *Orthopedics.* 2010;33(7):498

Dowling S, Spooner CH, Liang Y, et al. Accuracy of Ottawa ankle rules to exclude fractures of the ankle and midfoot in children: a meta-analysis. *Acad Emerg Med.* 2009;16(4):277–287

Koutures CG, Gregory AJM; American Academy of Pediatrics the Council on Sports Medicine and Fitness. Clinical report—injuries in youth soccer. *Pediatrics.* 2010;125:410–414

LaBella CR. Common acute sport-related lower extremity injuries in children and adolescents. *Clin Pediatr Emerg Med.* 2007;8:31–42

LaBella CR, Carl R. Preventing knee ligament injuries in young athletes. *Pediatr Ann.* 2010;39;714–720

Metzl JD. Managing sports injuries in the pediatric office. *Pediatr Rev.* 2008: 29:75–85

Metzl JD. Preparticipation examination of the adolescent athlete: part 1. *Pediatr Rev.* 2001:22:199–204

Metzl JD. Preparticipation examination of the adolescent athlete: part 2. *Pediatr Rev.* 2001;22:227–235

Rodenberg RE, Cayce K, Hall S. Your guide to a dreaded injury: the ACL tear. *Contemp Pediatr.* 2006;23:26–39

Stiell IG, Greenberg GH, McKnight RD, Nair RC, McDowell I, Worthington JR. A study to develop clinical decision rules for the use of radiography in acute ankle injuries. *Ann Emerg Med.* 1992;21(4):384–390

Stricker PR. *Sport Success Rx! Your Child's Prescription for the Best Experience.* Elk Grove Village, IL: American Academy of Pediatrics; 2006

Sullivan JA, Anderson SJ. *Care of the Young Athlete.* 2nd ed. Rosemont, IL: American Academy of Orthopaedic Surgeons, American Academy of Pediatrics; 2010

CHAPTER 105

Evaluation of Limp

Paul Bryan, MD

CASE STUDY

A 6-year-old boy who has a 2-day history of right knee pain and limp is brought to the office. No history of knee trauma, swelling, redness, or associated fever is present. The medical history is unremarkable. The boy is afebrile, and his height and weight are at the 10th percentile for age. Examination of the right leg reveals decreased abduction and internal rotation of the hip; the knee is normal. The boy limps when he walks and favors his right leg.

Questions

1. What is the differential diagnosis of painful and painless limp in children?
2. What is the differential diagnosis of knee pain in children?
3. What laboratory and radiographic tests are indicated in the evaluation of children with limp?
4. What is the appropriate management of children with suspected infectious causes of limp?

A limp is a gait disturbance that occurs when an effort is made to minimize weight bearing on an affected leg so that pain and instability are reduced. The disturbance may be secondary to muscle weakness, deformity, pain, or a combination thereof. Muscle weakness may be due to primary muscle disease, neurologic conditions, or disuse atrophy. Structural causes of limp include leg length discrepancy and joint stiffness, while painful causes of limp include trauma, synovitis, infection (ie, bone, joint, or soft tissue), or neoplasm. A limp can be a sign of significant underlying disease, and accurate diagnosis and appropriate management are essential to prevent potentially serious morbidity, including long-term disability.

Epidemiology

A limp may be due to pain originating in a leg or to pain referred from the abdomen or spine. Age often defines the diagnostic possibilities because certain disorders are seen more frequently in particular age groups. Infectious causes of limp occur more frequently in infants and young children, and noninfectious causes are more common in school-aged children and adolescents (Box 105-1).

Clinical Presentation

A painful limp usually has an acute onset and may be associated with systemic signs such as fever or irritability, especially when the etiology is infectious. Toddlers may simply refuse to walk or walk with a slow, cautious gait when they are in pain rather than limp. Non-painful limp often has an insidious onset and is commonly due to weakness (eg, muscular dystrophy) or deformity (eg, leg length discrepancy).

Box 105-1. Differential Diagnosis of Limp in Children

CHILDREN AGES 1–3 YEARS

Painful Limp

- Septic arthritis/osteomyelitis
- Transient synovitis
- Intervertebral diskitis
- Juvenile idiopathic arthritis (JIA)
- Neoplasia (leukemia, metastatic disease)
- Trauma (toddler's fractures)
- Child abuse

Painless Limp

- Developmental hip dysplasia
- Neuromuscular disease (cerebral palsy)
- Leg length discrepancy

CHILDREN AGES 4–10 YEARS

Painful Limp

- Septic arthritis/osteomyelitis
- Transient synovitis
- Trauma
- Legg-Calvé-Perthes disease (LCPD) (acute phase)
- Intervertebral diskitis
- JIA
- Sickle cell pain crisis
- Neoplasia (leukemia, primary bone tumor, metastatic disease)

Painless Limp

- LCPD (chronic phase)
- Developmental hip dysplasia
- Neuromuscular disease (cerebral palsy, muscular dystrophy)
- Leg length discrepancy

CHILDREN AND ADOLESCENTS AGES ≥11 YEARS

Painful Limp

- Trauma
- Septic arthritis/osteomyelitis
- Slipped capital femoral epiphysis (SCFE)
- Osgood-Schlatter disease
- JIA
- Sickle cell pain crisis
- Neoplasia (leukemia, primary bone tumor, metastatic disease)

Painless Limp

- SCFE
- Leg length discrepancy
- Neuromuscular disease (cerebral palsy, muscular dystrophy)
- Scoliosis

Pathophysiology

Normal gait has 2 phases: stance and swing. During the stance phase, either one or both feet are on the ground; during the swing phase, one foot is not touching the ground as the limb is moved forward. Stance phase is shortened in limp to decrease the amount of time spent in bearing weight on the affected side or to minimize instability.

Normal adult gait is smooth and efficient, requiring the coordinated actions of the muscles of the legs and pelvis. Normal gait in children varies according to age and developmental maturity. Toddlers typically walk with a broad-based, tiptoe, "bouncing" gait with arms abducted for balance. They may initiate the stance phase with either toe or heel strike. By 2 years of age, children should initiate the stance phase consistently with heel strike. Children who are 3 to 4 years of age should exhibit normal adult gait with reciprocating arm swing most of the time.

Several types of abnormal gaits are recognized. A shortened stance phase due to pain is characteristic of an **antalgic gait.** Weakness of the hip abductors (gluteus medius) leads to a **Trendelenburg gait,** where the pelvis dips down during stance phase, producing a swaying type of gait. A tiptoe or **toe-to-heel** gait is normal in children for several months after they learn to walk. Persistence of such a gait beyond 2 years of age is abnormal and may result from either idiopathic heel-cord contracture or contracture secondary to cerebral palsy.

Differential Diagnosis

Trauma is a frequent cause of limp in children and adolescents. Toddlers may simply refuse to walk and have an occult fracture, such as a **toddler's fracture.** This is an oblique or spiral fracture of the middle or distal tibia, which occurs after a fall or jump involving a twisting motion. Toddlers are at risk for such injuries because of their unsteady gait. Standard anteroposterior (AP) and lateral radiograph views can initially be normal, and oblique views may be helpful. Follow-up radiographs or a bone scan may be necessary to make the diagnosis. Older children will usually be able to recall a specific injury and localize pain to a specific area. Radiographs are usually obtained to determine if a fracture is present. Individuals who have tenderness over open growth plates should be splinted and warrant close follow-up even with normal radiographs, as there is a possibility of a Salter-Harris type I fracture, which occurs through the growth plate and may not be radiographically apparent.

Painless limp in toddlers may be due to **developmental hip dysplasia, cerebral palsy,** or **leg length discrepancy** (anisomelia). As a result of developmental hip dysplasia, children may have a Trendelenburg gait secondary to leg length discrepancy or to weakness of the hip abductors. Children with spastic cerebral palsy often walk on their toes because of increased tone or heel-cord contractures. Functional or apparent leg length discrepancies may result from pelvic obliquity or spinal deformity. Children with true leg length inequality compensate by either walking on tiptoe on the shorter side or bending the knee on the longer side; in either case, their gait is abnormal. Limb discrepancies may be managed with orthotics (eg, heel lifts) for mild cases, and surgical lengthening or shortening procedures may be necessary for more severe cases.

Transient synovitis of the hip is a benign self-limited inflammatory process involving the synovial lining and is one of the most common causes of limp in the young child. The exact cause of the inflammation is not known. There has been an association with certain upper respiratory infections, but no infectious agent has been identified. Trauma has also been implicated as a potential factor in initiating the inflammatory response because the contusion triggers a chemical synovitis. Age varies, but it typically affects children 3 to 8 years old. Individuals usually present with acute onset of unilateral hip pain associated with a limp. There can be referred pain to the anterior thigh or knee. Most children are either afebrile or have low-grade temperatures (<38.5°C [101.3°F]). The leg may be held in a position of abduction, flexion, and external rotation to reduce intracapsular pressure and associated pain. Symptoms are usually unilateral, but in up to 5% of cases there is bilateral involvement, often with one side being more symptomatic than the other.

Laboratory evaluation typically consists of complete blood cell count (CBC), erythrocyte sedimentation rate (ESR), and C-reactive protein (CRP). The laboratory results are usually within normal limits or slightly elevated. Radiographs are often obtained, which are usually normal or show signs suggestive of an effusion. An ultrasound is often performed to look for the presence of an effusion within the joint, which is often present in this condition. If an arthrocentesis is performed, the fluid in transient synovitis usually has a white blood cell (WBC) count of less than 50,000/mm^3 and a negative Gram stain. Individuals with normal laboratory values or with a fluid aspirate not suggestive of septic arthritis (when arthrocentesis has been performed) are typically managed with supportive care and close follow-up within 24 to 48 hours. Rest and nonsteroidal anti-inflammatory agents are the mainstays of therapy. Virtually all children recover within 3 to 10 days with no significant sequelae. Recurrence rates vary from 4% to 17% within the first 6 months following an episode of synovitis.

Septic arthritis occurs when there is an infection within the joint space. In children, this usually occurs in the face of bacteremia, with hematogenous spread to the highly vascular synovium. It can also occur from contiguous spread of an adjacent infection (eg, osteomyelitis) or by direct inoculation (eg, surgery or penetrating trauma). *Staphylococcus aureus* remains the most common pathogen identified across all age groups, with increasing incidences of community-acquired methicillin-resistant strains. Infants younger than 2 months can also be infected by neonatal pathogens, such as *Streptococcus agalactiae* (eg, group B streptococcus [GBS]) and gram-negative enteric organisms (eg, *Escherichia coli*). *Staphylococcus aureus, Streptococcus pyogenes, Streptococcus pneumoniae,* and *Kingella kingae* are the main organisms identified in the 2-month to 5-year age group. Children older than 5 years will usually have infections caused by *S aureus* or *S pyogenes. Neisseria gonorrhoeae* infections can be seen in sexually active adolescents.

Infants and children will often present with fever, decreased use of the affected extremity, limp, and refusal to walk. The most commonly affected joint is the hip, which is classically held in a position of abduction, flexion, and external rotation to reduce intracapsular pressure and associated pain. Passive range of motion typically elicits significant discomfort and resistance. Parents of infants may notice considerable crying with manipulation of the legs with activities such as diaper changing.

Subtle or early cases can often present a diagnostic challenge because there can be significant clinical and laboratory overlap with transient synovitis. Unfortunately there is no highly sensitive or specific laboratory test that can readily distinguish these 2 entities. Fever higher than 38.5°C (101.3°F) was shown to be the single best predictor of septic arthritis in one study, with no children diagnosed with transient synovitis having a temperature above 38.5°C. Other predictors include refusal to bear weight, ESR greater than 40 mm/hour, a CRP greater than 2.0 mg/dL, and serum WBC count greater than 12,000/mm^3. Unfortunately, with the exception of high fevers, one or more of these factors can also occur with transient synovitis. The presence of one of these 5 factors was associated with a probability of having septic arthritis of around 37%, while the presence of all 5 factors was associated with a probability of 98%. Imaging often consists of radiographs and ultrasound. Radiographs usually are non-diagnostic but may demonstrate joint-space widening suggestive of an effusion. Ultrasound will usually demonstrate the presence of an effusion.

Analysis of synovial fluid remains the gold standard for the diagnosis of septic arthritis, and arthrocentesis of any effusion under sedation or anesthesia is indicated if there is a clinical suspicion of septic arthritis. A WBC count greater than 50,000/mm^3 within the fluid aspirate is generally considered diagnostic of septic arthritis; however, elevated counts can be seen in certain rheumatologic conditions. The presence of bacteria on Gram stain of joint aspirate regardless of WBC count suggests infection. Routine cultures of joint aspirate as well as peripheral blood cultures should be sent. In addition, with the increasing recognition of *K kingae* as a causative agent in septic arthritis, joint aspirations should be directly inoculated into blood culture bottles to enhance isolation because this organism is difficult to recover with standard culture techniques. In most studies, only around 50% of joint aspirate cultures grew out an identifiable pathogen. In one recent study, close to 50% of the aspirates that were sterile on standard culture media grew out *K kingae* from blood cultures.

Complications occur in 10% to 25% of all cases, increasing when delays of 5 days or more have passed before initiation of therapy. These complications include abnormal bone growth, permanent limp, unstable articulation of the affected joint, and decreased range of motion.

Osteomyelitis is an infection of the bone that is typically caused by a bacterial organism. Close to 50% of pediatric cases of osteomyelitis occur in children younger than 5 years. Most cases of osteomyelitis in children occur from hematogenous deposition of bacteria into the bone marrow during a transient episode of bacteremia. Other cases may be caused from contiguous spread of an adjacent infection or direct inoculation. Osteomyelitis most commonly

begins in the highly vascularized metaphysis of long bones of young children. The femur, tibia, and humerus account for most cases. As with septic arthritis, *S aureus* remains the most common organism identified across all age groups. Other organisms include *S pyogenes*, *S pneumoniae*, and *K kingae*. Young infants can also be infected by neonatal pathogens such as GBS and enteric gram-negative organisms. Individuals with sickle-cell disease are commonly infected with *Salmonella*. Individuals who have suffered a puncture wound through the foot can be infected with *Pseudomonas aeruginosa*, resulting in osteochondritis.

Children often present with fever and pain at the affected site. Younger children may present with limp or refusal to bear weight. If there is subperiosteal spread, there may be erythema, warmth, and swelling at the affected site.

Laboratory tests can be supportive of a diagnosis of osteomyelitis, but are usually not specific. Typically a serum CBC, ESR, and CRP are obtained along with blood cultures. Leukocytosis may be present, but in more than half the cases, the WBC count can be normal. Inflammatory markers are elevated in up to 90% of cases. Blood cultures are positive in up to 55%. Radiographs are often normal or show only soft-tissue changes early in the course of the disease. Periosteal reactions and lytic lesions are usually not present until day 10 to 21 into the disease. Bone scans can be helpful in the preverbal child or in individuals who cannot localize their pain. Magnetic resonance imaging (MRI) has become the study of choice, with a reported sensitivity of 97%. It is very useful for distinguishing between bone and soft-tissue infections.

Diskitis refers to an inflammatory process involving the intervertebral disks. This disease typically occurs in children younger than 5 years. It occurs almost exclusively in the lumbar region, causing progressive limp, back pain, and refusal to walk. Most children are afebrile. It is thought to occur in younger children because of the presence of vascular channels in the cartilaginous region of the disk space as well as an abundant intraosseous arterial anastomoses. These vascular channels disappear with age. Laboratory studies are often nonspecific, with slight elevations in the peripheral WBC count and ESR. Radiographs are abnormal in most cases (75%), with decreased vertebral disk space and erosion of adjacent vertebral endplates being the most common abnormalities seen. Bone scans will demonstrate nonspecific increased marker uptake in the affected area. Computed tomography scans rarely provide a specific diagnosis and are not generally used. Magnetic resonance imaging will demonstrate characteristic inflammatory changes and allow for differentiation from other conditions, such as vertebral osteomyelitis.

The exact etiology of diskitis is not known, and the treatment is somewhat controversial. Several authors propose that it is the result of an infectious process and warrants antibiotic therapy. Others propose that it is simply a benign self-limited disease because most cultures are sterile and patients can recover without any antimicrobial therapy.

Legg-Calvé-Perthes disease (LCPD) is an idiopathic avascular necrosis of the femoral head. The exact etiology is unclear but involves some disruption in the vascular supply of the capital femoral epiphysis. This is most commonly seen in children 3 to 12 years old (median age 7 years). It is usually unilateral, but can be bilateral in up to 15% of cases. Children typically present with a chronic intermittent limp that can be either painful or painless. It is not uncommon for the child to be symptomatic for months before a diagnosis is made. Pain is usually worsened with internal rotation and abduction.

Laboratory tests are usually normal. Radiographs early in the course of the disease may either be negative or show widening of the joint space. In later stages, radiographic findings include an increased density and decreased size of the femoral head (necrosis), patchy areas of radiolucency near the epiphysis (fragmentation), and flattening of the femoral head (reconstitution).

Slipped capital femoral epiphysis (SCFE) is a displacement or slipping of the femoral head from the neck of the femur through the open physis (growth plate). This is the most common hip disorder affecting adolescents. It is more common in boys than girls and occurs more frequently among African Americans and Hispanics than whites. Typical age of onset is 9 to 16 years. Individuals are often noted to be overweight and frequently present with a chief complaint of knee pain. They will often have an antalgic gait. The foot is noted to be externally rotated in severe slips but may be neutral or intoed in mild slips. The examination of the knee will be normal without discomfort, despite the complaint of knee pain. Passive flexion of the hip will often result in obligate external rotation. There will usually be pain with internal rotation. An SCFE is stable when the individual can walk with or without crutches, an unstable SCFE occurs when the child cannot walk. Laboratory testing is not indicated. Radiographs of the hip in the AP and frog-leg positions reveal the diagnosis in approximately 80% of the cases. Both hips should be viewed because up to 20% of SCFEs are bilateral. Ultrasound in experienced hands has been shown to be an effective diagnostic tool (sensitivity of 95%). Computed tomography scan and MRI can both reveal the presence of a slip. The MRI is much more sensitive and can detect physeal widening in the pre-slip condition.

Osgood-Schlatter disease (OSD), or traction apophysitis of the tibial tubercle, is an overuse injury of the knee seen most commonly in adolescent athletes. Repetitive microtrauma causes partial avulsion of the patellar tendon at its insertion on the tibia. Individuals will typically present with a localized bony prominence, swelling, and tenderness over the tibial tubercle at the insertion of the patellar tendon. Radiographs are commonly performed to rule out other pathology and will typically demonstrate soft tissue swelling/edema of the skin and tissues, as well as ossific fragments within the tendon. Computed tomography, MRI, and ultrasound will show characteristic changes consistent with OSD, but are generally not indicated.

A limp can also result from certain systemic disease processes, such as **juvenile idiopathic arthritis, sickle cell disease** (SCD), and **neoplastic disease.** Juvenile idiopathic arthritis may involve multiple joints, and there is usually evidence of inflammation (eg, warmth, swelling/effusion, redness). The pain is usually worse in the morning and improves throughout the day. **Sickle cell disease** is now detected on newborn screen, and most patients know of their diagnosis. Acute pain crises with SCD can affect multiple areas,

resulting in significant discomfort, limp, and refusal to walk. Careful consideration for infectious etiologies (ie, osteomyelitis) is necessary in the highly febrile or ill child with SCD who presents with a limp or bone pain. In addition, SCD patients are at risk of avascular necrosis of the hip secondary to vasoocclusive episodes. Neoplastic disease processes such as leukemia or primary bone tumors (eg, Ewing sarcoma or osteosarcoma) can present with bone pain and limp. The presence of pallor, petechiae, disseminated lymphadenopathy, or hepatosplenomegaly may suggest the presence of leukemia. The peripheral CBC will usually show the presence of blasts and varying degrees of involvement of the various cell lines (ie, anemia, thrombocytopenia). Primary bone tumors may present with bony deformities or overlying soft-tissue swelling. Radiographs will often reveal characteristic bony lesions, which may require an MRI to ascertain involvement. Computed tomography scans may be necessary to look for metastases. Individuals may require referral to an orthopedist for biopsy to ascertain a definitive diagnosis and possibly for amputation. Referral to an oncologist will be necessary to initiate appropriate therapy, including possibly chemotherapy or radiation.

Evaluation

History

The history should focus on the time of onset of the limp, its chronicity, and the degree of disability it produces. Often a history of trauma is provided, even when a non-traumatic cause is present. Young toddlers are often falling as they learn how to walk, and parents will frequently relay some trivial or unrelated injury. Delayed motor development may be a sign of neuromuscular disease such as cerebral palsy, whereas a history of loss of motor milestones may indicate muscular dystrophy or spinal cord tumor. It is important to remember that pelvic pathology may be referred to the hip, and hip pathology is often referred to the knee or thigh.

Physical Examination

Physical examination begins with observation for any overt deformities (eg, leg length discrepancy, deformity, joint swelling). All joints should be palpated, and the presence of swelling, tenderness, erythema, or warmth should be noted. A thorough evaluation of the hips is essential in children with knee pain. The type of gait abnormality may be determined by observing children walk or run.

Children should also be examined both supine and standing, if possible. Standing children can be assessed for pelvic obliquity and spinal deformities. Range of motion of the hips, knees, ankles, and feet can be checked in supine children, comparing the affected side with the non-affected side. Deep tendon reflexes and muscle strength should be assessed, and leg length measurements should also be made as indicated. Children should be supine for a true measurement of leg length, taken as the distance from the anterosuperior iliac spine to the medial malleolus. A discrepancy of more than 2 cm is considered significant in adults. The significance of discrepancies can be confirmed by imaging studies.

Laboratory Tests

Laboratory procedures are usually necessary in children with an acute onset of limp. Complete blood cell count, CRP, and ESR are useful markers of systemic disease or significant inflammation. There can be significant overlap between the differing etiologies, and no single screening test reliably distinguishes between the various inflammatory and infectious causes of limp. Blood and local cultures (eg, joint or bone fluid) may be useful in the evaluation of suspected infectious entities. Additional testing for rheumatologic causes may be clinically indicated, such as antinuclear antibody or rheumatoid factor (see Chapter 144).

Imaging Studies

Radiographs are the most commonly used imaging study. Usually 2 views are obtained. Examination of the hip involves imaging in the AP view as well as the frog-leg position. Both hips should be radiographed for comparison and to assess for the presence of bilateral disease. Ultrasound is helpful if there is concern about an effusion within the joint space and can also be used to guide diagnostic and therapeutic interventions (eg, arthrocentesis). Computed tomography scan can sometimes provide useful information, but MRI is being used with increasing frequency because of its superior resolution and lack of radiation. Bone scans may be helpful in the early stages of disease when radiographs are typically normal or when there is difficulty establishing a localized area of involvement.

Management

The management depends on the etiology. Management of septic arthritis consists of surgical drainage and intravenous (IV) antibiotics. Empiric therapy typically consists of a semisynthetic penicillinase-resistant penicillin (eg, nafcillin or oxacillin). If there are high rates of community-acquired methicillin-resistant strains of S aureus in the region, then clindamycin or vancomycin may be necessary until sensitivities can be performed. The addition of a third-generation cephalosporin is indicated in the newborn period pending Gram stain and culture results or when N gonorrhoeae is suspected in adolescents. Length of therapy is typically 2 to 4 weeks of IV antibiotics. Prognosis is generally good with prompt diagnosis and management within 4 days of symptom onset.

Management of osteomyelitis also consists of IV antibiotics. Occasionally surgery may be indicated, particularly if there is a subperiosteal or soft-tissue abscess or sequestra present. Empiric antibiotic therapy consists of a semisynthetic penicillinase-resistant penicillin (eg, nafcillin or oxacillin). In areas where community-acquired methicillin-resistant organisms are of concern, clindamycin or vancomycin may be necessary. Neonates and individuals with SCD require the addition of a third-generation cephalosporin pending culture results. In individuals with a presumed pseudomonal infection, an extended spectrum β-lactam (eg, ceftazidime, cefepime, or piperacillin/tazobactam) plus an aminoglycoside are indicated. Four to 6 weeks of antibiotic therapy is recommended. Some studies have shown that switching to an oral antibiotic may be acceptable following a week of parenteral therapy if good compliance is likely, an organism has been identified, clinical improvement is noted, the patient is afebrile, and the inflammatory markers have begun to normalize. Oral dosages 2 to 3 times those normally recommended for non-bony infections are often used for β-lactam antibiotics. Other oral antibiotics (eg, clindamycin, trimethoprim-sulfamethoxazole, fluoroquinolones) have excellent bioavailability, and the usual oral dosages may be used. Consultation with an infectious diseases specialist is often indicated.

Supportive measures with nonsteroidal anti-inflammatory agents are generally indicated for the management of diskitis. Antistaphylococcal antibiotics should also be considered. A brace may be helpful for support and pain relief. Most patients recover without any complications.

Prompt referral to an orthopedist is indicated in cases of LCPD. The goal of treatment of LCPD is to maintain full joint mobility and prevent deformity of the femoral head. Bed rest and immobilization decrease the pain and help restore range of motion. Traction and abduction casts/braces are used to contain the femoral head within the acetabulum in an effort to maintain its spherical shape. Surgical correction of gross deformities of the femoral head may be necessary in severe cases.

Treatment for SCFE consists of surgical reduction and stabilization with placement of screws through the epiphysis. The screws are typically left in place and do not need to be removed. Non–weight bearing is maintained until early callus is seen on the posterior-inferior metaphysis and the pain has resolved. Gradual and progressive weight bearing is allowed, and progression to full weight bearing usually occurs 3 to 4 months after fixation. No running or jumping is allowed until the physis closes.

Treatment of OSD consists of rest, ice, nonsteroidal anti-inflammatory agents, and strengthening exercises of the quadriceps and hamstring muscles. Surgical treatment is rarely indicated and is reserved for those patients who do not respond to conservative therapy.

Prognosis

The prognosis depends on the etiology of the limp, rapid diagnosis, and appropriate therapy.

The prognosis is good in most cases of septic arthritis and osteomyelitis if the infection is diagnosed early and treated appropriately. Prognosis of osteomyelitis is usually good, with less than 2% of patients who receive at least 3 weeks of antibiotic therapy developing chronic osteomyelitis. Treatment of chronic disease can be difficult, often necessitating prolonged courses of antibiotics (up to 6–12 months) and multiple surgeries for debridement. Rare complications include disturbances in bone growth, limb length discrepancies, arthritis, abnormal gait, and pathologic fractures. Prognosis is also good if diagnosis occurs at a young age (<8 years old). The main complication is degenerative arthritis of the hip.

Prognosis of LCPD is related to the degree of femoral head involvement and age at onset of the disease. Children younger than 6 years have the best prognosis. The risk of development of degenerative arthritis in adulthood increases in children whose disease is more extensive and whose condition is diagnosed later (ie, after 8 years of age).

If patients with SCFE are untreated, the potential for further slipping of the femoral head remains until the growth plate closes. Potential treatment-related complications of SCFE include chondrolysis of the femoral head and acetabulum, avascular necrosis, and fracture at the site of pin placement. In general the prognosis is good and is based on the degree of slippage. The main complication is the development of avascular necrosis of the femoral head, which typically leads to degenerative hip disease later in life. This occurs in up to 15% of slips and is more common in an unstable SCFE. Only 7% of patients in the moderate-slip category have a poor outcome compared with 24% of patients in the severe-slip category.

In about 5% to 10% of cases, OSD may become chronic, with persistent swelling and tenderness. In such cases a radiograph may show the formation of an ossicle over the tibial tubercle; this ossicle may require surgical resection.

CASE RESOLUTION

In the case described at the beginning of the chapter, the child's history and physical examination seem to be consistent with LCPD. The child's knee pain is actually secondary to hip pathology. The diagnosis may have been missed if the physician had not examined the hips and noted the abnormality in range of motion. Both AP and frog-leg radiographs of the hips were taken, which showed widening of the joint space. Orthopedic consultation was obtained, and hospitalization for bed rest and ensured immobilization were recommended.

Selected References

Caird MS, Flynn JM, Leung YL, Millman JE, D'Itallia JG, Dormans JP. Factors distinguishing septic arthritis from transient synovitis of the hip in children. *J Bone Joint Surg.* 2006;88:1251–1257

Copely LAB. Pediatric musculoskeletal infection: trends and antibiotic recommendations. *J Am Acad Orth Surg.* 2009;17:618–626

Dahl MT. Limb length discrepancy. *Pediatr Clin North Am.* 1996;43:849–865

Do TT. Transient synovitis as a cause of painful limps in children. *Curr Opin Pediatr.* 2000;12:48–51

Dormans JP, Moroz L. Infection and tumors of the spine in children. *J Bone Joint Surg Am.* 2007;89:79–97

Fernandez M, Carrol CL, Baker CJ. Discitis and vertebral osteomyelitis in children: an 18-year review. *Pediatrics.* 2000;105:1299–1304

Frank G, Mahoney HM, Eppes SC. Musculoskeletal infections in children. *Pediatr Clin North Am.* 2005;52:1083–1106

Gutierrez K. Bone and joint infections in children. *Pediatr Clin North Am.* 2005; 52:779–794

Gholve PA, Cameron DB, Millis MB. Slipped capital femoral epiphysis update. *Curr Opin Pediatr.* 2009;21:39–45

Gholve PA, Scher DM, Khakharia S, et al. Osgood Schlatter syndrome. *Curr Opin Pediatr.* 2007;19:44–50

Henrickson M, Passo MH. Recognizing patterns in chronic limb pain. *Contemp Pediatr.* 1994;11:33–62

Hurley JM, Betz RR, Loder RT, Davidson RS, Alburger PD, Steel HH. Slipped capital femoral epiphysis. The prevalence of late contralateral slip. *J Bone Joint Surg.* 1996;78:226–230

Kocher MS, Mandiga R, Zurakowski D, Barnewolt C, Kasser JR. Validation of a clinical prediction rule for the differentiation between septic arthritis and transient synovitis of the hip in children. *J Bone Joint Surg.* 2004;86:1629–1635

Koop S, Quanbeck D. Three common causes of childhood hip pain. *Pediatr Clin North Am.* 1996;43:1053–1066

Laine JC, Kaiser SP, Mohammad D. High-risk pediatric orthopedic pitfalls. *Emerg Med Clin N Am.* 2010;28:85–102

Lehman CL, Arons RR, Loder RT, Vitale MG. The epidemiology of slipped capital femoral epiphysis: an update. *J Pediatr Orthop.* 2006;26:286–290

Loder RT. Controversies in slipped capital femoral epiphysis. *Orthop Clin North Am.* 2006;37:211–221

Luhman SJ, Jones A, Schootman M, Gordon EJ, Schoenecker PL, Luhman JD. Differentiation between septic arthritis and transient synovitis of the hip in children with clinical prediction algorithms. *J Bone Joint Surg.* 2004;86:956–962

MacEwen GD, Dehne R. The limping child. *Pediatr Rev.* 1991;12:268–274

Ranson M. Imaging of pediatric musculoskeletal infection. *Sem Muscuolskeletal Radiology.* 2009;13:277–299

Renshaw TS. The child who has a limp. *Pediatr Rev.* 1995;16:458–465

Reynolds RAK. Diagnosis and treatment of slipped capital femoral epiphysis. *Curr Opin Pediatr.* 1998;11:80–83

Schmit P, Glorion C. Osteomyelitis in infants and children. *Eur Radiol.* 2004; 14:L44–L54

Shah SS. Abnormal gait in a child with fever: diagnosing septic arthritis of the hip. *Pediatr Emerg Care.* 2005;21:336–341

Vazquez M. Osteomyelitis in children. *Curr Opin Pediatr.* 2002;14:112–115

Yagupsk P. *Kingella kingae:* from medical rarity to an emerging pediatric pathogen. *Lancet.* 2004;4:358–367

CHAPTER 106

Musculoskeletal Disorders of the Neck and Back

Carol D. Berkowitz, MD, and Andrew K. Battenberg, BS

CASE STUDY

A 4-week-old male infant is brought to the office by his mother, who complains that her son always holds his head tilted to the right. She reports that he has held it in this position for about 1 week and prefers to look mainly to the left. The infant is the 8-lb, 8-oz product of a term gestation born via forceps extraction, and he had no complications in the neonatal period. He is feeding well on breast milk and has no history of fever, upper respiratory symptoms, vomiting, or diarrhea.

On examination, the head is tilted toward the right side with limited lateral rotation to the right and decreased lateral side bending to the left. Except for the presence of a small mass palpable on the right side of the neck, the examination is within normal limits.

Questions

1. What laboratory or radiologic studies are indicated in infants with torticollis?
2. What is the differential diagnosis of torticollis in infants?
3. What are some of the common musculoskeletal abnormalities that may be seen in association with torticollis?
4. What are other common musculoskeletal problems in children and adolescents?
5. What is the current recommended management of children and adolescents with idiopathic scoliosis?

Children with disorders of the spine can present with deformity, back pain, or occasionally both. Non-traumatic congenital and developmental deformities of the spine are frequently encountered in pediatric practice. Torticollis and scoliosis are 2 of the most common disorders in children that present as spinal deformity. **Torticollis,** or wry neck, is a positional abnormality of the neck resulting in abnormal tilting and rotation of the head. **Scoliosis** refers to any lateral curvature of the spine that measures more than 10 degrees as determined by an anteroposterior (AP) radiograph of the spine. Scoliosis can be divided into 3 categories: infantile (birth–3 years), juvenile (3–10 years), and adolescent. **Back pain** is a far less common complaint in children than in adults. When such pain occurs in children, it usually signals the presence of organic disease. However, in adolescents, musculoskeletal strain is a common etiology.

Epidemiology

Some degree of spinal asymmetry is seen in about 2% to 5% of the population.

The most common type of **torticollis** seen in children is congenital muscular torticollis. The incidence is estimated to be between 1% to 2%, and is increased in breech presentations (1.8% vs 0.3% in vertex presentation). It is associated with developmental dysplasia of the hip (DDH) in as many as 10% to 20% of affected infants. Family history may be positive in up to 10% of cases.

Acquired torticollis is much more common in older children and is usually secondary to trauma or infection, including cervical lymphadenitis, retropharyngeal abscess, myositis, and even upper respiratory tract infections. Episodes of benign paroxysmal torticollis, which often begin in the first year of life and generally resolve by 5 years of age, may have a familial basis. An association with benign paroxysmal vertigo and migraines has been noted.

Infantile scoliosis is rare in the United States and usually spontaneously resolves. The prevalence of juvenile **scoliosis** among school-aged children is 3% to 5%. A right thoracic single curve is the most common curve seen by physicians. Seventy-five percent to 80% of cases of structural scoliosis are idiopathic, 10% are due to neuromuscular causes, 5% are congenital, and the remaining 5% to 10% are due to trauma or miscellaneous causes. Scoliosis that begins in childhood affects boys and girls equally, and affected boys actually outnumber girls during the first 3 years of life. However, idiopathic scoliosis that develops after the age of 10 years is more common in girls than boys, with a ratio estimated between 5 and 7:1. In children with cerebral palsy, the incidence of scoliosis is increased, and it is found in about 20% of all cases.

Back pain is quite uncommon in preadolescent children. Unlike in adults, where it is often difficult to identify the cause of back pain, most cases of back pain in children have an identifiable etiology.

Clinical Presentation

Although **torticollis** may be noted at birth, it usually manifests at 2 to 4 weeks of age. Infants with congenital muscular torticollis present with a characteristic head tilt toward the affected side with the chin pointing toward the opposite side; this positioning is secondary to unilateral fibrosis and contracture of the sternocleidomastoid muscle (Figure 106-1). Unrecognized or untreated cases of torticollis may present as plagiocephaly (see Chapter 70) or facial asymmetry during infancy. Benign paroxysmal torticollis of infancy may present as recurrent episodes of head tilt that may be associated with vomiting, ataxia, agitation, or malaise (Dx Box).

No obvious deformity may be noted in mild **scoliosis.** Asymmetry of shoulder heights, scapular prominence or position, and waistline or pelvic levelness may all be signs of scoliosis (see Dx Box) (Figure 106-2A). Back pain is reported in 25% of adolescents with idiopathic

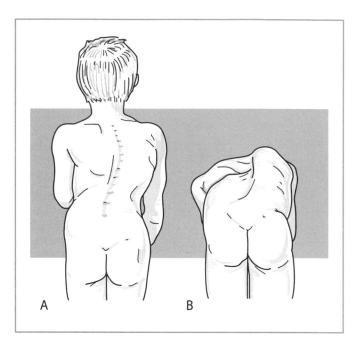

Figure 106-2. Scoliosis. A. Child with scoliosis (rear view). B. Child with scoliosis performing bend test.

scoliosis. Scoliosis may be detected during school-based screening programs or preparticipation sports physicals.

When pain is present, further examination for some other cause (eg, bone tumors, spondylolysis, spondylolisthesis) is warranted.

Preverbal children with **back pain** may present with limp or refusal to bear weight or walk.

Pathophysiology

Torticollis may be either congenital or acquired. The etiology of congenital muscular torticollis is unknown. It is believed to be due to intrauterine positioning or trauma to the soft tissues of the neck during delivery, which results in venous occlusion and ischemia of the sternocleidomastoid muscle. This leads to edema and degeneration of the muscle fibers with eventual fibrosis of the muscle body. Deformities of the face and skull may result if the condition is left untreated. Plagiocephaly (cranial asymmetry), with flattening of the face on the affected side and flattening of the occiput on the contralateral side, is seen most commonly.

Unlike kyphosis and lordosis, which are curves in the AP plane, **scoliosis** is a lateral curvature of the spine occurring in the frontal plane. Scoliosis can be either functional (nonstructural) or structural. In functional scoliosis, there is no fixed deformity of the spine and the apparent curvature disappears with lying down or with forward flexion. Individuals with leg length discrepancies appear to have scoliosis but have no spinal abnormality. Structural scoliosis may be idiopathic or caused by various underlying disorders. The cause of idiopathic scoliosis is unknown, and there appears to be a higher incidence of scoliosis in other family members. In addition, there are reports of lower levels of melatonin in patients with scoliosis, compared with age-matched controls. This finding has

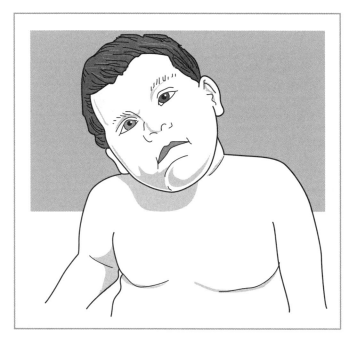

Figure 106-1. Torticollis. Infant with congenital muscular torticollis showing head tilt.

Dx Torticollis and Scoliosis

Torticollis
- Head tilt
- Limited range of motion of the neck
- Contracture of the sternocleidomastoid muscle
- Plagiocephaly (congenital torticollis)
- Firm, non-tender, mobile mass within the body of the sternocleidomastoid muscle (congenital torticollis)

Scoliosis
- Lateral curvature of the spine
- Some pain
- Back or truncal asymmetry

not been confirmed and its relationship to the scoliosis is unclear. Abnormalities of fibrillin have also been seen in some patients with scoliosis, a finding also reported in patients with Marfan syndrome. In structural scoliosis, as the spine curves laterally it forces the vertebrae to rotate, resulting in deformity of attached structures. For example, a "rib hump" may be produced due to scoliosis in the thoracic spine (see Figure 106-2B). Pelvic obliquity or flank prominence may be produced when the curvature is in the lumbar spine.

Differential Diagnosis

The differential diagnosis of congenital and acquired **torticollis** is presented in Box 106-1. Congenital muscular torticollis is the most common cause of congenital torticollis. Acquired torticollis is seen primarily in older infants and children, and may appear in association with nystagmus and head nodding, a clinical triad referred to as spasmus nutans. Cervical lymphadenitis is a common cause of acquired torticollis in children 1 to 5 years of age, whereas trauma to the soft tissues or muscles of the neck is seen more frequently in school-aged children. Acute episodes (eg, benign paroxysmal torticollis of infancy) must be differentiated from chronic conditions (eg, Sandifer syndrome, rheumatoid arthritis).

Box 106-1. Common Causes of Torticollis

Congenital
- Congenital muscular torticollis
- Pterygium coli (skin web)
- Occipitocervical spine anomalies (eg, Klippel-Feil syndrome)

Acquired
- Infectious
- Cervical lymphadenitis
- Retropharyngeal abscess
- Osteomyelitis of cervical vertebrae
- Traumatic
- Atlanto-occipital, atlas-axis (C1–C2), or C2–C3 subluxation
- Cervical musculature injury (spastic torticollis)
- Cervical spine fractures
- Neurologic
- Tumors (posterior fossa or cervical cord)
- Dystonic drug reactions
- Syringomyelia
- Ocular disturbances (strabismus, nystagmus)
- Other
- Spasmus nutans
- Sandifer syndrome (hiatal hernia with gastroesophageal reflux)
- Benign paroxysmal torticollis of infancy
- Rheumatoid arthritis
- Hysteria
- Soft tissue tumors of the neck

Functional or nonstructural **scoliosis** may be secondary to poor posture, leg length discrepancies, or muscle spasm. Structural scoliosis can be classified into idiopathic, congenital, neuromuscular, and miscellaneous forms (Box 106-2). Idiopathic scoliosis, which is by far the most common type of structural scoliosis, may be divided into 3 categories based on age: infantile (0–3 years), juvenile (3–10 years), and adolescent (>10 years). The adolescent form occurs most frequently, accounting for up to 85% of cases.

Congenital scoliosis results from anomalies of the spine such as hemivertebrae or failure of vertebral segmentation. The incidence of cardiac and renal anomalies is increased. Although neuromuscular scoliosis is most often seen in children with spastic cerebral palsy, it may also be apparent in other conditions, such as poliomyelitis, meningomyelocele, muscular dystrophy, Friedreich ataxia, and spinal muscular atrophy. The miscellaneous causes of scoliosis are uncommon and include trauma, metabolic disorders, and neurocutaneous diseases.

The most common causes of **back pain** in children may be classified into 5 categories (Box 106-3). When pain is significant enough that a child presents to the emergency department, common causes include trauma (25%), muscle strain (24%), sickle cell crisis (13%), idiopathic cause (13%), urinary tract infection (5%), and viral syndrome (4%). Other infectious causes, such as diskitis, occur much more frequently in children than adults. Because the spine of children is smaller and has greater flexibility and ligamentous strength, children have a lower risk of traumatic injury than adults. Common causes of back pain in adults, such as musculoskeletal back pain (ie, muscle strain) and herniated disks, are uncommon in children. Predisposed individuals often experience their first episode

---

Box 106-2. Common Causes of Scoliosis

Functional Scoliosis
- Poor posture
- Leg length discrepancies
- Muscle spasm
- Herniated disk
- Back injury

Structural Scoliosis
- Idiopathic
- Congenital
- Neuromuscular
- Miscellaneous
- Trauma (eg, fractures or dislocations of the vertebrae)
- Intraspinal tumors
- Metabolic disorders (eg, juvenile osteoporosis, osteogenesis imperfecta, mucopolysaccharidosis)
- Neurocutaneous syndromes (eg, neurofibromatosis)
- Marfan syndrome

Box 106-3. Common Causes of Back Pain in Children

Infectious
- Myalgias (eg, influenza)
- Diskitis (more common in children <5 years of age)
- Vertebral osteomyelitis (pyogenic, tuberculosis [Potts disease])
- Referred pain (pyelonephritis, pneumonia)

Inflammatory
- Rheumatologic diseases (juvenile rheumatoid arthritis, ankylosing spondylitis)
- Crohn disease/ulcerative colitis/psoriatic arthritis
- Disk space calcification

Neoplastic
- Primary vertebral and spinal tumors (eg, Ewing sarcoma, osteosarcoma, neuroblastoma)
- Metastatic disease (eg, neuroblastoma)
- Benign tumors (eg, eosinophilic granuloma, osteoid osteoma)

Developmental
- Spondylolysis, spondylolisthesis (adolescents)
- Scheuermann kyphosis (adolescents)

Traumatic
- Herniated nucleus pulposus (disk herniation)
- Ligamentous or muscle strain (eg, overuse syndromes)
- Compression fracture of vertebrae

Other
- Sickle cell crisis
- Osteoporosis (eg, rickets, osteogenesis imperfecta)
- Child abuse
- Psychogenic

Questions

Torticollis, Scoliosis, and Back Pain

Torticollis
- Is there any family history of torticollis?
- What type of delivery did the mother have (eg, cesarean or vaginal)? Were forceps required?
- When was the head tilt first noticed?
- Does the infant move his or her neck in all directions, or does he or she always prefer to look in one direction?
- Does the infant have any recent history of trauma to the head or neck area?
- Is the head tilt persistent or does it come and go?
- Has the infant been sick or febrile?
- Does the child have nystagmus or head bobbing?

Scoliosis
- Is there a family history of scoliosis?
- Have the parents noticed the curvature of the spine? If so, how old was the child when the condition was first noted?
- Has the curvature increased since it was first noticed?
- Does the child have any back pain?
- Has the child had any previous treatment for the condition?
- (If appropriate) Has the child begun menstruating?

Back Pain
- How long has the child had the pain?
- Where is the pain localized?
- Is the pain persistent or does it come and go?
- Does the pain radiate anywhere (eg, down the legs)?
- Is the child limping or having difficulty walking?
- Has the child lost any motor milestones (eg, skills such as walking or standing that he or she could previously perform)?
- What makes the pain better? What makes it worse?
- Has there been any recent history of trauma or has the child begun participating in a new sport or physical activity?
- Has the child had a fever?
- Has the child had any problems with bowel or bladder function?
- Is the child taking any medication?

---

of musculoskeletal back pain during adolescence or young adulthood, and children, as a whole, account for only 1% to 4% of all herniated disks.

Evaluation

History

A careful history may provide clues to diagnosis and etiology (Questions box). Back pain is reported in about 25% of adolescents with scoliosis.

Physical Examination

In children with suspected **torticollis,** a thorough examination with specific attention to the head and neck region should be performed. Limited head rotation toward the affected side with decreased lateral side bending to the opposite side may occur. During the first 4 to 6 weeks of life, a firm, non-tender mobile mass (or pseudotumor) may be palpated within the body of the sternocleidomastoid muscle; the mass gradually regresses by 6 months of age. Because torticollis is associated with DDH, the hips should be examined for stability.

A neurologic examination should also be performed to look for any neurologic deficits that may be signs of an underlying tumor. Fever or signs of inflammation point to infectious causes. Because torticollis may be secondary to visual disturbances such as strabismus, a careful eye examination is warranted. The presence of nystagmus or head nodding suggests spasmus nutans.

Screening for **scoliosis** should be part of the routine health maintenance examination of school-aged children and adolescents. Children should be examined with the back fully exposed. The posture should be observed. The presence of any skin lesions such as café-au-lait spots should be noted. Any midline skin defects such as dimples or hair patches should also be noted because they are often associated with underlying spinal lesions. The spine should be palpated for any signs of tenderness, and a complete neurologic examination should be performed.

The back should be observed for asymmetry of the shoulders, scapulae, or pelvis. Physicians should have children bend forward at the waist to an angle of 90 degrees. This maneuver accentuates the curvature of structural scoliosis and emphasizes the rotational deformity of the spine. For example, in thoracic scoliosis, a characteristic rib hump is apparent on the convex side of the curve. A scoliometer can be used to determine the degree of scoliosis. More than 7 degrees of angulation correlates with a Cobb angle of 20 degrees and warrants referral to an orthopedist.

Scoliosis is described in terms of the primary or major curve, which is predominantly thoracic. The major curve may be accompanied by a secondary or minor curve, which is predominantly lumbar and often compensates the primary curve. The location is defined by the apical vertebra (eg, T2–T11 = thoracic, T12–L1 = thoracolumbar), the direction of the curvature by the side of convexity, and the severity indicated by the degree of curvature as measured on the spinal radiograph. Curves greater than 15 degrees are abnormal. Mild scoliosis is defined as curvature of less than 20 degrees, moderate as 20 to 40 degrees, and severe as greater than 40 to 45 degrees.

The evaluation of **back pain** begins with observation of children's posture and gait. Any midline skin lesions should be noted. A thorough general physical examination is important because referred pain (eg, pancreatitis, pyelonephritis, nephrolithiasis) may be causing the symptoms in the back. The spine should be palpated for any signs of tenderness. A complete neurologic examination should be performed, and any motor or sensory deficits should be noted. The motor examination should emphasize evaluation of the hips and the lower extremities, including range of motion and strength.

Laboratory Tests

In cases of **congenital torticollis,** laboratory studies are rarely necessary. In acquired torticollis, if any infection is suspected, a complete blood cell count (CBC) and blood and local cultures may aid in the diagnosis.

No specific laboratory tests are required in the evaluation of idiopathic **scoliosis.** Specific laboratory studies may be performed in the evaluation of other forms of scoliosis as indicated by the history and physical examination (eg, a urine metabolic screen for suspected metabolic disturbances).

Laboratory assessment for **back pain** depends on the history and physical examination. A CBC, blood culture, and erythrocyte sedimentation rate may be useful in the evaluation of suspected infectious etiologies. Rheumatologic studies such as a rheumatoid factor or human leukocyte antigen typing may help in the diagnosis of rheumatologic conditions. If the back pain is of acute onset, studies such as a urinalysis or serum amylase would help determine if the pain is referred, for example, in pyelonephritis or pancreatitis.

Imaging Studies

Radiographs are generally not useful in children with suspected **torticollis** unless bony anomalies are suspected. Magnetic resonance imaging (MRI) of the sternocleidomastoid muscle mass may be considered if an underlying condition (eg, a branchial cleft cyst) is suspected. Computed tomography scan or MRI of the head or cervical spinal cord would be indicated if a neurologic tumor is suspected.

Routine radiographs are not required in the evaluation of all children with mild scoliosis (ie, minor degrees of curvature noted on physical examination). It may be best to obtain radiographs after orthopedic evaluation is complete. A standing AP spine radiograph is used to determine the location and direction of the curvature, measure the degree of asymmetry (Cobb angle), and evaluate the vertebrae. Repeat radiographs of the spine are used to follow the progression of the curvature over time. Because the risk of curve progression before skeletal maturity is a primary concern, hand and wrist radiographs should be taken to assess bone age in prepubertal children with scoliosis. Magnetic resonance imaging is recommended in individuals with rapid progression of their curve at more than 1 degree per month. Magnetic resonance imaging should include cervical, thoracic, and lumber spine to identify deformities such as an Arnold-Chiari malformation or a tethered cord.

As with scoliosis, routine radiographs are not indicated in all cases of **back pain.** Various radiologic studies may be ordered depending on the suspected diagnosis. Radiographs may be useful in the evaluation of suspected vertebral abnormalities such as spondylolysis and spondylolisthesis. However, these conditions may represent incidental findings and not be the source of the back pain. If diskitis is suspected, a bone scan may be more appropriate than radiographs. Similarly, a bone scan or MRI is useful in the evaluation of suspected vertebral tumors.

Management

Treatment of congenital muscular **torticollis** consists of **passive stretching exercises** of the neck. With the neck in a neutral position (ie, not hyperextended), the head is bent to one side so that the ear on the side opposite to the contracted muscle is brought to the shoulder, or the chin is lowered to touch the shoulder on the affected side. In addition, **changing the placement of the crib** in relation to the nursery door and **repositioning toys and mobiles** in the crib stimulate children to look toward the side opposite the preferred gaze. Torticollis resolves spontaneously in most infants. When the deformity persists beyond the age of 1 to 2 years, **surgical release** of the contracted muscle may be indicated.

Management of acquired torticollis depends on etiology. The evaluation and treatment of many of these conditions can be complex and often require consultation with specialists in head and neck surgery, neurology, and orthopedic surgery.

Management of **scoliosis falls into 3 groups: observation, bracing, and surgery. Observation** involves **close follow-up** with careful repeat examinations and radiographic studies. Children who have not undergone their rapid growth phase are at greatest risk of marked progression of their curve. The Risser sign is used to assess the degree to which skeletal maturation has progressed. The sign is based on the degree of ossification of the iliac apophysis, with a Risser 0 signifying no ossification and a Risser 5 representing full ossification. An initial consultation with an orthopedic surgeon is generally advisable, even in minor degrees of curvature. The goal of follow-up is early detection of curvature with implementation of treatment to prevent or reduce curve progression. Children with curves less than 20 to 25 degrees should be monitored for progression. Curves between 25 to 45 degrees do not require bracing in skeletally mature individuals (Risser 4 or 5) but should be braced (eg, with Milwaukee brace) in growing children. The goal of **bracing** is not to correct any existing curvature but to prevent further curve progression. The efficacy of bracing is determined by adherence to the regimen. **Surgery** (eg, the Harrington rod or posterior spinal fusion) may be indicated for children with curves greater than 40 to 45 degrees. These curves have a high likelihood of progression regardless of the patient's age and skeletal maturity. The development of pedicle screws has advanced the process of spinal fusion.

Although the management of **back pain** is diagnosis dependent, **rest** and **immobilization** are principles of treatment that apply in many instances. In the management of diskitis, antistaphylococcal antibiotics may be necessary in addition to immobilization. If spondylolisthesis and spondylolysis do not respond to rest and immobilization, operative stabilization may be required. In adolescents with low back pain related to muscular injury, conservative treatment, including bed rest, heat, and anti-inflammatory medications, may be tried for 1 to 2 weeks followed by a gradual return to normal activity. It is not advisable to institute such treatment in younger children without pursuing a more extensive evaluation or consultation with an orthopedic surgeon because the risk of serious disease is significant in this age group.

Prognosis

Congenital muscular **torticollis** responds to conservative management in about 90% of infants. The asymmetry of the face and skull also corrects over time once the contracture of the sternocleidomastoid resolves. Spasmus nutans, a condition that develops between 4 and 12 months of age, usually resolves spontaneously by 3 years of age.

The direction and location of the curvature in **scoliosis** do not change with age, but the degree of curvature may remain stable or progress. Factors associated with a high risk of curve progression include female gender, positive family history for scoliosis, younger age at diagnosis (especially before the adolescent growth spurt), and a larger curve at the time of diagnosis. In addition, a double curve is more likely to progress than a single curve, and a thoracic curve is more likely to progress than a lumbar curve. Left untreated, severe scoliosis can produce cardiopulmonary impairment or cosmetic deformity, which may lead to low self-esteem and poor body image. Decreased exercise tolerance has been reported in individuals with curves as small as 20 degrees. Individuals with infantile and juvenile scoliosis experience increased mortality from pulmonary and cardiac conditions during their 40s and 50s.

Most cases (80%–90%) of low **back pain** in adolescents and young adults resolve spontaneously in 2 to 8 weeks. It is important for patients to learn how to prevent recurrence by improving posture, learning how to lift heavy objects appropriately, and instituting a program of exercises to help strengthen the abdominal and back muscles.

CASE RESOLUTION

The history of the infant presented in the opening case scenario is consistent with congenital muscular torticollis. Physical examination helps confirm the diagnosis. The hips should be evaluated thoroughly because of the association of congenital muscular torticollis with DDH. A program consisting of neck stretching exercises and repositioning of interesting toys and objects in the infant's crib to the side opposite the preferred gaze should be instituted. The infant can be reevaluated in 2 to 3 weeks to monitor progress.

Selected References

Ballock RT, Song KM. The prevalence of nonmuscular causes of torticollis in children. *J Pediatr Orthop.* 1996;16:500–504

Boachie-Adjei O, Lonner B. Spinal deformity. *Pediatr Clin North Am.* 1996; 43:883–897

Cheng JCY, Au AWY. Infantile torticollis: a review of 624 cases. *J Pediatr Orthop.* 1994;14:802–808

Davis PJ, Williams HJ. The investigation and management of back pain in children. *Arch Dis Child Educ Pract Ed.* 2008;93:73–83

Epps HR, Salter RB. Orthopedic conditions of the cervical spine and shoulder. *Pediatr Clin North Am.* 1996;43:919–931

Epstein JA, Epstein NE, Marc J et al. Lumbar intervertebral disk herniation in teenage children: recognition and management of associated anomalies. *Spine.* 1984;9:427–432

Glancy GL. Advances in idiopathic scoliosis in children and adolescents. *Adv Pediatr.* 2007;54:55–66

Kautz SM, Skaggs DL. Getting an angle on spinal deformities. *Contemp Pediatr.* 1998;15:111–128

Lenke LG, Betz RR, Harms J, et al. Adolescent idiopathic scoliosis: a new classification to determine extent of spinal arthrodesis. *J Bone Joint Surg Am.* 2001;83A:1169–1181

Lowe TG, Edgar M, Marguiles JY, et al. Etiology of idiopathic scoliosis: current trends in research. *J Bone Joint Surg Am.* 2000;82A:1157–1168

Payne WK, Ogilvie JW. Back pain in children and adolescents. *Pediatr Clin North Am.* 1996;43:899–917

Ramirez N, Johnston CE, Browne RH. The prevalence of back pain in children who have idiopathic scoliosis. *J Bone Joint Surg Am.* 1997;79:364–368

Selbst SM, Lavelle JM, Soyupak SK, Markowitz RI. Back pain in children who present to the emergency department. *Clin Pediatr.* 1999;38:401–406

Stewart DG Jr, Skaggs DL. Adolescent idiopathic scoliosis. *Pediatr Rev.* 2006; 27:299–306

Gastrointestinal Disorders

CHAPTER 107

Vomiting

George Gershman, MD

CASE STUDY

A 6-week-old male infant who has been vomiting after each meal for 3 days is brought to the office. He is breast-fed, afebrile, and otherwise well. The history of the pregnancy and birth are normal. His birth weight was 3,500 g, and his current weight is 4,500 g. The physical examination is unremarkable. The mother nurses the infant in the office. Although he feeds hungrily and well, he vomits about 5 minutes after the feeding. The vomiting is projectile, and the vomitus shoots across the room. The vomitus contains curdled milk. On reexamination of the abdomen, a small mass is felt in the right upper quadrant.

Questions

1. What is the mechanism of vomiting, and how does it differ from regurgitation and rumination?
2. What are the common causes of vomiting in infants?
3. What are the common causes of vomiting in older children?
4. What is the significance of bilious vomiting?
5. What are the unique features of vomiting related to increased intracranial pressure?
6. What are some strategies for the management of vomiting in older children?

Vomiting is a common complaint of infants and children, and led Thomas Phaire to write, "Many times the stomake of ye child is so feble that it cannot retayne eyther meate or drynke" (*The Boke of Chyldren*, 1553). Vomiting is defined as the forceful ejection of the stomach contents through the mouth. The mechanism involves a series of complex, neurologically coordinated events under the control of the central nervous system (CNS). In contrast, regurgitation is the effortless bringing up of 1 or 2 mouthfuls of food without distress or discomfort. This is a frequent symptom of gastroesophageal reflux in infants (see Chapter 108). Rumination, a form of autostimulation, is the voluntary induction of regurgitation. It is most often noted in infants between the ages of 3 and 6 months. Rumination occurs in infants with developmental retardation or with a disturbed mother–infant relationship. It is said that affected infants always smell like vomitus, which is on the clothing, but that the vomiting is rarely seen because the presence of another person provides distraction.

Rumination should be considered in infants from deprived environments (eg, neglectful homes). Cases of rumination have been described in premature infants who were maintained in a neonatal intensive care unit after they no longer needed vigilant care from the nursing staff. Incubators, which were cut off from the outside environment, contributed to the isolation and subsequent rumination. The condition resolved once the infants were held and nurtured.

Epidemiology

Fifty percent of infants have spitting up or vomiting as an isolated complaint and less than 5% of these infants have significant underlying disease. Vomiting occurs less frequently in older children, who often experience acute, self-limited illnesses, such as gastroenteritis.

Clinical Presentation

Infants and children may present with vomiting as an isolated complaint or in association with other symptoms, including faintness, diaphoresis, sweating, pallor, tachycardia, fever, anorexia, abdominal pain, or diarrhea (Dx Box). When vomiting has persisted over a period, weight loss or failure to thrive (FTT) may occur. Neurologic symptoms, including headache and gait disturbances, may be noted in children with CNS problems. Other neurologic symptoms of altered muscle tone, lethargy, seizures, or coma in young infants suggest inborn errors of metabolism.

 Dx **Vomiting**

- Vomiting
- Nausea
- Abdominal pain
- Anorexia
- Diarrhea
- Headache
- Fever
- Lethargy

Pathophysiology

Vomiting is a reflex reaction that occurs in response to numerous stimuli: enteric infections, toxins, drugs, chemotherapy, radiation, etc. The final common pathway involves expulsion of food from the relaxed stomach into the mouth due to coordinated contraction of the abdominal wall, respiratory muscles, increased intra-abdominal and thoracic pressure, and relaxation of the lower and upper esophageal sphincters.

Anything that delays gastric emptying may be associated with vomiting. Gastric emptying may be retarded by a high-fat meal, swallowed mucus (eg, maternal mucus after birth, nasal mucus with an upper respiratory infection), fever, infection, and malnutrition. Delayed gastric emptying may develop with long-standing diabetes mellitus.

Vomiting can be divided into 3 phases: nausea, retching, and emesis. However, nausea may occur without retching and vomiting, and retching may occur without vomiting.

Nausea is a significant and difficult to define discomfort related to the sensation of a need to vomit. It can be produced by various stimuli (eg, bacterial toxins, drugs, intestinal distention, visceral pain, unpleasant memories, labyrinthine stimulation, noxious odors, visual stimulations, unpleasant taste, and increased cerebral pressure). Peripheral receptors in the stomach and the small and large intestines detect emetic stimuli; distention and contractions are recognized by mechanoreceptors and toxins are sensed by chemoreceptors. Emetic stimuli may also originate from the obstructed or inflamed bile ducts, peritoneal inflammation, mesenteric vascular occlusion, the pharynx, and the heart. Vagal pathways mediate emetic responses to a variety of peripheral stimuli. Most afferent vagal fibers project to the nucleus tractus solitarius and some to the area of postrema or the dorsal vagal motor nucleus. The serotonergic pathway plays the central role in nausea induced by peripheral stimuli.

The area postrema on the dorsal surface of the medulla close to the fourth ventricle is considered the chemoreceptor trigger zone to a variety of neurochemical stimuli. Bacterial toxins, drugs, toxic products of metabolic disorders, and radiation therapy may induce nausea by stimulation of numerous central receptors: dopamine D_2, muscarinic M_1, histaminergic H_1, serotonergic 5-HT3, and vasopressinergic subtypes located in the area postrema. However, afferent excitation of multiple brain sites, including nucleus tractus solitarius, the dorsal vagal and phrenic nuclei, the medullary nuclei controlling respiration, the hypothalamus, and the amygdala, is responsible for coordinated activities of various organs and muscles and the induction of retching and emesis.

Retching is the second phase of vomiting. It is produced by concurrent contractions of inspiratory thoracic, diaphragmatic, and abdominal muscles against the closed glottis. The generated high positive intra-abdominal pressure forces gastric contents into the esophagus and herniates the gastric cardia into the thorax. At this phase, the high negative thoracic pressure prevents emesis of gastric fluids.

Emesis is the final stage of vomiting. Synchronous contractions of the inspiratory and expiratory muscles generate high positive intrathoracic pressure sufficient to produce expulsion of gastric contents into the mouth. Oral propulsion of the vomitus is facilitated by the elevation of the hyoid bone and larynx. Airways are protected from aspiration by glottis closure. Elevation of the soft palate prevents passage of the vomitus into the nasal cavities. Hyperventilation may occur before emesis. During vomiting, breathing is suppressed.

With emesis, retrograde giant contractions originate from the middle of the small intestine. Intestinal contents move into the stomach causing enterogastric reflux. Within the stomach, the fundus remains flaccid, but the antrum and pylorus contract. Relaxation of the lower esophageal sphincter also occurs.

In children with pyloric stenosis, enterogastric reflux is prevented by hypertrophy of the pylorus. Projectile vomiting is facilitated by giant, often-visible contraction of the antrum and relaxation of the proximal stomach and low esophageal sphincter. Nausea is not associated with vomiting related to pyloric stenosis, and affected infants are frequently eager to eat immediately after vomiting.

Vomiting induced by increased intracranial pressure (ICP) is also not associated with nausea. In addition, such vomiting frequently occurs first thing in the morning on awakening and on an empty stomach. Regurgitation is a return of undigested food back up the esophagus to the mouth without the force and displeasure associated with vomiting. It could be manifested by visible spitting up after feeding or could be silent. Clinical evidence of regurgitation is not always associated with gastroesophageal reflux disease (GERD).

Differential Diagnosis

Vomiting could be a manifestation of gastrointestinal (GI), renal, metabolic, allergic, and CNS disorders. Some of them respond to medical management, and others mandate surgical intervention (Box 107-1). The presence of bile in the vomitus, referred to as bilious vomiting, is a serious sign, usually indicative of intestinal obstruction distal to the major duodenal papilla and of the need for surgical intervention. Bilious vomiting can also occur in children with pseudo-obstruction syndrome or acute pancreatitis and other conditions leading to paralytic ileus.

The presence of blood in the vomitus is another ominous sign and is discussed in Chapter 109.

The most common cause of vomiting is acute viral or bacterial gastroenteritis. Acute gastroenteritis is discussed in greater detail

Box 107-1. Differential Diagnosis of Vomiting in Infancy	
Medical Conditions	
• Gastroenteritis	• Inborn errors of metabolism
• Ingestion of maternal blood or mucus	• Congenital adrenal hyperplasia
• Overfeeding	• Parenteral infections (eg, otitis media, urinary tract infection)
• Food allergies	
Surgical Conditions	
• Atresia/stenosis of gastrointestinal tract	• Intussusception
	• Volvulus
• Pyloric stenosis	• Appendicitis
• Ulcers	

in Chapter 110. In cases that are not related to acute gastroenteritis, considering the age of the patient is the best approach to the differential diagnosis of vomiting.

Infants

Vomiting in neonates may be associated with the ingestion of irritants such as maternal blood or mucus. Either of these substances delays gastric emptying. Structural anomalies of the GI tract may also cause vomiting in neonates. The onset of symptoms is directly related to the level of obstruction, the higher the structural obstruction, the earlier the onset of vomiting. Lesions of the esophagus, such as esophageal atresia, may be evident in the delivery room, with an unsuccessful attempt to pass a nasogastric tube. Lower GI lesions, such as ileal atresia, may not present for several days. These lesions require surgical intervention. Infants with atretic lesions may also have a history of polyhydramnios or a single umbilical artery.

Overfeeding is the most common reason for spitting up in young infants. Frequently, infants who present with vomiting are actually experiencing spitting up or regurgitation. Overfeeding is less likely to occur in breastfed infants, because they have better control of their satiety. The physician should approach breastfed infants who are vomiting with care and concern.

Mothers of bottle-fed infants may feel that the volume of formula consumed by their infants is insufficient. Some non-nursing mothers feel the need to reinsert a nipple in the infant's mouth, and infants who are still interested in sucking (nonnutritive sucking) continue to feed, often exceeding the capacity of the stomach.

Food allergies are another common cause of vomiting during infancy. Infants with cow's milk formula intolerance may experience vomiting. At least 30% of these infants are also allergic to soy protein. Associated symptoms such as diarrhea, rhinorrhea, eczema, and growth failure frequently occur.

Gastroesophageal reflux is a common cause of regurgitation. It is described in detail in Chapter 108.

Achalasia is a rare cause of vomiting during infancy. It is defined as an absence of effective esophageal peristalsis and coordinated relaxation of the low esophageal sphincter. Ingested food that is unable to pass into the stomach may be regurgitated. Children with achalasia usually do not present until later in childhood, although they may have a prenatal history of polyhydramnios, a sign suggesting an abnormal swallowing pattern, even in utero.

Metabolic disorders, including inborn errors of metabolism and endocrine problems, may also be associated with vomiting. For example, children with galactosemia may present with vomiting as well as with jaundice, dehydration, cataracts, and hepatomegaly. Other inborn errors of metabolism include methylmalonic acidemia, disorders of the urea cycle, phenylketonuria, maple syrup urine disease, renal tubular acidosis, hypercalcemia, and diabetes insipidus. Some of these disorders induce symptoms suggestive of sepsis, such as lethargy and seizures.

Male infants with congenital adrenal hyperplasia (CAH) may present with vomiting and electrolyte disturbance, symptoms indicative of adrenal insufficiency. Affected male infants usually present at about 10 to 14 days of age with vomiting and hyperkalemia (which should not be attributed to hemolysis of the specimen); hyponatremia develops later. In females, CAH is usually detected in the newborn nursery because of ambiguous genitalia. Diagnosis of this potentially lethal condition is critical to ensure the institution of replacement therapy and survival of affected infants.

Vomiting may be induced by infection in parts of the body other than the GI tract. Most notably, urinary tract infections (UTIs) in infants may cause projectile vomiting, a symptom highly suggestive of pyloric stenosis. These infants are usually febrile and the diagnosis is considered when the urinalysis or culture is positive. Otitis media may also be associated with vomiting.

Vomiting, especially if unrelated to meals, may occur with increased ICP. In young infants, this suggests the possibility of an intracranial hemorrhage as occurs with abusive head trauma.

Pyloric stenosis, a condition caused by hypertrophy of the muscle surrounding the pyloric channel, is the most common surgical condition associated with vomiting in infancy. The condition affects males significantly more frequently than females and usually appears in infants between the ages of 2 weeks and 2 months. Factors that are known to increase risk of pyloric stenosis include being firstborn, male, and a greater birth weight, and early exposure to erythromycin. The emesis is projectile and non-bilious, and frequently contains curdled milk, which reflects delayed gastric emptying, a problem caused by failure of the hypertrophied pylorus to relax. Affected infants have an intact appetite and are eager to eat. In some infants, starvation leads to few bowel movements and constipation; in others there may be small, frequent, mucus-laden stools (starvation diarrhea) that represent succus entericus. If pyloric stenosis is not diagnosed promptly, infants may fail to gain weight or may exhibit FTT. Symptoms suggestive of pyloric stenosis may result from an antral web or duplication of the GI tract.

Children

Vomiting in children is frequently associated with gastroenteritis. Infections elsewhere in the body, particularly UTIs, streptococcal pharyngitis, and otitis media, are also associated with vomiting. Labyrinthitis presents with vomiting associated with dizziness. Older children with new-onset diabetes mellitus may present with vomiting. Vomiting may also appear in children who are already known to be diabetic. This is particularly true when ketosis is present. Slow gastric emptying (gastroparesis) is a complication of long-standing diabetes mellitus. Vomiting is also a component of peptic ulcer disease, which is described in more detail in Chapter 112.

Vomiting may be a major symptom of CNS-related problems, such as tumors, infections, hydrocephalus, malformations, and other causes of increased ICP. As previously noted, vomiting in CNS-related conditions is often unrelated to meals and may not be associated with nausea. Autonomic epilepsy and migraine headaches are also associated with vomiting. Cyclic vomiting is an unusual condition characterized by recurrent episodes of vomiting with intervals of complete wellness between attacks. Emotional upset can precipitate events, and there may be a history of migraine headaches.

Vomiting is one of the hallmarks of Reye syndrome, a disorder that involves an encephalopathy in association with fatty infiltration of the liver. The etiology of the condition is unclear, but the root of the disorder seems to be related to mitochondrial dysfunction. Affected children usually have a history of an antecedent viral illness, most commonly influenza or chickenpox. Following a period of recovery, they experience altered consciousness with vomiting. Hepatic enzymes and serum ammonia are elevated. Aspirin, which uncouples oxidative phosphorylation, is apparently linked to Reye syndrome, both epidemiologically as well as theoretically. There has been a marked reduction in the incidence of Reye syndrome related to the decrease in the use of aspirin and vaccination of children against varicella and influenza.

Certain medications, including theophylline, erythromycin, and digitalis, may also be associated with vomiting. Some of these medications cause transient relaxation of the lower esophageal sphincter and others affect the chemoreceptor trigger zone.

Familial dysautonomia, Riley-Day syndrome, a rare condition that affects Jewish individuals, results in vomiting. The disorder is inherited in an autosomal-recessive manner and consists of an imbalance in the autonomic nervous system. Children experience intractable vomiting in addition to excess perspiration, inability to produce tears, difficulty swallowing and chewing, and cold hands and feet. They also have hyperpyrexia and hypertension. These children require fluid replacement and management with antiemetics.

Surgical conditions such as appendicitis, gall bladder disease, and twisted ovarian cysts are discussed in Chapter 112.

Adolescents

Vomiting during the adolescent years may be caused by any of the previously mentioned conditions. In addition, adolescents may develop vomiting in association with intentional ingestion of illicit drugs or alcohol. Many adolescents have incorrect notions of the sexual activity needed to initiate pregnancy. Teenaged girls, who have been vomiting, especially for a time, should be evaluated for pregnancy, regardless of their disclosed sexual activity status.

Adolescents with eating disorders, particularly bulimia, vomit but may not disclose their vomiting. They may ingest emetics, such as ipecac, to help control their weight (see Chapter 133).

Evaluation

History

A complete history is essential for correct diagnosis (Questions Box). A positive family history of vomiting may suggest a diagnosis of food intolerance/allergy, gastroesophageal reflux or peptic ulcer disease, migraine, or familial dysautonomia.

Physical Examination

The examination shows the impact of vomiting on children's growth. The weight may provide evidence of the chronicity of the process; weight loss suggests a protracted course. Evidence of other infections,

---

Questions

Vomiting

- What is the nature of the vomiting (projectile, bilious, non-bilious)?
- How long has the child been vomiting?
- Are any symptoms such as fever, diarrhea, dizziness, or lethargy associated with the vomiting?
- What is the relationship of the vomiting to meals?
- Does the vomiting occur at night, indicating possible hiatal hernia and gastroesophageal reflux?
- Is there a family history of vomiting?
- Is the child taking any medications?
- Have any measures been taken to relieve the vomiting?

---

such as otitis media or pneumonia, may also be apparent. An abnormal neurologic examination would suggest a CNS process or an inborn error of metabolism. The fundi of the eyes should be assessed for the presence of papilledema or retinal hemorrhages. Nystagmus may be noted in children with labyrinthitis or CNS disturbances. The examination of the abdomen may show abdominal distention due to surgical or non-surgical conditions such as Hirschsprung disease; malrotation; adhesions after previous surgery; pancreatitis; celiac sprue; chronic idiopathic constipation; and abdominal, pelvic, or retroperitoneal masses.

Laboratory Tests

The laboratory assessment is determined by the differential diagnosis. If gastroenteritis or enterocolitis is suspected, an examination of the stools for leukocytes and occult blood is appropriate. Specimens for bacterial or viral cultures or viral antigen detection can be submitted. A complete blood cell count may support the diagnosis of infection or reveal signs of anemia. In breastfed neonates and infants, vomited blood should be evaluated using the Apt Downey test to determine whether it came from the mother or infant.

Electrolytes should be obtained in infants or children with a history of significant vomiting and may confirm dehydration, acid-base imbalance or electrolyte disturbance. Infants with pyloric stenosis who vomit stomach contents develop a hypochloremic-hypokalemic alkalosis. A urinalysis also may show evidence of dehydration as well as signs of a UTI. Tests for inborn errors of metabolism, such as urine for acid analysis, are appropriate if this is suspected.

Imaging Studies

Radiographic procedures, such as esophagram or upper GI series, are the procedure of choice for diagnosis of esophageal and duodenal atresia and intestinal malrotation. An abdominal ultrasound is most effective in the diagnosis of pyloric stenosis or intussusception. A flat plate of the abdomen may show stomach distention, a "double bubble" (air in the stomach and duodenum), or a paucity of intestinal air in cases of high-level obstruction. Consultation with a pediatric gastroenterologist may lead to additional diagnostic tests, such as endoscopic evaluation.

Management

The initial step in the management of vomiting infants or children is to ensure adequate hydration and integrity of the cardiovascular bed. This may require the administration of intravenous fluids. Oral rehydration is the mainstay of therapy in infants and children whose vomiting is related to gastroenteritis. Small, frequent feedings with clear fluids are better tolerated than large, infrequent feedings, although the latter may be necessary in infants with diarrhea because each feeding may result in a bowel movement. Antiemetics such as phenothiazines are discouraged in children because of the high incidence of side effects, including dystonic posturing. Drugs commonly used in pediatric practice include antihistamines, dopamine D_2, and serotonin 5-HT3 receptor antagonists. Oral ondansetron is frequently used as a single dose to manage the vomiting seen in acute viral gastroenteritis in the pediatric emergency department or as repeated doses for hospitalized children with other conditions associated with vomiting.

Further management depends on the diagnosis. Bacterial infections should be treated with the appropriate antibiotics. Surgical conditions, such as pyloric stenosis or intussusception, should be managed operatively. Inborn errors of metabolism require consultation with a geneticist and dietary manipulation. Congenital adrenal hyperplasia should be managed in consultation with an endocrinologist. This condition necessitates replacement hormonal therapy.

Prognosis

Most cases of acute vomiting resolve spontaneously or are readily managed once the underlying condition is diagnosed. The overall prognosis is therefore quite good.

Protracted vomiting may result in starvation and FTT, however. Severe vomiting may cause tears in the esophagus and lead to hematemesis. Obstructive causes of vomiting in infants respond to surgical intervention.

CASE RESOLUTION

The infant in the case history exhibits the signs and symptoms consistent with pyloric stenosis. The boy is a healthy, vigorous breastfed infant, and his weight gain of 1,000 g in 6 weeks (average: 25 g/d) is normal. The vomitus is curdled indicating that it has been in the stomach for more than 3 hours. Gastric emptying is delayed. The presence of a mass in the right upper quadrant is also consistent with the diagnosis. An ultrasound would confirm the finding. It would be equally appropriate to feed the infant nothing by mouth, start intravenous fluids, and obtain surgical consultation.

Selected References

Chandran L, Chitkara M. Vomiting in children: reassurance, red flag, or referral? *Pediatr Rev.* 2008;29:183–192

Chelimsky G, Czinn SJ. Peptic ulcer disease and gastritis. In: Lifschitz CH, ed. *Pediatric Gastroenterology and Nutrition in Clinical Practice.* New York, NY: Dekker; 2002:501–515

Chong SKF. Gastrointestinal problems in the handicapped child [gastroenterology and nutrition]. *Curr Opin Pediatr.* 2001;13:441–446

Freedman SB, Adler M, Seshadri R, Powell EC. Oral ondansetron for gastroenteritis in a pediatric emergency department. *N Engl J Med.* 2006;354:1698–1705

Gordon N. Recurrent vomiting in childhood, especially of neurologic origin. *Dev Med Child Neurol.* 1994;36:463–470

Gershman G. Approach to the child with gastroesophageal reflux. In: Osborn LM, DeWitt TS, First LR, Zenel JA, eds. *Pediatrics.* Philadelphia, PA: Mosby; 2005:658–665

Li BUK Nausea, vomiting and pyloric stenosis. In: Walker WA, Kleinman RE, Sanderson IR, Goulet OJ, et al eds. *Pediatric Gastrointestinal Disease, Pathophysiology, Diagnosis, Management.* 5th ed. Vol. 1. Philadelphia, PA: B. C. Decker; 2008:127–138

Murray KF, Christie DL. Vomiting. *Pediatr Rev.* 1998;19:337–341

CHAPTER 108

Gastroesophageal Reflux

Jeremy Screws, MD

CASE STUDY

A 22-month-old boy presents with a history of vomiting small amounts of food twice weekly. The emesis occurs most often after meals or periods of being very active. There does not seem to be any pain or discomfort with the vomiting. He has been otherwise healthy, with an uneventful course as an infant, good weight gain, and no hospitalizations. He has had mild respiratory symptoms beginning at 6 months with some nighttime cough and occasional wheezing. There is no history of pneumonia, dysphagia, or abdominal pain. Physical examination is normal, with no anemia or urinary tract disease noted on laboratory assessment.

Questions

1. What are the characteristics of gastroesophageal reflux (GER)?
2. What is the difference between GER and gastroesophageal reflux disease (GERD)?
3. What groups of children are at risk for GER?
4. What is the appropriate workup for an infant with suspected GER?
5. What is the appropriate management of infants and children with GER and GERD?
6. What is the natural history of GER in children?

Gastroesophageal reflux includes a spectrum of disease from physiological phenomena to pathologic disease. It involves the retrograde movement of gastric contents into the esophagus. Reflux episodes often follow meals and are brief. Gastroesophageal reflux may manifest as **regurgitation** to the oral pharynx with re-swallowing or vomiting with expulsion from the mouth. Gastroesophageal reflux is common in infants beginning at 2 to 3 months of age and resolving in most individuals by 18 months.

Although this process is common in the first year of life, it typically does not pose a problem unless it fails to resolve by 18 to 24 months. In contrast, GERD denotes a more severe pattern involving injury to the esophagus as well as the presence of extra-intestinal disease. This term is used when there are symptoms present such as pain, feeding or swallowing difficulties, cough, wheezing, or poor weight gain. Complications including pneumonia or esophagitis are also part of reflux disease. While GER may require only anticipatory guidance and monitoring, GERD necessitates further evaluation and medical therapy. Although GER and GERD are defined separately, there is sometimes confusion in the medical community. It must be emphasized that GERD involves symptomatic disease.

Epidemiology

Gastroesophageal reflux has a heterogeneous presentation, making it difficult to study longitudinally. We must be careful to make the distinction between GER and GERD as opposed to using these terms synonymously. Most infants with either condition who are brought for medical care will present by 6 months of age. Regurgitation occurs at least once daily in half of infants younger than 3 months and in nearly two-thirds of infants by 4 months. By 12 months only 5% of infants will continue to have symptoms. Gastroesophageal reflux disease is considerably less common, with the prevalence depending on the type of symptom studied. It is reported at less than 10%. Most infants with reflux will need little to no medical intervention.

High-Risk Groups

Patients with neurologic injury have a higher prevalence of GERD. The management of these individuals requires a more aggressive approach. They are more likely to have esophagitis or aspiration, and anti-reflux surgery should be considered early in the treatment regimen. Infants who have undergone repair of esophageal atresia also have more severe disease, with at least one-half requiring anti-reflux surgery. Chronic respiratory disease such as cystic fibrosis is associated with GERD. It is described in two-thirds of patients with asthma, but this association is controversial. It is not clear whether the altered physiology of these diseases causes reflux, or if reflux exacerbates the pulmonary dysfunction. Similar triggers for asthma and GERD are described, so it may be that they are coexisting and unrelated. Recent studies with intraluminal impedance monitoring (see Evaluation) show that non–acid reflux occurs frequently in asthmatics. This would help to explain the lack of success of therapy aimed at acid suppression in this group of patients.

Clinical Presentation

The most frequent presentation for infants with GER is recurrent vomiting that is non-forceful and small in volume (Dx Box). Vomiting typically occurs after feeding and does not seem to disturb the patient. Some parents report a link between fussiness or crying with feeding, but this is not reproducible in trials comparing

Dx Presenting Signs and Symptoms of Gastroesophageal Reflux Disease

- Regurgitation
- Vomiting
- Fussiness or sleep disturbance
- Poor weight gain
- Hematemesis or anemia
- Odynophagia or dysphagia
- Asthma/apnea/aspiration

symptoms with pH studies. Further symptoms such as poor weight gain, anemia, or swallowing difficulties are characteristic of GERD. Nighttime cough, asthma, and recurrent pneumonia are respiratory presentations that may be seen. Older children can have recurrent emesis but may also complain of chest or abdominal pain. The adult symptoms of heartburn and regurgitation with epigastric or chest pain may not be noted in children until 8 to 12 years of age. Sandifer syndrome is a rare presentation in infants, with characteristic paroxysmal movements involving arching of the back that may be mistaken for seizures.

Pathophysiology

There are many factors felt to be involved in the pathophysiology of reflux disease. Many of these change as the child grows. This helps explain the improvement in infant GER over time. Motility and pressure differentials between the esophagus and stomach control the flow of gas and liquid across the lower esophageal sphincter (LES). Refluxate is allowed into the distal esophagus multiple times daily in all ages by *transient lower esophageal sphincter relaxations*. Increased frequency or duration of these relaxations, rather than low LES pressure, is felt to be a major cause of GERD. Transient lower esophageal sphincter relaxations are mediated by a brain stem reflex involving the vagal nerve and the release of nitric oxide.

The position of the gastroesophageal junction and its relationship to the diaphragmatic crura play an important role. The opposed crura have a "pinchcock" action that works with the esophagogastric angle, or angle of His, to prevent reflux. As this angle becomes more open or obtuse, reflux may increase. Disruption of this anatomical association, as seen with *hiatal hernia*, predisposes individuals to reflux.

Relaxations of the LES that are too frequent or prolonged expose the esophageal mucosa to noxious material. Secretions from the esophagus and salivary glands neutralize the refluxate and sweep it into the stomach. Appropriate peristalsis of the esophagus is therefore necessary for clearance. Inflammation in the distal esophagus exacerbates this process by decreasing peristalsis. Position influences gravity, with the upright position favoring anterograde movement. The composition of the refluxate influences the damage that can occur. Hydrochloric acid, pepsin, bile acids, and pancreatic enzymes have all been implicated in mucosal injury. The mucosa must combat this exposure with its own defense.

Before food or secretions can move out of the esophagus, the stomach must be ready to accept it. The fundus normally relaxes without an increase in pressure. Dysfunction of this fundic accommodation or delay in gastric emptying can increase pressure in the stomach and exacerbate reflux. The volume of ingested feedings is noted to be a factor in infants. Based on the size of their stomachs, infants typically take twice the volume of older children. This leaves more material in the stomach at any given time, potentially increasing intragastric pressure.

Differential Diagnosis

A diverse group of symptoms, each with its own list of potential diagnoses, are associated with reflux disease. Regurgitation and vomiting are the most commonly reported symptoms. Many of the causes of vomiting in the newborn can be separated from reflux with a history and physical examination (Box 108-1). Forceful, bilious, or bloody emesis is not typical of reflux. Fussiness and crying are nonspecific symptoms with etiologies ranging from infantile colic to meningitis. Esophagitis has many other etiologies of which eosinophilic

Box 108-1. Common Non-Reflux Causes of Vomiting	
Infections	***Neurologic***
• Sepsis	• Hydrocephalus and shunt malfunctions
• Meningitis	• Subdural hematoma
• Urinary tract infection	• Intracranial hemorrhage
• Otitis media	• Tumors
Obstruction	• Migraine
• Pyloric stenosis	***Allergic***
• Malrotation	• Dietary protein intolerance
• Intussusception	***Respiratory***
Gastrointestinal	• Post-tussive emesis
• Eosinophilic esophagitis	• Pneumonia
• Peptic ulcer disease	***Renal***
• Achalasia	• Obstructive uropathy
• Gastroparesis	• Renal insufficiency
• Gastroenteritis	***Cardiac***
• Gall bladder disease	• Congestive heart failure
• Pancreatitis	***Other, Seen in Adolescents***
• Celiac disease	• Recreational drugs
• Pill esophagitis	• Alcohol
• Crohn disease	• Pregnancy
Metabolic/Endocrine	***Other***
• Galactosemia	• Overfeeding
• Fructose intolerance	• Self-induced vomiting
• Urea cycle defects	
• Diabetic ketoacidosis	
Toxic	
• Lead poisoning	

esophagitis must be considered. This condition presents more typically in the atopic child with dysphagia. It may also present with food impaction in the esophagus, which is secondary to strictures and a small-caliber esophagus. However, the pain and vomiting of eosinophilic esophagitis may mimic GERD. An esophageal biopsy reveals the presence of intra-epithelial eosinophils. Management focuses on dietary manipulation and the elimination of identified foods that the child is allergic to.

Evaluation

Separating the mildly symptomatic "happy spitter" from the child with very apparent, painful erosive esophagitis may not prove difficult. However, deciding how much vomiting is too much may prove vexing. The presence of certain risk factors in the initial history should prompt further evaluation. These factors include poor weight gain, food avoidance, respiratory disease, unexplained anemia or frank hematemesis, or significant chest or abdominal pain.

History

Targeted questions about the timing and volume of feedings and their relationship to regurgitation can help build the case for reflux. Specific attention should be paid to respiratory symptoms such as nighttime cough or previous episodes of pneumonia. Difficulties with feeding and swallowing should be outlined carefully. Gagging or dysphagia with different consistencies should be noted. Family history of reflux, especially as an infant, may be helpful. A history of atopy in the family, including asthma and food allergies, will assist when considering eosinophilic esophagitis. Clinical questionnaires, including the Infant Gastroesophageal Reflux Questionnaire, have been validated but do not predict prognosis or severity. They are more useful in the research setting.

Physical Examination

One should perform a full physical examination, including an observance of feeding. Neurologic deficits or delay should be noted. The abdomen should be carefully palpated for masses or distension. Growth parameters should be reviewed longitudinally and the child's body habitus, particularly the amount of subcutaneous tissue, should be noted.

Laboratory Tests

Most patients with reflux will need no laboratory testing. Urinary tract infections may present in infants with only vomiting so a urinalysis and culture is reasonable. Children with large volume emesis or weight loss should be assessed for acidosis or other electrolyte abnormalities. Markers of kidney and liver function are reasonable to obtain. If anemia is suspected based on the physical examination or the presence of hematemesis, hematologic studies should be obtained.

Intra-esophageal pH Monitoring

Currently measurement of the intra-esophageal pH for periods of 24 to 48 hours is considered the gold standard for the diagnosis of GERD. This is performed by placing a catheter transnasally into the distal esophagus to measure the intraluminal pH as the patient records the symptoms of interest, such as cough and pain. Meals are also recorded. Monitoring of pH can be performed safely in all age groups, and certain parameters of this study do correlate with esophagitis. It does not detect non–acid reflux, making its utility in linking respiratory disease to GERD questionable. It may be combined with multichannel sleep studies to investigate apnea or nighttime symptoms. A wireless device that attaches to the esophageal mucosa has been used in children. The device can be placed with or without endoscopy, but the size of the capsule may prohibit its use in smaller children.

Upper Gastrointestinal Series (UGI)

Contrast radiography of the upper gastrointestinal (GI) tract is often employed early in the evaluation of reflux. The utility of the test is not for screening; however, its sensitivity and specificity are both low. The brief duration of the examination misses episodes of reflux. Conversely, if episodes are seen it must be noted that the positioning of the patient and the pressure applied to the abdomen are not physiological. This test should be used only to identify anatomical anomalies that could cause vomiting, such as malrotation, esophageal or intestinal webs, pyloric stenosis, or hiatal hernia. Large volumes of refluxate to the level of the proximal esophagus or pharynx, if seen, are more likely to indicate GERD.

Scintigraphy

Nuclear medicine studies may be employed in the evaluation of reflux. In general they involve the administration of an age-appropriate feeding of technetium-labeled food. For infants this would be labeled formula at a volume that approximates a typical feeding. For older children this would include a mixed meal of liquids and solids. Scans are taken serially to mark the location of the tracer. There are 3 questions that can be answered with these studies. The first use of this method is to quantify the rate at which the stomach empties. This may be expressed as half time ($T_{1/2}$), which refers to the time taken to empty 50% of the tracer from the stomach. Alternatively, it may be expressed as percentage emptied at 90 minutes. For children younger than 1 year the $T_{1/2}$ should be less than 60 minutes for liquids. For older children a $T_{1/2}$ of 90 minutes has been accepted. The second use for scintigraphy is measurement of tracer in the esophagus, indicating a reflux episode. Shorter intervals between scans are required, and both acid and non–acid reflux are measured. As with the UGI, this test has a low sensitivity for reflux disease, making it unacceptable as a screening examination. However, the specificity is higher and multiple episodes may be supportive for the diagnosis of GERD. The third use for this modality is detection of aspiration. Delayed scans up to 24 hours later may be employed, which can show tracer in the pharynx or lung fields. This use is also limited due to low sensitivity. However, a positive test is helpful in linking reflux to pulmonary pathology.

Endoscopy With Biopsy

Endoscopy of the upper GI tract is moderately invasive but allows direct visualization of the esophagus. The presence and severity of esophagitis can be documented. Other disease processes causing esophagitis, including infection, *eosinophilic infiltration,* and Crohn disease, can be diagnosed. Biopsies should always be taken, even in the absence of macroscopic findings, as histologic esophagitis may be responsible for symptoms. Basal zone hyperplasia and increased papillary length are found in reflux esophagitis. Mucosal breaks are most suggestive of pathological reflux. Eosinophilic esophagitis may have specific endoscopic findings of linear or circular furrowing or white specks. However, the location and number of eosinophils on biopsy are necessary to separate this diagnosis from GERD. Traditional pH monitoring catheters or wireless devices can be placed at the time of endoscopy.

Multichannel Intraluminal Impedance

Impedance monitoring is increasing in clinical use as smaller, less expensive equipment becomes available. This technology involves the placement of a catheter transnasally into the distal esophagus, similar to traditional pH monitoring. However, these catheters have multiple sensors arranged from proximally to distally that can detect the flow of liquid or gas and determine the direction of movement of this bolus. Liquids moving from the distal catheter to the proximal (retrograde) catheter are noted to be reflux. Typically a pH sensor at the distal end is included so that boluses may be described as acid or non-acid. This study is especially attractive in small infants where frequent feedings buffer acidity and in respiratory diseases where non–acid reflux has been implicated. Normal values for all pediatric age groups are currently in press.

Management

Infants that are thriving with no symptoms other than regurgitation or vomiting will benefit primarily from alleviation of parental anxiety. Discussion involving the normal course and benign nature of GER may be all that is required. The infant should be followed for changes in feeding, weight, or respiratory complaints and the regurgitation should begin to resolve by the end of the first year. Referral to a pediatric gastroenterologist should be considered when there is poor weight gain or hematemesis, or when there is respiratory disease (coughing, wheezing, or apnea).

Lifestyle Changes

Life in recumbency has its disadvantages for infants, namely allowing the esophagus and stomach to reside at the same level. This concept has led to the use of positioning in infants. There are multiple positions used including prone, prone at a 30-degree angle, or supine at a 30-degree angle. The only proven position seems to be prone. Unfortunately this position has been associated with a higher rate of sudden infant death syndrome (SIDS) in infants. The practitioner must balance the risk of GERD with that of SIDS in the individual patient. The 30-degree supine position does not seem to be more effective in decreasing reflux than the flat supine position, but there is conflicting evidence on this point.

Infants with reflux are often put through "formula roulette." Cow's milk or soy-based formulas are employed and some progress to partially digested or elemental formulas. There is a select group of infants with regurgitation that have cow's milk protein intolerance who may respond to a 2-week trial of hypoallergenic formula. This is more likely in the patient with a family history of atopy. Nearly half of infants intolerant of milk protein will also exhibit symptoms with soy, thus protein hydrosylate formulations may be of more use. There is no indication for lactose-free cow's milk formulas in this patient population. Rice cereal may be used as a thickening agent. This does not change findings on esophageal pH monitoring, but it may decrease the frequency of regurgitation. Patients with poor weight gain will benefit from the increased caloric density of the thickened formula. One tablespoon of rice cereal per 2 ounces of formula will increase the content from 20 to 27 cal/oz. Increasing amounts of rice cereal will increase the viscosity and caloric density, but this also increases osmolarity. Excessively concentrated formulas may worsen vomiting. Nipples used with thickened formula will need to be tailored by crosscutting, but this may lead to increases in coughing or gagging. Formulas containing commercial "antiregurgitant" agents are now available. Although no more effective than rice cereal for regurgitation they do not increase the caloric density and may require less energy to pull from the nipple. This must be balanced with the unknown long-term risks of these newer ingredients as well as the increased cost.

Environmental and dietary factors have been studied in the older child and teenager. Currently only caffeine, chocolate, and spicy foods that provoke symptoms should be avoided. Obesity and exposure to tobacco smoke have also been implicated.

Medications

The pharmacologic agents that are used in reflux disease are felt to be safe and, therefore, sometimes used empirically without diagnostic confirmation (Table 108-1). Although this may be useful in adolescents for up to 4 weeks, it should be used with much caution in infants or young children. There is emerging evidence of harm from acid suppression, especially proton pump inhibitors (PPI). Acid suppression is the mainstay of treatment. The goal is to reduce exposure of the esophagus to acid. There are 3 main types of drugs that can be used: antacids, histamine-2 receptor antagonists (H2RA), and PPIs. The only clinically effective antacids are those that contain aluminum, which has been associated with bone and nervous system toxicity, especially in infants. Histamine-2 receptor antagonists inhibit acid production in the gastric parietal cell. They are effective in the healing of esophagitis; however, tachyphylaxis has been seen as early as 1 week after initiation. Further complicating this class of medications are side effects such as fussiness that may appear to be reflux symptoms. Cimetidine and famotidine have the most evidence for use in pediatrics.

Table 108-1. Pharmacologic Agents Used for Reflux Disease

Drug	Pediatric Dose	Adverse Effects
Cimetidine	20–40 mg/kg/d, divided 3–4 times per day	Hypotension, gynecomastia, reduced hepatic metabolism of other drugs, neutropenia, agranulocytosis, thrombocytopenia
Famotidine	0.5–1 mg/kg/d divided every day to twice per day	Headache, dizziness, constipation, diarrhea
Omeprazole	0.7–3.3 mg/kg/d divided every day to twice per day	Headache, diarrhea, abdominal pain, nausea, rash, vitamin B_{12} deficiency, constipation
Lansoprazole	15 mg (weight <30 kg) 30 mg (weight >30 kg)	Headache, nausea, constipation, diarrhea, abdominal pain, proteinuria, hypotension, elevated transaminases
Metoclopramide	0.1 mg/kg/dose 4 times per day before meals	Drowsiness, restlessness, dystonia, gynecomastia, galactorrhea
Erythromycin	3–5 mg/kg/dose 3–4 times per day before meals	Diarrhea, vomiting, cramps, antibiotic effect, pyloric stenosis

Proton pump inhibitors bond and deactivate hydrogen, potassium-adenosinetriphosphatase pumps and reduce meal-induced acid production. They should be taken 30 minutes prior to a meal so that the drug is in the bloodstream in the largest concentration at mealtime. Omeprazole and lansoprazole have been studied the most in children, although no PPI is approved for infants younger than than 1 year. Proton pump inhibitors may be used as the initial drug, or following failure by H2RAs. There are 2 approaches that are used in initiating these medications. **Step-up** therapy involves beginning with H2RAs or low-dose PPI and escalating therapy until symptoms have improved. **Step-down** therapy progresses from high-dose PPI to resolve symptoms then low-dose PPI or H2RA to maintain remission. Healing of esophagitis at higher doses takes 4 to 8 weeks, with symptoms resolving in this time frame. Histamine-2 receptor antagonists are more effective than PPIs in the fasting state. Therefore, they may be effective for nighttime symptoms that persist through high-dose PPI therapy when taken at bedtime.

There are emerging studies in children and adults showing adverse effects from long-term acid suppression. Up to 14% of patients can have side effects of headache, diarrhea, constipation, or nausea. Increased rates of community-acquired pneumonia gastroenteritis and necrotizing enterocolitis have been described. Adult studies have shown increased hip fractures and vitamin B_{12} deficiency, suggesting malabsorption secondary to hypochlorydria, but these have not been reproduced in children. Further studies are needed to understand the significance of these adverse effects, but we must use caution with empiric therapy when accurate testing such as pH studies or endoscopy is available.

Prokinetic agents are indicated in the patient with evidence of delayed gastric emptying. Effects on LES tone and esophageal peristalsis seem to be less important than accelerated gastric emptying. Cisapride, a mixed serotonergic agent, was the model drug for this class. It has been shown to improve reflux symptoms and pH parameters in infants. However, it has been associated with QT prolongation and arrhythmia with some deaths. The use of cisapride has been severely restricted since 2000. Other drugs in the group are less likely to improve reflux but are still widely used. Metoclopramide also has mixed serotonergic effects, in addition to anti-dopaminergic and cholinomimetic actions. Adverse effects including central nervous system complications limit the use of this drug. This drug now carries a black box warning from the US Food and Drug Administration. Erythromycin is a motilin receptor agonist that is also used less commonly in GERD. There is evidence that its use in pregnancy or in young infants may increase the risk of pyloric stenosis. Many interactions have been seen with this macrolide antibiotic, which also limits its use.

Barrier agents include sodium alginate, which is not readily available in the United States, and sucralfate, which contains aluminum. The former is not effective in most cases of GERD and the latter should be reserved for short-term treatment of erosive lesions in the esophagus.

Anti-Reflux Procedures

Patients that continue to have reflux on maximum medical therapy or those that have serious extra-esophageal manifestations such as recurrent aspiration or Barrett esophagus should be considered for surgery. Patients requiring long-term drug therapy may also be selected for surgery. The most popular procedure is the Nissen fundoplication. The laparoscopic approach to fundoplication is used widely and entails a full wrap of the fundus of the stomach around the esophagus to increase LES tone and create a more acute angle of His. More than 90% of patients remain symptom-free up to 11 years postoperatively. Complications including gas bloat, dumping syndrome, and dysphagia are reported at variable frequencies. Failure rates are higher in neurologically impaired children and those with esophageal atresia repair. There are several other fundoplication procedures that have variable degrees of wrapping.

Significant delay in gastric emptying may require an additional surgical procedure at the gastric outlet. Antroplasty or pyloroplasty enlarges the exit from the stomach. There is some theoretical concern that fundoplication itself results in accelerated gastric emptying. The additive effects of pyloroplasty might result in dumping of gastric contents into the duodenum too rapidly. This has not been shown to be a significant problem, and this procedure should be given strong consideration in infants or children with moderate or severe gastric-emptying delay noted clinically or by scintigraphy.

Endoscopic anti-reflux procedures have mixed results in adults. Endoscopic transesophageal plication involves placing sutures through the gastroesophageal junction, pleating the mucosa and reducing the size of this opening. Endoluminal application of radio-frequency energy has been used to remodel the tissue of the LES to reduce reflux episodes. Pediatric experience is limited. Other options include endoscopic placement of inert barriers into the tissue of the LES. All of these endoluminal techniques need further clinical data, especially in children, before they can be recommended broadly.

Prognosis

Complications arising from untreated GERD include esophagitis, Barrett esophagus, strictures, and esophageal adenocarcinoma. However, most infants with GER have a more favorable outcome. Regurgitation resolves in most children by 18 months and is absent by 24 months in 98%. There is some evidence that a portion of patients that become asymptomatic will continue to have abnormal histology in the esophagus at follow-up endoscopy. Therefore, it is unclear if the disease process continues into later childhood. Future studies that follow infants with reflux longitudinally into adulthood will be of great benefit. There is much to be learned in the area of non–acid reflux and its role in respiratory disease as intraluminal impedance becomes more widely used.

Children with persistent reflux symptoms into later childhood have a worse prognosis. Patients with a history of esophageal atresia repair or severe neurologic injury may have a poor prognosis, often requiring high-dose medication or anti-reflux surgery. They are more likely to suffer from complications of GERD.

CASE RESOLUTION

This toddler continues to have frequent emesis at almost 2 years of age with extra-esophageal manifestations including wheezing. He should be referred to a pediatric gastroenterologist for evaluation of GERD. He is unlikely to have spontaneous symptom resolution at this age.

Selected References

Michail S. Gastroesophageal reflux. *Pediatr Rev.* 2007;28:101–110

Orenstein S, Khan S. Gastroesophageal reflux. In: Walker WA, Goulet O, Kleinman RE, Sherman PM, Shneider BL, Sanderson IR, eds. *Pediatric Gastrointestinal Disease: Pathophysiology, Diagnosis, Management.* 4th ed. Hamilton, Ontario, Canada: BC Decker Inc.; 2004:384–399

Rudolph CD, Mazur LJ, Liptak GS, et al. Guidelines for evaluation and treatment of gastroesophageal reflux in infants and children: recommendations of the North American Society for Pediatric Gastroenterology and Nutrition. *J Pediatr Gastroenterol Nutr.* 2001;32(suppl 2):S1–S31

Vandenplas Y. Gastroesophageal reflux. In: Wyllie R, Hyams JS, Kay M, eds. *Pediatric Gastrointestinal and Liver Disease.* 3rd ed. Philadelphia, PA: Elsevier Inc.; 2006:305–325

Vandenplas Y, Rudolph CD, Di Lorenzo C, et al. Pediatric gastroesophageal reflux clinical practice guidelines: joint recommendations of the North American Society for Pediatric Gastroenterology Hepatology and Nutrition, European Society for Pediatric Gastroenterology Hepatology and Nutrition. *J Pediatr Gastroenterol Nutr.* 2009;49(4):498–547

CHAPTER 109

Gastrointestinal Bleeding

George Gershman, MD

CASE STUDY

A 4-year-old boy is evaluated for intermittent passing of bright red blood from the rectum for 2 weeks. Blood either coats the stool or appears as a spot after a bowel movement. The mother reports no vomiting, diarrhea, loss of appetite, weight loss, fever, or abdominal pain. The boy has no history of constipation, straining, or pain with defecation and is taking no medications. The family has no pets and has not traveled recently.

On physical examination, the boy is a well-appearing, energetic, interactive youngster. Weight and height are at the 75th percentile for age. The abdomen is soft, flat, and non-tender, and bowel sounds are normally active. No organomegaly or masses are evident. No rashes, bruising, or hemangiomas are present. No tags, fissures, or fistulas are seen on close visual inspection of the perianal area. Digital rectal examination reveals normal sphincter tone, and a small, mobile, pea-like mass is palpable in the rectal vault. A film of bright red blood is present on the glove after the examination. A complete blood cell count with platelet count and a prothrombin/partial thromboplastin time determination yield normal results.

Questions

1. What is involved in the assessment of children with gastrointestinal (GI) bleeding?
2. How are upper and lower GI tract bleeding differentiated?
3. What conditions usually account for upper and lower GI tract bleeding?
4. What management options are available for GI bleeding?
5. How does the physician decide what type of management is appropriate for each individual patient?

Bleeding from the GI tract in infants and children is always stressful and frightening for patients and their parents and challenging for a physician, especially if bleeding is severe.

Fortunately, life-threatening GI bleeding is rare in pediatric practice. However, a pediatrician or emergency department (ED) physician should be prepared to initiate effective resuscitation and diagnostic workup focusing on common age-specific causes of GI bleeding.

The primary goal of this approach is a reduction of morbidity associated with significant hemorrhage.

Epidemiology

The incidence of bleeding from the upper GI tract (upper GI bleeding) among infants and children is unknown. Clinical experience suggests that the incidence in children is significantly less than in adults. It is supported indirectly by epidemiological data from the United Kingdom and United States, which indicate that the incidence of upper GI bleeding in adults younger than 29 years is approximately 18 to 23 per 100,000 adults per year, which is almost 4 to 5 times lower than among older age groups. However, the risk of upper GI bleeding is higher (between 6.2% and 10.2%) in infants and children admitted to pediatric intensive care units.

Despite the fact that rectal bleeding is quite common in pediatric practice, the epidemiology of this problem is not well established.

According to published data, rectal bleeding was a chief complain of 0.3% of all visits to a tertiary ED during a 10-month period.

Clinical Presentation

There are 4 presentations of blood loss from the GI tract: hematemesis, melena, occult bleeding, and hematochezia.

Hematemesis is the term that applies to the vomiting of bright-red "fresh" blood or "coffee-ground" emesis of dark-brown "old" blood exposed to hydrochloric acid. Usually hematemesis reflects acute bleeding from the esophagus, stomach, or proximal duodenum. Swallowing of maternal blood in neonates, and epistaxis in older children, should be ruled out to avoid unnecessary invasive procedures.

Melena is defined as liquid, coal black, shiny, sticky, tarry, foul-smelling stool. It suggests bleeding from the upper GI tract. Occasionally the site of bleeding can be located in the ileum or right colon. However, in this case stool is black but not tarry. Melena suggests a minimum loss of 50 to 100 mL in adults or 2% of blood volume in children. Stool may remain black or tarry for a few days after massive hemorrhage even though active bleeding has ceased.

Occult bleeding implies the presence of an invisible quantity of blood in stool detected by a special technique. It is a synonym for chronic, recurrent losses of small amounts of blood, which often lead to severe microcytic anemia. The most commonly used technique for detection of blood in stool is the hemoccult stool test. This test is based on the chemical reaction of a dye (guaiac) with peroxidase-containing substances and hydrogen peroxide. It is not specific for presence of blood (hemoglobin) in stool.

False-positive results could be secondary to peroxidase activity in food products such as cantaloupe, radishes, bean sprouts, cauliflower, broccoli, grapes, and red meat or iron preparations. False-negative results of the hemoccult test are associated with prolonged colonic transient time and bacterial degradation of hemoglobin to porphyrin, which does not have peroxidase activity.

Hematochezia is the passage of bright red or maroon-colored blood from the rectum. This may be pure blood, bloody diarrhea, or blood mixed with stool. As a rule, it is a sign of lower GI bleeding from the distal colon or less frequently from the right colon or the distal ileum. Rarely hematochezia may occur in children with massive bleeding from the duodenum.

Pathophysiology

Compensatory responses to acute bleeding facilitate a restoration of depleted intravascular volume, maintenance of a normal cardiac output (CO) and adequate oxygenation of vital organs (brain, heart, lungs, and adrenal gland), and mobilization of internal energy stores.

Two parameters determine the degree of compensation: volume of blood loss and velocity of bleeding.

Mild Blood Loss (<15% of Circulatory Volume) or Class 1 Bleeding

Relatively slow blood loss of less than 15% of blood volume triggers (1) redistribution of depot blood from the venous system to systemic circulation and (2) shift of extracellular fluids into the vascular space. Adequate CO without changes in heart rate and blood pressure is maintained and there are no hemodynamic abnormalities. However, a rapid blood loss (even <10% of blood volume) may compromise CO and trigger tachycardia and other compensatory mechanisms to restore normal blood circulation.

Moderate Blood Loss (Between 15%–30% of Circulating Volume) or Class 2 Bleeding

Blood loss of more than 15% of blood volume leads to tachycardia, an increased systemic vascular resistance (SVR) due to activation of the sympathetic nervous system and hypothalamic-pituitary-adrenomedullary axis. In children, CO depends on heart rate rather than stroke volume due to smaller ventricular mass. With hemorrhage, tachycardia is the principal mechanism for maintenance of an adequate CO in pediatric patients; however, prolonged tachycardia increases myocardial oxygen demand and decreased diastolic-dependent coronary perfusion. This eventually leads to cardiovascular decompensation if fluid resuscitation is delayed or insufficient.

Normal blood pressure and adequate perfusion of vital organs in children with moderate bleeding is maintained by increased SVR and redistribution of blood from skin, muscle, splanchnic organs, and kidney to the brain, heart, lungs, and adrenal gland due to local production of adenosine, nitric oxide, and prostaglandins. Therefore, blood pressure is a poor indicator of cardiovascular homeostasis in children with moderate GI bleeding. In contrast, persistent tachycardia is the red flag of pending cardiovascular collapse.

Severe Blood Loss (>30% of Circulating Volume) or Class 3 Bleeding

Failure of compensatory mechanisms and decreased CO leads to hypotension and tissue hypoxia. Compensatory tachypnea contributes to respiratory alkalosis in the initial phase of severe bleeding. Tissue hypoxia compromises mitochondria functional capacity to generate energy as adenosine triphosphate. This leads to metabolic acidosis due to excessive production of lactic acid and cellular death.

Hypoperfusion of the kidney causes acute spasm of the preglomerular arterioles and acute tubular necrosis and renal failure. Hypoxia and excessive cytokine production can induce liver failure: sudden onset of jaundice due to hepatocellular necrosis, elevation of transaminases, coagulopathy, hypoglycemia, and encephalopathy. Myocardial ischemia is a common consequence of severe bleeding. Sepsis, thrombotic microangiopathy, and a systemic inflammatory response syndrome may occur in the late stages of uncontrolled or inadequately treated severe hemorrhage.

Evaluation

Initial assessment of the child with suspected GI bleeding should be focused on hemodynamic stability and clues for etiology of bleeding. Four major questions must be answered promptly.

1. Is the patient stable?
2. Is the bleeding real?
3. Where is the source of bleeding?
4. What is the best approach to hemostasis?

The first and the most important step in the initial assessment of the child with suspected GI bleeding is determination of hemodynamic stability. Box 109-1 outlines procedural management of GI bleeding, focusing on restoring hemostasis.

A prompt assessment of estimated blood loss and the degree of hemodynamic instability should be done using objective criteria, such as mental status, skin color, capillary refill, pulse, blood pressure, and orthostatic maneuvers (Table 109-1). Special attention should be focused on tachycardia and narrowed pulse pressure, which are the earliest signs of impending shock. Hypotension usually occurs in the late phase of shock in children and is an ominous finding. The value of the initial hematocrit may not accurately reflect the severity of blood loss. First, the hematocrit does not fall immediately with hemorrhage due to proportionate reductions of plasma and red cell volumes. Second, the hematocrit begins to fall due to compensatory restoration of the intravascular volume by the shift of extra vascular fluids into the vascular bed. This process begins shortly after the onset of bleeding; however, it is not complete for 24 to 72 hours. At this point, plasma volume is larger than normal and the hematocrit reaches its true nadir assuming that bleeding has stopped.

Box 109-1. Procedural Management of Gastrointestinal Bleeding

Endoscopic Hemostasis of Non-Variceal Bleeding

Indications

- Active bleeding from a gastric or duodenal ulcer
- Stigmata of recent bleeding: a non-bleeding visible vessel in the ulcer base and a densely adherent clot
- Bleeding arteriovenous malformation
- Bleeding after polypectomy

Methods

- Injection of vasoconstrictive agent
- Thermal coagulation
  - Bipolar coagulation
  - Heater probes
  - Argon plasma coagulation device
- Metal clips

Endoscopic Hemostasis of Variceal Bleeding

Indications

- Active bleeding from esophageal or gastric varices
- History of bleeding secondary to portal hypertension
- Failure of shunting procedure

Techniques

- Sclerotherapy
- Endoscopic variceal ligation

Polypectomy

Indication

- Juvenile polyps less than 3 cm
- Multiple polyps less than 2 cm

Table 109-1. Clinical Manifestations of Gastrointestinal Bleeding According to Blood Loss Volume

Symptoms and Signs	Blood Loss		
	<15%	15%–30%	>30%
Normal appearance	+	−	−
Anxiety	−	+	+
Disorientation	−	−	+
Lethargy	−	−	+
Tachycardia	−	++	+
Pallor	−	+	++
Livedo reticularis	−	+	++
Cold extremities	−	+	+
Capillary refill >2 seconds	−	+	+
Hypotension	−	−	+
Narrowed pulse pressure	−	+	+
Elevated diastolic pressure	−	+	−
Low diastolic pressure	−	−	+

Differential Diagnosis

There are 3 essential components of the diagnosis of GI bleeding

- Confirmation that bleeding is real
- Allocation of the bleeding area to the upper versus lower GI tract
- Detection of the specific cause of bleeding

Red staining of emesis or stool can be induced by cranberries, cranberry juice, cherries, strawberries, beets, tomatoes, candies, amoxicillin, phenytoin, and rifampin. Bismuth preparations, activated charcoal, iron, spinach, blueberries, and licorice can simulate bleeding by staining emesis and coloring stool black. An appropriate history, a normal physical examination, and guaiac-negative stool are sufficient to rule out a true bleeding episode.

It is important to remember that hematemesis and/or melena can be secondary to epistaxis. History of recent tonsillectomy and adenoidectomy, nasal allergies, dry environment, or nose-picking habits increases the probability of epistaxis. Thorough examination of the nose and oropharynx can help to establish the right diagnosis.

Detailed history and physical examination help narrow the diagnostic workup. For example, treatment with nonsteroidal anti-inflammatory drugs (NSAIDs) is a risk factor for acute gastric ulcers and bleeding from the stomach. Jaundice, hepatomegaly, spider hemangiomata, prominent vessels of the abdominal wall, or ascites are the signs of chronic liver disease and suggestive of portal hypertension. However, GI bleeding in a febrile child with hemodynamic instability and jaundice could be secondary to sepsis-related coagulopathy and acute ulcer of the stomach or the duodenum and cholestasis.

Careful assessment of the perineum can reveal the anal fissures, fistulas, or perianal inflammation.

If the source of bleeding is not obvious, the placement of a nasogastric tube is very useful. A tube with the largest bore tolerable should be placed for adequate gastric lavage: a 10F to 12F sump tube is a reasonable choice for small children; 14F to 16F for older patients. Room temperature saline is the optimal fluid for irrigation. Iced saline lavage is no longer recommended because it compromises platelet function at the bleeding site and may induce hypothermia (especially in infants) with subsequent clinically significant arrhythmia. A bloody or coffee ground aspirate indicates upper GI bleeding if epistaxis was ruled out. The absence of blood in the stomach does not exclude upper GI bleeding because the source of hemorrhage can be in the duodenum. The presence of coffee-ground fluid in gastric aspirate, which promptly clears by gastric lavage, suggests that bleeding has stopped. Failure to obtain clear return on gastric lavage indicates ongoing bleeding.

The results of blood tests give some clues to the nature of bleeding. Low hemoglobin and hematocrit with normal mean corpuscular volume (MCV) are typical for acute blood loss. An elevated blood urea nitrogen (BUN) suggests volume depletion and absorption of the blood proteins in the small intestine, which support the diagnosis of upper GI bleeding. Very low hemoglobin, hematocrit, and MCV in a hemodynamically stable patient is consistent with chronic GI blood loss.

Knowledge of common causes of GI bleeding in an age-specific group of children helps with the diagnostic strategy (Table 109-2).

In general, endoscopy is the method of choice for the diagnosis of the specific causes of acute and chronic GI bleeding related to mucosal and submucosal lesions of the GI tract. The choice of the particular type of endoscopic procedure is related to suspected pathology. Upper and lower GI endoscopy and enteroscopy are routine methods for diagnosis of such diseases as acute or peptic ulcers, esophagitis, gastritis, esophageal varices, vascular malformations, ulcerative colitis, Crohn disease, polyps, and other causes of GI bleeding. Capsule endoscopy is the new method with the unique ability to assess the entire small intestine. It is used for diagnosis of GI bleeding of obscure origin usually after negative results of conventional endoscopic procedures.

Table 109-2. Common Causes of Gastrointestinal (GI) Bleeding in Children

Age	Upper GI Bleeding	Lower GI bleeding
Neonates (0–30 days)	• Swallowed maternal blood • Stress ulcers/sepsis • Hemorrhagic gastritis • Hemorrhagic disease of the newborn	• Necrotizing enterocolitis • Midgut volvulus • Hirschsprung disease • Vascular malformation
Infants (30 days–6 mo)	• Cow's milk or soy protein allergy • Esophagitis • Prolapse gastropathy	• Anal fissure • Allergic proctitis or enterocolitis • Intestinal lymphoid hyperplasia • Intussusception
Infants and children (6 mo–6 y)	• Epistaxis • Esophagitis • Prolapse gastropathy • Portal hypertension • Drug-induced ulcers • Gastritis • Mallory-Weiss tear	• Anal fissures • Intussusception • Meckel diverticulum • Intestinal lymphoid hyperplasia • Polyps • Infectious colitis • Hemolytic uremic syndrome • Henoch-Schönlein purpura
Children and teenagers (7–18 y)	• Epistaxis • Drug-induced gastropathy and acute ulcers • Peptic ulcer • Esophagitis • Gastritis • Portal hypertension	• Infectious colitis • Ulcerative colitis • Crohn disease • Anal fissure • Polyps

Radiograph and abdominal ultrasound are useful for diagnosis of structural abnormalities such as intussusception, necrotizing enterocolitis, and malrotation.

Technetium (Tc)-99m pertechnetate scan is the diagnostic procedure of choice in children with suspected Meckel diverticulum. It is 85% sensitive and 95% specific.

A tagged red blood cell scan and angiography are alternative methods used in children with active GI bleeding of obscure origin, especially when vascular anomalies or hemobilia are suspected.

Age-Associated Causes of GI Bleeding

Neonates

In healthy breastfed neonates and infants, hematemesis could be caused by swallowed maternal blood. In such cases, careful examination of maternal breast and areola can lead to correct diagnosis. In addition, the Apt-Downey test can be useful especially in the first 3 to 4 weeks of postnatal life while concentration of fetal hemoglobin is still high. The test is based on the chemical reaction of adult hemoglobin with sodium hydroxide, which leads to a color change from bright red to yellow or crusty brown. Fetal hemoglobin is resistant to hydroxylation, and blood from the infant remains bright red.

Acute gastric or duodenal ulcers should be suspected in sick premature or full-term asphyxiated or septic newborns or patients with intracerebral bleeding, raised intracranial pressure, congenital heart disease, respiratory failure, or hypoglycemia. The typical scenario includes sudden onset of hematemesis or melena and signs of hemodynamic instability. Occasionally, severe upper GI bleeding can occur in healthy, full-term neonates within the first few days of life.

Gastrointestinal bleeding is a common manifestation of necrotizing enterocolitis (NEC).

The warning signs of NEC are abdominal distention, feeding intolerance with increased gastric residuals, mild diarrhea, hematochezia, or stool positive for occult blood.

Plain radiographs reveal nonspecific distribution of bowel gas, pneumatosis intestinalis, or gas in the portal vein, depending on the severity of bowel ischemia.

Rare causes of GI bleeding in the first month of life include Hirschsprung enterocolitis, midgut volvulus, duplication cyst, vascular malformation, and hemorrhagic disease of the newborn, particularly in breastfeeding neonates who did not receive vitamin K.

Infants Up to First 6 Months of Age

One of the leading causes of GI bleeding in infants younger than 6 months is cow's milk or soy protein allergy. The spectrum of symptoms includes recurrent vomiting, hematemesis, failure to thrive, and diarrhea with guaiac-positive stools or hematochezia.

Exclusively breastfeeding infants may develop similar symptoms on rare occasions. Elimination of cow's milk, eggs, peanuts, shellfish, and tree nuts from maternal diet may lead to resolution of allergic symptoms in the breastfeeding infant. For infants with persistent symptoms or whose mothers are unable to restrict their diet according to current recommendations and for formula-fed infants with cow's milk protein allergy, hypoallergenic (extensively hydrolyzed and free amino acid–based) formulas can be used to relieve the symptoms. Most infants with GI manifestations of cow's milk protein allergy will improve within the first 2 weeks of treatment.

An anal fissure is another common cause of bleeding in infants. The diagnosis is made by careful examination of the anus.

Intermittent rectal bleeding with streaks of frank blood mixed with normal-appearing stool can be secondary to intestinal lymphoid hyperplasia of the colon or terminal ileum. During endoscopy, multiple hemispheric smooth nodules of less than 4 mm can be found in clusters or diffusely throughout the GI tract. It results from an excessive reaction of the GI tract lymphatic tissue (lymphoid follicles and Peyer patches) to food-related or other antigens. Spontaneous regression of lymphoid follicles is quite common. In addition to parental reassurance, an elimination diet for breastfeeding mothers is a reasonable initial treatment. Feeding with extensively hydrolyzed protein formula is the next therapeutic step. Corticosteroid therapy is restricted to infants with a severe form of this disease: recurrent abdominal pain, significant anemia, persistent rectal bleeding, diarrhea, and failure to thrive. In such cases, immunodeficiency has to be excluded.

Esophagitis should be suspected as a cause of bleeding in infants with a history of recurrent emesis and interrupted feeding patterns associated with crying, irritability, or arching. The patients with repaired esophageal atresia with or without tracheoesophageal fistula are at higher risk of severe reflux disease and esophagitis. Bleeding induced by esophagitis is usually recurrent and not intensive. The patients may have hematemesis with streaks of blood or guaiac-positive stool.

Infants or older children can develop minor bleeding due to prolapse of gastric mucosa into the esophagus through the gastroesophageal junction (prolapse gastropathy). This condition is manifested by recurrent emesis with food and appearance of flecks of denatured blood at the end of vomiting. The presence of large amounts of frank blood or clots at the end of recurrent emesis suggests a more serious problem such as Mallory-Weiss tear.

Infants and Children Younger Than 7 Years

Several diseases have a higher incidence in this age group compared to other children.

The signs and symptoms of **portal hypertension** are a large-volume hematemesis; history of omphalitis associated with catheterization of the umbilical vein; presence of splenomegaly or hepatosplenomegaly; and other stigmata of chronic liver disease, such as jaundice, spider angiomas, caput medusa, and ascites. Esophageal varices are the most common site of bleeding in children with intrahepatic-sinusoidal and extrahepatic-presinusoidal forms of portal hypertension. Two-thirds of children with portal hypertension will bleed before 5 years of age. The diagnosis is based on the presence of esophageal or gastric varices or hypertensive gastropathy during an upper GI endoscopy.

Intussusception, which is more common in the first 2 years of life, is strongly considered in infants and children with sudden onset of severe, cramping abdominal pain intercepted with pain-free episodes and currant jelly stools. A lead point is often present in children older than 2 years. Diagnosis is confirmed by ultrasonography (positive: "concentric circles" or the "target-shaped" sign) or barium enema. Hydrostatic reduction of intussusceptions is successful in more than 90% of children.

Meckel diverticulum is the most common congenital anomaly in children. It is estimated that approximately 2% of infants have a remnant of the omphalomesenteric duct. However, less than 5% of children will develop complications, including GI bleeding. The predominant location of Meckel diverticulum is the distal ileum (40–60 cm above the ileocecal valve). Ectopic tissue is present in up to 80% of symptomatic patients. Gastric mucosa is the most common type of ectopia. The cause of bleeding is peptic ulceration at the junction of the ectopic gastric mucosa and normal ileum, the so-called marginal ulcer. Bleeding can be massive, but it may cease spontaneously secondary to contraction of the splanchnic vessels in response to hypovolemia. This phenomenon explains the intermittent nature of bleeding from Meckel diverticulum. Bleeding is usually painless, but sometimes coincides with recurrent abdominal pain.

The diagnostic procedure of choice is a Tc-99m pertechnetate scan.

Juvenile polyps may occur in as many as 1% of children, with peak incidence from 2 to 5 years of age. The common clinical presentation is recurrent, painless bleeding with a small amount of blood on formed stool. Diarrhea and tenesmus can occur when the polyp is large and located in the left colon.

Typical juvenile polyps are smooth, rounded, and red. Polyps of less than 1 cm are usually sessile; polyps larger than 1 cm have short or long stalks. Juvenile polyps are composed of normal and cystically dilated crypts embedded in an abundant lamina propria. Colonic mucosa adjacent to the large polyp has a distinguished, so-called chicken skin appearance. Colonoscopy is indicated due to the high incidence (almost 50%) of coexisting polyps in the descending and more proximal portions of the colon.

Endoscopic polypectomy is the treatment of choice. There is a general consensus that a single juvenile polyp is not a premalignant condition. Therefore, removal of a solid juvenile polyp is curative. Surveillance colonoscopy is not indicated unless the child develops a new episode of rectal bleeding.

Hemolytic uremic syndrome (HUS) should always be suspected in infants and toddlers with bloody diarrhea, which is present in three-quarters of children with epidemic HUS. In two-thirds of these children, *Escherichia coli* 0157:H7 can be isolated. Bloody diarrhea in HUS results from hemorrhagic colitis caused by the presence of endothelial damage produced by verotoxin and Shiga toxin and submucosal hemorrhages. Tenesmus is common. Diffuse, severe abdominal pain with peritoneal signs can occur.

The presence of the so-called thumbprinting sign on a barium enema or a computed tomography scan reflects a submucosal hemorrhage of the colon. Colitis-related symptoms last no longer than a week, followed by signs of hemolytic anemia and oliguria. Known GI complications of HUS are intussusception, pancreatitis, and intestinal obstruction. Small or large bowel perforation may occur during peritoneal dialysis, which may be performed to manage the acute renal failure that can accompany HUS.

Henoch-Schönlein purpura is most common in children younger than 7 years. The median age is 4 years. Henoch-Schönlein purpura should be suspected in children with sudden onset of severe diffuse abdominal pain, vomiting, and hematochezia following a viral illness during the winter and early spring and about a week after the appearance of purpuric-type skin lesions on the buttocks or lower extremities.

On rare occasions, GI manifestations may precede the skin rash. Severe anemia is uncommon. The small and large bowels have different degrees of hemorrhagic lesions. These may be apparent on a small bowel radiograph series or barium enema with coarsening of folds and thumbprinting. Abdominal pain and hematochezia are self-limited. Treatment with corticosteroids is controversial, although it may shorten the course of GI symptoms of abdominal pain by 1 or 2 days.

Children 7 Years and Older

The common causes of GI bleeding in this age group are listed in Table 109-2.

Drug-induced gastritis or acute ulcer should be strongly suspected in children treated with NSAIDs or oral steroids. The degree of bleeding ranges from mild to moderate. The typical clinical presentation is the sudden onset of abdominal discomfort followed by hematemesis or melena. Two types of lesions can occur: gastropathy or acute gastric ulcers due to alteration of the mucosal microcirculation and the mucosal cytoprotection related to suppression of local synthesis of prostaglandins. The incidence of NSAID-related GI bleeding is much higher in patients with *Helicobacter pylori* gastritis. Therefore, eradication of *H pylori* infection is recommended before long-term therapy with NSAIDs.

Although **peptic ulcer disease** (PUD) is relatively rare in pediatric patients, it accounts for at least a third of the cases of upper GI bleeding in school-aged children. Most bleeding ulcers are located in the duodenal bulb. At least 80% of bleeding episodes from duodenal ulcers cease spontaneously. However, if the bleeding is arterial, it may become life-threatening. Urgent endoscopy is necessary as soon as the patient becomes more stable after fluid resuscitation.

The risk factors for recurrent bleeding are large ulcer (>2 cm), location of the ulcer on the posteroinferior wall of the duodenal bulb, blood spurting from the base of the ulcer, a visible vessel, or an adherent clot. In these circumstances the risk of recurrent bleeding is relatively high even after initially successful endoscopic hemostasis and acid suppression with intravenous (IV) infusion of proton pump inhibitors. The most critical time for re-bleeding is the first 3 days following the initial hemostasis.

The risk of recurrent bleeding is minimal in children with a clear base ulcer or a pigmented spot sign, a small flat thrombus in the center of an ulcer. Endoscopic hemostasis is not indicated in these cases. Hemodynamically stable children without the endoscopically identified risk factors can be managed safely on an outpatient basis.

Colitis is the most common cause of rectal bleeding in older children and teenagers. Infectious colitis is by far more common than inflammatory bowel disease.

In general, bacterial colitis is an acute, self-limited disorder manifested by sudden onset of fever, tenesmus, and bloody diarrhea lasting from 5 to 7 days.

Chronic diarrhea (lasting ≥2 weeks) is usually associated with chronic inflammatory bowel disease. Rare causes of chronic infectious colitis are *Yersinia enterocolitica*, tuberculosis, *Entamoeba histolytica*, *Strongyloides stercoralis*, and opportunistic infections in immunocompromised patients.

Clostridium difficile colitis should be ruled out, especially in children treated with antibiotics or hospitalized patients.

Ulcerative colitis usually presents with insidious onset of diarrhea, nocturnal diarrhea, and subsequent hematochezia. Clinical manifestations of moderate to severe forms of ulcerative colitis include bloody diarrhea, abdominal cramps, urgency to defecate, malaise, anorexia with weight loss, intermittent low-grade fever, and some degree of anemia and hypoalbuminemia.

Crohn disease has a more indolent onset associated with abdominal pain, diarrhea, poor appetite, and weight loss. Diarrhea is not grossly bloody unless there is bleeding from an anal fistula or colitis that is diffuse or left-sided.

Differentiation between bacterial colitis and the early stage of chronic inflammatory bowel disease is always a challenge. A high index of suspicion and negative bacterial stool culture results, including *Yersinia* species and other rare pathogens, are essential parts of early diagnosis. The definitive diagnosis of chronic inflammatory bowel disease is based on the results of upper and lower GI endoscopy, including multiple biopsies.

Management

Resuscitation

It is imperative to initiate resuscitation of the hemodynamically unstable patient almost immediately before any diagnostic procedure is considered. Two large-bore peripheral IV lines or a central line should be placed and secured. Blood has to be typed and cross-matched and sent for baseline laboratory assessment of hemoglobin, hematocrit, MCV, platelet count, electrolytes, creatinine, BUN, liver enzymes, and clotting factors. Oxygen supplementation and large boluses of saline target restoration of circulation and tissue oxygenation. The volume of isotonic solution should be sufficient to improve tachycardia and reverse narrow pulse pressure. Blood transfusion is indicated for patients with

- Persistent tachycardia, abnormal pulse pressure, or orthostatic hypotension after replacement of 15% to 20% of blood volume with isotonic solution

- Estimated blood loss of 30% or more
- Hemoglobin 6 g/dL or less
- Uncontrolled bleeding
- Hemorrhagic shock
- Hemoglobin of 7 g/dL to 9 g/dL in children with chronic heart and lung diseases and signs of hypoxia

Packed red cells are the product of choice for replacement of blood loss. Matched whole blood is preferred for patients with massive bleeding. Fresh-frozen plasma is indicated for children with suspected or documented clotting factor deficiency including those with acute or chronic liver disease. Platelet transfusion is indicated in rare cases of severe bleeding with estimated blood loss of more than 50% of the patient's blood volume or children with active hemorrhage and platelet count less than 50,000/mm^3. Early blood transfusion is reasonable for children with active bleeding and known chronic heart or lung diseases. Monitoring of vital signs is a more accurate way to assess the effect of blood transfusion than monitoring of hematocrit soon after transfusion. It is reasonable to wait 6 hours before checking a posttransfusion hematocrit.

Octreotide (a synthetic somatostatin analogue) is effective adjuvant medical therapy of severe bleeding from esophageal or gastric varices. It should be given to the child with active hemorrhage and any evidence of chronic liver disease or previously diagnosed portal hypertension. The initial bolus of 1µg/kg of IV octreotide is followed by continuous infusion of octreotide 1µg/kg/hour. The dose can be increased every 6 hours up to 5 µg/kg/hour.

The definitive therapy of moderate to severe upper GI bleeding related to PUD or varices (esophageal or gastric) and lower GI bleeding from polyps or vascular malformation relies on endoscopic hemostasis.

Surgery should be reserved for children with severe uncontrolled bleeding from a known source or specific disorders, such as Meckel diverticulum.

Prognosis

The prognosis for infants and children with GI bleeding depends on the condition causing the bleeding. Early, aggressive treatment of the consequences of blood loss is essential to decreasing morbidity and mortality. Generally the prognosis is good, and overall mortality is less than 5%.

Selected References

Abd El-Hamid N, Taylor RM, et al. Aetiology and management of extrahepatic portal vein obstruction in children: King's College Hospital experience. *J Pediatr Gatsrenetrol Nutr.* 2008;47:630–634

Boyle JT. Gastrointestinal bleeding in infants and children. *Pediatr Rev.* 2008;29:39–52

Durno CAD. Colonic polyps in children and adolescents. *Can J Gastroenterol.* 2007; 21(4):233–239

Goyal A, Treem WR, Hyams JS. Severe upper gastrointestinal bleeding in healthy full-term neonates. *Am J Gastroenterol.* 1994;89:613–616

Kalach N, Bontems P, Koletzko S, et al. Frequency and risk factors of gastric and duodenal ulcers or erosions in children: a prospective 1-month European multicenter study. *Eur J Gastroenterol Hep.* 2010;22:1175–1181

Li Voti G, Acierno C, Tulone V, Cataliotti F. Relationship between upper gastrointestinal bleeding and non steroidal anti-inflammatory drugs in children. *Pediatr Surg Int.* 1997;12:264–265

Reveiz L, Guerrero-Lozano R, Camacho A, et al. Stress ulcer, gastritis, and gastrointestinal bleeding prophylaxis in critically ill pediatric patients: a systematic review. *Pediatr Crit Care Med.* 2010;11:125–132

Sagar J, Kumar V, Shah DK. Meckel's diverticulum: a systemic review. *J R Soc Med.* 2006;99(10):501–505

du Toit G, Meyer R, Shah N, et al. Identifying and managing cow milk protein allergy. *Arch Dis Child Pract Ed.* 2010;95(5):134–144

CHAPTER 110

Diarrhea

George Gershman, MD

CASE STUDY

An 8-month-old male infant is evaluated for a 2-day history of fever and blood-streaked, mucus-laden stools. His appetite is reduced, and he is only taking sips of diluted apple juice. He has had a single episode of vomiting. There are no ill contacts. On examination, the patient is irritable with a temperature of 102.2°F (39.0°C), a pulse of 180 beats/min, a respiratory rate of 58 breaths/min, and a blood pressure of 90/65 mm Hg. The mucous membranes are dry, the fontanelle is depressed, and the skin turgor is reduced. The abdomen is soft and bowel sounds are active.

Questions

1. What are the 4 major categories of diarrhea?
2. What are the common infectious agents that cause diarrhea in infants and children?
3. What are the characteristics of diarrheal stools caused by different etiologies?
4. What conditions lead to prolonged diarrhea in infants and children?
5. How is diarrhea managed in infants and children?

The word *diarrhea* is derived from Greek and means "to flow through." Diarrhea is characterized by increased volume of stool, which is associated with a looser consistency and an increased frequency of bowel movements. The frequency of defecation and consistency of stool vary from individual to individual. For example, wide variations in frequency of bowel movement may be seen under certain conditions such as breastfeeding. Some breastfed neonates have a bowel movement once a week, whereas others may pass stool up to 10 times a day.

Diarrhea has several causes, which include infection, inflammation, and exposure to foods and drugs that affect the absorption of water from the small and large intestines.

Epidemiology

Acute diarrhea is very common throughout the world. In the United States, acute gastroenteritis is second in frequency only to upper respiratory infections. According to the World Health Organization, 2.5 million children in Latin America, Asia, and Africa die annually from dehydration secondary to diarrhea. In contrast, approximately 400 children die from this condition in the United States each year. These children often come from lower socioeconomic classes.

In the United States, each child experiences an average of 0.9 episodes of diarrhea per year unless enrolled in a child care facility. In that case, the number increases to up to 3.2 episodes per year, a figure similar to that of children in developing nations. The leading cause of diarrhea in children in developing nations is infection with viruses, bacteria, or parasites. The severity of the infection is influenced by the underlying state of nutrition. An episode of acute gastroenteritis can precipitate severe malnutrition in marginally intact children. The fecal-oral route is the major path for the spread of infectious diarrhea. In developing nations, poor sanitation and contaminated

drinking water perpetuate the problem. In the United States, contaminated food supply, such as the contamination of eggs and poultry with *Salmonella,* is associated with the spread of bacterial gastroenteritis. Puppies have been found to be a reservoir of *Campylobacter.*

Definitions

Diarrhea is defined as stool weight more than 10 g/kg/day in infants and more than 200 g/day in older children.

Acute diarrhea comprises 2 criteria: (1) sudden onset and (2) resolution of diarrhea within 2 weeks.

Persistent diarrhea implies an acute onset of diarrhea that lasts at least 14 days. The definition is based on acute onset diarrhea that continues beyond the expected duration of an infectious etiology.

Chronic diarrhea is defined as diarrhea lasting at least 14 days and associated with specific causes (eg, celiac disease or inflammatory bowel diseases).

Clinical Presentation

The presenting symptoms include frequent, watery stools, which may contain blood or mucus. Affected children may experience fever, vomiting, bloating, and abdominal pain. Signs and symptoms of dehydration, such as decreased skin turgor, dry mucous membranes, depressed fontanel, diminished tearing, and tachycardia, may be present. Persistent diarrhea may be associated with weight loss and failure to gain weight at an appropriate rate (Dx Box).

Pathophysiology

The consistency of stool depends on the stool's water content. The movement of water through the wall of the intestine is always related to the movement of electrolytes, because no active transport of water occurs. The absorption of water is associated with the active

Dx **Diarrhea**

- Liquid stools
- Frequent stools
- Blood in stool
- Mucus in stool
- Fever
- Poor weight gain or weight loss
- Dehydration
- Vomiting
- Abdominal pain

transport of sodium, and the secretion of water is associated with the electrogenic transport of chloride. Regulatory mechanisms of water and electrolyte transport across the intestine require integration of the enteric nervous system, cells in the lamina propria, and epithelial cells. This complex system works through the generation of hormone peptides, active amines, arachidonic acid metabolites, and nitric oxide. The bulk of absorbed water crosses the intestinal epithelium between the cells (tight junctions) following the osmotic gradient generated by the transport of nutrients and electrolytes. Thus diarrhea is the reversal from the normal status of absorption to exaggerated secretion. This can be induced by 2 processes: (1) excessive osmotic load generated by ingestion of nonabsorbable sugars such as lactulose or malabsorption of lactose, or other nutrients, which generates an abnormal osmotic pressure inside the lumen of the intestine and water leak into the gut and (2) active secretion of enterocytes secondary to direct action of viral or bacterial products/toxins and different substances on the cells, particularly in the crypt areas.

Osmotic diarrhea occurs whenever digestion and/or absorption are impaired. In general, it is relatively small-volume diarrhea, which is dependent on oral intake and abolished with fasting. The most common causes of osmotic diarrhea are (1) malabsorption of carbohydrate due to excessive consumption (eg, concentrated formulas or carbonated beverages) or decreased production of brush-border enzymes or the presence of non-absorbable substances such as lactulose, sorbitol, or magnesium salts in the intestinal lumen; (2) decreased absorptive capacity of the intestine due to acute or chronic inflammation of the small bowel mucosa (eg, acute viral gastroenteritis, cow's milk protein allergy, bacterial overgrowth, giardiasis, or celiac disease); (3) lack of pancreatic enzymes or bile acid; and (4) decreased absorptive capacity of the small intestine secondary to congenital or acquired short bowel syndrome.

Recent data suggest that disruption of the differentiation of intestinal enteroendoscrine cells has profound effects on the nutrient absorption by the small intestine.

In general, nonabsorbed nutrients create an osmotic load that stimulates water leak into the intestinal lumen across the tight junction. In addition, unabsorbed nutrients, such as carbohydrates, are the substrate for fermentation by colonic bacteria with liberation of

short-chain organic acids, which create a secondary osmotic load in the large intestine and exacerbation of osmotic diarrhea.

Secretory diarrhea can be induced by any process, which creates a state of active intestinal secretion. In general, secretory diarrhea is associated with intestinal loss of large volumes of fluids, which continues despite cessation of eating. Secretory diarrhea can be induced by bacterial, viral (eg, rotavirus and HIV), or protozoon (*Cryptosporidium parvum* in immunocompromised children) infection or excessive secretion of several hormones and neuropeptides such as serotonin, histamine, cholecystokinin, etc. Secretory diarrhea is also seen with certain tumors, such as ganglioneuroblastoma, and congenital disorders of fluid and electrolyte metabolism, such as congenital chloride diarrhea. The classic example of secretary diarrhea is infection with enterotoxigenic *Escherichia coli* and *Vibrio cholerae*. Both bacteria produce toxins that bind to specific enterocyte membrane receptors and activate adenyl cyclase, and production of cyclic adenosine monophosphate (by cholera toxin and heat-labile toxin from enterotoxigenic *E coli*) or cyclic guanosine monophosphate (by heat-stable toxin produced by *E coli*). The ultimate pathway involves the opening of chloride channels and massive water loss. Secretory diarrhea is particularly common in the developing nations, where it is related to infection with organisms such as enterotoxin *E coli* and *V cholerae*. In the United States, the most common cause of secretory diarrhea is rotavirus infection. Vasoactive intestinal peptide-secreting tumors such as ganglioneuroma and neuroblastoma must be considered in the diagnosis in children with persistent secretory diarrhea.

In reality, both osmotic and secretory components are present in many cases of diarrhea.

Motility disorders such as Hirschsprung disease or pseudo-obstruction syndrome can be associated with persistent nonspecific diarrhea.

Inflammatory diarrhea occurs acutely with certain infections or chronic inflammatory bowel disease. **Steatorrhea** refers to the presence of an excessive amount of fat in the stools. Approximately 95% of the fat content of food should be absorbed. In infants younger than 12 months, 10% of ingested fat may appear in the stool. Fat malabsorption occurs with problems of the small intestine, including giardiasis, chronic liver and pancreatic disorders such as biliary atresia, and cystic fibrosis.

Differential Diagnosis

Acute Diarrhea

The major cause of diarrhea in children and infants in developed countries is **acute viral gastroenteritis.** The most common virus is rotavirus, which usually occurs during the winter months. The disorder was referred to as *winter vomiting syndrome.* Infants present with a history of antecedent mild upper respiratory symptoms, followed by fever and vomiting. Watery diarrhea, which is usually free of blood or mucus, then occurs. About 10% of infected infants have signs of otitis media. Dehydration may also occur secondary to rotavirus infection. It is typically mildly hypernatremic, with serum sodium values of about 150 mEq/L. Enteric adenovirus is the second most common viral pathogen causing diarrhea. In the summer months, enteroviral infections may produce similar diarrheal illness.

The most common **bacterial agents** associated with gastroenteritis in the United States are *Shigella, Salmonella,* and *Campylobacter. Aeromonas,* a common pathogen in developing countries, is recovered in less than 1% of cases of diarrhea in the United States.

Campylobacter produce signs of colitis, with blood and mucus in the stools. Patients are usually febrile and experience abdominal cramps. As a rule, children infected with *Shigella* are sicker, with higher levels of fever and more marked leukocytosis. In addition, infants and toddlers are particularly prone to seizures. Infection with *Salmonella* may also be associated with high fever. Stools may be mucus-laden, and inflammation of the small intestine may be evident. Parasitic infections, particularly with *Giardia lamblia, Entamoeba histolytica,* and *Cryptosporidium parvum,* may be associated with diarrhea and may follow a more protracted course. Infestation with these organisms does not usually result in fever.

Infectious conditions that do not affect the gastrointestinal (GI) tract (otitis media and urinary tract infection) may also be associated with diarrhea. Sixty percent of children with hepatitis A develop diarrhea in the first week of illness. Other conditions may also result in diarrhea. In newborns, infection with *E coli* may produce epidemic outbreaks of large, explosive, watery, green stools without blood. These outbreaks may result in closure of newborn nurseries. Watery stools may herald the onset of **necrotizing enterocolitis;** blood is usually present, however. Necrotizing enterocolitis most often affects preterm infants with respiratory distress syndrome. The pathogenesis of necrotizing enterocolitis remains largely unknown. One of the risk factors appears to be hypoxia and ischemia related to pulmonary immaturity. The mechanism of disease production seems to be related to hypoxia of the intestinal mucosa. Feeding intolerance, bloody stools, pneumatosis intestinalis, and air in the portal vein are the hallmarks of the disorder. Enterocolitis may also occur in infants with Hirschsprung disease. Adrenal insufficiency, as well as certain inborn errors of metabolism, such as galactosemia, may lead to diarrhea. In general, other symptoms such as vomiting occur. Infants may present in shock because of hypovolemia related to dehydration.

Food intolerance may result in diarrhea in infants as well as in older children. Overfeeding or the ingestion of large quantities of fruit juices, dried fruits, or sorbitol-containing products can produce osmotic diarrhea. Food allergies may also be associated with malabsorption. In infants, cow protein intolerance can produce diarrhea, growth retardation, anemia, hypoproteinemia, edema, respiratory symptoms, and eczema. Eosinophilia and elevated levels of immunoglobulin E are uncommon in infants with cow's milk protein allergy. Because 25% to 50% of cow protein–allergic children are also soy protein–allergic, symptoms of diarrhea may not abate when soy formula is offered. However, soy formula does help infants with lactase deficiency. Congenital lactose intolerance is an extremely rare disorder. Acquired lactase deficiency is fairly common, especially in certain racial groups; it is reported in 10% of whites, 70% to 80%

of African Americans, and 90% of Asians. The disorder is associated with diarrhea, cramping, bloating, and abdominal pain after consumption of lactose. The stool has an acid pH, floats because it contains air, and is positive for reducing substances. Lactase deficiency may occur following an episode of acute gastroenteritis, when the brush border of the small intestine has been disrupted.

Persistent Diarrhea

Infants and children may have a protracted course of loose stools following an episode of acute gastroenteritis.

Risk factors for persistent diarrhea are
- Caloric and protein malnutrition
- Vitamin A and zinc deficiency
- Prior infection such as measles
- Male gender and young age between 6 and 24 months
- Young maternal age

In most cases, no cause for persistent diarrhea can be detected, but infestation with *Shigella* or enterotoxigenic *E coli* may be a contributing factor. The possibility of infection with HIV should be considered in infants and children with protracted diarrhea, especially in geographic areas where disease prevalence is high. Certain children with acute diarrhea have such a modified diet (eg, clear fluids) that they develop starvation stools. These slimy, dark green or golden stools represent succus entericus, the secretion of the small intestine. Starvation stools do not have a fecal odor. Insufficient fat in the diet may contribute to starvation diarrhea.

Chronic Diarrhea

Inflammatory bowel disease, which occurs more commonly in older children and adolescents, is associated with chronic diarrhea. Ulcerative colitis presents with infiltration of the lamina propria with inflammatory cells, distortion of the glands, and crypt abscesses. Fever, weight loss, and anorexia are often present. Diarrhea is the hallmark of the disease, and patients experience tenesmus as well as mucus-laden and bloody stools. Inflammation always affects the rectum. It can be localized in the left colon (left-side colitis) or spread out through the entire large intestine (pancolitis).

Crohn disease may also lead to chronic diarrhea, although lower abdominal pain aggravated by defecation may be a more prominent part of the medical history. Affected individuals frequently experience extraintestinal manifestations of the disease, such as fever, anorexia, weight loss or growth retardation, recurrent stomatitis, uveitis, arthralgia and arthritis, and clubbing. Perianal disease, such as fistulas, may be noted in 30% of patients.

Irritable bowel syndrome may lead to chronic diarrhea in infants and children. Affected children do not suffer from diarrhea at night, which is the sign of infectious or secretory diarrhea. Partially formed first stool in the morning and increased frequency during the day is the classic history. Bowel movement tends to occur after each meal, suggesting a prominent gastrocolic reflex. Children may have 3 to 10 stools per day, which may be mucus-laden and contain undigested vegetable fiber. Alternating periods of constipation may occur. Affected children appear well throughout this illness, without weight loss, growth impairment, fever, leukocytosis, steatorrhea, or protein malabsorption. Their appetite remains good. Treatment of this type of chronic diarrhea involves the use of a high-residue diet to add bulk to the stool and thereby prevent small, frequent stools. Other conditions that lead to chronic diarrhea include intestinal polyposis; the use of certain medications, such as antibiotics; and the use of heavy metals, such as iron.

Chronic diarrhea may also be associated with **maldigestion**, as with cystic fibrosis, or **malabsorption,** as with celiac disease or gluten enteropathy.

Newborns with **cystic fibrosis** may present with meconium ileus or rarely with acute appendicitis. Failure to thrive is common among patients with cystic fibrosis despite the fact that many of them have voracious appetites. Stools are large, bulky, and foul-smelling secondary to the steatorrhea. Isolated GI complaints are reported in 15% to 20% of patients with cystic fibrosis, but most affected children are also prone to pulmonary infections. Rectal prolapse is another complication.

Celiac disease is related to an immunologic reaction to the gliadin portion of the wheat protein, gluten. This protein is also found in barley, rye, and oat. Characteristically, villous flattening is apparent on small intestinal biopsy. This flattening restricts the absorptive capacity of the intestine and leads to malabsorption. Children with the classic form of celiac disease have short stature, pale skin, sparse hair, protuberant abdomen, and wasted buttocks. In recent reports, subtle signs of celiac disease have been recognized and usually reflect the growth failure or anemia. Symptoms appear a few months after grains are introduced into the diet, usually between the ages of 9 and 12 months. Stools are mushy, bulky, and foul-smelling. Fat content in the stool may be 2 to 3 times the normal level.

Evaluation

History

A careful history should be obtained (Questions Box).

Physical Examination

Children should be assessed for the presence of dehydration as evidenced by altered vital signs, delayed capillary refill, decreased skin turgor, a sunken fontanelle, dry mucous membranes, and reduced tearing. Skin changes in the perianal area or evidence of diaper dermatitis would indicate the irritative nature of the stools. Perianal fissures may be present in Crohn disease. Evidence of growth retardation should be determined by assessing the growth parameters, particularly weight. Failure to gain weight over a period of months should trigger the workup of GI disorders such as chronic inflammatory bowel disease, celiac disease, or cystic fibrosis.

Laboratory Tests

Stool assessment, a major component of the evaluation, involves 4 steps. First, the stool is evaluated for its quantity as well as its gross appearance. Undigested pieces of fruits and vegetables in the stool

Questions

Diarrhea

- How long has the diarrhea been present?
- How frequent is the stooling?
- What is the consistency of the stools?
- Is stooling related to eating, which is a sign of osmotic diarrhea, or does it occur even if the child does not eat, which is a sign of secretory diarrhea?
- Do the stools contain any blood or mucus, which suggests a bacterial or parasitic infection?
- Is the child febrile?
- Does the child have any symptoms associated with the stooling problems?
- Does the child have a recent history of travel or exposure to animals?
- Is anyone at home ill?
- Has the child experienced any change in the frequency of urination, which is an important measure of the state of hydration?
- What is the child's diet now? What has it been?

of toddlers are often a sign of poor chewing. Small, thread-like bodies that resemble worms are concretions of bile and are common in the stool of infants. The change in stool volume with fasting can also be checked. Reduced volume in the face of fasting is consistent with osmotic diarrhea.

Second, the stool is subjected to chemical and microscopic analyses to detect the presence of unabsorbed nutrients such as carbohydrates and fats. The presence of carbohydrates may be detected using a small amount of stool liquified in about 1 mL of water. A Clinitest tablet is added to the sample, and a change in color from blue to green or orange is indicative of the presence of undigested carbohydrate. If the main source of dietary sugar is sucrose, as determined by the history, the specimen must be hydrolyzed by heating with hydrochloric acid. If the specimen sits around for too long, the presence of bacteria in the stool may break down the carbohydrate and lead to a false-negative result. The presence of fat can be determined both qualitatively and quantitatively. The stool may be examined under a microscope with just water or using a Sudan or Carmine red stain. If there are 10 or more globules of fat per high-power field, a quantitative fat analysis over a 3-day period should be undertaken. Ten percent of children with abnormal stool fat on microscopic assessment have a normal 3-day quantitative stool fat value. Quantification of fecal elastase-1 is an accurate alternative approach for diagnosis of exocrine pancreatic insufficiency in children with cystic fibrosis.

Third, the stool is examined for the presence of blood and leukocytes. Blood may be present in the stool but originates from excoriations in the diaper area rather than from the GI tract. To assess for leukocytes in the stool, the mucus component of the stool should be smeared on a glass slide and stained with methylene blue. More than 2 to 4 leukocytes per high-power field is abnormal and suggests a bacterial infection. The sensitivity of the fecal leukocyte test is 85% but the specificity is only 50% to 60%. Absence of leukocytes or erythrocytes in the stool signifies a very low probability of an invasive bacterial infection (predictive value of a negative test is 95%). A stool specimen should be submitted for culture and may be evaluated for ova and parasites. Stool analysis using Rotazyme will detect rotavirus. Fourth, stool is assessed for levels of sodium and potassium and stool osmolality to calculate the so-called ion gap (ion gap = stool osmolarity − [(Na+K) × 2]). Ion gap exceeding 100 mOsm/kg and low sodium concentration in stool (<40 mEq/L) is typical for osmotic diarrhea. On the contrary, ion gap equal to or lower than 100 mOsm/kg and sodium concentration in stool higher than 70 mEq/L is consistent with secretory diarrhea.

Additional studies, especially in the face of dehydration or fever, include serum electrolytes, complete blood cell count, urinalysis, and urine culture. Serological markers such as tissue transglutaminase and antiendomysial antibodies are good screening tests of gluten enteropathy. Upper GI endoscopy with a small bowel biopsy is indicated for confirmation of celiac disease or diagnosis of other causes of persistent or chronic malabsorptive diarrhea. Colonoscopy should be considered after consultation with a gastroenterologist if inflammatory bowel disease or familial polyposis is suspected.

Management

Initial management of children with gastroenteritis involves **adequate hydration and replacement of any fluid or electrolyte deficits** (see Chapter 66). Bolus therapy may be necessary in children with significant dehydration. Children with significant dehydration may require admission to the hospital and the administration of intravenous fluids. Less severely affected children may be managed as outpatients using oral rehydrating solutions such as Pedialyte or Infalyte. Alternatively, parents can be advised to make oral rehydrating solutions by using water (1 liter), sugar (4–8 teaspoons), and salt (½ teaspoon).

Dietary manipulation in the treatment of diarrhea is somewhat controversial. Traditionally, affected children have been placed on clear fluids for 1 or 2 days, with a gradual return to a more regular diet with time. A **BRAT diet** (bananas, rice or rice cereal, applesauce, tea or toast) was often recommended because of the intrinsic binding properties of the particular food. Recent studies recommend a full resumption of a normal diet, including dairy products, as the way to ensure adequate nutrition during the acute illness. A high-fat, low-carbohydrate diet accelerates improvement. A lactose-free diet is beneficial for infants and children with persistent diarrhea.

Antimicrobial therapy is indicated for infection with certain pathogens such as *Campylobacter, E histolytica, G lamblia,* and *Shigella.* Antimicrobial agents are used to treat *Salmonella* infection in certain populations such as neonates, immunodeficient children, and children with sickle cell anemia. **Antidiarrheal agents** are not usually recommended for the management of diarrhea in children. Diarrhea is believed to be the body's way of eliminating a toxic substance that has been ingested. In addition, the diarrhea often progresses in spite of the medication, which has its most binding effect after the illness has subsided, leading to constipation.

Children with chronic diarrhea secondary to a specific condition should be managed as dictated by the particular disorder.

Prognosis

Most cases of diarrhea in infants and children in the United States are self-limited and resolve without problems. More chronic cases may lead to malnutrition. Enteral feedings or hyperalimentation may be used to ensure a good outcome. Some children require consultation with a pediatric gastroenterologist.

CASE RESOLUTION

In the case history, the presence of blood and mucus in the stool suggests a bacterial etiology. The stool should be examined microscopically for leukocytes using methylene blue. Their presence supports a bacterial etiology. A stool specimen as well as a blood specimen should be sent for culture. Because the infant appears dehydrated (ie, sunken fontanelle, poor skin turgor, tachycardia), admission to the hospital should be considered to allow for rehydration and the administration of parenteral antibiotics.

Selected References

Gastanaduy AS, Beque RE. Acute gastroenteritis. *Clin Pediatr.* 1999;38:1–12

Grimwood K, Forbes DA. Acute and persistent diarrhea. *Pediatr Clin North Am.* 2009;56(6):1343–361

Guandalini S, Kahn SA. Acute diarrhea. In: Walker WA, Goulet OJ, Kleinman RE, et al, eds. *Pediatric Gastrointestinal Disease, Pathophysiology, Diagnosis, Management.* 5th ed. Philadelphia, PA: B.C. Decker; 2008:253–264

Guarino A, De Marco G. Persistent diarrhea. In: Walker WA, Goulet OJ, Kleinman RE, et al, eds. *Pediatric Gastrointestinal Disease, Pathophysiology, Diagnosis, Management.* 5th ed. Philadelphia, PA: B.C. Decker; 2008:265–274

Koletzko S, Osterrieder S. Acute infectious diarrhea in children. *Dtsch Arztebl Int.* 2009;106(33):539–548

Limbos MA. Approach to the child with diarrhea. In: Osborn LM, DeWitt TG, First LR, Zenel JA, eds. *Pediatrics.* Philadelphia, PA: Mosby; 2005:627–633

Pietzac MM, Thomas DW. Childhood malabsorption. *Pediatr Rev.* 2003; 24:195–206

Sondheimer JM. Office stool examination: a practical guide. *Contemp Pediatr.* 1994; suppl:5–14

Talusan-Soriano K, Lake AM. Malabsorption in childhood. *Pediatr Rev.* 1996; 17:135–142

Walker-Smith JA. Chronic diarrhea. In: Lifschitz CH, ed. *Pediatric Gastroenterology and Nutrition in Clinical Practice.* New York, NY: Dekker; 2002: 685–700

CHAPTER 111

Constipation

Doron D. Kahana, MD, and George Gershman, MD

CASE STUDY

A 6-year-old child is brought to the office by her mother who reports 6 months of episodic belly pain. The mother states that the child complains mostly in the afternoon and evening and rarely at night or morning. The pain will last a few minutes and is sometimes severe. She notes that her daughter vomited once and had soiled her underwear on a few occasions. She believes the child toilets daily but has not asked or supervised her directly. The mom reports that the toilet was plugged a few times after the child defecated. The child has a great appetite and eats an age-appropriate diet that is high in pastas, breads, cow's milk, and cheese. The child at times is gassy and looks bloated. Otherwise the child is healthy, growing and developing normally, and is in first grade. On examination, vital signs are normal, she is at the 75th percentile in height and 90th percentile in weight. On questioning the child as to the specific location of her pain, she points to her umbilicus. On deep palpation there is a firm mass in the left lower quadrant; it is non-tender and the abdomen is otherwise soft. A rectal examination reveals hard, dry stool in the vault. The rest of the examination is normal.

Questions

1. What is the definition of constipation?
2. How is the stooling pattern related to diet?
3. What diseases and medical conditions are associated with constipation?
4. How do familial factors influence stooling patterns?
5. What is the management of chronic constipation?

Introduction

Constipation is a common and significant complaint that accounts for approximately 3% of visits to pediatric clinics and up to 25% of pediatric gastroenterology visits. Clinically, it is defined by stools that are dry, hard, and/or difficult to pass. Reduced *frequency* of stooling is a common characteristic of constipation, but is not universal or definitive. The guidelines of the North American Society for Pediatric Gastroenterology, Hepatology and Nutrition define constipation as "a delay or difficulty in defecation, present for two or more weeks and sufficient to cause significant distress to the patient." Normal stooling frequency averages 3 to 4 per day during the first weeks of life and decreases to 1 to 2 per day with introduction of table foods by 1 year of age. After age 4 and into adulthood, normal stool frequency ranges from 3 per day to 3 per week.

Many factors influence the frequency of stooling in normal infants and young children, including diet, familial pattern of intestinal motility, personal sensitivity, hygiene habits, hydration status, variable stressors, and intake of medications. Exclusively breastfed infants may have long intervals (sometimes several days) between normal bowel movements.

Functional constipation is defined as constipation in the absence of organic disease; however, it is important to note that chronic constipation is also a condition that begets disease and, thus, must be treated appropriately. Constipation is one of a number of unique medical conditions that create a positive feedback loop; stool withholding results in worsening constipation as stretch receptors accommodate a distended rectum and contractile forces fail to result in complete evacuation.

In infancy, peristaltic motility may be weak or poorly coordinated, and the lack of physical mobility/ambulation requires the infant to exert a physiological effort (ie, Valsalva maneuver) to allow passage of stool. Parents may interpret "straining" as a sign of constipation despite the passage of soft, normal stools. Therapy in such cases, if necessary, is usually non-medical and involves manual stimulation of the anal sphincters and mobilization of the infant. Older infants and toddlers may have constipation secondary to food intolerance, such as cow's milk protein allergy, and removal of the inciting agent may result in complete resolution. Toilet training can prove to be a challenge, especially in constipated toddlers, and stressful parent–child interactions may result in resistance on the part of the child.

Commonly, chronic constipation in childhood is triggered by a painful evacuation that results in an unpleasant experience. School-aged children may elect to withhold stool because of fear of toileting outside the home or because of social stressors (eg, parental divorce, bullying). Assessment of the etiology of constipation requires a careful medical history to determine the age of onset, the characteristic of the stool, and the presence of contributing factors. After all, regular toileting is a sign of good health.

Epidemiology

Prevalence of constipation in infants is less than 3% and increases between the ages of 2 and 4 years. Onset often coincides with toilet training and dietary changes, as well as increased colonic transit time. Longer transit allows for more extensive colonic fermentation of food residue, salvage of micronutrients, and greater resorption of water, but it is associated with firmer, drier stools that may trigger abdominal and rectal discomfort. Defecation may become unpleasant and lead to stool withholding behavior.

Prevalence of constipation in infants and toddlers is equal among males and females, but it becomes 3 times more frequent in boys than in girls by age 5 years. Fecal soiling, or encopresis, a significant comorbidity, is reported in up to one-third of females and half of males with severe, chronic constipation (see Chapter 53).

Clinical Presentation

Infants often present with infrequent stooling. Some parents report facial grimacing and grunting during defecation as well as apparent discomfort or fussiness with bowel movements. History of delayed passage of meconium, recurrent vomiting, or poor weight gain indicates the need for further evaluation. Toddlers usually present complaining of abdominal pain and reporting the passage of hard or large stools. School-aged children may have fecal soiling, which usually represents overflow incontinence (only 10%–15% of all cases of encopresis are non-fecal retentive). Parents describe a stool withholding posture, where the legs are clamped together and the gluteal muscles are contracted in an effort to suppress defecation (Figure 111-1). Poor appetite and episodic vomiting in severe cases are secondary to a persistent sense of fullness from a dilated and impacted colon. Hydronephrosis, urinary tract infections, and enuresis are also associated with chronic constipation and an impacted colon.

Pathophysiology

What Is the Colon?

The colon is a muscular organ that processes dietary residue through bacterial fermentation, salvaging nutrients and reabsorbing more than 90% of the water that enters, and prepares stool for transient storage and eventual excretion (Figure 111-2). Fermented food residue produces gas (eg, hydrogen, methane) and short-chain fatty acids; the latter provide colonocytes with readily available fuel (via butyric acid) and enter the portal circulation for calorie salvage in the liver (eg, propionic and acetic acids). The fermentation process may release other micronutrients and vitamins and is thus an important component of colonic function.

Normal Physiology

Digested food normally takes about 2 to 6 hours to reach the cecum from the duodenum (gastric emptying half-time is normally 60–90 minutes). The propagation of food in the small intestine occurs via peristaltic waves called the migrating motor complex. Once chyme is in the cecum, peristalsis slows down and it may take several hours or days for it to be expelled as stool. The longer

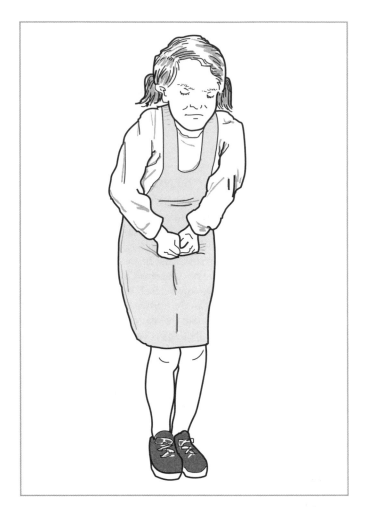

Figure 111-1. **Child exhibiting retentive posture.**

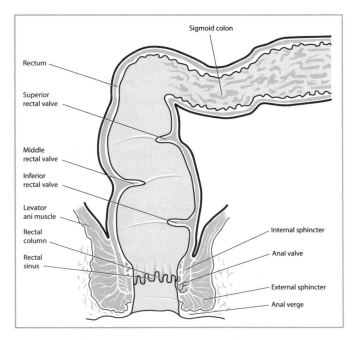

Figure 111-2. **Diagram of anus, rectum, and sigmoid colon.**

the transit time, the more extensive the water resorption and the more likely it is for the stool to be dry and hard. The rectosigmoid is the sensing organ that initiates the process of defecation and can store stool until it is socially acceptable to expel it. Contraction and emptying of the rectosigmoid is stimulated by eating, a process called the *gastrocolic reflex*. In the rectum, the pelvic floor muscles (levator ani, puborectalis) regulate fecal retention and defecation. The puborectalis suspends the rectosigmoid and imposes constraints that facilitate voluntary stool retention (continence). Continence is also promoted by contraction of the internal and external anal sphincters.

Defecation

The urge to defecate is signaled by the propulsion of feces from the sigmoid colon to the rectum. Distention of the rectum causes relaxation of the internal anal sphincter; the external anal sphincter and puborectalis must voluntarily relax under parasympathetic conditions. The pelvic floor muscles descend, permitting straightening of the anus and rectum (see Figure 111-2). Thus defecation is facilitated by squatting or sitting and by increasing intra-abdominal pressure. The urge to defecate can be consciously repressed by voluntary contraction of the external anal sphincter and likely subconscious sympathetic reflex inhibition and contraction of the puborectalis muscle. The process of defecation is learned early in childhood and remains spontaneous throughout life. The spontaneity of this process may be lost for a variety of reasons, including secondary to trauma, pelvic floor dysfunction (dyssynergia), pseudo-obstruction, or surgical resection.

The Vicious Cycle of Constipation

If the urge to defecate is suppressed, the rectosigmoid and eventually the entire colon will become dilated and impacted, and defecation may become difficult. The increased caliber of the colonic lumen makes contractions weaker and less effective in propagating stool. Moreover, the constipated child may become desensitized to rectal distention. Eventually, delayed defecation leads to formation of hard, bulky stool, which makes defecation difficult and painful. The child learns to tighten the external anal sphincter and gluteal muscles, pushing feces higher into the rectal vault and suppressing the urge to defecate—this is the vicious cycle of constipation (Figure 111-3). In children, the initiating event may be a painful evacuation, possibly after an acute illness (eg, cold, respiratory infection). Intentional and prolonged suppression of defecation is an important factor in the pathogenesis of chronic constipation.

Familial Factors

Some families are predisposed to constipation. Concordance for constipation is 4 times more common in monozygotic twins than dizygotic twins. It may be related to increased absorption of water or an unusually long or poorly motile colon. Poor sensitivity to a critical rectal volume or the need for a particularly large rectal volume may delay the initiation of defecation in genetically predisposed individuals.

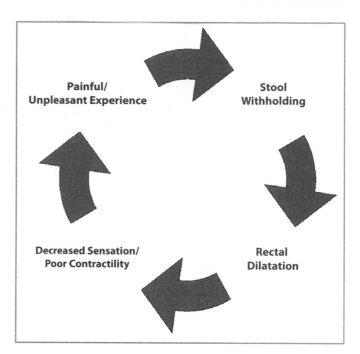

Figure 111-3. The vicious cycle of constipation.

Differential Diagnosis

The differential diagnosis of constipation can be divided into congenital versus acquired and then into the following etiologic categories: anatomical; neurologic; hormonal; infectious/toxic; drug-induced/metabolic; functional or other, such as genetic or allergic (Box 111-1). Functional constipation is supported by a characteristic history that includes poor dietary and hydration habits, stool withholding behavior, and a normal physical examination. Dietary history may reveal high consumption of cow's milk (>24 oz/day), cheese, or sugary fruit juice, as well as poor intake of fruits, vegetables, and whole grains. Stool withholding is most commonly seen in young, school-aged children and often is a product of a stressful environment such as a new sibling, a move, parental struggles, or a new school environment.

Chronic constipation that is resistant to medical therapy should not be ignored. Conditions such as Hirschsprung disease and congenital intestinal malrotation can present past the neonatal period and may lead to intestinal devastation (eg, volvulus and ischemia). Several conditions are particularly important to consider when evaluating constipation in infants, including Hirschsprung disease, hypothyroidism, anal stenosis/atresia, meningomyelocele (occulta), and cerebral palsy. Failure to pass meconium, or a delay in the passage of meconium (meconium ileus) beyond 24 hours, should also raise suspicion for a congenital or genetic aberration (eg, Hirschsprung, cystic fibrosis).

Hirschsprung disease is an intestinal motility disorder resulting from aganglionosis of the myenteric plexus that usually affects the rectosigmoid. However, the entire colon can be involved in a distal to proximal distribution. The severity of the disease and complexity of surgical treatment is directly proportional to the length of the affected colon. When ganglion cells are missing in the very distal

					Drug-Induced/	
Box 111-1. Differential Diagnosis of Constipation						
Anatomical	*Neurologic*	*Hormonal*	*Other*	*Infectious/Toxic*	*Metabolic*	*Functional*
• Anal stenosis • Imperforate anus • Ectopic anus • Postsurgical stricture	• Hirschsprung disease • Cerebral palsy • Hypotonia • Spina bifida (occulta) • Meningomyelocele • Sacral agenesis • Intestinal pseudo-obstruction syndrome	• Hypothyroidism • Panhypopituitarism • Multiple endocrine neoplasia • Pheochromocytoma	• Cystic fibrosis • Celiac disease • Cow's milk protein allergy	• Post-infectious ileus • Botulism	• Analgesics (opioids) • Antacids • Anticholinergics • Bismuth • Iron • Cholestyramine • Hypocalcemia • Hyperkalemia	• Dehydration • Stool withholding • Stress • Anxiety • Fear of painful evacuation

portion of the rectum, the disorder may resemble chronic idiopathic constipation, often recalcitrant to medical therapy. The prevalence of Hirschsprung disease is about 1 in 5,000 live births and may account for up to 3% of all cases of constipation referred to a gastroenterologist. Physical examination of a patient with Hirschsprung disease may reveal some degree of abdominal distention and an empty rectal vault. In infants, a rectal examination frequently induces explosive stool due to distention of the internal anal sphincter. Early recognition of this condition is important to prevent the development of toxic megacolon and enterocolitis, a condition that carries high morbidity and mortality. Hirschsprung disease may be seen in conjunction with syndromes such as trisomy 21, Smith-Lemli-Opitz, and Waardenburg syndromes, and several genetic mutations in the receptor tyrosine kinase gene *RET* have been described as responsible for the pathogenic mechanism.

Infants with hypothyroidism secondary to hypopituitarism may also present with constipation and are not diagnosed through the newborn screening process because of normal (ie, low) levels of thyroid-stimulating hormone. These children may either appear clinically normal or display some of the features of hypothyroidism (eg, large fontanel, umbilical hernia, coarse facies, macroglossia).

Anal stenosis, imperforate anus with a perineal fistula, or an anteriorly displaced anus may not be recognized immediately in the newborn period because the condition may be subtle. Anorectal malformations occur in about 1 in 7,000 live births, which reinforces the need for a perianal and rectal examination with every constipated child.

Severe constipation that begins prior to toilet training is more suggestive of an organic etiology, such as Hirschsprung, malrotation, or pseudo-obstruction. Pseudo-obstruction may present in older children with a history of intermittent constipation, abdominal distention, pain, nausea, and vomiting. Onset of constipation around the time of toilet training, when stooling had been normal in the past, suggests functional constipation.

Constipation may develop in some children in association with the use of medications such as iron or bismuth (Pepto-Bismol), codeine or other narcotics, chemotherapeutic agents (eg, vincristine),

and agents with anticholinergic properties (eg, pseudoephedrine, imipramine).

Evaluation

History

Commonly associated historical signs and symptoms of constipation include abdominal pain (especially during and after meals), abdominal distention, excessive flatulence, hard stools, dyschezia (painful evacuations), bright-red blood per rectum, toilet plugging episodes, and urinary symptoms (eg, enuresis, recurrent infections) (Questions Box). Overflow incontinence may mislead the clinician to a differential diagnosis for chronic diarrhea. Fecal soiling due to stool retention and overflow is noted in many children with severe, chronic constipation, although a complete physical examination in such a

---

Questions

Constipation

- What is the child's stooling pattern? How often does the child have a bowel movement? What is the appearance and consistency of the stool?
- What was the child's age when the problem began?
- What makes up the child's diet?
- Does the child take any medications?
- Does the child have any symptoms associated with constipation, such as recurrent abdominal pain? If so, how long have these been occurring?
- Has the child been sick recently with any illnesses that might cause constipation?
- Has the child recently experienced any changes in routine that could cause constipation?
- Is there a family history of constipation?
- How old was the child when he or she was toilet trained?
- Is there any bleeding with stooling?
- Is there pain with stooling?
- Have any remedies such as laxatives, enemas, or suppositories been used to relieve the symptoms?

setting should reveal both a stool mass in the lower left abdominal quadrant and an impacted colon or rectum on digital manipulation. As with all conditions that present with abdominal pain, it is important to screen for the presence of recurrent mouth sores, skin rashes, joint pain, weight loss, bloody or mucosy stools, incomplete evacuations, and tenesmus (rectal spasm accompanied by a strong urge to defecate, often with the passing of blood and/or mucus). Family history of inflammatory bowel disease, celiac disease, irritable bowel syndrome, constipation, and atopy (eg, food allergy) should also be noted with every child presenting with abdominal pain.

Physical Examination

The physical examination in cases of functional constipation is usually normal. If the child is complaining of abdominal pain, ask the child to indicate the area of greatest pain with one finger. In functional disease, the child most often will point directly to the umbilicus. Palpation may reveal a firm stool mass in the left lower quadrant that is classically non-tender. Consistency and color of the stool in the rectum will vary, but a hard and dry stool is strongly suggestive of stool impaction. An empty rectum should raise suspicion for an organic etiology. Digital manipulation followed by an "explosive" passage of stool is suggestive of Hirschsprung disease. The back of the child should be inspected for a sacral dimple or a hair tuft, especially in infants, as this may be a sign of occult spinal cord anomaly.

Signs of pallor, mouth sores, hepatosplenomegaly, arthritis, or skin rashes may suggest another underlying disease process.

Laboratory Tests

Malnourishment is possible if the child consumes a restricted diet (eg, more than 24 ounces of cow's milk or soda per day) or has a suggestive physical examination (eg, pallor, dry skin). Iron-deficiency anemia and mineral deficiencies (eg, calcium, zinc) are signs of poor nutritional intake. A lipid panel may reveal high triglycerides (from excessive sugar intake) and low high-density lipoprotein (from poor quality fat intake). Thyroid function may require evaluation in certain cases.

Imaging Studies

A flat plate of the abdomen is usually not indicated, but may help on a clinical level by showing the child and/or parents the significant amount of stool present. Anatomical studies such as a barium upper gastrointestinal series evaluate for malrotation, a congenital stricture, imperforate anus, or Hirschsprung disease. It is recommended for barium enema to be performed without a prior clean-out, in order to sensitize the study for the presence of a transitional zone.

Further Tests

Anorectal manometry and a suction rectal biopsy may be carried out by a gastroenterologist to help diagnose Hirschsprung disease; however, only a full-thickness rectal biopsy will confirm the presence or absence of aganglionosis and must be performed by a surgeon. Colonic manometry can also measure colonic peristaltic waves and help diagnose pseudo-obstruction and other dysmotility disorders.

Management

In the Primary Care Setting

Most cases of constipation can be evaluated and managed by primary care physicians. In functional constipation, the mainstay of management involves a 3-pronged approach of dietary therapy, behavioral modification, and medications (Figure 111-4).

Diets that predispose to constipation are rich in simple carbohydrates (eg, sugar), refined and processed carbohydrates (eg, pasta), saturated fat (eg, fried food), processed meat (eg, hotdogs), and dairy (especially milk and cheese). Dietary therapy should begin by decreasing the intake of these food items and increasing the intake of fruit, vegetables, whole grains, legumes, and tree nuts. Prune juice and fruit nectars (eg, pear, peach, apricot) may be supplemented and are well tolerated, effective, and may be mixed with the child's favorite drink. Most fruit, such as pears, papaya, and cantaloupe, as well as vegetables, roots, and tree nuts are high in beneficial fiber. Dried fruit (eg, raisins, cranberries) are rich in sorbitol and thereby cathartic. It is important to continuously introduce new food items to the diet, especially fruit and vegetables. Introduction of certain foods, such as whole grain breads and brown rice, may need to be gradual and require some adjustment, but will render life-long benefits (Box 111-2).

Behavior modification can also be challenging, but absolutely essential to breaking the vicious cycle. Teaching of proper "toilet hygiene" to the child should be done in a firm and consistent manner, and engaging the child with a sticker or star chart may help. In short, it is recommended that the child sit on the toilet once or twice daily for 8 to 10 minutes at a time, preferably after a meal (taking advantage of the gastrocolic reflex). Longer toilet sitting should be discouraged as it may lead to perianal disease such as a fissure or hemorrhoids. Even if the child fails to have a bowel movement with each toilet sitting, good toilet hygiene will make the experience a routine and hopefully help prevent further reluctance to use the toilet. Biofeedback is useful when available, especially

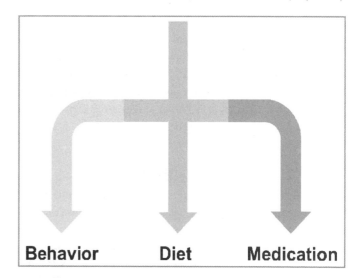

Behavior   Diet   Medication

Figure 111-4. **Three-pronged management of constipation.**

Box 111-2. Dietary Therapy in Chronic Constipation						
Avoid/Decrease			Introduce/Increase			
Simple/Processed Carbohydrates	Fat	Meat/Dairy	Fruit/Nectar	Dried Fruit	Vegetables/ Roots	Legumes/Tree Nuts/Seeds
• Sugar • Corn syrup • Soda • White bread • White rice • Pastries/biscuits • Pasta/macaroni • Potato/corn chips	• Fried food • Saturated fat • Trans fat • Animal fat • Gravy • Vegetable oil	• Processed meat • Red meat • Ground beef • Cold cuts • Cow's milk • Cheese • Cream	• Pears • Plums • Papaya • Peaches • Pineapple • Apples • Berries • Cantaloupe	• Prunes • Raisins • Apricots • Cranberries • Cherries • Dates	• Asparagus • Broccoli • Cauliflower • Carrots • Spinach • Yams • Parsnip • Celery • Beets	• Red beans • Garbanzo beans • Peas • Cashews • Almonds • Walnuts • Pistachios • Sunflower seeds • Flaxseed

in children with encopresis and/or paradoxical contraction of the external anal sphincter.

Medications are generally safe and largely over the counter (Box 111-3). The 2 most commonly used medications are polyethylene glycol (PEG-3350), a nonabsorbable high molecular weight synthetic polymer (non-fermentable), and lactulose, a nonabsorbable high molecular weight sugar (fermentable). Both work by helping the colon retain water and thus prevent the complete dehydration of stool. Lactulose is a prebiotic that is fermented into short-chain fatty acid and can beneficially lower stool pH; however, the process may cause gassiness and bloating in some patients and therefore dosing may need to be increased gradually. Suppositories or enemas are largely avoided nowadays, as is manual disimpaction, with high-dose polyethylene glycol administration showing equal efficacy with less invasiveness. Mineral oil is useful in lubricating hard stool and may decrease the pain associated with disimpaction; however, it should not be given to infants or neurologically impaired patients due to risk of aspiration and chemical pneumonitis. Dietary fiber supplements (ie, prebiotics), such as psyllium husk, guar gum, inulin, and fructans, are helpful for maintenance therapy. Probiotics, notably the strains *Lactobacillus reuteri, L plantarum, Bifidobacterium longum, B breve,* and *B animalis* subsp. *Lactis,* have also shown usefulness in the therapy of constipation.

The most important element in the management of functional constipation is persistence and longevity. Several months of therapy (eg, 6–12) are often needed and considered safe, as the colon needs to heal from a chronic injury in order to regain regularity. Dietary changes and toilet hygiene should be incorporated into a healthy lifestyle and practiced into adulthood.

When to Refer to a Gastroenterologist

Constipation that is resistant to medical therapy should not be ignored. Although uncommon, anatomical aberrations (eg, malrotation), Hirschsprung disease, and intestinal pseudo-obstruction may present after infancy and lead to toxic megacolon or intestinal/colonic volvulus, resulting in intestinal ischemia and devastation. These conditions may require surgical intervention and long-term follow-up and thus should be referred to a specialist.

Box 111-3. Pharmaceutical and Supplement Therapy in Constipation		
Osmotic Laxatives	Psyllium Husk	Prebiotics/Probiotics
• Polyethylene glycol • Lactulose • Magnesium hydroxide • Phosphate	• Bulking agents • Guar gum • Bran • Calcium polycarbophil • Methylcellulose	• Inulin • Fructo-oligosaccharide • *Lactobacillus reuteri, L plantarum* • *Bifidobacterium longum, B animalis, B breve*
Lubricant/Detergent	Stimulants	Enemas/Suppositories
• Mineral oil • Docusate sodium	• Senna • Bisacodyl	• Phosphate • Saline • Mineral oil • Glycerin

Special attention should be paid to infants with persistent constipation because of the high risk of serious conditions such as Hirschsprung disease or malrotation.

Prognosis

The prognosis varies with etiology. Functional constipation is usually amenable to routine management, but treatment failures are reported in 20% of children with functional fecal retention and some long-term studies suggest persistence of symptoms for 25% to 50% of children. A long delay in presentation increases the risk of poor clinical outcome. Age at presentation and stooling frequency are also strong predictors of clinical outcome. Relapse rate at 1 year, after a successful initial intervention, is less than 5%, but increases to 10% to 40% after 5 to 7 years, with significantly higher rates for women. Long duration of symptoms, poor self-esteem, and prior sexual abuse are among risk factors for a poor prognosis. Nonetheless, long-term studies largely show 2 important conclusions: (1) prolonged laxative use is important and (2) dietary and behavioral modifications are ultimately successful in weaning laxative use (Figure 111-5).

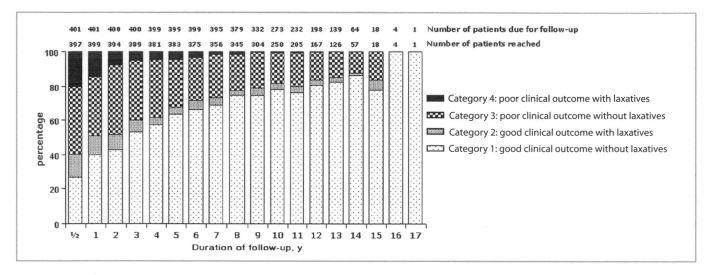

Figure 111-5. **Clinical outcomes of patients according to follow-up year, divided into the 4 defined outcome categories. Numbers in the upper row above the bars show the numbers of patients due for follow-up evaluation each year. Numbers in the second row show the numbers of patients reached for follow-up evaluation each year. (Reproduced from Bongers MEJ, van Wijk, Reitsma JB, Benninga MA. Long-term prognosis for childhood constipation: clinical outcomes in adulthood. *Pediatrics.* 2010;126:e156–e162.)**

CASE RESOLUTION

The child in the case scenario has functional constipation. The belly pain is visceral and related to gas distention and stool retention. The relation of her pain to meals is a reflection of the gastrocolic reflex. A single episode of vomiting may be coincidental and is not overly concerning. Soiling may occur with fecal impaction and overflow incontinence. Parents are often unaware of their children's toileting habits. Gassiness implies stool retention and fermentation in the colon. It is essential to note normal appetite and growth parameters. The rectal examination helps confirm the diagnosis. No further testing is necessary for this child at this point, and the primary care physician should initiate therapy.

Selected References

Abi-Hanna A, Lake AM. Constipation and encopresis in children. *Pediatr Rev.* 1998;19:23–31

Bae SH. Long-term safety of PEG-4000 in children with chronic functional constipation: a biochemical perspective. *Korean J Pediatr,* 2010;53(7):741–744

Baker SS, Liptak GS, Colletti RB, et al. Evaluation and treatment of constipation in children: summary of updated recommendations of the North American Society for Pediatric Gastroenterology, Hepatology and Nutrition. *J Pediatr Gastroenterol Nutr.* 2006;43:405–407

Bekkali N, van den Berg M, Dijkgraff MGW, et al. Rectal fecal impaction treatment in childhood constipation: enemas versus high doses oral PEG. *Pediatrics.* 2009;124:e1108–e1115

Biggs WS, Dery WH. Evaluation and treatment of constipation in infants and children. *Am Fam Physician.* 2006;73:469–477

Bongers MEJ, van Wijk MP, Reitsma JB, Benninga MA. Long-term prognosis for childhood constipation: clinical outcomes in adulthood. *Pediatrics.* 2010;126:e156–e162

Coccorullo P, Strisciuglio C, Martinelli M, et al. Lactobacillus reuteri (DSM 17938) in infants with functional chronic constipation: a double-blind, randomized, placebo-controlled study. *J Pediatr.* 2010;157:598–602

Croffie JM, Fitzgerald JF. Idiopathic constipation. In: Walker WA, Goulet OJ, Kleinman RE, et al, eds. *Pediatric Gastrointestinal Disease.* Hamilton, Ontario, BC: Decker; 2004

Del Piano M, Carmagnola S, Anderloni A, et al. The use of probiotics in healthy volunteers with evacuation disorders and hard stools. A double-blind, randomized, placebo-controlled study. *J Clin Gastroenterol.* 2010;44:S30–S34

Dupont C, Leluyer B, Maamri N, et al. Double-blind randomized evaluation of clinical and biological tolerance of polyethylene glycol 4000 versus lactulose in constipated children. *JPGN.* 2005;41:625–633

El-Hodhod MA, Younis NT, Zaitoun YA, Daoud SD. Cow's milk allergy related pediatric constipation: appropriate time of milk tolerance. *Pediatr Allergy Immunol.* 2010;21:e407–e412

Loening-Baucke V. Prevalence, symptoms and outcome of constipation in infants and toddlers. *J Pediatr.* 2005;146:359–363

Maffei HVL, Vicentini AP. Prospective evaluation of dietary treatment in childhood constipation: high dietary fiber and wheat bran intake are associated with constipation amelioration. *JPGN.* 2011;52(1):55–59

Plunkett A, Phillips CP, Beattie RM. Management of chronic functional constipation in childhood. *Pediatr Drugs.* 2007;9(1):33–46.

Raghunath N, Glassman MS, Halata MS, et al. Anorectal motility abnormalities in children with encopresis and chronic constipation. *J Pediatr.* 2011;158:293–296

Rubin G. Constipation in children. *Clin Evid.* 2004;11:385–390

CHAPTER 112

Abdominal Pain

George Gershman, MD

CASE STUDY

An 12-year-old boy has a 3-month history of intermittent abdominal pain. The pain is present prior to eating and is alleviated by food. The pain also occurs at night. As a result of his symptoms, the child has missed 1 to 2 days of school each week. The family moved to the area 6 months ago, and initially the child seemed to be adjusting to his new school and environment. In addition, the boy has a history of a 5-lb weight loss. He has a positive family history of abdominal pain; his father has been diagnosed with a peptic ulcer. On physical examination, the vital signs are normal. The weight is at the fifth percentile and the height is at the 25th percentile. There are no abnormal physical findings, and the patient is quiet and cooperative. The rectal examination is normal, and the stool is negative for occult blood.

Questions

1. What are the different types of abdominal pain?
2. What characteristics distinguish functional from organic abdominal pain?
3. What are the common organic causes of recurrent abdominal pain in children?
4. What are 2 etiologies for functional pain?

Abdominal pain is one of the most common symptoms of childhood. It may be acute or chronic. Acute abdominal pain resolves within 4 weeks from the onset of symptoms. Most children with acute abdominal pain have self-limiting conditions such as viral or bacterial gastroenteritis. However, a sudden onset of abdominal pain can be caused by serious, life-threatening conditions (eg, acute appendicitis, intussusception, or hemolytic uremic syndrome). Chronic abdominal pain is defined as pain that persists at least for 2 months. Most children with chronic abdominal pain suffer from so-called functional abdominal pain (FAP). The criteria for childhood FAP must include all of the following criteria: presence of abdominal pain at least once per week for 2 or more months prior to diagnosis; episodic or continuous nature of abdominal pain; insufficient criteria for other functional gastrointestinal disorders; and absence of anatomical abnormalities, and inflammatory and metabolic and neoplastic processes related to patient's symptoms. Children with FAP suffer equally from intermittent or continuous non-localized abdominal pain. Onset of pain is usually not associated with defecation. Children with FAP and loss of daily function fall into the category of FAP syndrome (FAPS). The term *functional abdominal pain* should not suggest that affected children are malingerers or their symptoms are fictitious.

An organic etiology is found in less than 10% of school-aged children with chronic or recurrent abdominal pain (RAP). However, failure to recognize and/or delayed therapy can have devastating effects.

Epidemiology

According to community- and school-based studies, up to 38% of children and adolescents experienced abdominal pain weekly, with up to 24% of children reporting symptoms persisting for longer than 8 weeks. Abdominal pain is the essential part of several functional gastrointestinal disorders such as irritable bowel syndrome (IBS), functional dyspepsia, and abdominal migraine, as well as organic disorders, which occur with variable frequency in different age groups.

Pathophysiology

There are 3 main reasons for acute or chronic organic abdominal pain: inflammation, distention of the viscera, and ischemia.

Abdominal pain can originate from abdominal viscera (visceral pain), parietal peritoneum, abdominal wall, retroperitoneal skeletal muscles (somatic pain), and extra-abdominal sites (so-called referred pain). Impulses of visceral pain are carried out primarily by small, unmyelinated, slow-conducting afferent C fibers incorporated into the autonomic sensory pathways. Each visceral organ receives dual sympathetic and parasympathetic innervations. Sensory fibers associated with the sympathetic nervous system traverse both pre-vertebral (celiac, superior, and inferior mesenteric ganglion) and paravertebral ganglion and terminate in the spinal cord. Sensory fibers contained in the vagus and pelvic nerves (parasympathetic branch of the autonomic nervous system) terminate in the brain stem and lumbosacral spinal cord respectively. Sensory fibers from visceral organs that connect with the spinal column terminate within the 4 to 5 spinal segments. This explains why visceral pain is poorly localized and often perceived along the midline as a dull or aching sensation. For example, the onset of acute appendicitis is usually manifested by pain in the periumbilical or epigastric areas before the pain migrates to the right lower quadrant. It is frequently accompanied by symptoms of autonomic disturbance (eg, nausea or pallor).

Somatic pain is induced by irritation of parietal peritoneum and supportive tissue. The signals from the pain receptors (nociceptors) are transmitted for the most part by rapid conducting myelinated A-delta fibers responsible for tactile, thermal, and chemical stimulation and discrimination of location and intensity of stimuli. As a result, somatic pain is well localized, intense, and sharp. The important characteristic of somatic pain is aggravation by movement. Therefore, the child with somatic abdominal pain is likely to lie still in contrast to the restless patient with visceral pain.

The classic example of referred pain is abdominal pain induced by inflammation of parietal pleura at the onset of pneumonia as the result of shared central projections of the parietal pleura and abdominal wall.

The location of abdominal pain is determined by the level of spinal cord connection with the corresponding visceral organs through the afferent sensory fibers. The structures of the foregut origin, such as distal esophagus, stomach, duodenum, liver, and pancreas, are innervated by the nerves that enter the spinal cord at the level T5 to T9 segments. Pain from these organs is perceived between the xiphoid and umbilicus. The structures related to the primitive midgut (small intestine, appendix, and right colon) project the afferent fibers to the T8 to T9 segments of the spinal cord. As a result, the associated pain affects the periumbilical area. The structures related to the embryonic hindgut, including the left colon and the rectum, share the innervations, which involve the spinal segments T10 to L1 and allocate the pain between the umbilicus and symphysis pubis.

Radiation of the pain may be helpful in diagnosis (eg, pain related to acute cholecystitis or biliary colic often refers to the area just under the inferior angle of the right scapula or above the right clavicle). Another example of referred pain is pain between the scapulas and middle back region in patients with pancreatitis.

The pathophysiology of functional abdominal pain is different from acute or chronic organic abdominal pain. The genesis of functional abdominal pain is related to abnormalities in the enteric nervous system and dysregulation of the brain–gut interaction. It is now believed that children with functional abdominal pain may have abnormal responses to the normal physiological functions related to meals as well as intestinal distention during peristalsis, associated hormonal changes, and psychological conditions like anxiety and parental separation.

Research data suggest that visceral hyperalgesia is the key element in the pathophysiology of functional abdominal pain. This theory implies sensitization of the various receptors associated with afferent innervation of the gastrointestinal (GI) tract by an infectious or allergic process or abnormal processing of afferent signals by the central nervous system.

Clinical Presentation

Children who experience abdominal pain may present with pain that may be characterized as persistent or intermittent, waxing and waning or steady and unrelenting, sharp or dull, and worsened or unaffected by movement. They may have associated complaints, including vomiting, diarrhea, constipation, fever, weight loss, headache, and anorexia (Dx Box).

Pain from distention of smooth muscle also waxes and wanes, is poorly localized, and is unaffected by motion. Distention of any hollow viscus, including the stomach, intestines, biliary tree, fallopian tubes, or ureters, can result in such symptomatology. A classic example of such pain is renal colic, where the patient is writhing because of the discomfort.

Dx Abdominal Pain

- Abdominal pain
- Abdominal wall rigidity
- Abdominal tenderness
- Vomiting
- Alterations in bowel sounds
- Diarrhea or constipation
- Anorexia
- Fever

Differential Diagnosis

In assessing the possible disease entities that may account for abdominal pain, patient age and duration of symptoms are the key differential components. The location of the pain may provide a clue to the etiology. Disease affecting the stomach is usually appreciated in the epigastrium. Duodenal problems are noted between the xiphoid and the umbilicus, small intestinal pathology is appreciated in the periumbilical area, and cecal inflammation may be felt from the epigastrium to McBurney point. Disease in the colon is less specifically noted but is usually felt in the hypogastrium. Bladder and colon problems may be suprapubic or sacral. Pain may also be referred to the back. Renal colic is also noted in the back, but more in a lateral or costovertebral angle (tenderness) site.

Acute and Chronic Abdominal Pain

Young Infants: Medical Conditions

A unique disorder of infants, **colic** has been referred to as paroxysmal fussiness of infancy (see Chapter 46). The onset of symptoms is usually between 2 and 4 weeks of age, with resolution by 3 to 4 months. Although recurrent abdominal pain seems to be present, abdominal pain has never been established as the cause of colic. Colic is characterized by fussiness and crying. Symptoms usually appear after feeding, particularly late in the day around dinnertime. Infants cry, clench their fists, and flex their legs. A gas–cry–air-swallowing cycle seems to occur. The symptoms may respond to a number of measures, including rhythmic motion and anti-gas medications. Infants with colic usually appear well otherwise and often have accelerated weight gain secondary to repeated feeding made in efforts to quiet them.

Abdominal pain may also occur with **food allergy,** particularly cow's milk protein allergy. Generally, symptoms such as vomiting, diarrhea, hemoccult-positive stools, failure to thrive, rhinitis, eczema, pallor, irritability, and a positive family history of allergies are associated with food allergies. Disaccharidase deficiency may result in abdominal pain, but diarrhea is also usually present.

Young Infants: Surgical Conditions

Intussusception occurs in infants 3 months of age and older. The child may have been previously well or have experienced a recent bout of diarrhea. Vomiting is reported in about 50% of patients, and pallor is frequently present. Lethargy is not an uncommon associated symptom. An etiology is noted in less than 2.5% of affected infants, although a lead point (lymphoma or Meckel diverticulum) may be found in 5% to 10% of older children. The intussusception most often involves the area around the ileocecal valve. Compression of the vessels within the bowel wall may lead to necrosis and gangrene. The presence of blood and mucus in the stools gives a "currant jelly" appearance, although the initial stool is often normal, having been the stool that was present in the rectum prior to the intussusception.

The abdominal examination of affected children may be benign except for pain over the area of the intussusception or may reveal the presence of a mass. Bowel sounds may be increased secondary to the obstruction. The rectal examination may reveal blood and the presence of a mass. Fever and leukocytosis may also be noted. A flat plate of the abdomen is usually nonspecific. Intussusception is diagnosed by abdominal ultrasound or barium enema. Hydrostatic reduction is the treatment of choice of intussusception. It is successful in almost 90% to 95% of children. Failure of hydrostatic reduction or associated complications are related to delayed diagnosis and severe edema and necrosis of the affected bowel.

School-Aged Children: Medical Conditions

Functional Abdominal Pain

As noted previously, most children with RAP suffer from functional gastrointestinal disorders (FGID). According to the clinical presentation, FGID can be subdivided into 5 categories: FAP, FAPS, functional dyspepsia, IBS, and abdominal migraine. Children with FAP usually do not have association of pain with eating, defecation, menses, or exercise. It is occasionally triggered by new environment, difficulties at school, or domestic problems. The pain is usually periumbilical and quite severe. It can be recurrent or continuous and may affect daily activity.

Irritable bowel syndrome in children is characterized by abdominal discomfort or pain associated with 2 or more symptoms: improvement after defecation, onset of pain associated with a change in frequency, and change in form of stool. Symptoms that cumulatively support the diagnosis of IBS are 4 or more stools per day or 2 or less stools per week, lumpy/hard or loose/watery stool, straining, urgency or feeling of incomplete evacuation, passage of mucus, bloating, or a feeling of abdominal distention. Children with IBS are often anxious and express multiple somatic complaints.

Although many children seem to outgrow the FAP and IBS, long-term follow-up studies suggests that a significant number remain symptomatic into adulthood.

Children with functional dyspepsia experience persistent or recurrent abdominal pain or discomfort centered in the upper abdomen (above the umbilicus). Pain is not relieved by defecation or associated with the onset of change in stool frequency or form. Dyspeptic symptoms may follow a viral illness. The pain is often relieved by medical inhibition of gastric secretion. Children with functional dyspepsia may suffer from nausea, early satiety, postprandial fullness, vomiting, and a sense of bloating.

Abdominal migraine is characterized by paroxysmal episodes of intense, acute periumbilical pain that lasts for one or several hours. Pain is often incapacitating. Children return to their usual state of health for weeks to months between the paroxysms of pain. When present, the pain interferes with normal activities and is often accompanied by pallor, anorexia, photophobia, headache, nausea, and vomiting. There is an increased incidence of maternal migraine in children with abdominal migraine.

As mentioned previously, an organic etiology is found in less than 10% of school-aged children with RAP. The alarming symptoms and signs of organic diseases are persistent right upper and right lower quadrant pain; pain that wakes the child from sleep; dysphagia; persistent vomiting; arthritis; perirectal disease; GI blood loss; nocturnal diarrhea; involuntary weight loss; deceleration of linear growth; delayed puberty; unexplained fever; and family history of inflammatory bowel disease, celiac disease, or peptic ulcer disease.

Peptic ulcers may develop in children in 3 situations. Acute infantile ulcers may occur in newborns secondary to stress and hypoxia. Stress ulcers may occur in children who are the victims of trauma, including burns and hypoxia (eg, after submersion). The routine use of histamine H_2 receptor antagonists or proton pump inhibitors has reduced the incidence of ulcers in hospitalized critically ill children.

The most common type of ulcers in children is acute, drug-induced ulcerations of the stomach and the duodenum due to nonsteroidal anti-inflammatory drugs or corticosteroids. Chronic or peptic ulcers may develop in prepubertal children and teenagers with no apparent precipitating factors. A positive family history of peptic ulcer disease is reported in 25% to 50% of affected children. Unlike the classic ulcer symptoms of adults, in which pain occurs on an empty stomach and is relieved by eating, children may find that ulcer-related pain is without a specific clinical pattern. Positive family history, microcytic anemia, and hemoccult-positive stools should raise a clinical suspicion and prompt referral of the child to the pediatric gastroenterologist. There is clear evidence linking ulcer disease and infection with *Helicobacter pylori* in adults. The relationship between *H pylori* and peptic ulcer disease in children is not so strong, though two-thirds of pediatric patients with endoscopic evidence of peptic ulcer disease have infection with *H pylori*.

Mesenteric adenitis may produce symptoms indistinguishable from appendicitis, although affected children may not be so ill-appearing. Nausea and vomiting and a history of an antecedent upper respiratory infection are often present.

Parenteral infections such as tonsillitis or pneumonia may present with fever and abdominal pain. In addition, hepatitis may result in pain and tenderness localized to the right upper quadrant in association with anorexia. Hepatitis in children is usually due to hepatitis A, and many infected young children are anicteric (see Chapter 114).

Pancreatitis produces abdominal pain that is often referred to the back. In the past, mumps was the most common cause of pancreatitis. Other infections such as hepatitis B, Epstein-Barr virus and coxsackievirus B, and *Mycoplasma pneumoniae* are the common infectious etiologies of acute pancreatitis.

Acute pancreatitis can be induced by some medications (eg, steroids, chemotherapeutic agents). Familial and recurrent forms of pancreatitis are also reported. Trauma, particularly from injuries sustained as a result of an impact against handlebars of bicycles, is a common cause. In children with pancreatitis and no apparent etiology, trauma related to child abuse should be considered.

Parasitic infestations, particularly with *Giardia lamblia,* may produce abdominal pain, often with bloating and diarrhea.

Genitourinary problems may result in abdominal pain. An abnormal urinalysis provides clues to the etiology. Renal stones occur infrequently in children, and boys are more often affected than girls. In two-thirds of affected children, stones are detected incidentally or in association with a urinary tract infection (UTI). Stones may be composed of calcium phosphate or oxalate, magnesium, uric acid, cystine, or xanthine. In addition to flank or abdominal pain, patients may also experience hematuria, fever, recurrent UTI, and persistent pyuria.

Hematologic and vascular disorders such as sickle cell disease, rheumatic fever, and Henoch-Schönlein purpura may also present with abdominal pain. Sickle cell anemia should be considered in African American children with abdominal pain. Pain may be related to vaso-occlusive events including bowel ischemia and splenic infarction or cholecystitis. Henoch-Schönlein purpura, which is also referred to as anaphylactoid purpura, is characterized by a hemorrhagic skin rash, joint pain, and renal abnormalities in addition to abdominal pain. This pain may result from a number of processes, including vasculitis and ischemia of the bowel wall, edema of the bowel wall, and intussusception of the small intestine.

Diabetes mellitus may lead to abdominal pain secondary to cramping of accessory muscles of respiration during a bout of ketoacidosis.

Acute intermittent porphyria is an uncommon cause of abdominal pain in children. The pain is often colicky and may be associated with constipation, nausea, and vomiting. Neurologic symptoms such as pain or paresthesia in the extremities may be present. Often symptoms are precipitated by the ingestion of medications (eg, barbiturates, sulfa drugs). Some antispasmodic medications, such as Donnatal elixir, contain phenobarbital and can precipitate an attack. The diagnosis is made by evaluating the urine for the presence of protoporphyrins.

Primary peritonitis is secondary to infection with *Streptococcus pneumoniae* and is seen in children with nephrotic syndrome, cirrhosis, and sickle cell disease, and in young girls with fever, abdominal pain, and vaginal discharge.

School-Aged Children: Surgical Conditions

Appendicitis is the most common surgical condition that produces abdominal pain in school-aged children. Appendicitis may even occur in newborns, where it is seen in association with conditions such as cystic fibrosis and Hirschsprung disease that lead to diminished passage of stool. The condition is frequently difficult to diagnose in children younger than 3 or 4 years for 2 reasons: (1) examination of such young children for pain is difficult and (2) symptoms are similar to those of acute gastroenteritis (ie, fever, abdominal pain, anorexia). Classically, patients complain of periumbilical pain that localizes to the right lower quadrant in 1 to 5 hours. They often have a low-grade fever, with a temperature of 100.4°F (38°C). Vomiting and increased urinary frequency may occur. Stooling is variable.

The physical examination may reveal guarding and localized pain as well as rebound tenderness. A positive psoas or obturator sign may be present, indicating inflammation of these muscles. Tenderness may also be noted on rectal examination. Leukocytosis over 10,000/mL is also usually present. A radiograph of the abdomen may reveal 1 of 4 signs: a fecalith in the appendix (appendicolith), air in the cecum (sentinel loop), blurring of the shadow of the psoas muscle, or edema of the abdominal wall on the right side. A chest radiograph is also useful to rule out the presence of pneumonia, which may produce symptoms that mimic appendicitis.

Meckel diverticulum may be responsible for abdominal pain in a number of ways. It may serve as the lead point for an intussusception, cause symptoms of ulcer disease (pain or hemorrhage) secondary to the presence of ectopic gastric mucosa, or become acutely inflamed as in appendicitis. Meckel diverticulum follows the rule of 2s: it affects 2% of the population, is 2 feet from the ileocecal valve, is 2 inches in length, and is 2 times more common in males than in females.

Adolescents

In female adolescents, **gynecologic problems** such as torsion of the ovary, mittelschmerz, dysmenorrhea, and pelvic inflammatory disease must be considered as causes of abdominal pain (see Chapter 98). In addition, pain may result from gall bladder disease secondary to cholelithiasis or cholecystitis. Cholelithiasis is also a consideration in previously pregnant adolescent patients with abdominal pain and fatty food intolerance.

Evaluation

History

A thorough history should be obtained (Questions Box). A detailed description of pain may suggest a specific etiology. For example, pain worsened by eating can occur in children with gastroesophageal reflux disease, gastritis, cholecystitis, or pancreatitis. Nocturnal pain or pain relieved by a meal is more common in children with peptic ulcer disease. Pain relieved by defecation is suggestive of IBS. Pain aggravated by defecation raises suspicion of chronic inflammatory

Abdominal Pain — Questions

- What is the nature of the pain? Is it sharp or dull, well or poorly localized, intermittent or relentless, worsened or unaffected by movement?
- How often does the pain occur?
- How long has the pain been present?
- Do any maneuvers, such as eating or lying down, reduce the symptomatology?
- Is the pain related to meals in any way? Is it worse after eating?
- Are any symptoms such as fever, weight loss, anorexia, vomiting, diarrhea, constipation, dysuria, or headache associated with the pain?
- Does anyone else in the family have similar symptoms?
- Does the pain occur at night and on weekends?
- Is there a history of travel?

bowel disease. Localization of abdominal pain is an important additional diagnostic clue; functional abdominal pain is usually localized along the midline or periumbilical area. Associated symptoms such as fever, weight loss, anorexia, vomiting, diarrhea, leukocytosis, and an elevated sedimentation rate also suggest an organic etiology.

Physical Examination

The physical examination should include an assessment of the severity of the pain. Children should be observed when they do not suspect that they are being watched. For example, a child who stands up and hops around when the physician leaves the room may have pain with a psychosomatic basis. Detection of abdominal tenderness may be ascertained during auscultation of the abdomen by pressing down with the stethoscope.

A rectal examination is also an integral part of the evaluation. In prepubescent girls with genitourinary symptoms or adolescent females, a genital assessment should be included.

Growth parameters should be evaluated for evidence of impairments, especially in children with RAP. Abnormal findings such as abdominal masses or perianal skin tags are clues to an organic etiology. Children who appear vigilant and keep their eyes open during the examination often have organic problems.

Laboratory Tests

The laboratory assessment is determined by the differential diagnosis. In general, laboratory tests include a complete blood cell count, a urinalysis, and an erythrocyte sedimentation rate (in recurrent cases). In children with suspected lactose intolerance, a hydrogen breath test is recommended by some physicians, although a trial of dietary manipulation or use of exogenous lactase (eg, Lactaid) may be more cost-effective. Other laboratory tests, such as serum amylase or liver function studies, are appropriate if pancreatitis or hepatitis is suspected. Detection of *H pylori* antigen in the stool supports the diagnosis of *H pylori*. Stool evaluation for occult blood and parasites is also helpful. Consultation with a gastroenterologist should be considered in patients suspected of having ulcer disease or inflammatory

bowel disease. Specialists may order diagnostic procedures such as endoscopy to arrive at the diagnosis.

Imaging Studies

In general, a flat plate of the abdomen should be obtained, especially if an acute surgical condition is suspected. Abdominal computed tomography can be useful in some children with right low quadrant pain to confirm the diagnosis of acute appendicitis. Abdominal ultrasound and a barium enema are indicated to diagnose intussusception. Technetium scans help detect Meckel diverticulum if ectopic gastric mucosa is present. Ultrasonography is useful in suspected cases of cholelithiasis and cholecystitis. It may also detect pancreatic edema or pseudocyst, hydronephrosis, or abdominal masses.

Management

Management depends on the suspected cause of the abdominal pain. Medical conditions warrant treatment with **pharmacologic agents.** Peptic ulcer disease requires H_2 blockers such as cimetidine, proton pump inhibitors such as omeprazole, or cytoprotective agents like sucralfate. Infection with *H pylori* is managed with a combination of different antibiotics with proton pump inhibitors and bismuth preparations. Urinary tract infections should be treated with antibiotics. Conditions such as appendicitis mandate **surgical intervention.**

The management of children with RAP is challenging. A 3-tiered empiric trial has been suggested for children in whom no distinct cause is identified. First, a high-fiber diet should be implemented. This helps alleviate the abdominal pain symptoms of children with IBS. Second, antacids, H_2 blockers, or proton pump inhibitors are used empirically to see if symptoms respond to decreased acid levels. Third, a trial of Lactaid or a lactose-free period may also be implemented. A low dose of tricyclic antidepressant (eg, amitriptyline 0.1mg/kg–0.2 mg/kg) has been used successfully in children with functional abdominal pain.

Prognosis

In general, the prognosis for children with acute abdominal pain is good, although it varies depending on the condition. In 30% to 50% of children with RAP, the symptoms resolve within 2 to 6 weeks of diagnosis. Thirty percent to 50% of affected children experience abdominal pain as adults, although the pain does not limit their activities. As adults, these individuals may experience IBS or other chronic nonspecific complaints, such as headache, backache, and chronic pelvic pain.

CASE RESOLUTION

In the case history, the boy has the classic symptoms of peptic ulcer disease. His symptoms are alleviated by eating and exacerbate at night. In addition, the family history is positive for peptic ulcer. Further evaluation may include a stool test for *H pylori* antigen, and referral to pediatric gastroenterologists for further workup, including upper GI endoscopy.

Selected References

Campo JV, Di Lorenzo C, Chiapetta I, et al. Adult outcomes of pediatric recurrent abdominal pain: do they just grow out of it? *Pediatrics.* 2001;108(1):e1

Chiou E, Nurko S. Management of functional abdominal pain and irritable bowel syndrome in children and adolescents. *Expert Rev Gastroenterol Hepatol.* 2010;4(3):293–304

Hyman PE, Milla PJ, Benninga MA, Davidson GP, Fleisher DF, Taminiau J. Childhood functional gastrointestinal disorders: neonate/toddler. *Gastroenterology.* 2006;130:1519–1526

Rasquin A, Di Lorenzo C, Forbes D, et al. Childhood functional gastrointestinal disorders: child/adolescent. *Gastroenterology.* 2006;130:1527–1537

Saps M, Seshadri R, Sztainberg M, et al. A prospective school-based study of abdominal pain and other common somatic complaints in children. *J Pediatr.* 2009;154:322–326

Vlieger AM, Benninga MA. Chronic abdominal pain including functional abdominal pain, irritable bowel syndrome and abdominal migraine. In: Walker's *Pediatric Gastrointestinal Disease: Pathophysiology-Diagnosis-Management.* 5th ed. Philadelphia, PA; B.C. Decker; 2008:715–728

CHAPTER 113

Jaundice

Melissa K. Egge, MD

CASE STUDY

A 2-month-old male infant is brought to the office for a routine well-child checkup. He was the product of a full-term, normal, spontaneous vaginal delivery, with a birth weight of 3,600 g. He has been feeding well, exclusively at the breast. Loose stools follow each feeding. On physical examination, the infant weighs 4,900 g. The examination is normal except that the boy appears jaundiced. On further questioning, the mother states that her son has been jaundiced since shortly after birth, and she feels that his appearance has not changed. The color of the stool is yellow.

Questions

1. What are the common causes of unconjugated hyperbilirubinemia in young infants?
2. What are the common causes of conjugated hyperbilirubinemia in young infants?
3. What are the usual causes of jaundice in older children and adolescents?
4. What is the appropriate management of hyperbilirubinemia in breastfed infants?

Jaundice is a condition that occurs when bilirubin reaches a level in the blood that makes it visibly apparent. In newborn infants, this level is 5 mg/dL. In older children and adolescents, jaundice becomes apparent at serum bilirubin levels of 2 mg/dL. The term **physiological jaundice** is used to denote the jaundice that normally occurs following birth. In full-term infants, bilirubin reaches its peak of about 6 mg/dL between the second and fourth days of life. Levels above 10 mg/dL are probably not physiological. Bilirubin generally returns to a normal level (<1 mg/dL) by 12 days of age. Premature infants experience their peak level of bilirubin, which may be up to 10 to 12 mg/dL, between the fifth and seventh days of life. Levels over 14 mg/dL are probably not physiological. Levels may be elevated in premature infants for up to 2 months.

Although physiological jaundice, a benign finding, affects all infants, other more serious disorders may present with similar symptomatology. The physician must be able to differentiate between these conditions to ensure appropriate intervention and management. New-onset jaundice in older children and adolescents is caused by other disorders.

Epidemiology

Jaundice is nearly universal in neonates because of the rapid turnover of red blood cells and the relative immaturity of the liver. Breast milk jaundice affects about 1% of breastfed infants. Various illnesses, particularly bacterial infections, also may precipitate jaundice in newborns. Neonatal cholestasis (conjugated hyperbilirubinemia), which is seen in a small number of cases of neonatal jaundice, is due to neonatal hepatitis or extrahepatic biliary atresia 45% of the time. Genetic and metabolic diseases now comprise approximately 45% of the cases of neonatal cholestasis that were previously known as idiopathic.

Jaundice occurs much less frequently in the post-neonatal period and is most often secondary to viral hepatitis (see Chapter 114).

Clinical Presentation

Children with jaundice have yellow skin, conjunctiva, and mucous membranes. In newborns, the coloration may not be appreciated by parents because of its gradual onset and the parents' inexperience. The finding may be apparent in otherwise asymptomatic infants during routine health maintenance visits. In addition to the yellow color, children with jaundice may also present with symptoms related to the cause of the jaundice, including vomiting, anorexia, failure to thrive, acholic (white) stools, dark urine, fatigue, and abdominal pain or fullness (Dx Box).

Dx Jaundice

- Yellow skin, mucous membranes, and conjunctiva
- Tenderness in the right upper quadrant of the abdomen
- Hepatomegaly
- Anorexia
- Acholic stools
- Vomiting
- Pruritus

Pathophysiology

Bilirubin, a red pigment found primarily in bile, forms from the breakdown of heme-containing compounds, mainly hemoglobin, but also muscle myoglobin, cytochromes, catalases, and tryptophan pyrrolase. Blockage along any point in the physiological or anatomical pathway may result in increased levels of bilirubin and the appearance of jaundice (Figure 113-1). After the breakdown of hemoglobin, unconjugated bilirubin is taken up by the hepatocyte plasma membrane carrier, bilitranslocase. Once within the hepatocyte, bilirubin is bound to intracellular proteins (Y proteins or ligandin). Uptake depends on hepatic blood flow and the presence of the necessary binding proteins. Once in the liver, unconjugated bilirubin is conjugated by the enzyme glucuronyl transferase. Conjugated bilirubin, which is water-soluble, can be eliminated through the kidneys. Following conjugation, bilirubin passes into the bile through the bile canaliculi. It then moves to the gastrointestinal (GI) tract, where some of it may be reabsorbed (enterohepatic circulation), or be acted on by bacteria to form urobilinogen and stercobilinogen, which may appear in the urine or stool, respectively.

In neonates, a number of factors contribute to physiological jaundice. Increased destruction of red blood cells occurs because the red blood cell survival in infants is only 70 to 90 days, as opposed to 120 days in older children. Hepatic uptake is lower, perhaps as a result of decreased levels of hepatic proteins as well as decreased hepatic blood flow. Levels of glucuronyl transferase do not reach adult values until the second week of life. These decreased levels of glucuronyl transferase mean that conjugation of bilirubin occurs at a slower rate.

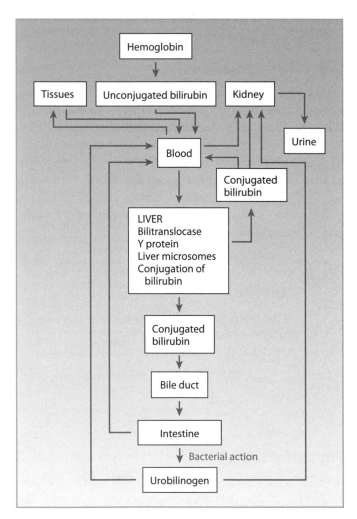

Figure 113-1. The bilirubin pathway.

In some infants, glucuronyl transferase levels remain low; these individuals remain prone to jaundice at times of illness, stress, and starvation (Gilbert syndrome). Some breastfed infants also experience prolonged jaundice. Jaundice in breastfed infants may be related to poor caloric or fluid intake, weight loss, slow passage of meconium, or the type or number of bacteria in the intestine. It is believed that some unknown substance in the mother's milk, perhaps pregnanetriol, blocks glucuronyl transferase. (See Chapter 24 for more information about breastfeeding.) Reabsorption of bilirubin is increased through the enterohepatic circulation because of the diminished number of bacteria in the GI tract in young infants.

In older children, similar mechanisms may act to cause an increase in the bilirubin level. Hemolytic anemias (eg, glucose-6-phosphate dehydrogenase [G6PD] deficiency or pyruvate kinase deficiency [PKD]) may lead to increased red blood cell destruction. Inflammatory or infectious processes involving the liver, such as hepatitis, may impair the ability of the liver to excrete bilirubin. Pharmaceutical and toxicological agents may also interfere with the ability of the liver to metabolize bilirubin.

Differential Diagnosis

The differential diagnosis of jaundice in children involves 3 criteria: (1) age; (2) the type of hyperbilirubinemia (conjugated or unconjugated); and (3) if the hyperbilirubinemia is conjugated, the nature of the obstruction (intrahepatic or extrahepatic). The latter 2 factors are particularly important in determining the etiology of jaundice in young infants. A diagrammatic representation of the differential diagnosis of jaundice in children is shown in Figures 113-2, 113-3, and 113-4.

Infants Younger Than 8 Weeks of Age

Unconjugated Hyperbilirubinemia

Jaundice occurs universally in all newborns, but marked elevation of bilirubin levels or presence of jaundice in the first 24 hours of life or beyond 2 weeks of age warrants assessment. When less than 15% of the total bilirubin is direct, unconjugated hyperbilirubinemia is present. This is best determined by measuring the levels of total and direct bilirubin in the blood. **Physiological jaundice** is associated with unconjugated hyperbilirubinemia. The hematologic workup of affected infants is normal. Jaundice related to inadequate breast milk intake is called *breastfeeding jaundice,* which may resemble physiological jaundice and occurs during the first week of life, whereas with *breast milk jaundice,* bilirubin levels rise during the second week of life when physiological jaundice is improving. In breastfed infants, levels may reach as high as 25 to 30 mg/dL. Breast milk jaundice usually peaks by the age of 4 weeks and can last up to 12 weeks.

Conditions associated with slow intestinal transit time and increased enterohepatic circulation, such as hypothyroidism, also may result in jaundice. As with physiological and breast milk jaundice, the hematologic workup is normal. High intestinal obstructions, such as pyloric stenosis, duodenal atresia, annular pancreas,

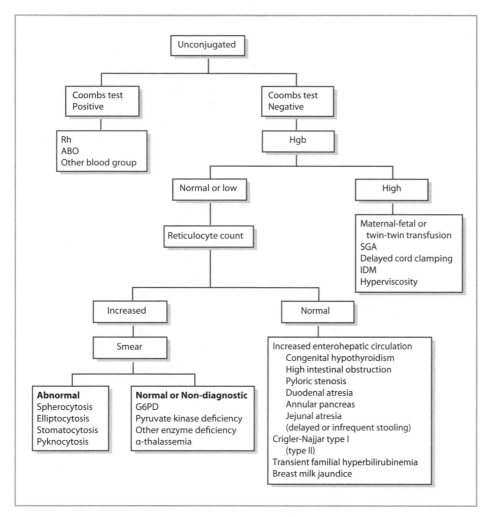

Figure 113-2. Differential diagnosis of jaundice in neonates (during the first 8 weeks of life). Unconjugated hyperbilirubinemia. G6PD, glucose-6-phosphate dehydrogenase; Hgb, hemoglobin; IDM, infant of diabetic mother; SGA, small for gestational age.

elevated hemoglobin is associated with jaundice include maternal-infant or twin-twin transfusions, infants who are small for gestational age, delayed clamping of the umbilical cord, infants of diabetic mothers, and infants with hyperviscosity syndrome.

Conjugated Hyperbilirubinemia

When more than 15% of the total bilirubin is direct, the jaundice is categorized as conjugated hyperbilirubinemia. Conjugated hyperbilirubinemia is always pathologic. Total parenteral nutrition is the most common cause of conjugated hyperbilirubinemia in the neonatal intensive care unit but does not usually present a diagnostic dilemma. The institution of oral feedings helps reverse the process. In other cases, determination of whether the problem is intrahepatic or extrahepatic is the major consideration. Some conditions of intrahepatic involvement represent a spectrum involving progression from inflammation of bile canaliculi (hepatitis) to their destruction (biliary atresia).

Inflammation of the hepatocytes is hepatitis. This disease may be caused by an infection in the liver or elsewhere in the body (eg, sepsis and urinary tract infections [UTIs] in young infants). Urinary tract infections are usually caused by *Escherichia coli*. The hepatic involvement resolves with appropriate antibiotic therapy of the primary infection.

and jejunal atresia, may lead to jaundice, perhaps because of starvation and decreased levels of glucuronyl transferase.

Crigler-Najjar syndrome type I involves an absence of glucuronyl transferase in which bilirubin levels can approach 50 mg/dL at birth. An indirect hyperbilirubinemia on the order of 20 mg/dL that persists beyond 2 weeks in the absence of hemolysis is indicative of the type II version of this syndrome. Because of very high bilirubin levels, type I disease may lead to kernicterus unless managed with exchange transfusion. Phototherapy, cholestyramine, and eventual liver transplantation are additional therapies. The disorder is inherited in an autosomal-recessive manner and is extremely rare.

Hematologic problems may also produce jaundice in the neonatal period. Such problems are most often associated with blood group (usually Rh or ABO) incompatibility between mothers and infants, but some minor blood group determinants can precipitate similar problems. Jaundice occurs in affected infants because of the rapid destruction of red blood cells. Other infants may have a hemolytic anemia such as spherocytosis. Jaundice may also occur if excess blood is present in the infant's system. Situations in which

Primary liver infection may be due to **TORCHS** (*t*oxoplasmosis, *o*ther agents, *r*ubella, *c*ytomegalovirus [CMV], *h*erpes simplex virus [HSV], HIV, *s*yphilis) agents, the most common culprits being CMV and HSV. Infants infected prenatally often have low birth weights, hepatosplenomegaly, petechial rashes, and ocular findings such as cataracts and chorioretinitis. Hepatitis A may cause an acute infection, but rarely manifests as jaundice in neonates. Hepatitis B is a possible etiology of neonatal cholestasis, and hepatitis C is usually an asymptomatic infection. **Other infectious causes** include enteroviruses, reovirus 3, parvovirus B19, human herpesvirus 6, adenovirus 2, *Listeria monocytogenes*, and tuberculosis. Differentiating among these conditions is usually done on the basis of culture, polymerase chain reaction, or serology. Certain physical and epidemiological findings may help to distinguish these entities, however. Syphilis is more common in the developing nations of the world. Jaundice may appear within the first 24 hours of life or be of later onset. Infection with *L monocytogenes* infection may be associated with the presence

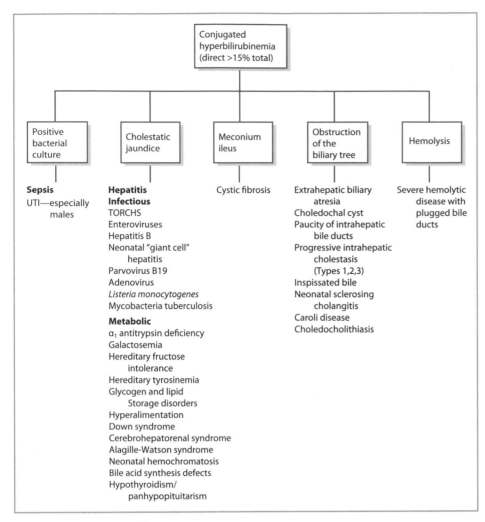

Figure 113-3. **Differential diagnosis of jaundice in neonates (during the first 8 weeks of life). Conjugated hyperbilirubinemia. UTI, urinary tract infection.**

of focal granulomas on the posterior pharynx. Similar granulomas in the liver are evident.

Metabolic diseases and **inborn errors of metabolism** may also lead to hepatitis. Most of these conditions are inherited in an autosomal-recessive manner. In addition to jaundice, infants may present with vomiting, irritability, lethargy, anorexia, hepatomegaly, hypoglycemia, failure to thrive, bleeding, or cataracts. Galactosemia may be detected through neonatal screening or may present earlier as *E coli* sepsis. Infants with hereditary fructose intolerance present after exposure to fructose, sucrose, or sorbitol. α_1-antitrypsin deficiency may account for 20% to 30% of cases of idiopathic neonatal liver disease and for 10% of neonatal cholestatic disease. Inborn errors of metabolism generally present with a direct hyperbilirubinemia, while inborn errors of erythrocyte metabolism (PKD or G6PD) present with an indirect hyperbilirubinemia.

Genetic conditions that lead to jaundice in newborns include hereditary tyrosinemia, infantile Gaucher disease, Niemann-Pick disease, and Wolman disease. Cystic fibrosis may also cause cholestatic jaundice because of the presence of inspissated bile in the bile canaliculi. Fifty percent of these infants have meconium ileus,

meconium peritonitis, or intestinal atresia. "Plugged" bile ducts may be seen with severe hemolytic anemia where bilirubin production is markedly elevated. Drugs may also induce intrahepatic cholestasis. A number of syndromes are associated with persistent intrahepatic cholestasis. Alagille syndrome (arteriohepatic dysplasia) is characterized by unusual facies, skeletal and cardiovascular anomalies, and a paucity of intralobular bile ducts. The incidence is 1 in 100,000 live births. Progressive familial intrahepatic cholestasis and bile acid synthetic defect, together with Alagille syndrome, account for cholestasis in 10% of affected neonates. Not surprisingly, as the etiologies for more of these cases are identified through genetic and pathologic testing, fewer cases are labeled *idiopathic neonatal hepatitis.*

Extrahepatic biliary atresia accounts for about 25% of cases of cholestasis in newborns. Obliteration of the biliary tree is apparent. Infants are often well until 3 to 6 weeks of age, when they develop conjugated hyperbilirubinemia. The incidence is 1 in 14,000 live births. It has been postulated that some primary insults such as α_1-antitrypsin, metabolic disorders, or viral infections such as CMV and HSV may incite biliary atresia. Choledochal cysts appear as dilatations of the biliary tree and obstruct the passage of bile.

Older Infants, Children, and Adolescents

The approach to the differential diagnosis of jaundice in older infants and children is similar to the process in young infants. Unconjugated hyperbilirubinemia is usually due to hemolysis, and the level of indirect bilirubin helps clarify the differential diagnosis. Patients whose indirect bilirubin is greater than 6 mg/dL may have **Crigler-Najjar syndrome type II** and respond favorably to phenobarbital. Patients with levels under 6 mg/dL may have hemolytic anemia. **Congestive heart failure (CHF)** and **hypothyroidism** may also produce unconjugated hyperbilirubinemia. **Gilbert disease,** a benign condition in which the bilirubin rises to about 5 mg/dL in response to stress and starvation, may result in jaundice. The prevalence of Gilbert syndrome, an autosomal-recessive disease, is 5%. **Drugs,** including rifampin and birth control pills, may also be associated with unconjugated hyperbilirubinemia.

Conjugated hyperbilirubinemia may result from 2 different processes: (1) cholestasis and (2) hepatocellular inflammation or injury. Signs of cholestasis are high levels of alkaline phosphatase (3 times

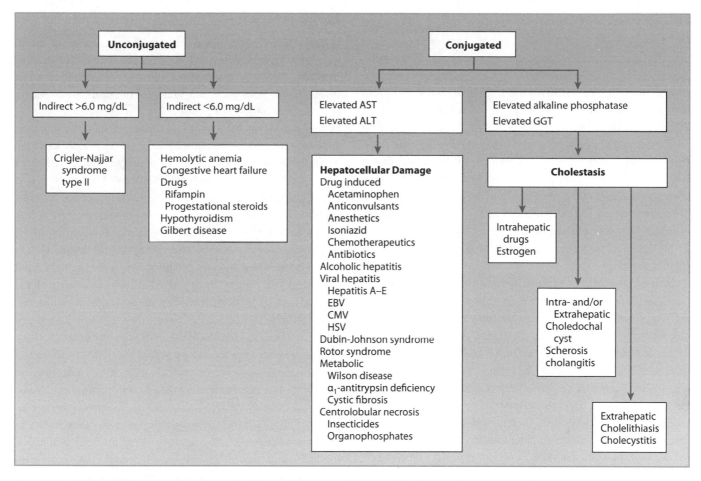

Figure 113-4. Differential diagnosis of jaundice in older infants, children, and adolescents. ALT, alanine aminotransferase; AST, aspartate aminotransferase; CMV, cytomegalovirus; EBV, Epstein-Barr virus; GGT, gamma-glutamyl transferase; HSV, herpes simplex virus.

normal), mildly to moderately elevated transaminases, and increased γ-glutamyl transpeptidase. Cholestatic jaundice, related to drugs (estrogens) and alcohol, may occur on an intrahepatic basis. **Byler syndrome** is a familial disorder characterized by intrahepatic cholestasis. Extrahepatic cholestasis is seen with cholelithiasis or other obstructions of the biliary tree. Cholelithiasis may occur in individuals with hemolytic anemia and in adolescents who are overweight or postpartum. Hepatocellular injury most often results from hepatitis (see Chapter 114), including infectious, alcoholic, and drug-induced hepatitis. Rarer disorders include Dubin-Johnson syndrome and Rotor syndrome. Metabolic diseases such as Wilson disease, α₁-antitrypsin deficiency, and cystic fibrosis should be considered in the differential diagnosis of every older child presenting with conjugated hyperbilirubinemia.

Evaluation

History

A careful history must be obtained (Questions Box).

Physical Examination

Patients should be evaluated for evidence of organomegaly, ocular anomalies, rashes, hearing deficits, and unusual facial features. The

---

Questions

Jaundice

- What associated symptoms are present?
- How long have the symptoms been present?
- Does the child have a fever, which may suggest the presence of an infection?
- What is the color of the stools (acholic stools suggest obstruction)?
- Does the child have a family history of jaundice or consanguinity?
- What makes up the child's diet? If the child is an infant, is he or she breastfed or bottle-fed?
- When did the parents first notice the jaundice?
- Has the child been jaundiced previously?
- Has the child been vaccinated against hepatitis A and B?
- Is there a history of foreign travel or shellfish ingestion?

---

unique facial features are pathognomic for certain genetic disorders such as Byler or Alagille syndromes. Rashes and lymphadenopathy are associated with certain infectious conditions, including congenital infections (TORCHS) in newborns and infectious mononucleosis in adolescents. Patients should also be checked for the presence of any cardiac anomaly, which may suggest a genetic syndrome or CHF.

Laboratory Tests

In the newborn nursery, noninvasive methods are used to measure the level of jaundice. The "jaundice meter" uses reflectance spectrophotometry to determine the skin color and correlates highly with serum bilirubin levels. An icterometer is another noninvasive method, which uses an acrylic plastic color chart that is placed against an infant's nose.

The aim of the laboratory assessment is to discover where the bilirubin metabolism is abnormal. The total bilirubin as well as the fractionated bilirubin levels should be determined. The presence of elevated levels of direct-reacting bilirubin represents conjugated hyperbilirubinemia. The demonstration of a yellow color to the foam of a shaken specimen of urine is a rapid test for conjugated hyperbilirubinemia. Urine test strips also readily detect conjugated bilirubin in the urine.

In children with unconjugated hyperbilirubinemia, a complete blood cell count with reticulocyte count and evaluation of the peripheral smear confirm hemolytic anemia. Serum haptoglobin levels are diminished in hemolytic disorders. In neonates, the Coombs test should be performed, and infant and maternal blood types should be determined. The hemoglobin should also be determined. A normal or low hemoglobin may be seen in the face of hemolytic anemia. An elevated reticulocyte count or an abnormal peripheral blood smear indicates hemolysis. Hemolytic anemias with abnormal peripheral smears include spherocytosis, elliptocytosis, stomatocytosis, and pyknocytosis (see Chapter 83).

In children with conjugated hyperbilirubinemia, tests should be performed to determine if infections such as bacteremia, UTI, congenital infection, or hepatitis are present. Evaluation for metabolic diseases should also be obtained by assessing the urine for the presence of reducing substances, organic acids, and bile acid metabolites. A sweat chloride test and α_1-antitrypsin level should be considered. The status of liver function can be determined by evaluating aspartate aminotransferase, alanine aminotransferase, γ-glutamyl transpeptidase, and alkaline phosphatase. To assess synthetic liver function, one should test prothrombin time, total protein, albumin, glucose, cholesterol, and ammonia.

Imaging Studies

The anatomy of the biliary tree can be evaluated using ultrasound. Choledochal cysts may be visualized using this modality. When a "triangular cord sign" is seen on ultrasound, the diagnosis of biliary atresia is almost certain. A triangular-shaped echogenicity demonstrates the atretic ductal remnant in the area cephalad to the portal vein bifurcation. Other imaging tests, including excretion studies (radioisotope scans) and cholangiogram, can be used to help differentiate hepatitis from biliary atresia. Consultation with a pediatric gastroenterologist may be appropriate.

Liver Biopsy

A histologic evaluation may be necessary if laboratory results have not defined an etiology. Detailed review by an experienced pathologist may be diagnostic and save the infant from an exploratory surgery.

Management

The management of jaundice depends on the cause of the condition. Physiological jaundice and jaundice secondary to breastfeeding frequently require no intervention. Primary prevention is the best strategy to combat breastfeeding jaundice. Educate the mother to initiate breastfeeding within 1 hour of life with continuous rooming-in, breastfeed every 2 to 3 hours, promptly respond to hunger cues, and prohibit supplementation with water or sugar water. However, if bilirubin levels are greater than 20, interrupting breastfeeding for 24 to 48 hours will successfully lower bilirubin levels, but support and counseling are mandatory to ensure that breastfeeding resumes. Studies suggest that the use of a casein hydrolysate formula such as Nutramigen may lead to a greater degree of reduction in the level of bilirubin than the use of a whey-predominant formula such as Enfamil. Some practitioners use **bilirubin-reducing lights,** but other clinicians believe that breastfed infants can tolerate bilirubin levels as high as 25 to 30 mg/dL without danger of kernicterus. Newer phototherapy techniques involve the use of woven fiberoptic pads that can be used in the home. Increasing the exposure of the infant to phototherapy by using standard phototherapy above and a fiberoptic pad below is more effective than either modality alone. Clinical trials are demonstrating the efficacy of a single intramuscular dose of Sn-mesoporphyrin in treating and preventing neonatal hyperbilirubinemia. Sn-mesoporphyrin, a **metalloporphyrin,** blocks heme oxygenase, the first step in the production of bilirubin. Sn-mesoporphyrin may be especially helpful in situations when blood transfusions are prohibited by the parents for religious reasons or when known hemolytic disease will put the infant at risk for kernicterus. Infants who are preterm, ill, or have jaundice as a result of hemolysis may be at a greater risk from elevated bilirubin levels. **Exchange transfusion** may be indicated in addition to placement under bilirubin-reducing lights. A rule of thumb: Preterm infants should receive exchange transfusions when the bilirubin reaches the infant's weight (eg, 11 mg/dL in a 1,100-g infant). Intravenous immunoglobulin may prevent the need for exchange transfusion in babies with hemolysis due to blood group or Rh incompatibility by reducing hemolysis.

Diet and nutrition can be an integral part to supporting an infant with conjugated hyperbilirubinemia. Medium-chain triglyceride formulas such as Pregestimil or Alimentum allow for absorption independent of bile acids. Supplementation with fat-soluble vitamins A, D, E, and K is also beneficial. If galactosemia is suspected, switch to soy formula pending results of the newborn screen.

Medications play a limited role in the management of jaundice. **Phenobarbital** may speed up the liver's excretion of bilirubin, even in cases of hemolytic anemia. This drug is also useful in the management of jaundice due to certain genetic conditions such as Crigler-Najjar syndrome type II. The appropriate **antibiotics** should be used to combat infections associated with jaundice. For relief of pruritus, ursodeoxycholic acid (15–30 mg/kg/day), or rifampicin may be offered.

Infants with biliary atresia may require **surgery.** Surgery links the surface of the liver to the intestinal tract, allowing for passage of bilirubin directly into the lumen of the small intestine. Adolescents with gallbladder disease may also require surgical intervention (ie, a cholecystectomy).

Prognosis

Most infants with elevated bilirubin levels have physiological jaundice or breast milk jaundice. The prognosis is excellent in these children. In recent years, concern has arisen about a recrudescence of kernicterus, including cases in breastfed, healthy term infants. Early discharge from the nursery and late follow-up may have contributed to this debilitating complication. Physicians should pursue an appropriate assessment of hyperbilirubinemia in jaundiced infants and not ascribe the symptoms to breastfeeding. Conditions other than physiological jaundice or breast milk jaundice may be less amenable to therapy and may require ongoing medical or surgical intervention. Children with metabolic abnormalities usually require lifelong nutritional intervention, those with hepatic disease may succumb to their hepatic dysfunction, and those treated with surgical correction of biliary atresia may have recurrent episodes of cholangitis leading to cirrhosis and the eventual need for liver transplantation.

In contrast, older infants, children, and adolescents with jaundice often have self-limited conditions that spontaneously resolve.

CASE RESOLUTION

In the case history, the infant is breastfed, which raises the possibility of breast milk jaundice. Fractionated bilirubin and hemoglobin determination are appropriate to assess the bilirubin level and confirm the absence of hemolysis. One approach to the diagnosis of breast milk as the etiology of the jaundice is to stop breastfeeding for a day or two to see if the bilirubin level decreases. (Sometimes an infant may not resume breastfeeding.) Biliary atresia or metabolic or infectious hepatitis should also be considered because of the infant's age.

The presence of normal-colored stools is reassuring, however, and makes biliary atresia less likely. The urine should be checked for the presence of reducing substances, which is a noninvasive way of evaluating the infant for galactosemia. The birth record should be obtained. Knowledge of the maternal and infant blood types would allow evaluation for mother–infant blood group incompatibility.

Selected References

Balistreri WF, Bezerra JA. Whatever happened to "neonatal hepatitis"? *Clin Liver Dis.* 2006;10:27–53

Farrant P, Meire HB, Mieli-Vergani G. Ultrasound features of the gall bladder in infants presenting with conjugated hyperbilirubinemia. *Br J Radiol.* 2000;73:1154–1158

Haber BA, Russo P. Biliary atresia. *Gastroenterol Clin North Am.* 2003;32:891–911

Kappas A. A method for interdicting the development of severe jaundice in newborns by inhibiting the production of bilirubin. *Pediatrics.* 2004;113:119–123

Maisels MJ. Neonatal jaundice. *Pediatr Rev.* 2006;27:443–454

Pashankar D, Schreiber RA. Jaundice in older children and adolescents. *Pediatr Rev.* 2001;22:219–225

Suchy FJ, Sokol RJ, Balistreri WF. *Liver Disease in Children.* 3rd ed. Cambridge University Press; 2007

Watchko JF. Identification of neonates at risk for hazardous hyperbilirubinemia: emerging clinical insights. *Pediatr Clin N Am.* 2009;56:671–687

CHAPTER 114

Viral Hepatitis

ChrisAnna M. Mink, MD, and Monica Sifuentes, MD

CASE STUDY

A 15-year-old boy is brought to the office with a 1-week history of intermittent fever, vomiting, diarrhea, and diffuse abdominal pain. His mother reports the appearance of "yellow eyes and skin" on the day before the visit. Her son was previously in good health, and he has not seen a physician in several years. He is taking no medications and has no known ill contacts. He has no history of recent travel outside the United States and denies any unusual food ingestions. Mom reports that he frequently eats at a local fast-food restaurant with his soccer team, but his family does not eat there. He has one ear piercing and denies sexual activity, drug use, or tattoos.

The physical examination is significant for a temperature of 101.4°F (38.6°C), pulse of 100 beats/min, and blood pressure of 110/63 mm Hg. The teen is a well-developed, well-nourished male with yellow skin and sclera.

The abdomen is soft, with mild diffuse tenderness, most notably over the right upper quadrant, and normal bowel sounds. The liver edge is palpated 5 cm below the right costal margin, and no splenomegaly is present. The rectal examination is normal, with guaiac-negative stool.

Questions

1. What are the most common causes of viral hepatitis in children and adolescents?
2. What is the appropriate evaluation for children and adolescents with suspected hepatitis?
3. What complications are associated with viral hepatitis?
4. What treatments are currently available for viral hepatitis, and how does treatment differ depending on the specific etiology?

Hepatitis is an inflammation of the liver that can occur as the result of an exposure to a toxin, such as a chemical or drug, or an infectious agent. Viruses are the most common cause of hepatitis in children and adolescents, and previously, most cases in the United States were the result of hepatitis A virus (HAV), hepatitis B virus (HBV), or hepatitis C virus (HCV). With the advent of routine immunization for pediatric and adolescent age groups for HAV and HBV, the incidence of both infections has dramatically declined. Routine immunizations have reduced the occurrence of infection, as well as complications and long-term consequences, especially for hepatitis B. All 3 of these unrelated viruses can produce an acute illness characterized by nausea, malaise, abdominal pain, and jaundice. Hepatitis B virus and HCV also can produce a chronic infection that is associated with an increased risk for chronic liver disease and hepatocellular carcinoma.

Other common viruses that can cause hepatitis in children are Epstein-Barr virus (EBV), cytomegalovirus (CMV), varicella-zoster virus (VZV), adenovirus, enteroviruses, and herpes simplex virus (HSV); however, their contribution to the overall morbidity and mortality associated with infectious hepatitis is minimal.

Epidemiology

In 2008 nearly 7,500 cases of viral hepatitis were passively reported in the United States to the Centers for Disease Control and Prevention. Most cases were due to HAV or HBV, and fewer than 900 were attributed to HCV. This reflects a more than 80% decline in HAV and HBV from the peak incidence in 1995. The number of cases of HCV is slightly increased. The total number of hepatitis cases is probably underestimated as a result of under-recognition and underreporting, but likely exceeds 25,000.

Although the incidence of HAV and HBV infections are declining, children younger than 15 years have the highest incidence of infectious hepatitis. Both genders are equally affected. Certain situations are associated with increased risk for infection with HAV. These include crowded living conditions, chronic care facilities, military institutions, prisons, child care centers, travelers to endemic areas, and high-risk sexual practices (eg, commercial sex workers and men who have sex with men). Poor personal hygiene and inadequate sanitation are also risk factors. In approximately 50% of hepatitis A cases, however, the source of infection is unknown. Hepatitis A is found worldwide, but specific locations are associated with an increased incidence of the disease, including Central and South America, Africa, the Mediterranean region, and Asia.

Groups at high risk for HBV infection include illicit parenteral drug users, commercial sex workers, men who have sex with men, heterosexuals with multiple sexual partners, health care workers, recipients of hemodialysis, household contacts of carriers of HBV, and immigrants from HBV-endemic areas. Individuals who live in crowded environments with poor hygienic standards, such as institutions for the developmentally disabled or correctional facilities, are also at risk for HBV infection. No risk factors are identified in 40% of cases. Worldwide, approximately 5% of the population (ie, 350 million people) is chronically infected with HBV. Areas with the highest incidence of hepatitis B include Southeast Asia, most of Africa, the Pacific Islands, China, and parts of the Middle East.

Approximately 10% to 15% of primary infections with HBV result in a chronic carrier state. The younger children are when they are infected with HBV, the more likely they are to become chronic carriers. Between 70% and 90% of infants born to infected mothers become carriers, and at least 50% of children infected before the age of 5 years become carriers. Boys have a greater risk of becoming carriers than girls, though the reason for this disparity is not known.

Hepatitis C virus accounts for 20% to 40% of all viral hepatitis in all age groups. High-risk individuals are recipients of transfusions of blood or blood products, recipients of organ or tissue transplants, intravenous (IV) drug users, health care workers with blood exposure, hemodialysis patients and, infrequently, sexual or household contacts of infected persons. No identifiable source can be found in at least 35% of cases. In the pediatric population, recipients of blood and blood products before 1992, clotting factor concentrates before 1987 (eg, hemophiliacs), dialysis patients, institutionalized children, and high-risk infants (eg, maternal history of IV drug abuse, sexually transmitted infections [STIs], or HIV coinfection) are most likely to be at risk for HCV infection.

Because hepatitis D only occurs as a coinfection with HBV, high-risk groups are the same, with the exclusion of health care workers and homosexual males. High prevalence rates occur in Eastern Europe, Central Africa, southern Italy, and the Middle East.

Hepatitis E virus (HEV) infection is endemic in developing countries such as Mexico, Central and Southeast Asia, North Africa, China, and India. No cases of HEV infection acquired in the United States have been reported. In endemic regions, HEV is the most common cause of symptomatic hepatitis in children. Young and middle-aged adults are most commonly affected, and HEV infection is especially severe for pregnant women.

Clinical Presentation

Children with acute hepatitis generally present with complaints suggestive of a "flu-like" illness, including fever, malaise, decreased appetite, nausea, and vomiting. They may also report diffuse abdominal pain. Unlike adults in whom jaundice is a common finding, pediatric patients, particularly infants and young children, are frequently anicteric. Hepatomegaly is often found on physical examination though not universally, and there may be varying degrees of right upper quadrant discomfort (Dx Box). A nonspecific macular

---

rash, papulovesicular acrodermatitis (Gianotti-Crosti syndrome), and arthralgias can also occur in the course of HBV infection.

Pathophysiology

Hepatitis A

Hepatitis A virus is a picornavirus composed of single-stranded RNA with only one serotype. The most common modes of transmission are through close personal contact and contaminated food and water. This generally occurs by fecal contamination and oral ingestion. Shellfish, such as raw oysters, clams, and mussels, are a frequent source of infection. Infected food handlers may also transmit the disease.

The average incubation period for hepatitis A is 28 to 30 days (range: 15–50 days). Peak viral secretion occurs before the onset of jaundice. The virus is shed in the stool 2 to 3 weeks before the onset of jaundice and up to 1 week after its appearance. However, most young children are anicteric, so infections often go unnoticed during this highly contagious period (Figure 114-1). The duration of illness is usually 2 to 4 weeks. A prolonged course or relapse occurs in 10% to 20% of adult cases. A chronic carrier state for HAV does not exist, though fulminant infections can occur. Lifelong immunity is conferred after a single infection. Mortality is rare, especially in children.

Hepatitis B

Hepatitis B virus is a double-stranded DNA virus in the Hepadnaviridae family. The disease is usually spread by contact with infected blood or blood products, but it can also occur through close interpersonal contact. Although hepatitis B surface antigen (HBsAg) is found in numerous body secretions (blood and blood products, feces, urine, tears, saliva, semen, breast milk, vaginal secretions, cerebrospinal and synovial fluid), only serum, semen, vaginal secretions,

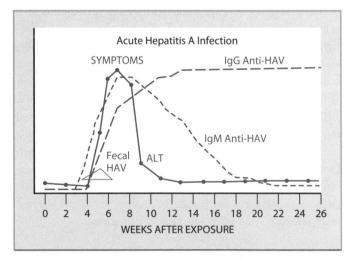

Figure 114-1. Course of acute hepatitis A infection. HAV, hepatitis A virus; Ig, immunoglobulin. (Reproduced with permission from Tabor E. Etiology, diagnosis and treatment of viral hepatitis in children. In: Aronoff SC, Hughes WT, Kohl S, Speck WT, Wald ER, eds. *Advances in Pediatric Infectious Diseases*. Chicago, IL: Year Book Medical Publishers; 1988.)

Dx Hepatitis

- Diffuse abdominal pain
- Nonspecific symptoms (fever, malaise, anorexia, nausea, and vomiting)
- Jaundice (not necessarily in all cases)
- Dark urine and light-colored stool
- Pain or tenderness over the liver area
- Hepatomegaly

and saliva have been proven contagious. No fecal-oral transmission occurs. Transmission is facilitated through percutaneous inoculation (eg, tattooing, IV drug use) and exposure of cuts in the skin and mucous membranes to contaminated fluids on objects such as razors and utensils. Sexual transmission occurs via semen, vaginal secretions, and saliva. Perinatal vertical transmission occurs in infants whose mothers are acutely infected or chronic carriers. Although the exact mode of transmission is unclear for household contacts, postnatal infection from household exposure has been reported.

The average incubation period for HBV infection is 3 to 4 months (range: 1–6 months). Figure 114-2 depicts the typical course of acute hepatitis B, along with the course of the chronic carrier state.

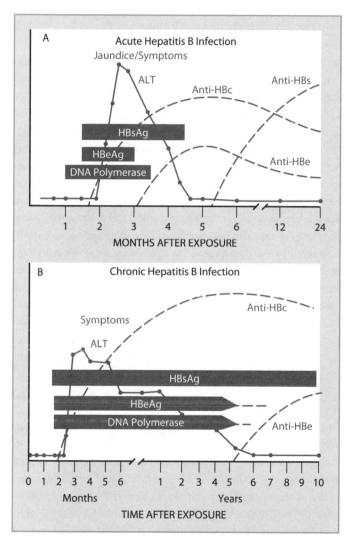

Figure 114-2. Course of hepatitis B infection. A. Acute hepatitis B infection. B. Chronic hepatitis B infection. ALT, alanine aminotransferase; HBc, hepatitis B core; HBe, hepatitis B e; HBeAg, hepatitis B e antigen; HBs, hepatitis B surface; HBsAg, hepatitis B surface antigen. (Reproduced with permission from Tabor E. Etiology, diagnosis and treatment of viral hepatitis in children. In: Aronoff SC, Hughes WT, Kohl S, Speck WT, Wald ER, eds. *Advances in Pediatric Infectious Diseases.* Chicago, IL: Year Book Medical Publishers; 1988.)

Hepatitis C

Hepatitis C virus is a single-stranded RNA virus in the *Flavivirus* family, and it is able to mutate rapidly, thus escaping detection by the host's immune system. Like HBV, HCV can be spread through contact with contaminated blood and blood products. Conditions associated with HCV infection in children and adolescents include hemophilia and hemoglobinopathies such as thalassemia and sickle cell disease (possibly due to increased exposure to blood products), a history of malignancy, administration of hemodialysis or solid organ transplantation, and IV drug use. Vertical transmission can occur, but seems to be infrequent (1%–5% of infants born to HCV-infected mothers). Contaminated immune globulin (Ig) administered between April 1, 1993, and February 23, 1994, has been implicated as a source of HCV infection. Transmission of infection via household and sexual contact has been demonstrated as well.

The incubation period is variable, ranging from 2 weeks to 6 months, and averages 6 to 7 weeks. Most affected children are anicteric as well as asymptomatic. If symptomatic infection is present, it is usually mild, insidious, and indistinguishable from infections due to HAV or HBV. Jaundice occurs in only 25% of patients. Fulminant hepatitis is extremely uncommon.

Hepatitis D

Acute delta hepatitis, or hepatitis D, is caused by a distinct single-stranded RNA virus that requires HBsAg for replication. Both the virus and a delta antigen are enclosed in an envelope of HBsAg. Transmission is similar to HBV, but vertical transmission is uncommon. Hepatitis D occurs either as a coinfection with HBV or a superinfection in a chronic carrier of HBV. Acute disease is usually more severe and carries a higher risk of fulminant hepatitis than hepatitis B infection alone.

Hepatitis E

Hepatitis E virus is caused by an enterically transmitted RNA virus. Transmission is primarily through contaminated drinking water and fecal-oral spread, especially during rainy or monsoon seasons in endemic areas.

The incubation period ranges from 2 to 9 weeks, with most cases of acute infection being self-limited. Mortality is low in endemic populations, except in pregnant women. Nearly all cases of HEV infection in the United States have been reported in travelers to endemic areas.

Differential Diagnosis

The differential diagnosis of hepatitis depends on the patient's age, possible exposures, and immunization history. Possible infectious causes in neonates include overwhelming bacterial sepsis, VZV, and congenital infections (TORCHES [toxoplasmosis, rubella, CMV, HSV, HIV, enteroviruses, and syphilis]), in addition to HBV infection. Perinatal transmission of HAV is rare. Genetic disorders and anatomical abnormalities causing biliary obstruction (eg, biliary atresia) should also be considered (see Chapter 113).

In older infants and children, in addition to HAV, HBV, and HCV, other viral etiologies include EBV, CMV, enteroviruses (including coxsackieviruses), adenovirus, VZV, HSV and, less commonly, rubella, rubeola, and HIV. Acute or chronic anemias such as sickle cell disease can also cause hepatomegaly and jaundice. Noninfectious conditions to consider include drug-induced hepatitis (eg, treatment with prescribed medications such as isoniazid or phenytoin); toxin ingestion (eg, acetaminophen, herbal remedies); and conditions such as cystic fibrosis, α_1-antitrypsin deficiency, Wilson disease, and other congenital disorders such as Caroli disease (intrahepatic dilation of the bile ducts).

In adolescents, viral etiologies to consider are similar to those listed for children. Other infectious processes to consider in the adolescent age group include biliary tract infections, bacterial sepsis, Fitz-Hugh–Curtis syndrome (liver inflammation associated with pelvic infections, especially with *Chlamydia trachomatis* and *Neisseria gonorrhea,* and *Mycoplasma hominis.*) The list of prescribed and illicit drugs that may cause liver toxicity is extensive and includes oral contraceptives, seizure medications, alcohol, inhalants, acetaminophen, and tetracycline.

Evaluation

History

A comprehensive history should be obtained in children of all ages (Questions Box). A dietary and travel history is essential, especially when considering HAV and HEV.

For young infants, a complete maternal and obstetrical history should be obtained and include the following questions: Does the mother have any history of IV drug use? Does the mother come from an area where hepatitis is highly endemic, such as Southeast Asia?

Questions

Hepatitis

- Does the child have any history of fever, malaise, anorexia, or weight loss?
- Has the child experienced any vomiting or diarrhea?
- Is any abdominal pain or discomfort present? If so, in what location?
- Are yellow eyes or any changes in skin color apparent? If so, for how long?
- Is the color of the urine dark and the stool light?
- What is the child's recent travel history?
- Has the child ingested any shellfish in the previous 1 to 2 months?
- Has the child been in contact with any individuals with hepatitis or jaundice (including sexual contacts)?
- Is the child taking any medications (eg, isoniazid)?
- Does the child have a history of transfusion with blood or blood products?
- Is the adolescent sexually active, or has the adolescent had any known exposure to sexually transmitted infections (STIs)?
- Does the adolescent have a history of intravenous (IV) drug use?
- Does the mother have a history of hepatitis, IV drug use, STIs, or multiple sexual partners?

Did the mother receive prenatal care? Was hepatitis B screening performed prenatally or at delivery? Did the mother have any known STIs or sexual contacts with hepatitis B–infected individuals, or did she have multiple sexual partners?

The physician should ask adolescents about sexual activity, STIs, and the number of sexual partners. In addition, it is important to inquire about parenteral drug use and tattoos.

Physical Examination

Most children with viral hepatitis are asymptomatic and generally do not present for medical evaluation. For symptomatic children, there are no clues on examination to aid in differentiating the causes. However, a complete physical examination should be performed to help rule out other etiologies. All vital signs should be recorded. The temperature is important, especially if children have a recent history of fever. In children who are vomiting, signs of dehydration (eg, tachycardia, evidence of orthostatic hypotension, dry mucous membranes, tenting of the skin, sunken eyes, and lethargy) should be noted. Growth parameters, particularly weight, should be obtained and compared with previous measurements if available.

The skin should be examined for jaundice; evidence of pruritus (eg, excoriations), which may be associated with elevated bilirubin; or a nonspecific rash. Icterus of the sclera, tympanic membranes, and palate should also be noted. The abdomen should be palpated for tenderness and organomegaly, particularly hepatomegaly. The liver span should also be determined by percussion because it will help monitor the patient's progress. Splenomegaly, which is not typically found in hepatitis, indicates a different diagnosis, such as leukemia, or another infectious cause, such as EBV or CMV. A rectal examination should also be performed to look for masses or blood in the stool, which may suggest a neoplastic etiology.

A neurologic examination is important to document any signs of encephalopathy from hyperammonemia, which occurs more commonly in chronic liver disease or fulminant hepatic failure.

Laboratory Tests

The initial laboratory tests needed are directed by the severity of illness in the child at presentation. At a minimum, these include liver function tests (LFTs) (alanine aminotransferase, aspartate aminotransferase, γ-glutamyltransferase, and total and direct bilirubin) and coagulation studies (prothrombin time [PT]/partial thromboplastin time). Monitoring PT is particularly useful because of its rapid turnaround time and predictive utility; if the value is greater than 3 seconds above the upper limit of normal (international normalized ratio >1.5), the prognosis is poor. Serologic testing for hepatitis A (HAV-IgM and HAV-IgG) and hepatitis B panel (HBsAg, HBs antibody, hepatitis B e antigen [HbeAg], HBe antibody, and hepatitis B core antibody) should also be performed. Diagnostic antibody patterns for HAV and HBV are shown in Figures 114-1 and 114-2.

Serum antibody to HCV (anti-HCV) should be sent, especially for individuals with risk factors for infection. A confirmatory test such as a recombinant immunoblot assay, which measures antibody to various regions of the HCV genome, is generally performed if a screening enzyme immunoassay (EIA) is positive, as false-positive EIAs may occur. Hepatitis C virus serologic assays detect IgG anti-HCV antibody; IgM tests are not available. Hepatitis C virus RNA polymerase chain reaction (PCR) has generally replaced the immunoblot for confirmatory testing, and PCR can also be use in other situations (eg, testing an immunocompromised individual who may not make antibodies). Serologic markers for hepatitis D (IgM and IgG anti-hepatitis D virus [HDV]) can be sent when concurrent HBV infection is evident. Isolation of the hepatitis D antigen in the liver, however, is the gold standard test for diagnosis of hepatitis D. Other serologic testing may be performed as indicated by history (eg, testing for syphilis with rapid plasma reagin for sexually active teens). A complete blood cell count and comprehensive metabolic panel may be needed in ill-appearing children, especially with signs of dehydration. A urinalysis for bilirubin should be done. In severe or complicated cases of viral hepatitis, additional testing such as liver biopsy or ultrasound may be indicated. For these cases, consultation with specialists in infectious diseases and hepatology is needed.

Management

For most cases of acute HAV, HBV, or HCV infection, therapy consists of **supportive care.** These illnesses are usually self-limited, and no specific therapy is indicated. Adequate nutrition and hydration are of primary importance. Therefore, the **intake of sufficient food and fluids** should be ensured. A low-protein diet during the acute phase of the illness may be considered. The use of **antipyretics** such as acetaminophen or ibuprofen for fever usually does not pose a problem in patients with mild disease and acutely elevated LFTs. However, because it is metabolized by the liver, it is preferable to limit the use of acetaminophen. Physical activity should be limited until patients feel better and LFTs return to normal. Children and adolescents can return to school when they are no longer jaundiced; they may also resume a normal diet at that time.

In children with more severe symptoms, IV hydration and an antiemetic may be indicated. Hospitalization is required for children who are moderately to severely dehydrated, are unable to tolerate fluids, or have evidence of fulminant liver failure. Treatment is aimed at correcting any metabolic abnormalities or electrolyte disturbances, including hypoglycemia. Coagulopathies should be corrected with vitamin K, fresh frozen plasma, and cryoprecipitate. Total parenteral nutrition may be required to maintain caloric needs.

Consultation with a pediatric gastroenterologist is important for management of children with acute fulminant liver failure or chronic, active hepatitis. Although no specific treatments are available for fulminant acute viral hepatitis, a few treatment options are now approved for treating children with chronic infection with HBV and HCV. Treatment options for both infections include immunomodulators such as interferon-α [IFN-α, available as IFN-α-2b and pegylated recombinant interferon-α-2a and anti-viral agents (eg, lamuvidine for HBV and ribavirin for HCV) generally given in combination regimens. Variables for choosing to treat and with what regimen depend on the child's age, underlying health status, and

degree of viral activity. All treatment regimens are associated with adverse effects. Most pediatric patients with chronic HCV infection are asymptomatic and do not usually warrant treatment.

Children and adolescents with HBV and HCV chronic infection and their parents should be counseled to avoid hepatotoxic medications and alcohol. Their parents should be informed of the possibility of transmission to others, and patients should refrain from donating blood, organs, tissue, or semen. In addition, sexually active adolescents should be informed of the possible risk to sexual partners. Toothbrushes and razors should not be shared among household contacts. Most children with chronic HBV and HCV should not be excluded from child care centers because of their infection. Possible reasons for exclusion of HBV-infected children include biting behaviors, bleeding disorders, and generalized dermatitis. Because children with chronic HBV and HCV infection are at risk for the development of serious liver disease, they should be followed regularly by their physician in conjunction with a pediatric gastroenterologist experienced in caring for these children.

Prevention

All children should routinely receive immunizations for HBV (starting as early as birth) and for HAV (starting at 12 months of age). For older children and adolescents, review of their immunization records should be performed at all medical encounters, and catch-up doses of hepatitis A and B vaccine should be provided. In the United States, some states require proof of HBV vaccination for school enrollment.

Hepatitis A

Routine **immunization** for children starting at the age of 12 months has been recommended by the Advisory Committee on Immunization Practices and American Academy of Pediatrics since late 2006. In 1995 target groups were given hepatitis A vaccine, which led to a more than 85% decline in disease incidence. **Hand washing** by food handlers, medical personnel, and child care workers is one of the primary methods for prevention of the spread of HAV. **Contact precautions** should be used for hospitalized patients for at least one week after onset of symptoms. Active immunization with hepatitis A vaccine and/or passive immunization with Ig is recommended as postexposure prophylaxis for all people who have had intimate exposure to infected individuals. The hepatitis A vaccine and Ig may be administered at the same time in different sites. Postexposure Ig is generally not indicated for contacts at school or work, but Ig is indicated for HAV-exposed infants younger than 12 months, as they are not candidates for HAV vaccine. The dose of Ig is 0.02 mL/kg within 48 hours of exposure, given no later than 2 weeks after exposure. Immune globulin is 80% to 90% effective in prevention of clinical HAV disease. Pre-exposure prophylaxis with vaccine and/or Ig is recommended for travelers to endemic areas. If the stay is less than 3 months, the dose of Ig is 0.02 mL/kg; for longer stays, the dose is 0.06 mL/kg every 5 months. Two inactivated hepatitis A vaccines have been licensed in the United States for use in children 12 months of age and older, as well as for adults. The vaccine efficacy is over 94%

for preventing clinical HAV disease. The 2 licensed vaccines seem to be interchangeable. Two doses of the vaccine are recommended and should be given initially and 6 to 12 months later. Combination vaccine against HAV and HBV (Twinrix, GlaxoSmith Kline) is licensed for individuals older than 18 years.

In addition to routine childhood immunization, specific other groups for whom hepatitis A vaccine is recommended include travelers to endemic areas who are older than 12 months of age, individuals with chronic liver disease, men who have sex with men, users of injection and illicit drugs, and those at occupational risk of exposure. Other potential recipients include child care center staff and attendees, hospital personnel, food handlers, and individuals with hemophilia.

Hepatitis B

Preventive strategies for hepatitis B include universal immunization of all infants beginning shortly after birth and pre-exposure and post-exposure prophylaxis. In addition, the vaccination of selected individuals at increased risk and "catch-up" vaccination for unimmunized adolescents, especially those at high risk, is recommended.

Passive immunization with **hepatitis B immunoglobulin (HBIG)** is recommended for infants born to known HBsAg-positive mothers or mothers whose status is unknown. Passive immunization is also recommended for susceptible individuals who are sexual partners of persons with acute hepatitis B infections, household contacts (including children <1 year who have received <2 doses of vaccine), and those who experience mucosal or percutaneous exposure to HBsAg-positive blood. Unimmunized victims of sexual assault or abuse should receive HBIG if the offender is known to be HBsAg-positive. Simultaneous active immunization with the hepatitis B vaccine is recommended in these cases.

Immunization with the hepatitis B vaccine (active immunization) is currently recommended for all infants, adolescents not previously immunized, IV drug users, men who have sex with men, children receiving blood or blood products regularly (eg, hemophiliacs), children in chronic care facilities, household contacts of chronic carriers, and health care professionals. The standard schedule consists of 3 doses. Infants should receive the first dose before discharge from the nursery or shortly thereafter, the second dose 1 to 2 months later, and the third dose at 6 to 18 months of age. Infants should not receive the 3rd dose before 6 months of age. Intervals for other individuals are similar.

Perinatal vertical transmission of HBV can be prevented by giving newborns HBIG (0.5 mL intramuscularly) within 12 hours after birth and hepatitis B vaccine concurrently (at a different site) prior to discharge. This practice prevents approximately 90% of chronic infections in infants born to mothers with HBsAg and HBeAg. Post-immunization serologic screening is recommended, however, for these infants at 1 year of age because approximately 5% become carriers despite appropriate preventive vaccination. Special schedules for active and passive immunizations against HBV should be consulted for premature infants who weigh less than 2,000 g.

Hepatitis C

No vaccine exists for the prevention of HCV infection. Because Ig is manufactured from plasma that is HCV-antibody negative, it is not recommended for prophylaxis.

Current recommendations include screening individuals with risk factors for HCV infection (see Pathophysiology), infants born to HCV-infected women, recipients of Ig between April 1993 and February 1994, and children with clinical hepatitis found not to have hepatitis A or B.

Hepatitis D

Prevention of HBV infection through universal vaccination is the most important means of controlling HDV infection.

Prognosis

The prognosis for children with viral hepatitis depends on etiology, as well as the child's age and underlying health status, at the time of infection. For HAV infection, the outcome is generally good, with an uneventful recovery. Infants and children infected with HBV, on the other hand, are at high risk of becoming chronic carriers, especially if infected at a young age. Approximately 25% of carriers develop chronic, active hepatitis, which often progresses to cirrhosis. In addition, the risk of developing hepatocellular carcinoma is 12 to 300 times higher in these patients compared with the rest of the population.

Chronic hepatitis also occurs with HCV infection, though it is unknown whether chronic infection and subsequent complications are higher for neonates. Autoimmune complications such as arthritis, serum sickness, and erythema multiforme are common with chronic disease. Approximately 70% of patients with acute HCV infection later develop chronic hepatitis, and 10% to 20% progress to cirrhosis and hepatic failure. Hepatocellular carcinoma has also been described in a small proportion of patients.

Likewise, complications of hepatitis D, such as cirrhosis and portal hypertension, are not uncommon. They occur more frequently than with hepatitis B alone and progress more rapidly. Infection with HEV does not result in a chronic condition. Fatal hepatitis A is a rare occurrence. The overall mortality associated with HBV, HCV, and HEV is also low (approximately 1%–2%), though HEV can be fatal in 20% of infected pregnant women. For hepatitis D, mortality it is more variable, ranging from 2% to 20%. Figures increase to 30% for HBV with coinfection with hepatitis D.

CASE RESOLUTION

In the case history, the teen has a classic presentation of viral hepatitis despite no history of travel to an endemic area. Statistics point to probable infection with hepatitis A, and exposure possibly occurred at the fast-food restaurant. Because he does not appear to be dehydrated or seriously ill, he can be managed as an outpatient. Serologic testing for hepatitis A, B, and C should be performed, in addition to LFTs and coagulation studies. The parents should be informed of the probable diagnosis and if confirmed as hepatitis A, all household contacts should receive hepatitis A vaccine and/or prophylaxis with Ig. They should also be educated regarding the infectivity of the disease and counseled about supportive therapy. Public health officials should be consulted for management of other individuals who were possibly exposed. The boy should have limited physical activity while symptomatic and he should be scheduled for a follow-up visit in a few days for repeat LFTs and coagulation tests. The prognosis is good.

Selected References

Advisory Committee on Immunization Practices; Fiore AE, Wasley A, Bell BP. Prevention of hepatitis A through active or passive immunization: recommendations of the Advisory Committee on Immunization Practices (ACIP). *MMWR Recomm Rep.* 2006;55(RR-07):1–23

American Academy of Pediatrics. Hepatitis A. In: Pickering LK, Baker CJ, Kimberlin DW, Long SS, eds. *Red Book: 2009 Report of the Committee on Infectious Diseases.* 27th ed. Elk Grove Village, IL: American Academy of Pediatrics; 2009:329–337

American Academy of Pediatrics. Hepatitis B. In: Pickering LK, Baker CJ, Kimberlin DW, Long SS, eds. *Red Book: 2009 Report of the Committee on Infectious Diseases.* 27th ed. Elk Grove Village, IL: American Academy of Pediatrics; 2009:337–357

American Academy of Pediatrics. Hepatitis C. In: Pickering LK, Baker CJ, Kimberlin DW, Long SS, eds. *Red Book: 2009 Report of the Committee on Infectious Diseases.* 27th ed. Elk Grove Village, IL: American Academy of Pediatrics; 2009:357–360

Broderick A, Jonas MM. Overview of Hepatitis B in Children. UptoDate. http://www.uptodate.com/online/content/topic.do?topicKey=pedi_hep/2866&selectedTitle=1%7E150&source=search_result. Accessed January 24, 2011

Centers for Disease Control and Prevention. Surveillance Data for Acute Viral Hepatitis—United States, 2008. http://www.cdc.gov/hepatitis/Statistics/2008Surveillance/index.htm

Curry MP, Chopra S. Acute viral hepatitis. In: Mandell GL, Bennett JE, Dolin R, eds. *Mandell, Douglas, and Bennett's Principles and Practice of Infectious Diseases.* 6th ed. Philadelphia, PA: Elsevier; 2005:1426–1441

Daniels D, Grytdal S, Wasley A; Centers for Disease Control and Prevention. Surveillance for acute viral hepatitis—United States, 2007. *MMWR Surveill Summ.* 2009;58:1–27

Kim WR. The burden of hepatitis C in the United States. *Hepatology.* 2002;36:S30–S34

Mast EE, Weinbaum CM, Fiore AE, et al. A comprehensive immunization strategy to eliminate transmission of hepatitis B virus infection in the United States: recommendations of the Advisory Committee on Immunization Practices (ACIP) part II: immunization of adults. *MMWR Recomm Rep.* 2006;55(RR-16):1–33

Schwimmer JB, Balisteri WF. Transmission, natural history, and treatment of hepatitis C virus infection in the pediatric population. *Semin Liver Dis.* 2000;20:37–46

Tovo PA, Lazier L, Versace A. Hepatitis B virus and hepatitis C virus infections in children. *Curr Opin Infect Dis.* 2005;18:261–266

Wasley A, Miller JT, Finelli L; Centers for Diseases Control and Prevention. Surveillance for acute viral hepatitis—United States, 2005. *MMWR Surveill Summ.* 2007;56:1–24

Wolff DC. Viral Hepatitis. http://emedicine.medscape.com/article/185463-overview. Accessed January 24, 2011

Neurologic Disorders

CHAPTER 115

Hypotonia

Kenneth R. Huff, MD

CASE STUDY

A 6-month-old girl is brought to the office because she does not reach for her toys anymore. The pregnancy was full term, but the mother remembers that the fetal kicking was less than with an older brother. Delivery was uncomplicated, and the infant fed well from birth. The girl began to show visual attention at 2 to 3 weeks, smiled socially at 1 month, and pushed up while prone at 2 months. Although she turned over at 4 months, she has not done this in the last month. She no longer reaches up to the mobile over her crib.

On examination, the girl lies quietly on the table and watches the examiner intently. Her growth parameters, including head circumference, are normal. After she has been undressed, it is apparent that she "seesaw" breathes (ie, abdomen rises with inspiration) and has a "frog-leg" posture. Her cranial nerve examination is normal except for head-turning strength. When she is pulled to a sitting position, her head lags far behind and her arms are straight at the elbows. She cannot raise her arms off the table. When a rattle is placed in her hands, she manipulates the toy, which she regards from the corner of her eye. Her deep tendon reflexes are absent, but her pain sensation is intact.

Questions

1. How is the level of nervous system involvement determined in infants with hypotonia? What levels of the nervous system are usually involved in the infant with hypotonia?
2. What is the significance of a loss of developmental milestones or abilities?
3. How are clinical management issues related to prognosis?
4. When is genetic counseling appropriate for children with hypotonia?

Infants with decreased tone are referred to as hypotonic or "floppy." Hypotonia is most simply defined as lower than normal resistance to passive motion across a joint, but is also suggested by abnormal posture. Although the lack of resistance may have other components (such as connective tissue abnormalities suggested by an unusual range of joint mobility, blue sclera, hyper-elastic skin, or Down syndrome features), muscle strength is a key component. Tone can be used as a surrogate indicator of strength in infants who cannot cooperate with resistance testing. Weakness can also be inferred from functional observations and the inability to sustain limbs against gravity or the lack of a withdrawal response of a limb to a painful stimulus. Identification of the level of the nervous system affected (eg, upper motor neurons, spinal cord, anterior horn cell, peripheral nerve components, myoneural junction, or muscle fibers) is most important in determining the etiology of hypotonia in infants and children. Only after this localization is the likely pathology defined in most cases.

Epidemiology

Hypotonia is not unusual in neonates, and non-neuromuscular causes of hypotonia are more common than neuromuscular conditions. Non-neuromuscular causes include hypoxic-ischemic encephalopathy and brain lesions related to premature birth, such as intraventricular hemorrhage and periventricular leukomalacia. Genetic abnormalities also are frequently present shortly after birth. Spinal muscular atrophy (SMA) is a common progressive genetic condition with an incidence similar to cystic fibrosis, about 1 in 5,000. Duchenne muscular dystrophy is the most common neuromuscular condition in childhood, with an incidence of 1 in 1,700 to 1 in 3,500 male births. The Duchenne gene has been found to spontaneously mutate in approximately 50% of the cases. Among nongenetic disorders, the incidence of acute postinfectious polyneuritis or Landry–Guillain-Barré syndrome is 2 to 8 per 100,000.

Clinical Presentation

Hypotonia in infants often presents as an unusual posture of the infant, diminished resistance to passive movements of limbs or trunk, or an excessive range of joint mobility. Hypotonic infants have delayed motor milestones, decreased movements, and poor head and trunk control (Figure 115-1). Older children may have decreased ability to resist with strength testing of individual muscle groups as well as impaired functional strength in sitting, standing, walking, climbing, or running (Dx Box). Swayback posture in standing may indicate hip girdle or proximal weakness. Pointed toes in the supine position may indicate an upper motor cause.

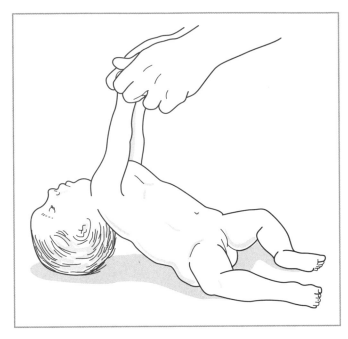

Figure 115-1. Hypotonic infant being pulled into sitting position. Arms are completely extended, head control is poor, and legs are abducted at the hip.

 Hypotonia

- Decreased resistance to passive movement of a joint
- Muscular weakness in older children
- Etiologic diagnosis related to the nervous system level of the lesion

Pathophysiology

Tone is a product of connective tissue structural elements, including ligaments, tendons, and joint capsules; muscle fiber number and integrity; and nerve fiber input to muscle. Nerve input to the muscle includes the number and myelination of axon fibers, trophic factors from the nerve, and the frequency of action potentials depolarizing the muscle membrane. The control of tone through the anterior horn cell is complex and involves more than just corticospinal tract (upper motor unit) but also other descending tract influences. Lesions of the neuromuscular apparatus (lower motor unit), which includes muscle, nerve, nerve sheaths, and anterior horn cell, can most directly decrease tone, but lesions of any of the other structures at many levels of the nervous system can also affect tone. The final common pathway of upper or lower motor unit modification of tone is through the gamma loop (fusimotor) system. Gamma motoneurons within the anterior horn of the spinal cord innervate the contractile muscle portions on each end of the intrafusal fiber and enhance the sensitivity of the sensory endings to stretch, which in turn transmit signals back to the alpha motoneurons in the anterior horn innervating the rest of the muscle. Different levels of the central nervous system (CNS) (motor cortex, thalamus, basal ganglia, vestibular nuclei, reticular formation, and cerebellum) can modify tone through their effect on the gamma motoneuron.

The nature of the lesion at different levels of the nervous system may be quite variable. For example, ultrastructural abnormalities occur in congenital myopathies, including those related to respiratory chain defects, anterior horn cell apoptosis occurs in SMA and may also occur with ischemic insults, and stripping of myelin by macrophages occurs with acute postinfectious polyneuritis.

Differential Diagnosis

Distinguishing clinical features in determining the level of the lesion in the nervous system include pattern of weakness, activity of muscle stretch reflexes, presence of fasciculations or sensory loss, cerebrospinal fluid findings, serum muscle enzyme levels, **electromyography (EMG)** pattern, nerve conduction studies, and histologic appearance of the muscle and/or nerve biopsy. It is useful when assessing the hypotonic child to separate upper motor neuron or brain causes from neuromuscular causes (Table 115-1). The former include perinatal hypoxia-ischemia, intracranial hemorrhage, and cerebral dysgenesis. These problems may present with hypotonia in infancy but later are evident as a static encephalopathy. A child with a CNS cause may have a below normal level or range of attention and may lack age-appropriate social skills. Seizures or hemiparesis also signify a likely CNS cause. Fine motor coordination, quality and repertoire of movements, and language may be affected in an older child. The deep tendon reflexes may be brisk or easily elicited. The Babinski

Table 115-1. Differential Diagnosis of Infantile Hypotonia	
Level	*Specific Lesion*
Cerebral hemisphere	Static encephalopathy related to perinatal or prenatal insults Dysgenesis (eg, Down syndrome) Degenerative conditions (eg, storage disease)
Spinal cord	Traumatic transection Dysraphism or other malformation
Anterior horn cell	Spinal muscular atrophy Poliomyelitis
Peripheral nerve	Leukodystrophy Type III hereditary sensorimotor neuropathy Acute polyneuritis (rarely occurs in infancy)
Myoneural junction	Myasthenia gravis Toxin (botulism or "mycin" antibiotic)
Muscle	Congenital structural myopathy Congenital myotonic dystrophy Congenital muscular dystrophy Mitochondrial myopathy
Systemic	Amino and organic acidopathies, hypercalcemia, renal acidosis, rickets, celiac disease, hypothyroidism, collagen disease, congenital heart disease

reflex may be dorsiflexor. In infants, fisting of the hands, scissoring of the extended legs on vertical suspension, and movement through postural reflexes such as the asymmetrical tonic neck reflex are clues to an upper motoneuron process. Serum muscle enzymes, EMG, nerve conduction, and muscle biopsy will all be normal if assessed. However, neuromuscular causes include congenital myopathy, SMA, muscular dystrophy, and acute postinfectious polyneuritis. A child with one of the neuromuscular causes for the hypotonia that don't involve cranial innervated muscles may have an interested and visually attentive facial appearance in the presence of severe weakness that allows only sparse or nearly absent limb movements. Deep tendon reflexes may be difficult to elicit or absent in many neuromuscular lesions.

Older children may display a different pattern of weakness that gives a clue to the level of involvement. If the weakness is preferentially in upper extremity extensor and lower extremity knee flexor, ankle dorsiflexor, and ankle everter muscle groups, the lesion may involve the upper motoneuron. Static bilateral hemiparesis may suggest severe hypoxemic-ischemic insult; diplegia may suggest periventricular leukomalacia in a former prematurely delivered infant. This differential weakness from CNS causes may be present and contribute to hypotonia for a long period before spasticity intervenes and affects tone. If the weakness involves limb agonist and antagonist muscles equally, however, it may represent a neuromuscular process. It should also be remembered that hypotonia can result from disorders with combined lesions in levels above the lower motoneuron and in the motor unit. Examples include Krabbe leukodystrophy, Pompe disease, and hypoxic-ischemic insults involving both the upper motoneuron and the anterior horn cell during the acute phase.

Evaluation

A methodical assessment using clinical and laboratory features in children to localize the lesion to a level of the nervous systems can help anatomically narrow a wide differential diagnosis (Table 115-2).

History

Particular areas of the history are especially important (Questions Box). Level of fetal movements relative to other pregnancies and possibilities of toxic or infectious fetal exposures should be obtained. Relatively decreased fetal movements may signify an early degenerative condition. Polyhydramnios can signal prenatal interference with swallowing. Birth events should be investigated for sources of possible trauma to the neonatal nervous system, such as prematurity or birth asphyxia. The physician should determine whether any developmental skills have been lost. Any associated loss of tone or strength could signify a progressive condition rather than a static problem as would occur with a birth injury. The acuity of the developing weakness also is an important clue in the differential diagnosis. Immediate-onset hypotonia accompanied by constipation, poor feeding, and other bulbar involvement may suggest botulism. Acute losses of tone and strength may also occur with enteroviral poliomyelitis, Landry–Guillain-Barré syndrome, myasthenia, and myositis. Relapsing-remitting courses of hypotonia may be seen with myasthenia, metabolic myopathies, and periodic paralysis in the older child. A progressive deterioration in intellectual functions might point to a leukodystrophy, storage disorder, or other degenerative disorders, such as one of the "Leigh syndromes," particularly if ataxia, brain stem symptoms, and respiratory dysfunction subsequently develop.

In addition, the family history should be determined. The presence of weakness or hypotonia in other family members, or the presence of early unexplained neonatal deaths in the family, may indicate a genetic or maternal basis for the patient's hypotonia.

Physical Examination

Dysmorphic features should be noted in developmentally delayed children with hypotonia because they may suggest cerebral dysgenesis in some instances (eg, the characteristic stigmata of Down syndrome) or neuromuscular conditions in other instances (eg, hypoplastic mandible, high-arched palate, thin ribs with deformed rib cage, or pectus excavatum). Poor feeding with small male genitalia in the neonate may suggest Prader-Willi syndrome. A large tongue with decreased growth parameters may point to hypothyroidism. Hepatomegaly may be seen with Niemann-Pick and Zellweger syndromes. Signs of brain dysfunction, such as lethargy, unresponsiveness to the environment, and lack of social skills, should be noted. The neonate who acutely develops signs like those of sepsis along with generalized hypotonia may have an inborn error of metabolism that is decompensating and requires emergent intervention. Age-appropriate cognitive abilities should be assessed as a measure of cerebral function. This assessment may range from primarily

Clinical Feature	Anatomical Site				
	Cerebrum	Spinal Cord	Anterior Horn Cell	Neuromuscular Junction	Muscle
Alertness	Decreased	Normal	Normal	Normal	Normal
Cry	Decreased	Normal	Normal/weak	Weak	Normal/weak
Eye movements	Sometimes abnormal	Normal	Normal	Abnormal	Normal
Tongue fasciculations	Absent	Absent	Present	Absent	Absent
Muscle bulk	Normal	Normal	Decreased	Normal	Decreased
Deep tendon reflexes	Normal/increased	Decreased/increased	Absent	Normal	Normal/decreased

Table 115-2. Approach to the Diagnosis of Hypotonia

Hypotonia

Questions

- Were the fetal movements of the child abnormal or less than those of previous pregnancies?
- Was the pregnancy full term? Was the delivery complicated?
- Does the mother, any siblings, or other family members suffer from a similar weakness?
- Has the child lost any developmental skills? Is the problem getting worse?
- If the weakness is worsening, how rapidly is it progressing?

observation of visual attention in very young infants to evaluation of language and academic skills in older children. Cranial nerve examination with regard to eye movements, facial strength, and presence of tongue fasciculations is important, especially in the differential diagnosis of many neuromuscular conditions. Ocular muscle involvement may be part of mitochondrial myopathies, myotubular myopathy, and myotonic dystrophy. Blindness and hyperacusis responses may suggest Tay-Sachs disease. Facial muscle involvement is common in some congenital myopathies and myotonic dystrophy but not a part of SMA. Sucking and swallowing difficulty is a feature of SMA, congenital myotonic dystrophy, myotubular and nemaline myopathies, neonatal myasthenia, and Prader-Willi syndrome, in addition to birth asphyxia.

Tone and strength should be examined carefully in both trunk and limbs with the head in the midline. Passive pronation, supination, flexion, extension, and gentle shaking of hands and feet can demonstrate hypotonia, as can the traction maneuver for head control, horizontal prone suspension for trunk tone, scarf sign and axillary suspension for shoulder girdle tone, and popliteal angle for lower extremity tone. In premature infants there is normally a caudal-rostral progression of tone development, particularly flexor tone, correlated with age up to 40 weeks term. Individual joint movements should be observed and agonist-antagonist strengths should be tested bilaterally to look for asymmetries and focal discrepancies. There may be a paucity of spontaneous limb movements, and breathing may be paradoxical with chest lowering and stomach rising due to primarily diaphragmatic strength. Severe respiratory compromise along with profound hypotonia may be features of neonatal spinal cord injury as well as congenital myopathies. A loss of pain sensation (evidenced by facial grimace following a painful stimulation below the neck) would suggest the former cause rather than the latter. The plantar response should be obtained particularly in older children. The presence of contractures is common in congenital muscular dystrophy and congenital myotonic dystrophy. The older child may have developed scoliosis from gravity effects on a weak spine. The absence of deep tendon reflexes and or presence of percussion myotonia should also be carefully noted. Sensory testing is important in suspected neuropathies, radiculopathies, and myelopathies. The responses to be observed are latency, limb movement (more than stereotyped triple flexion), facial grimace and cry, and habituation. In the case of a hypotonic neonate, the mother may also need to be

questioned and examined particularly for the presence of symptoms or signs of myotonic dystrophy or myasthenia gravis.

Observation rather than formal individual muscle testing is often easier and more revealing, particularly in infants and preschool-aged children. Useful activities to observe include walking, running, climbing stairs or stepping onto a stool, lying on the floor and coming to a standing position unassisted, smiling, closing the eyes tightly, and speaking. The ambulatory child may have a waddling gait from hip girdle weakness, genu recurvatum from quadriceps weakness, or talipes planus from foot weakness. Arising from a prone position on the floor the child may demonstrate the Gower sign by first getting to the hands and knees, then walking the feet forward to the hands, and finally "walking" the hands up the trunk to gain an upright position, rather than quickly rising from squatting without using the hands.

Laboratory Tests

One purpose of laboratory tests in children with neuromuscular conditions is to confirm the level of the nervous system involved (Table 115-3). **Serum creatine phosphokinase (CPK),** a screen for muscle fiber necrosis, should be requested when the history suggests a degenerative condition or the examination indicates the cause of the hypotonia is in the neuromuscular unit. Creatine phosphokinase is 10 to 100 times higher than normal in children with muscular dystrophy, and it may also be mildly elevated in female carriers of the mutant dystrophin gene in their first 3 decades of life. The serum CPK level may be less markedly elevated in children with inflammatory myopathies, such as dermatomyositis and polymyositis, and to some extent following muscle trauma. Severe hypotonia at birth can be a result of inborn errors of metabolism, such as peroxisomal disorders, non-ketotic hyperglycinemia, congenital lactic acidosis, organic acidemias, fatty acid oxidation disorders, maple syrup urine disease, molybdenum cofactor deficiency, and hyperammonemic syndromes, which can be screened using blood or plasma tests. The evaluation of the hypotonic depressed neonate should include an evaluation for infection (complete blood cell count and appropriate cultures) as well as an assessment of pH; blood gas; glucose; electrolytes; liver function tests; ammonia; amino acids in the blood; and sugars, organic acids, and ketones in the urine. Spinal

Table 115-3. Laboratory Tests Useful in the Diagnosis of Hypotonia Caused by Neuromuscular Lesions			
Test	**Anatomical Site**		
	Anterior Horn Cell	**Neuromuscular Junction**	**Muscle**
Muscle enzymes	Normal	Normal	Normal/increased
Tensilon test	Normal	Abnormal	Normal
Electromyography	Neuropathic	Decremental/incremental	Myopathic
Muscle biopsy	Group atrophy	Normal	Myopathic

fluid examination is sometimes helpful if there is an increase in white cells related to possible infection or inflammation or if there is an increased level of protein as seen in immune, storage, or necrotizing CNS conditions.

Useful information about the presence of neuropathic, myopathic, and neuromuscular junction disorders can be obtained from the nerve conduction velocity and EMG. Demyelinating neuropathies slow **nerve conduction** or produce signs of a segmental conduction block. If the problem is a motor neuropathy, an axonal neuropathy may have depressed amplitude of the nerve action potential or fibrillation potentials on EMG. In some myopathies, bizarre or small amplitude potentials and myotonia may be seen on EMG. Decremental response to stimulation and other abnormalities are evident with myasthenia gravis and neuromuscular junction blockade caused by the botulinum toxin. An intravenous (IV) edrophonium (Tensilon) test can confirm the diagnosis of myasthenia gravis in children with easy fatigability by history or on examination. Some neuromuscular conditions are associated with cardiomyopathies and, therefore, the electrocardiogram can help in diagnosis as well as bring to light potentially critical problems needing acute intervention such as heart conduction block.

When properly handled, the **muscle biopsy** gives useful diagnostic information about neuromuscular disorders that may cause hypotonia. A large portion of the tissue should be frozen for histochemical studies. Histochemistry can differentiate neuropathic changes from myopathic changes related to fiber type specificities as well as disclose structural abnormalities pointing to dystrophy or congenital myopathy. Histochemical stains can also give information about metabolic myopathic disorders. Another portion of the muscle should be fixed in glutaraldehyde for electron microscopy to determine if ultrastructural abnormalities such as those seen in specific congenital or mitochondrial myopathies are present.

Metabolic and molecular genetic studies can sometimes be done on blood or urine samples, such as thyroid functions if clinical suspicion of hypothyroidism persists, white blood cell enzymatic assays, very–long chain fatty acid profiles, lysosomal enzyme screens, plasma amino acid levels, and urine organic acid levels. However, if a genetic disorder is preferentially expressed in muscle tissue and direct gene analysis is not feasible, a muscle biopsy specimen can be analyzed. Tissue can be subjected to other specific expression analyses such as dystrophin protein levels, glycolytic enzyme activity, respiratory chain enzyme complex assays, carnitine levels, or fatty acid transport assays to confirm the diagnosis. Cytogenetic analysis may be useful when Down syndrome or other chromosomal aberrations are suspected and DNA methylation analysis is done when Prader-Willi syndrome is suspected as a cause of non-paralytic hypotonia. Blood sample molecular techniques, including use of specific nucleic acid probes, comparative genomic hybridization, copy number variance, and exon sequencing screens can sometimes be used to help make specific diagnoses for genetic disorders (eg, Duchenne or other X-linked muscular dystrophies, myotonic dystrophies, mitochondrial cytopathies, and SMA). Often these blood tests have eliminated the need for more painful electromyography or muscle biopsy.

Imaging Studies

A magnetic resonance imaging scan is often helpful in at least 4 situations: (1) when deficits in mental status, cognitive function, or attention are apparent in children with hypotonia; (2) when the neurologic examination suggests an upper motoneuron component to the weakness or hypotonia such as active deep tendon reflexes or persistent ankle clonus; (3) when a progressive congenital muscular dystrophy is suggested by both myopathic signs and CNS signs; and (4) when children have hypotonia as part of a multiorgan system dysgenesis such as with a chromosomal aberration, because of the relatively higher likelihood of a CNS component to the dysgenesis. A computed tomography scan is also sometimes helpful in evaluating the presence of calcification in brain structures as might occur in metabolic abnormalities or necrotizing brain insults if these are part of the clinical differential.

Management

Specific management depends on diagnosis but ranges from supportive respiratory measures to anti-inflammatory therapies to physical and orthopedic therapy and devices to improve function. Sometimes the potential for recovery is an important factor in determining the degree of aggressiveness in the clinical management and therapy sessions for children with neuromuscular conditions. An infant with a congenital myopathy may gradually increase in strength and should, therefore, receive intensive supportive care including long-term ventilatory support and gastrostomy feeding. On the other hand, the family of an infant with a rapidly degenerative terminal condition such as the severe infantile type of Werdnig-Hoffmann anterior horn cell disease may elect not to undertake respiratory support after they understand the course of the disease and lack of curative therapy. Such families continue to benefit from the ongoing information provided by the physician and the support of paramedical personnel and lay groups. Affected children can also benefit from palliative therapies and hospice care.

Children with profound weakness easily succumb to respiratory infections and have difficulty with recovery from anesthesia; therefore, they require vigilance on the parent's or caretaker's part and early intervention because they may need intense **respiratory support.** Children with long-term neuromuscular weakness can sometimes benefit from **orthopedic** procedures to improve limb function by joint stabilization or equalizing of muscle strengths across joints or scoliosis stabilization to prevent respiratory compromise. **Physical and occupational therapy** can accelerate recovery after procedures and maximize function.

Children with acquired acute hypotonic weakness (Box 115-1) may require therapies more directed at the underlying pathophysiological process. Acute postinfectious polyneuritis requires careful, frequent monitoring of respiratory status and artificial ventilation when significant loss of vital capacity has occurred. In addition, children should be considered for **plasmapheresis** when their condition rapidly worsens early in the course of the disorder. Intravenous immunoglobulin is an alternative therapy that may be particularly useful in a child too small for the venous access required for pheresis. Specific antisera are used for botulinum intoxication. Dysimmune myasthenia can be treated with anticholinesterase medication, IV immunoglobulin, and/or thymectomy when it is resistant or only partly responsive to immunosuppressive medication. In addition to the more acute disorders, chronic relapsing polyneuritis and myositis can be treated effectively with various anti-inflammatory agents including prednisone and immunoglobulin during periods of exacerbation. Suspected metabolic disorders can be managed with semi-focused metabolic therapy such as stopping a toxic nutrient; using a high-energy alternative nutrient (glucose); treating hyperammonemia with benzoate, phenylbutyrate, or arginine; dialysis; administering insulin to control hyperglycemia; reducing periods of catabolism; and supplementing vitamin cofactors and carnitine. Metabolic myopathies are still often empirically treated with thiamine, riboflavin, nicotinamide, coenzyme Q10, biotin, l-carnitine, succinate, vitamins C or K, and medium-chain triglyceride oil, using these in some cases based on tissue analysis.

Treatment and care of children with muscular dystrophy is presently directed individually toward maintaining mobility and preventing contractures through physical therapy, bivalved casts, braces, and surgical repair. Inactivity increases disability. Adjunctive corticosteroid therapy is useful in children with Duchenne dystrophy, but beneficial effects are temporary and must be weighed against steroid toxicity. Presently new therapies for providing dystrophin expression are under active investigation, including "exon skipping" promoting drugs and dystrophin gene fragment-carrying viral vectors. Many new hardware technologies (eg, long leg braces, electric wheelchairs, battery-operated ventilators, and noninvasive positive-pressure ventilation for some cases of respiratory insufficiency) have allowed affected children to overcome previously insurmountable disabilities.

Prognosis

Spinal muscular atrophy type I generally progresses to death over a couple of years, and Duchenne muscular dystrophy generally progresses to full time artificial ventilation over 15 to 20 years. However, the course of many genetic conditions can be quite variable and is related to different alleles at the disease gene locus, the position of the critical base pair substitution or deletion, or other loci that may have a modifying effect on either disease gene expression or the pathophysiology of the disease. For example, both the SMA and dystrophin genes have multiple abnormal modes of expression with widely different prognostic implications for disease course. The weakness of congenital myopathies usually slowly improves. Toxin-mediated infant botulism and immune-mediated disorders, particularly Landry–Guillain-Barré, generally have a good outcome although long-term supportive measures may be necessary.

CASE RESOLUTION

The 6-month-old girl in the case history was judged to have hypotonia caused by a neuromuscular condition, in part because of her alert appearance and absent deep tendon reflexes. Neuropathic abnormalities on electromyography and muscle biopsy were also present. A blood test for the survival motor neuron genes did not detect any normal sequences, confirming the diagnosis of spinal muscular atrophy type I. The family received genetic counseling, became involved in a support group, and eventually reached a decision to forego intubation when respiratory failure overtakes their daughter. The physician coordinated hospice services for the family.

Selected References

Dubowitz V. *Muscle Disorders in Childhood.* 2nd ed. Philadelphia, PA: W. B. Saunders; 1995

Fenichel GM. *Clinical Pediatric Neurology.* 5th ed. Philadelphia, PA: W. B. Saunders; 2005:149–170

Huff K. Approach to the child with weakness or paralysis. In: Osborne L, DeWitt T, First L, Zenel J, eds. *Pediatrics.* Philadelphia, PA: Elsevier; 2006

Leonard JV, Morris AA. Diagnosis and early management of inborn errors of metabolism presenting around the time of birth. *Acta Paediatr.* 2006;95:6–14

Sarnat H, Menkes J. Diseases of the motor unit. In: Menkes J, Sarnat H, Maria B, eds. *Child Neurology.* Philadelphia, PA: Lippincott; 2006

Swaiman K. Muscular tone and gait disturbances. In: Swaiman K, Ashwal S, Ferriero D, eds. *Pediatric Neurology Principals and Practice.* 4th ed. Philadelphia, PA: Elsevier; 2006

Volpe J. Neonatal hypotonia. In: Jones HR, Devivo D, Darras B, eds. *Neuromuscular Disorders in Childhood and Adolescence.* Philadelphia, PA: Butterworth Heinemann; 2003

CHAPTER 116

Headaches

Kenneth R. Huff, MD

CASE STUDY

A 12-year-old girl is brought in with a history of headaches. Although she has been sent home from school twice in the last 6 weeks, she has experienced headaches for at least a year. The last episode, 1 week ago, was typical. The headache began as a dull feeling over both eyes, radiated up to the top of her head, and eventually became pounding. She had no preliminary visual symptoms or other warning signs prior to the head pain. The episode began during an afternoon class after she had been outside on a hot, sunny day for physical education. The headache worsened after she walked home from school. Once she got home, she went to her room, drew the curtains, and lay down on her bed. She experienced some nausea and loss of appetite but no vomiting. She did not get up for dinner. She denied diplopia, vertigo, ataxia, or limb weakness, and her speech was observed to be articulate and coherent. She took two 80-mg children's acetaminophen tablets without significant relief but eventually fell asleep. The following morning she felt fine.

Between headaches, her behavior has not changed, and she has continued to make above-average grades. She has not experienced any major changes in her home environment. When initially questioned, her mother denied having migraines, but she admits to needing to lie down because of headaches about once a month. A detailed **neurologic examination of the girl is completely normal.**

Questions

1. What are the major types of headache?
2. How do the symptoms help differentiate the types?
3. How does family history influence the etiology and help in the management of the headache?
4. What is the appropriate treatment for the problem headache?

Headaches, which are very common in adolescents and older children, frequently prompt parents to bring their children to the physician's attention. The physician must differentiate headaches that are symptomatic of a progressive intracranial process from those that may possibly be intermittently disabling but do not necessitate surgery. The cornerstone of this determination is obtaining key historical information and noting abnormalities on examination of the nervous system. Decisions about management strategies are most influenced by etiology and, if it has become a chronic problem, the impact the headaches are having on the child's life.

Epidemiology

The contribution of "symptomatic" headaches (those related to tumors, vascular abnormalities, or meningitis) to the overall prevalence of headache is relatively small. Chronic recurrent headaches in children that are not related to a self-limited condition are frequently lumped together as migraine, which includes classic and common migraine. The prevalence of migraine that comes to a physician's attention is about 3% to 10% for all children, but as many as 30% of children by age 15 admit to having experienced a headache in the last year. Although initial headache symptoms begin most often between ages 6 and 12 years, many patients come to medical attention for the first time during adolescence, especially girls whose headache prevalence is double that of boys. Headaches are also commonly associated with trauma, acute intercurrent infection, or other systemic illness. A multigenerational family history of "sick headaches" is a frequent finding in the child with migraine. This history must be specifically elicited by the physician, however, because its significance is often discounted by the parents.

Clinical Presentation

Parents must interpret the nature and severity of their child's experience and symptoms, which may be difficult especially in younger children. Younger children may rarely complain of head pain or more commonly of stomachache or present with nausea or vomiting. Adolescents may report persistent, dull, aching, or pounding head pain. It may be increasing in intensity or frequency and be associated with neurologic signs, which may suggest an intracranial mass lesion, or the pain may be episodic, relatively stable in frequency over many months, and similar to that experienced by other family members either presently or in the past, which may suggest a migraine etiology (Dx Box). Classic migraine, which is relatively unusual in children, is distinguished from common migraine by the presence of an aura of specific sensory symptoms that precede the headache. Both types of headache may be associated with lethargy, slowness of movement and response, intolerance of intense sound or light, and loss of appetite.

Dx Headaches (Migraine)

- Head pain, often pounding in character, over the eyes, at the vertex, or in the occipital region
- Pain frequently accompanied by nausea, anorexia, photophobia, or phonophobia
- Pain sometimes preceded by visual symptoms such as scotomata
- Presence of trigger factors, including bright light, intercurrent illness, or stress
- Family history of headaches (often)

Pathophysiology

Pain fibers are carried in the trigeminal nerves from the scalp, skull, meninges, and vessel walls within the brain. Traction on these fibers or inflammation at the endings produces the pain that is associated with mass lesions or meningeal inflammation. The usual distinction between migraine and tension headache pathophysiology is more difficult to make in the younger child and may involve the types of trigger factors (Box 116-1) that occur at different ages. Several different mechanisms that involve one or more environmental factors may trigger headache in genetically predisposed individuals. The migraine generator probably resides in the brain stem and has input to the trigeminal nucleus. The pathogenic neurotransmitter at the nerve endings may be serotonergic (perhaps emanating from platelet stores), but release may be precipitated by a cascade of local cytokines, substance P, calcitonin gene-related peptide, and histamine in and around vessel walls leading to changes in vascular permeability and local swelling. The relative roles of genetic susceptibility and environmental agents are subjects of current investigation.

Box 116-1. Triggers of Migraine

- Glare, dazzle, bright sunlight, or fluorescent lighting
- Physical exertion, fatigue, lack of sleep, hunger
- Change in ambient temperature or humidity
- Allergic reactions, pungent odors
- Certain foods, alcoholic beverages, and cold foods or beverages
- Anxiety, stress, and worry
- Head trauma
- Menstruation and oral contraceptives
- Refractive errors (rare)

Differential Diagnosis

Acute Headaches

Emergent causes should be considered if headaches have an abrupt onset, develop rapidly, or are especially severe or if children describe them as a "thunderclap" or "the worst of my life." **Intracranial hemorrhage** from a ruptured aneurysm, an arteriovenous malformation or, rarely, as a secondary effect of hypertension is foremost on the list of such causes. If children have a condition that may potentially lead to stroke, such as coagulopathy, hemoglobinopathy, or heart disease, the stroke may become hemorrhagic and produce acute, severe headache.

Non-hemorrhagic meningeal irritation, such as the inflammation produced by bacterial or viral meningitis, may also cause acute headaches. These conditions may render patients confused and lethargic while still conscious and are often associated with fever. Both types of meningitis produce signs of meningeal irritation: nuchal rigidity (stiff neck) and Kernig and Brudzinski signs.

Chronic Progressive Headaches

Children with brain tumors, brain abscesses, or a block in cerebrospinal fluid (CSF) flow producing hydrocephalus frequently have a "crescendo" history of increasing severity or frequency of headaches. The headache may be consistently localized or may awaken the patient from sleep, presumably related to relative shift in intracranial traction forces due to gravity and the horizontal position. Many other children with brain tumors do not complain of a localized headache and may present with vomiting without headache as a prominent symptom. Idiopathic intracranial hypertension most often presents with headaches, and papilledema will be present when the eyes are examined. Standard imaging studies are normal, but CSF pressure is high when measured during a lumbar puncture. There may be a relationship to intracranial venous sinus obstruction in some cases. A serious sequela of idiopathic intracranial hypertension is an enlarging blind spot in visual fields and eventual loss of vision if pressure is not relieved. Therapies include CSF withdrawal, diuretics such as Diamox, and optic nerve fenestration or CSF diversion surgically.

Chronic Recurrent Headaches

The pain of **migraine headaches,** the most common chronic headache type, is dull in character, and if headaches are severe, patients shun other intense sensory stimuli. **Sinus infection** may be a cause of either chronically recurring headaches or acute headaches, especially if children relate that the pain is more facial than cranial. Symptoms of chronic nasal congestion, allergies, and postnasal drip may be associated with sinus headaches. Children with asthma also have recurring headaches possibly triggered by sinus involvement, generalized cytokine release, cerebrovascular smooth muscle reactivity, or medication side effect susceptibility.

Other types of headaches may recur. **Chronic daily headaches** (more than 15 headache days per month) in some cases may be transformed migraine or rebound headache due to abortive medication overuse. In other cases the history, though suggestive of migraine, is more consistent with **tension headaches** characterized by a feeling of a tightening band around the head; occurrence late in the day; and association with anxiety, depression, or a stressful environment. Adolescents, if they are susceptible individuals, may also have frequently recurring headaches due to irregular lifestyles such as not eating regularly or getting adequate sleep. **Posttraumatic headaches** may recur with gradually decreasing severity up to several months following head trauma. **Cluster headaches** are associated with lancinating pain, unilateral tearing, nasal stuffiness, and nighttime pacing, but are exceedingly rare in children.

Evaluation

History

Information should be obtained from patients, parents, and other caregivers concerning the quality, intensity, and location of the headache as well as other associated symptoms before and during the headache (Questions Box). The duration, clinical course, and conditions that evoke, intensify, or alleviate the pain are also important. It is useful to have children describe a typical episode (perhaps the most recent), including the circumstances of when and where the headache began and how it affected activities at the time. The degree to which the headache problem affects the child's lifestyle influences the management plan for chronic recurrent headaches.

Physical Examination

The blood pressure should be noted even though primary hypertension is an unusual cause of headaches in children. A thorough neurologic examination is needed to determine if findings suggest an emergent problem such as meningitis or potential neurosurgical condition such as intracranial hemorrhage, or brain tumor. The examination should assess for the presence of sinus tenderness by palpation, nuchal rigidity, funduscopic abnormalities such as papilledema or hemorrhages, and any focal neurologic signs. A brain tumor or other space-occupying lesion may present with ataxia and cranial nerve signs for a posterior fossa lesion; loss of visual fields or

hypothalamic dysfunction (endocrine abnormalities) for a suprasellar or third ventricular region lesion; and hemiparesis, hemisensory deficit, or language dysfunction for a cerebral hemispheric lesion. Personality changes or developmental regression should be especially noted. Increased intracranial pressure (ICP) may lead to papilledema, loss of upgaze, general hypertonicity, leg weakness, positive Babinski sign, spastic gait, loss of continence, or confusion or stupor owing to blockage of CSF by the tumor.

Rarely, children in the midst of a migraine headache may display confusion, aphasia, unilateral numbness or, less commonly, weakness, hemianopsia, or ophthalmoplegia. In these circumstances, the diagnosis of complicated migraine or a migraine syndrome is reached only after other diagnostic tests have eliminated more emergent conditions.

Laboratory Tests

If stiff neck is present and focal or lateralized neurologic signs are absent, an immediate CSF examination is indicated to diagnose the cause of meningeal inflammation. When hemorrhagic fluid is encountered, it is often useful to centrifuge a specimen to check for xanthochromia and to count cells in a subsequent sample to differentiate a traumatic spinal tap from subarachnoid hemorrhage.

Imaging Studies

Recent trauma, persistent vomiting, depressed alertness, crescendo history, change in pattern, or possibly even just recent onset of the headaches all may be indications for an immediate head magnetic resonance imaging (MRI) or computed tomography (CT) scan. Such decisions are also influenced by reliability of follow-up and ease of communication level with the child's caretaker. If signs or symptoms of increased ICP are apparent, a CT or MRI scan must be obtained to diagnose the etiology of the headaches. New focal or general neurologic signs also indicate the need for a CT or MRI scan. Cerebral angiography may be necessary in rare cases to locate a focal source of subarachnoid hemorrhage. Less emergent radiologic studies, but also including CT or MRI, are helpful with the diagnosis of chronic or recurrent sinus headaches.

Management

If a careful assessment has revealed no acute or progressive conditions, pain is not severe, frequency is low, duration is short, and effect on lifestyle or daily activities is minimal, the appropriate management is often just **reassurance.** Frequently, parental anxiety about a potential mass or hemorrhage far outweighs the morbidity produced by the headache symptom itself. Sometimes placing the child's headache problem in context with the parent's or other family member's headaches will help with reassurance, and sometimes in milder cases, non-pharmacologic or nonprescription medication strategies can be agreed on as a management plan. Education and sometimes a headache diary or log helps patients and their families take control and own their own problem (discern triggers and track intervention efficacy).

> ## Questions
> ### Headaches
>
> - Where is the child, what time of day is it, and what is the child doing when a typical headache or the last recalled headache begins?
> - Where is the pain located? How severe is the pain? How long does the pain last?
> - Is nausea, vomiting, or photophobia associated with the headache?
> - What does the child do after getting the headache? Does the episode require cessation of activities?
> - Does the child take any medication for the pain? If so, was it successful? What else, if anything, allows the child to feel better?
> - How long ago did the first headache occur? Are the headaches becoming more frequent or severe?
> - Have headaches ever awakened the child at night?
> - Have there been any changes in speech, vision, gait, or personality, or any loss of skills or abilities between headaches?
> - Does the child have any warning symptoms before the pain? Does unilateral visual loss, weakness or numbness, diplopia, confusion, or loss of consciousness occur with the headache?
> - How often does the child miss school because of a headache?
> - Do other members of the family have headaches? Do they ever need to lie down or do they take medicine for these headaches?

However, it may be apparent that the headaches have produced significant discomfort or an effect on lifestyle for the child and treatment is warranted (Table 116-1). Interventions should weigh side effects against effectiveness of treatment. A goal is a reduction in headache frequency, severity, duration, or disability with improved quality of life. Both pain and nausea may need treatment. **Symptomatic treatment** should be taken as soon after the onset of prodromal or headache symptoms as possible, and often the first choice should be an adequate trial of **acetaminophen or nonsteroidal anti-inflammatory drugs.** Headaches in adolescents are often helped by **isometheptene mucate.** For severe, recurrent headaches, serotonin receptor agonists are useful, and **sumatriptan and other triptans** have relatively tolerable but occasionally anxiety-provoking side effects and patients need to be informed about them as with any new medication. Dihydroergotamine or sumatriptan given intranasally are also effective abortive treatments and work faster than the tablets, but they may have a disagreeable taste if they should enter the posterior oropharynx. Refractory very severe headaches may respond to prochlorperazine (Compazine) or intravenous (IV) **dihydroergotamine** or **dexamethasone along with a bolus of IV fluids.**

The decision to begin a **prophylactic medication** should be based on the frequency and severity of the headaches. Again, the benefits of potentially controlling headache-related symptoms must be weighed against the risk of daily side effects. Anticonvulsants such as **valproic acid and topiramate** have been found to be successful anti-migraine agents. The β-blockers, including **propranolol,** have demonstrated efficacy as prophylactic agents. The antihistamine **cyproheptadine** has also been successful in many patients. **Amitriptyline** is an effective preventive treatment in older children and adolescents; a single bedtime dose should be used at first. A 1- to 2-week trial is necessary before concluding the initial treatment has been ineffective. Amitriptyline can be combined with propranolol if necessary. Calcium channel blockers, such as **verapamil,** and serotonin reuptake inhibitors, such as **fluoxetine,** may also be useful in older children and adolescents. Chronic daily headaches may be successfully treated with education, use of prophylactic medication, avoidance of analgesics because of rebound potential, and helping the children work their way back into a functional daily routine. Healthy lifestyle changes have been beneficial, particularly in adolescents, and biofeedback-assisted relaxation training has had

Table 116-1. Drugs Useful in Childhood Headaches	
Abortive (Symptomatic)	
Acetaminophen, PO	325–975 mg every 4 h (15 mg/kg/dose) (max: 5 doses/24 h)
Ibuprofen, PO	200–800 mg every 6 h (10 mg/kg/dose) (max: 40 mg/kg/24 h)
Naproxen, PO	5–7 mg/kg/dose every 8–12 h (max: 15 mg/kg/ 24 h [age >2 y])
Sumatriptan, SC, IN, or PO	6 mg SC or 5–20 mg IN or 25–100 mg PO (may repeat after 1 h SC, 2 h IN and PO) (max: 2 doses/24 h)
Ergotamine, PR	¼ rectal suppository (2 mg), repeat ¼ suppository every 30 min as needed (max: 4 mg/day [older children and adolescents])
Rizatriptan, PO	5–10 mg orally disintegrating or regular tablets (may repeat after 2 hours) (max: 3 doses/24 h)
Isometheptene mucate with dichloral-phenazone and acetaminophen, PO	1–2 caps at onset (may repeat every 1 h to 3–5 caps/day [adolescents])
Dihydroergotamine, IN or IV	4 mg IN (1 spray each nostril, repeat once after 15 min) or 0.25–1 mg at onset and 1 mg/h × 2 (max: 6 mg/wk [older children and adolescents])
Dexamethasone, IV Prochlorperazine, IV	4–16 mg single dose (0.25 mg/kg) or rapidly tapering every 6 h 5–10 mg single dose (older children and adolescents) 0.1–0.15 mg/kg/dose (younger children)
Prophylactic	
Propranolol	10–40 mg 2–4 times a day (max: 40–80 mg/24 h if ≤35 kg
	120–160 mg/24 h if >35 kg; no more than 320 mg/24 h)
Cyproheptadine	1–4 mg 2–4 times a day (0.25–0.5 mg/kg/24 h) (max: 16 mg/24 h)
Amitriptyline	10–75 mg at bedtime (max: 150 mg/24 h [older children and adolescents])
Verapamil	40 mg every 8 h (age 1–5 y); 40–80 mg every 8 h (age >5 y) (max: 240 mg/24 h)
Valproic acid	10–15 mg/kg/day initial, 30–60 mg/kg/day maintenance, divided twice a day or every day if ER (max: 60 mg/kg/day [follow clinical signs of toxicity and serum level])
Topiramate	50–200 mg/day divided twice a day after ramping from 25 mg twice a day over a few weeks
Fluoxetine	10 mg every morning initial (max: 40 mg/day [adolescents])

Abbreviations: ER, extended release; IN, intranasally; IV, intravenously; PO, orally; SC, subcutaneously; PR, rectally.

mixed results. If severe environmental stressors or psychological trauma is present as an ongoing headache trigger, patients may benefit from psychotherapy.

Prognosis

Many children with headaches have a good prognosis and do not require ongoing intervention after families are reassured of the benign nature of the problem. For other children, symptomatic medications are frequently effective. Prophylactic medication is necessary in a few cases. For patients receiving prophylactic therapy, periodic withdrawal of the medication should be attempted to establish that it is still necessary. Pediatric patients frequently experience remission of their headaches by late adolescence, and by adulthood, the incidence of headaches has decreased, particularly for males.

CASE RESOLUTION

In the case history, the child's symptoms and the circumstances of the headache suggest a diagnosis of migraine. No laboratory tests or imaging studies are necessary. The girl is begun on amitriptyline and instructed to keep a calendar of headache occurrences. She has 2 headaches in the first 2 weeks, which are aborted effectively with ibuprofen. Following these episodes, she has no further recurrences, and the amitriptyline is withdrawn successfully after 3 months.

Selected References

Ball AK, Clarke CE. Idiopathic intracranial hypertension. *Lancet Neurol.* 2006;5:433–442

Landy S. Migraine throughout the life cycle: treatment through the ages. *Neurology.* 2004;62(suppl 2):S2–S8

Lewis D. Headaches in infants and children. In: Swaiman K, Ashwal S, Ferriero D, eds. *Pediatric Neurology Principals and Practice.* Philadelphia, PA: Elsevier; 2006

Mack KJ. An approach to children with chronic daily headache. *Dev Med Child Neurol.* 2006;48:997–1000

Rothner AD. Pediatric headaches. *Semin Pediatr Neurol.* 2001;8:1–51

CHAPTER 117

Tics

Kenneth R. Huff, MD

CASE STUDY

An 8-year-old boy has unusual recurring behaviors that began 2 to 3 months ago. He stretches his neck or raises his eyebrows suddenly several times a day. Sometimes he is able to suppress these actions. The boy's parents report that in the last 2 years he has displayed several repetitive behaviors, including blinking, grimacing, rubbing his chin on his left shoulder, making a "gulping" sound, and sniffing. Originally they thought the sniffing was related to hay fever, but the boy has no other allergic symptoms. He does not use profane words. In conversations, he sometimes repeats the last phrase of a sentence that was just used whether by himself or someone else. In addition, he must touch each light switch in the hallway every time he leaves his room, and he must retie his shoelaces several times until they are exactly the same length. Although his schoolwork has not deteriorated, he has always had trouble completing tasks and finishing homework. Both his teacher and his best friend have asked about his strange behavior. His mother has a "psychological" problem with her son's gulping sounds (ie, they recur in her own mind), and she recalls that her father had a habit of frequently looking over one shoulder for no apparent reason.

Although during examination the boy does not exhibit any unusual behaviors, he raises his eyebrows twice and places his hand over his crotch several times while his parents are interviewed. Except for mild fine motor incoordination, the neurologic examination is normal.

Questions

1. What are the characteristics of tics?
2. What are the social implications of tics?
3. Should pharmacologic treatments be part of the management of tic disorders?
4. What other problems are associated with the tic disorder that also should receive intervention?

Tics are brief, abrupt, non-purposeful movements or utterances. They occur in a background of normal activity and are repetitive and involuntary but can be suppressed. Tourette disorder is a common etiology of tics in children. It is defined by multiple types of tics displayed over time. These include both motor tics and vocal tics produced by some sudden movement of air or saliva within the larynx, nasopharynx, or oropharynx, causing a perceptible sound. Tourette disorder frequently manifests solely as a nondisabling movement disorder but may also be associated with other neurobehavioral problems, which may include attention-deficit/hyperactivity disorder (ADHD), obsessive-compulsive disorder, mood and rage disorders, anxiety, and personality and conduct difficulties that may be more disabling than the tics.

Epidemiology

Tics are relatively common in children but often go unrecognized as a movement disorder. The onset of tics associated with Tourette disorder is generally between 5 and 12 years of age but can be as late as 21 years of age. The prevalence of tics is 5 times higher in males than in females. By various estimates, the Tourette disorder prevalence is between 0.1% and 3%, but many cases of Tourette disorder are familial, and other family members may have symptoms so mild that they never seek medical attention. In addition, some family members may have only non-tic manifestations of the syndrome, such as obsessive-compulsive symptoms, but data support a relationship between tics and obsessive-compulsive symptoms.

Clinical Presentation

Children with tics display sudden repetitive movements of the face, neck, shoulders, or hands in the context of normal behaviors, and normal behaviors are sometimes used to mask the tics. Sometimes tics can be suppressed for periods, such as when they would be embarrassing or during a time of intense physical activity, concentration, or performance, but they also may be worsened by stress or strong emotional feelings. Tics associated with Tourette disorder will vary in their manifestations over periods of weeks to months. Some examples of tics are blinking, eye rolling, grimacing, neck stretching, head turning or shaking, shoulder shrugging, and wrist flicking. Tics may either mimic normal, sometimes complex, movements or involve a series of orchestrated simple movements, such as sequential finger flexing, wrist bending, and arm stretching. Tics may include sudden repetitive sounds from the vocal apparatus (Dx Box). The sounds may include throat clearing, sniffing, sucking, or blowing. In addition, children with Tourette disorder may also have socially inappropriate words or gestures or repeat what they have just said or heard.

Children with Tourette disorder may have learning problems including easy distractibility and inability to finish schoolwork.

Dx Tics

- Sudden, brief uncontrolled movements
- Repetitive sounds from the vocal apparatus
- Behaviors occurring in the context of or mimicking normal behaviors but having no purpose

They also may have intrusive or repetitive thoughts, unfounded fears, or ritualistic actions that may involve touching, cleanliness or neatness, counting and exactness, symmetry or evenness, or irrational checking.

Classifications of tics according to the nature of the action can be helpful in understanding apparently widely different movements as being part of the same disorder because of ultimately shared central nervous system chemistry or circuitry (Box 117-1). Clonic tics are brief and dystonic tics are more sustained movements. In addition to simple tics, patients may rarely have other unusual behaviors (complex tics) including echopraxia (repetitive gestures), copropraxia (obscene gestures), and coprographia (obscene writing). Unusual speech patterns include irrelevant or nonsense words, palilalia

---

Box 117-1. Types of Tics Seen in Children With Tourette Disorder

Simple Tics
- Clonic
- Dystonic

Complex Tics
- Series of different or similar simple tics
- More complicated coordinated movement
- Copropraxia and coprographia

Vocal Tics
- Oropharyngeal, nasopharyngeal, or laryngeal sounds
- Consonants or syllables
- Meaningless or nonsense words or phrases
- Coprolalia
- Palilalia and echolalia

Sensory Tics

Box 117-2. Misconceptions in Diagnosing Tourette Disorder

- Attributing the unusual tic symptom to attention-getting or emotionally based behavior
- Diagnosing the episodic behavior as a seizure on the basis of inadequate historical information
- Attributing a vocal tic to an upper airway, sinus, or allergic condition
- Attributing an ocular tic to an ophthalmologic problem
- Requiring tics to be observed in the office before making the diagnosis
- Waiting for coprolalia to be present before making the diagnosis
- Assuming severe tics are necessary for the diagnosis, or assuming mild tics are a normal developmental phase

---

(repeating one's own words), echolalia (repeating another's words), and coprolalia (obscene speech). Many affected children describe a sensory tic, which is an indescribable, uncomfortable feeling that is relieved by a motor tic. Diagnosis is often delayed because of misunderstandings about the common and uncommon manifestations of Tourette disorder (Box 117-2).

Pathophysiology

Tics are thought to be generated from a functional abnormality in deep brain nuclei that might include the striate nuclei, the globus pallidus, the subthalamic nuclei, and the substantia nigra. The frontal cortex, thalamus, and limbic systems may also be involved.

Dopaminergic neurotransmission within these structures is likely to be part of the abnormal function because of one class of medication (stimulants) worsening the symptoms and another class (dopamine antagonists) effective as a treatment. In patients with Tourette disorder, the cerebrospinal fluid contains low baseline levels of homovanillic acid, a dopamine metabolite, which could result, as has been hypothesized, from a hypersensitive dopamine receptor. In addition, amphetamines and methylphenidate increase dopamine release, and in some instances, these agents precipitate tic symptoms. Haloperidol, an effective tic-suppressing medication, blocks the dopamine receptor and, therefore, may block a potentially hypersensitive receptor for dopamine. The observations of good clinical response with low doses of haloperidol and the finding of increased homovanillic acid levels remaining high long after disappearance of the neuroleptic drug due to receptor desensitization both support this hypothesis. The physiology may be more complex than that encompassed by this hypothesis, and other transmitters are probably involved as well because effective medications in other classes are also useful.

Recently an autoimmune hypothesis has been generated to explain an association of the sudden onset of tics and/or obsessive-compulsive symptoms with preceding group A streptococcal infections of the pharynx. This association has been termed PANDAS (pediatric autoimmune neuropsychiatric disease associated with streptococcus). It is intriguing that a clear relationship has been known for some time between the same bacteria and another movement problem, Sydenham chorea, but the evidence is conflicting and unconfirmed by large studies for the bacteria's role in common neuropsychiatric disease such as Tourette disorder or obsessive-compulsive disease and, therefore, routine screening has not been recommended.

Differential Diagnosis

The duration, frequency, and appearance of the movement and circumstances of occurrence of tics help distinguish them from several other episodic movement disorders. Myoclonus is a lightning-like, non-suppressible jerk of a small group of muscles, and chorea involves nearly constant, small amplitude movements of the fingers, hands, and feet that are often accompanied by grimacing movements of the face. Tremor is an oscillatory movement of an extremity or the head. Hemiballismus is an uncontrollable episodic throwing movement of an extremity. Hyperexplexia is a hyperactive startle response provoked by touch or sudden noise. Torticollis, or neck writhing, may be paroxysmal but is generally part of either a benign transient disorder or a chronic degenerative disorder, such as familial dystonia. Paroxysmal kinesigenic choreoathetosis, an unusual episodic condition precipitated by a sudden movement, is characterized by a twisted trunk and limb posture lasting a few seconds (longer than tics, generally) and not accompanied by loss of consciousness. Hypnagogic jerks and bruxism are persistent normal variant behaviors that occur in sleep.

Other repetitive behaviors are sometimes confused with tics. Compulsions are complex actions that are done against one's will or better judgment. Stereotypies are persistent repetitive senseless movements. Perseverative behaviors are continued activity after the cause for it has ceased. Self-injurious behaviors are usually biting or banging of a body part during periods of agitation. Addictive behaviors occur with psychological dependence due to a reward system. Habits are fixed practices established by repetition. Mannerisms are stereotyped movements or habits peculiar to an individual and part of their personality. Anger outbursts are sudden emotion-generated behaviors occurring with relatively little provocation.

Tic disorders are sometimes divided into 3 groups: (1) **simple transient tics,** which are monomorphic (always the same appearance over a period of months), last less than 12 months, and may be caused by particular environmental situations or psychological states; (2) **chronic tics,** which last longer than 12 months but are a single type; and (3) the **tics of Tourette disorder** (Box 117-3). However, all 3 types of tic disorders are sometimes found in the same family.

Box 117-3. Conditions Necessary for Diagnosis of Tourette Disorder

- Multiple motor and vocal tics variably manifested over time
- Tics present for at least 1 year
- Onset of tics before 21 years of age
- Tics not due to another known condition or substance

Evaluation

History

A thorough history should be taken when evaluating children with potential tic disorders. The physician should find out as much as possible about the duration, circumstances of occurrence, and frequency of the movements (Questions Box). Parents may imitate the behavior or, if possible, bring in a videotape of the child's behavior. This may give the physician more telling information than verbal descriptions. The physician should describe suggested tic behaviors because the parent may not be aware these behaviors may be tics.

Questions

Tics

- How long and how often has the child been displaying the unusual behaviors?
- In what circumstances do the unusual behaviors occur? For example, do the behaviors occur when the child is eating or sleeping, engrossed in an activity, or excited? Or do they occur when attention is on the child or after a startle or other triggering behavior?
- Can the parents or other caregivers imitate the child's unusual behavior?
- Is the child having difficulty at school (cognitively or socially)?

Physical Examination

Frequently tics are not seen by the physician when observing the child directly because the child is able to suppress them, but the physician may still be able to see the child's tics. The physician might be able to observe the child unobtrusively while the child and family are still in the waiting room. The child can be observed for tics "out of the corner of one's eye" during the course of the parent interview and examination. As part of the examination, a screen of cognitive abilities and fine-motor coordination should be included because of the comorbidity of ADHD and other learning disabilities and associated fine motor dysmaturity.

Laboratory Tests

There are no definitive diagnostic or supportive laboratory tests for Tourette disorder or for confirming the presence of tics. Children with atypical or ambiguous movement disorders should be screened for potential metabolic abnormalities, including routine determinations of calcium, magnesium, glucose, liver function enzymes, and ceruloplasmin levels (for Wilson disease). Thyroid function tests may also be requested if there are other signs or symptoms of thyroid dysfunction.

Imaging Studies

Imaging has been largely used in research evaluations of Tourette disorder patients where it has demonstrated volumetric increases in primarily right frontal white matter and the anterior parts of the corpus callosum in magnetic resonance imating (MRI) studies, reduced right basal ganglia activity in single-photon emission computed tomography studies, and increased right caudate and frontal cortex activity in functional MRI studies during tic suppression. These imaging modalities have not yet proven clinically useful in the care of individual patients, however.

Management

Goals of management should include (1) reduction in the frequency of tics during critical circumstances with a minimum of medication side effects and (2) attention to the other coexisting learning or behavioral disabilities. Before physicians prescribe drug treatment, they must consider the severity of the tic disorder and its potential or actual production of psychosocial disability or lack of it. Some children do not need medication for the movement disorder, and they and their families can be reassured by an understanding of the problem. Other patients may experience remission for weeks or months, during which they can reduce or discontinue their medications. Several classes of drugs are useful in the treatment of tic disorders. A first-line medication because of its relatively good efficacy, side-effect profile, and convenience is the **Catapres** transdermal skin patch containing clonidine, an α_2-adrenergic agonist. Dosage is titrated using the minimally effective size and strength of the patch. Guanfacine, an oral formulation in the same class, is also effective. The atypical antipsychotics, particularly risperidone, have also been effective with sometimes less sedation or potential for extrapyramidal side effects than tranquilizing dopamine blockers. Another useful medication is the neuroleptic **pimozide** (Orap). An electrocardiogram is recommended before beginning this medication because it has been associated with prolonged QTc. Concomitant use of inhibitors of CYP3A liver metabolism should not be given. **Haloperidol** has been useful in divided doses starting as low as 0.5 mg/day up to 2 to 6 mg/day. Children should begin with a low dose that is then titrated up to maximum efficacy or development of intolerable side effects. A potential disadvantage of haloperidol and other antipsychotics such as fluphenazine is cognitive sedation and the small possibility of tardive dyskinesia. **Botulinum toxin type A** injections may be useful for isolated persistent tics occurring in "needle-accessible" locations. Behavioral approaches including habit reversal training may be viable alternatives in some cases.

Treatment for children with Tourette disorder should be multimodal and prioritize, address, and monitor all problematic aspects of the syndrome (Box 117-4). Children with Tourette disorder should be assessed for learning disabilities including ADHD. Interventions may include organizational aids, homework time management, reduction in potential environmental distractions, and more **individualized instruction**. **Pharmacologic therapy** may include the Catapres patch, a tricyclic antidepressant, atomoxetine, or a stimulant. Long-acting methylphenidate or mixed amphetamine salt preparations are not necessarily contraindicated in children with Tourette disorder; these drugs do not worsen tics in all patients. Children with Tourette disorder are also susceptible to obsessive-compulsive symptoms. **Fluoxetine, sertraline,** and **clomipramine** are most useful for this comorbid problem.

Children with Tourette disorder and their families also frequently benefit from **lay educational materials** about the disorder. **Support groups** composed of other families that have children with the syndrome and local chapters of the Tourette's Syndrome Association may help. Referral for psychological or psychiatric counseling for patients and their families may be necessary because in its severe form, Tourette disorder may be socially devastating and may provoke secondary frustrations, low self-esteem, depression, and other emotional problems as well as the primary psycho-behavioral difficulties that may be part of the syndrome.

Box 117-4. Therapies Useful in Tourette Disorder

Tics
- Clonidine (Catapres transdermal patch): α_2-adrenergic agonist
- Risperidone (low dose) serotonin dopamine receptor antagonist
- Haloperidol (low dose): dopamine receptor blocker
- Pimozide (Orap): dopamine receptor blocker
- Fluphenazine: dopamine receptor blocker
- Guanfacine (Tenex): α_2-adrenergic agonist

Attention-Deficit/Hyperactivity Disorder and Learning Disability
- Clonidine (Catapres transdermal patch): α_2-adrenergic agonist
- Methylphenidate: if tics are not worsened
- Atomoxetine: norepinephrine transporter inhibitor
- Desipramine: tricyclic antidepressant
- Education interventions: individualized or small-group instruction

Obsessive-Compulsive Disorder
- Fluoxetine (Prozac): serotonin uptake inhibitor (non-tricyclic)
- Clomipramine (Anafranil): tricyclic antidepressant

Depression and Adjustment Problems
- Psychotherapy (individual and family)
- Imipramine: tricyclic antidepressant
- Support group

Prognosis

The prognosis in most children with tics is good. Less than 20% of adults and older children who were symptomatic in grade school continue to manifest clinically significant tic symptoms. Some symptomatic children, however, have ongoing problems with a productive educational experience or developing appropriate peer relationships. Therefore, according to the severity of these issues early in childhood, the physician must individualize the management strategy to achieve a favorable prognosis later when educational and social problems may be harder to reverse. Because the movements may change or even remit over long periods, the psychological adjustments become very important in the long-term prognosis.

CASE RESOLUTION

The boy in the case history is diagnosed as having Tourette disorder. After a discussion with his family about the disorder, he is treated with Catapres patches. A questionnaire is sent to his teacher concerning ADHD symptoms at school. At a 6-week follow-up visit, he has fewer tics and is doing better in school (classroom situation of 15 students for most of the day).

Selected References

Coffey B, Shechter R. Treatment of co-morbid obsessive compulsive disorder, mood, and anxiety disorders. *Adv Neurol.* 2006;99:208–221

Dale R. Post-streptococcal autoimmune disorders of the central nervous system. *Dev Med Child Neurol.* 2005;47:785–791

Denckla M. Attention-deficit hyperactivity disorder (ADHD) comorbidity: a case for "pure" Tourette syndrome? *J Child Neurol.* 2006;21:701–703

Erenberg G. The relationship between Tourette syndrome, attention deficit hyperactivity disorder, and stimulant medication: a critical review. *Semin Pediatr Neurol.* 2006;12:217–221

Huff K. Approach to the child with movement disorders. In: Osborn L, Dewitt T, First L, Zenel J, eds. *Pediatrics.* Philadelphia, PA: Elsevier; 2005:770–777

Leckman JF, Bloch MH, Scahill L, King RA. Tourette syndrome: the self under siege. *J Child Neurol.* 2006;21:642–649

Piacentini J, Chang S. Behavioral treatments for tic suppression: habit reversal training. *Adv Neurol.* 2006;99:227–233

Robertson M. Tourette syndrome, associated conditions and the complexities of treatment. *Brain.* 2000;123:425–462

Snider LA, Swedo SE. PANDAS: current status and directions for research. *Mol Psychiatry.* 2004;9:900–907

Zinner SH, Mink JW. Movement disorders I: tics and stereopathies. *Pediatr Rev.* 2010;31:223–233

Dermatologic Disorders

CHAPTER 118

Acne

Monica Sifuentes, MD

CASE STUDY

A 15-year-old adolescent male comes to your office for a preparticipation sports physical. He is healthy and he has no questions, complaints, or concerns.

The adolescent is well developed and well nourished, with normal vital signs, including blood pressure. The physical examination is entirely normal except for the skin. Multiple closed comedones (whiteheads) are noted along the hairline. Erythematous papules and pustules are present across the forehead and over both cheeks. Scattered open comedones (blackheads) are located over the nose and cheeks as well. The chest and back are clear, with no lesions.

Questions

1. What is the pathogenesis of acne vulgaris?
2. What are some contributing factors in the development of acne?
3. What are the different types of acne lesions?
4. What management options are available for the treatment of mild, moderate, and severe acne in adolescents?
5. What are the indications for the use of isotretinoin?
6. What is the prognosis for adolescent patients with acne?

Acne vulgaris is a common condition that most frequently occurs in adolescents. The spectrum of disease varies among individuals and is caused by a variety of factors. Regardless of the etiology and extent of acne, the disease can be devastating to adolescents both physically and psychologically. Primary care physicians should, therefore, acknowledge acne as a medical problem, even when patients do not mention it initially, and should treat the condition as a chronic disease.

Epidemiology

Most cases of acne that require treatment occur in individuals 9 to 19 years of age, although the condition can also affect young infants and adults. Boys and girls are equally affected, but the condition is usually more severe in males and typically lasts longer in females. Certain individuals may be genetically susceptible to acne. Caucasian teens are more likely to have acne than African American and Asian teens. Certain cultural practices, such as the use of oil-based hair care products by some African Americans, also can lead to a specific pattern of lesions along the forehead and temporal areas (pomade acne). Estimates indicate that more than 85% of adolescents in the United States are affected with acne and that more than $1 billion is spent annually on acne treatments. And although acne is generally believed to be a pubertal event, a fair number of young adults continue to manifest lesions after 25 years of age.

Several factors contribute to the development of acne-like eruptions. Internal agents include endogenous hormones (eg, androgens, progesterone) and specific drugs (eg, progestin-only contraceptives, isoniazid, phenytoin, corticosteroids, anabolic steroids, lithium-containing compounds). External agents include skin bacteria, especially *Propionibacterium acnes;* industrial chemicals (eg, petroleum, animal and vegetable oils); oil- or wax-containing cosmetics; greasy sunscreen or suntan preparations; and local pressure from objects such as headbands, shoulder pads, helmets, or chin straps. Excessive perspiration and emotional stress also can aggravate acne. Specific foods such as chocolate, caffeine-containing soda, pizza, and french fries have not been shown to cause or worsen acne, although this is controversial.

Clinical Presentation

The lesions of acne vulgaris primarily affect the face, especially the cheeks, forehead, and chin; the chest, the back; and the shoulders. Lesions can be non-inflamed or inflamed (Dx Box). Non-inflamed lesions, or comedones, can be opened or closed to the environment. Closed comedones (whiteheads) are small, flesh-colored bumps, and open comedones (blackheads) contain central, dark material. Inflamed lesions are typically erythematous papules, pustules, or nodules and may be more cystic in appearance.

 Dx **Acne**

- Occurrence predominantly during puberty
- Lesions more severe in males
- Location on face, chest, back, and shoulders
- Non-inflamed, open comedones (blackheads) or closed comedones (whiteheads)
- Inflamed papules or pustules
- Nodules, cysts, or scarring may be present
- Possible exacerbation premenstrually or related to stress

Lesions are generally concentrated in the centrofacial areas or "T-zone" early in the course of acne. The T-zone includes the forehead, nose, and chin areas, which are rich in sebaceous glands. Over time, lesions can develop in other areas of the body, such as the neck, chest, shoulders, and back.

Pathophysiology

Although the exact etiology of acne remains unclear, the pathogenesis of acne involves certain processes that occur within the pilosebaceous unit.

1. **Abnormal follicular keratinization.** The earliest change in the formation of acne occurs in the horny cells that line the sebaceous follicle. A disturbance in the differentiation of these cells leads to excessive shedding of the cells into the lumen. Impaction of the follicle occurs as these horny cells stick together.

2. **Overproduction of sebum.** The sebaceous gland is highly responsive to hormonal stimulation, namely androgens. With the rise in androgens during puberty, hypertrophy of the sebaceous gland occurs, and the production of sebum is increased. The flow of sebum is obstructed by the above follicular hyperkeratosis, resulting in retention of all material.

3. **Proliferation of *P acnes*.** The overproduction of sebum in acne provides a ripe environment for the proliferation of *P acnes,* an anaerobic diphtheroid that, along with *Staphylococcus epidermidis* and *Pityrosporum ovale,* is part of the microflora of the sebaceous follicle. In addition, *P acnes* possesses a lipase that hydrolyzes sebum triglycerides into free fatty acids. These acids irritate the follicular wall and cause inflammation.

4. **Inflammation.** The expulsion of sebum into the dermal layer of the skin occurs as a result of the rupture of the pilosebaceous follicle. This initiates an inflammatory process and the formation of inflammatory lesions such as pustules and cysts. In addition, *P acnes* produce biologically active extracellular materials, which increase the permeability of the follicular epithelium. The bacterium also produces chemotactic factors that are responsible for the migration of inflammatory cells to the area.

5. **Comedones.** The above processes can lead to a number of noninflammatory and inflammatory lesions (Table 118-1). Comedones are early noninflammatory lesions made up of sebum, horny cells, and bacteria. They can be closed or open. A **closed comedo,** or **whitehead,** is a dilated plugged sebaceous follicle that is closed to the surface of the skin. An **open comedo,** or **blackhead,** occurs as a result of dilatation of the follicular orifice at the surface of the skin and open communication with the outside environment. The dark color at the surface of the skin, however, is not dirt and may be from a number of processes such as oxidation of melanin in the horny cells, interference with the transmission of light through compacted epithelial cells, or the presence of certain lipids in sebum.

Table 118-1. Classification of Acne	
Category	*Physical Findings*
Grade I	Noninflammatory acne → open and closed comedones Closed comedones then lead to any of the next 3 levels of inflammatory acne
Grade II	Early inflammatory acne → presence of comedones and papules (obstructed follicles)
Grade III	Moderate, localized inflammatory acne → pustules or larger, more inflamed papules
Grade IV	Severe, more generalized inflammatory acne → cystic, nodular lesions

6. **Pustules** and **papules** are inflammatory lesions. Pustules lie in the superficial epidermal layer of the skin, and papules occur in the lower dermal layer. Because of their deeper location, they are often accompanied by a more severe inflammatory reaction, and scarring may result. **Nodules** or **cysts** are suppurative inflammatory lesions located deep within the dermis. Associated with the most severe form of acne, nodules are the result of deep pustules that rupture and then become lined with epithelium. When nodules are present, significant scarring can be a major problem.

Evaluation

History

The primary historical issues to explore in patients with acne vulgaris are both medical and psychological (Questions Box). From a medical standpoint, practitioners should determine how long the acne has been present and if the condition has ever been treated. Psychological aspects should include questions to assess the patient's overall self-esteem. Expectations regarding treatment and recovery also should be assessed at the initial visit before therapy is begun.

Physical Examination

The physical examination should focus on the primary sites of acne: face, chest, back, and shoulders, although the entire skin should be inspected closely at the first visit. Individual lesions should be checked for signs of inflammation and infection at each follow-up visit. Their distribution also should be recorded along with their response to treatment. The presence or absence of scarring should be assessed as a measure of the severity of acne and a predictor of outcome. Young women with very irregular menses and obesity should be examined for hirsutism, which might indicate excessive adrenal or ovarian androgen production as a contributor to the development of acne.

Laboratory Tests

In general, no laboratory studies are needed either at the time of the initial evaluation or during the treatment of mild to moderate acne. If there is a history of abnormal menses and evidence of hirsutism

Acne

Questions

Medical Aspects

- How long has the adolescent had acne?
- Has the adolescent ever received treatment for acne?
  - — How long did treatment continue?
  - — What treatment methods were used?
  - — For what reasons was the therapy discontinued?
- Is the adolescent currently using any treatment products?
  - — Do the lesions seem to be getting better or worse?
- If the acne has never been treated, is treatment desired?
- Do any activities, medications, or environmental agents seem to exacerbate the lesions?
- Does the adolescent have a family history of acne?
- Is the adolescent taking any oral medications
- Does the adolescent have any other medical conditions?

Psychological Aspects

- Is the adolescent bothered by the lesions?
- Is the adolescent embarrassed about his or her appearance? If so, does this embarrassment prevent the adolescent from participating in certain activities?
- Is the adolescent ever ridiculed by his or her peers because of the acne?

For postpubertal females

- Does the acne worsen prior to menses?
- Are menses regular?
- Is there any evidence of hirsutism?
- Is the adolescent sexually active?
- Is she using any hormonal contraception?

or virilization in the adolescent female, a free testosterone, early morning cortisol and 17-hydroxyprogresterone, and serum dehydro-cpiandrosterone sulfate (DHEAS) levels are indicated to differentiate between the various causes of hyperandrogenism. In the case of severe acne when isotretinoin is indicated, several pretreatment studies are necessary. A complete blood cell count, liver function tests, and a fasting lipid profile are recommended. In addition, a pregnancy test must be performed prior and to within 2 weeks of starting isotretinoin in female adolescents. These studies should be obtained in consultation with a dermatologist, who is generally responsible for prescribing isotretinoin.

Management

The general management of acne begins with counseling and should include patient education regarding the pathophysiology of the condition to dispel any myths regarding its etiology and treatment. In addition, the patient's motivation should be assessed to better individualize therapy. Realistic expectations regarding duration of therapy and likely outcome of treatment should be reviewed with the teenager. Parental involvement helps optimize care in cases of severe acne.

All adolescents with acne should follow these general recommendations:

1. Wash skin with mild soap and water once or twice daily. Frequent washing will not improve acne and may irritate the skin.
2. Use cosmetics, sunscreens, and moisturizers sparingly or switch to oil-free products that indicate they are noncomedogenic.
3. Avoid picking at lesions and excessive scrubbing, especially with abrasive cleansers. Traumatizing acne lesions may contribute to scar formation.
4. Note that dietary modifications generally are not indicated.
5. Use sunscreen and restrict ultraviolet therapy.
6. Follow the prescribed regimen carefully (Table 118-2) and understand that long-term treatment is often required.

Table 118-2. Treatment of Acne[a]	
Classification	**Recommended Treatment Regimen**
Grade I (mild)	Benzoyl peroxide (BP) 2.5%–5% every other day or at bedtime May increase to twice a day, if no response and tolerated, and/or topical retinoid at bedtime
Grade II (mild-moderate)	BP and/or topical retinoid as above plus topical antibiotics once or twice a day if inflammation present, or topical combination product (BP combined with antibiotic) and/or topical retinoid at bedtime
Grade III (moderate)	BP in the morning and topical retinoid at bedtime plus oral antibiotic
Grade IV (severe)	Above treatment for grade III acne, plus referral to a dermatologist for consideration for treatment with isotretinoin

[a]Courtesy of Victor C. Strasburger, MD.

The specific therapies prescribed depend on the severity and duration of the acne, the type of lesions, and patients' ability to comply with the proposed treatment regimen. The patient's skin type should be taken into consideration when selecting the appropriate vehicle for the active ingredient, such as a cream, gel, lotion, solution, or ointment. Oily skin types tend to respond better to gels or solutions, whereas creams, lotions, and ointments are better for dry skin. The most effective regimens include topical products such as benzoyl peroxide, retinoic acid, and antibiotics; systemic antimicrobials; hormonal agents; and isotretinoin. Most often, however, combination therapy is used and later modified according to the patient's response. Physicians should remember to discuss with the adolescent that the acne often looks worse before it gets better and that the treatment is long-term. Noticeable improvement usually takes at least 6 to 8 weeks.

Topical Therapy

Several topical products are available for the treatment of acne. **Benzoyl peroxide (BP)** is bactericidal for *P acnes* and acts as a comedolytic agent as well. It should be considered as the first line of therapy for the management of both comedonal and mild inflammatory acne. Although over-the-counter products are available, the more effective gel preparations are preferable and available by prescription. The lowest concentration possible should be used initially (eg, 2.5% or 5% concentration). Higher concentrations may be used in cases in which the trunk or back are involved, however, increasing the concentration does not necessarily increase its efficacy and may just result in more irritation.

Therapy should be initiated gradually, especially if used in combination with retinoic acid, because BP is inherently irritating and drying. Initially, a thin application should be used once a day every other day, and the frequency should be increased as tolerated. Allergic contact dermatitis rarely develops, but if it does, treatment must be discontinued. A nonacnegenic, noncomedogenic sunscreen is recommended as well to protect against the photosensitivity associated with BP usage.

Tretinoin or retinoic acid (Retin-A, Avita) is the mainstay of therapy for noninflammatory or comedonal acne. This vitamin A derivative reduces microcomedo formation by normalizing follicular keratinization and decreasing the adhesiveness of horny cells shed into the follicular lumen. It also has some anti-inflammatory effects. It is available by prescription as a gel, cream, or liquid in several different concentrations. Recently, microsphere technology has become available, which is less irritating and allows the medication to be delivered slowly at higher concentrations. It seems to be as effective as the older formulations.

Like BP, retinoic acid can be very irritating and may cause some erythema, peeling, stinging/burning, and dryness, which are thought to be dose-dependent. Therefore, therapy should be initiated cautiously with a cream or gel, which is less potent and drying than the liquid preparation. To further reduce irritation, patients should be instructed to wash with a mild soap no more than 2 times a day and to wait at least 20 to 30 minutes for the skin to dry completely before applying the product. Physicians often recommend that patients apply retinoic acid before bedtime rather than in the mornings, which tend to be more hectic for the average teenager. A small, pea-sized dot of tretinoin should be used each time and divided into 3 smaller dots on the skin before rubbing a thin film gently to most of the face, concentrating on the affected areas but also applying it to some of the less affected skin. Patients also should be cautioned against excessive sun exposure while using retinoic acid because this agent lowers the sunburn threshold. Combined daily treatment with BP is warranted in cases of mild inflammatory acne; however, because BP inactivates tretinoin, the 2 drugs cannot be applied simultaneously. Most clinicians recommend BP in the morning and tretinoin at night.

Adapalene (Differin) and tazarotene (Tazorac) are 2 relatively new third-generation topical retinoids that have been used in the treatment of acne. Adapalene is less irritating and has been shown to be more photostable than tretinoin; however, it is not approved for children younger than 12 years. It is available in an alcohol-free gel, cream, or solution. Tazarotene, originally created for the treatment of psoriasis, is the most effective of the topical retinoids, but is more expensive and irritating than the other retinoids, and there are concerns about its teratogenicity. It is therefore not widely prescribed for the treatment of acne.

Azelaic acid (Azelex), a naturally occurring derivative from wheat, has both antibacterial and anti-keratinizing activity. It inhibits the growth of *P acnes* and has an antiproliferative effect on keratinocytes. Although less potent than tretinoin, azelaic acid may be useful in patients with mild to moderate inflammatory and comedonal acne who cannot tolerate topical tretinoin or BP because it seems to be less irritating. Pruritus, burning, stinging, tingling, and erythema have been reported, however. It is available by prescription as a 20% cream and should be applied twice daily.

Antibiotic Therapy

Both topical as well as systemic antibiotics can be used in the treatment of mild to moderate inflammatory acne. The choice of which to use usually depends on the extent of skin involvement and severity of inflammation. **Topical antibiotics** are often useful in patients with mild inflammatory lesions that are unresponsive to BP or retinoic acid alone. Such antibiotics act by inhibiting the growth of *P acnes* and reducing the number of comedones, papules, and pustules. Erythromycin, tetracycline, and clindamycin are available as topical preparations. The **erythromycin gel** is most popular; the recommended dosage is twice daily. Allergic reactions from topical formulations rarely occur. Compared with systemic antibiotics, topical preparations have fewer systemic side effects because of decreased absorption. Topical antibiotics alone are not recommended as monotherapy because resistance generally develops with prolonged use and the therapeutic response can take a while. Both erythromycin and clindamycin are available in combination with benzoyl peroxide and are very effective against *P acnes;* however, combination preparations are generally more costly.

Systemic antibiotics are the mainstay of therapy in patients with nodular or cystic inflammatory acne and in patients who have not responded to topical antibiotics or who have inflamed lesions involving the trunk as well as the face. However, systemic agents have not been shown to be effective with comedonal acne. The success of oral antimicrobial therapy relates to the suppression of *P acnes* and the inhibition of bacterial lipases. As a result, free fatty acids and other by-products are reduced, thereby decreasing inflammation.

Tetracycline and its derivatives **(doxycycline and minocycline)** are the preferred first-line oral antibiotics for the treatment of moderate to severe inflammatory acne. Alternatives include amoxicillin, co-trimoxazole, and trimethoprim. Other systemic antibiotics such as erythromycin have been used in the past; however, antibiotic resistance is now a problem. In addition, clindamycin is used much less frequently because of its associated side effects like pseudomembranous colitis. Doxycycline and minocycline are particularly beneficial when lesions fail to respond to tetracycline. However, tetracycline and doxycycline are not recommended in children younger than 9 years or in pregnant females. The most common side effects include candidal vaginitis, especially in females who also take oral contraceptives (OCPs); gastrointestinal (GI) disturbances; and photosensitivity. The ultimate goal of oral antibiotic therapy is use of the minimum dose to control lesions and minimize side effects. Most patients require prolonged or frequent intermittent courses of oral antibiotics, however, before remission occurs. In general, the dose of the antibiotic and the dosing interval should not be reduced before a significant clinical effect is seen, which may take 6 to 8 weeks. At that time the dose of the oral antibiotic may be gradually tapered and topical antibiotic treatment may be substituted.

Hormonal Therapy

Hormonal therapy is indicated in menstruating females who are unresponsive to other forms of treatment and who are candidates for isotretinoin. Oral contraceptives antagonize the action of circulating androgens by increasing the production of sex-binding globulin, which decreases biologically active free testosterone. In addition there is decreased androgen production by the ovaries through feedback inhibition of pituitary gonadotropin secretion. Clinical improvement in inflammatory lesions has been reported with ethinyl estradiol (35 μg) and the progestin norgestimate (Ortho Tri-Cyclen) and ethinyl estradiol/drospirenone (Yasmin). In general, OCPs must be taken for 2 to 4 months before any improvement is seen, with relapses occurring if treatment is discontinued. Ortho Tri-Cyclen and Estrostep have been approved by the US Food and Drug Administration (FDA) specifically for their antiandrogen effects, although other OCPs have shown similar efficacy in reducing acne lesions.

Specific endocrine disorders such as polycystic ovarian syndrome and the metabolic syndrome also may exacerbate acne and should be investigated in female adolescents with a history of oligomenorrhea, hirsutism, obesity, and insulin resistance. In these cases, hormonal therapy will treat the hyperandrogenism as well as the accompanying acne by decreasing adrenal androgen production.

Systemic Therapy

Because sebaceous glands are androgen-dependent, antiandrogens such as spironolactone can reduce sebum production, and therefore improve acne. However, this therapy is generally reserved for adult females. Doses range from 100 to 200 mg/d; however, lower doses may also be effective. Several months of spironolactone therapy are needed for maximum benefit, with prolonged therapy often required. Gynecomastia occurs not infrequently. Agranulocytosis is a rare complication.

Isotretinoin Therapy

Isotretinoin (Accutane, Claravis, Sotret, Amnesteem), a systemic oral analog of vitamin A, is currently the most effective treatment available for severe nodulocystic acne that is resistant to conventional therapy. This agent is also useful in patients with a propensity for scarring. It influences all aspects of acne formation: sebum secretion, follicular keratinization, and inflammatory responses. For patients with severe forms of inflammatory acne, isotretinoin has been hailed as a "miracle drug", despite its many side effects.

Given the numerous potentially serious adverse effects of the drug, referral to a dermatologist is strongly recommended for patients who require isotretinoin therapy. The most significant of these adverse effects is teratogenicity, although other issues include dryness and chapping of the skin and mucous membranes, musculoskeletal effects, GI issues, neurologic problems, and hematologic abnormalities. Isotretinoin can also elevate triglyceride levels, particularly in patients with diabetes mellitus, obesity, alcohol abuse, and familial hyperlipidemia. There also are psychiatric concerns regarding isotretinoin use, including aggressive and/or violent behavior, and an increased risk of depression or suicide, which has led to additional black box warnings by the FDA. Although an association has not been confirmed to date, clinicians are advised to be aware of the coexistence of a mental health disorder when prescribing isotretinoin and are urged to monitor patients closely for a psychiatric referral if indicated.

To minimize fetal exposure to isotretinoin, a special restricted distribution program called iPLEDGE is now administered by the FDA for physicians and pharmacists who prescribe systemic isotretinoin. This computer-based risk management program includes specific educational materials as well as policies and procedures that must be read and signed by the prescribing physician. In addition, informed consent is required of all patients for whom the medication is being prescribed. Two forms of birth control for female patients and documentation of a negative pregnancy test also is required prior to dispensing of the medication. An identifying qualification sticker also must be affixed to all isotretinoin prescriptions indicating the prescribing physician is appropriately registered with the FDA distribution program. Monthly follow-up by the prescribing dermatologist is mandatory.

Prognosis

Fortunately, most uncomplicated cases of acne (approximately 90%) resolve by the third decade of life. For those individuals with nodulocystic lesions, however, acne and significant scarring can continue to be a problem. Therefore, early and aggressive treatment is imperative.

CASE RESOLUTION

In the case history, the adolescent should be offered treatment for his mild to moderate comedonal and inflammatory acne. This may include BP, retinoic acid (Retin-A), and topical antibiotics. The common side effects of the medications (eg, dry skin, peeling) should be reviewed, and the teen should be instructed to use a noncomedogenic sunscreen. A follow-up appointment should be arranged after 3 to 4 weeks to assess compliance with and tolerance of the treatment regimen.

Selected References

Goldsmith LA, Bolognia JL, Callen JP, et al. American Academy of Dermatology Consensus Conference on safe and optimal use of isotretinoin: summary and recommendations. *J Am Acad Dermatol.* 2004;50:900–906

Haider A, Shaw JC. Treatment of acne vulgaris. *JAMA.* 2004;292:726–735

Koblenzer CS. The emotional impact of chronic and disabling skin disease: a psychoanalytic perspective. *Dermatol Clin.* 2005;23:619–627

Krowchuk DP. Managing adolescent acne: a guide for pediatricians. *Pediatr Rev.* 2005;26:244–255

National Campaign to Control Acne. Secaucus, NJ: Thomas Professional Postgraduate Services; 2003

Paller AS, Mancini AJ. Disorders of the sebaceous and sweat glands. *Hurwitz Clinical Pediatric Dermatology: A Textbook of Skin Disorders of Childhood and Adolescence.* 3rd ed. Philadelphia, PA: W. B. Saunders; 2006:185–195

Smith JA. The impact of skin disease on the quality of life in adolescents. *Adolesc Med.* 2001;12:343–353

Strasburger VC. Acne: what every pediatrician should know about treatment. *Pediatr Clin North Am.* 1997;44:1505–1523

Tom WL, Friedlander SF. Acne through the ages: case-based observations through childhood and adolescence. *Clin Pediatr* 2008;47:639–651

Witchel SF. Hyperandrogenism in adolescents. *Adolesc Med.* 2002;13:89–99

Yan AC. Current concepts in acne management. *Adolesc Med.* 2006;17:613–637

Zaenglein AL, Thiboutot DM. Expert committee recommendations for acne management. *Pediatrics.* 2006;118:1188–1199

CHAPTER 119

Disorders of the Hair and Scalp

Ki-Young Suh, MD; Kathy K. Langevin, MD, MPH; and Noah Craft, MD, PhD

CASE STUDY

A 6-year-old child presents with a 1-month history of a swelling on the right side of her scalp that is associated with hair loss. She has previously been in good health, and she has no history of fever. On examination, she is afebrile, has normal vital signs, and appears well. An area of nontender, boggy swelling 2 × 2 cm with associated alopecia is apparent over the scalp in the right temporal area. Small pustular lesions are scattered over the involved area. Generalized scaling of the scalp and occipital adenopathy are evident.

Questions

1. What are the common causes of circumscribed hair loss in children?
2. What are the common causes of diffuse hair loss in children?
3. What are the common causes of scalp scaling in children?
4. What features distinguish tinea capitis from alopecia areata?
5. What is the treatment for tinea capitis? Is there a role for topical antifungal agents?

Disorders of the scalp may be either congenital or acquired during childhood or adolescence. Conditions may be further classified according to the presence or absence of hair loss (alopecia), whether the hair loss is diffuse or circumscribed, and whether the hair loss results in scarring of the scalp.

Epidemiology

Acquired circumscribed hair loss is more commonly seen than diffuse hair loss. Most cases of acquired circumscribed hair loss result from tinea capitis, alopecia areata, or trauma due to traction or trichotillomania.

Tinea capitis is a fungal infection of the scalp most often caused by the dermatophytes *Microsporum canis* or *Trichophyton tonsurans*. *Trichophyton tonsurans* accounts for most cases in the United States, but in a given geographic area, the etiologic fungus may change over time. Tinea capitis, which is less common in infants and postpubertal adolescents, is seen primarily in school-aged children between the ages of 3 and 7 years. Prevalence is estimated to be between 3% and 13% in the pediatric population. Boys are affected more often than girls with *M canis*, though both are affected equally in epidemics caused by *T tonsurans*. African American and Latin American children are more vulnerable to infection. Human-to-human transmission is more common with *T tonsurans*, an anthropophilic fungus. Children who handle dogs or cats, which harbor *M canis*, a zoophilic fungus, are susceptible to infection. Carriers are most commonly adults exposed to affected children, and carriers are considered contagious. Up to 60% of affected children are asymptomatic. Tinea capitis can result in localized patches of hair loss and can result in scarring if the infection becomes inflammatory.

Alopecia areata is believed to be an organ-specific autoimmune disorder with a prevalence of 158 per 100,000 persons, occurring equally in males and females. Family history is positive in 10% to 50% of affected patients. Although alopecia areata may develop at any age, it is rare before the age of 1 year, and 40% to 50% of cases develop alopecia areata before the age of 21 years. It may be seen in association with atopic dermatitis, Down syndrome, and other autoimmune diseases.

Trichotillomania, or compulsive pulling at the hair, may be seen in association with other impulse disorders such as thumb sucking and nail biting (see Chapter 51). It results in hair loss due to self-induced trauma. Usually the scalp hair is involved, but eyebrows or eyelash hair may also be affected. Although trichotillomania may be seen at any age, onset is usually between the ages of 5 to 12 years. It is more commonly seen in girls and women rather than boys and men and in children rather than adults. **Traction alopecia** is more commonly seen in females whose hair-grooming practices result in excessive tension and trauma to the hair.

Clinical Presentation

Children may present with specific complaints, including localized baldness, pruritus, scaling, or inflammation (Dx Box). Occasionally, lymphadenopathy, particularly in the occipital area, is the major presenting symptom.

Pathophysiology

An understanding of the physiology of the normal hair growth cycle helps in the evaluation of hair and scalp disorders. The scalp of an average human being contains about 100,000 hairs. Individuals with

Dx Disorders of the Hair and Scalp

- Circumscribed or generalized hair loss (alopecia)
- Scaling
- Pruritus
- Erythema of the scalp
- Localized or generalized swelling of the scalp
- Occipital adenopathy

blonde hair generally have 10% more hairs and those with red hair have 10% less. Healthy terminal hair grows an average of 0.3 mm per day or approximately 1 cm per month.

The hair follicle is responsible for most disturbances of hair growth because the hair shaft itself is a nonliving structure. Normal hair growth is a cyclical process composed of 3 stages. The anagen phase, the period of active hair growth, lasts for an average of 3 years (range: 2–6 years). Normally, about 85% to 90% of scalp hair is in this phase at any one time. The catagen phase, the transition period, lasts for about 10 to 14 days. The telogen phase, the final resting phase, lasts for about 3 to 4 months. About 13% of scalp hairs are in this phase at one time. The average individual loses about 100 to 150 telogen hairs per day. The normal hair cycle results in replacement of each scalp hair every 3 to 5 years.

Tinea capitis is a communicable infection and can be acquired via interpersonal contact, contact with infected animals, and via fomites. There are 3 patterns of hair invasion. In endothrix infections (eg, *T tonsurans*), the fungus produces chains of spores within the hair shaft. In ectothrix infections (eg, *M canis*), spores are present around the exterior of the hair shaft. Favus, the most severe form of tinea capitis, demonstrates hyphae and air spaces within the hair shaft. This is usually caused by *Trichophyton schoenleinii*, a less common etiologic organism. Though dermatophytes have a relatively short incubation period (up to 3 weeks) they are viable in fomites for months. Subcutaneous invasion in conjunction with an exaggerated host response can result in kerion.

Alopecia areata is thought to be due to aberrant expression of class I human leukocyte antigens on early anagen follicles resulting in T lymphocyte recognition of these normally immune hairs. There follows an immunologic attack causing premature telogen. The hairs then break easily at the surface of the scalp. The hairs at the margins of alopecia are easily plucked and they have an "exclamation mark" appearance with the proximal end thinner than the distal end.

Differential Diagnosis

While some hair disorders can be easily recognized clinically, the differential diagnosis can be challenging at times. Familiarity with the appearance of these conditions is critical. The Internet can be valuable in providing access to images of many dermatologic conditions. Some sites such as VisualDx (accessible at www.visualdx.com) display pictorial representations and allow for searching by features such as by hair loss patterns, symptoms, exposures, skin color, scalp location, age, immune status, and many other factors.

Scalp Disorders Without Associated Hair Loss

These conditions are divided into those disorders seen most often in neonates and young infants and those seen more frequently in children and adolescents (Box 119-1). **Caput succedaneum,** a generalized edema involving the soft tissues of the scalp, and **cephalhematoma,** a subperiosteal hematoma, are 2 of the most common lesions of the scalp that occur during the neonatal period. A cephalhematoma does not extend beyond the suture lines of the affected bone, which distinguishes it from caput succedaneum. Both conditions result from birth trauma and generally resolve spontaneously within a few weeks to months without further complications.

Box 119-1. Common Disorders of the Scalp Without Associated Hair Loss

Neonatal Period and Early Infancy
- Birth trauma to the scalp (eg, caput succedaneum, cephalhematoma)
- Scalp abscess (at fetal scalp electrode site)
- Herpes simplex infection
- Cradle cap/seborrheic dermatitis
- Atopic dermatitis[a]
- Scabies

Childhood and Adolescence
- Seborrheic dermatitis[a]
- Atopic dermatitis[a]
- Head lice (pediculosis capitis)
- Psoriasis[a]

[a]May occur with or without associated hair loss.

Other neonatal scalp conditions include infections such as **scalp abscess** and **herpes simplex virus (HSV) infection**. Scalp abscess occurs most commonly as a complication of scalp electrode placement and has an incidence of 0.4% to 4.5%. The infectious agents are usually flora of the cervix and vagina. Management depends on the severity of the infection (eg, associated cellulitis or signs of systemic involvement). Although most cases are self-limited, the abscess can be complicated by intracranial infection. Herpes simplex virus infections of the scalp are not uncommon in neonates; 85% of neonatal HSV infections occur at time of delivery and the scalp usually has the longest contact with the cervix, one of the sites for transmission of infection. Herpes lesions are typically vesicular, but petechial, purpuric, or bullous lesions may also be apparent. Skin lesions typically develop at 1 week of life but may be present at birth or develop as late as 3 weeks later.

Atopic dermatitis and **seborrheic dermatitis** are the 2 most common diagnoses of scalp scaling among infants and children younger than 10 years. **Seborrheic dermatitis** is a red, scaly eruption that occurs mainly on the scalp (otherwise known as cradle cap), face, and postauricular and intertriginous areas (see Chapter 121). It is often seen in infants younger than 2 years. Additionally, the scale, often termed *dandruff* in children 2 to 10 years, is usually seborrheic dermatitis, and this is seen more in African American children. Unlike atopic dermatitis, seborrheic dermatitis is generally non-pruritic. Occasionally the inflammatory process is severe enough to result in diffuse hair loss. Psoriatic lesions of the scalp and Langerhans cell histiocytosis can mimic seborrheic dermatitis. Skin biopsy may be required for definitive diagnosis. It is often seen in conjunction with adenopathy of the head and neck without associated tinea infection.

Atopic dermatitis on the scalp is also characterized by erythema and scaling of the scalp, and it can overlap with seborrheic dermatitis. Atopic dermatitis on the scalp can be associated with significant pruritus with rubbing and scratching that result in the secondary effects of crusting and lichenification. Severe atopic and seborrheic dermatitis, as well as psoriasis, can result in **tinea amiantacea** (not a fungal infection), which usually presents as a localized, thick, adherent, white or gray scale.

Head lice (pediculosis capitis) are an extremely common childhood infestation that affects girls more often than boys and is most common in children aged 3 to 11 years. Lice are spread by direct contact with infected individuals or infested clothing, combs, or other hair accessories. Pruritus is the primary symptom along with erythema and scaling, with secondary impetigo being common. The viable ova or nits may be visible as small, oval, tan to brown specks found most commonly in the hair above the ears and the nape of the neck. Hatched eggs are clear to white. Generally, only the ova closest to the scalp are viable. They are difficult to remove.

Scabies, a pruritic infestation commonly seen in children, generally does not affect the scalp, except in infants, the elderly, and the immunocompromised. On the scalp of infants, 2- to 3-mm erythematous papules are seen, with overlying excoriations and, often, secondary bacterial infection.

Scalp Disorders Associated With Hair Loss

Box 119-2 lists the common scalp disorders associated with hair loss. When evaluating hair loss in children, it is important to determine whether the loss is diffuse or circumscribed.

Nevus sebaceus is a congenital lesion that mainly occurs on the face and scalp, occurring in about 3 of 1,000 neonates. These lesions are characteristically hairless. In addition, they are usually solitary, well-circumscribed plaques on the scalp, yellow-orange in color, and ovoid to linear in shape. Nevus sebaceus can be associated with a small risk of malignant transformation, namely basal cell carcinoma, at a rate of less than 1% before the age of 18 years. Other growths within nevus sebaceus may also occur at a rate of approximately 1%. Therefore, regular monitoring or consideration of excision should be part of the management. Because of the relatively low risk and low metastatic potential, it is reasonable to postpone excision until later in life. **Aplasia cutis congenita** is a congenital skin defect with localized areas of epidermal, dermal, and/or subcutaneous tissue loss. Lesions can occur anywhere on the body, but most are found along the midline of the scalp. At birth, the lesions usually appear as punched out, round or oval defects that may have an overlying thin, glistening membrane. Erosion, ulceration, or a scar due to healing in utero can also be seen. A "hair collar" often surrounds the lesion.

Aplasia cutis congenita is a result of many possible etiologies, and it can be an isolated defect or in association with other congenital defects such as cleft lip or palate, syndactyly, or multiple other anomalies. Small defects generally heal well, whereas larger defects may require surgical excision and eventual skin grafting. Preoperative imaging studies may be required for extensive, severe cases.

Tinea capitis, a fungal infection of the scalp, is one of the most common causes of acquired hair loss in children. This condition is characterized by patchy alopecia with broken-off hairs and scaling of the scalp. *Trichophyton tonsurans* infection sometimes appears as a series of black dots within the affected area due to the presence of fragmented hairs. The diagnosis can be difficult in children with either diffuse scalp scaling or a diffuse pustular eruption without significant alopecia. Occasionally, an intense hypersensitivity response may result in a boggy swelling of the scalp known as a **kerion.** The surface of the kerion may be smooth or covered with small pustules, mimicking a bacterial infection. Uncomplicated tinea capitis leaves no scars, but kerions or favus may result in permanent, scarring hair loss.

Alopecia areata, which frequently leads to hair loss, is characterized by well-defined areas of complete hair loss without associated scaling, irritation, or inflammation of the scalp. Hairs at the periphery of bald patches can usually be easily plucked. The most common presentation is that of one or more round or oval bald patches. A less common subtype is the ophiasis pattern, in which hair loss is present in a band along the periphery of the temporal and occipital scalp. Associated nail defects, including nail pitting (most common) and ridging, may be seen. Occasionally, alopecia totalis (loss of all scalp hair) or alopecia universalis (loss of all body and scalp hair) may result.

Common traumatic causes of alopecia in children are traction alopecia and trichotillomania. **Traction alopecia** often occurs along the margins of the hairline secondary to having the hair pulled back in tight ponytails or braids. Short, broken hairs and follicular papules may be seen. Chronic, prolonged traction can result in permanent, scarring alopecia. **Trichotillomania** is a self-induced form of traction alopecia in which children twist or pull out their hair either consciously or subconsciously (see Chapter 51). Hair pulling is generally believed to occur in a younger population and usually resolves with minimal or no intervention needed. Trichotillomania is now classified in *Diagnostic and Statistical Manual of Mental Disorders, Fourth Edition,* in the habit and impulse disorders category. Hair is generally plucked in a wave-like fashion across the scalp or centrifugally from a starting point. The occiput is generally spared. Trichotillomania may mimic other types of alopecia, but the diagnosis can usually be made on the basis of the bizarre patterns of hair loss with hairs broken at differing lengths. Children occasionally eat the hairs as they are pulled out, resulting in the formation of a **trichobezoar** (hair ball) in the stomach.

Discoid lupus erythematosus, lichen planus, and **secondary syphilis** are uncommon causes of localized hair loss from the scalp in children. The patches of alopecia in discoid lupus erythematosus often appear hypopigmented with hyperpigmentation at the periphery. Because adnexal structures are involved in discoid lupus, scarring alopecia is commonly seen. Lichen planus, an idiopathic inflammatory disease of skin and mucous membranes, can result in both scarring and non-scarring alopecia. Secondary syphilis lesions appear as "moth-eaten" patches of alopecia that are non-scarring.

A variety of structural defects, endocrine and metabolic disorders, and toxins may be associated with diffuse loss of scalp hair (Box 119-2). **Intrinsic structural defects of the hair** may cause hairs to break, thus resulting in failure of hair growth. In some forms of **ectodermal dysplasia,** the number of hair follicles is reduced or the follicles are altogether absent, giving the appearance of sparse or thinning hair. Many of the ectodermal dysplasias have abnormalities of the teeth, nails, and sweat glands. **Monilethrix** is an autosomal-dominant condition that can appear in isolation or in association with other anomalies. Microscopic evaluation of hairs show a "beads on a string" appearance due to alternating nodes and internodes

---

Box 119-2. Common Disorders of the Scalp With Associated Hair Loss

CIRCUMSCRIBED HAIR LOSS

Congenital
- Aplasia cutis congenita
- Nevus sebaceus
- Epidermal nevus

Acquired
- Tinea capitis
- Alopecia areata
- Traction alopecia
- Trichotillomania
- Discoid lupus erythematosus
- Secondary syphilis
- Herpes simplex virus
- Lichen planus

DIFFUSE ALOPECIA

Congenital
- Congenital hypothyroidism
- Hair shaft defects (eg, Menkes syndrome, monilethrix)
- Ectodermal dysplasias and other genetic syndromes

Acquired
- Seborrheic dermatitis
- Psoriasis
- Telogen effluvium
- Anagen effluvium (secondary to toxins or chemicals)
- Endocrine (eg, diabetes mellitus)
- Hypothyroidism-hypoparathyroidism-hypopituitarism
- Medication-induced (isotretinoin)
- Androgenic alopecia (eg, male pattern baldness)
- Loose anagen syndrome

Other
- Nutritional (eg, acrodermatitis enteropathica, malnutrition, iron deficiency, rickets)
- Systemic lupus erythematosus

---

resulting in fractures between the nodes. Pili torti can be seen in several syndromes including **Menkes syndrome (kinky hair syndrome).** Affected patients have twisted hair leading to premature breakage and, thus, chronically short hair. There is often baldness at sites of friction.

Telogen effluvium is a common cause of diffuse hair loss that may occur 2 to 4 months after a variety of events, including pregnancy, discontinuation of oral contraceptives, severe febrile illness, medications, severe diets, or significant emotional stress. Hair loss results from the abrupt conversion of numerous scalp hairs from the anagen (growth) phase to the telogen (resting) phase. Loss of more than 150 hairs per day is considered abnormal. Patients may complain of losing several hundred hairs a day, but the occurrence of clinically significant baldness is rare. Estimates indicate that individuals must lose about 25% of their hair before thinning becomes clinically apparent. The hair loss may continue for several weeks, but complete regrowth usually occurs within 6 to 12 months. **Anagen effluvium** results in the loss of growing hairs due to a sudden cessation of the growing phase. It occurs most commonly after systemic chemotherapy.

Loose anagen syndrome is a disorder in which the anagen hair follicle is anchored improperly, resulting in easy, painless plucking of the hairs. This can result in patchy diffuse hair loss or focal areas of alopecia. This is a familial condition, with fair-haired females more commonly affected. Often, these children will not need a haircut through early childhood. The hair is expected to spontaneously become normal by the teenage years without treatment.

Evaluation

History

The age of the child guides the differential diagnosis, because some lesions are more common at one age than another. See the Questions Box to review pertinent history that may be helpful in diagnosis.

Questions

Disorders of the Hair and Scalp

- Is the child losing any hair?
- If so, is the child losing hair from all over the scalp or only from localized areas on the scalp?
- Has the child lost any body hair (eg, eyebrows, eyelashes) in addition to the scalp hair?
- How long has the child been losing hair?
- Is the scalp pruritic or scaling?
- Have the parents noticed the child twisting or pulling the hair?
- Is the child's hair often in ponytails or braids?
- Has there recently been any significant stress in the child's life?
- Do any pets live in the home?
- Is the child taking any medications?
- Is anyone else in the home or anyone in close contact with the child having similar symptoms?

Physical Examination

The scalp should be examined to see if the hair loss is diffuse or circumscribed and whether scalp hairs can be plucked easily. Signs of irritation, inflammation, or scaling of the scalp should also be noted, as well as the presence of adenopathy, nail changes, or hair loss elsewhere on the body.

Wood light examination of the scalp for fungus is helpful if positive. A negative examination does not rule out the possibility of fungal infection, however, because *T tonsurans,* the most common cause of tinea capitis in the United States, does not fluoresce. *Microsporum canis* fluoresces yellow-green under the Wood light.

Laboratory Tests

Laboratory assessment is useful in some cases. If fungal infection is suspected, a KOH examination should be performed by the primary care physician. Scales and broken hairs can be obtained from involved areas by brushing, scraping (eg, with a No. 15 scalpel blade), plucking, or rubbing a moistened 4" × 4" gauze over affected areas and then removing broken hairs and scale from the gauze with forceps. The scrapings should be placed on a glass slide, dissolved in KOH solution, heated gently, and examined under the microscope. Hyphae and spores within the hair shaft (eg, *T tonsurans* infection) or surrounding the hair shaft (eg, *M canis* infection) should be noted.

In addition to microscopic examination, fungal cultures are recommended in all cases of suspected tinea capitis. Brushings using either a moistened sterile cotton swab or a sterile brush as used in Pap smears will yield the most reliable results. Hair or scalp scrapings are inoculated onto Sabouraud agar or dermatophyte test medium (DTM). Within 5 to 14 days, a distinctive growth seen on the Sabouraud agar or a color change from yellow to red in the DTM confirms the diagnosis. A negative KOH examination and fungal culture, in addition to a lack of inflammation and scaling, may be required for differentiating trichotillomania or alopecia areata from tinea capitis.

The diagnosis of telogen effluvium is usually suggested by the history and counting the number of hairs lost each day. If the diagnosis is in question, the patient may be referred to a dermatologist for examination of the involved hair roots via biopsy and determination of the anagen-telogen ratio, which is usually about 85:15. A telogen count of more than 25% is considered to be diagnostic of telogen effluvium. The ratio of anagen to telogen hairs is normal in trichotillomania.

A more extensive laboratory workup may be required if the hair loss is persistent or the history or physical examination is suggestive of systemic disease (see Box 119-2). Studies that may be considered include liver function tests, thyroid function studies, a serum Venereal Disease Research Laboratory test, antinuclear antibodies, and serum electrolytes.

Management

Management depends on the diagnosis. Herpetic infection in a newborn requires immediate attention and systemic antiviral therapy because the risk of systemic infection is significant. Scalp electrodes and vacuum-assisted vaginal deliveries should be avoided in neonates with mothers known to have HSV infections because these can increase the rate of infection transmission. Currently cesarean section delivery remains the standard of care, though most cases of herpes simplex in infants are in those born to mothers without known infection at time of delivery.

Children suspected of nevus sebaceus should be referred to a dermatologist. Excision may be considered, not only because of the risk, albeit low, of secondary neoplastic changes, but also because these lesions can become more prominent and warty in appearance and friable during puberty and adulthood.

Seborrheic dermatitis can persist into the pubertal years, contrary to previously held belief. Cradle cap, the greasy form of seborrheic dermatitis, can be treated with simple skin care measures such as bathing and the use of moisturizing emollients. Gentle shampoos, low-potency corticosteroids and, if needed, 2% ketoconazole cream can resolve most cases. Past infancy, seborrheic dermatitis may be treated with **shampoos containing tar, pyrithione zinc, ketoconazole, or selenium** in rotation. Topical, mild corticosteroid solutions can be used if pruritus is significant.

Head lice may be treated with **pyrethrin products,** such as permethrin 1% cream rinse (Nix) or the prescription 5% cream typically used for scabies. Other medications such as malathion and ivermectin can also be effective. All topical medications should be used twice, 1 week apart, regardless of package insert information. A fine-toothed comb or tweezers may be required after rinsing to remove the ova or nits of head lice. Other alternative treatments have been unsubstantiated, such as using mayonnaise or petroleum jelly. Heat, such as that associated with blow-drying the hair, also kills a large percentage of the lice.

Permethrin 5% cream is the preferred scabicide. It should be applied from head to toe in infants younger than 2 years, and from neck to toe for those older than 2 years, for 8 to 12 hours, washed off, and repeated in 1 week. Permethrin 5% cream can be used in infants as young as 2 months and pregnant women. For these patients, sulfur 6% ointment can be used. For both scabies and lice, the treatment of fomites is also important. Clothing, bed linens, and towels should be washed in hot water and machine-dried in high heat. Fomites that cannot be laundered should be sealed in plastic for 48 to 72 hours.

Oral griseofulvin administered for at least 6 to 12 weeks has been the long-held treatment of choice for **tinea capitis.** Although griseofulvin can have many side effects, including gastrointestinal disturbances, hepatotoxicity, and leukopenia, it is generally well tolerated by children and is available in suspension form. Hematologic, renal, and liver function studies can be monitored in children on high doses or prolonged treatment. Higher dosing is occasionally required due to increasing resistance. Care should be made to use proper dosing when using micronized (20–25 mg/kg) or ultra-micronized (10–15 mg/kg) griseofulvin. Newer antifungal agents are also being used with great success, often for shorter durations than griseofulvin, which can increase compliance. **Itraconazole** can be given as either continuous or pulse therapy and is also available as a solution. **Fluconazole,** also available as solution, is usually administered for 3 to 6 weeks or at a higher dose once weekly for 8 to 12 weeks. **Terbinafine,** available in tablets or granules, has also been effective at shorter treatment times than griseofulvin. Monitoring of blood cell counts and liver and renal function are recommended monthly before and during treatment. Ketoconazole is contraindicated in this population due to its potential for adverse effects, especially in light of other available agents. Generally, longer courses of treatment are needed for *M canis* infection. Topical antifungal agents are not effective on the scalp for treatment of tinea capitis because the hair follicle must be penetrated, requiring the use of systemic therapy. Twice-a-week shampooing with ketoconazole or selenium sulfide shampoos has been shown to reduce carriage of spores and reduce infectivity. A course of oral **prednisone** may be required in conjunction with an oral antifungal if a kerion is present to minimize discomfort and permanent, scarring hair loss. Children with kerions are often misdiagnosed as having a bacterial infection of the scalp and treated with oral antibiotics. However, the pustules in kerions are generally sterile, and even when secondary bacterial infection is present (eg, about 30%–50% of patients), antibiotics do not alter the course of the condition.

Children believed to have alopecia areata should be referred to a dermatologist immediately. Therapy for **alopecia areata** consists of **both topical and intralesional corticosteroids,** topical anthralin, or minoxidil. Topical immunotherapy with a sensitizer such as squaric acid has also been used for the treatment of extensive alopecia areata. Occasionally oral steroids can be tried for extensive or rapidly progressing disease. Many psychosocial factors should be considered when treating children with this condition. Children with severe forms of the disease may benefit psychologically from wearing a wig. The National Alopecia Areata Foundation is available as a support group for affected children and their families.

Prognosis

Common disorders of the scalp, such as seborrheic dermatitis, head lice, and tinea capitis, generally respond well to treatment and rarely result in long-term sequelae. The course and prognosis of alopecia areata are quite variable and may be difficult to predict. Generally, the prognosis for regrowth is good if hair loss has occurred in only a few patches. The prognosis is usually poorer with younger age at onset, positive family history, nail involvement, and an ophiasis (band-like)

pattern of hair loss. It is important to pursue further workup if a condition does not respond to therapy because it is critical that a condition such as Langerhans cell histiocytosis, a mimicker of seborrheic dermatitis, not be missed. Many of the hair disorders are a result of syndromes that will not respond to therapy and, thus, education for patients and their families is important.

CASE RESOLUTION

The child presented in the case scenario exhibits physical findings of a kerion. Diagnosis can be made clinically on the basis of the appearance of the lesion. The diagnosis is established by microscopic evidence of hyphae and culture confirmation. Treatment with oral antifungals and possibly oral steroids should be initiated. Carriers should also be identified and treated. The child should be examined in 4 weeks to ascertain the response to therapy and check for any adverse reactions.

Selected References

Chosidow O. Clinical practices. Scabies. *N Engl J Med.* 2006;354:1718–1727

Harrison S, Sinclair R. Optimal management of hair loss (alopecia) in children. *Am J Clin Dermatol.* 2003;4:757–770

Honig PJ. Treatment of kerions. *Pediatr Dermatol.* 1994;11:69–71

Hordinsky M. Alopecias. In: Bolognia JL, Jorizzo JL, Rapini RP, eds. *Dermatology.* St Louis, MO: Mosby; 2003:1033–1050

James WD, Berger TG, Elston DM. *Andrews' Diseases of the Skin.* 10th ed. Toronto, Ontario, Canada: Elsevier, Inc.; 2006:298–299, 483–485, 749–751

Kakourou T, Uksal U; European Society for Pediatric Dermatology. Guidelines for the management of tinea capitis in children. *Pediatr Dermatol.* 2010;27:226–228

Koot RW, Reedijk B, Tan WF, De Sonnaville-De Roy van Zuide. Neonatal brain abscess: complication of fetal monitoring. *Obstet Gynecol.* 1999;93:857

Meinking TL, Burkhart CN, Burkhart CG. Infestations. In: Bolognia JL, Jorizzo JL, Rapini RP, eds. *Dermatology.* St Louis, MO: Mosby; 2003:1321–1326

Möhrenschlager M, Seidl HP, Ring J, Abeck D. Pediatric tinea capitis: recognition and management. *Am J Clin Dermatol.* 2005;6:203–213

Nield LS, Keri JE, Kamat D. Alopecia in the general pediatric clinic: who to treat, who to refer. *Clin Pediatr.* 2006;45:605–612

Pierson D, Randel C, et al. Benign epidermal tumors and proliferations. In: Bolognia JL, Jorizzo JL, Rapini RP, eds. *Dermatology.* St Louis, MO: Mosby; 2003:1711–1712

Rosen H, Schmidt B, Lam HP, et al. Management of nevus sebaceus and the risk of basal cell carcinoma: an 18-year review. *Pediatr Dermatol.* 2009;26:676–681

Sybert VP, Zonana J. Ectodermal dysplasias. In: Bolognia JL, Jorizzo JL, Rapini RP, eds. *Dermatology.* St Louis, MO: Mosby; 2003:906–913

Weinder EJ, McIntosh MS, Joseph MM, et al. Neonatal scalp abscess: is it a benign disease? *J Emerg Med.* 2009 [Epub ahead of print]

Williams JV, Eichenfield LF, Burke BL, Barnes-Eley M, Friedlander SF. Prevalence of scalp scaling in prepubertal children. *Pediatrics.* 2005;115:e1–e6

CHAPTER 120

Diaper Dermatitis

Ki-Young Suh, MD; Kathy K. Langevin, MD, MPH; and Noah Craft MD, PhD

CASE STUDY

A 6-month-old infant has a 3-day history of a rash in the diaper area. The mother has been applying cornstarch, but the rash has gotten worse and has spread to the inner thighs and the abdomen. The infant has no history of fever, upper respiratory tract symptoms, vomiting, or diarrhea. He was seen in the emergency department 1 week ago for acute gastroenteritis, which has since resolved. On examination, a poorly demarcated, shiny, erythematous rash is noted over the convex surface of the buttocks, lower abdomen, and genitalia, with relative sparing of the intertriginous creases. The rest of the physical examination is within normal limits.

Questions

1. What are the common causes of rashes in the diaper area (diaper dermatitis)?
2. What are the features that distinguish one type of diaper dermatitis from another?
3. What systemic diseases may present with diaper dermatitis?
4. What are some common treatments for diaper dermatitis?

Diaper dermatitis is used to describe a wide variety of skin disorders that present with a rash in the area covered by the diaper. The most familiar form of diaper rash, irritant contact diaper dermatitis, is one of the most common skin disorders of infants and young children. Other infectious and inflammatory processes in the diaper area can also result in dermatitis. Successful management requires making the correct diagnosis and identifying the etiology and associated factors.

Epidemiology

Diaper dermatitis is the most common dermatologic disorder in infancy, with a peak incidence at 9 to 12 months of age, though some reports have shown a high incidence in the first month of life. Prevalence in infants is estimated at anywhere from 7% to 35%. This disorder is not limited to infants and small children but to any individual who wears diapers, though the incidence in adults is unknown.

Clinical Presentation

The lesions of diaper dermatitis primarily affect the skin of the buttocks, gluteal cleft, lower abdomen, perineum, and proximal thighs. **Irritant contact dermatitis,** the most common type of diaper dermatitis, appears as erythema and scaling papules and plaques or poorly demarcated, glistening erythema over the convex surfaces, with relative sparing of the intertriginous folds (Figure 120-1A). Candidal infection is another common form of diaper dermatitis and is characterized by a beefy red, sharply demarcated plaque with white scale at the border and/or small, satellite papules and pustules along the margins. Candidal infections may be primarily

concentrated within the skin folds (Dx Box) (Figure 120-1B). Other etiologic causes of diaper dermatitis can be challenging to distinguish from one another but can usually be differentiated by their distribution and response to therapy.

Dx Diaper Dermatitis

- Urinary or fecal incontinence requiring diaper wearing
- Erythematous rash over anogenital region
- Associated gastroenteritis, antibiotic therapy, or oral thrush

Pathophysiology

Many factors are involved in the pathophysiology of irritant diaper dermatitis. Prolonged contact with moisture, urine, feces, or irritating chemicals plays an important role in the initiation of these disorders. Friction generated as the infant tries to move around may further aggravate the condition and lead to maceration of the skin. Secondary infection, most often with *Candida albicans,* may be seen in many cases.

The cause of irritant diaper dermatitis is multifactorial, with prolonged exposure to moisture resulting in fragile skin and a compromised protective barrier, leading to increased irritant penetration and potential growth of microorganisms. Fecal enzymes (proteases, lipases, and urease) also weaken this barrier. Friction from a diaper can easily abrade this fragile skin. Diapers clearly play a role in this disorder; societies where diapers are not worn do not see this condition. Ammonia produced by bacterial breakdown of urea is no longer believed to be the causative factor in cases of irritant diaper dermatitis.

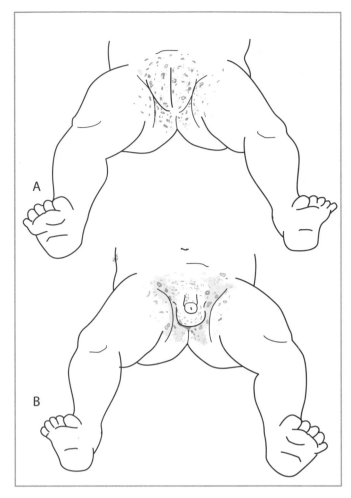

Figure 120-1. Diaper dermatitis. A. Diaper dermatitis secondary to contact. Convex surface areas are affected. B. Diaper dermatitis secondary to *Candida*. Intertriginous areas are affected, and satellite lesions are present.

Differential Diagnosis

While most cases of diaper dermatitis can be easily recognized clinically, the differential diagnosis can be challenging at times or when the condition fails to respond to therapy. Familiarity with the difference in appearance of these conditions is critical. The Internet can be valuable by providing access to images of many dermatologic conditions. Some sites such as VisualDx (accessible at www.visualdx.com) display a pictorial representation and allow for searching by features such as rash morphologies, symptoms, exposures, skin color, body location, and many other factors.

Diaper dermatitis is a general term to refer to a rash that occurs in the area covered by the diaper. Therefore, a specific diagnosis based on the etiology of the diaper dermatitis is important. The differential diagnosis of diaper dermatitis is presented in Box 120-1.

Irritant contact dermatitis, the most common cause of diaper dermatitis, is most prominent on the skin of the buttocks, perineum, lower abdomen, and proximal thighs. The skin of the creases is relatively unaffected. Exposure to proteolytic enzymes and irritant chemicals in the face of excessive heat or moisture is believed to lead to this condition. Friction with the diaper at sites of contact may

---

aggravate it. Such a rash is poorly demarcated and can give the skin a glistening, red appearance.

Granuloma gluteale infantum is a possible complication of irritant diaper dermatitis, presenting with violaceous nodules and plaques on the buttocks, vulva, scrotum, and perineum. Though alarming in appearance, these are benign and will resolve once the dermatitis is cleared, though scarring can result. The development of granuloma gluteale infantum does not necessarily correlate with the severity of the preexisting irritant dermatitis. **Jacquet erosive dermatitis** is another potential complication when the irritant dermatitis is severe. This form is characterized by small, well-demarcated erosions or ulcers that can also feature elevated borders. With chronic irritant dermatitis, children may also develop **perianal pseudoverrucous papules and nodules,** which are small bumps characterized by a flat-topped, moist, smooth, shiny surface. All 3— granuloma gluteale infantum, Jacquet's erosive dermatitis, and perianal pseudoverrucous papules and nodules—are considered to be on a disease continuum as less common manifestations of irritant contact dermatitis.

Candidiasis, due to infection with *C albicans,* typically begins in the creases (intertriginous areas) and then spreads to other surfaces. Sometimes associated with oral thrush, candidiasis is also a common sequela of systemic antibiotic therapy. The rash appears as bright, beefy red plaques with sharp, raised borders and many small satellite papules, vesicles, and pustules along its margins, often with desquamation. *Candida albicans* can be a cause of secondary infection of already inflamed skin as well as a primary causative factor in some cases of diaper dermatitis. Recurrent candidal diaper dermatitis can be associated with candidal colonization of the gut and oral cavity.

Seborrheic diaper dermatitis, like candidal diaper dermatitis, also primarily affects the intertriginous areas of the groin. The lack of pruritus, manifest as sleeping and feeding well, distinguishes it from atopic dermatitis. The rash has a characteristic salmon-colored, greasy appearance with a yellowish scale, though it can be acutely inflamed. Satellite lesions can be seen. Seborrheic dermatitis of the face, scalp (including postauricular areas), neck, trunk, and proximal extremities is usually seen in association with seborrheic dermatitis of the diaper area.

Allergic contact dermatitis is a less common cause of diaper dermatitis but should be considered in patients who do not respond to standard therapeutic interventions. Allergens can be from the chemical makeup of the diaper itself or from topical preparations such as soaps, emollients, and baby wipes that are applied to the diaper area. For example, rubber additives such as mercaptobenzothiazole found in the elastics of disposable diapers have been shown to cause allergic diaper dermatitis on the hips and outer buttocks, a distribution reminiscent of a cowboy's gunbelt holster and hence the nickname "Lucky Luke" dermatitis. Other allergens to consider are emulsifiers in topical preparations, fragrances, disperse dye, and preservatives.

Bacterial infections can cause diaper dermatitis. **Impetigo,** especially bullous impetigo, is a not uncommon eruption in the diaper area. It is more commonly observed in neonates, often as epidemics. Bullous impetigo is caused by *Staphylococcus aureus* and is toxin-mediated. The rash presents as vesicles on the diaper area, as well as the trunk and face. These enlarge into 3- to 5-cm bullae that easily rupture, leaving superficial erosions with thick, honey-colored crusts. There can be associated systemic symptoms of fever and diarrhea. Perianal bacterial disease can result from group A beta-hemolytic streptococcus or *S aureus.* Classically, perianal streptococcal dermatitis manifests as well-demarcated, bright red, tender patches. Rectal bleeding and painful defecation may also be noted.

Congenital syphilis can present with diaper dermatitis findings in 30% to 60% of those born with this infection. Initially, there is usually a bright erythematous morbilliform eruption that fades to a coppery color, often with scaling. Pustules can develop later. Buttocks, face, extremities, palms, and soles are generally affected.

Diaper rashes that seem to persist despite seemingly adequate therapy should raise suspicion for other systemic diseases. Though less common, these include psoriasis, atopic dermatitis, zinc deficiency, biotin deficiency, and Langerhans cell histiocytosis. **Psoriasis** may occur anywhere on the body, but lesions typically occur on the scalp, face, elbows, and knees. In infants, generally between 2 to 8 months of age, psoriasis may involve the diaper area. Lesions elsewhere on the body are typically well-circumscribed, erythematous plaques with a thick, silvery scale. However, psoriatic lesions in the diaper area may be difficult to differentiate from seborrheic dermatitis or candidal infection. Plaques are brightly erythematous and sharply demarcated. Skin biopsy, family history of psoriasis, or nail involvement may help confirm the diagnosis.

Atopic dermatitis is rare in the diaper area, even in infants who have lesions elsewhere on the body. The relative sparing of the diaper area is perhaps a result of the increased moisture of the skin in this area. (See Chapter 121 for a discussion of atopic dermatitis.)

Zinc deficiency can cause dermatitis in a characteristic periorificial distribution (mouth, nose, ears, eyes, and anogenital area) and distal extremities. Zinc deficiency may result from an inherited defect called acrodermatitis enteropathica or develop secondary to insufficient intake or malabsorption such as in patients with cystic fibrosis. **Acrodermatitis enteropathica** is a rare, autosomally recessive inherited disorder with mutations in *SLC39A* resulting in defective zinc transporters in the small intestine. In breastfed infants, the disease becomes manifest shortly after weaning, whereas in bottle-fed infants, signs and symptoms appear days to weeks after birth. Afflicted infants are irritable and listless and present with diarrhea, failure to thrive, and skin lesions in the previously mentioned distribution featuring erythematous bullous and pustular lesions as well as dry, red, scaly patches. Candidal and *S aureus* superinfection can occur. Treatment consists of oral zinc supplementation. Biotin deficiency, as well as several other nutritional deficiencies, can present with identical skin findings, and treatment is with supplementation of the deficient nutrient.

Langerhans cell histiocytosis refers to a group of disorders characterized by proliferation of histiocytes, a progenitor cell in the bone marrow. Members of this group include Letterer-Siwe disease and Hand-Schüller-Christian disease, eosinophilic granuloma, and congenital self-healing reticulohistiocytosis. Skin lesions may involve the scalp and flexural areas of the perineum, axilla, and neck. The lesions appear as small, pink to tan scaling papules and pustules that can coalesce; ulceration may be apparent in the inguinal crease with secondary impetiginization (honey-colored crusting caused by *S aureus* superinfection). The rash is most often confused with that of seborrheic dermatitis. Diagnosis can be confirmed by skin biopsy.

Evaluation

History

A thorough history should be obtained (Questions Box). Candidal diaper dermatitis should be suspected if oral antibiotic therapy has recently been used.

> **Diaper Dermatitis** **Questions**
>
> - When did the rash begin?
> - Does the rash resolve and then recur?
> - Is the rash pruritic?
> - Is the infant feeding, sleeping? Is he/she irritable?
> - Have any home remedies or previous treatments been used? Which ones?
> - Does the child have a family history of atopic dermatitis or psoriasis?
> - Is the child taking antibiotics now or has the child used them recently?
> - What type of diapers is used?
> - How frequently are the diapers changed?

Physical Examination

On physical examination, the presence of skin lesions elsewhere on the body should be noted. This is particularly important in the case of a persistent, resistant, or recurrent diaper rash, where systemic diseases such as psoriasis must be considered. The distribution of the rash within the diaper area itself may provide clues to the diagnosis. Candidal and seborrheic dermatitis occur primarily in the creases, whereas irritant contact dermatitis usually affects the convex areas of the skin with relative sparing of the intertriginous areas. Streptococcal disease manifests primarily as marked perianal erythema.

Laboratory Tests

Although the diagnosis of candidal diaper dermatitis is usually evident clinically, microscopic examination of skin scrapings with KOH may be performed to establish the diagnosis. Typically, budding yeast with hyphae and/or pseudohyphae is seen. The diagnosis of perianal streptococcal disease or bullous impetigo may be confirmed by bacterial cultures from the perianal area or bullous lesions, respectively. Biopsies may be warranted for recalcitrant diaper dermatitis. Other laboratory studies may be carried out to investigate for suspected nutritional deficiencies.

Management

The mainstay of therapy for irritant diaper dermatitis is prevention, requiring **good hygiene,** which involves keeping the diaper area clean and dry. Gentle but thorough cleansing of the diaper area is necessary when stool is present and can be done with water alone or water and mild soap. The area should then be patted dry and allowed to air-dry completely if possible or dry with the use of cotton balls. Cleansing frequently with harsh soaps or scrubbing too vigorously can further irritate skin that is already damaged and inflamed.

In addition, the diaper should be **changed frequently.** The diaper area should be exposed to as much air as reasonably possible (eg, by allowing the infant to sleep without a diaper). Cloth and regular disposable diapers are not as effective as superabsorbent gel diapers in decreasing moisture. Although **dusting powders** such as cornstarch or talc minimize friction and talc does not enhance the growth of yeast on skin, concern about pulmonary effects from inhalation precludes their routine use even in the absence of any skin inflammation. **Moisture-resistant barrier ointments or creams** such as zinc oxide or petrolatum are very helpful in reducing irritation. The role of hygiene in all forms of diaper dermatitis cannot be overemphasized. Topical application of medicated creams and ointments is not effective in the presence of poor hygiene.

Irritant contact dermatitis usually responds to the above-described hygienic measures and the application of barrier ointments and low-potency **topical corticosteroids** such as 0.5% or 1% hydrocortisone ointment or cream. Seborrheic dermatitis usually resolves spontaneously but can also be treated with low-potency topical corticosteroids. Candidal diaper dermatitis responds to **topical antifungal creams** such as nystatin, miconazole, or clotrimazole. In addition, a low-potency corticosteroid may be required if inflammation is severe. Oral antifungal therapy is usually not indicated,

though may be needed in cases of recurrent candidiasis. Oral antibiotic therapy usually clears perianal streptococcal or staphylococcal disease, but the relapse rate is high. The topical antibiotic mupirocin may be used to treat bullous impetigo only if the lesions are superficial, few, and isolated. Oral antibiotics (eg, cephalexin or clindamycin) may be required for more extensive bacterial infections. Combination topical medications containing both a corticosteroid and an antifungal should not be recommended routinely because they usually contain high-potency corticosteroids. When topical steroids and antifungals are used in conjunction with barrier ointment, the medication should be applied before the barrier ointment.

When the more common causes of diaper dermatitis, such as irritant contact dermatitis, *Candida,* or seborrheic dermatitis, do not respond to conventional therapy, further workup must be initiated because there may be an underlying systemic disease manifesting as diaper dermatitis; some of these can be life-threatening.

Prognosis

Although recurrence of diaper dermatitis is common, the usual varieties respond well to measures aimed at keeping the diaper area clean and dry and to medicated creams.

CASE RESOLUTION

The infant presented in the case scenario has irritant contact dermatitis. He has a recent history of gastroenteritis, and stool is known to be particularly irritating to the skin. Treatment includes keeping the diaper area clean and dry with frequent diaper changes, use of superabsorbent diapers, and fastidious toilet, as well as topical application of a low-potency corticosteroid ointment or cream and a barrier ointment such as zinc oxide after bathing.

Selected References

Fritsch PO, Reider N. Other eczematous eruptions. In: Bolognia JL, Jorizzo JL, Rapini RP, eds. *Dermatology.* St Louis, MO: Mosby; 2003:216–217

Heath C, Desai N, Silverberg NB. Recent microbiological shifts in perianal bacterial dermatitis: *Staphylococcus aureus* predominance. *Pediatr Dermatol.* 2009;26:696–700

James WD, Berger TG, Elston DM. *Andrews' Diseases of the Skin.* 10th ed. Toronto, Ontario, Canada: Elsevier, Inc.; 2006:360–361, 483–485

Robson KJ, Maughan JA, Purcell SD, et al. Erosive papulonodular dermatosis associated with topical benzocaine: a report of two cases and evidence and granuloma gluteale, pseudoverrucous papules, and Jacquet's erosive dermatitis are a disease spectrum. *J Am Acad Dermatol.* 2006;55:S74–S80

Scheinfeld N. Diaper dermatitis: a review and brief survey of eruptions of the diaper area. *Am J Clin Dermatol.* 2005;6:273–281

Smith WJ, Jacob SE. The role of allergic contact dermatitis in diaper dermatitis. *Pediatr Dermatol.* 2009;26:369–70

Ward DB. Characterization of diaper dermatitis in the United States. *Arch Pediatr Adolesc Med.* 2000;154:943–946

CHAPTER 121

Papulosquamous Eruptions

Ki-Young Suh, MD; Kathy K. Langevin, MD, MPH; and Noah Craft, MD, PhD

CASE STUDY

A 6-month-old female infant presents with an erythematous, confluent, slightly raised and scaly rash on the cheeks. The extremities are also covered with a fine papular rash. The infant has had some scaling behind the ears and on the scalp since early infancy, but the symptoms have recently increased. The mother has been applying baby oil to the scalp to relieve the scaliness. Except for some intermittent rhinorrhea, the infant has otherwise been well. Immunizations are deficient; she received only the first set when she was 2 months old. The family history is positive for bronchitis. The infant's weight is at the 75th percentile, and the height is at the 50th percentile. Vital signs are normal. The physical examination is normal except for the presence of the rash.

Questions

1. What are the characteristics of papulosquamous eruptions?
2. What are the common conditions associated with papulosquamous eruptions in children?
3. What are the appropriate treatments for the common papulosquamous eruptions?
4. When should children with papulosquamous eruptions be referred to a dermatologist?

Rashes, a common problem in children, can be classified in ways that help to establish a diagnostic approach. First, rashes are assessed in terms of appearance, whether macular (flat), papular (raised), squamous (scaly), vesicular (fluid-filled), or bullous (large, fluid-filled). Next, the extent of the rash is determined. Rashes may be described as generalized or localized. Location is also important. The site of a localized rash may be consistent with certain diagnoses, for instance, diaper dermatitis. Pruritus is an important distinguishing feature. Other systemic symptoms must also be taken into consideration. Rashes may be a primary skin condition or may be a manifestation of an underlying infection or reaction to a precipitating agent.

Papulosquamous eruptions, the subject of this chapter, are rashes characterized by scaly papules and plaques. Eczema is a poorly defined group of skin disorders characterized clinically by scale, and histologically by spongiosis, and makes up a large component of the papulosquamous disorders. The etiology of many papulosquamous eruptions is unknown, and the clinical appearance of lesions is the reason they are classified together.

Epidemiology

Although a large number of conditions may cause papulosquamous eruptions in children, a select number of diagnoses account for most problems. One of the most common causes of papulosquamous eruptions in children is atopic dermatitis. Atopic dermatitis has become increasingly more common, and the prevalence in school-aged children in the United States is estimated to be between 10% to 20%. Positive family history is often elicited. Though the severity of atopic dermatitis generally improves with age, lifelong dry, itchy skin, in varying degrees of severity, is not uncommon. Seborrheic dermatitis is another common eczematous skin rash seen in the pediatric population. Though most commonly described in infants younger than 3 or 4 months, it can occur in all pediatric age groups. It is estimated to have a prevalence of up to 5%, encompassing both the pediatric and adult populations, though higher in adults with males more commonly affected. It is generally more severe during the winter months.

Scabies is likely the most common cause of worldwide papulosquamous eruptions and is frequently encountered in both general pediatric and dermatology settings. The prevalence is much greater in developing countries and in situations where populations are forced into close proximity (eg, during wars or incarcerated individuals). Family members and close contacts are at greatest risk of infection.

Clinical Presentation

Papulosquamous eruptions consist of skin-colored to erythematous raised, scaly papules and plaques that may involve the face, trunk, or extremities. The lesions can be pruritic, and scratching may lead to crusting or secondary infection. Sometimes multiple family members are affected (Dx Box). Chronicity and repeated manipulation, may lead to thickening or lichenification of involved skin.

Pathophysiology

The pathophysiology of atopic dermatitis has not been definitively established. Recent evidence suggests that mutations in the filaggrin gene, which is responsible for much of the skin barrier function, may play a large role in atopic dermatitis. However, it seems to be a multifactorial disease with variable expression, influenced by environmental factors. Inheritance of this disease is associated with atopy, made up of the triad of atopic dermatitis, allergic rhinitis, and asthma. The disorder is attributed largely to skin barrier function; however, immune dysfunction and reactivity of nerves and blood vessels may also be involved. Initially, the disease is characterized by Th1 cytokine predominance, but later in chronic disease, there is activation of the Th2 immune pathway with a resultant synthesis of cytokines, including IL-4 and IL-5, causing elevated immunoglobulin (Ig) E levels, eosinophilia, and diminished cell-mediated immunity. Elevated IgE is reported in 43% to 82% of patients with atopic dermatitis.

Like atopic dermatitis, the etiology of seborrheic dermatitis remains unclear. There is believed to be an association with the yeast *Malassezia furfur,* though whether this organism is causative has not been established. It is widely accepted that this yeast has some role in seborrheic dermatitis, which is further substantiated by the improvement of this skin condition with antifungal agents. Individuals with seborrheic dermatitis that is severe or extensive may have some sort of immune dysfunction, as in uncontrolled HIV and AIDS.

The inflammatory response in scabies is triggered by an infestation with a mite, *Sarcoptes scabiei.* The adult female burrows under the skin and lays 60 to 90 eggs. After 2 weeks, the eggs become adults. Affected individuals may be asymptomatic on first exposure. Up to 2

to 6 weeks after infestation, the host's immune system becomes sensitized to mites or scybala (mite feces), resulting in systemic pruritus and rash. In most individuals the rash associated with scabies is an allergic phenomenon and does not represent mites at each eruptive papule on the body.

Differential Diagnosis

While many papulosquamous eruptions are easily distinguishable clinically, the differential diagnosis can be challenging at times. Familiarity with the appearance of these conditions and their differentiating features is critical. The Internet can be valuable by providing access to images of many dermatologic conditions. Some sites such as VisualDx (accessible at www.visualdx.com) display pictorial representations and allow for searching by features such as rash morphologies, symptoms, exposures, skin color, body location, age, immune status, and many other factors.

Most conditions that are associated with papulosquamous eruptions in children include atopic dermatitis, seborrheic dermatitis, contact dermatitis, psoriasis, pityriasis rosea, lichen planus, lichen striatus, scabies, and fungal infections of the skin.

Eczema is a general term that is used to denote a type of papulosquamous eruption. The most common eczematous conditions seen in children are atopic eczema or dermatitis, seborrheic dermatitis, and contact dermatitis. **Atopic dermatitis** is a disorder of infancy and childhood and may persist into adulthood. More than half of affected individuals are symptomatic by 1 year, and 90% of cases have their onset by 5 years of age. The area of involvement changes with age. In infancy, the face, scalp, and extensor surfaces are involved, often in areas where the infant can relieve itching by rubbing, and the diaper area is often spared (Figure 121-1A). By childhood, the more typical pattern seen in adulthood becomes prominent with involvement of the neck and antecubital and popliteal fossae. Adults

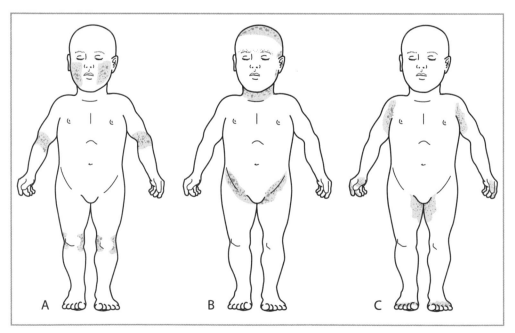

Figure 121-1. Typical distribution of papulosquamous eruptions in children. A. Atopic dermatitis: usually located on cheeks, creases of elbows, and knees. B. Seborrheic dermatitis: usually located on scalp, behind ears, thigh creases, and eyebrows. C. Scabies: usually located on axillae, webs of fingers and toes, and intragluteal area.

tend to have greater extremity involvement, along with the head and neck. Clinically, xerosis (dry skin), erythema, and a pruritic papular eruption are apparent. Scratching and rubbing lead to crusting, weeping, and eventually lichenification. Changes in color, including hypopigmentation and hyperpigmentation, may also occur. Hypopigmented areas with fine scale that are usually noted on the face are called pityriasis alba (considered to be the mildest form of atopic dermatitis). Xeroderma, or dry skin, is a frequent coexisting condition. Ichthyosis vulgaris, characterized by dirty-appearing excessive scaling and hyperlinear palms, is seen in half of patients affected with atopic dermatitis. Lesions around mucosa (Dennie-Morgan lines in the infraorbital fold under the eye and cheilitis around the mouth) may also be seen. Symptoms of other atopic conditions, such as allergic rhinitis, asthma, or food-related allergies, will occur in many of these patients.

Seborrheic dermatitis, which frequently develops during the first 3 months of life, is characterized by scaly papules or confluent scaly plaques, particularly of the scalp. Scalp eruptions in infancy are referred to as cradle cap. Seborrheic dermatitis has a predilection for areas with a high density of sebaceous glands, such as the scalp, face, ears, presternal chest, penis, and intertriginous areas, including the folds of the diaper region (Figure 121-1B). The red or pink papules and plaques may have a greasy quality. Secondary infections may occur with *Candida,* particularly in the intertriginous areas. Seborrheic dermatitis is usually not exceedingly pruritic, and this feature can be used to distinguish between it and atopic dermatitis. The intertriginous involvement and the onset shortly after birth also differentiate these 2 types of dermatitis. Severe seborrheic dermatitis can be associated with an immune deficiency, most commonly in HIV-infected patients.

Irritant or allergic contact dermatitis occurs when individuals come into physical contact with an irritant or a specific allergen, respectively. Irritant dermatitis is caused by direct cytotoxic effect, while allergic contact dermatitis is a delayed type IV hypersensitivity response to an allergen. Though their etiologies are different, they typically have a similar clinical appearance. Individuals usually develop well-defined erythematous vesicles, papules, or plaques, often with scale, and can have oozing and subsequent lichenification. Diaper dermatitis is one of the most common types of irritant dermatitis in the pediatric population (see Chapter 120). Rhus dermatitis (poison ivy/oak) and nickel allergy are 2 common types of allergic contact dermatitis seen in this population. It remains controversial whether atopic dermatitis is a risk factor for allergic contact dermatitis. However, children with atopic dermatitis may have more exposure to sensitizers, in conjunction with a damaged epithelial barrier, putting them at risk.

Plaque-type psoriasis, a chronic papulosquamous skin condition manifested most commonly as well-defined erythematous papules and plaques with silvery scale, is a not uncommon disease of childhood, with females more frequently affected. About 40% of adult patients with psoriasis report having the disease in childhood. It most commonly affects the scalp in the pediatric population as well as the face and intertriginous areas. Infrequently, a young infant may develop psoriasis in the diaper area. Guttate psoriasis features smaller scaly papules and is usually precipitated by group A streptococci infection in the pharynx or perianal area. Pruritus is variable, but not prominent. Classically, psoriatic lesions can develop at sites of trauma (scratches and cuts), known as the Koebner phenomenon.

Pityriasis rosea is a self-limited papulosquamous eruption that is frequently seen in adolescents. The lesions tend to be round or ovoid and classically have a symmetrical distribution on the trunk extending downward from the midline at a 45-degree angle. Classically, there is a larger "herald patch" preceding the eruption by a few days to weeks. It should be duly noted that the classic presentation is not always present—many patients cannot recall a herald patch and the pattern over the trunk is commonly haphazard. It is generally self-limited and resolves in 1 to 2 months. It is pruritic in about one-quarter of those affected. Though the etiology is unknown, recent evidence suggests that human herpesvirus 7 infection is associated with most cases, and some patients may have a viral prodrome preceding the rash.

Lichen planus is an uncommon papulosquamous eruption in the pediatric population. It is characterized by pruritic, polygonal, pink to purplish flat-topped papules overlying Wickham striae; white scale can be seen. Etiology is also unknown, though hepatitis C, as well as other viruses, as a causative factor has been proposed. Flexor surfaces are usually affected and these lesions can Koebnerize.

Lichen striatus is an asymptomatic lichenoid eruption consisting of flat-topped papules that are skin color to slightly hyperpigmented. The lesions develop along the lines of Blaschko and may be arranged in a curvolinear distribution. This eruption spontaneously resolves over months to years. It is mostly commonly seen between 9 months to 9 years of age. The etiology is unknown.

Scabies may resemble atopic or seborrheic dermatitis in infants and young children. The lesions may be papules, pustules, or vesicles. The characteristic burrow, which is only 3- to 10-mm long, is often difficult to appreciate unless certain diagnostic maneuvers are undertaken. The lesions are most often noted on the skin of the hands and feet, including the palms and soles in infants and young children. Intertriginous areas such as the intragluteal region, groin, and finger webs are commonly infected (Figure 121-1C). In infants, the face and head may be involved. Scratching and secondary infection may alter the appearance of the rash. Reddish-brown nodules may be characteristic of more chronic infection. In institutionalized or immunosuppressed individuals, extensive mite infection can occur, resulting in thick, greasy-appearing, yellowish scale and crusts over the extremities and trunk, a condition referred to as *crusted scabies.*

Fungal infections (eg, tinea corporis and tinea pedis) commonly appear as papulosquamous eruptions. Commonly, the lesions assume a characteristic morphology, with scaly papules grouped in a circle or coalesced into a plaque with central clearing.

Evaluation

History

A thorough history should be obtained (Questions Box). The presence of a rash in other family members suggests a contagious condition such as scabies or a familial disorder such as atopic dermatitis. An onset in the first few weeks of life is consistent with seborrheic dermatitis. It is important to determine if any medications have been used because these may modify the appearance of the rash. In addition, certain medications can cause a rash themselves, though these tend to be more morbilliform in appearance (see Chapter 122). Pruritus should be noted. Asking about lesions developing at sites of previous trauma can aid in diagnosing eruptions that Koebnerize, such as psoriasis and lichen planus.

Questions

Papulosquamous Eruptions

- How long has the child had the rash?
- What did the rash look like when it first appeared?
- Are other family members affected?
- Have any medications been used to treat the rash or any been given prior to the onset of the rash?
- Is pruritus present?
- Does the child have any other symptoms such as wheezing or rhinorrhea?
- Does the child have a history of any contact between the affected skin and any irritating substance?
- Has the child been febrile?

Physical Examination

The physical examination helps define the exact nature of the eruption and its distribution, which is often the clue to its etiology. The entire body should be examined, and particular attention should be paid to the intragluteal region and web spaces between fingers and toes. Certain rashes have characteristic appearances. For example, a circular cluster of scaly papules with central clearing signifies tinea corporis or the herald patch of pityriasis rosea. The presence of burrows characterizes scabies. Burrows appear as a 3- to 10-mm grayish-white line (only about 1 mm wide). Vesicles, pustules, and nodules may also be present in scabies.

It is also important to distinguish if any secondary lesions, such as linear excoriations, are present. Secondary infections are also important to diagnose and treat because they can complicate many of the papulosquamous eruptions.

Associated cutaneous features can also aid in diagnosis. Hyperlinear palms, keratosis pilaris (erythematous 1- to 2-mm folliculocentric papules often on lateral upper arms, anterior thighs, and cheeks), and perioral/periocular lichenified papules are often seen in children with atopic dermatitis.

Overall health, including height, and weight should be assessed. Failure to thrive in conjunction with eczematous skin changes should raise the suspicion for an immunodeficiency.

Laboratory Tests

Certain diagnostic tests may help clarify the etiology of certain papulosquamous eruptions. In children with atopic dermatitis, approximately 30% may have coexisting food allergies and 70% may have coexisting respiratory allergies. Food allergies tend to develop during early infancy whereas respiratory allergies may develop during childhood. While it is important to identify food (and later on, environmental) allergies via skin or radioallergosorbent/immunoCAP testing, which measures allergen-specific IgE (Chapter 80), parents must understand that food allergies **infrequently** cause or exacerbate atopic dermatitis. Based on misperceptions on the role of food allergies in atopic dermatitis, parents may on their own institute dietary restrictions for their child, which often results in gross undertreatment of the skin itself and may even lead to dangerous levels of malnutrition. Therefore, proper referral and counseling are especially important in infants who have both atopic dermatitis and food allergies. Patch testing may identify allergens causing contact dermatitis. Serologic IgE may or may not be elevated in children with atopic dermatitis.

The burrow of the mite that causes scabies may not be readily apparent. Scrapings with mineral oil are most commonly done today to help identify the mite, eggs, or feces (scybala)—any of these are diagnostic. Multiple burrows or web spaces are scraped. Scrapings of skin also assist in diagnosing candidal or tinea infections. These scrapings should be mixed with 10% to 20% KOH, which facilitates the dissolution of epithelial debris and allows for identification of the spores or hyphae.

If a secondary bacterial infection is suspected, cultures of the skin are indicated. Most of the papulosquamous eruptions are diagnosed clinically and no other specific diagnostic tests, short of a skin biopsy, assist in the diagnosis.

Management

The management is determined by the diagnosis.

Management of atopic dermatitis hinges on skin barrier function and the reduction of dryness and irritation with **vigilant skin care.** There has been debate whether frequent short baths daily versus bathing infrequently is more beneficial. It is most crucial that these patients bathe for short times only, applying cleansers only to the face, groin, and other soiled areas. The cleanser should be soap-free or the soap should be nonirritating, nondrying, and perfume- and dye-free. Children should pat dry after bathing with immediate application of either emollient or medication. Thick emollients such as petroleum jelly or other greasier ointments are preferable. In general, moisturizer from a jar tends to be more hydrating than that from a pump. For school-aged children, using greasier emollients at night under pajamas and then thinner emollients during the day may increase compliance. Sunflower seed oil is an inexpensive emollient that can be used after morning bathing for daytime use. Avoiding scratchy clothing such as wool can be helpful, as can humidifiers in the winter to prevent excessive environmental dryness. The humidifiers should be cleaned regularly to prevent mold buildup, and a cool mist is considered safer to prevent burns.

Topical steroids are used to treat various papulosquamous eruptions, especially during flares. These drugs are the mainstay of therapy designed to minimize inflammation. The agents usually prescribed in cases of atopic as well as seborrheic dermatitis are triamcinolone 0.025%, 0.1%, and hydrocortisone 1% creams or ointments. Though ointments allow for better penetration and, often, less irritation, they are often disliked for their greasy texture, minimizing its usefulness because they are not applied regularly. The weaker hydrocortisone should be used for the face and groin and the higher strengths in areas of thicker skin. Chronic use should be discouraged to avoid skin atrophy. Parents can be educated on applying the medication to the appropriate areas for 1 to 2 weeks for flares, with maintenance use on weekends or 2 days per week. Sometimes brief courses of systemic steroids may be needed during more severe exacerbations, but if a patient is requiring oral steroids regularly, a referral to a dermatologist may be needed to consider other treatments such as systemic immunomodulators or ultraviolet (UV) therapy, both used for atopic dermatitis and psoriasis. Oral steroids may be required for rhus contact dermatitis, one of the more common forms of allergic contact dermatitis, and should be given for 2 to 3 weeks to prevent flaring.

For scaly scalp psoriasis, seborrheic dermatitis, and atopic dermatitis, several treatments can be used. For pruritus and inflammation, a topical steroid in gel, liquid, or foam vehicle can be applied. Mineral oil can help loosen scale, but needs to be washed out using an anti-seborrheic shampoo to prevent buildup. It should be massaged gently onto the scalp and allowed to sit for several minutes before rinsing. Fluocinolone oil or steroid shampoos can be used effectively for scalp psoriasis as well.

Tacrolimus and pimecrolimus are topical calcineurin inhibitors, which can be used as steroid sparing agents, most often in mild cases of atopic dermatitis, seborrheic dermatitis, and inverse psoriasis (intertriginous). As of January 2006, a black box warning was placed on these 2 medications because there have been rare cases of skin cancer and lymphoma among patients using these drugs. The causal relationship for this warning was not well defined and, thus, many dermatologists still prescribe these medications in conjunction with topical steroids for their patients. As stand-alone agents, they are not as effective as steroids for more severe cases and are substantially more expensive.

In psoriasis, topical steroids are often used in conjunction with **calcipotriene** ointment or cream. **Tar** and **anthralin** are still used today as adjunctive topical treatments, though are falling out of favor due to their messy quality and more favorable alternatives.

Antihistamines may play a role in reducing the pruritus, especially at bedtime due to their sedating effect. Hydroxyzine and diphenhydramine work well in the evenings. For daytime, fexofenadine, cetirizine, or loratadine are less-sedating choices. Regular use of antihistamines during a flare can help to break the itch-scratch cycle often observed in children with atopic dermatitis. The other conditions can have variable degrees of pruritus for which antihistamines can be useful. Clipping fingernails decreases the risk of skin trauma after scratching.

Antibiotics are indicated if secondary infection is present. The most common pathogen involved is *Staphylococcus aureus*. Staphylococcal antigens also exacerbate the inflammation of atopic dermatitis. Treatment with antistaphylococcal systemic antibiotics such as cephalosporins may be needed for more widespread secondary infections. Topical antibiotics such as mupirocin may be used in localized secondary infections. Streptococcal-associated guttate psoriasis should also be treated with appropriate antibiotics.

Seborrheic dermatitis is generally treated with a combination of products including topical keratolytics, corticosteroids, and antifungals (see also Chapter 119). The seborrheic dermatitis of infancy can be treated with topical shampoos containing selenium sulfide and gentle sloughing of the scaly lesions using a soft brush or cloth. Topical calcineurin inhibitors have anti-inflammatory properties without skin atrophy side effects, but are generally reserved for periorbital or recalcitrant cases due to the cost of the medications.

If children with atopic dermatitis develop infection with herpes simplex (eczema herpeticum), they should be treated with **acyclovir.** Involvement of the nasal tip is concerning for eye involvement and warrants an ophthalmology consult. If involvement is severe, the patient may need to be hospitalized for intravenous antiviral therapy. Children with atopic dermatitis are also prone to viral infections resulting in warts and molluscum contagiosum, and these should be managed accordingly.

Coinfection with *Candida*, which occurs with seborrheic dermatitis and psoriasis, requires the use of topical medications such as **nystatin, clotrimazole, or miconazole.** Antifungal shampoos may also help in reducing the scaling due to fungal agents such as *Pityrosporum*. Tinea corporis also responds to topical antifungal agents. Tinea capitis will require systemic antifungals (see Chapter 119).

The treatment for pityriasis rosea remains controversial, especially because it is a self-resolving condition. There are several studies demonstrating effectiveness of **acyclovir, erythromycin,** or **UV therapy** to speed recovery.

There are several medications used to treat scabies. The current preferred product is 5% **permethrin** cream. It is approved for infants 2 months or older, although its safety and efficacy has been reported in a 23-day-old infant. It should be applied from head to toe in infants and from neck to toe in small children and adults, left on for 8 to 12 hours, then rinsed off. **Lindane,** which has been used for more than 50 years and previously used worldwide, is a 1% cream. Because of concern about the percutaneous absorption of lindane and its potential neurotoxicity, it is no longer widely used and is not available in some areas. Oral **ivermectin** is also a successful scabicide. A single dose of 200 µg/kg, then repeated in 1 week, can be used in children weighing more than 15 kg and women who are not pregnant or breastfeeding. All scabicides should be re-administered 7 days after initial treatment. The effective elimination of scabies necessitates that all affected household members be treated simultaneously and that bed linens and clothing be washed in hot water. Patients should be warned that the pruritus of scabies often takes several weeks to subside and can be treated supportively with steroids and antihistamines.

Prognosis

In general, the prognosis for children with papulosquamous eruptions is excellent with appropriate management, which is contingent on accurate diagnosis. Both atopic dermatitis and seborrheic dermatitis tend to improve as children get older. However, chronic problems such as hand dermatitis, which can be exacerbated by occupational exposures, can become a significant problem in patients with atopic dermatitis. Children with significant atopic dermatitis should be counseled against careers with frequent wet work, such as hairdressers, hospital workers, or food service. It is also critical to counsel families that maintaining atopic dermatitis with the prevention of flares is the primary goal and is more important than having perfect skin. Families of children with severe atopic dermatitis can have difficulty in maintaining a good quality of life for these patients, and the entire family structure can suffer as chronic care can be challenging. Children with atopic dermatitis frequently face remissions and exacerbations, particularly associated with seasonal changes. Prevention and maintenance must be stressed. It is advisable that patients with recalcitrant eczema have further workup with an allergist to eliminate triggers.

Many of these eruptions, such as lichen striatus and pityriasis rosea, are self-limited and only need symptomatic treatment. Psoriasis has a more chronic course, and early diagnosis and treatment can help to reduce the disease severity and progression. Chronic disease such as atopic dermatitis and psoriasis can be psychologically challenging for children because they can often be ridiculed at school and excluded from activities for unfounded fears of contagiousness. The teachers may need to be educated as well and emotional and psychological support provided for these children.

Scabies and tinea will improve with appropriate management and education to prevent recurrence.

CASE RESOLUTION

The infant's presentation in the case history is characteristic of atopic dermatitis. The baby experienced the onset of symptoms as a young infant (most atopic patients develop symptoms after 2 months of age). Atopic dermatitis can often affect the head and face of young patients. Xerosis is also apparent.

The most important discussion with the mother should be on good skin care. The mother should be advised that although she may use the baby oil to loosen the scale on the scalp, she should shampoo afterward with a mild antiseborrheic shampoo to prevent buildup. A mild topical steroid, such as hydrocortisone 1% ointment, may also be recommended though chronic use should be dissuaded. If skin scrapings reveal secondary infection with *Candida*, an antifungal cream should be added to the regimen; if a secondary bacterial infection is suspected, a culture should be taken and treatment with either topical or systemic antibiotics initiated. Short baths with a mild cleanser and regular application of emollients is critical.

The mother should also be educated on potential flares with vaccinations and infections, as well as with climate changes. It is important that the infant catch up on her vaccinations, but cautioning the mother about a potential flare can prevent distress.

Selected References

Clayton TH, Wilkinson SM, Rawcliffe C, et al. Allergic contact dermatitis in children: should pattern of dermatitis determine referral? *Br J Dermatol.* 2006;154:114–117

Eichenfield LF, Friedlander SF. Coping with chronic dermatitis. *Contemp Pediatr.* 1998;15:53–66

Gupta AK, Bluhm R, Cooper EA, et al. Seborrheic dermatitis. *Dermatol Clin.* 2003;21:401–412

Kang K, Postr AM, Nederost ST, et al. Atopic dermatitis. In: Bolognia JL, Jorizzo JL, Rapini RP, eds. *Dermatology.* St Louis, MO: Mosby; 2003:199–214

Lewkowicz D, Gottlieb AB. Pediatric psoriasis and psoriatic arthritis. *Dermatol Ther.* 2004;17:364–375

Nelson JS, Stone MS. Update on selected viral exanthems. *Curr Opin Pediatr.* 2000;12:359–364

Peterson CM, Eichenfield LF. Scabies. *Pediatr Ann.* 1996;25:97–100

Sidbury R, Poorsattar S. Pediatric atopic dermatitis: should we treat it differently? *Dermatol Ther.* 2006;19:83–90

Williams JV, Eichenfield LF, Burke BL, Barnes-Eley M, Friedlander SF. Prevalence of scalp scaling in prepubertal children. *Pediatrics.* 2005;115:e1–e6

CHAPTER 122

Morbilliform Rashes

Kathy K. Langevin, MD, MPH, and Noah Craft, MD, PhD

CASE STUDY

A 10-month-old infant girl is brought to the office with a history of rhinorrhea, cough, and fever for 3 days prior to the onset of a confluent, erythematous rash. The rash started on her face. She has been irritable, and her eyes are red and teary. Her immunizations include 3 sets of diphtheria, tetanus, and acellular pertussis, polio, rotavirus, *Haemophilus influenzae* type b, conjugated pneumococcal, and hepatitis B vaccines. No one at home is ill. The girl was seen in the emergency department 2 weeks before because she caught her finger in a car door. On physical examination, the girl's temperature is 102.2°F (39°C). A confluent eruption of erythematous macules and papules is evident on the face, trunk, and extremities. Rhinorrhea and conjunctivitis are also present.

Questions

1. What are the common causes of febrile macular/papular or morbilliform rashes in children?
2. What features distinguish one disease from another?
3. How does a child's nutritional status affect their reaction to certain exanthem-inducing viruses?
4. What are the public health considerations concerning viral exanthems in children?

Exanthems are skin findings resulting from an underlying disease. More than 50 different viruses, in addition to bacteria and *Rickettsia*, have been identified, though viruses tend to be the leading cause. In children, these exanthems are most commonly macular, papular, or mixed. The rash of measles is described as morbilliform, and this adjective is used to describe similar-appearing eruptions of macules and papules. Frequently these rashes are seen in conjunction with fever, and additional symptoms include myalgias, rhinorrhea, conjunctivitis, headache, gastrointestinal (GI) complaints, and lymphadenopathy. The exanthems of various underlying viruses can also be seasonal. Although many of the common childhood illnesses of the past are now prevented by immunizations, not all segments of the population are adequately immunized. In addition, some children are not eligible for immunization because of their young age. Allergic reactions to medications, particularly antibiotics, may also result in similar eruptions and can be accompanied by symptoms of low-grade fever and pruritus. Differentiating viral exanthems from allergic reactions may be difficult in febrile children who have been empirically started on antimicrobial agents.

Epidemiology

In most children, the viruses that cause exanthems produce mild disease without significant morbidity or long-term sequelae. Of greater concern to the public health is the risk of potential spread through the population. Morbilliform eruptions are a common presenting complaint, particularly in certain age groups and at certain times of the year.

Measles, also known as rubeola, is caused by an RNA virus, and has markedly decreased in the United States since the live vaccine was introduced in 1963. It is transmitted by direct contact with infectious droplets or by airborne spread. In temperate climates, it is most frequently seen in the winter and spring. In the pre-vaccine era, measles was a significant cause of morbidity and mortality. Periodic resurgences have occurred, particularly among unimmunized preschoolers, older adolescents, and young adults. In addition, young infants are also at risk because of decreased levels of passively transferred maternal immunity related to lack of maternal natural infection or immunization. Vaccine-related immunity apparently wanes more rapidly in mothers than does naturally acquired immunity. Because of the increased number of cases in preschoolers and in children with primary vaccine failure who received the vaccine appropriately, the 2-dose recommendation by the American Academy of Pediatrics was implemented in 1989, though there continue to be cases each year. Measles is no longer endemic in the United States but continues to be imported. The incubation period of measles is about 10 days. Individuals are infectious from about 3 to 5 days before the onset of rash until 4 days following its appearance.

Rubella is also caused by an RNA virus and is no longer considered endemic in the United States, with less than 15 cases annually. Sporadic outbreaks are reported, generally in foreign-born or underimmunized persons, but about 10% of US-born individuals older than 5 years are considered to be susceptible. The peak incidence is in the late winter to spring, and it is likely transmitted via direct or droplet contact from nasopharyngeal secretions. Though generally a mild disease, its most serious manifestation is congenital rubella syndrome, which may develop in the offspring of infected pregnant women, with the greatest risk of congenital defects during the first trimester. The incubation period is 14 to 23 days.

Erythema infectiosum, also called fifth disease, is most commonly seen in children 4 to 10 years of age during late winter to early spring. Most adults have antibodies indicating previous infection. The disease is caused by an acute infection with parvovirus B19, a DNA virus, and spread through respiratory secretions, percutaneous exposure to blood or blood products, and vertical transmission from mother to fetus. The incubation period is generally 4 to 14 days but may be up to 21 days.

Roseola infantum, also known as exanthem subitum, generally affects children from 6 months to 2 years of age, as maternal antibodies are protective until the age of 6 months. The illness is due to infection with human herpesvirus (HHV) 6 or 7, though HHV-6b, a DNA virus, is most commonly the etiologic agent. The virus is shed in the saliva, even among healthy, previously infected infants. Almost all children are seropositive by the age of 4. Reactivation is possible though not common, and there is no seasonal pattern. The incubation period for HHV-6 is likely 5 to 15 days and is unknown for HHV-7.

Enteroviruses are the most common cause of exanthems in the summer and fall. They are all RNA viruses of the picornavirus group and include coxsackieviruses (groups A and B), echoviruses, and enteroviruses. Infection is spread through fecal-oral and respiratory routes as well as via fomites. There is also vertical transmission. Infection is more common in young children and in those with poor hygiene. The incubation period is usually 3 to 6 days.

Kawasaki disease, an acute self-limited vasculitis, is of uncertain etiology, although an infectious cause is suspected due to epidemics occurring usually in the winter and spring. Most patients are between 6 months and 5 years of age. Males outnumber females by a ratio of 1.5:1. The incidence of the disorder among Asians is higher than in other populations, suggesting genetic factors play a role. The incubation period is unknown.

Gianotti-Crosti syndrome, also known as papular acrodermatitis of childhood, has historically been associated with hepatitis B infection. In the United States, it is believed to be a host response to multiple viral infections including, but not limited to, hepatitis A and B, Epstein-Barr virus (EBV), measles, and the enteroviruses. It is seen most frequently in children 1 to 6 years of age.

Scarlet fever is a cutaneous reaction to several erythrogenic exotoxins produced by group A streptococcus (GAS) via delayed-type hypersensitivity. It is transmitted through respiratory secretions. Scarlet fever is usually seen in young children between 1 to 10 years with pharyngitis. It occurs most commonly in cooler climates during the late fall, winter, and early spring. The incubation period is 2 to 5 days.

Rocky Mountain spotted fever (RMSF) is caused by *Rickettsia rickettsii,* an intracellular organism. Infection is transmitted by the bite of *Ixodes* ticks, which are both reservoirs and vectors of the organism. It can be seen throughout the United States, with most cases seen in the southern states. Children younger than 15 years are most commonly infected. Highest incidence of infection is seen between April and September. The incubation period lasts from 2 to 14 days.

Clinical Presentation

Morbilliform eruptions may involve the face, trunk, or extremities. The eruption is usually erythematous, and the lesions are flat or slightly raised. Occasionally, lesions within the mouth, referred to as enanthems, are evident. Most children are febrile (Dx Box) and may have other symptomatic complaints.

Dx Morbilliform Rashes

- Macular, papular, or combined rash
- Fever
- Enanthems (lesions in the mouth)
- Lymphadenopathy
- Respiratory symptoms
- Gastrointestinal symptoms

Pathophysiology

The mechanism for development of a rash is variable. In some cases, the rash is the reaction of the body to infection or to the presence of a toxin. In general, the sequence involves exposure to an infectious agent and then acquisition of the agent most commonly through droplet infection or fecal-oral contamination. The agent, usually a virus, then replicates, perhaps in the reticuloendothelial system. Lymph nodes enlarge, reflecting the involvement of the reticuloendothelial system. Associated viremia may be present.

In Kawasaki disease, vasculitis affects multiple organ systems. Various cytokines and autoantibodies play a role in the inflammatory response. In a toxin-mediated rash (eg, scarlet fever), previous exposure to the toxin is believed to sensitize the individual.

Differential Diagnosis

While many exanthems can be easily recognized clinically, the decreased frequency of many of these usual childhood diseases means that physicians encounter these conditions less frequently than in the past. Familiarity with the appearance of these conditions is critical to diagnosis. The Internet can be valuable by providing access to images of many dermatologic conditions. Some sites such as VisualDx (accessible at www.visualdx.com) display pictorial representations and allow for searching by features such as rash morphologies, symptoms, exposures, skin color, body location, age, immune status, and many other factors.

Morbilliform exanthems are associated with several infectious diseases, such as measles, rubella, erythema infectiosum, roseola, enterovirus infections, Gianotti-Crosti syndrome, Kawasaki disease, scarlet fever, and RMSF. Drugs can also cause eruptions similar to those caused by the aforementioned diseases.

The rash associated with **measles** is preceded by the 3 "Cs" of cough, coryza, and conjunctivitis in addition to fever, which last for several days before the eruption of the exanthem. Lesions on the buccal mucosa, called Koplik spots, are well-circumscribed white-gray papules (Figure 122-1) that appear during the prodrome and resolve

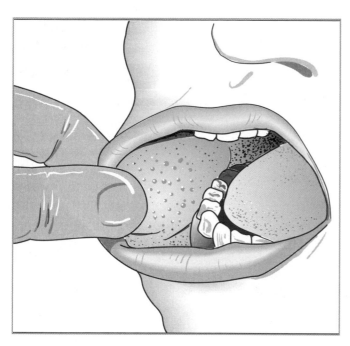

Figure 122-1. Koplik spots.

after 3 to 4 days. This enanthem, though rare, is pathognomonic for measles. The measles rash itself usually begins on the head, particularly behind the ears and around the margin of the scalp, and then spreads cephalocaudally. After 2 to 3 days, the eruption becomes confluent and copper-colored, fades in the order it appeared, and then may desquamate.

Measles is not generally associated with systemic lymphadenopathy. The major complications of measles in children in developed nations are pneumonia, encephalitis, and secondary bacterial infections. In developing nations, death usually results from respiratory and neurologic complications, often in those with marginal nutritional status especially vitamin A deficiency. In individuals who were initially immunized with killed measles vaccine (1963–1968), acquisition of measles results in atypical measles, generally more severe than regular measles, and characterized by acute high fever, myalgias, and cough. A papular, vesicular, or hemorrhagic eruption that begins peripherally follows a few days later. Lobar pneumonia is usually present, and associated findings include hepatosplenomegaly and weakness.

Rubella produces a relatively minor illness in children, although adults, particularly women, may experience a painful arthritis. Up to half of infections are asymptomatic. There can be a prodrome of fever, headache, conjunctivitis, and upper respiratory symptoms. The eruption consists of fine erythematous macules and papules that become near confluent, starting on the face and progressing caudally to the trunk, resolving after 3 days. Lymphadenopathy, particularly of the postauricular or suboccipital nodes, is characteristic of the disease. Forschheimer spots are pinpoint rose-colored macules that can develop on the soft palate in patients with this infection. Congenital rubella syndrome results in multisystem anomalies that can follow maternal infection and is part of the TORCH congenital infections (toxoplasmosis, other agents [hepatitis B, coxsackievirus,

syphilis, varicella-zoster virus, HIV, parvovirus B19], rubella, cytomegalovirus, herpes simplex).

Erythema infectiosum (EI) is characterized by a distinctive eruption that may be preceded by mild prodromal symptoms including low-grade fever, headache, myalgias, and malaise. The eruption generally occurs 7 to 10 days after the prodrome. The facial rash consists of erythematous patches on the cheeks with sparing of the nasal bridge and periorbital areas. This "slapped-cheek" appearance generally fades after several days and is considered the first stage of the illness. In the second stage the extremities may develop a lacy reticulated rash of macules and papules 1 to 4 days later that can be pruritic. Palm and sole involvement is rare. This usually lasts about a week but may have recurrences over several weeks in the third stage, with triggers such as activity, sunlight, emotional stress, and hot baths. Most children are only mildly ill and may attend school, but children with underlying hematologic disorders may experience aplastic crises because of the affinity of parvovirus B19 for developing red blood cells. Immunocompromised children are also at risk for chronic anemia. Pregnant females may transmit this infection to their fetuses, which can result in fetal hydrops, growth retardation, isolated pleural and pericardial effusions, and fetal loss. Adults with parvovirus infection frequently develop arthritis, though only 10% of children experience this symptom. Neurologic disturbances including encephalitis and neuropathies may follow parvovirus infection, though this is rare. **Papular-purpuric gloves and socks syndrome (PPGSS)** is a self-limited acute eruption linked to parvovirus B19 infection. It occurs usually in the spring and summer, characterized by often-painful edema and erythema and progressing to purpuric macules and papules with a sharp line of demarcation at the wrists and ankles. A nonspecific enanthem of petechiae and erosions can occur. Symptoms of myalgias, lymphadenopathy, anorexia, and fatigue may follow the rash. The exanthem generally resolves after 1 to 2 weeks with no residual sequelae.

Roseola infantum usually causes a fairly mild illness in children, though there can be associated complications. Defervescence usually accompanies the rash, which consists of fine, non-pruritic, blanchable, pink macules or papules with a surrounding halo that generally appear first on the trunk, and then spread centrifugally. Some may develop an enanthem consisting of erythematous papules on the soft palate and uvula called Nagayama spots. Periorbital edema can also be seen. On average, the rash evolves over 12 hours and usually resolves by 2 days. Infants may appear sickest during the prodromal phase, when the fever is high (temperature: often ≥103°F [39.5°C]), and infants are irritable as a result. Fever generally lasts 3 to 5 days and can be accompanied by upper respiratory symptoms and lymphadenopathy. Seizures during the febrile period can occur in up to 15% of primary infections. Workup to rule out sepsis is often warranted.

The skin eruptions associated with **enterovirus infections** are highly variable. They may be distinct and characteristic, such as hand-foot-and-mouth disease (HFMD), most commonly associated with coxsackievirus A16 and enterovirus 71 (see Chapter 123). However, many of the enteroviral exanthems are less distinctive and have a generalized morbilliform appearance. Neurologic complications associated with enteroviral infections include aseptic meningitis and encephalitis and have been reported in infections with coxsackievirus B and enterovirus 71. Other systems affected by enteroviral infections include respiratory, GI, ophthalmic, and cardiac.

The rash of **Kawasaki disease** is also highly variable; it may be morbilliform, urticarial, scarlatiniform, or resemble erythema multiforme. During the first week of illness, there may be desquamation of the perineum. The diagnosis of Kawasaki disease requires fever (generally >39°C [lasting at least 5 days]) and 4 out of the 5 following findings: (1) bilateral non-purulent conjunctivitis; (2) changes in the oropharyngeal mucosa including fissured lips, oral erythema, and strawberry tongue; (3) changes in the extremities such as erythema/edema or desquamation; (4) cervical lymphadenopathy with one node measuring at least 1.5 cm in diameter; and (5) the exanthem described previously. Irritability, abdominal pain, and diarrhea are not uncommon. Incomplete Kawasaki disease can be diagnosed when only 2 of the additional criteria are met, thus the practitioner should consider this diagnosis when persistent high fever and only 2 or 3 of the above symptoms are present. The major complication of Kawasaki disease is coronary artery abnormalities, and males and those younger than 12 months are at increased risk.

The exanthem of **Gianotti-Crosti** syndrome consists of monomorphic, pink- to skin-colored, usually non-pruritic papules on the face, buttocks, and extremities, with sparing of the trunk. There is often a prodrome of fever and upper respiratory symptoms with associated generalized lymphadenopathy and hepatosplenomegaly. The exanthem fades after 2 to 3 weeks but can last up to 2 months.

Scarlet fever is primarily a disease of childhood. The onset is marked by sudden high fever, headache, vomiting, malaise, and sore throat. Within 12 to 48 hours, erythema develops on the neck, chest, and axillae. The rash quickly becomes generalized to a sandpaper-like rash of fine red papules on an erythematous background. Linear accentuation in the axillary, antecubital, and inguinal folds is known as Pastia lines. The face is flushed, except around the mouth (circumoral pallor). There is pharyngeal injection with exudate developing after a few days. The tongue is initially white with prominent red papillae (Figure 122-2), known as strawberry tongue. As the scarlet fever rash resolves, desquamation begins in 7 to 10 days, lasting up to 6 weeks.

The rash of **RMSF** begins as blanchable pink macules or papules that evolve into petechial or purpuric non-blanching lesions. They begin on the wrists and spread centripetally. The palms and soles are almost always involved. The exanthem is preceded by symptoms of fever, headache, and malaise. Gastrointestinal symptoms such as nausea, vomiting, and diarrhea can be present. The rash generally develops 2 to 3 days after the prodrome.

Morbilliform rashes are the most common type of cutaneous **drug eruption.** They generally begin as erythematous macules and papules on the trunk that then spread to the extremities symmetrically. There is usually concurrent eosinophilia. Pruritus and low-grade fever can also be present, often confounding the diagnosis. Though most drug rashes begin 1 to 2 weeks after starting the drug,

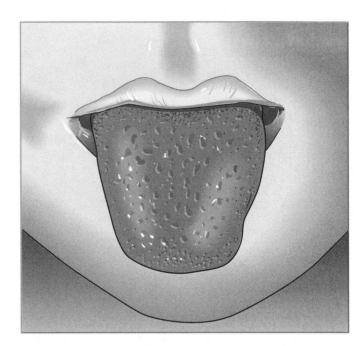

Figure 122-2. **Strawberry tongue.**

an eruption may develop after a drug has been discontinued. After stopping the offending medication, the rash usually resolves over 1 to 2 weeks, but there can be progression to Stevens-Johnson syndrome or toxic epidermal necrolysis. The underlying pathogenesis of many of these drug rashes continues to be unknown; however, current studies indicate a cell-mediated pathogenic mechanism.

Infection with **EBV** is associated with rash in young children and in adolescents on antibiotics, usually ampicillin or amoxicillin. The eruption is morbilliform, and the lesions may be erythematous or copper-colored. Fever, upper respiratory symptoms, lymphadenopathy, hepatosplenomegaly, and facial and peripheral edema, including unilateral periorbital edema, may be noted. The rash is likely due to an immunological interaction between the infectious agent and the drug.

Evaluation

History

A thorough history should be obtained (Questions Box).

Physical Examination

The focus of the physical examination is to help define the characteristics of the eruption such as location, extent, and degree of coalescence. The presence of any associated physical findings such as fever, lymphadenopathy, enanthem, desquamation, rhinorrhea, conjunctivitis, organomegaly, or central nervous system (CNS) symptomatology should be determined.

Laboratory Tests

Laboratory assessment may be helpful in certain conditions, though most of these diagnoses are made clinically. Serologic testing is most valuable for defining a community outbreak of a specific disease such as measles. In most viral exanthems, the results of serologic studies are not available until the condition has resolved and the patient has recovered. Tests may include acute and convalescent titers for specific viruses. Alternatively, immunoglobulin (Ig) M levels of antibodies against certain infections may be used to document that the infection was recent. Polymerase chain reaction may also be useful. Isolating the virus can confirm the diagnosis, but is often difficult to obtain. Because neutropenia and lymphocytosis characterize many viral illnesses, such findings are not helpful in differentiating specific causal agents. Lymphocytosis, with characteristically atypical lymphocytes, distinguishes EBV infection. Although a heterophile antibody test is usually positive in older children and adolescents, it may be nonreactive in young children, where infection is documented by specific EBV serology.

Pregnant women with suspected parvovirus B19 infection should have IgM and IgG levels drawn. If infection is confirmed, serial ultrasounds should be performed to monitor for symptoms of hydrops fetalis. Confirming diagnosis of rubella in a pregnant woman is also important because of the potential risk of congenital rubella syndrome.

Kawasaki disease is associated with elevation in markers of inflammation, including leukocytosis, thrombocytosis, elevated erythrocyte sedimentation rate, and C-reactive protein, though no test is diagnostic. Sterile pyuria is noted in 70% of the cases. Scarlet fever is characterized by leukocytosis. Eosinophilia can also be seen after a few weeks in up to 20% of patients. Laboratory confirmation, either via rapid streptococcal test or throat culture, should be done to confirm that the pharyngitis is due to GAS, not a virus. If the pharyngitis has resolved, serologic studies such as antistreptolysin O provide evidence of the recent infection.

A 4-fold or greater change in titer between acute and convalescent serum as determined by indirect immunofluorescent antibody assay is diagnostic for RMSF. Many patients will have thrombocytopenia, leukopenia, anemia, and hyponatremia. In general, any child presenting with headache, fever, and possible exposure to tick bite should be evaluated for this disease.

Imaging Studies

An echocardiogram to check for evidence of coronary artery aneurysm is a mandated part of the evaluation in Kawasaki disease, both during the acute phase and with serial repeat examinations, more frequently and earlier in those at high risk. Long-term cardiac management is required for those with identified coronary artery abnormalities. Ultrasound, if performed in children with suspected Kawasaki disease who present with symptoms of an acute surgical abdomen, may reveal hydrops of the gallbladder.

Management

The management of most viral exanthems is supportive and symptomatic. Hydration is critical because GI complaints of diarrhea are often associated. Antihistamines should be used for symptoms of pruritus in addition to regular use of emollients. Painful oral lesions can be treated with topical analgesics. In cases where complications such as encephalitis or pneumonia develop, hospitalization is indicated. Spread of infection such as measles to susceptible contacts can be reduced through the use of vaccine within 72 hours of exposure, or immunoglobulin within 6 days. Measles vaccine should be administered after the Ig in children who have been exposed. The measles, mumps, rubella vaccine is administered for the 2-dose vaccine series in children at about 12 months of age and again at 4 years. Measles, mumps, rubella, varicella is no longer available in the United States. HIV infection is not a contraindication to measles vaccination. In developing nations, administration of vitamin A is recommended to all children with measles if vitamin A deficiency is present in the community and mortality from measles is 1% or greater. Antibiotic therapy should be initiated if bacterial coinfection is suspected but should not be started empirically. The management of Kawasaki disease includes the administration of intravenous IG (IVIG) and aspirin, which should be started within 10 days of onset of fever. The current recommendation is to administer a single dose at 2 g/kg given as an infusion over 10 to 12 hours. Periodic echocardiograms are also required in these patients with close monitoring by a cardiologist. Measles and varicella vaccinations should be deferred for 11 months in any patient receiving IVIG.

If there is a concern for hepatitis in patients with Gianotti-Crosti syndrome, workup should be initiated.

Control measures are important because most morbilliform exanthems are due to infectious agents. Children with postnatal rubella should be kept from school or child care facilities for 1 week after onset of rash. Those with congenital rubella syndrome are considered contagious for 1 year, and caregivers must be educated. Females receiving rubella vaccine should not become pregnant for 28 days following vaccination. Hand hygiene is an important control measure that should be used to minimize spread of many of these viruses.

Vigilant education about the importance of immunizations is vital to reducing the impact of diseases such as measles and rubella. Though the number of cases in the United States is low, importation of these viruses from other countries mandates continued widespread vaccination.

Pregnant women infected with parvovirus B19 with ultrasound suggestive of hydrops fetalis should be referred to a tertiary care facility because intrauterine blood transfusions have proven successful. Routine exclusion of pregnant women from the workplace where erythema infectiosum has been identified is not recommended because the virus is transmitted before the onset of rash and is, thus, unlikely to be effective. Patients with aplastic crisis and chronic parvovirus infection may be contagious for extended periods and require longer periods of precautions. In addition, patients with PPGSS are considered infectious when clinical symptoms of their eruption are present. Patients with aplastic crises may need transfusions, and IVIG has been used successfully in immunocompromised patients with chronic infection. However, most cases of EI do not require absence from school or treatment beyond supportive care.

Treatment with doxycycline is the drug of choice for infection with *R rickettsii*. Penicillin within 10 days of onset of symptoms is used to treat scarlet fever as a result of GAS pharyngitis to prevent the development of rheumatic fever. Erythromycin can be used in patients allergic to penicillin.

Prognosis

The prognosis for most morbilliform rashes of childhood is generally good, with full resolution of symptoms unless children are very young, have congenital disease, have an underlying condition, or develop long-term complications. In some young infants, viruses that cause exanthems may produce severe complications such as pneumonia and encephalitis. Subacute sclerosing panencephalitis is a late-onset, rare, and serious degenerative CNS disease that occurs as a complication of measles infection. Some patients with roseola may develop chronic neurologic sequelae, but most cases are benign. The prognosis for Kawasaki disease is usually favorable with appropriate management. Up to 25% of untreated children and a fraction of those who have been treated may develop coronary artery aneurysms, sometimes with symptoms remaining silent for years. Kawasaki disease is the leading cause of acquired heart disease in children in the United States. In patients with severe infection with RMSF, long-term neurologic complications can be seen.

CASE RESOLUTION

The infant in the case scenario has the classic symptoms of measles. Normally such a young infant would not yet have received immunization against measles because the first dose is administered at 12 to 15 months of age with the second dose at 4 to 6 years of age. Immunoglobulin will likely not modify the disease in this patient because her rash is near confluent, suggesting exposure more than 6 days ago. She should be evaluated for evidence of complications, including pneumonia. Unimmunized household contacts, as well as pregnant women and other contacts younger than 1 year, should receive IG. Treatment is supportive.

Selected References

American Academy of Pediatrics. *Red Book: 2009 Report of the Committee on Infectious Diseases.* 28th ed. Pickering LK, Baker CJ, Kimberlin DW, Long SS, eds. Elk Grove Village, IL: American Academy of Pediatrics; 2009

Gable EK, Liu G, Morrell DS. Pediatric exanthems. *Prim Care.* 2000;27:353–369

Halpern AV, Heymann WR. Bacterial diseases. In: Bolognia JL, Jorizzo JL, Rapini RP, eds. *Dermatology.* St Louis, MO: Mosby; 2008:1081

Mancini J. Exanthems in childhood: an update. *Pediatr Ann.* 1998;27:163–170

Mancini AJ, Shani-Adir A. Other viral diseases. In: Bolognia JL, Jorizzo JL, Rapini RP, eds. *Dermatology.* St Louis, MO: Mosby; 2003:1255–1269

Marin M, Broder KR, Temte JL, Snider DE, Seward JF; Centers for Disease Control and Prevention. Use of combination measles, mumps, rubella, and varicella vaccine: recommendations of the Advisory Committee on Immunization Practices (ACIP). *MMWR Recomm Rep.* 2010;59(RR-3):1–12

Meissner HC, Strebel PM, Orenstein WA. Measles vaccines and the potential for worldwide eradication of measles. *Pediatrics.* 2004;114:1065–1069

Nelson JS, Stone MS. Update on selected viral exanthems. *Curr Opin Pediatr.* 2000; 12:359–364

Newburger JW, Takahashi M, Gerber MH, et al. Diagnosis, treatment, and long-term management of Kawasaki disease: a statement for health professionals from the Committee on Rheumatic Fever, Endocarditis, and Kawasaki Disease, Council on Cardiovascular Disease in the Young, American Heart Association. *Pediatrics.* 2004;114:1708–1733

Pinna GS, Kafetzis DA, Tselkas OI, Skevaki CL. Kawasaki disease: an overview. *Curr Opin Infect Dis.* 2008;21(3):263-270

Romano A, Demoly P. Recent advances in the diagnosis of drug allergy. *Curr Opin Allergy Clin Immunol.* 2007;7(4):299-303

Scott LA, Stone MS. Viral exanthems. *Dermatol Online J.* 2003;9:4

Yawalkar N. Drug-induced exanthems. *Toxicology.* 2005;209:131–134

Zaoutis T, Klein JD. Enterovirus infections. *Pediatr Rev.* 1998;19:183–191

CHAPTER 123

Vesicular Exanthems

Kathy K. Langevin, MD, MPH, and Noah Craft, MD, PhD

CASE STUDY

A 2-year-old toddler is evaluated for a 2-day history of fever (temperature: 103.1°F [39.5°C]), runny nose, decreased appetite, and a rash over the abdomen. The boy has had no previous known exposures to chickenpox (varicella) and no history of varicella vaccination. He attends child care daily. No one at home is ill. The boy is currently taking no medications except for acetaminophen for fever, and he has no history of dermatologic problems. On physical examination, the heart rate is 120 beats/min, the respiratory rate is 20 breaths/min, and the temperature is 100.4°F (38.0°C). The toddler's overall appearance is nontoxic. The skin examination is significant for a few scattered erythematous vesicular lesions over the abdomen and one erythematous papule on the back. The rest of the examination is normal.

Questions

1. What are the most likely causes of vesicular exanthems in febrile children?
2. How can types of vesicular rashes be differentiated on the basis of patient history?
3. What are the key historical questions to ask?
4. What is the natural course of varicella?
5. What treatment options are available for children with varicella? What options are available for other vesicular exanthems?

Exanthems are generalized, erythematous rashes that are due to an underlying disease. They are most frequently caused by viral or bacterial infections, though they can also be due to noninfectious etiologies. Infectious eruptions are most commonly morbilliform in the pediatric population, but they can have variable manifestations, including vesicular, bullous, petechial, and purpuric eruptions. Vesicles are elevated, fluid-filled lesions that measure 1 cm or less in diameter. Bullae are quite similar, only larger in size. Vesicles often lose their initial morphology quickly because they can break spontaneously or coalesce into bullae. They can arise de novo or from macules or papules. Vesicles may be discrete, grouped, generalized, or linear, depending on their etiology, and their specific distribution is often helpful in formulating a differential diagnosis.

Epidemiology

Epidemiological factors can help differentiate infectious from non-infectious etiologies. Patient age, season of the year, presence or absence of similar cases in the community, regular attendance at child care or school, and lower socioeconomic class, which may contribute to exposure, should all be considered. Gender and ethnicity are usually less informative but can help distinguish certain diseases causing exanthems.

Primary varicella-zoster virus (VZV), or chickenpox, is a herpesvirus and one of the most common vesicular exanthems seen in childhood. In the pre-vaccine era, 90% of children in the United States were infected before the age of 10, with 3 to 4 million cases annually. Males and females are equally affected. Most reported cases are in children younger than 10 years, although the percentage of infections in adolescents and young adults has increased since the routine administration of the varicella vaccine. It is primarily transmitted person to person by airborne spread of aerosolized viral particles from vesicles of infected persons. It may also be transmitted through respiratory secretions, from contact with zoster lesions, and vertically from mother to fetus. It is extremely infectious and transmission to susceptible household contacts approaches 80%. The incubation period ranges from 10 to 21 days, but varicella can develop between 1 to 16 days of life in newborns delivered to mothers with active disease around the time of delivery.

Herpes simplex virus (HSV) is a DNA virus, with HSV-1 and HSV-2 affecting most adults worldwide. Herpes simples virus 1 infections generally occur outside the genital area while HSV-2 infects the anogenital area. However, there has been an increase in the prevalence of extragenital HSV-2. Neonatal infection is generally acquired at delivery from an infected mother who is often unaware of her infection. Herpes simples virus 1 is typically transmitted by direct contact with oral secretions or lesions and HSV-2 from direct contact with infected genital secretions. Shedding of viral particles can occur in the absence of active infection. The incubation for HSV infections is 2 days to 2 weeks.

Hand-foot-and-mouth disease (HFMD), as well as herpangina, are due to enteroviral infections. Hand-foot-and-mouth disease is most commonly due to infection with coxsackievirus. Coxsackievirus groups A and B have been implicated in herpangina. Enteroviral infections occur most commonly in summer and early fall. The incubation period for most enteroviruses is between 3 to 6 days.

Bullous impetigo is a less common form of impetigo than the non-bullous forms. Bullous impetigo is most frequently seen in the summer and is transmitted by direct person-to-person contact, possibly via fomites as well. It is caused by coagulase-positive *Staphylococcus aureus,* mostly due to phage group 2, and is a localized reaction to exfoliative toxin released by the bacteria. It affects mostly neonates, infants, and younger children.

Infections caused by scabies or fungi can cause vesicular eruptions as well. Scabies is transmitted during prolonged close contact with an infested individual. Scabies has an incubation period of 4 to 6 weeks in patients without previous exposure. Reexposed patients develop symptoms a few days after repeat exposure. Tinea pedis is a common infection worldwide, though less so in children. It is acquired via contact with infected skin scales and in damp areas where the fungi reside. Tinea capitis, a common fungal infection in children (see Chapter 119), does not result in a vesicular rash, but like tinea pedis, can result in a dermatophytid or id reaction that is vesicular. The incubation period of fungal infections is unknown.

Dyshidrotic eczema is a disease that can occur in children with chronic eczematous dermatitis or atopic dermatitis, but can occur in non-atopic children as well. Rhus dermatitis is the prototypical allergic contact dermatitis, which develops about 1 to 3 days after exposure to plants such as poison ivy, poison oak, and poison sumac. Linear papules and vesicles are seen at points of contact between the plant antigen and the skin.

Clinical Presentation

Vesicular exanthems are eruptions of distinctive lesions that are raised and fluid-filled (Dx Box). They may be located anywhere on the child's body and, depending on the etiology, may or may not be pruritic. Other symptoms that may accompany such rashes include fever, upper respiratory symptoms, and gastrointestinal and central nervous system (CNS) involvement.

Dx **Vesicular Exanthems**

- Raised, fluid-filled vesicles on the skin
- Lesions may be pruritic
- Possible associated fever, upper respiratory infection symptoms, myalgias
- History of affected contacts
- Lesions on mucous membranes

Pathophysiology

Vesicles and bullae arise from a cleavage at various levels of the skin either within the epidermis (intraepidermal) or at the epidermal-dermal junction (subepidermal). Sometimes the 2 types of lesions can be differentiated based on the amount of pressure required to collapse the lesion, especially if the lesion is a large bulla. In addition, the thickness of the wall of a bulla can be estimated by its translucency or flaccidity. A biopsy of the lesion, however, is the only way to reliably differentiate between the 2 areas of separation, though this will not necessarily provide the diagnosis. Specific changes occur in the epidermis depending on the etiology of the vesicular exanthem. For example, with certain viral infections such as herpes simplex, varicella, and herpes zoster, a "ballooning degeneration" of epidermal cells occurs.

In bullous impetigo, the vesicles and bullae are caused by staphylococcal exfoliative toxin, which cause the keratinocytes in the granular layer of the epidermis to split apart. There are no bacteria seen within the blister cavity and a few inflammatory cells can be present.

The rash due to scabies infestation is the result of a hypersensitivity reaction to the proteins of the parasite. In vesicular lesions, there is spongiosis, or intercellular edema, in the epidermis caused by the mite, which can result in a vesicle. Spongiosis also leads to vesicle formation in dyshidrotic eczema, though the pathogenesis of this disease is not known. Dyshidrotic is a misnomer because this disease is not related to sweat gland dysfunction or occlusion. Spongiosis is also present in id reactions and allergic contact dermatitis.

Differential Diagnosis

While many vesicular eruptions are easily distinguishable clinically, the differential diagnosis can be challenging at times. Familiarity with the appearance of these conditions and their differentiating features is critical. The Internet can be valuable by providing access to images of many dermatologic conditions. Some sites such as VisualDx (accessible at www.visualdx.com) display pictorial representations and allow for searching by features such as rash morphology, symptoms, exposures, skin color, body location, age, immune status, and many other factors.

Primary VZV infection (chickenpox) consists of an average of 300 vesicles with the greatest concentration of lesions on the head and trunk, though it can be generalized. Lesions exist in various stages of resolution, progressing from erythematous macules and papules that then evolve into vesicles and, eventually, pustules that then crust and heal normally without scarring. Characteristically, the vesicle has been described as a "dewdrop on a rose petal." Associated prodrome includes malaise and mild fever, and is usually present. Symptoms tend to be more severe in older patients. Fetal infection during the first or early second trimester can result in fetal demise or in congenital varicella syndrome, consisting of limb hypoplasia, cutaneous scarring, ophthalmic abnormalities, and CNS defects. Infection acquired from 5 days pre-partum to 2 days postpartum can also be fatal because of the absence of protective maternal antibodies. Bullous varicella can result when *Staphylococcus aureus* infects the vesicles of chickenpox, with greater chance for scarring.

Herpes zoster, a reactivation of a latent infection with the VZV, can also cause a vesicular rash. The virus, which rests dormant in neuronal cells, travels along the nerves when reactivated and becomes released into the skin. It is generally a disease of older people, though children can be affected. In zoster, the lesions are grouped unilaterally in the distribution of 1 to 3 sensory dermatomes. It can be quite painful, and postherpetic neuralgia can last for months. In immunocompromised patients, the rash of zoster can become disseminated.

Disseminated HSV in an infant is usually due to HSV-2, is very severe, and is often accompanied by skin findings. In children and adolescents, HSV-1 gingivostomatitis and perioral vesicles are the most common clinical findings. A prodrome of parasthesia with recurrent infection is not uncommon. There can also be an ulcerative enanthem. Herpes simplex virus persists for life in the sensory ganglia and, when reactivated, results in single or grouped vesicles, often on the vermilion border with an erythematous base. Triggers include stress, ultraviolet exposure, and fever. Genital lesions are more frequently due to HSV-2, but the prevalence of genital infection due to HSV-1 is increasing.

Hand-foot-and-mouth disease is associated with a brief, mild prodrome of fever, malaise, and mouth pain. The exanthem consists of erythematous macules and papules with a central gray vesicle. Generally, the volar surfaces of the hands and feet, as well as the buttocks, tend to be involved. The concomitant enanthem is seen on the tongue, buccal mucosa, palate, uvula, and anterior tonsillar pillars. In herpangina, patients acutely develop fever, malaise, headache, and neck pain. There is a painful enanthem of small grayish-white vesicles on the soft palate, uvula, buccal mucosa, pharynx, and tonsils. These ulcerate with a surrounding red halo.

Impetigo is the most common bacterial skin infection in children. In bullous impetigo, there can be associated fever, weakness, and diarrhea, though there are often no systemic symptoms. Small vesicles enlarge rapidly into flaccid bullae that easily rupture. These lesions can be generalized and can arise from normal-appearing skin.

Parasites such as the tiny mite *Sarcoptes scabiei* can cause an intensely pruritic, generally papular eruption, though vesicular lesions can occur. Commonly, secondary excoriations are seen (see Chapter 121). In older children and adults, interdigital folds, flexor wrists, waistline, trunk, and genital area are more commonly affected. A linear burrow is pathognomonic but often difficult to identify clinically. Patients younger than 2 years have involvement predominantly of the head, neck, palms, and soles. In this age group, the eruption is more likely to be vesicular (Box 123-1). Arthropod bites can also result in isolated and scattered vesicles.

Fungal pathogens that cause tinea pedis include *Trichophyton rubrum*, *Trichophyton mentagrophytes*, *Trichophyton tonsurans,* and *Epidermophyton floccosum*. Infection can directly cause a scaly or vesicular rash or can result in a hypersensitivity reaction to the fungi, presenting as vesicles on the palms, soles, sides of the fingers, and occasionally on the extremities and trunk. *Trichophyton mentagrophytes* can cause vesicles and bullae on the medial foot. It can be associated with an id reaction, in which deep-seated pruritic vesicles develop secondary to tinea infection elsewhere. An id reaction, most commonly on the hands, face, and trunk, can also result from tinea capitis, usually caused by *T tonsurans* and *Microsporum canis,* though it does not cause a vesicular exanthem on its own.

The clinical appearance of dyshidrotic eczema can be identical to that of an id reaction or fungal infection and consists of "tapioca," pearl-like, deep-seated vesicles frequently on the palms and soles, as well as the lateral sides of the fingers that are extremely pruritic.

Box 123-1. Common Causes of Acute Vesicular Exanthems
Infectious
Viral
• Varicella-zoster virus
• Herpes simplex virus
• Enterovirus
Bacterial
• *Staphylococcus aureus*
Fungal
• *Trichophyton rubrum*
• *Trichophyton mentagrophytes*
• *Trichophyton tonsurans*
• *Microsporum canis*
• *Epidermophyton floccosum*
Infestations
• *Sarcoptes scabiei*
• Arthropod bites
Noninfectious
• Allergic contact dermatitis
• Dyshidrotic eczema
• Id reaction

Secondary impetiginization (bacterial superinfection) is common. Cases can be acute and recurrent, as well as chronic.

A delayed type 4 hypersensitivity reaction secondary to contact with plants of the genus *Toxicodendron* is a common cause of allergic contact dermatitis. The main allergen in these plants is a catechol. Rhus dermatitis causes a classic linear vesicular rash (see Chapter 121). Contact with other allergenic substances may also produce a vesicular rash and such substances include nickel, rubber compounds, fragrances, and preservatives in cosmetics.

The differential diagnosis of acute vesicular exanthems can also be organized according to the distribution of the lesions. Distinctive locations as well as specific patterns are important to consider in each individual case. The presence or absence of fever can assist in developing the appropriate differential (Figure 123-1). Epidemiological, as well as historic, information may suggest the diagnosis. For example, known exposure to VZV (chickenpox) 10 to 21 days prior to a vesicular eruption facilitates diagnosis of this disease. A history of hiking, camping, or other outdoor activities suggests possible contact with poison ivy or poison oak.

In addition, the presence of a specific prodrome can often be elicited with primary or recurrent herpes simplex. Pain on swallowing often occurs with enteroviral infection. A history of similar lesions lessens the likelihood of acute primary infection and suggests a chronic condition such as the recurrent disorder pompholyx (dyshidrotic eczema).

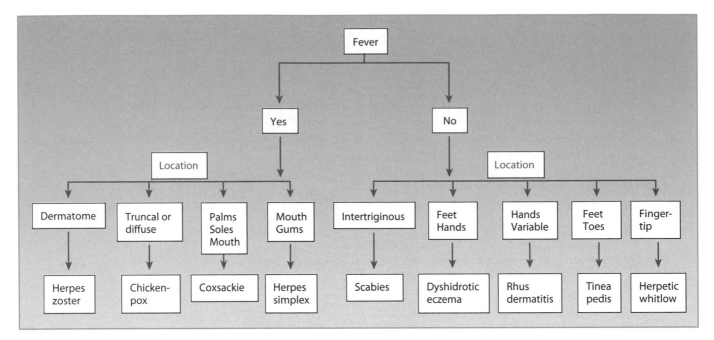

Figure 123-1. **Approach to the evaluation of vesicular eruptions.**

Evaluation

History

A thorough history should be obtained (Questions Box). Practitioners must inquire about the current state of general health, as well as the specific details about the eruption.

Questions

Vesicular Exanthems

- How long has the child had the rash? Where is it located?
- Does the child have associated symptoms such as fever, runny nose, cough, or sore throat?
- Does the child have nonspecific symptoms such as decreased appetite?
- If the child has any symptoms accompanying the rash, did these develop at the same time as the rash?
- Is there any reason to suspect that the patient is relatively immuno-compromised from chronic steroid use, chemotherapy, or an acquired immunodeficiency?
- Does the child have a history of similar lesions?
- Does anyone else in the family have a similar rash?
- Has the child been camping or hiking in the woods?
- Are there pregnant contacts?

Physical Examination

Although the physical examination focuses on the skin, other aspects of the examination are helpful diagnostically. Vital signs should be taken to verify the presence or absence of fever. The oropharynx should be examined closely for any lesions on the tongue, gingiva, buccal mucosa, palate, anterior tonsillar pillars, and posterior pharynx. The lips should also be examined for any evidence of vesicular lesions that may occur with a primary or recurrent herpes simplex infection.

Patients should be completely unclothed to permit a thorough examination of the skin. The distribution of the lesions should be noted. Physicians should determine whether the vesicles are grouped in a particular dermatomal distribution, as with zoster (shingles), or more generally distributed and in various stages of development, as with varicella. A linear distribution may suggest contact with poison ivy or poison oak. Physicians should also note the following: Do the lesions include or exclude the palms and soles? Are the buttocks involved? Are the lesions concentrated on one specific part of the body, such as the feet and toes or the hands? Are the sizes of the lesions uniform? If not, are other larger bullous-like lesions present in addition to vesicles?

It is also helpful, if at all possible, to examine the skin of family members for similar lesions.

Laboratory Tests

Few, if any, laboratory studies are usually needed in healthy children with vesicular eruptions because the diagnosis is often made clinically. A Tzanck smear showing multinucleated giant cells that contain intranuclear viral inclusions may be useful in making a preliminary diagnosis of HSV or VZV. Direct fluorescent antibody and polymerase chain reaction are rapid and sensitive methods to diagnose VZV and HSV.

Definitive confirmation of scabies can be made by microscopic examination of skin scrapings from suspicious lesions. The presence of the adult mite or ova, larvae, nymphs, or feces (scybala) is diagnostic. For children with suspected tinea pedis, a skin scraping mixed with potassium hydroxide can be performed and examined under the microscope. Fungal cultures can also be taken.

Management

The mainstay of treatment for most vesicular eruptions is parent and child education as well as reassurance. For example, most varicella, HSV, gingivostomatitis, HFMD, and herpangina infections are self-limited and no treatment except parental reassurance and education regarding adequate hydration is necessary. These diseases can, however, be quite serious, as the recent epidemic of enterovirus-71 in Asia did result in death in severe cases. Depending on the etiology of the vesicular rash, immunocompromised children such as those with HIV or AIDS and patients who are receiving chemotherapeutic agents or systemic corticosteroids may require specific intervention.

Topical agents such as calamine lotion, oatmeal soaks, or Aveeno baths should be used in children with intense pruritus or multiple lesions. Topical products, which are potentially sensitizing (eg, diphenhydramine-containing agents) should be used cautiously and discontinued if the condition is not improving. Cool, wet compresses with plain water or aluminum acetate (Burow solution) can be quite soothing in cases of rhus dermatitis, scabies, or tinea pedis.

Antipyretics (acetaminophen) may be used to treat otherwise healthy children with varicella. Aspirin-containing medications should be avoided in children with varicella because of the association with Reye syndrome. Oral analgesics may also be indicated for symptomatic relief of pain associated with herpetic gingivostomatitis or enterovirus mouth lesions.

Oral antihistamines (diphenhydramine or hydroxyzine) may be used in children with varicella or scabies for treatment of pruritus. These drugs are also helpful in allergic contact dermatitis (rhus dermatitis) and dyshidrotic eczema. Though the sedating antihistamines are generally more effective, non-sedating antihistamines can also be used in the daytime, particularly for the more chronic dyshidrotic eczema.

Steroids may be effective in the control of some vesicular rashes; however, the practitioner must first be certain the lesions are not secondary to varicella or herpes simplex. In certain cases, steroids may be used in infectious diseases, such as eczema herpeticum, but in conjunction with antiviral therapy, and under close monitoring. Topical steroids can be used for outbreaks of vesicles of dyshidrotic eczema, reserving oral steroids for severe outbreaks. In severe cases of rhus dermatitis, a course of systemic steroids, such as prednisone, 1 to 2 mg/kg/d, may be warranted and generally requires at least 2 to 3 weeks of therapy. Use of an oral histamine-2 blocker such as ranitidine or famotidine can help prevent gastritis as a complication of oral prednisone.

Oral acyclovir is not recommended routinely for the treatment of uncomplicated varicella in otherwise healthy children, but should be considered when the risk of developing moderate to severe disease is increased. According to the American Academy of Pediatrics (AAP) Committee on Infectious Diseases, acyclovir should be considered in patients older than 12 years; those with chronic cutaneous or pulmonary disorders; those receiving chronic or short, intermittent courses of corticosteroids (systemic or aerosolized); or those receiving salicylates long term. Oral or intravenous (IV) acyclovir may also be warranted in pregnant women infected with varicella. Acyclovir is most effective if initiated within the first 24 hours of the exanthem though the impacts on symptoms may be minimal. (See the AAP 2009 *Red Book* for further details and specific recommendations regarding immunocompromised children and the role of VariZIG.)

Additional recommendations for children with varicella include keeping fingernails short in young children to prevent superinfection of lesions from scratching. Children should drink plenty of fluids to avoid dehydration. Patients are considered contagious from 1 to 2 days prior to the onset of the rash until the lesions are all dried and crusted (usually 5–7 days after the rash develops), at which time they may return to school. In children with persistent or recurrent fever, secondary complications should be considered. A significant association between primary varicella injection and invasive group A beta-hemolytic streptococcal infection has been recognized and should be considered in the child with fever on or beyond the fourth day of the illness. There is a possible association between ibuprofen treatment and increased severity of GAS superinfection, thus ibuprofen should be avoided for the treatment of fever due to varicella. In infants greater than 28 weeks' gestational age born to mothers with varicella infection 5 days pre-partum, disease severity can be mitigated by placentally transmitted maternal antibody to the virus.

Treatment with acyclovir for zoster, or shingles, can heal lesions more rapidly and provide pain relief. It is possible that the varicella vaccine may reduce the risk of developing zoster. Since 2006, the recommendation is for 2 doses of varicella vaccine as immunity appears to wane and sporadic outbreaks occur. Incidence of varicella zoster infection has decreased by 80% since universal use of the live attenuated vaccine in healthy children.

Persons with frequent, generally more than 6 per year, outbreaks of HSV, may benefit from suppressive therapy with acyclovir. Herpetic whitlow is an HSV infection on the fingertip as a result of direct autoinoculation from oral or genital lesions. Treatment is not usually indicated. Herpes gladiatorum and herpes rugbiaforum are cutaneous HSV infections on the skin of wrestlers and rugby players, respectively. While it does not require treatment with antiviral agents such as acyclovir, athletes should not be engaged in person-to-person contact when herpes lesions are present. Eczema herpeticum is HSV infection in children with underlying atopic dermatitis or other underlying skin disease that results in rapidly progressive widespread vesicles that then erode and crust. There can be significant fever and irritability, and severe infection may warrant hospitalization for treatment with IV acyclovir. Treatment with topical calcineurin inhibitors (eg, tacrolimus) is contraindicated.

Localized bullous impetigo in otherwise healthy patients can be treated with topical mupirocin 2% or retapamulin 1% ointments. More widespread or complicated infections require **oral antistaphylococcal therapy** with agents such as amoxicillin and clavulanate (Augmentin), erythromycin, or cephalexin (Keflex). Recurrent disease should warrant workup for carriage and treatment if needed. Local knowledge of methicillin-resistant *S aureus* rates and bacterial cultures should be considered. For the treatment of tinea pedis, topical **antifungal agents,** in powder, cream, or ointment formulations, can be effective when applied twice daily until clear. Discomfort can be alleviated with cool water or Burow solution soaks. Tinea pedis can be difficult to control. Its treatment is centered on meticulous foot hygiene. Because careful foot care is often not a priority for most patients, complete eradication is not realistic. Patients should be instructed to wash their feet and change their socks when they return from school, dry their feet completely, avoid occlusive shoes, and wear open-air shoes or sandals whenever possible. Topical antiperspirants may be needed (aluminum chloride). Cotton socks are recommended. In severe or refractory cases, an oral antifungal preparation such as griseofulvin, terbinafine, or itraconazole may be prescribed for an extended period. Tinea capitis also requires oral antifungal therapy (see Chapter 119). For the treatment of scabies, see Chapter 121.

Prognosis

Overall, the prognosis for vesicular exanthems is good, with most children recovering in 1 to 2 weeks, depending on the etiology. Secondary infections can occur with varicella, however, and should be suspected in children with persistent or recurrent fever. Additional complications in non-immunosuppressed patients include bacterial superinfection of the skin, pneumonia, CNS involvement, Reye syndrome, glomerulonephritis, and arthritis. Complications from HSV infections include conjunctivitis, keratitis, and encephalitis.

Secondary infections with skin flora can be a complication of any of these skin conditions because denuded lesions allow for superinfection. In addition, many of these rashes can be pruritic, resulting in open, excoriated skin.

CASE RESOLUTION

In the case presented at the beginning of this chapter, the toddler has a classic presentation of primary varicella (chickenpox). Management should include symptomatic treatment with acetaminophen and antihistamines, along with topical preparations such as calamine lotion and oatmeal baths. The parent should be instructed regarding the natural course of this infection and be informed that the infection is highly contagious. In addition, symptoms indicating possible complications, such as persistent or recurrent fever, circumferential redness or swelling of the lesions, and shortness of breath, should be reviewed with the parents.

Selected References

American Academy of Pediatrics Committee on Infectious Diseases. *Red Book: 2009 Report of the Committee on Infectious Diseases.* 28th ed. Elk Grove Village, IL: American Academy of Pediatrics; 2009

Chayavichitsilp P, Buckwalter JV, Krakowski AC, Friedlander SF. Herpes simplex. *Pediatr Rev.* 2009;30:119–130

Dyer JA. Childhood viral exanthems. *Pediatr Ann.* 2007;36:21–29

Gershon AA. Varicella-zoster virus infections. *Pediatr Rev.* 2008;29:5–11

Kim KH. Enterovirus 71 infection: an experience in Korea 2009. *Korean J Pediatr.* 2010;53(5):616–622

Lopez AS, Guris D, Zimmerman L, et al. One dose of varicella vaccine does not prevent school outbreaks: is it time for a second dose? *Pediatrics.* 2006; 117:e1070–e1077

Mancini AJ, Bodemer C. Viral infections. In: Schachner LA, Hansen RC, eds. *Pediatric Dermatology.* St Louis, MO: Mosby; 2003

Mancini AJ, Shani-Adir A. Other viral diseases. In: Bolognia JL, Jorizzo JL, Rapini RP, eds. *Dermatology.* St Louis, MO: Mosby; 2008:1219–1222

Scott LA, Stone MS. Viral exanthems. *Dermatology Online J.* 2003;9:4

Yang LPH, Keam SJ. Spotlight on Retapamulin in impetigo and other uncomplicated superficial skin infections. *Am J Clin Dermatol.* 2008;9(6):411–413

The New Morbidity

CHAPTER 124

Autism Spectrum Disorders

Robin Steinberg-Epstein, MD

CASE STUDY

The mother of 18-month-old twin boys is concerned because one twin is not talking as much as his twin sibling. They are both very active. She feels that even though the child is quiet, he is very smart. He likes to figure out how things work. He seems very sensitive to sounds and covers his ears around loud noises. He loves music and even knows which CD his favorite song is on. He will play with his sibling, but doesn't seem interested in other children.

In your office both boys are very active. It is difficult to get an adequate examination, because this child is screaming the whole time. While both children have stranger anxiety, the twin about whom the mother is concerned seems to have extreme stranger anxiety. He otherwise appears well.

Questions
1. What are autism spectrum disorders (ASDs)?
2. How do ASDs differ from language delay?
3. How do you evaluate a child for ASDs?
4. Where can a clinician refer a patient with an ASD?
5. What types of treatment are available?
6. Should a child suspected of having an ASD receive further immunizations?

Autism spectrum disorders are characterized by impairment in communication, social interaction, and odd behaviors/interests. According to the *Diagnostic and Statistical Manual of Mental Disorders* (4th edition text revision), a person with autistic disorder must meet 6 of 12 possible criteria across 3 primary domains: social interaction, communication, and restrictive or repetitive behaviors. These disturbances must originate prior to age 3 and cause significant degrees of impairment (Box 124-1).

Autism spectrum disorders include autistic disorder, Asperger syndrome, Rett syndrome, and pervasive developmental disorder not

---

Box 124-1. Diagnostic and Statistical Manual of Mental Disorders (DSM-IV-TR) Diagnostic Criteria for Autistic Disorder[a]

A. A total of six (or more) items from (1), (2), and (3), with at least two from (1) and one or more from (2) and (3):

  (1) qualitative impairment in social interaction, as manifested by at least two of the following:

   (a) marked impairment in the use of multiple nonverbal behaviors such as eye-to-eye gaze, facial expression, body postures, and gestures to regulate social interaction

   (b) failure to develop peer relationships appropriate to developmental level

   (c) a lack of spontaneous seeking to share enjoyment, interests, or achievements with other people

   (d) lack of social or emotional reciprocity

  (2) qualitative impairment in communication as manifested by at least one of the following:

   (a) delay in, or total lack of, the development of spoken language (not accompanied by an attempt to compensate through alternative modes of communication such as gesture or mime)

   (b) in individuals with adequate speech, marked impairment in the ability to initiate or sustain a conversation with others

   (c) stereotyped and repetitive use of language or idiosyncratic language

   (d) lack of varied, spontaneous make-believe play or social imitative play appropriate to developmental level

  (3) restrictive repetitive and stereotyped patterns of behavior, interests, and activities, as manifested by at least one of the following:

   (a) encompassing preoccupation with one or more stereotyped and restricted patterns of interest that is abnormal either in intensity or focus

   (b) apparently inflexible adherence to specific, nonfunctional routines or rituals

   (c) stereotyped and repetitive motor mannerisms (hand or finger flapping or whole body movements)

   (d) persistent preoccupation with parts of objects (wheels, doors, lights)

These symptoms result in significant or abnormal functioning in at least one area (social interaction, social language, or symbolic/imaginative play) with onset prior to age 3.

[a] Reprinted with permission from American Psychiatric Association. *Diagnostic and Statistical Manual of Mental Disorders*. 4th ed. Text rev. Washington, DC: American Psychiatric Association; 2000.

otherwise specified. While the criteria differ somewhat, all of these disorders have in common an impairment in social communication and repetitive or unusual interests of varying degrees. Because these disorders require similar management and treatment, and there is some subjectivity in assessing the level of impairment, many choose to use the term *autism spectrum disorder* to incorporate all those who are significantly affected by its symptomatology.

Epidemiology

As recently as 1999 the prevalence of this disorder was thought to be 1 in 2,500. More recent numbers from the Centers for Disease Control and Prevention (2009) cite 1 in 110 children. This amounts to 1.5 million Americans. The incidence is rising by almost 15% a year. Boys are affected approximately 4 times as often as girls, which equates to 1 in every 70 boys. However, affected girls are often more impaired. Autism is considered the fastest-growing developmental disability. This increase is, in part, the result of an understanding of a broader phenotype.

Clinical Presentation

Autism spectrum disorders are truly a spectrum of social communication deficits. While there is a certain set of behaviors that defines the disorder, any child may have any combination of the symptoms that lead to the same result—severe and incapacitating social deficits. Furthermore, the challenges that face this population are more than just developmental delays. Their behaviors are aberrant and odd.

Many children with autism have difficulty with eye contact and body posture. Even those who have some eye contact often do not use their eyes to convey a social message. They may look out of the corner of their eyes, focus only on the lips of the speaker, or only look infrequently. In other words, they may make eye contact, but at the wrong time. They may talk to you with their bodies facing away from you. They may not gesture to help clarify intention.

While some children have limited communication, some offer too much information. They may be quick to talk to you about things they are interested in, but are not able to talk to you about your interests. They seem socially insensitive. As younger children they are often entertained by their own interests for long periods. Some have limited need for relationships, yet others desire interaction but do not understand how to initiate or maintain interactions. While many of these children are nonverbal, some repeat or echo what they hear from movies, television, or nearby conversation. Others seem able to converse, but have trouble with social banter. It is important not to be deceived by a child who interacts or hugs, but only on his own terms.

Autistic children often have a fascination with patterns. The pattern may be in the form of household routines, or patterns within a particular subject area. This may manifest in an obsession for sameness and resistance to change or in an obsessive need to know everything about a particular topic. Many know all there is to know about such favorite topics as Thomas the Tank Engine or dinosaurs from the Jurassic period, but cannot answer a question such as, "How are

you?" or "What is your name?" They may be upset by a road detour or a furniture rearrangement. Some of these children, out of an incredible ability to recognize patterns, will be able to read as early as 2, even though they are unable to speak functionally and cannot comprehend what they read.

A significant portion of children have difficulty with sensory processing. This takes the form of problems with smells, tastes, sounds, sights, and touch. This symptom may be manifest in the need to taste everything including nonfood items, covering ears in loud situations, or an inability to tolerate tags in clothing.

There is a huge variation in cognitive ability. The severity of autism is independent of cognitive ability. While a significant portion of those with autism are mentally retarded, many are of normal intelligence and even gifted.

Parents often raise behavioral concerns. It is important to recognize red flags and behaviors that demand further evaluation (Boxes 124-2 and 124-3). In other words, there are certain classic symptoms, but be mindful of the child that is just unable to connect with others. Clinicians should rely on their own instinct. Inconsistent symptoms are the hallmark of this disorder. Some parents of children with autism describe a phenomenon whereby the children are developing normally until 12 to 15 months of age and then suddenly lose skills or stop progressing. This is particularly concerning.

Pathophysiology

There are numerous proposed etiologic possibilities for the origins of autism, from the inbreeding of computer "whizzes" to exposure to microwaves. However, no consistent explanation or pattern has emerged. We do know that the structure of the brain is different, but why?

Box 124-2. Red Flags (Common Aberrant Behaviors Associated With Autism)

- Decreased eye contact (common, but NOT universal)
- Only wants to be cuddled on his terms
- Areas of unusual knowledge—recognizes entire alphabet by 2, all types of dinosaurs by 4, names of all Thomas trains, interest in fans or spinning items
- More interested in how things work than with playing
- Unusual sensitivities—oversensitive to hearing, bright lights, shirt tags, new foods, new places
- Smelling or licking nonfood items
- Repeating words instead of answering questions or answering off topic
- Difficulty interacting with other children
- Plays amongst children, not with them
- Resistance to change, "very independent"
- "In his own world"
- Lines things up
- Unusual hand movements or jumping when emotional
- Things have to be a certain way
- Odd tone of voice (prosody)
- Increased pain tolerance

Box 124-3. Absolute Indications for Referrals

- Not babbling or gesturing (pointing, waving) by 12 months
- No single words by 16 months
- Absence of 2-word non-echolalic phrases by 24 months
- ANY loss of ANY language or social skills at ANY age requires immediate evaluation.

---

[a] Filipek PA, Accardo PJ, Baranek GT, et al. The screening and diagnosis of autism spectrum disorders. *J Autism Dev Disord.* 1999;29:439–484.

Up to 10% of those with autism have another medical condition (Box 124-4) that might have led to this disorder. However, this leaves 90% without an etiology.

Genetics seems to play a role in the development of autism. There is a risk of the disorder among siblings of up to 8%, which is more than 10 times the risk in the normal population. Family members are more likely to exhibit social deficits, anxiety, or depression than are family members who do not have a relative with the disorder. Several candidate chromosomes have been suggested as being associated with this disorder, but no one loci is responsible for this disorder.

It is also important to realize that up to 30% of children with autism have abnormalities on electroencephalogram (EEG). This may point to the structural abnormalities in the autistic brain but does not seem to account for the disease itself. The epileptiform changes should be evaluated by a neurologist to determine if medication is indicated.

Several environmental markers have also been suggested as being linked to autism, but none has proved credible. Major epidemiological studies both within the United States and internationally have examined the roles of vaccinations, diet, and thimerosal preservative in the development of this disorder. None of these studies has found proof to support these theories. Children with ASD should receive routine health maintenance including all recommended immunizations. There are noted associations such as older paternal age, prematurity, and jaundice.

Differential Diagnosis

Very few entities present with impairment in the same 3 domains as those that are affected by autism. There are a limited number of disorders that mimic autism (Box 124-5). On the other hand, there are several disorders that commonly occur with autism (Box 124-6) and, if not identified, will make treatment more difficult.

Evaluation

There is not one diagnostic test, blood or otherwise, that will confirm the diagnosis of autism. The diagnosis is based on history and the interaction with the child.

History

Regular developmental surveillance and screening should be part of every well-child evaluation, especially between ages 9 and 30 months. The American Academy of Pediatrics recently suggested adding a 30-month visit for developmental screening in an attempt to

---

Box 124-4. Medical Conditions Associated With Autism

- Epilepsy
- Fragile X
- Tuberous sclerosis
- Prader-Willi syndrome
- Visual or auditory impairment syndrome
- Down syndrome
- Cerebral palsy
- Neurofibromatosis
- Congenital rubella

Box 124-5. Disorders That May Mimic Autism

- Hearing impairment
- Global developmental delay
- Tourette disorder and comorbidities
- Selective mutism
- Reactive attachment disorder
- Lead ingestion
- Sensorimotor integration dysfunction
- Severe auditory processing/language deficit
- Severe anxiety
- Severe attention-deficit/hyperactivity disorder
- Brain trauma
- Childhood onset schizophrenia

Box 124-6. Disorders That Can Occur With Autism

- Tuberous sclerosis
- Congenital blindness
- Global developmental delay
- Chromosomal abnormalities (Down syndrome, fragile X syndrome, Prader-Willi syndrome, etc)
- Phenylketonuria
- Epilepsy
- Elevated lead level
- Congenital infections
- Brain trauma
- Bipolar disorder
- Neurofibromatosis
- Congenital profound hearing loss
- Tourette disorder
- Landau-Kleffner syndrome
- Inborn errors of metabolism
- Anemia
- In utero exposure to drugs/alcohol
- Depression/anxiety
- Attention-deficit/hyperactivity disorder

capture atypical development to target for early intervention. Special attention should be given to a child who has a sibling with autism or a child whose parent or caregiver has expressed concern. Several screening tools can be used, including the Parents' Evaluation of Developmental Status (PEDS), Ages and Stages Questionnaire (ASQ), or the Brigance. The Modified Checklist for Autism in Toddlers (M-CHAT) is another excellent screening tool (moderate sensitivity and high specificity) to identify both developmental and social competency skills which, when deficient, may be associated with autism. These screening tools are quick and easy and can be filled out by the parent in the waiting area or with minor assistance from office personnel.

Once you suspect that a child has a developmental difference, it is important to gather as much information as possible. Thorough birth and medical histories are important in helping to understand if early experiences may predispose this child to any deficits.

Family history is also important because this disorder is presumed to be genetic. Furthermore, it may help to consider other etiologies. Family structure will help to determine if abuse, neglect, or maternal depression play any role in the child's delay. However, autism is NOT due to poor parenting.

Developmental history is the most important part of the history. It is important to probe all 4 areas of developmental milestones: fine motor, gross motor, language, and social development (see Chapter 27). Again, we expect more significant delays in language and social interaction, but you may see delays in all components of development. Additionally, probing for abnormal behaviors specific to autism helps distinguish this disorder from others. See the Questions Box for some suggestions that may help elicit information relevant to a diagnosis of autism in a toddler, but you must adjust the history depending on the age of the child. Always include early language milestones. Be aware that children with autism tend to have splinter skills. These are skills that may be normal or above developmental level for age. Don't let these skills distract you from probing areas of suspected delay.

Finally, parents and physicians often fall victim to common myths and excuses regarding development (Box 124-7) because it is not easy for many parents to discuss or admit delays. These myths, while they sound plausible, are not substantiated and only serve to further delay onset of intervention.

Physical Examination

A thorough physical examination with special attention directed to the growth parameters, neurologic examination, dysmorphic features, and neurocutaneous stigmata are essential to a complete evaluation. Height, weight, and head circumference should be plotted. Keep in mind that 25% of children with autism have a head circumference greater than the 97th percentile. That is not to say that everyone with a large head has autism, only that it is an associated feature. Those with Rett syndrome have a head circumference that may arrest by 5 months of age. Of course, in utero infections may predispose to a small occipitofrontal circumference and developmental concerns.

Questions

Autism

Questions to Ask Parents

- Does he seem to hear you? Did he have a hearing test in the neonatal period?
- Does he make noises? If so, what kind?
- When did he say his first word after "mama" and "dada"? Does he have 2-word phrases?
- Are there any other behaviors that concern you?
- Can he scribble? Has he lost any skills? Does he line things up?
- When did he first walk? What does he like to play with?
- Do tags on the back of clothes bother him?
- Is he interested in other children? What does he do if he sees another child in a park?
- When do you first remember him pointing with one finger?
- Does he play peek-a-boo? Will he try to engage you?
- Does he talk into a play phone?
- Does he eat a variety of foods?
- Does he turn when you call him?

Questions to Ask Yourself as the Clinician

- Are there any complicating historical factors that may predispose this child to a developmental problem?
- Is this merely personality variation, or does this represent delays and aberrant behavior?
- Is this a language delay or are you concerned about more social or odd behaviors?
- What should be done to evaluate?
- What types of intervention would be helpful?

Box 124-7. Common Excuses for Unusual Behaviors

1. We speak 2 languages at home. (By age 3 in a bilingual home, language should follow a normal progression. Social and unusual behaviors should always follow a normal trajectory.)
2. He is a boy. (This is accounted for in the range of normal.)
3. He is a twin. (If one twin is autistic, the other twin has a great risk of being autistic or delayed.)
4. He is the first child. (No evidence that firstborns speak late.)
5. He is the baby. (No evidence that last borns speak late.)
6. He is having a bad day.
7. He watches too much television. (Neglect can lead to delays, but these children still need intervention.)

These are NOT reasons to delay evaluation!

Detecting subtle physical signs such as clinodactyly, simian crease, or a high-arched palate, while not diagnostic, are somewhat helpful in raising suspicion for neurodevelopmental delays. A Wood light evaluation may be helpful in uncovering neurocutaneous stigmata.

A series of dysmorphic features like a thin upper lip, flat philtrum, and upturned nose might suggest a syndrome such as fetal alcohol syndrome. Hypotonia is a common finding amongst children with autism, but might suggest an inborn error of metabolism. One must also check reflexes because degenerative disorders, such as muscular dystrophy, can present with language delay.

One of the most useful examinations in the office is to simply have a conversation with an older child or to play with a younger child. Bring out bubbles and engage in a popping game. Watch the child's eyes and his interaction with you and with his parent. Pretend the otoscope is a phone that rings, pick it up, talk briefly, and pass it to the child. Watch his response. Does he play with you or just with the bubbles or neither? Does he display repetitive flapping when excited?

Laboratory Tests

No single laboratory or radiologic evaluation will make the diagnosis. However, some tests are helpful to rule out comorbid conditions. If the child has not had an audiological evaluation, then this is step one. However, do not wait for the audiology results before referring the patient for help. From a medical perspective, a tiered approach to the workup is often helpful. The first tier would include laboratory studies such as a high-resolution karyotype and a DNA test for fragile X. In those with global developmental delay or regression (or when indicated), consider a lead level, carnitine profile, plasma homocysteine levels, serum amino acids, urine organic acids, thyroid evaluation, and vision evaluation. Consider ammonia, lactate, and pyruvate on those with a severe presentation. An EEG would be appropriate if concerns of seizures are present. Check the results of the newborn screen. The yield of this evaluation is anticipated to be low (approximately 4%), but if positive, may aid in the diagnosis of a specific comorbidity.

A relatively new test, chromosomal microarray (comparative genomic hybridization), has been found to yield 3 times the detection rate of chromosomal alterations as compared to the high resolution karyotype. Replacing the high resolution karyotype with this test would improve detection to over 7%. It is expected that this test will become part of the new standard.

Tier 2 would include an evaluation aimed toward specific rare diseases. Some consideration might be given to chromosomal 15 methylation, MECP2 (methyl CpG binding protein 2 [in females]), PTEN (phosphatase and tensin homolog deleted on chromosome 10), fibroblast karyotype if pigmentary abnormalities are noted, sterol profile, guanidinoacetate urine analysis (only in males), or other associated genetic evaluations. Current literature would suggest that evaluations for autism yield an etiology 15% of the time.

Imaging Studies

If there is a history of regression, microcephaly, or the presence of focal findings suggestive of central nervous system malformations, consider a magnetic resonance imaging (MRI) test. Otherwise, obtaining an MRI is considered low yield. Children with regression, more significant involvement, or behavior suspicious of a seizure should receive an EEG. While positron emission tomography and single-photon emission computed tomography scans will show abnormalities, they are not considered specific enough for either diagnosis or to direct care. There are no present indications for their use in an individual child with autism. They are used primarily in the research setting.

Management

Making the diagnosis is sometimes challenging, but early diagnosis is critical in changing ultimate outcomes. Early diagnosis and intervention can reduce cost of lifelong care by two-thirds.

For children younger than 3 years, refer to the local governmental agency in addition to speech/language and occupational therapy, which is covered by their health insurance. In most states there exists a government-sponsored early intervention program for children 0 to 3. This agency is responsible for the evaluation and behavioral/educational/therapeutic interventions for children with suspected delays. This should lead to a comprehensive diagnostic evaluation and placement in an intensive intervention program. Therefore, once a hearing test has been completed, a referral to such an agency is the next step. It takes on average 6 months from the time a child is seen in a physician's office to when those services are obtained. Therefore, it is important to identify children before age 2 ½ years. Make that referral!

For children older than 3 years, the responsibility belongs to the local school system. So even though a child is not yet school-aged, their local school district is responsible for both the evaluation and interventions necessary to appropriately remediate this child. However, the clinician should check with local resources to ensure that such a system exists in the respective state. Be aware that between ages 3 and 21 years, each child is entitled to a free and appropriate education guaranteed under the federal mandate known as the Individuals with Disabilities Education Act. This program should be comprehensive and individualized to each child's needs. After a thorough assessment, the school will meet with the parents to develop an Individualized Education Plan.

Most children with autism require at least speech and language services, occupational therapy, and social skills training. Many require a one-on-one aide in a mainstream class, and others benefit from special education services in the form of pullout or a special day class. Augmentation can be created privately. Some states have mandated that medical insurance support these additional, yet necessary, services, but in others it is the sole responsibility of the parent.

Interventions

Autism is a neurologic condition that can improve with intensive **multimodality interventions.** This improvement is slow. There are no quick solutions, magic medications, or diets to "cure" autism. Behaviors like impulsive aggression, repetitive behaviors, resistance to change, and obsessive behaviors are frequently targeted by systematic interventions. Furthermore, some basic social learning behaviors can be shaped with different types of intervention. There are a number of different techniques (Box 124-8) based on different psychological principles that may be used to help improve the difficulties associated with autism.

Box 124-8. Techniques Used for Treatment

Floor Time

This intervention uses personal relationships and play in the child's area of interest to draw the child through increasingly complex developmental tasks.

Applied Behavioral Analysis

Applied behavioral analysis strives to achieve pre-learning skills such as eye contact, imitation, sitting, and following simple directions using the principles of conditioning and behavioral psychology. In a 1:1 fashion a child is trained to respond in a predetermined way using a specific curriculum and reinforcers.

Behavioral Analysis

This method uses close study of behaviors, determining antecedent triggers and consequences, such as a tantrum. The goal is to substitute acceptable responses, such as using words, and increases rewards for substituted behaviors.

Pivotal Response Training

This strategy uses principles of behavior analysis but also uses the child's interests and internal drives to motivate. The hope is to generalize the skills from a therapy room to a variety of environments. Children with autism often have difficulty performing the same previously mastered skill in a new setting.

Picture Exchange Communication System

This system uses pictures that the nonverbal child can use to show a caregiver what they want.

Treatment/Education of Autism and Communication Handicapped Program

This is a complete program that incorporates the child into a large autism community. The goal is toward autonomy and uses many methods based on cognitive therapeutic principles.

Social Stories

These are often used as a complementary strategy. These stories describe in detail basic social skills in different scenarios.

Speech and language services are a vital component of intervention. The initial goal is to help establish communication. In higher-functioning children who already have established language, this service is vital for the establishment and development of prosocial language—eye contact, inferences, understanding jokes, and the more subtle aspects of language. Social skills groups are often used to teach appropriate social responses in a semi-naturalistic environment.

Occupational therapy is often necessary to help with both fine motor skills and the processing of sensory information. This can be helpful in easing transitions. There is not a great deal of research to support its use for sensory concerns, but it is a widely accepted premise that sensory exposure helps children who have either an oversensitive or an undersensitive sensory system.

Special education in the form of an aide, classroom pullout, or special day class is often necessary to help with commonly associated learning disabilities. Children with autism can have a full array of learning difficulties. Commonly associated learning difficulties

are in reading comprehension, written expression, specific math disability, and auditory comprehension.

Under the law, these services should occur in the least restrictive and most appropriate environment.

Pharmacotherapy

The mainstay for treatment of autism remains behavioral. Medications do not seem to help the core symptoms of autism. However, almost 2 of 3 of these children receive medications for behaviors that, despite intensive behavioral intervention, continue to obstruct progress or become dangerous.

Only 2 drugs are US Food and Drug Administration–approved for use in this population; risperidone and aripiprazole are approved for the agitation associated with this disorder. On the other hand, there are many other targeted behaviors for which medications are used. The choice to use medication is not a simple one. It should be directed toward the emotion or psychological function causing the symptom. The most common medications include selective serotonin reuptake inhibitors and stimulants. However, research and clinical experience tells us that children with autism are more sensitive to side effects and at lower doses. Therefore, the choice and direction of medication management in this population is often best guided by a developmental-behavioral pediatrician, neurologist, or child psychiatrist (see Chapter 126).

Alternative Treatments

A variety of alternative treatments have been suggested. Secretin injections, dietary restrictions, chelation, high-dose vitamins, antifungals, and neuron injections are just some of the interventions considered in this realm. Some of these methods reported anecdotal improvement; others are dangerous and have resulted in death. None of these methods is considered traditional or the standard of care because there are minimal empiric data to support their use.

Prognosis

Many children show dramatic improvements with early intervention. Unfortunately, others show minimal improvement. Therefore, all children need intensive interventions. Some prognostic indicators such as IQ, early and intensive interventions, and a supportive family bode well. Obtaining an accurate IQ is often challenging. The major determinant of ultimate outcome seems to be progress in a comprehensive, early intervention program for 2 years, prior to age 5. Having little or no language by age 6 is a poor prognostic indicator. Therefore, the goal remains focused on early identification, intensive treatment, and advocacy for children to receive such interventions with ongoing support.

The intensive early intervention programs have only been available since about 1995. Autistic children have now moved into the mainstream. In spite of receiving early intervention, these children continue to have problems with transitions, more complex social interactions, and higher-level organization tasks. Therefore, physicians must continue to advocate for and support these families through the years.

Many adults with autism also continue to require significant support. They may require sheltered living and work environments, safety monitoring, ongoing medical support and, depending on severity, institutionalization.

Another significant portion of autistic children attend college, get married, and have children. This portion is difficult to quantify because these numbers are changing very rapidly and the true number of children with this disorder has yet to be realized.

CASE RESOLUTION

The child described in the vignette was evaluated by a developmental pediatrician and the local governmental agency where he received a comprehensive assessment by a multidisciplinary team. The diagnosis was confirmed and his brother was also noted to have a language delay. They were both placed into an early intervention program. The primary patient was placed in a one-on-one structured teaching environment for 4 months. After significant improvement, he was moved to a therapeutic preschool setting that emphasized generalization of his newly acquired skills, speech therapy, occupational therapy, and social skills. His brother received speech therapy 2 times a week. Both are due to start a regular kindergarten class in the fall with ongoing speech and social support. The primary patient has been placed on a stimulant medication to control hyperactivity and problems with attention.

Selected References

Aman MG. Treatment planning for patients with autism spectrum disorders. *J Clin Psychiatry.* 2005;66(suppl 10):38–45

American Academy of Pediatrics Council on Children With Disabilities, Section on Developmental Behavioral Pediatrics, Bright Futures Steering Committee, Medical Home Initiatives for Children With Special Needs Project Advisory Committee. Identifying infants and young children with developmental disorders in the medical home: an algorithm for developmental surveillance and screening. *Pediatrics.* 2006;118:405–420

American Psychiatric Association. *Diagnostic and Statistical Manual of Mental Disorders.* 4th ed. Washington, DC: American Psychiatric Association; 1994

Autism Society. www.autism-society.org

Barbaresi WJ, Katusic SK, Voigt RG. Autism: a review of the state of the science for pediatric primary health care clinicians. *Arch Pediatr Adolesc Med.* 2006;160:1167–1175

Centers for Disease Control and Prevention. Evaluation of a methodology for a collaborative multiple source surveillance network for autism spectrum disorders—Autism and Developmental Disabilities Monitoring Network, 14 Sites, United States, 2002. *MMWR Surveill Summ.* 2007;56(SS01):29–40

Centers for Disease Control and Prevention. Prevalence of autism spectrum disorders—Autism and Developmental Disabilities Monitoring Network, six sites, United States 2000. *MMWR Surveill Summ.* 2007;56(SS01):1–11

Centers for Disease Control and Prevention. Prevalence of autism spectrum disorders—Autism and Developmental Disabilities Monitoring Network, 14 sites, United States, 2002. *MMWR Surveill Summ.* 2007;56(SS01):12–28

Courchesne E, Carper R, Akshoomoff N. Evidence of brain overgrowth in the first year of life in autism. *JAMA.* 2003;290:337–344

Filipek PA, Accardo PJ, Baranek GT, et al. The screening of autism spectrum disorders. *J Aut Dev Discord.* 1999;29:439–484

Jarbrink K, Knapp M. The economic impact of autism in Britain. *Autism.* 2001;5:7–22

Madsen KM, Hviid A, Vestergaard M, et al. A population-based study of measles, mumps, and rubella vaccination and autism. *N Engl J Med.* 2002;347:1477–1482

Richardson A, Montgomery P. The Oxford-Durham study: a randomized, controlled trial of dietary supplementation with fatty acids in children with developmental coordination disorder. *Pediatrics.* 2005;115:1360–1366

Attention-Deficit/ Hyperactivity Disorder

Andrew J. Barnes, MD, MPH, and Iris Wagman Borowsky, MD, PhD

CASE STUDY

Cody, a 10-year-old boy, has visited a primary care clinic annually for well-child care, seeing different pediatricians each time. After failing all subjects during the first half of fourth grade, his teacher asks his mother to see if Cody's doctor can do anything to help him at school. When the appointment is made, the clinic obtains standardized attention-deficit/hyperactivity disorder (ADHD)-specific behavioral rating scales from Cody's parents and teachers. Prior to the visit, the pediatrician reviews these rating scales and Cody's medical history. She discovers that at Cody's 6-year well-child visit, a colleague documented, "likely has ADHD, medication is indicated." The medical records indicate that the family deferred starting stimulant medication and were told to follow up as needed. There is no further mention of ADHD. Cody also has a history of several urgent care and emergency department visits for minor unintentional injuries.

Questions

1. What are the primary symptoms of ADHD? What other conditions should be considered in the differential diagnosis of ADHD?
2. What other psychiatric disorders or neurodevelopmental disabilities commonly coexist with or mimic ADHD?
3. What is the appropriate evaluation of children with suspected ADHD?
4. What treatment modalities are useful in the management of ADHD?
5. What is the role of primary care in the long-term management of ADHD?

The core symptoms of ADHD are inattention, impulsivity, and hyperactivity. The *Diagnostic and Statistical Manual of Mental Disorders, Fourth Edition (DSM-IV)* diagnostic subtypes of ADHD are (1) predominantly inattentive type, (2) predominantly hyperactive/impulsive type, and (3) combined type. Most children and adolescents with the disorder have the combined type, exhibiting symptoms of both inattention and hyperactivity/impulsivity. Growing evidence suggests that differentiating such subtypes has little bearing on prognosis or treatment; with *DSM-5*, ADHD diagnostic criteria and categorical nosology are likely to change.

The diagnosis of ADHD is based solely on clinical judgment, requiring documentation of at least 6 of 9 behaviors from the inattentive and/or hyperactive/impulsive *DSM-IV* domains (Box 125-1). Some symptoms of ADHD must be present before 7 years of age, and present symptoms must persist in at least 2 major contexts of the child's life (eg, home and school) for at least 6 months. These symptoms must be more frequent and severe than those typically seen in children of the same developmental age and must impair the child's developmental competence, learning, and/or social interactions. The symptoms should not be better explained by another condition (such as anxiety or autism). If impairing symptoms occur at sub-diagnostic levels and/or are associated with a *DSM-IV* exclusionary condition such as autism, a diagnosis of ADHD-Not Otherwise Specified should be made. Treatment, however, is symptomatic and not specific to subtype.

Transient behavioral variations and problem-level ADHD-like symptoms that are not frankly disordered are best classified using the framework of *DSM-Primary Care (DSM-PC)* instead of *DSM-IV* (eg, "Hyperactive/Impulsive Developmental Variation—Middle Childhood: The child plays active games for long periods. The child may occasionally do things impulsively, particularly when excited.").

Epidemiology

Attention-deficit/hyperactivity disorder is the most common neurobehavioral disorder in children. An estimated 4% to 12% of school-aged children have ADHD, and there is a 3:1 predominance of boys in community samples. Over the past 2 decades, ADHD diagnoses have increased; it remains unclear whether this represents a true increase in incidence, secular changes in diagnostic criteria and practices, sociocultural bias, and/or effects of unspecified environmental factors.

Box 125-1. *DSM-IV-TR* Criteria for Attention-Deficit/Hyperactivity Disorder[a]

Diagnostic Criteria for ADHD

A. Either 1 or 2

1) Six (or more) of the following symptoms of **inattention** have persisted for at least 6 months to a degree that is maladaptive and inconsistent with developmental level:

Inattention

a) Often fails to give close attention to details or makes careless mistakes in schoolwork, work, or other activities

b) Often has difficulty sustaining attention in tasks or play activities

c) Often does not seem to listen when spoken to directly

d) Often does not follow through on instructions and fails to finish schoolwork, chores, or duties in the workplace (not due to oppositional behavior or failure to understand instructions)

e) Often has difficulty organizing tasks and activities

f) Often avoids, dislikes, or is reluctant to engage in tasks that require sustained mental effort (such as schoolwork or homework)

g) Often loses things necessary for tasks or activities (eg, toys, school assignments, pencils, books, or tools)

h) Is often easily distracted by extraneous stimuli

i) Is often forgetful in daily activities

2) Six (or more) of the following symptoms of **hyperactivity-impulsivity** have persisted for at least 6 months to a degree that is maladaptive and inconsistent with developmental level:

Hyperactivity

a) Often fidgets with hands or feet or squirms in seat

b) Often leaves seat in classroom or in other situations in which remaining seated is expected

c) Often runs about or climbs excessively in situations in which it is inappropriate (in adolescents or adults, may be limited to subjective feelings of restlessness)

d) Often has difficulty playing or engaging in leisure activities quietly

e) Is often "on the go" or often acts as if "driven by a motor"

f) Often talks excessively

Impulsivity

g) Often blurts out answers before questions have been completed

h) Often has difficulty awaiting turn

i) Often interrupts or intrudes on others (eg, butts into conversations or games)

B. Some hyperactive-impulsive or inattentive symptoms that caused impairment were present before 7 years of age.

C. Some impairment from the symptoms is present in 2 or more settings (eg, at school [or work] or at home).

D. There must be clear evidence of clinically significant impairment in social, academic, or occupational functioning.

E. The symptoms do not occur exclusively during the course of a pervasive developmental disorder, schizophrenia, or other psychotic -disorder and are not better accounted for by another mental disorder (eg, mood disorder, anxiety disorder, dissociative disorder, or personality disorder).

Code Based on Type

314.01 Attention-Deficit/Hyperactivity Disorder, Combined Type: if both criteria A1 and A2 are met for the past 6 months

314.00 Attention-Deficit/Hyperactivity Disorder, Predominantly Inattentive Type: if criterion A1 is met but criterion A2 is not met for the past 6 months

314.01 Attention-Deficit/Hyperactivity Disorder, Predominantly Hyperactive, Impulsive Type: if criterion A2 is met but criterion A1 is not met for the past 6 months

314.9 Attention-Deficit/Hyperactivity Disorder Not Otherwise Specified

[a] Reprinted with permission from American Psychiatric Association. *Diagnostic and Statistical Manual of Mental Disorders.* 4th ed. Text rev. Washington, DC: American Psychiatric Association; 2000.

Clinical Presentation

Children with ADHD have problems with selective attention and mental stamina for non-rewarding or non-preferred activities. They often make careless mistakes or fail to pay attention to details. They may be easily distracted and have difficulty starting tasks and concentrating on tasks long enough to complete them. Stopping a preferred activity can also be problematic, and caregivers often note that their children with ADHD over-focus or "get lost" in their favorite activities, such as videogames, drawing, or reading. Difficulties following instructions and organizing tasks and activities are also characteristic of ADHD. Poor impulse control manifests as difficulty waiting one's turn, frequently blurting out responses at inappropriate times, and interrupting or intruding on others. Symptoms of hyperactivity include fidgetiness, excessive talking at inappropriate times, difficulty remaining seated or playing quietly, and subjective feelings of restlessness in adolescents. Difficulties with social relationships and low frustration tolerance are also commonly seen in children with ADHD.

Pathophysiology

The etiology of ADHD is unknown. Genetic, prenatal/perinatal, and neurologic factors may play a role. Family studies indicate that first-degree relatives of children with ADHD have a risk of ADHD that is 5 times greater than normal controls. In addition, measures of behavior and attention are more alike in monozygotic twins than in same-gender dizygotic twins. The most widely confirmed gene association with ADHD is the 7-repeat allele of the D_4 dopamine receptor gene that, while found in about 30% of the general population, is found in 50% to 60% of those with ADHD. Prenatal and perinatal risk factors that have been associated with ADHD include in utero exposure to alcohol or cigarettes; extreme prematurity; brain injury or stroke; and severe early deprivation, neglect, and maltreatment.

Attention-deficit/hyperactivity disorder is currently conceptualized as a neurodevelopmental-behavioral disorder. Patients with frontal lobe lesions have long been known to exhibit severe and intractable inattention, hyperactivity, disinhibition, and impulsivity. Recent neurodevelopmental research suggests that frontal and prefrontal regions of the brain are involved in executive functions, including organizing, planning, sequencing, selective attention, impulse inhibition, the ability to stick to a plan yet change it as needed (set maintenance), the ability to self-talk through internal rules, and working memory. A number of recent studies, some longitudinal, show delayed maturation (myelination) and abnormal activation/inactivation of critical prefrontal circuits and fronto-striatal reward-motivation circuits in children and adolescents with ADHD compared to controls. Dopamine and norepinephrine are involved in neurotransmission within these brain pathways, and the prefrontal cortex is rich in catecholamine receptors. Psychostimulants that target ADHD symptoms increase the availability of these neurotransmitters in the brain. Stimulants seem to primarily increase activity in key areas of the striatum, such as the ventral tegmental area, in turn activating the prefrontal cortex and executive functions.

Differential Diagnosis

The symptoms of ADHD can be seen in a variety of other conditions (Box 125-2). Sensory deficits, especially hearing impairment, can imitate attention deficits. Attention-deficit/hyperactivity disorder symptoms are often a component of autism spectrum disorders and other neurodevelopmental conditions, such as neurofibromatosis, co-occurring with typical features of the respective diagnoses, such as impaired social communication in autistic children. Lead and other heavy metals have dose-related detrimental effects on behavior and development; likewise, chronic iron deficiency can result in or mimic ADHD. Seizure disorders, such as petit mal (absence) or partial complex seizures, may be misdiagnosed as predominantly inattentive-type ADHD. Other neurologic disorders that can present with symptoms of ADHD include Wilson disease and adrenoleukodystrophy; however, focal, sometimes progressive neurologic deficits of acute-to-subacute onset are the hallmarks of these rare conditions. Certain medications, such as high-dose corticosteroids, phenobarbital, and theophylline, may cause ADHD-like mental status effects, as can recreational drugs of abuse, including inhalants and marijuana. Hyperthyroidism can cause the hyperactive symptoms of ADHD, but other signs of increased metabolism, such as elevated heart rate, tremors, or weight loss, should be apparent. Exposure to alcohol or drugs in utero has been associated with subtle difficulties with learning and attention as the child develops. Congenital infections, central nervous system infections in early childhood, and traumatic brain injuries may produce behaviors similar to those seen in ADHD. Severe and/or chronic psychosocial-environmental problems, such as family stresses, marital discord, unemployment,

---

Box 125-2. Differential Diagnosis of Attention-Deficit/Hyperactivity Disorder

- Developmental delay
- Learning disability
- Language disorder
- Sensory deficiencies (eg, hearing or vision impairment)
- Autism spectrum disorders
- Seizure disorder
- Neurogenetic syndromes (eg, Neurofibromatosis type I)
- White matter disorders
- Iron deficiency
- Environmental toxins (lead)
- Side effects of medication (eg, phenobarbital)
- Hyperthyroidism
- Congenital infection
- In utero exposure to drugs or alcohol
- Previous brain insult (eg stroke, trauma, infection)
- Family stresses
- Ineffective parenting
- Psychiatric disorders
  — Conduct disorder
  — Oppositional disorder
  — Anxiety disorders
  — Affective disorders (depression, bipolar illness)
  — Personality disorders (aggression, antisocial behavior)
  — Substance abuse

---

poverty, homelessness, trauma/maltreatment, substance abuse, and ineffective parenting (eg, overly-permissive or overly-authoritarian) can also masquerade as, co-occur with, and/or exacerbate ADHD.

Children with ADHD have an increased prevalence of co-occurring psychological pathology, which can magnify the core symptoms of the disorder. These include oppositional defiant disorder (35%), conduct disorder (26%), depressive disorders (18%), anxiety disorders (26%), Tourette disorder and tics, speech and language disorders, and specific learning disabilities, such as dyslexia and dyscalculia. In adolescents and young adults, aggression, delinquency, and other antisocial behaviors, as well as substance abuse, are often seen together with untreated or undertreated ADHD.

Evaluation

Children and adolescents with symptoms of inattention, hyperactivity, academic or social underachievement, or impulsivity should be evaluated first by a primary care clinician, ideally one with whom the child has enjoyed continuity of care. A complete evaluation of this nature is best accomplished with plenty of time for face-to-face review of records and a comprehensive history and examination; 90 to 120 minutes is a suggested minimum amount of time to do this effectively and correctly, usually necessitating several appointments spaced apart by days or weeks.

History

The diagnostic evaluation of ADHD should begin with multiple informants (caregiver[s], child, sibling[s]) giving a comprehensive medical history that includes details of the child's problem behaviors, their antecedents, and their outcomes and consequences (Questions Box). The clinician should find out how these informants perceive and handle the child's behavioral problems and, in turn, how the child responds. Social/family stresses and the home-school environment should be described and evaluated, and school reports and report cards reviewed. Interviewing the child alone provides an opportunity to better understand his or her thoughts, feelings, insight, judgment, self-image, and developmental status; however, children generally have poor insight into their ADHD symptoms and are generally not considered reliable informants for *DSM* ADHD symptoms. Interviewing caregivers alone and talking with teachers over the phone before or after the visit can be very helpful and alleviate some of the burden on the child of what is often initially a problem-oriented discussion about him or her. The clinician should inquire about the child's difficulties, developmental strengths and competencies, adaptive strategies, stress management, self-regulation, protective factors, and adjustment.

Historical information should cover all *DSM* criteria (see Box 125-1). Parents and teachers may report the child's behaviors using an ADHD-specific questionnaire or rating scale that includes these (eg, Vanderbilt scales), which can be found in the American Academy of Pediatrics (AAP) toolkit *Caring for Children With ADHD: A Resource Toolkit for Clinicians.* Non–ADHD-specific developmental screening tools do not replace this type of comprehensive ADHD assessment because their sensitivity and specificity for ADHD are diagnostically inadequate.

The clinician should evaluate for coexisting conditions that would warrant further investigation. This is where broad screening tools, such as the Child Behavior Checklist and Behavior Assessment Scales for Children, can be useful. For example, frequent sadness or isolation would suggest depression, and persistent negative, hostile, and defiant behavior toward authority would suggest oppositional-defiant disorder. The AAP toolkit for clinicians includes both a scale specific to ADHD behaviors and a broader scale for possible coexisting conditions.

Physical Examination

The child's weight, height, and head circumference should be plotted on a growth curve and the pattern of growth evaluated; pubertal status should be recorded. Children should be examined for congenital anomalies, syndromic stigmata, or dysmorphic features, such as fetal alcohol facies or café-au-lait skin macules. A musculoskeletal evaluation should be done to document bulk, strength, tone, gait, station, and fine and gross motor coordination; a neurologic examination should include assessment of the cranial nerves, sensation including hearing and vision, balance and proprioception, and repetitive movements, tics, or tremors. The psychiatric and behavioral status examination should include an assessment of the child's mental status, affect, mood, insight, judgment, social-emotional reciprocity, joint attention, speech/language and communication, memory, fund of knowledge, and thought content and processes.

Observing the child's behavior during the office visit is crucial, with the caveat that many children with ADHD do not appear grossly hyperactive or inattentive in the office. Interaction between the child and his or her parents should be observed and documented nevertheless. The clinician should note how the child does with complex parental and examiner instructions, directives, and questions, and how parents deal with any "misbehavior." Does the child cooperate and comply with the examination, and does he or she seem motivated to change? How well does the child relate to adults? The clinician should watch the child play (eg, draw, play with toys) and note the child's organization of activities, attention span, distractibility, and motor activity.

Laboratory Tests

Diagnostic tests, such as specific neuropsychological or psychiatric metrics (eg, IQ tests), are not indicated for initial ADHD evaluations and should be guided by selected findings on the history and physical examination. Psychometric testing or standardized school district tests may show that a discrepancy exists between the child's raw abilities (IQ) and academic progress in one or more areas (achievement scores or grades); in this case, a referral for psycho-educational testing to rule out specific learning disabilities is indicated. Referral for further evaluation of speech, hearing, and vision should also be

---

Questions

Screening for Attention-Deficit/ Hyperactivity Disorder

- History of Presenting Complaint (from multiple informants)
  - What concerns do you have about his/her development, behavior, or learning?
  - How is he/she doing in school academically and socially?
  - Is he/she happy in school?
  - Has your child been held back in any grade, suspended, dropped out, or considered dropping out?
  - How often does he/she have problems completing home chores, class work, or homework?
  - How often does he/she have major problems controlling his or her behavior at home, in school, or with friends?
  - How often is behavior management, self-regulation, and/or discipline difficult at home or school?
  - What are the antecedents and consequences for problem behaviors at home and/or school? What discipline techniques have been tried and what effects did each have?
- Perinatal, Developmental, Academic, and Medical History
- Psychological History and Previous Treatments
- Social and Environmental History
- Family History (focused especially on immediate family ADHD, school problems, developmental delays, conduct problems; cardiac, musculoskeletal, neurological, or psychiatric conditions)

done as indicated. Blood tests, such as hematocrit, lead level, and thyroid hormone, likewise, are only indicated if there are relevant signs or symptoms. Additionally, computerized continuous performance tasks designed to measure vigilance or distractibility have low sensitivity and specificity and fail to adequately differentiate children with ADHD from controls.

Brain imaging (eg, magnetic resonance imaging or positron-emission tomography) currently has no role in the evaluation of ADHD. Despite their utility in population-level studies, such measures cannot yet accurately differentiate between the brains of individuals with and without ADHD. An electroencephalogram or neurologic consultation is indicated only if absence or partial complex seizures are suspected by history or physical examination.

Management

Treatment of ADHD must be multimodal, continuous, and longitudinal, recognizing that ADHD is a chronic condition. Family education should emphasize the strengths of children and families, and address parental concerns. Families should be aware that children with ADHD often experience functional impairments in academic achievement, self-esteem, social skills, peer status, unintentional injuries, and family functioning. The clinician can ease parents' guilt by explaining the neurodevelopmental basis of ADHD and assuring that ADHD is not the result of insufficient parenting. Children who discover that their problems are not their fault may feel that a heavy burden has been lifted from their shoulders. However, both parents and children may find it difficult to accept that the child has a chronic disorder. Support groups such as Children and Adults with ADHD (CHADD) (www.chadd.org) may be helpful for families. Clinicians should work together with the child, family, and school personnel to specify appropriate target outcomes. They should then monitor the child for target behaviors and adverse effects. If target outcomes are not met, the clinician should reevaluate the initial diagnosis, use of available treatments, adherence to the plan, and potential for coexisting conditions.

Behavior Management

The goals of behavior management are to modify the child's physical and social environment at home and school in order to influence positive behavioral change. Behavioral modification techniques include rewards for the target outcome behaviors (eg, verbal praise hugs; points or stars on a chart that can be traded for material objects or a desired activity, such as a game or special time with a parent) and punishments for unacceptable behaviors (eg, time out, loss of a privilege, extra chores, or reduction in allowance). Acceptable and unacceptable behaviors should be clearly defined and measurable, and rewards and punishments should be spelled out in a contract drawn up with the child. The strongest behavioral interventions follow immediately after a behavior (eg, immediate praise when a child follows a command after the first time it was given). If rewards or punishments are used over time, parents and teachers must be creative in periodically varying the rewards and penalties. Management of overactive children who have difficulty focusing attention, following

rules, and controlling impulses can be challenging for both parents and teachers. The best results come from praising and reinforcing positive behaviors and ignoring negative behaviors unless they are dangerous or intolerable. Using praising and ignoring in combination can be very successful. Parent commands should be clear and countable (eg, "You need to go upstairs to brush your teeth before the egg timer goes off in 3 minutes."). Because children with ADHD can have difficulty carrying out multistep commands, it is best to set them up for success by giving clear, doable, single-step commands. Behavior management in combination with medication management can be extremely effective. Potential benefits of behavioral therapy when used concurrently with medication include improved scores on some academic measures, improved behavior, and decreased anxiety symptoms. Interventions such as play therapy, psychotherapy, and cognitive therapy have no documented efficacy in managing core ADHD symptoms, but may be indicated for common co-occurring conditions such as anxiety, conduct disorder, and depression. Approaches that target executive function training and cognitive-emotional self-regulation may be useful adjuncts as well.

Educational Interventions

The pediatrician can improve the child's educational experience by contacting the child's teachers and even attending school conferences and special education meetings. While most children with ADHD can be managed in the regular classroom, special education in a smaller, more focused setting may be indicated for behavioral or academic difficulties. Teachers can use specific strategies to help children with ADHD focus their attention and follow directions in the classroom (Box 125-3). Behavioral therapy should be integrated into the classroom, focusing on a child's strengths and minimizing stigma. Teachers and caregivers who are most successful in working with children with ADHD are able to set firm limits and discipline children without anger or frustration, while at the same time remaining flexible enough to recognize when a change in tactics or even "rolling with it" is necessary. Caregivers of children with ADHD can request needed classroom accommodations through Section 504 of the Americans with Disabilities Act, and children whose ADHD symptoms lead to significant learning deficits may qualify for an Individualized Education Plan through the Individuals with Disabilities Educational Act. A letter from a primary

---

> ### Box 125-3. Strategies for Managing Children With Attention-Deficit/Hyperactivity Disorder in the Classroom
>
> - Seat children where distractions are minimized and teachers can see how and when children are paying attention.
> - Cue children discretely or nonverbally to remind them to refocus their attention.
> - Give clear, succinct, 1- to 2-step directions, and repeat them frequently and patiently.
> - Break up work periods by allowing children to get up and move around (eg, handing out papers, cleaning chalkboard).

care clinician documenting a child's health impairments, developmental risks, and academic limitations attributable to ADHD can go a long way in helping to ease this process for families and schools.

Because children with ADHD are easily provoked into misbehavior and are prone to clashes with peers, they can also benefit from closer supervision in unstructured school areas such as the playground, cafeteria, halls, and bus. Programs designed to improve social competence and peer relationships (eg, group social skills training, therapeutic recreational activities) may also be helpful.

Pharmacotherapy

Research has shown that psychostimulant medication with and without behavioral therapy is efficacious in reducing the core symptoms of ADHD. Furthermore, there is some evidence that these effects translate into an increased ability to follow rules, improved classroom behavior, and improved relationships with peers and parents; impacts on higher-order executive functions are less predictably attained. Effects of stimulant medication on learning are not well studied. Caution should be used when treating children younger than 5 years or weighing less than 20 kg with stimulant medication because many pharmaceutical stimulant preparations have narrower therapeutic windows on a per-kilogram basis for children of smaller stature.

Psychostimulants are the most commonly used agents for ADHD and, by far, the most evidence-based. Currently available stimulants include short-acting (3–6 hours), intermediate-acting (6–8 hours), and long-acting (10–12+ hours) formulations of methylphenidate and amphetamines (Box 125-4). Studies have found few, if any, differences between the efficacy of methylphenidate and dextroamphetamine, but some children will respond better to one or the other.

Box 125-4. Stimulant Medications

Methylphenidate
- Short (Ritalin, Metadate, Methylin)
- Intermediate (Ritalin SR, Metadate ER, Methylin ER)
- Extended release (Concerta, Metadate CD, Ritalin LA, Focalin XR, and transdermal [Daytrana])

Amphetamine
- Short (Dexedrine, Dextrostat)
- Intermediate (Adderall, Dexedrine)
- Extended release (Adderall-XR, Vyvanse)

Stimulants affect behaviors within 30 minutes and affect attention (eg, for a school subject like math) within 1.5 hours after administration. There is little evidence of tolerance to stimulants over time, but short-term tolerance occurs so that blood levels must increase during the day to maintain efficacy. Long-acting stimulants, such as Concerta, produce increasing plasma concentrations throughout the day, eliminate the need to take medication at school, and may persist during after-school homework time. A transdermal delivery system (Daytrana) is now available for children aged 6 to 12 years.

The most common side effects of stimulant medications are decreased appetite, stomachaches, headaches, delayed sleep onset, and jitteriness, occurring in 4% to 10% of children. Transient motor tics may occur while on the medication (or an existing chronic tic disorder or Tourette disorder exacerbated or unmasked). At higher doses, stimulants may negatively influence height velocity and may slightly decrease predicted adult height. While dosing of stimulant medication is based on individual variation in response, researchers have found that children generally do better on a maximized tolerable dose of stimulant medications, which is body-weight dependent, rather than the lowest dose that shows a clinical effect. The best stimulant dose for an individual child is thus the dose that produces near-complete symptom remission while producing acceptable side effects (eg, appetite suppression is usually tolerable whereas growth suppression is not). For this reason, it is recommended that clinicians do a controlled open-label titration trial of multiple dosages of a single agent using a systematic method. For example, one might use either long-acting methylphenidate in 18, 36, and 54 mg dosages, or long-acting amphetamine in 10, 20, and 30 mg dosages in 1-week blocks, with teacher- and parent-completed *DSM*-based scales (such as the Vanderbilt or Conners) at the end of each week. The clinician can then use these scales to develop a medication management plan with the family. Published guidelines, such as the Texas Medication Algorithm Project, can aid the clinician in this regard.

Once the medication dosage is stable and helpful, often after 2 to 4 visits over 1 to 2 months, follow-up should occur at least every 3 to 4 months, with particular attention to emerging developmental competencies, self-mastery, and improvement in targeted goal behaviors. Such visits should minimally include an interim history, weight, height, blood pressure, and scales of clinical response from caregivers and teachers.

If a particular stimulant does *not* produce symptom remission at all or only does so with severe or intolerable adverse effects, the clinician should systematically try 1 or 2 other stimulants because 70% to 80% of children can achieve complete remission of symptoms in this manner. If 2 or 3 psychostimulants are not effective or produce unacceptable side effects, other medications can be used. Atomoxetine (Straterra) is a non-stimulant medication that selectively inhibits the norepinephrine transporter. Atomoxetine is approved for children older than 6 years, has once-daily dosing, should be titrated to an effective weight-based dose, and often takes 1 to 6 weeks to produce effects; adverse effects can include gastrointestinal upset and mood irritability. α_2-agonists such as clonidine (Catapres) and guanfacine (Tenex, Intuniv) are often useful as adjuncts for children with poorly controlled hyperactivity/impulsivity or comorbid tics, although few children with ADHD achieve adequate symptom remission on α_2-agonist monotherapy. Tricyclic antidepressants and bupropion can have positive effects on ADHD symptoms for some children, although again are rarely used as monotherapy. Pemoline (Cylert) is generally not used because of the potential for fatal hepatotoxicity. Modafinil, mood stabilizers, antiepileptics, and atypical antipsychotics are generally not indicated in the treatment of ADHD in the primary care setting.

Complementary and alternative medicines, such as vitamins, dietary restrictions, and occupational therapy/sensory integration, are used by 54% of parents, but only 11% discuss these with their child's clinician. Primary care practitioners are challenged to help families safely navigate the limited evidence available on such therapies' risks and benefits. For example, melatonin is often helpful for comorbid sleep disorders prevalent in children with ADHD, and the Feingold Diet is said to alleviate hyperactivity by eliminating artificial flavors, colors, and preservatives in the diets of children sensitive to these putative effects. There is no evidence, or negative evidence, for some popular holistic approaches, such as Behavioral Optometry. Finally, while there may be neurobehavioral toxicity associated with low doses of various environmental toxins, particularly in young children, pediatricians are encouraged to emphasize primary prevention; there is no role for chelation in this context.

Prognosis

Attention-deficit/hyperactivity disorder is a chronic condition, persisting into adolescence and adulthood in about two-thirds of affected children. Overall, adults who had un- or under-treated childhood ADHD complete less schooling, hold lower-ranking occupations, have lower self-esteem and more social-skill deficits, and exhibit more antisocial behavior and alcohol and drug abuse. However, ADHD does not preclude attaining high educational and vocational goals, and more than half of adults with childhood ADHD no longer meet full *DSM-IV* criteria. Hyperactivity usually greatly diminishes or resolves in high school or early adulthood; some young adults experience a bothersome sense of inner restlessness. Attention problems and impulsivity may continue to varying degrees. Adults with ADHD may choose occupations that match their strengths and minimize limitations (eg, on-the-road salesperson vs desk job accountant). While some adults with ADHD choose to continue medication, others may function well without medication.

CASE RESOLUTION

Cody's primary care clinic reorganized their system of care to leverage the core concepts of the **medical home** to improve the care for children with chronic conditions, including ADHD. One of the clinic's nurses, Karen, has been trained to coordinate referrals to behavioral health and other specialists as indicated, communicate and coordinate care with schools and community services, and monitor adherence and response to treatments.

During Cody's visit, the pediatrician confirms the diagnosis of ADHD and probable comorbid anxiety using AAP practice guidelines and standardized criteria. She educates Cody and his family about multimodal evidence-based interventions for these conditions and introduces the family to Karen and the medical home model of care. Karen follows up with the family by phone 1 week later as planned and learns that they are reluctant to start Cody on any medicine. She guides Cody's parents to voice their preferences and cultural perspectives on possible interventions and then assists them in making another appointment with the same pediatrician, ensuring continuity of care. At the next visit, the pediatrician uses motivational interviewing to help the family find agreement on a watchful waiting approach with close, continuous school and home follow-up by Karen and at least quarterly visits with the same pediatrician. One month later, following a behavioral crisis at school, Cody's parents request an urgent appointment with same-day access. The pediatrician reviews recent parent and teacher behavioral rating scales at the point of care (gathered by Karen the prior week) and reiterates the available first-line treatment options. The family agrees to pursue an open titration trial of stimulant medication for ADHD symptoms and referral to a therapist for evaluation and possible treatment of the anxiety symptoms. Another clinic visit is scheduled in 1 month, while Karen follows up weekly with parents, teachers, and therapists.

Selected References

American Academy of Pediatrics Committee on Quality Improvement, Subcommittee on Attention-Deficit/Hyperactivity Disorder. Clinical practice guideline: diagnosis and evaluation of the child with attention-deficit/hyperactivity disorder. *Pediatrics.* 2000;105:1158–1170

American Academy of Pediatrics Committee on Quality Improvement, Subcommittee on Attention-Deficit/Hyperactivity Disorder. Clinical practice guideline: treatment of the school-aged child with attention-deficit/hyperactivity disorder. *Pediatrics.* 2001;108:1033–1044

American Academy of Pediatrics Task Force on Coding for Mental Health in Children. Wolraich ML, Felice ME, Drotar D, eds. *Diagnostic and Statistical Manual for Primary Care (DSM-PC) Child and Adolescent Version.* Elk Grove Village, IL: American Academy of Pediatrics; 1996

American Psychiatric Association. *Diagnostic and Statistical Manual of Mental Disorders.* 4th ed. Text rev. Washington, DC: American Psychiatric Association; 2000

American Psychiatric Association. DSM-5 Development Web Site. Proposed Revisions: 314.0x: Attention Deficit/Hyperactivity Disorder. May 20, 2010. www.dsm5.org/ProposedRevisions/Pages/proposedrevision.aspx?rid=383

August GJ, Winters KC, Realmuto GM, Fahnhors T, Botzet A, Lee S. Prospective study of adolescent drug use among community samples of ADHD and non-ADHD participants. *J Am Acad Child Adolesc Psychiatry.* 2006;45:824–832

Barkley RA. Major life activity and health outcomes associated with attention-deficit/hyperactivity disorder. *J Clin Psychiatry.* 2002;63(suppl 12):10–15

Bright Futures in Practice: Mental Health—Volume II, Tool Kit. www.brightfutures.org/mentalhealth/pdf/tools.html

Children's Medication Algorithm Project: Attention-Deficit/Hyperactivity Disorder. www.dshs.state.tx.us/mhprograms/adhdpage.shtm

Learning Disabilities Online. www.ldonline.org

Molina BS, Hinshaw SP, Swanson JM, et al. MTA at 8 years: prospective follow-up of children treated for combined-type ADHD in a multisite study. *J Am Acad Child Adolesc Psychiatry.* 2009;48:484–500

Pliszka S, American Academy of Child and Adolescent Psychiatry (AACAP) Work Group on Quality Issues. Practice parameter for the assessment and treatment of children and adolescents with attention deficit/hyperactivity disorder. *J Am Acad Child Adolesc Psychiatry.* 2007;46:894–921

Rojas N, Chan E. Old and new controversies in the alternative treatment of attention-deficit hyperactivity disorder. *MRDD Res Rev.* 2005;11:116–130

Swanson J , Kramer H, Hinshaw S, et al. Clinical relevance of the primary findings of the MTA: success rates based on severity of ADHD and ODD symptoms at the end of treatment. *J Am Acad Child Adolesc Psychiatr.* 2001;40:168–179

Texas Consensus Conference Panel on Pharmacotherapy of Childhood Attention Deficit Hyperactivity Disorder. The Texas Children's Medication Algorithm Project: revision of the algorithm for psychopharmcotherapy of attention-deficit hyperactivity disorder. *J Am Acad Child Adolesc Psychiatry.* 2006;45:642–657

CHAPTER 126

Psychopharmacology in Children

Robin Steinberg-Epstein, MD, and Kenneth W. Steinhoff, MD

CASE STUDY

An 8-year-old girl has been diagnosed with high-functioning autism. The local developmental-behavioral pediatrician has recommended treating her anxiety and inattention with atomoxetine. The girl's mom is very hesitant. She trusts you and wants your opinion.

Questions

1. How does one assess the safety and appropriateness of psychotropic medications?
2. What kind of blood tests are used to maximize safe administration and how often are they performed?
3. What is the evidence that psychotropic medications are overprescribed?
4. What are the usual side effects of commonly used psychotropic medications?

Psychopharmacologic agents are now used with greater frequency in the pediatric population. Approximately 50% of children and adolescents will, at some point before age 18, meet criteria for a psychiatric diagnosis. Almost a quarter of children will have substantial impairment as a result of those symptoms. Unlike antibiotics or other medications used in children, psychopharmacologic agents are used daily and for extended periods. Furthermore, it is important to recognize that there is a dearth of evidence-based information supporting the use of many medications in children, including psychotropics. Therefore, most of these medications are used in an **off**-**label** fashion. The medical community must then rely on published data (often in adult subjects), clinical experience, and expert consensus to guide medication choice, dose, and management. This often provokes parental anxiety and sparks numerous concerns from families who don't understand that the US Food and Drug Administration (FDA) label limits the claims a manufacturer can make but does not limit a clinician's use of medications. Furthermore, families are often anxious because clinicians rely almost exclusively on history and structured behavioral observation, which is the most important "test" for most of these disorders. Unfortunately, there is a national shortage of pediatric subspecialists trained to choose, monitor, and manage these medications for children. It is, therefore, necessary for pediatricians to be familiar with the various medication classes and the controversies facing families of affected children.

Pediatricians need to understand the principles guiding the use of these medications and to become familiar with some of the more frequently used psychopharmacologic agents. The most used classes of medication in children include **stimulants, selective norepinephrine reuptake inhibitors (SNRIs), selective serotonin reuptake inhibitors (SSRIs),** and **atypical neuroleptics,** also known as **serotonin-dopamine antagonists (SDAs).** This information can also be useful in helping families navigate this confusing maze.

The decision to use psychopharmacologic agents should not be made without considerable thought. Medication should be an integral part of a comprehensive treatment program that addresses the academic, behavioral, medical, and developmental needs of the child. The decision to place a child on any agent should be based on significant dysfunction as well as discussion and full disclosure of potential risks and benefits with both parents and child. Rating scales should be employed and target symptoms identified as a means of monitoring medication benefit. A medication trial, once undertaken, should be carefully monitored, methodically addressing both adverse events and effectiveness. It is generally best to change one agent or dose at a time, followed by structured observation (eg, rating scale[s]) to determine the effect of the change. Therefore, one usually begins with **monotherapy,** optimizes the dose, and assesses risks and benefits before developing a more complex regimen. Such a trial necessitates frequent visits and discussion with the administering physician. Given current scientific information and clinical experience, the use of psychopharmacologic agents in young children (<5 years) should be reserved for extraordinary circumstances.

It should come as no surprise that children are not little adults. Pharmacokinetics in children is affected by increased rates of metabolism in their relatively larger livers, a faster glomerular filtration, and variable fatty tissues. Some children, therefore, require a larger dose than those used for adults. Conversely, perhaps due to size, fat distribution, and other explanations, a much smaller, and seemingly ineffective, dose may be enough. There is little correlation between blood level and treatment response for most agents. Furthermore, some medications have a duration of effects that well exceed their **half-life** (atomoxetine), but for others (such as stimulants) their effect diminishes despite having a significant blood level. Additionally, for most agents (such as stimulants and SDAs) there is no correlation with milligrams per kilogram. Frequent clinical monitoring and communication with parent and family are vital to understanding medication benefit and adherence.

Psychostimulants

Psychostimulants (see Chapter 125) are the most studied psychotropics used in pediatrics. These medications are used to treat the hyperactivity, inattention, and impulsivity seen with **attention-deficit/hyperactivity disorder (ADHD)** and disturbances of attention seen in other disorders (**autism, traumatic brain injury, depression,** etc). Stimulants are also used in the treatment of **narcolepsy.** Over the past decade many new delivery systems have been developed with differing durations of action, which help to cater to the specific lifestyle needs of the patient. Much work has been done to determine optimal blood level delivery leading to the most consistent effect. Overall, the duration of action and clinical efficacy are more relevant than the blood level in this class of medication.

The mechanism of action of these agents is to increase **dopamine** and **norepinephrine** in the synapse. Overall, this enhances activity in the **prefrontal cortex** of the brain responsible for attention, focus, and **executive function** (organization and planning).

There is substantial evidence in multisite, double-blind, placebo-controlled studies (eg, Multimodal Treatment Study of Children With Attention-Deficit/Hyperactivity Disorder) to support the first-line use of these medications in the treatment of school-aged children and adolescents with ADHD. There is evolving evidence (Preschool ADHD Treatment Study) to support the use of these drugs in preschoolers. There is a growing body of evidence to support their use in autism, albeit at lower doses and with a lower threshold for side effects.

Parents have a variety of concerns related to stimulants, much of which is propagated by the media; however, NOT treating ADHD results in significant comorbidities and risks for negative outcomes. Nonetheless, several areas of controversy exist, and often become a primary focus for hesitant parents. Understanding the facts can help to demystify these medications for parents. For example, a risk of substance abuse has long been linked with stimulant medication. There is a substantial body of evidence to show that the use of stimulant medication does **not** lead to an increased risk of later substance abuse. In fact it is the untreated ADHD, linked with the development of maladaptive behaviors, which places adolescents at a higher risk of substance abuse. The hypothesis is that treatment of ADHD with stimulant medication will actually reduce substance abuse and a whole host of other potential negative outcomes such as early tobacco use, undesired pregnancy, motor vehicle crashes, etc. More long-term studies will be needed to clarify this issue.

Another frequently raised concern includes the association between stimulants and an increase in sudden unexpected deaths. This would obviously raise discomfort for any parent. However, scrutiny over these statistics by the FDA actually revealed a lower incidence of sudden unexpected deaths in those on stimulants compared with the unmedicated population. Those who died tended to have an underlying cardiac defect. This led to the FDA recommendation (2006) that those persons with **preexisting cardiac conditions** not use stimulants and those families with a history of cardiac structural defects or sudden unexpected death receive an echocardiogram and cardiac clearance prior to starting medication.

Height suppression has also historically been raised as a concern with these medications. Numerous studies have tried to answer this question. A recent longitudinal study (over 10 years) supports an initial growth suppression emphasized in the first 3 years, which appears to resolve over the remaining 7. Parents can be further reassured that if there is height suppression it seems to be minimal, in the range of 1.5 cm. It is better to have a high school graduate who is slightly shorter than a taller dropout. Finally, parents believe that their children will be "zombies" on medication. Children who are overmedicated can appear glassy-eyed and overly passive, but good communication and interaction between families and doctors will quickly alleviate this problem. Additional information regarding these medications may be found in Chapter 125.

Selective Norepinephrine Reuptake Inhibitors

The SNRIs presently include one medication that is frequently used in children: **atomoxetine** (Strattera). Atomoxetine is used in both the treatment of ADHD and for the **inattention** and **anxiety** associated with autism.

The mechanism of action for atomoxetine is to block the reuptake of norepinephrine in the synapse. This may have a direct effect on enhancing the signal-to-noise ratio in the brain and may also ultimately lead to an increase in dopamine in the prefrontal cortex of the brain. Unlike stimulant medications, atomoxetine avoids the nucleus accumbens so that it has no abuse liability.

Atomoxetine was originally studied as an antidepressant, but early investigation did not yield robust antidepressant effects. Marketed as providing "continuous symptom relief," a careful duration of action study shows little effect on core ADHD symptoms after 9 hours, but some possible other small effects (compliance) may last slightly longer. Its attractiveness stems from its identity as an FDA-approved **non-stimulant**. Although usually less effective than stimulants, it has a different side-effect profile and may show slight mood benefits.

Research shows that this medication, which is FDA approved for ADHD, is effective in treating symptoms of this disorder for a given individual, but in groups of people is not as effective as the stimulant medications. Atomoxetine generally has a 60% response rate (measured by 25% reduction in ADHD ratings) compared with a 70% to 80% response (measured by 30% reduction in ADHD ratings) found in stimulant medications. Furthermore, 3 different head-to-head studies with stimulants have demonstrated atomoxetine as less effective on average; however, some individual patients do well with this medication. It should especially be considered in cases of stimulant failure (poor tolerance and/or poor effect of a trial on a methylphenidate preparation and a trial on an amphetamine preparation), worries about substance use and diversion, exacerbation of tic disorder with stimulants, and the presence of comorbid anxiety or autism.

This medication is not without **side effects**. The side effects are very similar to the traditional stimulants with the added concerns of drowsiness, dizziness, and cough. Furthermore, atomoxetine carries a warning citing a slightly increased risk of suicidal thought similar to the SSRIs. It is not associated with tic exacerbation. Response to this medicine is more like that of an antidepressant, in that it may take 4 to 6 weeks to see the full impact of a particular dose. The dosage range is 0.5 mg/kg to 1.8 mg/kg. Those on the autistic spectrum tend to respond at lower doses and with a lower threshold for adverse side effects.

There have been a few reports of a serious **idiosyncratic reaction** suggesting liver failure. These patients were on FDA-approved doses of atomoxetine for several months. They had vomiting, jaundice, and elevated liver enzymes. These findings resolved off medication and returned with reexposure to the drug. This led to an FDA warning to consider potential liver failure in a vomiting patient on atomoxetine.

In consideration of both the stimulants and SNRIs, the American Academy of Pediatrics and the American Academy of Child and Adolescent Psychiatry recommend stimulants and SNRIs as first-line treatments for ADHD. There is no indication that blood or urine tests need to be monitored for either class of medication. Improvement, adverse event, and adherence monitoring using rating scales should occur regularly—at least every 3 months (once dose and agent have been optimized).

Parents often want to know if these medications can be used intermittently and stopped as soon as possible. Stimulants and SNRIs have their best results when administered 7 days a week and without large breaks. Longitudinal studies suggest that while some symptoms may resolve over time, significant impairment from even a small number of symptoms persists into adulthood for 60% to 70% of those diagnosed with ADHD. Therefore, many people may continue on medication for a number of years. To assess for continued benefit, a break from medication should be attempted annually. It is beneficial to reoptimize doses and agents throughout treatment. As children grow larger they often need higher doses. However, as compensatory mechanisms develop and some symptoms subside, some patients may require less medication. "Holidays" from medications has no established intrinsic value on their own and should only be recommended for children with significant medication side effects such as substantial weight loss. If a parent is requesting a **drug holiday** it is a signal that the parent may need to review the value of the medication. A discussion should ensue as to whether the parent and child continue to see benefit, the patient is having troubling side effects, or the medication at any dose is not helpful with concerning symptoms. Consider that atomoxetine, once stopped, needs time to rebuild in the system.

Selective Serotonin Reuptake Inhibitors

The SSRIs (Table 126-1) are frequently used in children and adolescents to treat a variety of depression- and anxiety-based symptoms (Box 126-1). Similar to the SNRIs, the SSRIs block presynaptic reuptake of serotonin after it is released into the synapse, thereby enhancing serotonin activity in the synapse. Empirical evidence has established their benefit in the treatment of depressive disorders and anxiety disorders.

Medication is NOT a substitute for therapeutic support. As a matter of fact, most clinical guidelines recommend psychotherapy as first-line treatment for most anxiety and depressive disorders in children. Biologic intervention should only be undertaken if psychotherapy progress is minimal or impairment severe. **Obsessive-compulsive disorder** (OCD) is a unique anxiety disorder that typically requires higher doses of SSRIs but is also responsive to a specific form of cognitive-behavioral therapy that includes exposure response prevention.

Medications are chosen based on side-effect profile and half-life. Due to a significant placebo effect and a lack of multiple, large, highly powered studies in children, only a few have any FDA approval in children (Table 126-1). There are numerous studies that may not meet strict scientific criteria, but taken together with vast clinical experience and consensus imply reasonably well-tolerated and

---

Box 126-1. Disorders Treated by Selective Serotonin Reuptake Inhibitors

- Depression
- Obsessive-compulsive disorder
- Generalized anxiety disorder
- Separation anxiety disorder
- Panic disorder
- Selective mutism
- Post-traumatic stress disorder
- Autism
- Bulimia

Table 126-1. Selective Serotonin Reuptake Inhibitors					
Generic	*Product*	*FDA Pediatric Approval*	*Suggested Pediatric Dose, mg*	*Half-life*	*Time Steady State, days*
Fluoxetine	Prozac	Depression/OCD	2.5–60	4–6 d	28–35
Sertraline	Zoloft	OCD	12.5–200	26 h	5–7
Fluvoxamine	Luvox	OCD	12.5–100 bid	15 h	5–7
Paroxetine	Paxil	None	5–30	21 h	5–10
Citalopram	Celexa	None	5–40	36 h	7
Escitalopram	Lexapro	Depression	2.5–20	27–32 h	7

Abbreviations: bid, twice a day; FDA, US Food and Drug Administration; OCD, obsessive-compulsive disorder.

beneficial effects of these medications. Studies have consistently found SSRIs to be more effective and safer than the tricyclic antidepressants as a treatment for depression.

These drugs are metabolized via the liver through the **cytochrome P450 system.** There are individual enzyme variations that lead to variable metabolism of any of the many medications that travel through these pathways. Overwhelming this system may lead to inhibition and buildup of medications or facilitated rapid metabolism of others. Thus monitoring of all medications metabolized via this pathway is necessary. Reduced metabolism of the SSRIs may lead to **serotonin syndrome**—a relatively rare response to a flood of serotonin—presenting with confusion, hypomania, restlessness, diaphoresis, shivering, tremor, hyperreflexia, and diarrhea. This syndrome often goes unrecognized and these patients may find their way to a pediatrician's office or emergency department (ED). Occasionally, the combination of an SSRI with an atypical antipsychotic or stimulant may precipitate such a response.

Many children with anxiety or depression go on to experience intermittent exacerbations throughout life. This does not mean that they should stay on these medications forever. Present recommendations support an initial 6- to 12-month treatment period with the SSRI that provided response. If the symptoms return after discontinuation, the next trial should last 2 years. Finally, if the symptoms again return, then this suggests longer-term treatment. Occasionally, symptoms will not respond the next time the same agent is used.

Selective serotonin reuptake inhibitors are generally well tolerated with mild transient side effects such as gastrointestinal symptoms, headache, increased motor activity, or insomnia. One needs to monitor for less common side effects like disinhibition, a phenomenon of increased impulsive behaviors in association with SSRIs that is usually dose related. Those with autism are particularly susceptible to this response.

There are no specific recommendations on dose other than to start low and go slow. Typically effects may be seen between 1 and 4 weeks. The value of increasing the dose (except in the case of OCD) versus continuing on at the same dose versus changing agents is not clear until a patient has been treated for at least a month. See suggested dosage ranges in Table 126-1.

Some have suggested that these medications are **addictive.** This relates to the appearance of withdrawal symptoms on sudden cessation. Abruptly stopping medications that have a shorter half-life such as paroxetine and sertraline may lead to flu-like symptoms including body aches and vomiting. A child may present to their primary care provider with flu-like symptoms, not recognizing a connection between the symptoms and having skipped their medications for several days. The onset and severity of symptoms is proportional to the dose and duration of use and inversely proportional to the half-life. Occasionally, these children end up hospitalized for vomiting and dehydration. Simply readministering their skipped dose alleviates the symptoms. A planned taper should take 4 to 6 weeks.

Again, controversy follows these medications. In 2004 the FDA created a black box warning advising that children and adolescents on SSRIs should be monitored for worsening depression, agitation, and suicidality, particularly in the early stages of treatment. This warning came out of an FDA meta-analysis showing an increased risk of suicidal ideation in depressed teens soon after starting the medications. No completed suicides occurred. This prompted an FDA recommendation to see children placed on SSRIs weekly for a month, then bimonthly for a month, then monthly and, ultimately, at longer regular intervals. This expectation was felt to be impractical for clinicians in practice. Therefore, these recommendations have recently been relaxed to incorporate physician judgment. It is advised to monitor each individual patient carefully, but the potential for benefit usually outweighs the risks. These concerns should NOT detract from the importance of these medications.

The FDA warning led to a decrease in prescriptions of SSRIs, which resulted in the first increase in the suicide rate since the FDA SSRI approval. The FDA warnings should serve only to increase awareness, not be a contraindication. An increase in suicidality has not been noted in adolescents with isolated anxiety or autism. Selective serotonin reuptake inhibitors serve a vital role in helping children paralyzed by anxiety, obsession, and depression to lead more normal lives.

Atypical Antipsychotics (Serotonergic Dopamine Antagonists)

The **atypical antipsychotics** or **second-generation antipsychotics** (Table 126-2), also known as **SDAs,** are medications with dopamine D2 and serotonin 5-hydroxytryptamine type 2 antagonism. These newer medications offer a lower risk of both **extrapyramidal side effects** like **dystonia; akathisia,** a feeling of restlessness; tremor; tardive dyskinesia; and hyperprolactinemia compared with the conventional antipsychotics. However, these medications carry significant cardiometabolic risks. Although initially billed as a safer alternative to traditional antipsychotics, some have suggested that these newer medications merely substitute one set of severe side effects

Table 126-2. Serotonin-Dopamine Antagonists (Atypical Antipsychotics)			
Generic	*Product*	*FDA Pediatric Approval*	*Dose*
Risperidone	Risperdol	Agitation with autism, schizophrenia, mania, and bipolar disorder	.25–10 mg/day
Olanzepine	Zyprexa	None	2.5–20 mg/day
Quetiapine	Seroquel	None	12.5–250 mg bid
Ziprasodone	Geodon	None	20–120 mg/day
Aripiprazole	Abilify	Agitation with autism, schizophrenia, mania, and bipolar disorder	.5–30 mg/day

Abbreviations: bid, twice a day; FDA, US Food and Drug Administration.

for another. These medications offer benefits for severe behaviors that are not responsive to other intervention.

While often used off-label, these medications are incorporated into best practice clinical guidelines for psychotic depression, schizophrenia, bipolar disorder, oppositional defiant disorder, conduct disorder, agitation in mental retardation, Tourette disorder, stuttering, and autism. The only diagnoses for which an atypical antipsychotic has pediatric approval are schizophrenia, bipolar disorder, mania, and agitation associated with autism. Therefore, while these medications often lack enough empiric evidence to be validated for all the indications mentioned, clinical consensus by experts recommend judicious use in treating children with serious mental illness after other forms of intervention have failed or in cases of severe psychosis or aggression. These medications should NOT be used to promote weight gain, as a sedative or sleep aid, or as a treatment for ADHD.

Medications are chosen based on clinical experience and side-effect profile. These medications are not innocuous. They must be used with full disclosure to parents. The most common side effects are listed in Box 126-2. The severity of some of the side effects deserve discussion. The SDAs, with possibly the exception of aripiprazole, have caused significant increases in weight, glucose, and lipids, and decreases in sensitivity to insulin, otherwise known as *metabolic syndrome.*

Box 126-2. Serotonin-Dopamine Antagonists: Potential Side Effects	
• Weight gain	• Dry mouth
• Sedation	• Headache
• Dizziness	• Cataracts (in dogs)
• Hypotension	• Increased liver function tests
• Prolongation of QT interval	• Decreased triiodothyronine, thyroxine
• Metabolic syndrome (hyperglycemia and increased lipids)	• Extrapyramidal side effects
	• Akathisia (sense of restlessness)
• Constipation	

There have been transient elevations of **prolactin** among recipients of these medications. The clinical significance of this increase is unclear. Weight gain frequently accompanies these medications and must be monitored. A prolonged QT interval on electrocardiogram (ECG) is rarely noted and has not been associated with death, but remains a clinical concern.

Risperidone is the best studied medication of its class for children. However, the studies on which its FDA approvals hinged exposed side effects, most notably weight gain. Therefore, anticipatory counseling regarding diet management is routinely recommended. Another important finding indicated that a small but significant number of children with agitation and autism were successfully able to stop treatment after 6 months, suggesting that a trial off medication may be warranted in those patients with agitation and autism successfully treated for 6 months.

Neuroleptic malignant syndrome is a rare, potentially life-threatening complication of neuroleptics that is extremely unlikely with the newer generation of medication. However, due to its lethality and its potential presentation to a pediatric office or ED this entity should be mentioned. Neuroleptic malignant syndrome is characterized by hyperthermia, autonomic instability, diaphoresis, "lead pipe" rigidity, increased creatine phosphokinase due to rhabdomyolysis, and delirium. It may occur at any point during treatment with these medications.

There is no set agreement on appropriate monitoring of these medications in children. Most conservative suggestions include following body mass index (BMI) at each visit, after 6 weeks, and again each 9 to 12 months checking complete blood cell count, a comprehensive chemistry including liver function tests, triiodothyronine, thyroxine, HbA1c, prolactin, fasting glucose, and lipid levels, especially in overweight children or in families with a history of diabetes mellitus. An ECG prior to starting medications, 1 month after baseline, and biannually are only necessary for children on ziprasidone to monitor the QT interval. Children are often sent to the primary care provider to obtain these tests and to monitor BMI.

As with any medication, psychotropic agents are sometimes misprescribed. By and large, however, psychopharmacologic agents are still underused in the treatment of many disorders. Hopefully, new and ongoing research will help physicians recognize mental illness in children and substantiate and refine the use of such medications in their care.

Careful thought and discussion of target symptoms as well as side effects will help physicians choose the best medication and treatment plan. It will also prepare parents to observe both the positive and negative response to medication.

While this chapter goes into significant detail on side effects, it is critical to understand that the diseases being treated are often incapacitating. Informed consent and parent/child involvement are vital in medication choice. Pediatricians have an extremely influential voice in supporting compliance. Therefore, knowledgeable guidance is crucial in helping parents make an uncomfortable and difficult decision that may ultimately lead to dramatic improvements in quality of life.

CASE RESOLUTION

You empathize with the parents over this decision but are able to explain that this medication is a reasonable and safe one to try. The patient starts the medication and experiences some nausea in the first few days. With your reassurance, this resolves. Her mom calls a few weeks later to thank you for your advice and to let you know that while her daughter still has difficulties from the autism, she seems to be somewhat less anxious and is functioning better at school.

Selected References

American Academy of Pediatrics Subcommittee on Attention-Deficit/Hyperactivity Disorder and Committee on Quality Improvement. Clinical practice guideline: treatment of the school-aged child with attention-deficit/hyperactivity disorder. *Pediatrics.* 2001;108:1033–1044

Biederman J, Spencer TJ, Monuteaux MC, et al. A naturalistic 10-year prospective study of height and weight in children with attention-deficit hyperactivity disorder grown up: sex and treatment effects. *J Pediatr.* 2010;157(4):635–640

Centers for Disease Control and Prevention. Prevalence of autism spectrum disorders—autism and Developmental Disabilities Monitoring Network, United States, 2006. *MMWR Morb Mortal Wkly Rep.* 2009;58(SS10):1–20

Filipek PA, Steinberg-Epstein R, Book TM. Intervention for autism spectrum disorders. *NeuroRx.* 2006;3:207–216

Greenhill L, Kollins S, Abikoff H, et al. Efficacy and safety of immediate-release methylphenidate treatment for preschool children with ADHD. *J Am Acad Child Adolesc Psychiatry.* 2006;45:1284–1293

Hammad TA, Laughren T, Racoosin J. Suicidality in pediatric patients treated with antidepressant drugs. *Arch Gen Psychiatry.* 2006;63:332–339

March J, Silva S, Petrycki S, et al. Fluoxetine, cognitive-behavioral therapy, and their combination for adolescents with depression: Treatment for Adolescents With Depression Study (TADS) randomized controlled trial. *JAMA.* 2004;292:807–820

McCracken JT, McGough J, Shah B, et al. Risperidone in children with autism and serious behavior problems. *N Engl J Med.* 2002;347:314–321

Merikangas KR, He JP, Burstein M, et al. Lifetime prevalence of mental disorders in US adolescents: results from the National Comorbidity Survey Replication (NCS-A). *J Am Acad Child Adolesc Psychiatry.* 2010;49(10):980–989

MTA Cooperative Group. A 14-month randomized clinical trial of treatment strategies for attention-deficit/hyperactivity disorder. *Arch Gen Psychiatry.* 1999;56:1073–1086

www.Nationalautismcenter.org. Study accessed 12/2010.

Pediatric OCD Treatment Study (POTS) Team. Cognitive-behavior therapy, sertraline, and their combination for children and adolescents with obsessive-compulsive disorder: the Pediatric OCD Treatment Study (POTS) randomized controlled trial. *JAMA.* 2004;292:1969–1976

Pliszka SR. AACAP Workgroup on Quality Issues: practice parameters for the assessment and treatment of children and adolescents with attention deficit hyperactivity disorder. *J Adolesc Child Psychiatry.* 2007;46:894–921

Sadock B, Sadock V. *Kaplan and Sadock's Synopsis of Psychiatry.* 9th ed. Philadelphia, PA: Lippincott Williams & Wilkins; 2003

US Food and Drug Administration Center for Drug Evaluation and Research Psychopharmacologic Drugs Advisory Committee. Sparlon (Provigil/Modafinil) Cephalon Inc. NDA 20-717 (S-109) [PowerPoint presentation]. www.fda.gov/ohrms/dockets/ac/06/slides/2006-4212S1-01-01-FDAMannheim.ppt

Walkup JT, Albano AM, Piacentini J, et al. Cognitive-behavioral therapy, sertraline, or a combination in childhood anxiety. *N Engl J Med.* 2008;359(26):2753–2766

Wigal T, Wigal S, Shanklin A, Kapelinski A, Steinberg-Epstein R. ADHD in preschoolers: a diagnosis or just a "phase"? *Consult Pediatr.* 2008;(suppl):S2–S8

CHAPTER 127

Physical Abuse

Melissa K. Egge, MD, and Sara T. Stewart, MD

CASE STUDY

A 6-month-old male infant arrives at the emergency department after becoming limp and nonresponsive at home. The mother states that her son was fine when she left him in the care of her boyfriend before going to the store for cigarettes. When she returned 1 hour later, he was asleep, but then he seized and stopped breathing. The infant is being ventilated by bag-valve-mask ventilation. On examination, the infant is pale and limp. The heart rate is 50 beats/min and the blood pressure is 130/80 mm Hg. There are no external signs of injury.

Questions

1. What are the major lethal injuries associated with physical abuse of children?
2. What are the types of injuries seen in physically abused children?
3. What are the presenting signs in children with head injuries?
4. What are the legal obligations of physicians in the area of child abuse?

Physical child abuse was first described in the pediatric literature in 1962 by Kempe et al in their classic paper on the **battered child syndrome.** Child abuse or maltreatment takes many forms, including physical abuse; **failure to thrive** (Chapter 129); **sexual abuse** (Chapter 128); **emotional abuse; prenatal exposure to substances** such as drugs and alcohol (Chapter 131); and **pediatric condition falsification (also referred to as medical child abuse),** a complex disorder previously known as Munchausen syndrome by proxy in which parents confabulate or create a medical condition in their children.

The nature and extent of inflicted injuries are variable and may include **bruises, burns, fractures, lacerations, internal hemorrhage,** and **ruptures.** Physicians must be aware of the legal obligations related to the suspicion of child abuse. They must assess the nature of the injuries, initiate appropriate medical therapy, and determine if the history offered is consistent with the medical findings.

Epidemiology

It is estimated that the rate of childhood victimization in the United States is 10 per 1,000, and that approximately 15% to 20% of these children suffer some form of physical abuse. Certain factors are associated with physical abuse. Most victims are young children; two-thirds are younger than 3 years and one-third are younger than 6 months. Caring for young children is frequently demanding, so crying infants and toilet-training toddlers are particularly at risk for abuse. Factors such as **lower socioeconomic class, substance abuse, poor parenting skills,** and **domestic violence** place children at increased risk for abuse.

Clinical Presentation

Children who have been physically abused present with injuries that range from non-severe to lethal (Dx Box). Visible bruises, **bites,** and burns may be noted. Children may also have symptoms related to fractures, such as crying or refusal to walk or move an extremity. More severely injured children may present with seizures, apnea, shock, or cardiopulmonary arrest.

Dx Physical Abuse

- Bruises
- Bites
- Burns
- Fractures
- Intracranial hemorrhage
- Intra-abdominal hemorrhage
- Apparent life-threatening event
- Retinal hemorrhage
- History that changes
- Injuries not explained by history

Pathophysiology

Injuries in children who experience physical abuse are the result of direct trauma inflicted on the children. Abusive parents often have unrealistic expectations of their children, leading to frustration and abuse when the child does not meet the expectations. Parents who have often been victims of abuse themselves know only corporal punishment as a disciplinary modality. These parents often exhibit poor impulse control; they do not intend to harm their children but desire to alter their children's behavior. As a result, sometimes the outcome is unexpected.

Head injuries, the most deadly form of abuse, may result from either a direct blow to the head or from rotational head movement (eg, shaking). Classically, a crying infant is vigorously shaken and suffers **diffuse axonal injury** or **intracranial hemorrhage.** In particular, subdural hemorrhage may occur from rupture of the bridging veins. The infant may also become apneic either during or after the trauma. Seizures, cerebral edema, hypoxic brain injury, and retinal hemorrhages may also occur. Such injuries are frequently associated with a fatal outcome or long-term damage to the central nervous system.

Abdominal trauma is the second most common cause of fatal child abuse and is typically due to a direct blow to the abdomen. Skeletal fractures result from multiple different types of traumatic forces to the bones. Rib fractures are most classically associated with the head trauma of shaking and are due to compression of the ribs by the hands that are holding the infant or child.

Differential Diagnosis

When evaluating children with physical injuries, the major differentiation is the distinguishing of injuries that are **intentional** or **abuse-related** from those that are **unintentional.** Practitioners should be suspicious of changing histories, histories that are inconsistent with the injuries sustained, and histories that do not match the developmental capabilities of the child. Unwitnessed injuries in young children, particularly pre-ambulatory infants, should also be suspect.

Bruises, burns, and fractures may be intentional or unintentional. Normal ambulatory children sustain bruises over bony prominences such as the forehead, elbows, and shins with unintentional, accidental trauma. Bruises over soft areas such as the cheeks or the pinnae of the ear, as well as bruises on protected areas such as the inner thighs or neck, are more suggestive of inflicted trauma. Injuries to the oral mucosa may result from efforts at forced feeding or occlusion of the mouth in an effort to silence crying. **Retinal hemorrhages** in infants most often result from intentional head trauma, such as shaking. They may also be due to other medical conditions that can usually be discerned from the history and physical examination and by consultation with an ophthalmologist. Ideally, a pediatric ophthalmologist performs indirect retinal examination of dilated eyes within 24 hours of the patient's admission (Box 127-1).

Children may be intentionally burned by being immersed in hot water or having hot objects such as irons or cigarettes held against them. Children who are immersed in hot water develop circumferential burns that may envelop an entire extremity. Such a burn is usually in a glove or stocking pattern, or in a doughnut pattern on the buttocks. These burns are distinct from splash or spill burns, which take on an irregular drip pattern. In distinguishing inflicted from accidental burns, a scene investigation is often helpful to measure the water temperature in the home water heater and determine the length of time required to reach that temperature in the location of the alleged incident. Families should be advised that their water heaters be set to 120°F to prevent accidental scald injuries.

Box 127-1. Causes of Retinal Hemorrhages	
• Inflicted head trauma	• Hypo- or hypernatremia
• Unintentional head trauma (rare)	• Vasculitis
• Birth trauma	• Papilledema
• Retinopathy of prematurity	• Hypertension
• Blood dyscrasias	• Cytomegalovirus retinitis
• Leukemia/lymphoma	• High-altitude illness
• Meningitis/sepsis	• Carbon monoxide toxicity
• Extracorporeal membrane oxygenation (ECMO)	• Osteogenesis imperfecta
	• Glutaric aciduria

Long bone fractures (especially humerus and femur) should be suspect, particularly in preverbal or pre-ambulatory children. Certain fractures, such as **classic metaphyseal lesions, rib, sternum,** and **scapula fractures,** are highly suggestive of inflicted trauma.

Numerous medical conditions may mimic abuse. Bullous impetigo may resemble burns. A coagulopathy may lead to multiple bruises. Leukemia, thrombocytopenia, and aplastic anemia are also associated with bruising. Osteogenesis imperfecta or rickets may result in multiple fractures. Bone cysts and osteoporosis due to inactivity from multiple causes (eg, cerebral palsy, paralysis, and meningomyelocele) may predispose to the development of pathologic fractures.

Evaluation

Children who present with injuries need to be evaluated with a careful history and complete physical examination. Infants with altered mental status, apnea, or seizures should be evaluated in a similar manner because their symptoms may be secondary to intracranial injury.

History

The history should focus on an explanation for the medical findings (Questions Box) and, in infants and toddlers, a thorough developmental history should be included. Children should be interviewed alone if they are of an appropriate age. Physicians should determine if other risk factors, such as domestic violence or substance abuse, are present.

Questions

Physical Abuse

- What caused the injury?
- Was the child healthy until the injury occurred?
- Has the child sustained similar injuries in the past?
- Is there a family history of any conditions that would account for easy bruisability or fragility of the bones (eg, von Willebrand disease, osteogenesis imperfecta)?
- Is the child developmentally normal? What are the child's motor skills?
- Who was with the child when the injury occurred?
- What was done immediately after the injury? Was medical care sought?

Physical Examination

A child's state of hygiene and growth parameters should be noted, and the physical examination should be comprehensive. The location, color, and size of bruises, abrasions, lacerations, or other skin trauma should be recorded. Dating of bruises is imprecise because the degradation rate of hemoglobin, and therefore the rate of color change, is influenced by the depth and extent of the bruise and by the child's health and nutritional status. Large blue-brown spots, which occur commonly on the back and buttocks in darker-skinned children, are termed *mongolian spots* or *congenital dermal melanocytosis.* These should not be mistaken for bruises.

Medical providers should also note any skin findings that resemble characteristic patterns of inflicted skin trauma, such as slap marks to the face or gag marks around the mouth. Pinch marks can also be seen on the genitalia of a toilet-training toddler. Belts, cords, and blunt objects may leave patterned marks on the skin after a child is hit with the object. Bite marks are composed of indentations, bruises, or breaks in the skin that reflect the configuration of teeth that is unique to the perpetrator (Figure 127-1). Inflicted burns may also assume a characteristic pattern depending on the mechanism of injury (Figure 127-2).

The extremities, skull, and ribcage should be carefully examined to detect the presence of skeletal trauma. Findings such as decreased range of movement, tenderness, swelling, redness, or bruising may be associated with an underlying bone fracture. These findings are not always present, however, particularly if the fracture is in its healing stages.

Practitioners should be aware that infants with head or abdominal injuries may also present with no external signs of trauma. Those with head injury may have seizures, apnea, vomiting, increased crying, or altered mental status, often with no explanation as to the etiology. The retina should be evaluated for hemorrhages in these children. Children with abdominal injuries may present in shock or with symptoms such as vomiting, abdominal pain, or distention. They may have a rigid abdomen with guarding and decreased bowel sounds. Inflicted abdominal injuries may include hematomas of the bowel wall, bowel perforations; or trauma to the liver, spleen, pancreas, or kidneys.

Laboratory Tests

Children who present with bruises should have a hematologic assessment with a complete blood cell count (CBC) and differential (including a platelet count), a prothrombin time, and a partial thromboplastin time. Cultures from lesions may help differentiate infection from burn injury.

Children with fractures should be assessed with a chemistry panel (including blood urea nitrogen and creatinine), calcium, phosphorus, and alkaline phosphatase levels.

Children with suspected abdominal trauma should be evaluated with a CBC, urinalysis, liver function studies, amylase, and lipase. These studies may demonstrate anemia secondary to hemorrhage, hematuria from renal injury, or elevated liver or pancreatic enzymes due to solid or hollow viscus organ trauma (see Chapter 63).

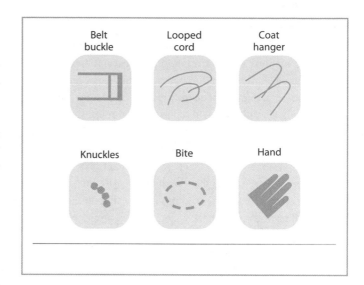

Figure 127-1. Patterned bruises associated with inflicted trauma.

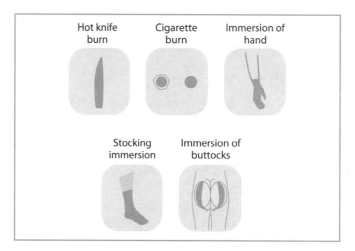

Figure 127-2. Patterned burns associated with inflicted trauma.

Imaging Studies

Children younger than 2 years who are suspected victims of physical abuse are at the highest risk of having an inflicted skeletal fracture. For this reason, this group of patients should be evaluated with a radiographic skeletal survey to identify any acute or healing fractures that may be present. Bone scintigraphy is also useful in detecting occult fractures and may be useful in conjunction with the skeletal survey. Follow-up skeletal survey in 2 weeks can also be useful to assess for fractures that were not noted at the time of the initial films.

If there is concern that children have suffered non-accidental head trauma, they should be evaluated with a computed tomography (CT) scan and magnetic resonance imaging. The combination of these modalities is particularly helpful in dating intracranial bleeding (see Chapter 64).

Abdominal radiographs may demonstrate air-fluid levels from dysmotility, distended loops of bowel, or free air under the diaphragm. Abdominal and pelvic CT scans may show bowel or solid organ disruption or hemorrhage.

Management

The management of children who are suspected victims of abuse focuses on medical stabilization and psychosocial investigation. Injuries should be treated in the appropriate manner. Children with extensive internal injuries frequently require admission to an intensive care unit. Consultation with appropriate surgical specialists in neurosurgery, orthopedics, or general surgery should be obtained.

The psychosocial assessment of the family often requires the expertise of a social worker. Further assessment may require an in-home evaluation such as that conducted by law enforcement or child protective services. All 50 states require that physicians who suspect child abuse report these suspicions to appropriate agencies. Physicians do not have to be certain of the abuse.

These mandated agencies pursue the investigation and provide supportive family services as needed. Children may be removed from their homes and placed in foster homes to ensure their safety. Cases of suspected abuse are usually evaluated in court to determine the safety of the children's environment, the ability of parents to care for their children, and the criminal culpability of suspected perpetrators. Physicians may be expected to offer testimony in such hearings.

Prognosis

The prognosis is variable. Some children succumb to inflicted injuries before coming to medical attention, and others sustain permanent neurologic damage. Even in cases in which the physical well-being of children is ensured, their mental and emotional well-being is often significantly impacted, requiring intensive and ongoing mental health care.

Recent longitudinal studies in adults have shown a link between adverse childhood experiences and health problems in adulthood.

Prevention

Practitioners should preemptively discuss with families those developmental stages that are at higher risk for parental frustration and subsequent child abuse, including infant colic, toddler potty training, and tantrums. Infant crying is the most common trigger for abusive head injury. A pediatric provider may offer guidance in handling these difficult situations and should assess the parents' coping skills with such behaviors when they arise. Pediatricians should also inquire about stressors particular to each family, such as unemployment, mental health issues, social isolation, and intimate partner violence. Support systems for the family should be identified and positive attributes praised.

CASE RESOLUTION

The case study describes a classic case of non-accidental trauma. The infant was left alone with an individual with limited parenting skills. The infant has evidence of increased intracranial pressure, and may have traumatic axonal injury or intracranial hemorrhage. The infant is intubated, given anticonvulsants, and admitted to a pediatric intensive care unit. Consultation with neurosurgery, ophthalmology, and social services is obtained. Appropriate imaging studies and skeletal surveys are performed when the infant is sufficiently stabilized, and the child is ultimately diagnosed with subdural hemorrhage, retinal hemorrhages, and rib fractures.

Selected References

Dubowitz H, Bennett S. Physical abuse and neglect of children. *Lancet.* 2007;369:1891–1899

Felitti VJ, Anda RF, Nordenberg D, et al. Relationship of childhood abuse and household dysfunction to many of the leading causes of death in adults: the Adverse Childhood Experiences (ACE) Study. *Am J Prev Med.* 1998;14:245–258

Flaherty EG, Stirling J. American Academy of Pediatrics Committee on Child Abuse and Neglect. Clinical report—the pediatrician's role in child maltreatment prevention. *Pediatrics.* 2010;126:834–841

Gerber P, Coffman K. Nonaccidental head trauma in infants. *Childs Nerv Syst.* 2007;23:499–507

Jenny C, American Academy of Pediatrics Committee on Child Abuse and Neglect. Evaluating infants and young children with multiple fractures. *Pediatrics.* 2006;118:1299–1303

Kellogg ND, American Academy of Pediatrics Committee on Child Abuse and Neglect. Evaluation of suspected child physical abuse. *Pediatrics.* 2007;119:1232–1241

Kempe CH, Silverman FN, Steele BF, Droegemueller W, Silver HK. The battered child syndrome. *JAMA.* 1962;181:17–24

Levin AV. Retinal hemorrhages: advances in understanding. *Pediatr Clin North Am.* 2009;56:333–344

Offiah A, van Rijn RR, Perez-Rossello JM, Kleinman PK. Skeletal imaging of child abuse. *Pediatr Radiol.* 2009;39:461–470

Reece RM, Christian C, eds. *Child Abuse: Medical Diagnosis and Management.* 3rd ed. Elk Grove Village, IL: American Academy of Pediatrics; 2008

Shipman K. Mental health treatment of child abuse and neglect: the promise of evidence-based practice. *Pediatr Clin North Am.* 2009;56:417–428

Swerdlin A, Berkowitz C, Craft N. Cutaneous signs of child abuse. *J Am Acad Dermatol.* 2007;57:371–392

CHAPTER 128

Sexual Abuse

Sara T. Stewart, MD

CASE STUDY

A 4-year-old girl is brought to the emergency department with the complaint of vaginal itching and discharge. Her past health has been good, and she has no medical problems. She lives with her biological parents and her 2-year-old brother.

On physical examination, the vital signs are normal and the child is well except that the genital area is swollen and erythematous and a green vaginal discharge is present. The girl is interviewed briefly but denies that anyone has touched her. The mother states that she has never left her daughter unattended and is angered by the questions.

Questions

1. What are the anogenital findings in prepubescent and postpubescent children who may have experienced sexual abuse?
2. What behavioral problems are common in children who have been sexually abused?
3. What are the pitfalls in disclosure interviews of children who have been sexually abused?
4. What is the significance of sexually transmitted infections (STIs) in children who have been sexually abused?

Child sexual abuse is the involvement of children and adolescents in sexual activity that they cannot consent to because of their age and developmental level. An age disparity exists between the victims, who are younger, and the perpetrators, who are older. The intent of the abuse is the **sexual gratification** of the older individuals, and the abusive incident(s) may or may not include physical contact. Sexual abuse may include acts of **oral, genital,** or **anal** contact by or to a child and may involve acts such as **exhibitionism** or involvement in **pornography.** It is differentiated from "sexual play" by the difference in the developmental levels of the participants and the coerciveness of the behavior.

Sexual abuse has been recognized with increasing frequency since the 1980s, in part because medical knowledge about the anogenital anatomy in both molested and non-molested prepubescent children has expanded. Technical advances have altered the manner in which these children are evaluated. In particular, the colposcope, with its potential for magnification and photographic or videotape documentation, has been valuable. Parental awareness and school-based programs have led to increased disclosures about abuse as well as a greater willingness on the part of adults to believe these disclosures.

Patient interviews are another key component of the assessment process that has been shaped by continued research in the field. Nonleading, open-ended questions are asked by interviewers as few times as possible and, when available, these questions are asked by specialized forensic interviewers.

Epidemiology

Approximately 17 in 1,000 children are thought to be victims of child maltreatment per year in the United States, and 10% of these are victims of sexual abuse. Exact figures on the prevalence of child sexual abuse are not readily available because they depend on reports of a condition that may not come to medical attention for many years. Anonymous surveys indicate that about 20% to 25% of women and 10% to 15% of men have been sexually abused before reaching adulthood.

Victims of sexual abuse come from all socioeconomic and ethnic groups. Girls experience sexual abuse at a rate 5 times that of boys. Some investigators believe that the statistics for boys are falsely low because boys are generally reluctant to disclose their abuse. Men are more commonly the perpetrators than women, and at least 20% of perpetrators are adolescents. Frequently, the sexual abuse has been occurring for several years. Perpetrators are usually known by the victims, and recent national data showed that 37% of perpetrators were biological parents, 23% were nonbiological parents, and 40% were other individuals. The mean time from onset of abuse to disclosure is 3 years. Sometimes children are not ready to disclose but the abuse is discovered accidentally because the victims develop symptoms, such as vaginal discharge or functional complaints.

Clinical Presentation

Most cases of child sexual abuse come to the attention of authorities after the child **discloses** the abuse. There may or may not be associated physical or behavioral complaints. Physical symptoms in the anogenital area may include **bleeding, pain, swelling, dysuria, vaginal discharge,** or **difficulty stooling.** More often, however, children have no specific anogenital symptoms. Instead, they have nonspecific complaints such as headache, abdominal pain, or vague systemic symptoms such as fatigue (Dx Box).

Dx   Child Sexual Abuse

- Anogenital erythema
- Anogenital bleeding
- Genital discharge
- Anogenital scarring
- Behavioral symptoms (eg, encopresis, enuresis)
- Disclosure of abuse
- Somatic complaints (eg, abdominal pain, headache)
- Sexually transmitted infections
- Sexualized behavior
- Pregnancy (adolescents)
- Delinquency, promiscuity (adolescents)

Behavioral changes may also be noted as these children respond to the stress of their victimization and their environments. These changes may include **sleep disturbances, hyperactivity, enuresis, encopresis, decreased appetite,** and **depression.** Sexually abused adolescents may manifest **school failure, delinquency**, and **suicide** attempts. Children may also respond with sexual behavior or sexual knowledge that is considered to be inappropriate or excessive for age.

Psychophysiology

Children suffer sexual abuse after becoming **entrapped.** They may be enticed with promises of rewards or presents, or may be made to feel special or grown up by being allowed to engage in adult behavior. Some children do not regard the sexual experiences as threatening but rather as a means by which they can obtain the love they crave. Only when they grow older do they realize that these sexual relationships were not normal or appropriate.

Other children are **coerced** into sexual activity with threats of physical harm. Once they have acquiesced, they are maintained in the relationship with threats of reprisal if they disclose the abuse. Children feel both guilty and responsible for what has happened. This sense of responsibility for family disruption is often perpetuated by the legal system, which may remove the children from their families or may place the offending family member in custody.

Lastly, some children enter into sexual relationships out of **curiosity.** They too become entrapped, particularly because they were initially willing to participate.

As a child reacts to an abusive experience, it is common to feel a need for secrecy. As a result, disclosures of abuse are often delayed, and when they do occur, the child often provides the information incrementally over time. Children may also recant their disclosures about abuse; such recantations are not considered to reliably indicate that the abuse did not occur.

Differential Diagnosis

A number of medical conditions that involve the anogenital area may be mistaken for acute or chronic changes due to sexual abuse (Box 128-1).

Box 128-1. Conditions Mistaken for Sexual Abuse

Genital	*Anal*
• Accidental trauma	• Inflammatory bowel disease
• Lichen sclerosus et atrophicus	• Hemorrhoids
• Urethral prolapse	• Anal abscess associated with neutropenia
• Labial adhesions	• Perirectal abscess
• Congenital malformations	• Perianal streptococcal infection
• Hemangioma	

Children may sustain accidental blunt or **penetrating** injuries to the genital area. The most common of these are **straddle injuries** that occur from falls. Pain and bleeding are the most common symptoms with these injuries, and the labia majora, labia minora, or periurethral areas are typically affected. The hymen is unaffected.

Genital bleeding is also a frequent complaint in girls with **urethral prolapse,** a condition that is reported most often in prepubescent African American girls between 4 and 8 years of age. These girls have a protuberant mass extruding from the urethra. The condition is of uncertain etiology but it is not related to abuse.

Lichen sclerosus et atrophicus is a less common dermatologic condition that can also be confused with the sequelae of sexual abuse. In this condition, there is typically atrophic, hypopigmented skin in a figure eight configuration in the anogenital area with associated macules, papules, and hemorrhagic blisters. The skin changes may be misinterpreted as scarring from prior abuse and because the atrophic skin is easily traumatized, findings may also be confused with recent abuse. One factor that may differentiate this condition from injuries related to sexual abuse is that the hymen is unaffected in lichen sclerosis et atrophicus.

Labial adhesions occur most commonly in toddlers and may be confused with scarring from prior sexual abuse. The adhesions develop as the result of inflammation in the genital area of a prepubertal (hypoestrogenic) female. There can be multiple causes of the inflammation, including poor hygiene, recurrent vulvovaginitis, and trauma. The presence of labial adhesions is not a specific indicator of past sexual abuse.

Congenital malformations may also affect the anogenital area. **Failure of midline fusion** along the median raphe can have the appearance of denuded skin and may be confused with an abrasion or superficial laceration of the area. This failure of fusion is a congenital finding, however, and there is no bleeding as with a traumatic injury. Other congenital malformations include hemangiomas that may bleed and be mistaken for traumatized tissue. These hemangiomas are most often noted in infants younger than 2 to 3 years, and they usually regress with time.

Medical conditions may also affect the perianal area and may be mistaken for abuse. **Crohn disease** may lead to fissures, fistulas, perirectal abscesses, or tags. In general, Crohn disease affects older children and produces other symptoms such as fever, weight loss, and stooling problems, or extraintestinal symptomatology. Perirectal abscesses may occur in patients with neutropenia, sometimes as the presenting complaint of leukemia. Hemorrhoids occur rarely in children, and their presence should raise concern about intra-abdominal venous congestion.

Conditions causing **vaginal discharge** (Box 128-2) may be related to sexual abuse, particularly if they are secondary to STIs such as **gonorrhea** or *Chlamydia* infection. Other agents, including *Candida, Shigella,* and **group A beta-hemolytic streptococci,** may produce similar symptoms, yet not be sexually acquired. The streptococci may produce a painful erythematous rash in the perianal area, which is frequently misdiagnosed as secondary to trauma or sexual abuse.

Box 128-2. Conditions Associated With Vaginal Discharge

- Gonorrhea
- *Chlamydia*
- *Trichomonas*
- Bacterial vaginosis
- Candidiasis
- Shigellosis
- Group A beta-hemolytic streptococcus infection
- Vaginal foreign body

Evaluation

The extent and urgency of the evaluation is in part dependent on whether the allegations involve an acute abusive episode or one that occurred in the past. An acute abusive episode (one that has occurred within the previous 72 hours) warrants an immediate assessment for evidence that may otherwise be lost within hours.

History

When a child presents with a physical finding, statement, or behavior that raises the concern of possible sexual abuse, it is important for the examiner to ask carefully thought out, non-leading questions to determine whether the level of suspicion has been reached such that the examiner is mandated to report the concern to a child protective services agency. Beyond that, an attempt should be made to minimize the number of times that the child is questioned about the abuse-related incidents. It is also important to establish sufficient medical history to address any pressing clinical issues. Such a history should include a review of systems, menstrual history, sexual activity history, past incidents of abuse, and any prior genital trauma or medical procedures of the anogenital area. A psychosocial history should also be obtained, as behavioral problems, depression, anxiety, suicidality, homicidality, and other issues requiring mental health expertise are common in sexually abused children (Box 128-3).

Because most victims of sexual abuse have a normal physical examination, the history is often of primary importance in the case. As a result, the child must also be interviewed by someone with

Box 128-3. Problems Reported in Sexually Abused Children

- Enuresis
- Encopresis
- Sexualized behavior
- Pseudomaturity
- Vaginal discharge
- Sleep disturbances
- Suicide
- School failure
- Delinquency (adolescents)
- Promiscuity (adolescents)

professional expertise in the areas of interviewing and child sexual abuse. This individual may be a physician, or it may be a social worker, psychologist, rape counselor, or specialized detective or district attorney. The interview should be structured to include open-ended questions such as, "Tell me what happened" (Questions Box). Interview tools such as drawings or anatomically detailed dolls may be used but are best left to experts with experience in these controversial modalities. Statements that children make should be recorded in the medical record as close to verbatim as possible.

Questions
Child Sexual Abuse

- Can you tell me what happened?
- Has anything like this happened before? If so, what happened the first time?
- Who did this to you?
- Has anyone else done this to you?
- How often has this happened?
- Where were other people (eg, your mother) when this happened?
- Did you tell anyone? Who? What did they do?

Physical Examination

It is helpful for the examiner to be familiar with the normal **anogenital** anatomy of prepubescent children. The anatomy of boys remains constant throughout childhood, except for the increase in size of the penis and testes and the appearance of pubic hair during adolescence. Figure 128-1 shows the normal anogenital anatomy of girls, which changes from infancy through adolescence. All girls are born with a hymen, which is thick and full and covers the hymenal orifice in newborns. As maternal hormones regress, the hymen becomes thinner and more translucent, frequently taking on an annular or crescentic configuration. When puberty begins, the hymen once again becomes thickened, scalloped, and full. Careful examination of the hymen may involve positioning a child in not only the supine frog-leg position, but also the prone knee-chest position (Figure 128-2). For a variety of reasons there are frequently no genital abnormalities noted on examination in victims of sexual abuse. Penetration of the hymen in postpubertal adolescents may result in stretching without tearing of the tissue, and in prepubescent children, hymenal transections may heal with little residual evidence of the trauma. Many types of abuse (eg, orogenital contact, fondling) commonly leave no

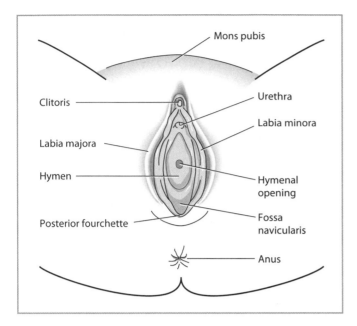

Figure 128-1.   Normal anogenital anatomy of prepubescent girls.

visible findings. The medical examiner must therefore realize that a normal anogenital examination does not preclude sexual abuse.

In cases of acute molestation, evidence of injury may be readily apparent, particularly if the examination is performed with the assistance of magnification such as **colposcopy,** or enhancing agents such as toluidine blue, which is preferentially taken up by exposed endothelium. Injuries that may be noted include **ecchymoses, petechiae, active bleeding, abrasions,** and **lacerations.** Those due to penile penetration commonly involve the hymen in the 6 o'clock position and the area of the posterior fourchette (see Figure 128-1).

The evaluation of children who have been molested in the past or on a chronic basis is more problematic. Many injuries heal with little residual scarring. Scarring that does occur may appear as a notch or concavity in the contour of the hymenal edge. The pattern of blood

vessels may also be interrupted, and areas of increased or decreased vascularity may be apparent. Sometimes a marked reduction in the amount of hymenal tissue is present in an area of prior trauma.

Male genitalia are less often injured by sexual abuse. More often the injuries seen in prepubescent boys, as well as in some girls, involve changes in the perianal area. The incidence of these changes in all children who have been sodomized is unknown but is believed to be low. When changes do occur, they may appear as scars, tags, or irregularities in perianal rugae and anal tone.

Laboratory Tests

When the molestation has occurred within 72 hours of the examination and the mechanism of injury could have resulted in deposition of body fluids on the child, **forensic evidence** should be collected as required by law enforcement. This evidence usually involves samples of vaginal washings and dried secretions, which are evaluated for the presence of DNA in an effort to identify the perpetrator. Clothing that was worn at the time of the assault should also be submitted since it is frequently positive for DNA evidence. **Forensic packages,** which are referred to as **rape kits** and are distributed by law enforcement agencies, have specific instructions concerning the appropriate collection of samples.

Approximately 5% to 10% of sexually abused children acquire an **STI** as a result of the abuse. Because of this, any child with a history of genital, oral, or anal penetration; a sibling with an STI; an assailant with a history of an infection; or a child, sibling, or assailant with signs or symptoms of an STI must undergo a laboratory evaluation for possible infection. If testing is indicated, cultures should be obtained from the involved body areas (vagina or urethra, rectum, throat). At a minimum, a child with genital discharge should be evaluated for *Neisseria gonorrhoeae*, *Chlamydia trachomatis*, and *Trichomonas vaginalis*. The presence of these infections in a prepubertal child, in the absence of perinatal transmission, is indicative

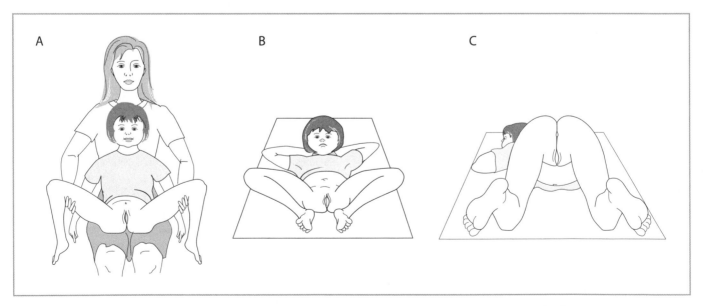

Figure 128-2.   Various positions for an anogenital examination in a prepubescent girl. A. Seated on the mother's lap. B. Supine, frog-leg position. C. Prone, knee-chest position.

of prior close genital contact. Most frequently this is due to sexual abuse. It is impossible to determine the etiology of vaginal discharge based only on its clinical characteristics.

All tests for STIs in prepubertal children should be evaluated in a reliable laboratory because of the legal implications of venereal infections in young children. Culture is considered to be the gold standard for diagnosing gonorrhea and *Chlamydia* in this setting because of its specificity. While newer nucleic acid amplification tests (NAATs) may have higher sensitivity in some settings, there are limited data on their use in prepubertal children so they should not be used as the sole method of evaluation. A positive NAAT should be confirmed by culture or by a second nucleic acid test targeting a different DNA sequence.

Testing for HIV, syphilis, hepatitis B, and hepatitis C should be performed if signs or symptoms of the diagnosis are present, if another STI is detected, if the perpetrator is known to be infected, or if the patient/family wishes to undergo the testing. Genital warts can be diagnosed clinically, and any lesions suspicious for herpes simplex virus types (HSV) 1 or 2 should be cultured and typed. While culture remains the gold standard for diagnosing HSV infection, serologies for HSV type-specific glycoprotein G antigens may be helpful if culture is not available. Lastly, pregnancy testing should be considered in any postpubertal girl.

Management

The management of children who have been sexually abused has 3 major components.

1. Any medical problem sustained as a result of the abuse, such as traumatic injuries, must be addressed. In addition, STIs should be managed (Table 128-1). See Chapter 97 for a more extensive discussion of STIs in adolescents. Adolescents who have been the victims of an acute assault should be offered pregnancy counseling, STI prophylaxis, and emergency contraception as medically indicated.

2. The emotional well-being of patients must be ensured. In cases of acute assault, crisis intervention is mandatory. If children have been the victims of chronic or prior sexual abuse, referral to appropriate counseling services should be done.

3. The physician must report the incident of sexual assault or abuse to the appropriate agencies, as mandated by the laws of the locality in which the physician practices. The physician may be required to testify in court about particular findings and whether abuse occurred. Testifying may be intimidating. It is helpful for the physician to review the medical records ahead of time and to discuss this information with the attorney who issues the subpoena to the physician.

Prognosis

Several factors influence the prognosis in cases of child sexual abuse, including the relationship of the perpetrator to the child, chronicity of the abuse, support following the disclosure, and preexisting psychosocial conditions. Physical injuries are usually nonexistent

Table 128-1. Management of Sexually Transmitted Infections in Children

Infection	Medication	Dose
Neisseria gonorrhoeae	Ceftriaxone	250 mg IM × 1 dose
	Cefixime (age >8 y, weight ≥45 kg)	400 mg PO × 1 dose
Chlamydia	Azithromycin	20 mg/kg PO × 1 dose (max: 1 g)
	Erythromycin (weight <45 kg)	50 mg/kg/d divided QID × 14 days
	Doxycycline (age >8 y, weight ≥45 kg)	100 mg PO BID × 7 days
Herpes genitalis	Acyclovir	1,200 mg/d divided TID × 7–10 days (max: 80 mg/kg/d)
Trichomonas	Metronidazole	15 mg/kg/d divided TID × 7 days OR 2 g PO × 1 dose (weight ≥45 kg)
Bacterial vaginosis	Metronidazole	15 mg/kg/d divided TID × 7 days OR 2 g PO × 1 dose (weight ≥45 kg)
Syphilis	Benzathine penicillin	50,000 U/kg, single IM dose (max: 2.4 million U)

Abbreviations: BID, twice a day; IM, intramuscularly; PO, orally; QID, 4 times a day; TID, 3 times a day.

or minor, and healing occurs with minimal residual evidence. In most cases, psychological counseling is indicated. Such counseling is beneficial, and emotional recovery is not only possible but likely to occur in a supportive environment.

Studies of **adverse childhood experiences** have shown that child sexual abuse is associated with an increased risk of medical, psychological, and social problems in adulthood.

CASE RESOLUTION

In the case history presented at the beginning of this chapter, the mother claims that no one has access to her child, but the girl's symptoms strongly suggest an infection with *Neisseria gonorrhoeae*. Secrecy about abuse is very common. Both the child and the mother should be interviewed by a skilled person. Cultures for gonorrhea should be carefully collected and sent to the most reliable laboratory. Antibiotic therapy may be initiated if the child is symptomatic. The case may be referred immediately to social services and law enforcement agencies if there is a disclosure. Alternatively, if the child denies the abuse, the referral may be deferred pending laboratory confirmation of the diagnosis.

Selected References

Adams JA. Guidelines for medical care of children evaluated for suspected sexual abuse: an update for 2008. *Curr Opin Obstet Gynecol.* 2008;20:435–441

Centers for Disease Control and Prevention; Workowski KA, Berman SM. Sexually transmitted diseases treatment guidelines, 2010. *MMWR Recomm Rep.* 2010;59:1–110

Chadwick DL, Berkowitz CD, Kerns D, McCann J, Reinhart MA, Strickland S. *Color Atlas of Child Sexual Abuse.* Chicago, IL: Year Book Medical Publishers; 1989

Dube SR, Anda RF, Whitfield CL, et al. Long term consequences of childhood sexual abuse by gender of victim. *Am J Prev Med.* 2005;28:430–438

Finkel MA. Medical aspects of prepubertal sexual abuse. In: Reece RM, Christian CW, eds. *Child Abuse: Medical Diagnosis and Management.* 3rd ed. Elk Grove Village, IL: American Academy of Pediatrics; 2008:269–320

Girardet RG, Lahoti S, Howard LA, et al. Epidemiology of sexually transmitted infections in suspected child victims of sexual assault. *Pediatrics.* 2009;124:79–85

Holmes WC, Slap GB. Sexual abuse of boys. *JAMA.* 1998;280:1855–1862

Johnson CF. Child sexual abuse. *Lancet.* 2004;364:462–470

Kaufman M; American Academy of Pediatrics Committee on Adolescence. Care of the adolescent sexual assault victim. *Pediatrics.* 2008;122:462–470

Kellogg N; American Academy of Pediatrics Committee on Child Abuse and Neglect. The evaluation of sexual abuse in children. *Pediatrics.* 2005;116:506–512

Shapiro RA, Makoroff KL. Sexually transmitted diseases in sexually abused girls and adolescents. *Curr Opin Obstet Gynecol.* 2006;18:492–497

Staller KM, Nelson-Gardell D. A burden in your heart: lessons of disclosure from female preadolescent and adolescent survivors of sexual abuse. *Child Abuse Negl.* 2005;29:1415–1432

Werner J, Werner MCM. Child sexual abuse in clinical and forensic psychiatry: a review of recent literature. *Curr Opin Psychiatry.* 2008;21:499–504

CHAPTER 129

Failure to Thrive

Carol D. Berkowitz, MD

CASE STUDY

A 2-year-old girl is brought to the office because of her small size. She was born at term but weighed only 2,200 g (less than fifth percentile) and measured 43 cm (less than fifth percentile). The mother is a 30-year-old gravida V para IV aborta I who smoked during pregnancy but denies using alcohol or drugs. She received prenatal care for only 2 weeks prior to delivery, and she claims to have felt well.

The child's physical health has been good. She is reported to be normal developmentally but speaks only 4 to 5 single words. She has not yet started toilet training.

The family history for medical problems, including allergies, diabetes, and cardiac and renal disease, is negative. The mother is 5 feet (152 cm) tall, and the father is 5 feet, 4 inches (163 cm) tall. The girl has 3 siblings, aged 5 years, 4 years, and 3 years, who are all normal. The father is no longer in the household. The mother is not employed outside of the home, and she receives public assistance.

She states that frequently there is not enough food in the home, although she receives food stamps.

On physical examination, the girl is less than the fifth percentile in height and weight. Although she is very active, she does not use any understandable words. The rest of the examination is normal.

Questions

1. What are the key prenatal factors that affect the growth of children?
2. How can caloric adequacy of a diet be assessed?
3. How do parental measurements affect their children's stature?
4. What are the behavioral characteristics of infants with environmental failure to thrive (FTT)?
5. What are some strategies to increase caloric intake of infants and children?

Failure to thrive can be defined as the failure of children to grow and develop at an appropriate rate. The term is most often applied to infants and toddlers younger than 3 years. Failure to thrive is not a disease or even a diagnosis but represents a sign that a child's size or rate of growth is below expected. The term FTT first appeared in the pediatric literature in 1933 and was used for children whose growth impairment related to a suboptimal environment. Prior to 1933 the condition was referred to as **cease to thrive.** The terms **growth deficiency, growth impairment, undernutrition,** and **inadequate growth** are sometimes used interchangeably. Historically, FTT has been divided into 2 distinct categories, **organic** and **nonorganic.** In organic FTT, an underlying **medical problem,** such as cystic fibrosis or congenital heart disease (CHD), is believed to contribute to the failure to grow at an appropriate rate. In nonorganic FTT, also referred to as **environmental deprivation,** inadequate growth is attributed to lack of nourishment and a non-nurturing home environment. Some clinicians use the term FTT exclusively to mean environmentally related growth impairment. It is important to recognize that many children with growth problems have both organic and environmental components, a condition sometimes referred to as *multifactorial* or *mixed* FTT.

The diagnosis of FTT is entertained when the growth parameters of children as plotted on a standardized curve are below the fifth percentile in height or weight. Children who are above the fifth percentile may also be diagnosed with FTT if the rate of growth has decelerated and 2 major percentiles (eg, decreased from the 75th percentile down to the 10th percentile) have been crossed within 6 months (Dx Box). Studies have shown, however, that between birth and 6 months of age approximately 39% of healthy infants cross 2 major percentiles on the weight for age curve (either up or down) as did up to 15% of children between 6 and 24 months of age. Similar trends were noted for length. Physicians should, however, carefully track these infants to be certain that such changes are related to the child's genetic disposition and not an environmental or medical problem.

Dx Failure to Thrive

- Weight below fifth percentile
- Height below fifth percentile
- Weight for height below fifth percentile
- Rate of growth lower than expected
- Delayed developmental milestones
- Disturbed interactional skills

The challenge for the physician caring for the child with FTT is to determine the etiology of the problem, which may not be readily apparent. Nonspecific, nondirected laboratory tests are not helpful because their yield is low and their cost is high. The evaluation of small, underweight children requires a careful history and physical examination as well as an assessment of mother–infant interactions. A home visit helps because it permits evaluation of the mother–infant relationship in a more natural setting and an assessment of the family's economic and food resources.

Epidemiology

The prevalence of FTT varies in different segments of the population. **Poverty** puts children at risk for **undernutrition,** and 12% of Medicaid recipients are less than the third percentile in weight. **Child neglect** can lead to FTT but is not a necessary component; approximately 60% of cases of child abuse are reported for child neglect. Several other factors may contribute to variations in growth. All of these are not the result of a pathologic process but may reflect variations in individual genetic potential.

Environmentally related FTT may occur in different family settings. In some families, an **acute depressive episode** in the mother is the key component (see Chapter 19). Family living conditions are good, and the educational background of the mother is adequate. The depressive episode may be related to a loss that occurred during the pregnancy or shortly after delivery or to peripartum depression, a distinct entity. The mother is too depressed to interact effectively with her children. In other families **financial resources** are marginal. The mother may be **chronically depressed** and the father involved in alcohol or substance abuse. Domestic violence frequently occurs (see Chapter 138). Spacing between children is less than 18 months, and the number of children is often the same as the age of the oldest child. The mother is too overwhelmed to meet the needs of the children. A third type of family also involves a mother who is depressed and has experienced losses, usually of a chronic nature. Her financial and educational backgrounds are adequate, but she views one of her children (the one who now presents with FTT) as bad or evil and the source of all her problems. As a result, an individual child is singled out, and the neglect is intentional.

Clinical Presentation

Children with FTT present with **low weight, short stature, poor appetite,** or **failure to gain weight or grow taller.** Sometimes parents may express concern, and at other times teachers may detect children's growth problems. Some children with FTT are diagnosed during a health maintenance visit or when they are being evaluated for another medical problem, such as a febrile illness. Following a child longitudinally will give the physician a better sense of the child's growth pattern and a clue to the etiology of observed growth impairments. When nutrition is suboptimal, weight tends to decrease first, followed by length and ultimately head circumference.

Pathophysiology

The common pathway for the development of FTT in both organic and nonorganic cases is **insufficient calories** to sustain growth (Box 129-2). Caloric intake may be inadequate for several reasons. Some factors are societal, specifically poverty and inadequate access

---

> ### Box 129-2. Factors Affecting Calories Available for Growth
>
> | *Insufficient Intake* | *Increased Loss* |
> |---|---|
> | • Poverty | • Malabsorption |
> | • Inadequate access to food | *Increased Needs* |
> | • Improper formula preparation | • Congenital heart disease |
> | • Eating difficulties | • Chronic lung disease |
> | • Vomiting | |

---

to food. Other factors may involve increased caloric needs. Certain chronic conditions are characterized by increased caloric expenditure (eg, some forms of chronic lung disease) or increased loss of ingested food (eg, diarrhea or malabsoprtion syndromes).

In environmentally related FTT, a disturbed mother–infant interaction is believed to contribute to reduced caloric intake and any associated gastrointestinal symptoms (ie, vomiting). Although various disturbances in mother–FTT infant dyads have been described, maternal depression is the most common maternal feature noted in environmentally related FTT. Infants withdraw after unsuccessful attempts to interact with nonresponsive mothers, and infants become apathetic and disinterested in food. Alternatively, overactive mothers, some of whom have a bipolar (manic-depressive) disorder, are out of synchrony with their infants. The infants become agitated, especially during feedings, and cannot feed and frequently vomit. These infants, who may interact with persons other than their mothers, usually do well in other environments.

Older children with long-standing environmental deprivation have **disturbed hypothalamic-pituitary functioning.** The etiology of this dysfunction is uncertain but has been attributed to sleep disturbances with an effect on levels of growth hormone.

Differential Diagnosis

The growth of children with FTT may be impaired with regard to weight, height, head circumference, or any combination of growth parameters. If weight is the only abnormal parameter, inadequate caloric intake is probably the major problem. If height is reduced and the weight is appropriate or high for height, the diagnosis may be short stature rather than FTT. Small head circumference in the face of low growth parameters suggests a central nervous system (CNS) basis for the growth delay. It is important to determine if children's skills are developmentally appropriate when determining the etiology of FTT. Affect and interactional skills should also be noted. Environmentally deprived infants are apathetic and noninteractive. They appear hypertonic and may be diagnosed with cerebral palsy or have features suggestive of infantile autism, but their symptoms resolve with a change in surroundings.

The most common causes of short stature include **familial short stature** and **constitutional delay.** Children with familial short stature are small because the parents are short. Except for a deceleration in growth, which usually occurs between the ages of 6 and 18 months, children with constitutional delay appear healthy. They have a delayed bone age that is comparable to their height age (the age when their height is at the 50th percentile), however. In children with either familial short stature or constitutional delay, growth parameters at birth are usually normal.

Children with low growth parameters at birth may have been premature or have suffered from **intrauterine growth restriction (IUGR).** Most studies support the notion that well premature infants exhibit catch-up growth (head circumference by 18 months, weight by 24 months, and height by 40 months). Ill preterm infants may not demonstrate such **catch-up growth,** either because of increased caloric needs related to residual medical problems (eg, bronchopulmonary dysplasia) or impaired nutritional intake resulting from certain conditions (eg, cerebral palsy). Overall, 15% of infants who are classified as IUGR or **small for gestational age (SGA)** do not exhibit catch-up growth. There is significant evidence now that IUGR may be associated with insulin resistance and subsequent propensity to obesity and metabolic syndrome. Disturbances in leptin, gherlin, and adiponectin have also been described. This recent finding has significant implications for the management of these infants vis a vis their nutritional intake. It is postulated that some individuals are "programmed" to be slighter and smaller, and nutritional interventions to achieve a more average weight have deleterious effects down the line.

Children who are **SGA** may have suffered any of several in utero insults that affect postnatal growth, including exposure to cigarettes, alcohol, and illicit drugs. In addition, maternal infection with such diseases as rubella may result in a congenital infection in infants with subsequent growth impairment.

A number of other conditions may lead to disturbed growth, including endocrine disorders, skeletal dysplasias, food allergies, and malabsorption. These conditions occur less frequently and are usually more readily apparent as children undergo the evaluation for the growth problem.

Evaluation

History

Careful questioning about certain topics provides clues to diagnosis in about 95% of cases. The physician should learn about the pregnancy and delivery, children's medical and dietary history, and the family history.

It is important to obtain a history of the pregnancy and delivery (Questions Box: Pregnancy and Delivery). The infant's birth weight and gestational age are key pieces of information. Low birth weight is said to account for 20% to 40% of short children from low-income families. It is helpful to confirm that the neonatal screen for genetic and metabolic diseases was normal. Recurrent spontaneous abortions suggest that mothers may have an underlying problem such as a balanced chromosomal translocation that leads to fetal wastage. Mothers who have experienced repeated losses may have difficulty bonding with subsequent infants. The physician should determine whether mothers used cigarettes, alcohol, or drugs during the pregnancy by asking mothers questions beginning with the phrase "How

---

Questions

Pregnancy and Delivery

- Was the pregnancy planned?
- How did the mother feel when she learned that she was pregnant?
- Was the infant wanted?
- Was prenatal care obtained?
- How many times has the mother been pregnant?
- Is there a history of abortions, either spontaneous or therapeutic?
- How much did the mother drink during the pregnancy, if at all?
- How much did the mother smoke during the pregnancy, if at all?
- How much did the mother use drugs (either prescribed or illicit) during the pregnancy, if at all? Which drugs did she use?
- Did the mother take any medications during the pregnancy?
- Did the mother have any rashes or illnesses during the pregnancy?
- Has the mother felt depressed, sad, or hopeless?
- Has the mother felt little interest or pleasure in doing things?
- Was the infant term or premature?
- How much did the infant weigh at birth?

---

much?" Any medications taken by the mother may affect the subsequent growth of the infant.

A review of children's medical history may also provide a clue to the etiology of FTT (Questions Box: Medical and Family History). It is essential that the physician obtain as many of the previous growth parameters as possible to determine whether children are small but growing at a normal rate or if their rate of growth is too slow. Previous illnesses should be assessed because these events may interrupt growth temporarily. Certain complaints may indicate underlying organic disorders, and recurrent infections raise the possibility of a congenital or acquired immune disorder including infection with HIV. A history of easy fatigability may be a clue to CHD. Although most children with CHD grow normally, growth problems may occur with congestive heart failure, some forms of cyanotic heart disease, and complex atrial septal defects, especially if associated with pulmonary hypertension. Children with urinary incontinence may have renal disease that interferes with their growth. The presence of seizures may be a sign of a CNS problem that makes it difficult to obtain adequate nutrition. Some children with seizures are heavily medicated and are too sleepy to eat.

Questions

Medical and Family History

- Is the child's growth rate normal or slow?
- Has the child had any previous illnesses (eg, gastroenteritis, recurrent pneumonia)?
- Does the child tire easily?
- How tall are the parents?
- Are there any medical problems that run in the family?

A family history as well as a **social history** is important to obtain. Determination of parental heights, which is best accomplished by measuring the parents, is critical. This is particularly important in children with short stature. Specific **mid-parental height curves** allow the physician to determine if a child's height is appropriate given the parental stature.

A nutritional assessment is an essential part of the history. The physician or another member of the health care team, such as a dietician, can perform this assessment. The dietary history can be determined either by using a **24-hour recall** of children's intake during the previous day or a prospective **3-day diary,** in which parents record the kinds and quantities of foods their children eat. This nutritional information can be used to find ways to alter children's diet to ensure adequate and balanced meals.

Physical Examination

The essential component of the physical examination is determination of growth parameters. Calculation of the **body mass index** (BMI = weight [kg] divided by height [m]^2) is useful in children older than 2 years. Children with a low BMI are suffering from undernutrition. Short children with a normal BMI are not. Infants younger than 2 years should be plotted on a weight-for-length curve to determine their degree of undernutrition or overnutrition. The World Health Organization has developed and distribued growth curves for children up to 24 months of age. These curves are felt to reflect optimal rather than average growth having been developed from a longitudinal study of healthy breastfed infants. These curves can be accessed at www.cdc.gov/mmwr/preview/mmwrhtml/rr5909a1.htm. Measuring arm circumference and triceps skinfold thickness is also useful and provides information about body composition that is not obtained by height and weight. Children should also be evaluated for dysmorphic features (eg, limb length discrepancies in Russell-Silver syndrome). It is important to remember that children with Down syndrome grow at different rates than other children, and separate standardized curves for assessing these children are available (see Chapter 37). Separate curves are also available for children with Turner and Williams syndrome. The presence of one major congenital anomaly or 2 minor anomalies suggests the existence of other anomalies. The incidence of growth hormone deficiency is reportedly higher in children with cleft lip and palate. Children with heart murmurs may have FTT related to CHD or to a syndrome such as Williams syndrome, in which the heart disease is but one feature.

Infants with environmentally related FTT exhibit certain **behavioral characteristics** that are easy to recognize. They refrain from making eye contact and exhibit **gaze** avoidance. Infants are not cuddly and do not like being held. When held, they may arch their backs in an effort to avoid the holder. Their muscles seem tense, and they are often considered to be hypertonic. These children may also exhibit specific disabilities including oromotor dyspraxia and sensory-motor disorder, and they may demonstrate food texture aversion or difficulty with chewing and swallowing **(sensory food aversion).** Children with neurologic disabilities often exhibit difficulties with oral skills. Children who have negative early experience with eating may have what has been termed *posttraumatic feeding disorder.*

Psychosocial Assessment

The evaluation of children with FTT and their families entails a detailed psychosocial assessment to determine what environmental factors may be affecting children's growth. Such an assessment is helpful even if the FTT has an organic basis, because chronic disease affects family functioning. This evaluation can be carried out by a primary care physician, social worker, or psychologist. The key is to query the caretaker about living conditions, adequacy of food supply, and economic resources.

Laboratory Tests

Routine laboratory tests appropriate for any pediatric health maintenance visit should be obtained in children with FTT if these studies have not been performed recently. Such tests include hemoglobin, lead level (screening as determined by risk factors and geographic area), and urinalysis. Other laboratory tests should be determined by the findings on history and physical examination. There is no recommended uniform diagnostic evaluation for FTT. Evaluation for endocrinopathies, such as hypothyroidism or growth hormone deficiency, should be carried out in children whose bone age is less than their height age or who have symptoms of these disorders. Genetic consultation or chromosomal assessment should be performed in children with dysmorphic features or in families with a history of fetal wastage.

Imaging Studies

Radiographs to determine bone age are useful in children with short stature that is not related to parental heights. Children with constitutional delay have a bone age that is consistent with their height age.

Management

Any recognized underlying medical problem, for instance nephrogenic diabetes insipidus, should be managed appropriately. Children with IUGR who are not demonstrating catch-up growth may be candidates for growth hormone therapy. Consultation with pediatric endocrinology is warranted.

Adequate Caloric Intake

Ensuring that children receive appropriate caloric intake is essential. The caloric intake, which averages 120 to 150 cal/kg/d for most infants, should be based on children's ideal rather than actual weight (see Chapter 23). For infants on formula, the physician should review the exact preparation of formula with the mother. Overly diluted formula results in an unusually large intake volume with a lack of weight gain. For infants who are breastfed, the physician should observe a feeding session to be certain that mothers have an adequate milk supply and infants are able to suck and swallow appropriately (see Chapter 24). Infants should be weighed before and after feeding. Some infants with FTT have neurologic problems that prevent them from sucking and swallowing consistently without becoming fatigued.

Children who are slow feeders may require **formula concentration** (Table 129-1). These infants may also receive added calories in the form of Polycose (glucose polymer) or oil such as medium-chain triglycerides mixed in the milk. Older children may be placed on supplemental feedings such as PediaSure or instant breakfast drinks, prepared with whole milk. These drinks are a less expensive form of nutritional supplementation than PediaSure and are well tolerated. Up to 24 oz/d of the breakfast drinks can be consumed, and are given in addition to, not in place of, a balanced diet.

Table 129-1. Concentration of Infant Formula to Increase Caloric Intake		
Concentrated Infant Formula (13-oz can)		
Formula (oz)	**Water (oz)**	**Calories (cal/oz)**
13	13	20
13	10	23
13	8	25
Powdered Formula		
Formula (scoops)	**Water (oz)**	**Calories (cal/oz)**
1	2	20
5	8	25

Mothers should be advised that many children preferentially tolerate 6 small meals a day rather than 3 large ones. In addition, parents should be told that access to non-nutritional foods such as cookies adversely affects children's appetites. Excess consumption of fruit juices should also be limited because it decreases the intake of other foods and may induce diarrhea. The physician should inform parents regarding foods that can be added to children's diets to increase caloric intake. These foods include powdered milk, cheese, sour cream, avocado, and peanut butter. Often children have a few favorite foods. Though food variety is appealing to adults, many children prefer a small number of nutritious foods. They should be allowed to consume these foods freely.

Children with neurologic disorders and associated problems with chewing and swallowing may need chronic gavage feeding or be fed through a gastric feeding tube.

Parenting Issues

Some parents need more help about appropriate child-rearing practices than the physician can provide. They should enroll in parenting programs that address multiple aspects of the parenting process. Mothers with substance abuse problems may need to participate in drug treatment programs. Other caregivers may need individual counseling for depression or emotional problems. A nurturing father has an important role in caring for an infant, particularly if a mother is experiencing postpartum depression.

In some middle-class families, mealtime has evolved into a battle of control. Some children find that food is supplied in a manner more conducive to its consumption at school rather than at home. Parents should be counseled about avoiding conflicts about meals with children because the children win simply by closing their mouths. Parents should be encouraged to allow toddlers independence around mealtime.

Families may also require supplementary services to ensure that food supplies are adequate and financial resources are sufficient. Such services include Supplemental Nutrition Assistance Program (SNAP, formerly food stamps); Supplemental Food Program for Women, Infants, and Children (WIC); and Temporary Assistance for Needy Families (TANF).

Regardless of the individual needs of the family, it is critical that the physician craft a therapeutic alliance with the child's caregivers.

Home Visitation

Home visitation services provide useful diagnostic information and help parents implement advice. Such information may include lack of access to running water, overcrowding, and inadequate food resources. Home visitation may be available in the community through the use of public health nurses or private visiting nurse agencies. These nurses should interact with the primary care physician so that families' compliance with treatment recommendations can be determined.

Child Protective Services

Involvement by **child protective services** (CPS) may be necessary if parents are unable to comply with medical recommendations, if children do not grow, or if there is intentional neglect on the part of families. In some families with children with FTT, the home environment is not safe for the children and they require placement elsewhere. Families in which one child is singled out as "bad" and is intentionally neglected need immediate referral to CPS, and some families overwhelmed by multiple problems including parental substance abuse also need such a referral (see Epidemiology).

Hospitalization

Hospitalization is occasionally necessary if infants with FTT are severely malnourished and food must be given in a controlled environment. Concern about refeeding syndrome can be addressed in the inpatient setting. In addition, these infants may have intercurrent illnesses that require inpatient care. In addition, health care professionals may determine that the home environment is unsafe and that no other placement, such as foster care, is available.

Children with either organic and environmentally related FTT usually gain weight in the hospital. Thus the hospitalization of children with FTT simply to demonstrate appropriate weight gain in a different environment is considered neither appropriate nor cost-effective. Some insurance companies will not reimburse hospitals for inpatient management of children with FTT. Additionally, some children with environmentally related FTT do not gain weight in the hospital because they are subjected to many diagnostic tests that interfere with nutritional intake (eg, receiving nothing orally), and they acquire nosocomial infections.

Prognosis

Many children with FTT respond dramatically to change in diet or in environment. Improvement in affect and cognitive functioning frequently follows nutritional improvement. These children grow and achieve and maintain normal stature. With early intervention, cognitive abilities also can be fully realized. Even when intervention has been delayed, catch-up growth and development are expected, although 25% to 30% may have weight and occasionally height below the fifth percentile. Continued monitoring for residual psychosocial or neurodevelopmental disabilities is appropriate even after growth has normalized. School performance and cognitive outcome in children who have experienced FTT is poorer than in children who have not experienced FTT. It is unclear if this association is related to early iron deficiency anemia, lack of calories or other micronutrient deficiencies, or psycho-environmental deficits.

CASE RESOLUTION

In the case scenario presented, the full-term infant had a low birth weight, which suggests IUGR. Although the mother reports using no alcohol or drugs, such denial is not uncommon. The child's growth pattern should be determined to see if the rate of growth has changed recently, and the BMI should be calculated to check for both undernutrition and short stature. A mid-parental height curve should be used to determine if the child's short stature is related to the parents' short stature. Intervention should involve mobilizing resources for the child and family to ensure adequate food and financial and emotional support.

Selected References

Berkowitz CD. Failure to thrive: a comprehensive approach. *Fam Pract Recertification.* 2004;26:41–59

Black M, Dubowitz H, Krishnakumar A, Star RH Jr. Early intervention and recovery among children with failure to thrive: follow-up at age 8. *Pediatrics.* 2007;120:59–69

Block RW, Krebs NF; American Academy of Pediatrics Committee on Child Abuse and Neglect and the Committee on Nutrition. Failure to thrive as a manifestation of child neglect. *Pediatrics.* 2005;116:1234–1237

Cook J, Frank D, Berkowitz C, et al. Food insecurity is associated with adverse health outcomes among human infants and toddlers. *J Nutr.* 2004;134:1432–1438

Drotar D, ed. *New Direction in Failure to Thrive: Research and Clinical Practice.* New York, NY: Plenum Press; 1985

Frank DA, Drotar D. Failure to thrive in child abuse: medical diagnosis and management. In: Reece RM, ed. *Child Abuse: Medical Diagnosis and Management.* Philadelphia, PA: Lea & Febiger; 1994:298–324

Gahagan S. Failure to thrive: a consequence of undernutrition. *Pediatr Rev.* 2006;27:e1–e11

Graham EA. Economic, racial, and cultural influence on growth and maturation of children. *Pediatr Rev.* 2005;26:290–294

Jaffe AC. Failure to thrive: current clinical concepts. *Pediatr Rev.* 2011;32:100–108

Kessler DB, Dawson P. *Failure to Thrive and Pediatric Undernutrition. A Transdisciplinary Approach.* Baltimore, MD: Paul H. Brookes Publishing Co.; 1999

Mei Z, Grummer-Strawn LM, Thompson D, Dietz WH. Shifts in percentiles of growth during childhood: analysis of longitudinal data from the California Child Health and Development Study. *Pediatrics.* 2004;113:e617–e627

Oates RK, Kempe RS. Growth failure in infants. In: Helfer ME, Kempe RS, Krugman RD, eds. *The Battered Child.* 5th ed. Chicago, IL: The University of Chicago Press; 1997:374–391

CHAPTER 130

Fetal Alcohol Syndrome

Melissa K. Egge, MD

CASE STUDY

A 6-year-old male is brought into the clinic by his maternal aunt who expresses concerns about her nephew's behavior that are echoed by his kindergarten teacher. The teacher has reported that the child has a limited attention span and is often disruptive in class. The child's growth parameters have remained at the third percentile since birth. He has a smooth philtrum, thin upper lip, and short palpebral fissures.

Questions

1. What are the diagnostic criteria outlined by the Centers for Disease Control and Prevention (CDC) for fetal alcohol syndrome (FAS)?
2. What is the differential diagnosis of the facial characteristics of FAS?
3. What typical behavioral and learning problems do children with FAS experience?
4. What therapeutic interventions are appropriate to recommend for children with FAS?

Fetal alcohol syndrome refers to a clinical diagnosis that requires careful evaluation by an experienced clinician to recognize the physical, behavioral, and cognitive abnormalities in an affected child. Diagnosis may be made at birth, but the condition is often not diagnosed until school age. Fetal alcohol syndrome has been recognized in the medical literature for decades and in historical literature for centuries; however, fine-tuning the criteria for diagnosis has been an ongoing process. Although several groups have created guidelines to help analyze children with FAS, the CDC in 2004 published broad-based criteria (Box 130-1) that are helpful for a number of reasons. First, they educate clinicians and caregivers about the wide spectrum of phenotypes that manifest after prenatal alcohol exposure. Second, using the most recent CDC criteria for FAS, the greatest number of potentially affected children is captured in the hopes that earlier intervention with a wider scope of services may be provided. Criteria must be met in all 3 categories of facial features, growth problems, and central nervous system abnormalities. For cases in which FAS is suspected but diagnostic criteria are incompletely met, the term fetal alcohol spectrum disorders (FASD) may be used to couch the findings, especially when maternal alcohol exposure is confirmed. The next step will be establishing criteria for FASD. However, at this time the term is not intended for diagnostic purposes but rather a descriptor of recognized phenotypes along a spectrum leading up to FAS.

Part of the difficulty in delineating a phenotype for alcohol exposure is that the degree of exposure is variable during embryogenesis (and organogenesis): quantity ingested, concomitant drug exposures, malnutrition, and individual genetic responses to exposure. This wide variability in degree of exposure and individual response leads to a multitude of clinical presentations.

Box 130-1. Centers for Disease Control and Prevention Diagnostic Criteria for Fetal Alcohol Syndrome

Requires all 3 of the following:
1. Facial features—all 3 required
   a. Palpebral fissure length ≤10th percentile for age/race
   b. Smooth philtrum rank 4–5
   c. Thin upper lip rank 4–5
2. Growth parameters—at least 1 required at any age (not height for weight)
   a. Height ≤10th percentile
   b. Weight ≤10th percentile
3. Central nervous system abnormalities—at least 1 of the following
   a. Structural—1 required
      i. Head circumference (OFC) ≤10th for age, sex
      ii. Brain abnormality by imaging
   b. Neurologic
      i. Seizures
      ii. Measured delay in motor skills
      iii. Abnormal neuro exam not attributed to another condition
   c. Functional—1 required
      i. Cognitive delay or global developmental delay (<3rd percentile)
      ii. Deficits in ≥3 functional domains (<16th percentile)
         1. Cognitive
         2. Executive function
         3. Motor function (fine and/or gross)
         4. Attention-deficit/hyperactivity disorder symptoms
         5. Deficits in social skills
         6. Other (sensory, memory, language, etc)

Adapted from: Bertrand J, Floyd RL, Weber MD, et al. *National Task Force on FAS/FAE: Guidelines for Referral and Diagnosis.* Atlanta, GA: Centers for Disease and Prevention: 2004:1–50

Epidemiology

Prenatal alcohol exposure is much more common than the number of diagnosed cases of FAS. It has been estimated by surveys of women of childbearing age that approximately 15% engage in regular consumption of alcohol and 2% are binge drinkers. Although estimates of children affected by FAS vary by region and population, an estimated 1 in 1,000 live births would meet criteria for diagnosis. The estimate jumps 10-fold when certain high-risk groups are the focus. Approximately 1 in 100 children in foster care and nearly that many (3–9/1,000) Native American children meet criteria for diagnosis of FAS. If one includes children who meet some but not all FAS criteria, the prevalence is 1 in 100 or greater.

Pathophysiology

Alcohol is a teratogen, and like other teratogens its effect on the developing fetus depends on several factors, many of which are difficult to record. While it is important to ask about the timing, quantity, and pattern of prenatal alcohol exposure, it is often difficult to obtain an accurate history. In addition, due to genetic differences in women's abilities to metabolize ethanol by alcohol dehydrogenase, each baby receives a unique "dose" during gestation. Also individualized is each woman's nutritional intake and use of other drugs or medications. Alcohol acts as a toxin to cause damage and apoptosis to neurons in the fetal brain. Alcohol also inhibits proper migration, development, and functioning of cells during embryogenesis, contributing to structural anomalies in multiple organ systems, such as the kidney, heart, and brain.

Clinical Presentation

Signs and symptoms of FAS may be recognized at birth or not until later in childhood. At birth, an infant may present with asymmetrical intrauterine growth restriction, small for gestational age, head circumference disproportionately smaller than the body, or appropriate for gestational age. A variety of birth defects have been associated with fetal alcohol exposure, and many of these have been demonstrated in animal models. Newborns may exhibit signs of withdrawal either from alcohol or concomitant drug exposure. With time, the infant may demonstrate failure to thrive or poor weight gain due to poor nippling. In toddlerhood, developmental delays may be recognized by a caregiver or during developmental screening questions by a primary care provider. As children approach school age, teachers may report behavioral concerns and poor school performance. Concerns such as distractibility, hyperactivity, and difficulty processing multistep directions may be raised in school. In addition, children may exhibit signs of fine motor delay, such as difficulty tying shoes or fastening buttons. Age-appropriate social skills are lacking in affected children, who often fail to develop "street smarts." They take the blame, succumb to peer pressure, and are oblivious to social norms. Approaching the teen years, the classic facies may become less distinctive.

Diagnosis

Facial Dysmorphia

There are 3 classic facial features required for the diagnosis of FAS. The characteristics are typical of midface hypoplasia and include short palpebral fissures, smooth philtrum, and thin upper lip. Other facial characteristics, such as epicanthal folds and flat nasal bridge, may be present but are not required for diagnosis. In order to accurately measure the palpebral fissures, the child should look directly up while the distance between the endocanthion and the exocanthion is measured. Palpebral fissure length (PFL) must be less than 2 standard deviations below the mean for a diagnosis of FAS.

There are lip-philtrum guides created by the University of Washington for Caucasians and for African Americans accounting for ethnic differences in contour of lips (Figure 130-1). The images are ranked 1 through 5, with 5 representing the most affected phenotype: thinnest lip and smoothest philtrum. When the child is neither Caucasian nor African American a best approximate is used. In order to properly use the lip-philtrum guides, the child's face should be relaxed, or the lip and philtrum will appear thinner and smoother. The clinician should evaluate the child's face within a specific horizontal planar view to avoid the illusion of a thinner lip. There are guidelines on how to use the images published on the University of Washington's FAS Web site at http://depts.washington.edu/fasdpn/.

Growth Problems

The criteria for deficiencies in growth may involve the child's weight or length or both at any time. With the CDC criteria, one may qualify to meet criteria for growth problems based on birth or postnatal measurements. The child's weight or length must be less than or equal to the 10th percentile for age and sex. It is important, however, to evaluate other organic and environmental etiologies of short stature or poor weight gain, such as poor nutrition. Considerations for small head circumference are accounted for in the central nervous system (CNS) abnormalities.

CNS Abnormalities

The criteria for neurologic problems may be met several ways as children manifest an array of cognitive, behavioral, and developmental deficits. Criteria for structural abnormalities are met by a head circumference at the 10th percentile or lower at any age or 3% or less when the child's weight and height are less than 10%. An experienced neuroradiologist may detect an abnormally small cranial structure, such as the cerebellum or corpus callosum, on magnetic resonance imaging. Manifestations of structural abnormalities include seizure activity not attributed to another cause or other focal deficits. Other functional CNS abnormalities may not be recognized until the child enters school and is compared to peers.

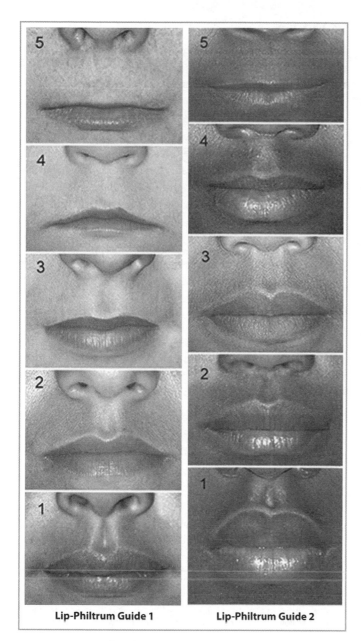

Lip-Philtrum Guide 1   **Lip-Philtrum Guide 2**

Figure 130-1. Lip philtrum guidelines for Caucasians and African Americans. Reproduced with permission from Susan Astley.

Table 130-2. Syndromes With Facies Resembling Fetal Alcohol Syndrome

Syndrome	Long or Smooth Philtrum	Thin Upper Lip	Small Palpebral Fissures
Cornelia de Lange	X	X	
Aarskog	X		
Williams	X		X
Dubowitz			X
Toluene embryopathy	X	X	X
Brachmann–de Lange	X		
Fetal hydantoin effects			
Noonan			
Fetal valproate	X	X	
Maternal phenylketonuria effects	X	X	X
Floating-Harbor	X		
Opitz	X		X

Differential Diagnosis

The hazards of using a "gestalt approach" to diagnosing FAS can lead to inappropriate stigmatizing labels and missed opportunity to diagnose another genetic disorder, which may carry a different prognosis. Several syndromes share facial features of FAS (Table 130-2). Fetal alcohol syndrome should be considered a diagnosis of exclusion when in utero alcohol exposure cannot be confirmed.

Evaluation

It is important that appropriately trained professionals assess the child for each component of diagnosis, but initial data should be gathered prior to referral.

History

A confirmed history of maternal alcohol consumption is not required for diagnosis, according to the CDC guidelines, but should be documented if available. A detailed developmental history is important to document, including feedback from teachers or child care providers.

Physical Examination

As detailed previously, measurement of the PFL and ranking of the child's philtrum and upper lip should be documented. Both current and previous height, weight, and head circumferences should be plotted on an appropriate growth chart. Also, any additional physical features may be recorded to support diagnosis.

Diagnostic Studies

Imaging studies to screen for cranial malformations are not currently recommended unless the child is experiencing some focal neurologic deficits or seizure activity. Similarly, targeted imaging of other organ systems is warranted when there are signs of an abnormality (ie, murmur would warrant an echocardiogram).

Consultation with a geneticist may be appropriate to rule out other disorders with similar phenotype (Box 130-2).

Management

Once a diagnosis related to alcohol exposure is suspected by a clinician, the referral process should begin. A dysmorphologist or experienced clinician may do the detailed measurements of the PFL and rank the facial features. Depending on local resources, a multidisciplinary team evaluation is ideal. A child psychologist or developmentalist can assess age-appropriate skills and need for therapeutic

Box 130-2. Physical Findings and Malformations Associated With Prenatal Alcohol Exposure

Cardiac
- atrial or ventricular septal defects, aberrant great vessels, and tetralogy of Fallot

Skeletal/Extremity
- shortened 5th digits, clinodactyly (curved 5th digit), radioulnar synostosis, Klippel-Feil syndrome, flexion contractures, hemivertebrae, camptodactyly (flexion contracture of digit), scoliosis, short metacarpals, short/webbed neck, hockey stick palmar crease

Renal
- aplastic, dysplastic, hypoplastic kidneys
- Ureteral duplications hydronephrosis horseshoe kidneys

Ocular
- strabismus refractive problems secondary to small globes ptosis
- retinal vascular anomalies

Auditory
- conductive hearing loss neurosensory hearing loss

Skin
- Hemangiomas, Hypoplastic nails

GU
- Hypoplastic labia majora

Facial features that are common but not required for diagnosis
- "Railroad track" ears
- Epicanthal folds
- Flat nasal bridge
- Cleft lip

intervention. Only validated instruments should be used to test developmental capabilities. When delays are detected, referral to appropriate therapies should be initiated through early intervention services. An individualized education plan (IEP) may be requested of the school by a caregiver who retains the child's educational rights. Public schools may provide occupational, physical, and speech therapies and social skills training. A psychiatrist may select therapies and medications particular to a child's unique mental health needs (see Chapters 125 and 126). Social workers are integral to providing support and additional resources to the family. As teens approach adulthood, referrals to vocational training and programs to transition young adults to independent living are important.

Prognosis

Unfortunately, many of the neurotoxic effects of alcohol on the developing fetus have lasting sequelae. Early interventions may improve but not correct cognitive deficits and associated mental health issues of aging children and adults with FAS. The mental health disorders are thought to be due to adverse childhood experiences (ridicule, harassment, failures) related to their behavioral and cognitive deficits. Some of the mental health disorders include oppositional defiant disorder, conduct disorder, depression, adjustment disorders, anxiety disorders, substance abuse, and sleep disorders. Unfortunately, many adults with FAS have failed to finish high school, and become unemployed or incarcerated. A fraction of adults with FAS will require assisted living arrangements.

CASE RESOLUTION

This child meets diagnostic criteria for FAS. It is recommended to the caregiver that she initiate obtaining "educational rights" over her nephew so she can request an IEP from his school's administration. An assessment for attention-deficit/hyperactivity disorder (ADHD), such as the Connor's Rating Scale, Vanderbilt, or another standardized measure for ADHD, should be given to the caregiver and teacher to each evaluate the child. Prescription for stimulant medications may be warranted in conjunction with behavioral therapy. Depending on local resources, the caregiver and child may be referred for psychotherapy, including parent–child interactive therapy where his aunt may be coached on how to deal with his behaviors in the most positive, effective manner.

Selected References

American Academy of Pediatrics Committee on Substance Abuse and Committee on Children With Disabilities. Fetal alcohol syndrome and alcohol-related neurodevelopmental disorders. *Pediatrics.* 2000;106(2):358–361

Bertrand J, Floyd RL, Weber MD, et al. *National Task Force on FAS/FAE: Guidelines for Referral and Diagnosis.* Atlanta, GA: Centers for Disease and Prevention: 2004:1–50

Bonthius DJ, Olson HC, Thomas JD. Proceedings of the 2006 annual meeting of the fetal alcohol spectrum disorders study group. *Alcohol.* 2006;40:61–65

Fetal Alcohol Syndrome Diagnostic and Prevention Network: http://depts.washington.edu/fasdpn/

Goodlet CR. Fetal alcohol spectrum disorders: new perspectives on diagnosis and intervention. *Alcohol.* 2010;44:579–582

Riley EP, McGee CL. Fetal alcohol spectrum disorders: an overview with emphasis on changes in brain and behavior. *Exp Biol Med* (Maywood). 2005;230(6):357-365

CHAPTER 131

Infants of Substance-Abusing Mothers

Sara T. Stewart, MD

CASE STUDY

An infant is born by emergency cesarean section because of abruptio placentae. The mother is a 29-year-old gravida VI para IV aborta II with a history of crack cocaine and heroin abuse during pregnancy. The infant is 36 weeks' gestation. The birth weight is 2,400 g, and the length is 43 cm. The physical examination is normal. The infant does well for the first 10 hours but then develops jitteriness, with irritability, diarrhea, sweating, and poor feeding. A urine toxicology test on the infant and mother are positive for cocaine.

Questions

1. What complications affect infants secondary to maternal substance abuse during pregnancy?
2. What withdrawal symptoms do newborn infants experience as a result of maternal substance abuse during pregnancy?
3. What typical behavioral and learning problems are found in infants and children whose mothers abused illicit substances during pregnancy?
4. What are the appropriate management strategies for infants who have experienced in utero drug exposure?

Maternal substance abuse during pregnancy places infants at risk for a number of medical, psychosocial, and developmental problems. The particular problems experienced by infants depend on the drug (or drugs) to which they have been exposed; many infants have been exposed to multiple drugs in addition to cigarettes and alcohol. The long-lasting effects of alcohol exposure are well established, but the effect of newer drugs is less well defined. Illicit drugs change in their popularity, form of use, and availability at different points in time.

The environment into which children are born also affects their health and development. Environments where substance abuse is common are frequently suboptimal for normal growth and development due to (1) the impact of substance abuse on parenting; (2) fragmentation of families; (3) domestic violence; (4) incarceration of significant family members; (5) illnesses, including HIV infection; (6) limited financial resources; (7) homelessness or substandard housing; (8) unemployment; (9) child abuse and neglect; and (10) limited access to health care. Because of these environmental issues, many drug-exposed infants are cared for by foster parents or nonparental family members. These factors also make it difficult to determine, in a given child, which problems are due to the drug exposure versus the accompanying environmental conditions. This differentiation is of less significance to the practitioner than to the researcher or epidemiologist because the practitioner will care for the problems that drug-exposed children manifest regardless of etiology.

Epidemiology

Approximately 10% of women between the ages of 15 and 44 years report having used illicit substances in the past month. While data collected via maternal self-report are typically an underestimate of prevalence, one national survey reported that 5.2% of women used illicit substances while pregnant. The highest rate of use was among pregnant adolescents aged 15 to 17 years, as 22% reported illicit drug use in the past month. The same survey also found that 12% of women reported drinking alcohol and 16% reported smoking cigarettes while pregnant. Meconium analysis has demonstrated not only extensive differences in the prevalence of in utero drug exposure among hospitals, but has also shown differences in the substances of choice in different geographic areas. While polysubstance abuse is the most common clinical scenario in all communities, national data on the primary drug of choice for pregnant teens admitted for substance abuse treatment has shown changes over the past 15 years. Primary alcohol abuse has decreased by 50%, primary cocaine abuse has decreased by 66%, primary methamphetamine abuse has increased by 4.4%, and primary marijuana abuse has increased by 2.4%.

Clinical Presentation

Many of the different substances that women use while pregnant can result in similar sequelae in the infant or child. In utero growth restriction, irritability, disordered eating or sleeping, and hypertonicity may be seen in newborns and infants. Older children may have developmental delays, symptoms of attention-deficit/hyperactivity disorder (ADHD), learning disabilities, or behavioral difficulties such as oppositional or impulsive behavior. Newborns that have been prenatally exposed to opiates such as heroin or methadone may manifest symptoms of neonatal abstinence syndrome (drug withdrawal). These symptoms may include respiratory, gastrointestinal (GI), or nervous system effects such as apnea, tachypnea, emesis, diarrhea, irritability, hypertonicity, tremors, seizures, temperature instability, and sneezing. Symptoms often occur within 72 hours of birth, but due to the long half-life of methadone, symptoms of methadone withdrawal may take up to 5 days to develop.

Alcohol and cocaine have been associated with birth defects as well. Abnormalities such as absent limbs, cardiac defects, genitourinary anomalies, ocular anomalies, and microcephaly have been reported with cocaine exposure. Alcohol has been associated with a spectrum of effects, termed *fetal alcohol spectrum disorders (FASD)*. Within this spectrum, a subset of patients fit the well-defined criteria for a diagnosis of fetal alcohol syndrome (FAS). These criteria include facial dysmorphology, growth deficiency, and neurodevelopmental abnormality. The presence of 3 sentinel features in the facial dysmorphology is the most sensitive and specific diagnostic finding for FAS. These features include a flat philtrum, thin upper lip, and short palpebral fissures. The spectrum of neurodevelopmental problems includes diagnoses such as microcephaly and seizures, as well as many types of developmental, cognitive, and behavioral difficulties. Also included within FASD is a category for alcohol-related birth defects. This category includes anomalies such as congenital heart defects, skeletal deformities, renal anomalies, hearing loss, ophthalmologic abnormalities, and cleft lip and palate.

Pathophysiology

Drugs used by pregnant women may affect infants in 3 different ways: (1) the drugs may be addictive and result in symptoms of withdrawal during the neonatal period, (2) they may be toxic and lead to impaired functioning and neurodevelopmental problems, and (3) they may be teratogenic and cause congenital anomalies and a dysmorphic appearance. The ultimate effects of the drugs are due to a complex interaction of environmental and genetic influences that have variable effects depending on the timing of the prenatal exposure. Differences in the maternal metabolism of drugs lead to differences in fetal exposure to toxins, and genetically determined differences in fetal susceptibility to the toxins lead to a spectrum of effects in exposed children. During gestation, the effects of drug exposure also vary depending on the timing of exposure. Each organ has a unique period of susceptibility as it forms during the first trimester. Prenatal substance exposure during this time period is more likely to result in organ malformation. The second and third trimesters primarily involve organ growth, cell differentiation, and functional maturation of organs, so exposure during this time period is

more likely to result in growth abnormalities or functional difficulties. The specific effects of the different substances on the developing fetus can be understood in terms of their biochemical properties.

In utero exposure to opiates such as heroin and methadone results in physiological addiction. These drugs bind to opiate receptor sites in the brain and GI tract. When the drugs are no longer present after birth, the newborn experiences withdrawal. Animal models have also found that prenatal exposure to opiates can lead to decreased density of cortical neurons and decreased development of neurons.

Cocaine and its metabolites cross the placenta and concentrate in amniotic fluid. Cocaine is toxic and teratogenic, and it interferes with 3 neurotransmitter pathways in the brain. (1) Cocaine blocks the reuptake of norepinephrine. This is associated with tachycardia, hypertension, diaphoresis, and an increased incidence of preterm labor. Diffuse vasoconstriction may affect the placenta and lead to anomalies such as placental infarcts or abruptio placentae. The fetus may also be affected by the vasoconstriction and its resultant hypoperfusion and ischemia, and may develop anomalies such as atresia of the GI tract, stroke, or absent limbs.

(2) Cocaine decreases the reuptake of dopamine. This effect is apparent in cocaine-using mothers who have decreased appetite and subsequent poor nutrition during pregnancy. Stereotypical behavior, hyperactivity, euphoria, confidence, and heightened sexuality may be associated with sexual promiscuity and increased risk of acquiring HIV and sexually transmitted infections (STIs). (3) Cocaine decreases serotonin reuptake, leading to decreased sleep. The sleep cycle of cocaine-exposed infants is often disrupted.

Methamphetamine is commonly manufactured from ephedrine or pseudoephedrine, and has greater central nervous system (CNS) penetration than its metabolite, amphetamine. It has direct toxic effects on the CNS and causes increased release and decreased reuptake of dopamine, norepinephrine, and serotonin. These neurotransmitter alterations result in symptoms that are similar to those described for cocaine. There is limited published data on the incidence of teratogenesis as a result of in utero methamphetamine exposure, but recent data show that exposed newborns are at risk of being born small for gestational age.

Direct effects of methamphetamine use are dose- and frequency-dependent in the adult user. It has been shown to have cardiovascular, pulmonary, renal, and hepatic toxicity. Higher dose and increased frequency have also been associated with psychosis and with toxicity to subcortical structures. More recent data have also noted subcortical white matter and gray matter changes in prenatally exposed children.

Reports have documented the occurrence of withdrawal symptoms within days after birth in alcohol-exposed neonates, but the more common effects of prenatal alcohol exposure are direct cellular toxicity and teratogenesis. The specific mechanism by which alcohol and its metabolites damage fetal tissues is unknown, but it has been shown to affect CNS neuronal migration and synaptogenesis. For a given level of alcohol intake, the precise level of fetal exposure to the metabolites is likely to vary among women, depending on maternal genetic makeup and the resulting variability in alcohol metabolism. The timing of the exposure during different periods of development can also lead to different teratogenic effects on the fetus. Exposure during the first trimester may affect organogenesis or craniofacial development, and exposure in the second and third trimesters can cause poor growth and neurotoxicity. Maternal alcohol use may also be associated with poor nutrition, resulting in poor delivery of nutrients to the fetus.

Phencyclidine (PCP) has sympathomimetic effects, including increases in blood pressure, heart rate, respiratory rate, deep tendon reflexes, and tone. In addition, PCP has cholinergic effects, causing sweating, flushing, drooling, and pupillary constriction. Infants exposed to PCP in utero do not exhibit these symptoms, however, but display neurologic and developmental disorganization.

Differential Diagnosis

The major differential diagnoses relate to the symptomatology produced by the abused substance or substances (Dx Box). Neonates exposed to addictive substances, most commonly opiates such as methadone and heroin, may present with symptoms of withdrawal (Box 131-1). Irritability and jitteriness may be symptoms of drug withdrawal or direct drug neurotoxicity, but may also be due to hypoglycemia, hypocalcemia, hypomagnesemia, and sepsis. Seizures occur in 1% to 3% of heroin-exposed infants, and the differential diagnosis for neonatal seizures includes intracranial hemorrhage, hypoxic-ischemic encephalopathy, CNS infection, CNS malformation, and metabolic disorders. Gastrointestinal symptoms such as vomiting or diarrhea may be confused with reflux, formula intolerance, obstruction, or infectious gastroenteritis.

Dx Infants of Substance-Abusing Mothers

- Symptoms of withdrawal (see Box 131-1)
- Congenital anomalies
- Developmental delay and behavioral disorders
- Growth retardation
- Sexually transmitted infections

Dysmorphic appearance may also be the result of alcohol or drug exposure. Fetal alcohol syndrome is the most clearly defined dysmorphic syndrome related to maternal substance abuse during pregnancy. In making such a diagnosis, other genetic disorders that may have overlapping findings should be considered as well.

Failure to thrive (FTT) may also be a presenting complaint in infants or children with a history of in utero drug or alcohol exposure. (See Chapter 129 for a discussion of the differential diagnosis of FTT.) It is important to consider maternal substance abuse in all patients who have been diagnosed with FTT, particularly if they were born small for gestational age.

Older children may present with a wide range of neurodevelopmental and behavioral problems. Common behavioral complaints

Box 131-1. Symptoms of Neonatal Abstinence Syndrome

• Irritability	• Vomiting
• Jitteriness	• Diarrhea
• Tremors	• Apnea
• Hypertonicity	• Tachypnea
• Seizures	• Sweating
• Mottling	• Poor feeding
• Temperature instability	• Sleeping difficulties

include impulsivity, inattention, hyperactivity, and antisocial behavior. While many of these symptoms have been correlated with prenatal drug exposure, postnatal environmental factors such as continued parental substance abuse, violence, inconsistent or poor parenting, and foster care placement are also significant contributors. As a result, it may be difficult to clearly determine the precise etiology of developmental and behavioral problems in a drug- or alcohol-exposed child.

Maternal substance abuse should be considered in all infants who present with STIs such as syphilis, hepatitis B, hepatitis C, and HIV.

Evaluation

History

The possibility of maternal substance abuse should be considered in the face of certain maternal risk factors. These factors include the absence of prenatal care, evidence of poor maternal nutrition, poor maternal weight gain, presence of STIs, symptoms of acute intoxication, abruptio placentae, precipitous delivery, and a history of domestic violence.

Infants who manifest symptoms of withdrawal should be evaluated for the possibility of maternal substance abuse. This assessment involves an appropriate history as well as a toxicological evaluation. Mothers disclose their drug history to varying extents, depending on the circumstances of the interview. If mothers are concerned about the health and well-being of their infants and do not fear legal repercussions, they are more likely to discuss their drug use. An appropriate drug history should be obtained in a nonjudgmental manner (Questions Box). Studies have shown that the use of a structured questionnaire rather than a cursory interview increases the incidence of reported substance abuse by 3- to 5-fold.

Physical Examination

Infants should be assessed for common complications related to maternal substance abuse. They should undergo a full physical examination to check for the presence of any malformations. Growth measurements should be noted, and physicians should determine if evidence of growth impairment or microcephaly is present. Premature infants should be monitored for problems related to prematurity, such as intraventricular hemorrhage and necrotizing enterocolitis. Assessment for signs of neonatal abstinence syndrome should be done in the days after birth (see Box 131-1). Neurologic

Questions

Infants of Substance-Abusing Mothers

- Did the mother use any substances such as alcohol, cigarettes, marijuana, or prescription and illicit drugs during the pregnancy?
- Has she ever used these substances? Is she currently using these substances?
- If so, how much? How frequently? By what route? To what extent is she trying to abstain?
- Is the mother at risk for sexually transmitted infections? Has she ever been tested?
- Did the mother have prenatal care? When did the care start?
- What is the status of other children in the family?
- Does the father abuse alcohol or drugs?

and developmental status should be assessed and monitored at each visit. Abnormalities such as hypertonicity, coarse tremors, and extensor leg posture are frequently noted in the newborn period, and disturbances in both fine and gross motor coordination may persist through the toddler years.

Laboratory Tests

In addition to obtaining a toxicological history, screening for drugs should also be performed. The legal guidelines for screening mothers for drugs vary in different localities. In general, if clinical symptoms indicate a need, infants can be screened on medical grounds without specific parental consent because the information obtained is important in the care of the infant. Screening of the mother's urine without her consent is more problematic, however, because of the potential legal implications of a positive test.

Testing is most commonly performed on urine samples, which are typically able to detect an exposure within the prior 3 days. It is important to realize that a negative screening test does not rule out the possibility of exposure within this window of time, however, as a drug's metabolite may be present but not to the level of the test's detection threshold. Newer tests include meconium analysis, which is more sensitive and specific than urine, and is able to detect exposures in the second and third trimesters. Recent data indicate, however, that its greatest sensitivity lies with exposures beyond 24 weeks' gestation. Analysis of newborn hair samples can also detect exposures occurring during the third trimester. At present, there is limited ability to determine precisely when an exposure occurred during gestation, other than according to the broad detection windows discussed here in conjunction with maternal self-report on the timing of drug use.

Most screening tests of urine, meconium, and hair samples use immunoassay techniques, which are inexpensive and sensitive, but not very specific. False-positive results may be obtained for multiple illicit substances. Common scenarios include a positive amphetamine screen in a patient who has taken over-the-counter medication containing ephedrine or pseudoephedrine, or a positive opiate screen in a patient who is using cough medicine with dextromethorphan. For this reason, and because of the potential legal implications of a positive result in this setting, it is strongly recommended that positive immunoassay results be confirmed with further testing of the sample via gas chromatography/mass spectrometry.

Further evaluation in the neonatal period should include an evaluation for the presence of STIs, particularly HIV, hepatitis B, hepatitis C, and syphilis.

Imaging Studies

There is no routine imaging recommended based solely on a history of in utero substance exposure. Instead, imaging should be directed by symptomatology. For example, infants with a heart murmur and a history of prenatal alcohol exposure warrant a cardiac evaluation and possible echocardiography. Also, infants with prenatal drug exposure and abnormal neurologic examinations should have a thorough neurologic evaluation, which may include neuroimaging.

Management

In the neonatal period, the management of drug-exposed infants requires attention to associated conditions such as prematurity, in utero growth restriction, and in utero infection with STIs.

Irritability and crying may occur either from withdrawal or as the result of drug toxicity on the CNS. These infants may respond to swaddling, a soothing voice, or a quiet environment as a means to reduce the symptoms. Some exposed infants may have slow or disordered feeding and may require evaluation by an occupational therapist or nutritionist as well.

The assessment of a newborn's withdrawal symptoms is typically done using a standardized scoring tool to assist in the documentation of symptom severity. Once scores reach a threshold level, pharmacologic treatment may be required. For opiate-exposed infants, treatment with an opiate such as methadone, diluted tincture of opium, or paregoric is particularly helpful. Paregoric, once commonly used to treat symptoms of withdrawal, is now used less frequently because of the presence of alcohol and benzoic acid in the preparation. Phenobarbital is also commonly used in cases of polydrug exposure. Diazepams are useful for symptoms related to alcohol withdrawal or to rapidly reverse symptoms of opioid withdrawal. Problems with using diazepam relate to the presence of sodium benzoate in the preparation, which can displace bilirubin from albumin. Medications should be tapered over time, allowing infants to outgrow the dosage.

Social service is also a key component of management. In many jurisdictions, child protective services must be notified of positive toxicological tests on newborn infants or their mothers. Likewise, infants who display symptoms of neonatal drug withdrawal may also have to be reported to these agencies. These agencies are generally responsible for performing a home assessment and determining the adequacy of the home environment. In some cases, infants may be assigned to foster homes. Parents may be ordered to participate in drug treatment programs and parenting classes.

After the newborn period the focus of management is on the provision of **well-child care and developmental monitoring.** Attention should be paid to physical growth and administration of immunizations. If a sensory impairment or neurodevelopmental delay is apparent, children should be referred to appropriate community agencies. Federal programs that operate under the Individuals with Disabilities Education Act provide interventional services for disabled and at-risk children 6 years of age and younger.

Symptoms of ADHD or other behavioral problems in older children may require intervention, with recommendation for specific school programs as well as pharmacologic treatment. Regular assessments of school performance should be obtained from children's teachers. Standardized neurodevelopmental tests should be administered at periodic intervals to ensure appropriate progress.

Prognosis

Many infants, particularly those exposed to alcohol in utero, suffer long-term sequelae and disability. Most commonly, these effects are subtle but can have far-reaching impact for the child. Remedial educational programs help, but do not cure, the problems. Recent studies have shown that for drug-exposed children, the environment in which they are raised is a significant factor affecting their ultimate outcome. A stable, nurturing environment minimizes the many adverse effects of prenatal drug exposure and promotes normal neurodevelopment by enforcing the acquisition of skills and knowledge.

CASE RESOLUTION

The case history presented highlights the typical features of the drug-exposed infant. Management includes testing for hepatitis B, hepatitis C, syphilis, and HIV and administering medication such as phenobarbital if the irritability does not respond to swaddling or other measures. The situation should be reported to child protective services to ensure an assessment of the infant's home environment.

Selected References

Davies JK, Bledsoe JM. Prenatal alcohol and drug exposures in adoption. *Pediatr Clin North Am.* 2005;52:1369–1393

Lester BM, Lagasse LL. Children of addicted women. *J Addic Dis.* 2010;29:259–276

Lozano J, Garcia-Algar O, Vall O, de la Torre R, Scaravelli G, Pichini S. Biological matrices for the evaluation of in utero exposure to drugs of abuse. *Ther Drug Monit.* 2007;29:711–734

Manning MA, Hoyme HE. Fetal alcohol spectrum disorders: a practical clinical approach to diagnosis. *Neurosci Biobehav Rev.* 2007;31:230–238

Nguyen D, Smith LM, Lagasse LL, et al. Intrauterine growth of infants exposed to prenatal methamphetamine: results from the infant development, environment and lifestyle study. *J Pediatr.* 2010;157:337–339

Osborn DA, Jeffery HE, Cole MJ. Sedatives for opiate withdrawal in newborn infants. *Cochrane Database Syst Rev.* 2005;3:CD002053

Pollard I. Neuropharmacology of drugs and alcohol in mother and fetus. *Semin Fetal Neonatal Med.* 2007;12:106–113

Shankaran S, Lester BM, Das A, et al. Impact of maternal substance use during pregnancy on childhood outcome. *Semin Fetal Neonatal Med.* 2007;12:143–150

Substance Abuse and Mental Health Services Administration. 2009 national survey on drug use and health. http://oas.samhsa.gov/nsduhLatest.htm

CHAPTER 132

Substance Abuse

Monica Sifuentes, MD

CASE STUDY

A 17-year-old adolescent male is brought to your office by his father with a chief complaint of chronic cough. You have followed this patient and his siblings for several years and know the family quite well. The father appears very concerned about "this cough that just won't go away." The adolescent is not concerned about the cough, however, and reports no associated symptoms such as fever, sore throat, chest pain, or sinus pain. You ask the father to step out of the room for the rest of the interview and the physical examination.

On further questioning, the patient reports that he smokes a few cigarettes a day and has tried marijuana as well as cocaine. He denies regular use of these substances, but reports exposure to these drugs at parties and when he hangs out with "certain friends." The adolescent is now in the 11th grade, attends school regularly, and thinks school is "OK." His grades are average to above average, but he thinks he might fail history this semester. Although he used to play baseball, he dropped out last year. He hopes to get a part-time job at a local fast-food restaurant this summer if his parents let him. Currently he is sexually active and uses condoms occasionally. He denies suicidal ideation and exposure to any firearms.

On physical examination, he appears well developed and well nourished with an occasional dry cough. He is afebrile, and his respiratory rate, heart rate, and blood pressure are normal. Pertinent findings on examination include slight conjunctival injection bilaterally and mild erythema of the posterior pharynx. No tonsillar hypertrophy is apparent. The rest of the examination is within normal limits.

Questions

1. What are the most common manifestations of substance use and abuse in adolescents?
2. What are the risk factors associated with substance abuse in adolescents?
3. What other conditions must be considered when evaluating adolescents with a history of chronic substance abuse?
4. What laboratory evaluation, if any, should be considered in adolescents with suspected substance use or abuse?
5. What are the specific consequences, if any, of short-term and long-term use or abuse of substances such as alcohol, marijuana, cocaine, opiates, and hallucinogens?

Primary care practitioners are in a unique position to educate patients, particularly young teenagers, about substance use and abuse through primary prevention and anticipatory guidance. Opportunities for education include health maintenance visits, the preparticipation sports physical, and during the encounter for an acute injury or illness. More importantly, given their long-standing relationship with families, primary care providers can identify and treat a substance abuse problem as it develops and assist patients and their families with the appropriate referrals and local resources.

Ideally, all preadolescent and adolescent patients should be questioned and counseled about the use of illicit drugs, alcohol, and tobacco at each health maintenance visit (see Chapters 6 and 33). Unfortunately, this occurs inconsistently because most health care professionals often feel uncomfortable opening Pandora's box, or simply do not have the resources to intervene. Time constraints, unfamiliar billing codes, and difficulty maintaining confidentiality for sensitive services in a busy office or clinic make screening for substance use a major challenge. Primary care practitioners thus lose a valuable opportunity to adequately assess adolescents for substance abuse and provide them with the necessary guidance to ensure their future health and well-being.

Substance use can be defined as the use of or experimentation with illicit drugs, alcohol, or tobacco. Illicit drugs include marijuana; cocaine; amphetamines; hallucinogens such as lysergic acid diethylamide (LSD), mescaline, and psilocybin, which is found in *Psilocybe mexicana* mushrooms; opiates; and phencyclidine (PCP). **Substance abuse** refers to the chronic use of mind-altering drugs in spite of adverse affects. **Addiction** is the term applied to compulsive and continued use of a substance in the face of these adverse consequences. The substance may produce physical dependence or symptoms of withdrawal when it is discontinued.

Epidemiology

Current Trends and Prevalence Rates

A wide range of substances are currently being used by adolescents in the United States. Alcohol, tobacco, and marijuana are clearly the more common and most popular substances and serve as "gateway drugs" to more serious drug use. Several surveys tracking adolescent substance use and abuse are conducted annually in the United States to identify high-risk behavior among 8th to 12th graders. The 3 most well-known of these surveys are Monitoring the Future administered annually by the University of Michigan for the National Institute on Drug Abuse of 8th, 10th and 12th grade students; the Youth Risk Behavior Surveillance (YRBS) survey conducted biannually by the Centers for Disease Control and Prevention (CDC) of students in grades 9 through 12; and the National Household Survey on Drug Abuse and Health, a computer-assisted interview of residents 12 years and older conducted in the home. It is important to remember that most statistics do not include the estimated 15% to 20% of students who drop out of high school before their senior year.

In a recent survey of graduating high school seniors (2009 YRBS), approximately 80% admitted to **alcohol** use at some time during their life. Just over half (51%) of students reported drinking alcohol during the month preceding the survey, and 3% to 5% admitted that they used alcohol daily. Binge drinking has probably contributed most to the overall morbidity and mortality associated with alcohol use in adolescents and young adults. Among high school seniors in the class of 2009, one-third reported having 5 or more drinks in a row at least once during the previous 2 weeks. Although **tobacco** use among adolescents decreased from 1975 to 1993, 2009 data from the CDC reveal that approximately 20% of teenagers nationwide still report current cigarette use. Eight percent of adolescents smoked a half a pack or more cigarettes per day in 2009 compared with 11% in 2005 and 19% in 1977. Among students nationwide who smoked cigarettes and are younger than 18 years, 14% report buying them themselves in a store or gas station. Nationwide current smokeless tobacco use (eg, chewing tobacco, snuff, or dip) and cigar or cigarillo use is 9% and 14%, respectively. As expected, its use is much higher among males than females.

Marijuana is the most commonly used illicit psychoactive substance. In 1993, 35% of high school seniors reported ever having used marijuana, and in 1997, this figure increased to more than 50%. Current estimates from the 2009 Youth Risk Behavior Surveillance System (YRBSS) report this figure to be approximately the same at 46%, with nearly 25% reporting marijuana use one or more times during the month preceding the survey. Daily use of marijuana has been reported in 5% of high school seniors.

The use of other substances among adolescents had generally taken a downward trend in the late 1980s and early 1990s; however, figures are increasing again. This is known in the substance abuse literature as "generational forgetting" as adverse effects of specific drugs fade over the years. Reportedly, approximately 9% of high school graduates in 1997 tried cocaine, with approximately 4% having used it in the previous month. These figures remain unchanged more than 20 years later in 2009. The 1991 prevalence rate for LSD usage was 5%, and its use has shown no appreciable decline in the past 10 years. In fact, LSD use among teens has increased significantly and may be more widespread than cocaine use among high school students. According to the latest YRBS 2009 survey, 10% of

high school seniors nationwide had tried LSD or another hallucinogenic drug. Lifetime amphetamine use among 12th graders was 4% in 2009 and ranged from 2.3% to almost 8% across state surveys. In addition, nationwide ecstasy use was reported as approximately 7%.

Concurrently, the reported use of over-the-counter (OTC) nonprescription stimulants that contain caffeine or phenylpropanolamine has increased. Other substances used to "get high," such as inhalants, are often used by younger students (preteens). Nineteen percent of ninth graders surveyed by the CDC in 1997 reported having sniffed or inhaled substances to become intoxicated compared with 13% in 2009. Dextromethorphan is one of the most recent OTC products to be abused by adolescents secondary to its hallucinogenic effects and easy accessibility. Recent studies report an increasing trend in its abuse, particularly in teens younger than 18 years. Additionally, prescription drugs such as Oxycontin, Percocet, Vicodin, Adderall, Ritalin, and Xanax are reported to have been taken by 20% of teenagers in 2009 without a doctor's prescription one or more times during their life.

Although not considered an illicit substance by some, anabolic steroids are abused by some adolescents, mostly males, to increase muscle size and strength. In 1997 approximately 3% admitted to using them at some time in their lives. More recently, studies indicate as many as 5.5% of high school students participating in sports use anabolic steroids (6.6% males, 3.9% females). The 2009 nationwide figure per the CDC is 3.3%, however these figures vary across state and local surveys from 2% to 7%.

Demographics

In general, adolescent males use illicit drugs more than females do, with a few exceptions. Males are more likely to use anabolic steroids, but females reportedly use amphetamines, barbiturates, tranquilizers, and OTC diet pills more than their male counterparts. In addition, although annual prevalence rates for overall alcohol use show little gender difference, adolescent males have a higher rate of heavy or binge drinking. Tobacco usage is essentially the same for both genders, except for smokeless tobacco and cigars where males predominate.

Non–college-bound adolescents are more likely to use illicit substances than their college-bound counterparts, and these adolescents are also more likely to use drugs more frequently. There is no difference, however, between the 2 groups in the rates of ever having tried illicit substances. Binge drinking also continues to escalate among older adolescents and young adults attending college. The specific influence of parental education, socioeconomic status, and race, or ethnicity on the use and abuse of illicit substances is difficult to determine since many other factors such as genetics and the environment contribute to drug use and addiction.

Risk Factors and Risk Behaviors

Although alcohol and tobacco are considered licit or lawful drugs, it is illegal for minors to purchase and use alcohol and tobacco in the United States. Alcohol and tobacco use, however, often begins during adolescence, and sometimes during the preteen years. The strongest predictor of drug use by youth is having friends who use drugs (alcohol, tobacco, or other substances) regularly. In addition, it has been shown that the more risk factors identified, the greater the risk of substance abuse in the teenager.

Several factors are important precursors (risk factors) to drug use during adolescence. These include association with drug-using peers; attitudinal factors, such as favorable attitudes regarding drug use in the family and low religiosity; poor school performance or academic failure, often beginning in the late elementary years; young age of initiation of alcohol or drug use; presence of a conduct disorder; environmental factors, such as the prevalence of drug use in a given community; a family history of alcoholism or drug use; poor parenting practices; high levels of conflict within the family; minimal bonding between parents and children; and early and persistent problem behaviors during childhood such as untreated attention-deficit/hyperactivity disorder (ADHD).

It has been well documented in the literature that early age of onset of alcohol and tobacco use is predictive for the use of other drugs, the use of a greater variety of drugs, and the use of more potent agents. Additionally, the use of alcohol at an early age is associated with future alcohol-related problems such as lifetime alcohol dependence and abuse. The early initiation of alcohol also results in greater sexual risk-taking behavior during adolescence (unprotected sexual intercourse, exposure to multiple sexual partners, being drunk or high during sexual intercourse, and increased risk of pregnancy) as well as academic problems and delinquent behavior later in adolescence. Long-term effects during young adulthood include employment problems, criminal and aggressive behavior, and continued substance abuse.

The role of the media and technology in adolescent alcohol and tobacco use has been the subject of much discussion over the last 10 years. A number of studies have confirmed that exposure to television and movie smoking is one of the key factors that prompt teens to smoke, and that preteens whose parents forbid them from viewing R-rated movies are less likely to begin smoking or drinking. One prospective study revealed that exposure to R-rated movies or having a television in the bedroom significantly increased the risk of initiating smoking for white teenagers. Additionally, watching more movie depictions of alcohol use is strongly predictive of drinking onset and binge drinking in adolescents in the United States. Advertising also contributes to the depiction of alcohol and tobacco use as normative activities. In fact, it has been reported that advertising may be responsible for up to 30% of adolescent alcohol and tobacco use.

Clinical Presentation

Adolescents who are involved in substance abuse may present to the physician in several different ways. Illicit substance use might be uncovered during the routine interview for an annual health maintenance visit or preparticipation sports physical. Alternatively, the adolescent might have physical complaints including chronic cough, persistent allergies, chest pain, and fatigue. Chronic conditions such as asthma may be worsening despite appropriate therapy in the adolescent smoking tobacco or marijuana.

Abdominal tenderness may be noted on physical examination and found to be associated with gastritis, hepatitis, or pancreatitis. The adolescent also recently may have been in a motor vehicle crash, involved in other trauma, or their parents may complain of the teen's frequent mood swings, irritability, or erratic sleep patterns.

Pathophysiology

Although several theories have been proposed to explain why casual substance use develops into abuse and addiction in some adolescents, the most critical factor seems to be the presence of underlying psychopathology. Adolescents who have untreated major depressive disorders, ADHD, or schizophrenia, for example, may use mood-altering substances to treat unpleasant feelings of dysphoria and low self-esteem. Although initially used as a temporary measure, this method of self-medication makes chronic use with some substances more likely.

It is well known that genetic influences play a role in adult use and abuse of alcohol; however, less evidence exists regarding adolescents. What is known is that families and parental attitudes play a significant role in the development of alcohol and other drug use in teens. Permissive attitudes toward alcohol and drug use by parents or guardians and parental or older sibling drug use predict greater drug and alcohol use in the adolescent.

Differential Diagnosis

The differential diagnosis for symptoms and behaviors associated with substance abuse includes underlying psychiatric disorders. Affective, antisocial, and conduct disorders as well as ADHD can be the primary or secondary condition in adolescents who are abusing drugs. Like adults, adolescents may be using illicit drugs to self medicate. The pharmacology and toxicity of the illicit substances most commonly used by adolescents are summarized in Table 132-1.

Evaluation

History

The interview should be conducted in a private, quiet area to minimize interruptions. If parents have accompanied adolescents, they should be politely asked to leave the room after they have had an opportunity to express their concerns and after issues of confidentiality are addressed in the presence of both parties. This avoids further awkward moments when parents may ask what was disclosed during the interview with their teenager. After parents have left the room, issues regarding confidentiality and privacy should be reviewed once again with the patient. Special circumstances, such as a disclosure of sexual or physical abuse and/or possible suicide ideation or homicidal intent, that dictate that confidentiality be broken also should be discussed (see Chapter 6).

The interview should then proceed in a casual, non-pressured fashion. Initial inquiries should cover less-threatening general topics such as school, home life, and outside activities, including activities

Table 132-1. Pharmacology and Toxicity of Substances Commonly Used by Adolescents[a]

Substance	Pharmacology	Effects	Toxicity
Nicotine	Potent psychoactive drug, acting on receptors in CNS to produce effects: stimulation, relaxation, focuses attention		**Non-tolerant individuals** Weakness, nausea, vomiting Feeling unwell
Marijuana	Active ingredient (Δ^9-tetrahydro-cannabinol) rapidly absorbed into bloodstream from inhaled smoke	**Low dose** Euphoria, relaxation, time distortion, auditory and visual enhancement **High dose/toxic** Mood fluctuations, hallucinations, paranoia, psychosis	**Acute** Panic attacks, psychosis (rare) **Chronic** Short-term memory impairment, amotivational syndrome, reduced sperm counts
Alcohol	Causes nerve cell membranes to expand and become more "fluid"—interfering with neuronal conduction Interference of neurotransmitters	**Mild** Disinhibition, euphoria, mild impaired coordination, mild sedation **Moderate** Increased sedation, slurred speech, ataxia	**Severe** Confusion, stupor, coma, respiratory depression
Cocaine	Increased release and decreased reuptake of biogenic amines causing CNS and peripheral nervous system stimulation Local anesthesia Vasoconstriction	Produces a sense of well-being and heightened awareness, decrease in social inhibition, intense euphoria	Delirium, confusion, paranoia, hypertension, tachycardia, hyperpyrexia, mydriasis
Stimulants Amphetamines Crystal methamphetamine Ecstasy	CNS stimulation (sympathomimetic)	Heightened awareness Restlessness and agitation, decreased appetite Low doses increase ability to concentrate	Hypertension, hyperthermia, seizures, stroke, coma, arrhythmias
Hallucinogens LSD Mescaline Mushrooms	Inhibits release of serotonin	Distortions of reality—perceptual alterations, "synesthesias" common (eg, "hearing" smells)	Paranoia, flashbacks, psychosis, depression
Phencyclidine	Dissociative anesthetic with analgesic, stimulant, depressant, and hallucinogenic properties	Dissociative anesthetic Dose-dependent euphoria, dysphoria, perceptual distortion	Psychoses; aggressive, violent behavior; depression; seizures, rhabdomyolysis
Opiates Opium Heroin Methadone	Binds to opioid receptors in CNS, causing CNS depression	Sedative analgesics Euphoria followed by sedation, somnolence	Respiratory depression, CNS depression, miosis, bradycardia, hypotension, arrhythmia, seizures, rhabdomyolysis
Sedatives Benzodiazepines Barbiturates	CNS depression, binds to specific receptor that potentiates GABA	Sedation Anxiety reduction	Similar to opioid intoxication
Anabolic steroids	Bind to androgen receptors at cellular level, stimulate production of RNA and protein synthesis	Euphoria Increased irritability and aggressiveness Induction of mental changes at high doses	Psychosis
Inhalants	CNS stimulation and excitement, progressing to depression	Euphoria, hallucinations, psychosis	Respiratory depression, arrhythmia, seizures, sudden sniffing death syndrome (sudden death secondary to arrhythmia)

Abbreviations: CNS, central nervous system; GABA, γ-aminobutyric acid; LSD, lysergic acid diethylamide.

[a] Data from Schwartz B, Alderman EM. Substances of abuse. *Pediatr Rev.* 1997;18:206–214, and Joffe A, Blythe MJ, eds. Mental health, psychotropic medications, and substance abuse. *Adolesc Med.* 2003;14:455–466.

with friends. **HEADDSSS** (*h*ome environment, *e*mployment and education, *a*ctivities, *d*iet, *d*rugs, *s*exual activity/sexuality [including a history of sexual abuse or assault], *s*uicide/depression, and *s*afety) allows for a thorough review of the essential components of the psychosocial history (see Chapter 6).

Some practitioners prefer to use questionnaires to obtain this background information. A questionnaire is given to patients to fill out while they are waiting to be seen, and the responses are reviewed privately during the actual visit (Box 132-1). Controversy exists regarding the role of such questionnaires, primarily concerning the truthfulness of answers, because parents may be with the teenager as he or she is attempting to complete the form.

More specific questions related to the use of alcohol and tobacco as well as illicit substances should be asked after general subjects have been discussed (Questions Box). If adolescents seem wary of answering these questions, it may be helpful to initially inquire about their friends. Questions should be phrased with the assumption that the responses will be affirmative (eg, How many beers do your friends drink in a week? And you, do you drink the same amount?). It is hoped that this less-threatening approach invites more honest answers. An assessment of the risk of suicidal behavior is also indicated. Further questions relevant to substance abuse are given in Box 132-2.

Because many clinicians do not have unlimited time to interview adolescents and obtain all of the details at one visit, another approach has been developed to efficiently screen for drug and alcohol problems using 3 questions: (1) Have you *ever* smoked a cigarette? (2) Have you *ever* had an alcoholic drink? and (3) Have you *ever* used marijuana or any other drug to get high? The thinking is that by using the word "ever" the clinician is asking a clearer question. Additional screening is recommended for any teenager who answers "yes" to any of these 3 initial questions. Six questions, known as the CRAFFT questions, are then reviewed to further screen the adolescent for drug and alcohol problems (Box 132-3). The teen receives 1 point for each "yes" answer; a total score of 2 or more indicates a high risk for a substance abuse problem and the need for additional follow-up as well as a referral to a mental health professional. The validity of this tool with adolescents has been reported in the literature and is well supported.

Physical Examination

Positive findings on physical examination are rare, especially in adolescents who use alcohol or other substances only occasionally. In adolescents with a history of chronic substance abuse, however, certain physical findings may be present.

All vital signs should be reviewed. Tachycardia and hypertension occur primarily with acute intoxication with cocaine or stimulants such as amphetamines. The current weight also should be recorded and compared with previous values, and any significant weight loss should be noted. The skin should be examined closely for track marks, skin abscesses, or cellulitis, especially if patients admit to using drugs intravenously. Findings consistent with hepatitis (hepatomegaly and jaundice) may be present in these individuals. The presence of diffuse adenopathy, thrush, leukoplakia, seborrheic dermatitis, or parotitis should raise the suspicion of HIV infection.

Box 132-1. Questionnaire Items Relevant to Substance Abuse[a]		
1. Do you smoke cigarettes?	Y_____	N_____
2. Do you smoke marijuana?	Y_____	N_____
3. Do you often feel "bummed out," down, or depressed?	Y_____	N_____
4. Do you ever use drugs or alcohol to feel better?	Y_____	N_____
5. Do you ever use drugs or alcohol when you are alone?	Y_____	N_____
6. Do your friends get drunk or get high at parties?	Y_____	N_____
7. Do you get drunk or get high at parties?	Y_____	N_____
8. Do your friends ever get drunk or get high at rock concerts?	Y_____	N_____
9. Do you ever get drunk or get high at rock concerts?	Y_____	N_____
10. Have your school grades gone down recently?	Y_____	N_____
11. Have you flunked any subjects recently?	Y_____	N_____
12. Have you had recent problems with your coaches or advisers at school?	Y_____	N_____
13. Do you feel that friends or parents just do not seem to understand you?	Y_____	N_____

[a] Reproduced with permission from American Academy of Pediatrics. *Substance Abuse: A Guide for Professionals.* Schonberg SK, ed. Elk Grove, IL: American Academy of Pediatrics; 1988.

Questions

Adolescent Substance Abuse

- Do any of the adolescent's friends drink alcohol, smoke marijuana or tobacco, or use any other drugs?
- What drugs, including alcohol and tobacco, are currently being used by the adolescent? For how long and how frequently?
- In what environments does the adolescent use these substances?
- Has the adolescent ever blacked out or been arrested while under the influence of drugs or alcohol?
- Has drug or alcohol use ever interfered with school, work, or other social activities?
- Has drug or alcohol use adversely affected relationships with family, friends, or romantic partners?
- Has the patient ever had sexual encounters while under the influence of drugs or alcohol?
- Does the adolescent ever use drugs or alcohol to feel better or to for get why he or she feels sad?
- Do the adolescent's parents use alcohol, tobacco, or illicit drugs?

Upper respiratory symptoms such as chronic nasal congestion, long-lasting "colds" and "allergies," and epistaxis can occur with chronic inhalation of cocaine. Signs of nasal congestion, septal perforation, and wheezing may be noted on examination. In addition, smoking crack cocaine can cause chronic cough, hemoptysis, and chest pain.

<table>
<tr><td colspan="2">

Box 132-2. Open-Ended Questions Intended to Provide a Basis for Further Exploration of Advanced Substance Abuse[a]

1. What do your friends do at parties? Do you go to the parties? Do you drink? Get drunk? Get high?
2. Do you drive drunk? Stoned? Have you ridden with a driver who was drunk or stoned? Could you call home and ask for help? What would your parents say? Do?
3. Do you go to concerts? Do you drink there? Do you get high? Who drives after the concert?
4. After drinking, have you ever forgotten where you had been or what you had done?
5. Have you recently dropped some of your old friends and started going with a new group?
6. Do you feel that lately you are irritable, "bitchy," or moody?
7. Do you find yourself getting into more frequent arguments with your friends? Brothers and sisters? Parents?
8. Do you have a girlfriend/boyfriend? How is that going? Are you having more fights/arguments with him/her lately? Have you recently broken up?
9. Do you find yourself being physically abusive to others? Your brothers/sisters? Your mother/father?
10. Do you think your drinking/drug use is a problem? Why?

[a] Reproduced with permission from American Academy of Pediatrics. *Substance Abuse: A Guide for Professionals.* Schonberg SK, ed. Elk Grove, IL: American Academy of Pediatrics; 1988.

</td><td colspan="2">

Box 132-3. The CRAFFT Questions: A Brief Screening Test for Adolescent Substance Abuse[a,b]

C	Have you ever ridden in a CAR driven by someone who was "high" or had been using alcohol or drugs?
R	Do you ever use alcohol or drugs to RELAX, feel better about yourself, or fit in?
A	Do you ever use alcohol or drugs while you are by yourself (ALONE)?
F	Do you ever FORGET things you did while using alcohol or drugs?
F	Do your FAMILY or FRIENDS ever tell you that you should cut down on your drinking or drug use?
T	Have you ever gotten into TROUBLE while you were using alcohol or drugs?

[a] Reprinted with permission from Knight JR, Sherritt L, Shrier LA, Harris SK, Chang G. Validity of the CRAFFT substance abuse screening test among adolescent clinic patients. *Arch Pediatr Adolesc Med.* 2002;156:607–614. © Children's Hospital Boston, 2009.
[b] Two or more "yes" answers suggest that the adolescent may have a significant problem with abuse or dependence, and warrants an additional assessment.

</td></tr>
</table>

Smoking marijuana over long periods can result in similar findings. Gynecomastia can be seen with use of anabolic steroids, marijuana, amphetamine, and heroin. In the adolescent female using anabolic steroids, there may be signs of virilization, such as a deep voice, hirsutism, and male pattern baldness. The detailed neurologic evaluation is probably the most important part of the examination. Any abnormalities in memory, cognitive functioning, or affect should be noted. Chronic marijuana use is sometimes accompanied by an amotivational syndrome.

Acute intoxication with some drugs such as cocaine may lead to delirium, confusion, paranoia, seizures, hypertension, tachycardia, arrhythmias, mydriasis, and hyperpyrexia. Acute PCP intoxication produces abnormal neurologic signs, tachycardia, and hypertension. Findings such as central nervous system and respiratory depression, miosis, and cardiovascular effects (eg, pulmonary edema, orthostatic hypotension) are consistent with opiate overdose. However, signs and symptoms of acute intoxication are generally seen in the emergency department setting rather than in the primary care provider's office or clinic.

Laboratory Tests

Routine drug screening in the evaluation of possible substance abuse is not recommended and generally not indicated. Specific laboratory studies should be performed only in those patients who are known substance abusers and enrolled in a drug treatment program to monitor for abstinence; required by court order; or in patients with an acute presentation of altered mental status, intoxication, or abnormal neurologic findings, such as may be seen in an emergency department setting. In the office setting, these symptoms are frequently absent, and urine or serum studies to "check" for drug use are not warranted nor useful.

If these tests are performed, they require the adolescent's consent. The results should not be shared with anyone other than the patient, unless the patient gives permission or the substance found is the cause of an acute medical condition. According to the American Academy of Pediatrics and the Society for Adolescent Medicine, obtaining a urine drug test without the consent of the adolescent undermines the physician–adolescent relationship and the development of a meaningful, trusting relationship at this critical time in the patient's life. Drug testing should not be performed simply to allay parental anxiety or confirm suspicions regarding possible substance abuse for a parent, teacher, or athletic coach.

If urine is obtained for drug testing, it is critical that it is not contaminated or diluted and that the provider be familiar with the particular laboratory performing the drug test as well as the reported sensitivity and specificity of each test. Urine testing is available to detect marijuana and its metabolites, cocaine, amphetamines, PCP, opiates, barbiturates, and benzodiazepines. Blood levels can be obtained for alcohol, marijuana, cocaine, amphetamines, barbiturates, and benzodiazepines. Although salivary or urinary concentrations of cotinine and nicotine concentrations can also be performed, these measurements are primarily used in research studies.

Testing for specific inhalants is not routinely done. The deleterious effects of these substances on the hematologic, liver, and renal systems can be evaluated by performing a complete blood cell count, liver function tests, prothrombin time and partial thromboplastin time, and blood urea nitrogen and creatinine.

Management

One of several approaches to the problem of substance use and abuse can be chosen depending on the adolescent's degree of risk-taking behavior and drug involvement, the provider's relationship with the adolescent and their family, the adolescent's desire to change their behavior, and the family's awareness of the problem.

Anticipatory Guidance

If preadolescents or adolescents and their peers are not participating in any high-risk behaviors including tobacco, alcohol, or drug use, pediatricians should provide patients with age-appropriate anticipatory guidance. This should include information regarding safety issues, consequences of alcohol and tobacco use, and exposures to illicit drugs. Adolescents should be praised and encouraged to continue their current behavior but should be invited to return to the office if they have any questions or problems. This may be particularly helpful for patients whose daily environment exposes them to high-risk situations for drug use.

Early Intervention

Primary care practitioners should provide early intervention guidance to preadolescents or adolescents who are engaging in occasional high-risk behavior but whose substance use does not interfere with or disrupt their daily lives. Such use implies only occasional or casual use of illicit substances by patients or peers. This scenario is the most challenging since many adolescents as well as their parents perceive occasional alcohol or drug use as "experimental" or a phase of "normal teen behavior" and therefore may trivialize any advice given by the pediatrician. Interventional guidance involves discussing potential risks created by the adolescent's current behavior. For example, individuals who drink alcohol or smoke marijuana at parties have an increased risk of involvement in a motor vehicle crash afterward either as the driver or passenger. Another common scenario involves alcohol intoxication and poor judgment with regard to sexual behavior. All teens should be made aware of the possible consequences of their unsafe behavior especially if their occasional drug use has progressed to more regular use in risky situations.

Specialized Programs

Preadolescents or adolescents who are routinely using drugs but are clearly motivated to stop can often be managed by primary care physicians. Many of these teenagers began using illicit substances at an older age, have a fairly good relationship with their families, have supportive relationships with friends who do not use drugs, and have continued to do well in school and participate in other outside activities. Practitioners initially should identify the problem and establish whether the adolescent desires to change their behavior. Then practitioners should meet with families, develop an appropriate strategy for treatment intervention, and follow the adolescents periodically in the office. Timely and consistent reinforcement by the primary care physician is necessary, especially in the beginning of treatment. Referral to outpatient programs, such as Alcoholics Anonymous or Narcotics Anonymous, also may be indicated. Appropriate community resources for the teenager as well as family should be reviewed.

Mental Health or Treatment Programs

Referral to a mental health or specialized treatment program (drug detoxification center) is indicated for adolescents who continue to use drugs despite office treatment by the primary care practitioner and adverse effects on their daily lives and relationships. In addition, those teenagers who are suspected to have a concomitant psychological or psychiatric condition should be referred immediately for psychiatric evaluation. Other criteria for specialty treatment programs include a long history of drug abuse, a serious life-threatening event in conjunction with substance abuse (eg, attempted suicide or motor vehicle crash), familial strife, or persistent involvement with a drug-dependent crowd. Primary care practitioners should become familiar with local inpatient programs and residential substance abuse treatment facilities in their community. Although the selection of a program is often dictated by financial resources, it is very important to select an appropriate one for both the adolescent as well as the family. Guidelines exist to aid practitioners in the selection process for both public and private facilities. These guidelines include total abstinence, appropriate professionals with expertise in drug abuse, familial involvement in the program, family therapy, and appropriate outpatient follow-up.

Prevention Programs

Prevention programs have been developed to assist and influence the decisions young people make about the use of illicit substances. Current programs focus on multiple aspects of the lives of children and adolescents. Programs may involve individual decision-making, self-esteem, and basic education regarding drugs. They frequently emphasize communication skills, family values and dynamics, parenting skills, and positive peer associations. Structured curricula also have been created for use in the schools, and community outreach programs have been organized by groups such as local police departments. The actual effectiveness of each type of program is a subject of controversy, but they are all aimed at somehow preventing the initial or continued use of illicit substances in children and preteens.

Prognosis

It is difficult to assess the outcome for adolescents who undergo treatment for substance abuse because definitions of success vary. For some teenagers, success implies periods of sobriety, for others it means complete abstinence, and for still others it is abstinence in addition to recovery from other contributing problems. Specific outcome data that are available, however, reveal that abstinence rates are positively correlated with regular attendance in a support group and parental participation in these groups. In addition, general success rates range from 15% to 45%, depending on short- or long-term assessments. As expected, there is a lifetime potential for relapse among all substance abusers.

CASE RESOLUTION

In the case presented, the adolescent is at high risk for substance abuse given his drug-using friends, tobacco use, possible school failure, and recent change in extracurricular activities (ie, dropping out of baseball). The findings on physical examination also are consistent with his smoking history. The physician should review these risk factors with the teenager and acknowledge the difficulty in removing one's self from such an environment. The adolescent's motivation to change his behavior should be assessed, and referrals to special intervention programs can be discussed. Regardless of the outcome, the physician should continue to see the teenager at an agreed-on interval to monitor his ability to quit smoking and high-risk behavior.

Selected References

American Academy of Pediatrics Committee on Sports Medicine and Fitness. Adolescents and anabolic steroids: a subject review. *Pediatrics.* 1997;99:904–908

American Academy of Pediatrics Committee on Substance Abuse. Alcohol use by youth and adolescents: a pediatric concern. *Pediatrics.* 2010;125:1078–1087

American Academy of Pediatrics Committee on Substance Abuse. Indications for management and referral of patients involved in substance abuse. *Pediatrics.* 2001;106:143–148

American Academy of Pediatrics Committee on Substance Abuse. *Substance Abuse: A Guide for Health Professionals.* Schydlower M, ed. Elk Grove Village, IL: American Academy of Pediatrics; 2002

American Academy of Pediatrics Committee on Substance Abuse. Testing for drugs of abuse in children and adolescents. *Pediatrics.* 1996;98:305–307

American Academy of Pediatrics Committee on Substance Abuse. Testing for drugs of abuse in children and adolescents: addendum—testing in schools and at home. *Pediatrics.* 2007;119:627–630

American Academy of Pediatrics Council on Communications and Media. Children, adolescents, substance abuse, and the media. *Pediatrics.* 2010;126:791–799

Anderson SL, Schaechter J, Brosco JP. Adolescent patients and their confidentiality: staying within legal bounds. *Contemp Pediatr.* 2005;22:54–64

Barangan CJ, Alderman EM. Management of substance abuse. *Pediatr Rev.* 2002;23:123–131

Bryner JK, Wang UK, Hui JW, Bedodo M, MacDougall C, Anderson IB. Dextromethorphan abuse in adolescence. *Arch Pediatr Adolesc Med.* 2006;160:1217–1222

Eaton DK, Kann L, Kinchen S, et al. Youth risk behavior surveillance—United States, 2009. *MMWR Surveill Summ.* 2010;59:1–142

Gray KM, Upadhyaya HP, Deas D, et al. Advances in diagnosis of adolescent substance abuse. *Adolesc Med.* 2006;17:411–425

Heyman RB. Screening for substance abuse in the office: a developmental approach. *Adolesc Med.* 2009;20:9–21

Hollman D, Alderman E, Adam HM. Substance abuse counseling. *Pediatr Rev.* 2007;28:355–357

Kaul P, Coupey SM. Clinical evaluation of substance abuse. *Pediatr Rev.* 2002;23:85–94

Knight JR, Sherritt L, Shrier LA, Harris SK, Chang G. Validity of the CRAFFT substance abuse screening test among adolescent clinic patients. *Arch Pediatr Adolesc Med.* 2002;156:607–614

Kulig JW; American Academy of Pediatrics Committee on Substance Abuse. Tobacco, alcohol, and other drugs: the role of the pediatrician in prevention and management of substance abuse. *Pediatrics.* 2005;115:816–821

Levy S, Knight JR. Helping adolescents to stop using drugs: role of the primary care clinician. *Adolesc Med.* 2008;19:83–98

Levy S, Knight JR. Office management of substance abuse. *Adolesc Health Update.* 2003;15:1–9

Monitoring the Future. www.monitoringthefuture.org

Rimsza ME, Moses KS. Substance abuse on the collage campus. *Pediatr Clin North Am.* 2005;53:307–319

Rodgers PD, Copley L. The nonmedical use of prescription drugs by adolescents. *Adolesc Med.* 2009;20:1–8

Sanchez-Samper X, Knight JR. Drug abuse by adolescent: general considerations. *Pediatr Rev.* 2009;30:83–93

Weddle M, Kokotailo P. Adolescent substance abuse. Confidentiality and consent. *Pediatr Clin North Am.* 2002;49:301–315

Wilson CR, Sherritt L, Gates E, Knight JR. Are clinical impressions of adolescent substance abuse accurate? *Pediatrics.* 2004;114:e536–e540

CHAPTER 133

Eating Disorders

Monica Sifuentes, MD

CASE STUDY

A 16-year-old adolescent female is brought to the office by her mother because she feels that her daughter is too thin. The mother complains that her daughter does not eat much at dinner and always says she is not hungry. Recently the girl bought diet pills that were advertised in a teen magazine. She claims that the pills are supposed to help her gain weight, so she doesn't understand why her mother is so upset. She says she feels fine and considers herself healthy.

The girl is a 10th-grade student at a local public school and attends classes regularly, although her friends are occasionally truant. She is involved in the drill team, the swim team, and the student council. She has many friends who have "nicer" figures than she does. Neither she nor her friends smoke tobacco or use drugs, but they occasionally drink beer at parties. The girl is not sexually active and denies a history of abuse. Her menstrual periods are irregular; the last one was approximately 6 weeks ago.

She currently lives with her mother, father, and 2 younger siblings. Although things are "OK" at home, she thinks her parents are too strict and don't trust her. They have just begun to allow her to date.

Her physical examination is significant for a thin physique and normal vital signs. On the growth chart, her weight is at the 15th percentile and her height at the 75th percentile, giving her a body mass index of 17 (10th percentile). The remainder of her physical examination is unremarkable.

Questions

1. What are the common characteristics of disordered eating in adolescents?
2. What are the important historical points to include when interviewing patients with suspected eating disorders? And which teens are considered at risk?
3. How is the diagnosis of anorexia nervosa (AN) and bulimia nervosa (BN) made?
4. What is the treatment plan for adolescents with eating disorders?
5. What are the medical complications of AN and BN?
6. What is the prognosis for these conditions? How can primary care practitioners help improve the outcome?

Eating disorders are complex problems that are sometimes difficult to diagnose based on strict *Diagnostic and Statistical Manual of Mental Disorders, Fourth Edition, Text Revision* criteria (Box 133-1). Adolescents may have partial or atypical forms, a combination of both AN and BN, or an underlying affective component that confuses the issue. They may not display a blatant refusal to eat, but may instead exhibit subtle characteristics of disordered eating: constant dieting, obsession with a certain physical exercise, or irregular menstruation. In addition, preoccupation with physical appearance and weight is not uncommon or necessarily pathologic in today's Western society. Both the fashion industry and media promote the idea that thinness and beauty are interrelated. Thus typical adolescents who long to be accepted by peers and who are learning to develop a sense of independence and control are prime targets for the development of eating disorders. The primary care physician is in a unique position to recognize individuals at risk, appropriately screen those teenagers with specific behaviors, and provide early intervention to prevent the development of a full-blown eating disorder (Box 133-2). The overall goal is to decrease the life-long medical and psychological morbidity and mortality associated with this condition in adolescents.

Epidemiology

In general, eating disorders are most common among white females and in more affluent communities. Although they occur in many other settings, in previous years they were nearly unheard of in lower socioeconomic groups, among ethnic minorities, or in children younger than 12 years. Today they can be seen in all ethnic, cultural, and social backgrounds in the United States as well as in other developed countries. In addition, males make up an estimated 5% to 10% of all patients with eating disorders.

Although dieting behavior among adolescents and young adults is not uncommon, true AN has a prevalence of approximately 0.5% to 1% in these individuals. Estimates have ranged from 1% to 10% in high-risk groups such as upper- and middle-class white females. Less than 5% of these cases are males, with a female-male ratio of 9:1. The age of onset is usually during early or middle adolescence (age 12–16 years). However, AN has been reported to have a second peak later in adolescence, and it has become increasingly more common for children and younger teens to be dissatisfied with their weight and concerned with body image. Studies have been reported in middle-income elementary school girls where significant body and weight dissatisfaction were noted with increasing grade. Skipping meals and desserts, fasting, and vomiting were all reported specifically to lose weight. Unfortunately, the goal for many of these young girls is not to be of normal weight, but to be underweight.

The prevalence of BN is approximately 1% to 4%, although some studies report that as many as 8% of adolescents and college women and 0.4% of men are bulimic. The age of onset tends to be later than for AN, with symptoms beginning during late adolescence (age 17–20 years) and young adulthood. Females outnumber males by a factor of 5.

Several other behavioral and affective disorders have been associated with AN and BN. These include major depression and other mood disorders in patients as well as first-degree relatives, alcoholism and substance abuse, other addictive behaviors (eg, laxative abuse), poor impulse control and anxiety disorders, and obsessive-compulsive personality. In addition, suicidal behavior (attempts) is more likely in individuals with BN as are reports of an increased incidence of family members with substance abuse and dependence disorders.

Mild variants of eating disorders, which do not meet full diagnostic criteria, occur in approximately 5% to 10% of postpubertal females. Additionally, more than half of junior high and high school girls have dieted at some time, many repeatedly.

Clinical Presentation

Patients with eating disorders usually present with complaints related to weight loss or failure to gain weight and often are referred to the primary care provider by concerned parents, well-intentioned friends, informed coaches, or school personnel. Many adolescents also present with secondary amenorrhea noted during an annual examination. Sometimes an underlying psychiatric condition such as obsessive-compulsive disorder (OCD) is the grounds for the medical referral. Occasionally patients with eating disorders are hospitalized because of complications such as electrolyte disturbances related to diuretic use, hematemesis from induced vomiting, or syncope from hypovolemia.

Pathophysiology

Anorexia Nervosa

Although several factors predispose individuals to the development of AN, this condition has no single cause (Box 133-3). Longitudinal studies clearly point to a significant role of inappropriate dieting behavior in the pathogenesis of an eating disorder. However, because not all dieters develop an eating disorder, other significant risk factors must be involved. Current theory suggests that a complex relationship exists among multiple factors, and that genetic-environmental interactions along with the adolescent's personal experiences (epigenetics) contribute to the etiology of AN.

Biological Factors

It has been postulated that the normal increase in adipose tissue with the onset of puberty creates a special problem for some females. An eating disorder may develop as an attempt to control or combat this normal pubertal weight gain with the initiation of dieting behavior. Preexisting hypothalamic dysfunction also has been implicated as a contributing factor to AN. In addition, changes in neurotransmitter levels have been shown to occur with initial vomiting or dieting. These changes may then lead to specific psychiatric symptoms that may perpetuate disordered eating. However, recent data with neuroimaging studies have shown that most of the physiological disturbances resolve with normalization of the patient's body weight. In addition, a pre-morbid disturbance in the neurotransmitter serotonin has been speculated to be a risk factor for the development of both AN and BN. Serotonin controls appetite by creating a sensation of fullness or satiety. In addition, it is known to have an effect on sexual and social behavior, mood, and stress responses. Although further studies are needed to confirm the exact role of this hormone in the development of an eating disorder, it has been shown that decreases in this brain neurotransmitter have been associated with impulsivity, aggression, and depression.

Leptin, a circulating hormone produced in adipose tissue, also seems to have a significant role in mediating the neuroendocrine effects of AN. Decreased concentrations of leptin are seen with reduced body fat stores as a result of decreased caloric intake and energy deficits. Paradoxically, leptin levels also appear to contribute to physical hyperactivity (compulsive exercise, restlessness), which is often seen in patients with AN despite their inadequate metabolic intake.

Genetic Factors

A genetic predisposition to anorexia has been shown in studies of monozygotic twins. The incidence of the disorder is increased in sisters and other female relatives of patients with AN.

Personal Characteristics

In general, patients with anorexia are described as obsessive-compulsive personality types, perfectionists, and overachievers. They also display low self-esteem and high anxiety levels despite their successes. They are the "model daughters" who have never caused any previous problems given their compliant, self-sacrificing, non-assertive nature.

There is an increased association between AN and major depression as well, and many studies of women have shown that first-degree relatives of patients with AN have higher rates of depression than the general population. However, many depressive symptoms in patients with AN improve with the restoration of body weight. Therefore, some of these clinical features of depression also may be secondary to the adolescent's state of malnutrition or starvation.

Familial Influences

Researchers have noted that certain family dynamics may serve to initiate and perpetuate AN, although it is no longer believed that family dysfunction is the main cause of disordered eating. Typically, however, the family is overprotective and rigid, with the mother often enmeshed in her daughter's life. Conflict resolution tends to be poor, and an inability to express feelings within the family is often evident. Multiple case-control studies have shown there is a higher rate of both AN and BN in relatives of patients with eating disorders. This may be due to inheritance patterns of personality traits as well as comorbid mood and anxiety disorders.

Social/Environmental Pressures

Both the media and Western industrialized societal standards are believed to play a role in "setting the stage" for the development of an eating disorder. Affluent communities are especially at risk for this. Within these social circles, thinness, food, eating, and obsessive exercise can become the prime focus of daily activity.

In addition, young women become caught in what has been labeled a "slender trap" in which thinness is equivalent to attractiveness and success. Food restriction or purging is a means of attaining thinness. An inability to maintain thinness equals failure. Role models in the media, such as fashion models and actresses, also serve as ideals by which young people create their standards.

Other Influences

Involvement in particular extracurricular activities, such as ballet and gymnastics, may contribute to the development of AN in females. For male athletes, such influences include participation in sports such as wrestling, in which maintaining a given weight is important and dieting is used to achieve that weight. Chronic medical conditions, such as diabetes mellitus or inflammatory bowel disease (IBD), also may contribute to the development of an eating disorder.

Bulimia Nervosa

Several theories have been proposed to explain the etiology of BN but, similar to AN, no single etiology has been confirmed. Most likely multiple factors contribute to the development of this eating disorder, and it is the complex interaction between these factors at a particular developmental point in an older adolescent's life that leads to this condition.

Biological, psychological, familial, and societal influences are thought to contribute to the development of BN in older teenagers and young adults. Among other issues, adolescent and parental obesity are both risk factors for BN as are early menarche, early sexual experiences, and a history of childhood sexual or physical abuse that occurs in conjunction with a comorbid psychiatric condition. More importantly, dieting has been documented as an important risk factor in this age group.

Familial dysfunction and high levels of conflict also have been associated with BN. Unlike with AN, conflict might be discussed openly but negatively within the family, and there may be an inadequate expression of emotions that may lead to a lack of parental warmth and concern. Thus the relationship between the parent and teenager is distant rather than enmeshed. The adolescent generally has a low level of self-esteem, high impulsivity, and body image dissatisfaction. Additionally, parents and relatives have a high rate of affective and eating disorders as well as alcoholism.

Differential Diagnosis

It is important to differentiate AN from BN, although occasionally this distinction may be difficult to make if patients display behavior consistent with both conditions. In addition, approximately 50% to 60% of patients with eating disorders have associated comorbid psychiatric disorders. Major affective disorders to consider include depression, bipolar disorder, and OCD. Anxiety disorders and substance abuse also are commonly seen, although the latter is more strongly associated with BN.

Other diagnoses to consider when evaluating patients for AN include IBD, malabsorption, celiac disease, diabetes mellitus, malignancies, Addison disease, hyperthyroidism or hypothyroidism, hypopituitarism, tumors of the central nervous system (CNS), and substance abuse, particularly with amphetamines and crack cocaine. Superior mesenteric artery syndrome is another important condition to consider in the differential diagnosis; however, it also can be a consequence of an eating disorder.

Evaluation

History

A complete medical history including a detailed review of systems should be obtained from all adolescents with suspected eating disorders to rule out the multiple other conditions in the differential diagnosis of weight loss. The primary care provider then should interview the patient alone and focus on establishing the diagnosis of disordered eating by addressing more specific issues related to food, eating behaviors, dieting, exercise, and body image (Questions Box). (See Steinegger in Selected References for a detailed discussion of interviewing techniques to use in patients with a suspected eating disorder.) The severity of both the medical and nutritional aspects of the condition should be determined initially, followed by a psychosocial evaluation. Inquiries should focus on symptoms associated with complications such as dysphagia secondary to esophagitis from recurrent vomiting, constipation from fluid restriction, or muscle weakness associated with emetine toxicity from chronic ipecac use. Although rarely seen by the primary care provider at the initial visit when the diagnosis of an eating disorder is made, recognition of serious medical complications is paramount to determining the urgency of further care.

Interviewing an adolescent with an eating disorder can be quite challenging; however, a thorough psychosocial assessment should be performed after a discussion about confidentiality has occurred with the adolescent and her parents. The **HEADDSSS** format (*h*ome environment, *e*mployment and education, *a*ctivities, *d*iet, *d*rugs, *s*exual

activity/sexuality, *s*uicide/depression, *s*afety) is useful to direct the psychosocial interview from general topics to more sensitive ones (see Chapter 6). Particular attention should be paid to the adolescent's overall functioning at home, with friends, and at school; the presence of other comorbid psychiatric disorders such as depression or anxiety; and a history of suicidal ideation or sexual/physical abuse. Out-of-control behavior as a result of substance abuse also should be assessed. The use of psychological testing/questionnaires to assess cognition and depression may be beneficial, depending on the comfort level of the primary care practitioner with these tools. Otherwise, consultation with a mental health professional is warranted.

A detailed menstrual history also must be obtained from females because secondary amenorrhea is frequently present in patients as

---

Eating Disorders — Questions

- Have there been any changes in the adolescent's weight? What is the most, and least, the adolescent has ever weighed? When did these weights occur, and for how long?
- How does the adolescent feel about how he or she looks? Is there anything he or she would like to change? How long has he or she been feeling this way?
- How much does the adolescent want to weigh?
- How often does the adolescent weigh himself or herself?
- What is a typical day of eating like, including eating times, types of foods, beverages, amount consumed, and portion size?
- What did he or she eat yesterday (24-hour dietary recall)?
- Does the adolescent have any food restrictions? Is the teenager a vegetarian? Does he or she count calories? Binge eat?
- Does the adolescent hide or throw away food?
- How does the adolescent and his or her friends handle weight control?
- What does the adolescent do when he or she feels "fat"? Does the adolescent vomit to lose weight? How often does this occur? Triggers?
- Has the adolescent or any of his or her friends ever used diuretics, diet pills, ipecac, enemas, or laxatives to lose weight or compensate for overeating?
- Does the adolescent exercise? If so, what type and how often? Is he or she stressed if they miss a workout?
- In what sports or dance activities, if any, does the adolescent participate?
- For females, are menstrual periods regular? Last menstrual period? Age at menarche?
- Does the adolescent have any other symptoms associated with complications of eating disorders?
- Does the adolescent have any depressive symptoms, such as sleeping problems or fatigue that can accompany eating disorders?

For Patients With Bulimia Nervosa

- When do binges occur?
- What are the precipitating factors?
- What happens specifically during a typical episode?
- Does the adolescent use drugs or alcohol?
- Is there a history of depression or attempted suicide?

an early sign of AN secondary to decreased body fat. Menses may be irregular or absent with BN as well. A family history of eating disorders, substance abuse, or psychiatric disease should be reviewed with the teenager and confirmed by the parent.

A dietary history should be obtained from the adolescent as well as the parents independently and should focus on any dietary restrictions or aversions. This may be difficult initially since the patient often does not believe he or she has a problem with food. A 24-hour dietary recall can be an important place to begin the assessment.

Physical Examination

In both conditions, the patient should undress, wearing only underwear, for the physical examination. This prevents any bulky clothes from hiding the true body habitus. The height and weight should be plotted on a growth chart, and the body mass index (BMI) should be calculated (BMI = weight [kg]/height [m2]). Delayed growth or short stature also should be noted because it can occur with severe malnutrition as well as other systemic conditions. Vital signs, including blood pressure, should be recorded. Evidence of cardiovascular instability can be manifested by tachycardia, bradycardia, or orthostatic hypotension. The patient also may be hypothermic as a result of her overall malnutrition. The general appearance and affect of the patient must be noted. Adolescents with full-blown AN are often emaciated with an obvious loss of subcutaneous tissue, and they may appear apathetic, anxious, or have a flat affect. Patients with BN may be mildly obese or of normal weight with a full-appearing facies secondary to parotid and submaxillary swelling, a complication of frequent purging. In most cases, however, the teen appears "normal" at the initial visit.

Physical findings in patients with **anorexia nervosa** are consistent with a "state of hibernation." Hypothermia, orthostatic hypotension, bradycardia, and lanugo (downy hair) on the arms and back are seen. The palms and soles may be yellow secondary to hypercarotenemia, and pigmentation of the chest and abdomen may be increased as a result of malnutrition. Thinning or loss of pubic and scalp hair as well as dry skin also may be seen. The breasts should be examined carefully for sexual maturity rating (SMR) (Tanner Staging) as well as galactorrhea. The presence of galactorrhea, along with a history of amenorrhea, warrants further investigation for a prolactinoma. Of note, patients with AN may have interrupted or delayed pubertal development. A cardiac murmur must be noted and further evaluated because one-third of patients with anorexia have mitral valve prolapse. The abdomen should be palpated for tenderness or masses, and may be scaphoid in appearance. Bowel sounds are often decreased in patients with anorexia, and stool may be palpated secondary to constipation. The presence of pubic hair (genital SMR) also should be noted. A rectal examination should be performed for any evidence of bloody stool, which is a finding consistent with IBD. The extremities should be evaluated for coldness, mottling, or edema. Finally, a complete neurologic examination, including a mental status evaluation, should be performed to exclude any signs of a CNS lesion or endocrine disorder.

In patients with **bulimia nervosa,** specific physical findings, if any, are often associated with dehydration and electrolyte imbalances that occur as a result of chronic vomiting or laxative abuse. Vital signs should be reviewed for tachycardia, sinus bradycardia, and orthostatic hypotension; their presence indicates hemodynamic instability. The patient also may be hypothermic. The skin should be inspected on the dorsum of the hand over the knuckles for scratches, scars, or calluses from self-induced vomiting (Russell sign). Petechiae and subconjunctival hemorrhages also may be seen as a result of severe retching. The oropharynx should be inspected for dental caries, enamel erosion, or discoloration as well as for parotid hypertrophy. In addition, palatal scratches or mouth sores can be seen. The abdomen should be palpated for epigastric tenderness or mid-abdominal pain. Positive findings may be due to esophagitis, gastritis, or pancreatitis.

From a musculoskeletal standpoint, any muscle weakness or cramping should be appreciated and may indicate an electrolyte abnormality. Edema of the extremities may be seen in laxative abusers and should be noted.

Laboratory Tests

Box 133-4 lists the laboratory studies necessary in the evaluation of patients with **AN.** A complete blood cell count may be helpful because leukopenia, anemia and, rarely, thrombocytopenia can be found with this disorder. Electrolytes (sodium, potassium, chloride, and carbon dioxide) and blood urea nitrogen are important especially if patients use diuretics, laxatives, or ipecac. Serum calcium and phosphorous must be monitored, especially in the "refeeding" phase of treatment. The erythrocyte sedimentation rate may be low with anorexia and high with IBD or some other inflammatory process. Normal liver function tests aid in excluding other causes of weight loss. Some endocrine tests help differentiate a hormonal problem from AN, especially in patients with primary or secondary amenorrhea (see Box 133-4). An electrocardiogram (ECG) allows practitioners to diagnose QTc prolongation, heart block, and arrhythmias. In addition, an ECG is indicated in patients with electrolyte abnormalities, or with a history of significant purging or weight loss.

Laboratory abnormalities in **BN** reflect the type and extent of purging behavior of adolescents. Box 133-4 summarizes the necessary laboratory studies for patients with BN.

Radiographic studies, such as computed tomography of the head or magnetic resonance imaging of the brain, are indicated if the diagnosis of an eating disorder is uncertain. Bone density studies such as a DEXA (dual-energy x-ray absorptiometry) scan are not performed routinely except in adolescents with amenorrhea of greater than 6 to 12 months. An upper and lower gastrointestinal series may be warranted in patients with esophageal complaints or if IBD is a strong consideration. The performance of other procedures, however, should be based on the individual case.

Box 133-4. Initial Laboratory Assessment for a Patient with an Eating Disorder

Anorexia Nervosa

- Complete blood cell count, erythrocyte sedimentation rate
- Serum electrolytes (Na, K, Cl, CO_2)
- Blood urea nitrogen/creatinine
- Serum glucose
- Serum calcium, phosphorous, magnesium, zinc
- Serum protein, albumin, cholesterol
- Liver function tests
- Endocrine labs (perform in patients with amenorrhea)
  — Urine pregnancy test
  — Follicle-stimulating hormone
  — Luteinizing hormone
  — Estradiol
  — Thyroid function tests: thyroid-stimulating hormone/T_4/T_3
  — Prolactin
- Urine pH and urinalysis
- Electrocardiogram

Bulimia Nervosa

- Serum electrolytes (Na, K, Cl, CO_2)
- Serum glucose
- Serum calcium, phosphorous, magnesium, zinc
- Blood urea nitrogen/creatinine
- Serum amylase
- Urine pH and urinalysis
- Electrocardiogram

Management

It is the role of primary care practitioners to recognize when inappropriate dieting and weight loss become an obsession for adolescents and when abnormal behaviors develop for maintenance of obvious malnutrition. When treating patients with eating disorders, physicians must first establish trust and, in doing so, patients should be reassured that practitioners are not attempting to remove all control by trying to make the adolescent "fat." The goal is to create a therapeutic alliance between the clinician, adolescent, and family to restore and maintain the patient's health and well-being. Depending on the severity of symptoms and the comfort level of the physician in monitoring the early medical, nutritional, and psychological issues, the adolescent may be followed by the primary care practitioner in conjunction with a registered dietitian, family therapist, and mental health professional (psychologist or psychiatrist). Early in the treatment course, the primary physician must be willing to follow the patient frequently (as often as once or twice a week if necessary). If the practitioner wishes to refer the patient to an experienced multidisciplinary team of specialists, it is important that the primary provider remain involved in the care of the teenager.

A consensus must be reached between the adolescent and pediatrician regarding the minimum acceptable weight given the patient's age, height, pubertal stage, premorbid weight, and previous growth.

This should be done with the assistance of a registered dietitian who is experienced in working with children and teenagers with eating disorders. Unlike with adults, weight restoration in the adolescent also must take into account normal growth needs. An agreement that describes goals of treatment and maintenance of health should then be established between the adolescent and all members of the treatment team. Weight gain must be the initial priority, especially in adolescents with AN as long as the patient is otherwise medically stable and does not require inpatient hospitalization. Details regarding this nutritional regimen, which includes a stepwise increase in daily caloric intake, amounts of protein to be ingested, daily fat intake, and treatment goal weights, should be developed by the dietitian and reviewed with the adolescent and his or her family in conjunction with mental health support and close medical follow-up. Early nutritional rehabilitation and timely medical stabilization are essential to correct the cognitive deficits associated with disordered eating.

Family and individual counseling is an important part of the overall therapeutic plan. Patients with disordered eating often try to hide their illness and generally are in denial regarding their abnormal eating patterns and the degree of weight loss. Parents, too, may be in denial or simply unaware of the extent of their teenager's condition. The primary care provider must work cooperatively with mental health colleagues to provide the necessary psychological and psychiatric services for their patient. Although extremely difficult, patients must begin to acknowledge their behaviors and accept the need for assistance before effective mental health intervention can occur. This also allows the adolescent to assert himself or herself and remain in control. Support groups also may be beneficial and frequently are an important component of a day-treatment program (day hospitalization, partial hospitalization) for those adolescents with eating disorders who require more intensive outpatient care but not an inpatient hospitalization or residential program. Day-treatment programs are generally less costly and may be more accessible than traditional hospital-based programs.

Pharmacotherapy with agents such as the selective serotonin-reuptake inhibitors (SSRIs) are generally not prescribed in adolescents with AN, except to treat comorbid conditions like depression and anxiety. Several studies have shown, however, that these same medications can be effective in patients with BN by decreasing binge-eating and purging behaviors. Serotonin/norepinephrine-reuptake inhibitors and tricyclic antidepressants are also an option.

Numerous studies have shown that eating disorders are best treated by an interdisciplinary professional team experienced in the care of children and adolescents with eating disorders. This team generally consists of the primary care provider, an adolescent medicine specialist with expertise in caring for patients with eating disorders, a psychologist or psychiatrist, a nutritionist, and a social worker. Ideally, the team is available to offer both inpatient as well as outpatient services, although most cases are managed in an outpatient setting. Criteria for inpatient admission should be established by the team and reviewed with patients and their families.

Medical complications of eating disorders are well established and listed in Box 133-5. Inpatient treatment is required for less than 75%

Box 133-5. Medical Complications of Eating Disorders[a]

Associated With Purging Behavior

- Fluid and electrolyte imbalances (from laxative abuse and vomiting)
- Irreversible cardiac muscle damage (from ipecac toxicity)
- Esophagitis, dental erosions, Mallory-Weiss tears (from chronic vomiting)
- Renal stones (from dehydration)
- Amenorrhea, hypoestrogenemia, osteopenia (from decreased body mass index [BMI])

Associated With Caloric Restrictive Behavior and Weight Loss

- Electrocardiogram abnormalities: low voltage, sinus bradycardia, sinus tachycardia segment depression (from electrolyte abnormalities), prolonged QTc
- Cardiac arrhythmias, including supraventricular beats and ventricular tachycardia, with or without exercise
- Mitral valve prolapse
- Pericardial effusion
- Delayed gastric emptying, slow gastrointestinal motility, constipation, bloating, fullness, abnormal liver function tests (from fatty infiltration of the liver)
- Increased blood urea nitrogen, increased risk of renal stones, total body depletion of sodium and potassium
- Refeeding syndrome (from extracellular shifts of phosphorous)
- Leukopenia, anemia, thrombocytopenia
- Amenorrhea, hypoestrogenism, osteopenia (from decreased BMI)
- Growth retardation, pubertal delay
- Cognitive deficits
- Cortical atrophy, seizures

[a] Modified from American Academy of Pediatrics Committee on Adolescence. Identifying and treating eating disorders. *Pediatrics.* 2003;111:204–211.

---

ideal body weight, continued weight loss despite intensive outpatient treatment, or a history of rapid weight loss. Refusal to eat or body fat less than 10% also are criteria for hospital admission. Other indications include cardiovascular compromise, such as bradycardia (<50 beats/min during the day or <45 beats/min at nighttime), orthostatic hypotension, or altered mental status; evidence of persistent hypothermia (<35.6 °C [96.08°F]); suicidal or out-of-control behavior; intractable vomiting; electrolyte disturbances or uncompensated acid-base abnormalities; hematemesis; and significant dehydration as evidenced by systolic blood pressure lower than 90 mm Hg. Cardiac arrhythmias, including prolonged QTc, also require inpatient monitoring. Rarely does confirmation of the diagnosis warrant an inpatient stay. The goal of hospitalization is to correct medical complications, document appropriate weight gain, and establish healthy and safe eating habits. Hospital admission also has been shown to improve the long-term prognosis of children and adolescents with eating disorders.

Prognosis

Overall, the outcome for patients with eating disorders is variable, with the recovery of some patients after minimal intervention and the development of more chronic problems in others. Binge eating, for example, may replace food restriction. Most studies report the prognosis as more favorable if the patient's condition is identified early and treated rapidly and aggressively. Predictors of poor outcome for AN include very low body weight at the time of initial treatment, long duration of illness, a concomitant personality disorder, a dysfunctional parent–child relationship, and a compulsion to exercise. For BN, factors found to be predictive of poor outcome include longer duration of illness at presentation, severity of eating pathology and frequency of vomiting, pre-morbid obesity, associated comorbid disorders such as personality disorder or substance abuse, and suicidal behavior. A family history of alcoholism also has been reported as a poor prognostic factor for BN.

The mortality rate for adolescents with AN is approximately 2%. Higher numbers were reported in the past when adult and adolescent data were combined. Exact figures for BN have not been determined, although it has been quoted as being similar to that of AN. The most common cause of death in both disorders is suicide. Medical causes are often due to cardiac arrhythmias from electrolyte abnormalities.

CASE RESOLUTION

In the case history presented at the beginning of this chapter, the girl does not meet the strict criteria for the diagnosis of AN, but her preoccupation with dieting and weight is worrisome. Concerns about her eating and dieting behaviors should be discussed with the teenager alone and then together with her family. Both the patient and her family should be strongly encouraged to seek treatment. She should be referred to a mental health professional and nutritionist for further evaluation, with the emphasis on healthy eating and the continued support and involvement of the primary care physician. She should be followed frequently until her weight and eating behaviors have reached the mutually agreed upon goal among all professionals involved in her care, after which she should continue to be seen at regular intervals.

Selected References

American Academy of Pediatrics Committee on Adolescence. Identifying and treating eating disorders. *Pediatrics.* 2003;111:204–211

American Academy of Pediatrics Committee on Sports Medicine and Fitness. Medical concerns in the female athlete. *Pediatrics.* 2000;106:610–613

Bachrach LK, Sills IN; American Academy of Pediatrics Section on Endocrinology. Bone densitometry in children and adolescents. *Pediatrics.* 2011;127:189–194

Butryn ML, Wadden TA. Treatment of overweight in children and adolescents: does dieting increase the risk of eating disorders? *Int J Eat Disord.* 2005;37:285–293

Fisher M. Treatment of eating disorders in children, adolescents, and young adults. *Pediatr Rev.* 2006;27:5–16

Fisher M, Golden NH, Jacobson MC, eds. The spectrum of disordered eating: anorexia nervosa, bulimia nervosa, and obesity. *Adolesc Med.* 2003;14:1–173

Fisher M, Golden NH, Katzman DK, et al. Eating disorders in adolescents: a background paper. *J Adolesc Health.* 1995;16:420–437

Hillman JK. 'Just dieting' or an eating disorder? A practical guide for the clinician. *Adolesc Health Update.* 2001;13:1–9

Katzman DK. Medical complications in adolescents with anorexia nervosa: a review of the literature. *Int J Eat Disord.* 2005;37:S52–S59

Levine RL. Endocrine aspects of eating disorders in adolescents. *Adolesc Med.* 2002;13:129–144

Phillips EL, Pratt HD. Eating disorders in college. *Pediatr Clin North Am.* 2005;52:85–96

Rome ES, Ammerman S, Rosen DS, et al. Children and adolescents with eating disorders: the state of the art. *Pediatrics.* 2003;111:e98–e108

Rosen DS; American Academy of Pediatrics Committee on Adolescence. Identification and management of eating disorders in children and adolescents. *Pediatrics.* 2010;126:1240–1253

Steinegger C, Katzman DK. Interviewing the adolescent with an eating disorder. *Adolesc Med.* 2008;19:18–40

Steiner H, Lock J. Anorexia nervosa and bulimia nervosa in children and adolescents: a review of the past 10 years. *J Am Acad Child Adolesc Psychiatry.* 1998;37:352–359

CHAPTER 134

Body Modification: Tattooing and Body Piercing

Monica Sifuentes, MD

CASE STUDY

A 16-year-old girl comes to your office for her annual physical examination. Although previously healthy, the mother is concerned that her daughter seems irritable and unwilling to participate in recent family events. The adolescent is currently in 10th grade at a local public school, gets As and Bs in most subjects, is a member of the volleyball team, and has just begun working at a movie theater part-time. Both of her parents are employed and the adolescent gets along well with her 19-year-old sister, who is currently in college, and her 14-year-old brother. She has many friends in the neighborhood as well as at school.

You interview the adolescent alone and learn that she occasionally smokes marijuana, has tried cocaine on one occasion, and attends parties where many people are drinking alcohol. She has been sexually active in the past but is not currently. She denies depression and describes her mood as generally happy, except when she is forced to spend what she believes is excessive time with her family instead of friends.

On physical examination the adolescent's height and weight are in the 50th percentile for age. Her body mass index is 21. Vital signs are normal. You note a small tattoo at her right hip area. The girl's mother is unaware of its presence according to the teen. She obtained it a few months prior while visiting her sister in college.

Questions

1. What is the epidemiology of body modification in adolescents and young adults?
2. What is the motivation for obtaining tattoos and body piercing in this age group, and is there an association with high-risk behavior?
3. What techniques are used to place tattoos and perform body piercing?
4. What adverse consequences can be seen following body modification, and what should be done to treat them?
5. How can the primary care provider assist an adolescent to make a safe and healthy decision regarding body modification?

Body modification is the practice of permanently altering one's appearance and historically has been practiced in many cultures for thousands of years. This includes tattooing, body piercing, scarification, and branding. Although much less common than tattooing and body piercing, scarification is the use of various techniques to produce scars on the skin. It is described as a more "intense" form of body modification and has been reported to be more appealing to darker pigmented individuals or those seeking a more dramatic result. The practice of body modification should be differentiated from "cutting," which is a disorder of self-mutilation that can be seen in adolescents suffering from anxiety, depression, or abuse and is beyond the scope of this discussion (see Chapter 50).

Although in the past body modification has been associated primarily with the disenfranchised such as criminals, gang members, or psychiatric patients, it is now a common occurrence in mainstream society. **Body art** is seen in most clinical settings serving youth and young adults as well as in middle schools, high schools, and on college campuses. Additionally, it is not uncommon to encounter a teenager with multiple tattoos and body piercings or to evaluate an adolescent for a possible complication of the procedure. Whether described as a rite of passage, expression of their own individuality, or desire to join a particular peer group, obtaining a tattoo or body piercing has become a widespread experience during adolescence and young adulthood and therefore should be added to the primary care provider's list of issues to review during the routine health maintenance visit.

Epidemiology

It is currently estimated that 13% to 25% of the general population has a tattoo in the United States. However, because tattooing was reportedly the sixth fastest-growing retail business in 1996, these figures are probably a gross underestimation. Surveys conducted in outpatient clinics and on school and college campuses confirm that approximately 10% to 13% of teens ages 12 to 18 years have a tattoo. In one particular study of more than 2,000 US high school students, 55% expressed interest in obtaining a tattoo regardless of its permanence or the students' academic success in school. In addition, it has been reported in the literature that half of new tattoos are in women and that many are obtained while in college.

Body piercings are more common in adolescents and young adults, and some experts speculate that this may be because the procedure is not permanent, allowing the individual to remove the jewelry at any time. In one study among college students, 45% had undergone body piercing and 22% had tattoos both with and without piercings. Other studies that include younger adolescents attending an outpatient adolescent clinic report approximately 27% of teens with body piercing and 13% with a tattoo.

The motivation for obtaining body art also has been reviewed in the literature, with most studies confirming the adolescent's search for uniqueness and desire to enhance their independence and self-identity. For some teenagers, it is seen as a form of decoration or it fulfills a desire for peer acceptance and can solidify group membership. Tattoos in particular can be seen as a quest to permanently document a relationship with an individual or group. Despite popular belief, studies do not confirm that most adolescents obtain a tattoo or body piercing impulsively while under the influence of illicit drugs or alcohol. In fact, many older teens and young adults report taking quite a while to decide whether to obtain a tattoo or piercing.

Parental involvement and permission to have a tattoo placed or body piercing performed is variable for many teenagers. In most cases, parents are not consulted prior to the procedure, although in many states parental consent is required by law, and tattooing of minors is prohibited. However, current legislation is not consistently enforced and, in many states, tattooing and body piercing have different regulations.

Clinical Presentation

Tattoos can be found on any area of the body and, depending on the talent of the artist and the desire of the client, can be simple and one color or very elaborate with many colors. In general, amateur tattoos are less intricate and are considered more risky because they are often not performed under ideal circumstances, following antiseptic techniques or with conventional pigments and applicators. Unconventional pigments include charcoal, India ink, and mascara. Pencils, pens, sewing needles, and other sharp objects, including guitar strings, may be used to apply the dye for a self-administered tattoo.

The most common site for piercing is high on the pinna of the ear. Regular lobular ear piercings are not generally included in the context of body modification because they occur commonly at any age. Other body sites that are pierced include the tragus of the ear, eyebrows, tongue, nose, nasal septum, lip, navel, and nipples. Intimate or genital piercings also can be seen in both males and females. The foreskin, penis, scrotum, clitoris, perineum, and labia are all common areas for intimate piercings. Although specific data by gender are not available, it is reported that more men than women tend to obtain genital piercings.

Technique, Application, and Safety Standards

Tattoos

The process for applying a professional or commercial tattoo is fairly standardized, although different tattoo parlors may have their own individual practices. In general, the client selects a design and the tattoo is stenciled or drawn on the skin. The skin is then cleansed with an antiseptic solution, and petroleum jelly is placed on the site. Most professionals use an electric tattoo gun, which is similar to a dental drill, that holds one or several needles in a needle bar that punctures the skin a few millimeters deep and up to several thousand times a minute. The pigment reaches the level of the dermis via the solid bore needle(s), and blood and serosanguineous fluid are wiped away as tattoo placement continues. When the tattoo is completed or the session is finished, an antiseptic ointment is applied, and a bandage is placed over the site.

The client is instructed to remove the dressing in 24 hours and to keep the area moist with an antibiotic ointment. Additionally, clients may place Keri lotion or vitamin E oil over the healing tattoo several times a day. The area should be cleansed with a mild soap and patted dry (not rubbed). If aftercare instructions are followed carefully, most tattoos heal in approximately 1 to 2 weeks.

Ideally the application process uses inks that are poured into one-time use disposable containers and needles that are disposed of after each client. However, although the pigments are subject to US Food and Drug Administration regulation, the tattooing process itself and the use of the inks are not regulated. In addition, certain pigments may not be approved for intradermal use and have been known to contain lead, mercury, and arsenic.

The practice of universal precautions is required by state and local regulatory agencies and advocated by specific educational groups such as the Alliance of Professional Tattooists (APT), a nonprofit organization established in 1992 to promote standards for professional and associate tattooists and develop guidelines for consumers to evaluate the safety of a tattooist. Membership in APT is voluntary and requires that the professional tattooist participate in a health and safety seminar and have at least 3 years of full-time experience at a consistent location. Despite these efforts and standards, however, specific areas of concern regarding the tattoo industry remain and include unlicensed tattoo artists and establishments, the presence of unregulated ingredients in the pigments, inconsistent cleaning of equipment between clients, an inability to reliably sterilize all parts of the equipment despite good efforts, and infrequent inspections of tattoo parlors by regulatory agencies.

Body Piercing

The process for body piercing is generally less complicated than tattooing and depends, in part, on the site to be pierced. The client chooses the jewelry and body part to be pierced, the area is cleaned with a topical antiseptic, and a large hollow needle is brought through the skin. The jewelry is then brought through the hole following the needle and sealed with a bead, bar, or metal disc. Because the procedure is relatively quick, topical anesthetics are usually not required.

While earlobe piercings are relatively straightforward, they are commonly performed using a "piercing gun" at a local mall, cosmetic shop, or kiosk. Because the stud is driven through the earlobe via the gun rather than through a hollow tube manually, the tissue ends up torn rather than pierced. Additional concerns regarding the piercing gun include inconsistent and informal training of personnel, an inability to sterilize all parts of the gun, and embedded earrings and ear backs. The gun cannot be adjusted for the thickness of other tissues, so although it is a popular method for earring placement, this tool is not recommended for sites other than the earlobe.

The immediate aftercare of piercing varies by the site pierced. For example, local skin discoloration and a non-malodorous serous exudate can occur with piercings of the nares or navel. Tongue or lip piercings have been associated with significant swelling for several days following the procedure. In addition, a yellow-white fluid secretion can occur that can mimic an infection to the unfamiliar examiner. Clients with oral piercings are generally instructed to dissolve ice in their mouths immediately post-piercing to help with pain and swelling, treat further discomfort with a nonsteroidal anti-inflammatory agent, and elevate the head when sleeping.

Healing times greatly vary depending on the body site. In general, sites with greater vascularity and exposure, such as the face and tongue, tend to heal faster than those through cartilage, which is poorly vascularized. Areas of the body that are subject to movement also have slower healing times. For example, the tongue may take 1 to 2 months to heal, the nasal septum 2 to 3 months, and the tragus of the ear 3 to 4 months. High-ear piercings through the cartilage also can take 3 to 4 months to heal. Navel piercings have the longest healing time (up to 12 months) because of friction and moisture from clothing and often are associated with the most complications.

As with tattooing, not all states have regulations and safety standards in place for body piercing and, if they do exist, local governing bodies do not consistently enforce them. Universal precautions should be strictly practiced, and adolescents need to be familiar with these guidelines as well as know how to find a reputable piercer prior to obtaining body art.

Because no formal training programs exist for piercers, many learn by video or apprenticeship. In general, practitioners in studios have completed an apprenticeship and have more training than those in cosmetic shops, malls, or ear-piercing kiosks. They also are more experienced in piercing sites other than the ears and may be a member of the Association of Professional Piercers (APP). The APP is a nonprofit organization dedicated to the education, health, and safety of body piercing for the public. It has developed self-regulatory policies for the industry, standards for membership in their organization, and annual conferences on health and safety issues. Membership includes at least 1 year of piercing experience, documented training in blood-borne pathogens and cardiopulmonary resuscitation, and certification in first aid. Members also must show

photographic proof of a medical-grade autoclave in the piercing studio and send in spore test results from the autoclave. To help document this, a detailed video of the studio is required along with copies of all aftercare education given to clients. Once this process is completed, the member receives a certificate to mount in the studio.

Current legislation regarding minors and piercing is regulated by individual states, and in some states, such as California, there is an exclusion of ear piercing performed with "piercing guns" from the definition of body piercing. With regard to minors, the APP requires that the parent or legal guardian as well as the minor show proof of identification prior to signing the consent form for body piercing. In addition, nipple or genital piercings are not performed on anyone younger than 18 years.

Evaluation

History

All teenagers should be interviewed alone, after their parent or legal guardian has had an opportunity to discuss their concerns with the health care provider (see Chapter 6). A visible tattoo or body piercing allows the health care provider to inquire about the circumstances surrounding the body art at the beginning of the interview in contrast to body art noted in an inconspicuous area of the body during the physical examination. Whether parental consent was obtained prior to the procedure should be addressed directly because this issue could be a basis for familial conflict both currently and in the future. The type of facility where the tattoo or piercing was obtained should be reviewed, along with whether universal precautions were followed. A general review of systems should be performed to exclude systemic conditions such as viral hepatitis as well as any other complications related to obtaining the tattoo or piercing. Specific questions about the area of the body that has been pierced also should be reviewed (Questions Box). For example, the teenager with a tongue piercing should be asked if he or she has problems with mastication, swallowing, loss of taste or movement, or permanent numbness.

It has been reported that amateur or self-administered tattoos are associated with increased psychosocial problems including substance abuse at a younger age, hard drug use, lower academic achievement (ie, grades), and a greater number of tattoos overall.

Other studies have shown, however, that not all adolescents and young adults with tattoos or body piercing engage in high-risk behavior (Box 134-1). Successful academic achievement and close family support have been reported in both tattooed and non-tattooed college students. Despite the fact that they are permanent, more than 50% of academically successful high school students with consistently good grades have reported an interest in tattoos.

Whether body art is seen as an expression of individuality, rebellious behavior, or succumbing to peer pressure, the presence of a tattoo or body piercing on an adolescent probably warrants an in-depth psychosocial assessment for both risk-taking behavior and possible exposure to a viral infection such as hepatitis C.

Questions

Tattoo and Body Piercing

- When was the tattoo or body piercing obtained?
- Did the teenager obtain the parent or legal guardian's consent prior to obtaining the tattoo or piercing?
- Is the adolescent satisfied with the tattoo or piercing?
- Was the tattoo or body piercing placed by a professional?
- Where was the studio located? Was it licensed? Was it clean "like a medical facility"?
- Did the tattooist or piercer wash their hands before gloving? Use new disposable gloves? Open all equipment in front of the teen?
- For tattoos, did the tattooist remove a sterile needle and tube set from a new envelope? Did he or she pour new ink in a new disposable container?
- For body piercing, did the piercer use individually wrapped sterile needles? Did he or she use a method not involving a piercing gun?
- Did the teen receive aftercare education, including written material?

Physical Examination

The routine physical examination in most adolescents with a tattoo or body piercing is completely normal unless there has been a past complication with the tattoo or piercing or there is a current problem. Poor aftercare and hygiene can prolong healing time in body piercings. In addition, smoking can delay the healing time associated with oral piercings. If the teen has recently had a tongue piercing performed, a larger barbell will be seen through the tongue. Larger barbells initially are placed with tongue piercing to accommodate the swelling associated with the procedure. Later the barbell is replaced with a shorter rod.

Both infectious and noninfectious complications from tattoos and body piercings can be seen and are listed in Box 134-2. While local infection occurs in only approximately 5% of tattoos, infectious complications have been reported in as many as 30% of body piercings. Signs of infection include erythema, warmth, swelling, and pain at the site, in addition to drainage in some cases. Rarely, a fluctuant, fluid-filled mass is seen if an abscess has developed.

Because some of the noninfectious complications can be related to the type of metal found in the jewelry, knowledge of this specific information is useful with body piercing. Only jewelry made from surgical stainless steel, titanium, solid 14k or 18k gold, or solid platinum should be used to avoid allergic dermatitis. Certain metals such as nickel, cobalt, and chromium have been associated with the development of contact dermatitis in sensitive individuals. Permanent makeup also has been reported to cause severe allergic contact dermatitis that can take from months to years to completely heal. The reported reactions included tenderness, itching, and "bumps" at the site of the permanent makeup application. Hypersensitivities to dyes or pigments from a professional tattoo also can appear as an erythematous outline of the original work. This also can occur with temporary tattoos from henna, which is approved as a hair dye and not for use on the skin. Its use has been associated with severe contact dermatitis, especially if an additive containing phenylenediamine is mixed with the henna to give the normal red-brown paste an additional black and blue color.

Keloids and hypertrophic scars can appear as a flesh-colored mass at the area of the tattoo or piercing and differ in their timing and resolution. A hypertrophic scar generally appears within 6 weeks of the tattooing or piercing, is confined to the margins of the wound, and has a tendency to regress spontaneously. In contrast, a keloid may present as long as 1 year after the initial wound, often grows beyond the border of the wound, and persists. Keloids are seen primarily in African American and Asian patients and can cause an itching or burning sensation that may prompt referral for removal.

Box 134-1. The Association Between Body Modification and High-Risk Behavior in Teens

Numerous studies have been conducted to explore the association between high-risk behavior and body modification in adolescents. To date, while there are no definitive answers, research has shown

- Adolescents with tattoos and/or body piercings were more likely to have engaged in risk-taking behaviors and at greater degrees of involvement than those without either. Risk-taking behaviors included disordered eating behavior, gateway drug use (cigarettes, alcohol, and marijuana), hard drug use (cocaine, crystal methamphetamine, and ecstasy), sexual activity, and suicide. Additionally, violence was associated with males having tattoos and with females having body piercings. Gateway drug use was associated with younger age of both tattooing and body piercing. (Carroll ST, Riffenburgh RH, Roberts TA, Myhre EB. Tattoos and body piercings as indicators of adolescent risk-taking behaviors. *Pediatrics.* 2002;109:1021–1028.)
- Adolescents with body modification had 3.1 times greater odds of problem substance use compared with those without body modification. (Brooks TL, Woods ER, Knight JR, Shrier LA. Body modification and substance use in adolescents: is there a link? *J Adolesc Health.* 2003;32:44–49.)
- Tattooing was significantly associated with older age, living in a single-parent household, and lower socioeconomic status. There also was greater involvement in sexual intercourse; higher levels of substance abuse in themselves as well as their peers, increased violent behaviors, and school problems. (Roberts TA, Ryan SA. Tattooing and high-risk behavior in adolescents. *Pediatrics.* 2002;110:1058–1063.)
- A correlation between body piercing in teens and increased rate of sexual intercourse, smoking, marijuana use, school truancy, running away, suicidal ideation/attempts, and peer substance use. (Armstrong ML, Roberts AE, Owen DC, Koch JR. Contemporary college students and body piercing. *J Adolesc Health.* 2004;35:58–61.)

Box 134-2. Complications of Tattoos and Body Piercing: Infectious and Noninfectious

Tattooing Complications

Infectious

Bacterial etiologies

- Local skin infections
  — Superficial pyodermas
  — *Staphylococcus aureus*
- Systemic infections
  — Syphilis
  — *Mycobacterium tuberculosis*
  — *Mycobacterium leprae*
  — Chancroid
  — Tetanus
  — Endocarditis

Viral etiologies

- Human papillomavirus
- Hepatitis B and C
- HIV

Noninfectious

- Hypersensitivity to dyes or pigments
- Allergic granulomas
- Malignant melanoma and basal cell carcinoma at tattoo site
- Keloid formation
- Swelling and burning during magnetic resonance imaging

Body Piercing Complications

Infectious

Bacterial etiologies

- *S aureus*
- *Pseudomonas aeruginosa*
- Group A beta-hemolytic streptococcus
  — Cellulitis
  — Septic arthritis
  — Acute glomerulonephritis
  — Erysipelas
  — Endocarditis
- *M tuberculosis*
- *Clostridium tetani*

Viral etiologies

- Hepatitis B and C
- HIV

Noninfectious

Body jewelry, in general

- Artifact on radiographs

High-ear piercing

- Pinna deformity

Tongue piercing

- Airway obstruction
- Chipped/cracked teeth
- Interference with mastication/swallowing
- Permanent numbness
- Articulation disorders
- Loss of taste/movement
- Oral mucosa inflammation

Lip piercing

- Injury to salivary ducts
- Aspiration of jewelry

Navel piercing

- Allergic dermatitis

Nipple piercing

- Trauma/avulsion of nipple

Genital piercing

- Tissue inflammation in sexual partner
- Scarring
- Interruption of urinary flow (in males)

Laboratory

In general, laboratory studies are not necessary if the adolescent is not engaged in high-risk behavior and is certain that universal precautions were followed when the tattoo or piercing was placed. In most cases, however, the teen may be uncertain and not remember the details. If this is the case, a serum test for viral hepatitis B and C should be obtained because it has been reported that hepatitis C virus is found in approximately 30% of people with tattoos compared with 3.5% of people without them. Additionally, an antibody test for HIV should be sent as it continues to be a major public health concern with regard to the industry. However, there have been no definitive documented cases of HIV transmission from tattooing or body piercing in the literature to date.

A serum test for syphilis also should be sent because unlike HIV, transmission of this and other sexually transmitted infections has been reported from tattooing or piercing.

If there is evidence of abscess formation such as what may be seen with perichondritis, a specimen of the purulent fluid should be obtained and sent for culture and antimicrobial sensitivities.

Management

Although not ordinarily requested by most adolescents, tattoo removal or modification is available for the patient that no longer wants their tattoo or is unhappy with its current appearance. Even with the newer techniques, however, tattoo removal is difficult, and only about 70% of tattoos can be completely cleared because of impurities in tattoo pigments, different ink densities and depths, and the presence of certain metals in the dyes. More importantly, the cost for tattoo removal is not negligible; while the cost for tattoo placement might be $50 to $100, it can cost as much as $1,000 for its removal. Techniques for removal include laser treatments, dermabrasion, salabrasion (using a salt solution), scarification, and surgical removal using tissue expanders. Camouflaging also can be performed: a new pattern is made using skin-toned pigments or the tattoo is modified and made into another one. For instance, the name of a person can be incorporated into a new tattoo of an animal. Certain nonprofit organizations also offer tattoo removal to ex-gang members as a part of their employment and educational services.

Although it seems counterintuitive, removal of jewelry is not recommended if a piercing appears infected. The concern is that, without a wick or surgical drain, any potential space left at the site when the jewelry is removed could result in the development of an abscess. Instead, the adolescent should be instructed to leave the jewelry in place to allow drainage of the wound, use warm compresses, and clean the area with an antimicrobial soap and water. The use of topical antibiotic ointments is controversial because they can be occlusive and contribute to delayed healing.

Oral antibiotic coverage against skin staphylococcus and streptococcal species should be administered if the tattoo or piercing appears superficially infected and other measures have not been effective. More aggressive treatment is required if the piercing site involves the cartilage such as with high-ear piercings. Auricular infections can occur even after the use of strict antiseptic techniques and may appear a few weeks after the initial piercing. The cartilaginous helical area of the ear is particularly prone to infection because it is poorly vascularized and takes a long time to heal. Additional antimicrobial coverage against *Pseudomonas aeruginosa* is essential in these cases, along with diligent follow-up to monitor the initial response to oral antibiotic therapy. Currently, oral fluoroquinolones offer good anti-pseudomonal as well as anti-staphylococcal coverage and penetrate cartilage well. Inpatient hospitalization for intravenous antimicrobial therapy and subsequent drainage of the site may be required for moderate or unresponsive infections. Early recognition of perichondritis and its appropriate treatment are essential to prevent the development of a persistent infection as well as to minimize a permanent auricular deformity. In addition, timely consultation with a plastic surgeon or otolaryngologist early in the course of the suspected infection is recommended for early incision and drainage of a perichondrial abscess, appropriate wound care, and possible reconstruction of any disfigurement.

Role of the Primary Care Provider

For the adolescent who has not yet obtained a tattoo or piercing, or who already has one and is contemplating the placement of another, education is essential. The practitioner should inquire where the adolescent plans to have the procedure performed and educate them regarding what key questions to ask and how to find a reputable studio. Additional information such as the APT and APP Web sites should be shared with the teenager, and written materials that contain the safety guidelines should be given to the adolescent at the visit. Teenagers are often reluctant to ask their health care providers for information about obtaining tattoos and piercings and almost never contact them if they believe they may have a complication associated with tattooing or piercing. Instead, they tend to ask their peers or contact the establishment where the tattoo or piercing was initially placed. Primary care providers should be a nonjudgmental resource during health maintenance visits to ensure the adolescent's continued health and safety. Additionally, the appearance of an uncommon medical condition such as unexplained hepatitis, endocarditis, or toxic shock in the adolescent patient warrants careful consideration of a possible complication related to tattooing or body piercing.

Prognosis

Most teens experience no adverse effects from body modification. Complications, while uncommon, are usually amenable to medical management. Risk-taking behavior that may occur in conjunction with body modification may carry long-term sequelae.

CASE RESOLUTION

Because the presence of one tattoo puts this adolescent at risk for obtaining another, the primary care provider should review safety guidelines for obtaining a tattoo and body piercing with the adolescent and offer the teenager educational material and/or Web site references to reinforce the discussion. The immunization status of the teenager also should be checked, with particular attention to tetanus and hepatitis A and B. Additionally, while alone with the teenager, the provider should review their concern regarding the adolescent's current high-risk behavior and its possible consequences. It also may be worthwhile to begin a discussion with the teen about telling her parents about the tattoo before they find out inadvertently.

Selected References

Armstrong ML, Caliendo C, Roberts AE. Genital piercings: what is known and what people with genital piercings tell us. *Urol Nurs.* 2006;26:173–179

Armstrong ML, Roberts AE, Owen DC, Koch JR. Contemporary college students and body piercing. *J Adolesc Health.* 2004;35:58–61

Association of Professional Piercers. www.safepiercing.org

Association of Professional Tattooists. www.safe-tattoos.com

Beers MS, Meires J, Loriz L. Body piercing: coming to a patient near you. *Nurs Pract.* 2007;32:55–60

Braverman PK. Body art: piercing, tattooing, and scarification. *Adolesc Med.* 2006;17:505–519

Brooks TL, Woods ER, Knight JR, Shrier LA. Body modification and substance use in adolescents: is there a link? *J Adolesc Health.* 2003;32:44–49

Carroll ST, Riffenburgh RH, Roberts TA, Myhre EB. Tattoos and body piercings as indicators of adolescent risk-taking behaviors. *Pediatrics.* 2002;109:1021–1028

Jervis PN, Clifton NJ, Woolford TJ. Ear deformity in children following high ear-piercing: current practice, consent issues and legislation. *J Laryngol Otol.* 2001;115:519–521

Larzo MR, Poe SG. Adverse consequences of tattoos and body piercings. *Pediatr Ann.* 2006;35:187–192

Laumann AE, Derick AJ. Tattoos and body piercing in the United States: a national data set. *J Am Acad Dermatol.* 2006;55:413–421

Meltzer DI. Complications of body piercing. *Am Fam Physician.* 2005; 72:2029–2034

More DR, Seidel JS, Bryan PA. Ear-piercing techniques as a cause of auricular chondritis. *Pediatr Emerg Care.* 1999;15:189–192

Nicoletti A. Teens, tattoos and body piercing. *J Pediatr Adolesc Gynecol.* 2004;17:215–216

Roberts TA, Ryan SA. Tattooing and high-risk behavior in adolescents. *Pediatrics.* 2002;110:1058–1063

Stewart GM, Thorp A, Brown L. Perichondritis—a complication of high ear piercing. *Pediatr Emerg Care.* 2006;22:804–806

Straetemans M, Katz LM, Belson M. Adverse reactions after permanent make-up procedures. *N Engl J Med.* 2007;356:2753

CHAPTER 135

Childhood Obesity

H. Mollie Greves Grow, MD, MPH, and Lenna Liu, MD, MPH

CASE STUDY

A 10-year-old girl is brought to your office by her mother to discuss concerns about the child's weight, which is 59 kg (130 lb). Her height is 140 cm (55 in), giving her a body mass index (BMI) of 30 kg/m² (>95th percentile for age). The rest of the physical examination, including vital signs, is normal. The mother, who also is overweight, says she doesn't want her daughter to "end up like me." The patient says she gets teased at school for being "fat". The history reveals that this patient is an only child who lives with her single mother in low-income housing in a large urban city. The mother works the day shift as a nurse's aide at a nearby nursing home. Because the mother is often tired, meals are simple and frequently consist of prepackaged foods such as pastries for breakfast and frozen dinners for supper. At school, the girl buys her lunch, which usually includes whole milk, a processed entrée, and a dessert. After school, the girl goes home, where she watches television and snacks on chips and soda until her mother arrives home from work. The mother does not allow her daughter to play outside because the neighborhood is unsafe.

Questions

1. How is obesity defined and measured, and what are some pitfalls in measurement?
2. How do genetic susceptibility and environment interact to influence a person's risk for obesity?
3. What are the complications of obesity?
4. What is the role of primary care providers in addressing childhood obesity?
5. How can obesity be treated?

Childhood obesity is of significant concern because overweight children are more likely to become overweight adults and are at increased risk for multiple chronic conditions. In addition, being obese carries a tremendous psychosocial toll for affected adults and children, as it remains one of the most stigmatized conditions. Obese children are often shunned by peers at school, feel isolated, and have fewer friends, while obese adolescents complete less schooling, go on to have lower household incomes, and are more likely to live in poverty than their non-obese counterparts. The primary care provider is usually the first (and frequently only) resource available to families to help screen for, inform about, and initiate treatment for childhood obesity.

Defining obesity presents certain challenges. Ideally, a measure of obesity would correlate with adiposity and predict morbidity and mortality. Body mass index (weight in kilograms/[height in meters]²) is the best and most widely used surrogate measure for obesity, but does not completely correlate with adiposity for all individuals. Standards for adults have established a BMI of 25 or greater as overweight and 30 or greater as obese, based on increased risk of morbidity and mortality above these levels. While BMI is the current preferred method for assessing degree of obesity in children, other criteria are also used (Dx Box). Experts classify children at 85% to 95% of BMI-for-age as **overweight** and those greater than 95% of BMI-for-age as **obese**. Since BMI is not a direct measure of adiposity, it is important to recognize that children who meet the BMI criteria for overweight and obesity will not all have adverse health effects of their weight status. A general helpful rule of thumb is that the higher the BMI goes above the 95th percentile, the greater likelihood of adverse health effects. The BMI category with the most rapid increase in risk for adverse health affects is BMI above the 99th percentile, which is associated with the most comorbidities (at that point switching to a BMI number, like adults, is often used). The BMI changes as children grow older due to changes in their proportion of bone mass and lean-to-fat tissue composition. After about 1 year of age, BMI-for-age values begin to decline and continue to do so during the preschool years until the BMI reaches a minimum around 5 to 6 years of age, before rising throughout the remainder of childhood, into adolescence and adulthood. This phenomenon of increasing BMI after the nadir in the preschool years is referred to as **adiposity rebound**. Early adiposity rebound (age <4.8) is a predictor of later obesity, and can be used clinically to identify children at risk.

Dx Obesity

- Body mass index ≥95th percentile for age (≥85 percentile = overweight)
- Weight-for-height ≥95 percentile
- >120% of ideal body weight for height and age

Epidemiology

The prevalence of obesity is on the rise in developed countries. Between 1980 and 2000, the percentage of overweight children and adolescents in the United States tripled, reaching 17.1% in 2003 to

2004. Since then, no significant increases have been seen overall among the US youth population, except for increases in the highest BMI group (>97th percentile). Hispanics, African Americans, and Native Americans are disproportionately affected. Prevention and treatment of obesity is important to avoid health risks that affect the individual and are costly to society as a whole. In the United States, the overall spending associated with overweight and obesity was $93 billion in 2002 dollars, half of which was publicly financed through Medicare or Medicaid.

Clinical Presentation

Obese children usually present to the physician in 1 of 2 ways. The parents or the child may come in concerned that the child is overweight. The physician must then consider the growth parameters and BMI-for-age to make an appropriate determination of the child's overweight status. The more common presentation involves parents who do not recognize that their child is overweight, and in fact may believe that being "pudgy" is a sign of health. The lack of awareness of their child's risk may particularly affect parents during the time of the adiposity nadir (ie, the preschool and early school age years), when early intervention to improve energy balance might yield the most benefit. Measurement of the child's height and weight and determination of the BMI-for-age is important at all ages to identify children who are overweight or obese, or gaining weight more rapidly than expected; it is especially critical during early childhood when outward appearances may be most unreliable. Seeing change in percentiles is particularly helpful to differentiate children who may be healthy and who grow steadily along a higher BMI curve, such as those 5% at the 95th percentile who are naturally in the high BMI range but are not actually "overfat."

Pathophysiology

Our understanding of the pathophysiology of obesity continues to evolve. Certain neurohormones affect appetite, satiety, and the balance between fat storage and energy production. In the end, obesity results when energy intake exceeds expenditure. The storage of excess calories was an advantage to our ancestors who faced intermittent food shortage; however, in our current setting where the environment provides highly palatable, convenient foods that are high in calories (but low in nutrients) and opportunities for physical activity are more limited, this predisposition to store excess calories has contributed to increasing rates of obesity.

It is known from twin and other studies that susceptibility to obesity is influenced substantially by **genetics.** Yet the magnitude of recent increases in obesity rates suggests the genetic susceptibility interacts with an **"obesogenic" environment** that facilitates unhealthy behaviors. National surveys indicate that Americans are consuming more calories now than they were 35 years ago. This trend is most related to increasingly widespread and easily available calorically dense foods in larger portions than ever before. A smaller but also important contribution of the population weight gain comes from less physical activity and more sedentary lifestyles. The reasons for this are myriad and include changes in transportation patterns, shifts in the workforce to less manual jobs, and automation of household work. Children have decreased opportunities for activity owing to safety concerns; parental work habits; the availability of television, computers, and other electronic toys; and reduced availability of physical education in school and after-school programs.

Differential Diagnosis

Most children who present to physicians as overweight have primary obesity (resulting from excessive caloric intake and low activity levels). Only a small proportion of overweight children will have an organic cause, although many parents may initially inquire about an organic etiology. A thorough history including review of systems, physical examination, and evaluation of growth parameters will help differentiate primary from organic obesity in most cases. While children with primary obesity tend to have normal or increased height-for-age, children with an organic etiology, such as hypothyroidism, are typically shorter than normal or have a delayed rate of linear growth. Certain genetic syndromes, such as Prader-Willi syndrome, pseudohypoparathyroidism, and Laurence-Moon-Biedl syndrome, are associated with obesity. However, children with these syndromes have other findings, such as developmental delay, dysmorphic features, and short stature, which are usually identifiable during the physical examination. While there may not be an organic cause of weight gain initially, there is evidence that weight gain can be exacerbated by acquired diagnoses, such as sleep apnea, that develop as complications of obesity.

Evaluation

History

The history should include the age of the child, parental weight, and lifestyle information (Questions Box). Knowledge of a child's birth weight and gestational age may be helpful. Full-term babies weighing more than 9 lbs are at increased risk of obesity. Prematurity is also a risk factor for subsequent obesity, possibly related to early metabolic effects of rapid "catch-up" weight gain after birth. Breastfeeding has been found to be somewhat protective against obesity in many epidemiological observational studies. A diet history, such as the 24-hour recall method or alternatively use of screening questions filled out by the parent in the waiting room, can be helpful to understand the dietary factors contributing to the child's overweight status as well as to identify areas for potential change. In addition, a history of signs or symptoms of complications of obesity should be elicited. For example, a teen may complain of hip pain suggestive of a slipped capital femoral epiphyses (SCFE). There may be a history of snoring, or apneic pauses followed by gasping for breath during sleep, and daytime sleepiness indicating sleep-disordered breathing and necessitating further evaluation for obstructive sleep apnea (OSA). A history of irregular menstrual periods is useful in the evaluation for polycystic ovary syndrome (PCOS).

Questions

Obesity

Open-ended questions to engage (lifestyle and family changes rather than targeting the child)

- How concerned is the parent/child about the child's weight?
- How has current weight affected their life (eg, teasing, difficulty exercising or with sleep)?
- What is the parent/family already doing to help the family with healthy eating and activity?
- Specific probes to learn more about the child's usual daily activities and home environment
  — Who cares for the child during the day? (Home-based child care provided by grandparents or other family members is associated with increased risk of overweight.)
  — How often does the child get to be physically active (ie, recess, physical education class, after school, on weekends)?
  — Where are there opportunities to add more activity (ie, to or from school, on weekends, playing sports or recreation, with parents)?
  — How much time does the child spend watching TV, playing video games, or using the computer?
  — On a typical day, starting first thing in the morning, what does the child eat?
  — How often does the family go to fast-food restaurants or go out to eat?
  — Who does the shopping and food preparation? Are there financial, time limitations?
  — What kitchen facilities are available at home?

Questions to set a mutual agenda

- What are some things the parent/family would like to change for healthier eating and activity?
- Who might support the parent/family in making changes?

Some additional questions for older children/adolescents include
  — Has the child tried to lose weight before? How?
  — Is the child/teen depressed?
  — Has the child/teen participated in fad dieting? Fasting? Laxative use? Diuretic use?
  — Has the child/teen used drugs to lose weight (illicit, over the counter, or prescription)?
  — Has the child/teen used nutritional supplements for weight loss?
  — Has the child/teen ever binged? Purged?
  — Does the child/teen use tobacco? Alcohol?

Physical Examination

The accurate measurement of height and weight using appropriate equipment and plotting growth parameters on a BMI chart should be essential components of every well-child visit. The revised 2000 growth curves (developed by the US National Center for Health Statistics and available at www.cdc.gov/growthcharts) enable the physician and other health providers to evaluate BMI-for-age (for children ≥2 years) relative to other children of the same gender. Prior to age 2 years, the clinician should use the World Health Organization weight-for-length curves (see Centers for Disease Control and Prevention Web site at www.cdc.gov) to assess proportional growth. Children should also be examined for any dysmorphic features suggestive of an underlying genetic syndrome.

The clinician should assess for potential complications of obesity when examining the overweight child. While many complications of obesity do not manifest until adulthood, overweight children are at risk for a number of conditions, including hypertension, hyperlipidemia, type 2 diabetes, nonalcoholic fatty liver disease, OSA, and orthopedic problems such as Blount disease and SCFE. One-third to one-half of obese children will have evidence of **metabolic syndrome,** a cluster of traits that include hyperinsulinemia, obesity, hypertension, and hyperlipidemia. The higher the BMI-for-age, the greater the risk that the child or teen will have metabolic complications. Blood pressure should be accurately measured with an appropriate-sized cuff (larger cuffs are needed for overweight youth) and compared with age-based standards. The physician should be alert for additional physical findings. The skin should be examined for striae and acanthosis nigricans, the velvety pigmented lesion commonly found on the neck or axilla, which is associated with insulin resistance in overweight children. Skin findings of hirsutism and acne in obese adolescent girls may indicate the presence of PCOS. The musculoskeletal examination should assess for Blount disease (severe tibial bowing), SCFE, or other degenerative joint diseases. Tanner stage should be assessed for evidence of premature puberty.

Laboratory Tests

If a genetic condition is suspected, an evaluation by a geneticist is indicated and high-resolution karyotype and other genetic tests, as directed by the suspected syndrome may be considered. For the rare cases in which an underlying endocrinologic disorder is suspected, thyroid function studies and/or cortisol levels may be considered. Laboratory studies to evaluate for potential complications of obesity are recommended starting at age 10 years, or before if there are specific concerns such as severe obesity (eg, >99th percentile BMI-for-age), or a strong family history of type 2 diabetes or hyperlipidemia. Children age 10 years and above with a BMI above the 95th percentile (and for those above the 85th percentile with family or other risk factors), are recommended to have fasting glucose and a fasting lipid panel. Some experts also recommend checking liver enzymes and fasting insulin levels. If the fasting glucose is abnormal, a glucose tolerance test is indicated. Children with a history of sleep-disordered breathing should be referred for a sleep study. Higher rates of nutritional deficiencies reported among overweight youth have included vitamin D, calcium, and iron, so screening for these should be considered based on dietary history and other risk factors.

Imaging Studies

Radiologic studies are indicated when orthopedic complications of obesity such as Blount disease or SCFE are suspected. An echocardiogram for evaluation of ventricular hypertrophy is a consideration in children with long-standing hypertension (left ventricle may be affected) or OSA (right ventricle may be affected).

Management

Since not all children who are obese will go on to be obese adults, a **staged approach** is now recommended in treating childhood obesity. The pediatrician's first task is to help prevent obesity through identifying risk and using patient-directed counseling to promote healthy target behaviors (and avoid unhealthy ones). Risk is largely determined by the child's age and history of parental obesity; however, race/ethnicity may also play a role. Obese children younger than 3 years without obese parents are at low risk for future obesity. These children should be monitored but, for the most part, do not require intervention. Between the ages of 3 and 5 years, parental obesity substantially increases the risk of a child becoming an obese adult. The chance of adult obesity in an obese preschooler with at least one obese parent is above 60%. In older children, the child's own obesity is an increasingly important predictor of adult obesity, regardless of whether the parents are obese. The probability that an overweight child older than 6 years will be obese as an adult is 50%, regardless of parental obesity status. Children determined to be at high risk for future obesity require close surveillance and intervention by the clinician.

Once a child has been identified as overweight, the **recommended stages of obesity treatment** are

- Stage 1 "Prevention Plus:" Initial treatment in the primary care office focuses on behavioral strategies for eating and activity changes to address causes of energy imbalance.
- Stage 2 (if no improvement within 3–6 months after Stage 1): "Structured weight management" involving specific targeted goal behaviors for eating, activity, and reducing sedentary time, and should include self-monitoring in the office or another setting for individual or group treatment.
- Stage 3 (if no improvement within 3–6 months after Stage 2): "Comprehensive multidisciplinary management" in pediatric weight management center or equivalent program.
- Stage 4 (for patients with BMI above 99th percentile or more severe comorbidities): "Tertiary Care Intervention" in a tertiary care facility that oversees more targeted medical weight loss and may offer surgical approaches.

The core of child obesity treatment focuses on behavior and lifestyle modification, the aims of which are to reduce BMI through sustainable and appropriate healthy eating and physical activities that do not lead to disordered eating or inappropriate body image. Throughout assessment and management of obesity, primary care clinicians need to help families recognize the importance of physical fitness and overall health, not just body size, and that the whole family needs to be involved. In addition, clinicians should monitor children and teens for inappropriate focus on weight or engaging in unhealthy weight loss practices including laxative abuse, induced vomiting, and fasting (see Chapter 133).

The initial weight change goal in caring for the prepubertal overweight child is slowing weight gain or maintaining weight during normal linear growth. If more advanced treatment is indicated, the goal may move to weight loss, but not more than 1 pound per month

is recommended for ages 2 to 5 years. Youth ages 12 to 18 years (or postpubertal) may start at any of the 4 treatment stages, depending on severity and readiness to change. Initial treatment goals for the older age group may be slowed weight gain or weight loss. The weight loss recommendation is not more than 2 pounds per month above age 5. As a quaternary intervention, surgical treatments for obesity are available for teenagers in some centers, but due to cost, complications, and side effects, they are reserved only for those with extreme obesity already resulting in health problems.

Box 135-1. Brief Motivational Interviewing (MI) Approach to Child Obesity Management

Goal: Through nonjudgmental questions and reflective listening, elicit a realistic plan for addressing child's weight/health consistent with family's values and goals.

Use: Basic MI Skills or "OARS"

O: Open-ended questions
(eg, those starting with "How…", "What…", or "Tell me about…")

A: Affirmations
(eg, "You are already doing a good job with…")

R: Reflections
(eg, "It sounds like you would like some help with changing…")

S: Summaries
(eg, "Let me see if I can summarize our discussion and plans between now and the next visit…")

Steps: Basic approach in 15 minutes

1. Assess body mass index (BMI), inform parent/patient, elicit response
   eg, "Your child's BMI is in a range where we start to be concerned about extra weight causing health problems. What concerns, if any, do you have about his/her weight?"

2. Set agenda: assess what they have already done, their goals for change, possible target behaviors
   eg, see sample Questions Box above

3. Assess motivation and confidence to make the changes
   eg, "On a scale of 1–10 with 10 being highest, how important are the changes we have talked about for you? Why are you an 'x' [number they chose] and not a 'y' [lower number]?"

4. Ask about ways to implement their plans/goals
   eg, "Who can help you with your plans? What will help you be successful? How have you been able to make a change in the past?"

5. Summarize: review plans (including follow-up), express confidence in the family, offer further help
   eg, "Let's summarize our discussion today. You have planned to _____ and this is important to you because_____. You will get some help from _____ to be successful. This sounds like a plan that can work. I know you can do it if you set your mind to it. I suggest we meet again in 1 month to check in. I look forward to hearing about how well you are doing. At that time we can discuss other ways I might be able to help, like a referral to a nutritionist or an exercise program."

Clinicians can feel most successful and efficacious in managing obesity if they tailor recommendations for the individual child and family, and access available community resources. **Motivational interviewing** techniques (Box 135-1) can be helpful in determining and promoting a family's readiness to make changes to address weight concerns. For families that are less ready, the clinician's role can be more focused on understanding values and current barriers, ordering appropriate testing to help families assess risk, checking back in frequently, and providing encouragement while respecting autonomy. For more ready families, the clinician's role moves into actively eliciting from the patient and parent what they consider to be important and feasible lifestyle changes, and how they want to go about reaching their goals. Because it is difficult to modify habits and behaviors related to food and activity, patients and their families require ongoing support and attention from their primary care providers and additional clinical and community resources as they attempt to integrate and maintain healthy behaviors in their lives. Engaging with the family to elicit solutions and problem-solve barriers is more likely to yield positive results than blanket advice or recommendations. Even if well-intentioned, clinician recommendations are unlikely to be implemented if they are inconsistent with a patient's and family's values, culture, and/or resources. For example, a child's participation in an after-school sports program may not be a realistic option if a family cannot afford the fees or transportation to and from the program is not available; instead, a school-based after-school program or an evening or weekend class at a community center with their parent might be an option.

In preventing and treating childhood obesity, clinicians must also recognize the gaps between knowledge and behavior: Understanding that good nutrition and physical activity are important does not necessarily translate into healthy eating or regular exercise. For example, a parent may know to limit fat and sugar but may still buy a lot of processed foods because of convenience or price, or because of not knowing how to prepare healthier foods. Alternatively, some families may have food insecurity or have periods of time with inadequate food that may lead to overeating inexpensive, energy-dense foods. These families should be connected with nutrition assistance programs (eg, Special Supplemental Program for Women, Infants, and Children [WIC], Supplemental Nutrition Assistance Program [formerly known as food stamps]). Most families need additional education on appropriate serving sizes, healthful food preparation, interpreting food labels, and making healthy food choices among the many mixed nutrition messages in the media. Given time limitations to provide this kind of support in primary care office visits, referral to a dietitian or nutrition classes through WIC can be an initial step in providing the education and planning needed for families to change eating habits. Dieticians can be particularly useful for motivated families in providing ideas to plan healthful daily meals and snacks.

Since the options for actively treating childhood obesity are currently limited in the primary care setting, it is critically important for clinicians to be aware of what treatment programs are available in

---

Box 135-2. 10 Guidelines to Help Families Toward a Healthier Lifestyle

1. Learn about the child's and family's usual diet and activity pattern so that you can elicit ideas about helpful changes they are interested in and capable of making.
2. Promote "5-2-1-0" simple guidelines for healthy living: 5 fruits and vegetables a day, 2 hours or less of screen time, 1 hour or more of physical activity, and 0 sugar-sweetened beverages per day.
3. Encourage intake of more "natural" foods such as fruits and vegetables (fresh or frozen). Limit processed and prepackaged foods and snacks (which have added sugar that overweight/obese children/teens don't need), by keeping them out of the house as much as possible.
4. Set family guidelines on recreational screen time or "seat time" with a goal of less than 2 hours a day including TV, videos, and computers.
5. Keep TVs out of children and teens' bedrooms (easier to do if providers help educate about not putting them there in the first place).
6. Promote "fitness over fatness": Incorporate physical activity into the child's and family's daily routine with a goal of 60 minutes per day. Find sports or activities that the child enjoys and can master.
7. Teach healthy beverages for all ages: milk and water is all we need. For children older than 1–2 years, change to 1% or fat-free milk. Limit milk to 16 to 20 oz per day after the first year of life. If parents serve juice, limit to less than 4 oz per day for toddlers and 6 oz for older children. Limit soda to special occasions (like a birthday).
8. Limit eating out, especially at fast food restaurants.
9. Have regular family meals cooked at home.
10. Encourage appropriate portion sizes for family members based on need (teach parents to respond to hunger cues when children are infants and toddlers).

---

the local area and take full advantage of these. Successful, evidence-based programs are now increasingly available to help children attain a healthier weight. To date, the most efficacious programs are moderate intensity family-based behavioral treatment, generally of 3 to 12 months' duration. Clinicians can play an active role in referring to structured treatment programs by being a knowledgeable source of information and helping families learn about and become interested in these programs. Families often need support and encouragement from a trusted provider to participate. If structured overweight treatment programs are not available in the local area, the clinician can recommend and refer to structured physical activity programs, such as at local YMCAs or community centers, which can help patients improve physical fitness and lower metabolic risks related to obesity, even if not leading to weight loss per se.

A basic set of guidelines that clinicians can use to help families move toward a healthier lifestyle are listed in Box 135-2. Items on this list are evidence-based from the standpoint that families who have implemented these generally have children with healthier weight. Some involve fairly simple changes, such as reducing the intake of sugar-sweetened beverages, or switching to a lower-fat milk. Other suggestions may require more knowledge or motivation to implement successfully. Many Web Sites provide excellent educational resources for families such as the US Department of Agriculture Food and Nutrition Service "MyPlate" (www.ChooseMyPlate.gov) and *Dietary Guidelines for Americans* published every 5 years (www.healthierus. gov/dietaryguidelines), Nemours Health (www.kidshealth.org), and the Let's Move campaign (www.letsmove.gov) initiated by First Lady Michelle Obama.

There are no quick fixes to the management of obesity. Appetite suppressing medications are neither recommended nor approved for use in children and teens. Their use in adults has also proved hazardous. Metformin, which is used in some obese teens, is indicated to address the insulin resistance in patients with metabolic syndrome.

Given the complexity of managing obesity, there are increasing options for clinical tools and additional training for pediatric providers. Resources include the American Academy of Pediatrics (AAP) and other specific online curricula (eg, Health and Obesity Prevention and Education curriculum available to providers at no cost by requesting materials from hopeproject@ucsd.edu).

Prevention

Prevention of obesity is our best option for reversing the growing epidemic of obesity and obesity-related comorbidities. Prevention of obesity should be a priority for all clinicians who care for children and should focus on 3 broad areas: (1) anticipatory guidance starting in infancy on healthful eating, minimizing screen time, and providing access to regular physical activity with an emphasis on promoting overall health; (2) early intervention for families whose children are at higher risk for developing obesity; and (3) advocacy for public health measures to increase opportunities for healthful eating and regular physical activity within our communities. Pediatric providers can take an active role to improve obesity trends in supporting changes in school and child care institutions, communities, and national policies (see resources available through the AAP at www.aap.org/obesity).

Prognosis

Without intervention, the average American life expectancy is currently projected to decrease, owing to the increasing incidence of diseases associated with obesity such as diabetes. Poor diet and sedentary lifestyles rival smoking as a preventable cause of premature death. Obese children who remain obese into adulthood are at greatly increased risk for all of the complications of obesity. However, there is hopeful evidence that early intervention at the family and community levels can change this trajectory. Pediatric providers continue to improve rates of BMI screening and referral; those who have had training in obesity, management are even more likely to implement current recommendations. Globally, more and more providers and organizations are taking an active role in preventing and treating childhood obesity and treatment options continue to evolve and improve. The fact that current childhood obesity rates in the US have stabilized may be a positive sign for the future.

CASE RESOLUTION

The opening vignette describes an obese girl. She is at substantial risk for remaining obese into adulthood based on her present weight and her mother's history of obesity, as well as social and economic risk factors. Working with a dietitian, the mother and her daughter learn about simple changes for healthy diets. They begin to plan meals and snacks that include fruits and vegetables and can be prepared in advance. The girl starts making her own lunch each night before school. The mom changes her grocery shopping: she buys 1% milk instead of whole milk, and she stops buying cookies, chips, and soda, except as an occasional treat. A social worker helps find an after-school program at the nearby YMCA. The patient starts attending and, with some special attention from the coach, finds she enjoys basketball and would like to try out for the school team next year. The mother wants to exercise more, and so the girl and her mother plan after-dinner walks around the track at the local high school.

Over the next 6 months, you follow the girl and her mother closely. The most recent growth parameters show that the girl has maintained her weight at 59 kg but has grown 5 cm to 145 cm, giving her a body mass index of 28. The mother has lost 5 lb during this period, and both are excited about continuing their new lifestyle.

Selected References

American Academy of Pediatrics Committee on Nutrition. Policy statement: prevention of pediatric overweight and obesity. *Pediatrics.* 2003;112:424–430

American Academy of Pediatrics Council on Sports Medicine and Fitness and Council on School Health. Policy statement: active healthy living: prevention of childhood obesity through increased physical activity. *Pediatrics.* 2006;117:1834–1842

Barlow S; American Academy of Pediatrics Expert Committee. Expert committee recommendations regarding the prevention, assessment, and treatment of child and adolescent overweight and obesity: a summary report. *Pediatrics.* 2007;120:S164–S192

Daniels SR, Arnett DK, Eckel RH, et al. Overweight in children and adolescents: pathophysiology, consequence, prevention and treatment. *Circulation.* 2005;111:1999–2012

Dietz WH, Lee J, Wechsler H, Malepati S, Sherry B. Health plans' role in preventing overweight in children and adolescents. *Health Aff (Millwood).* 2007;26:430–440

Division of Nutrition and Physical Activity: Research to Practice Series No. 4: Does breastfeeding reduce the risk of pediatric overweight? Atlanta, GA: Centers for Disease Control and Prevention; 2007

Freedman DS, Mei Z, Srinivasan SR, Berenson GS, Dietz WH. Cardiovascular risk factors and excess adiposity among overweight children and adolescents: the Bogalusa Heart Study. *J Pediatr.* 2007;150:12–17

Institute of Medicine, Committee on Prevention of Obesity in Children and Youth. *Preventing Childhood Obesity: Health in the Balance.* Washington, DC: National Academy of Sciences; 2004

Klein JD, Sesselberg TS, Johnson MS, et al. Adoption of body mass index guidelines for screening and counseling in pediatric practice. *Pediatrics.* 2010;125:265–272

Ogden, CL, Carroll MD, Curtin LR, Lamb MM, Flegal KM. Prevalence of high body mass index in US children and adolescents, 2007–2008. *JAMA.* 2010;303:242–259

Whitlock EP, O'Connor EA, Williams SB, Beil TL, Lutz KW. Effectiveness of weight management interventions in children: a targeted systematic review for the USPSTF. *Pediatrics.* 2010;125:e396–e418

CHAPTER 136

Divorce

Carol D. Berkowitz, MD

CASE STUDY

A 7-year-old girl who has been your patient for 5 years is brought in by her mother with abdominal pain that occurs on a daily basis and is not associated with any other symptoms. The pain is periumbilical. In obtaining the history, you learn that the father has moved out of the home and the parents are planning a divorce. The mother believes that her daughter's symptoms may relate to the impending divorce, and she wants to know what else to expect.

Questions

1. What are the problems faced by children whose parents are undergoing divorce?
2. What are the age-related reactions of children in families undergoing divorce?
3. What is the role of pediatricians in counseling families undergoing divorce?
4. What anticipatory guidance can be offered about custody and remarriage?
5. How can pediatricians help stepfamilies adjust?

Divorce represents the **"death"** of a marriage, and in some ways may be more devastating for children than the death of a parent. When a parent dies, that parent becomes idealized in the mind of children, but when parents divorce, the noncustodial parent is often devalued. In fact, each parent is frequently devalued by the other. For children, parents are no longer the idealized figures that they once were. The challenge for pediatricians is to maintain a neutral position. This may be particularly difficult because much of the contact has been with one parent rather than the other, usually the mother.

Pediatricians play a specific role in managing children going through a parental divorce because other resources are few. **Extended families** are no longer as available to provide help. Religious institutions have often failed to assume a counseling role in this area; some religions view divorce unfavorably. Most families do not seek out mental health services unless the problems are overwhelming. Therefore, it is important for pediatricians to become involved in anticipatory guidance of families undergoing divorce. This guidance focuses on preparing children and families for times ahead. In addition, practitioners serve as child advocates. The parents themselves are so consumed by their emotional turmoil that they are often not available or are not even aware of the stress and trauma their children are experiencing. Physicians should be aware of the effect of the divorce on children and their subsequent psychological development. In addition, pediatricians can help as new families form, assisting the transition of caretakers into the role of stepparents.

Epidemiology

Divorce affects nearly 50% of marriages though the rate recently has decreased to closer to 40% attributed in part to the decrease in the marriage rate. **Ethnic differences** exist; 38% of European American compared with 75% of African American children's parents divorce prior to the children's 18th birthday. The US Office of National Vital Statistics reported 1,045,289 divorces for 2009, a figure that is lower than the actual number of cases because California, Georgia, Hawaii, Louisiana, and Minnesota do not report their data. Divorce usually occurs in the first 14 years of marriage (mean: 7.8 years). Approximately 1 million children per year are affected by divorce. Nearly one-third of all children live in households in which parents are divorced or remarried. Children between the ages of 3 and 8 years are the major age group affected. Children involved with parental divorce take 2½ to 3 years to regain their equilibrium and master a sense of control. Divorce usually results in a decline of **economic resources** to mothers and children. In the first year after divorce, income is reduced to 58% of the pre-divorce level. Even after 5 years, income for mothers and children is only 94% of the pre-divorce amount; for intact couples, income has risen to 130% during that period. Decreased income is often associated with multiple moves to more affordable housing along with change in schools and loss of friends. More affordable neighborhoods may not provide the same resources and environment to which the children were previously accustomed.

Types of custody include **single-parent custody, joint custody, joint legal custody,** and **joint physical custody,** where parents have physical access to the child with equal frequency. **Birds-nest custody** is joint custody where children remain in the home and parents take turns moving in and out. Many states now allow for joint custody. Joint custody is associated with higher levels of involvement by the biological father, increased child support payments, and greater paternal satisfaction. Issues of **remarriage** and **stepsiblings** are also important. Eighty percent of divorced men and 75% of divorced women remarry, and 40% of these remarriages end in divorce. As a result of the high rate of remarriage, 1 in 3 children in the United States has a stepparent. Eighty-six percent of stepfamilies include the biological mother and a stepfather. Children in stepfamilies often have to readjust to differing roles in differing households and differing relationships between their biological parents, stepparents, biological siblings, and stepsiblings.

Psychophysiology

The experience that children have following parental divorce is influenced by many factors, including the individual child's **temperament** and **personality.** An easygoing child with strong self-esteem and a positive outlook fairs better than the child with a difficult temperament and less positive personality traits. The reaction to divorce also depends, to a large extent, on the age of the child (Table 136-1). In general, children do not have the cognitive ability to understand the meaning of divorce until they are 9 or 10 years of age. The experience is also different for children without siblings, "onlies." Not only do they lack brothers or sisters with which to commiserate, they may also experience parental "overconcern" manifested by being asked repeatedly how they are feeling and how they are doing. Studies have demonstrated that the negative effect of parental divorce on adolescent academic performance is mitigated by increased sibship size.

Table 136-1. Children's Reaction to Divorce	
Age	*Symptoms*
2½–4 y	• Regressive behavior
3½–5 y	• Aggressive behavior
5–6 y	• Whiny, immature behavior
6 y–adolescence	• Disequilibrium • Depression • Somatic complaints • Poor school performance

Children up to the age of 2 years experience **sleeping** and **feeding disturbances,** as well as spitting up and clinginess. Between the ages of 2½ and 4 years, children usually manifest **regressive behavior.** They become needy and dependent, and their behavior is characterized by irritability, whining, crying, fearfulness, increased separation anxiety, and sleep problems. Both aggression and regression, particularly in the area of toilet training, may develop. One-third of children in this age group continue to exhibit regressive behavior 1 year after divorce.

Preschool-aged children between the ages of 3½ and 5 years often show more aggressive patterns of behavior with hitting, biting, and temper tantrums. Regressive behavior may also be seen. Young children feel particularly responsible for their parents' divorce (ie, the parents are divorcing the child). At this point in development, children experience what Piaget has referred to as an egocentric way of thinking. Self-blame, decreased self-esteem, and a high level of fantasy, particularly about parental reunion, are apparent. Approximately 1 year after divorce, 65% of these children still show decreased levels of functioning.

Children who are 5 to 6 years of age are often **depressed** and may exhibit immature behavior. Girls in this age group seem to handle a divorce more poorly than boys. Two-thirds of girls are less well-adjusted 1 year after the divorce, as opposed to only about one-fourth of boys. These children seem moody and daydream. They may also be whiny and have temper tantrums.

School-aged children between the age of 6 years and adolescence seem to experience profound disequilibrium, with feelings of shame, anger, and loneliness. This anger may be manifested by antisocial behavior. Older children also talk about an overwhelming feeling of sadness and grief. Their somatic complaints include headache, abdominal pain, and an increase in symptoms of preexisting medical conditions such as asthma. Sometimes the somatic complaints of children, particularly those in the school-aged group, are attributed by one parent to the poor living conditions at the other parent's household.

It is important for physicians to anticipate that 50% of children involved in parental divorce show a deterioration in their school performance. Therefore, the school should be notified about the divorce and changes in family structure. Decreased school performance is attributed to decreased ability to concentrate, sadness, and depression.

Parental divorce is particularly difficult for adolescents, who describe it as "extraordinarily painful." The experience is worse for younger adolescents. During the first stages of divorce, they experience a personal sense of abandonment and a loss of parental love. Older adolescents are concerned about their future potential as marital partners. They also feel anxious about financial security, especially money for college. **De-idealization** of both parents is precipitous. Adolescent girls do better than boys early on, but this reverses with time. This pattern is referred to as a **sleeper effect** or **delayed effect,** with girls subsequently feeling rejected and unattractive as they reinterpret their parents' divorce with their additional maturation. Divorce during adolescence sometimes leads to **precocious sexual activity** or risk- or thrill-seeking behavior. Studies suggest that paternal involvement following the divorce reduces the risk of alcohol abuse. Adolescents from divorced families are more likely to experience teenaged parenthood. Adolescent girls from divorced families are less likely to succeed academically than girls from families where there has not been a divorce. In addition, the adolescent may turn to alcohol or drug use to help cope with the stress of parental divorce. Boys may engage in illegal activities such as burglary.

Differential Diagnosis

Children who present with complaints including headache, abdominal pain, enuresis, and poor school performance should always be assessed for environmental factors that may be contributing to their symptomatology. When evaluating a child with suspected **somatic complaints,** it is appropriate to consider organic etiologies.

Many parents who are undergoing a divorce do not appreciate the impact the divorce is having on their children. They are often caught up in their own personal feelings and are not aware of their children's symptomatology. In addition, divorcing parents actually experience a deterioration in their physical and mental well-being, and divorced mothers have an increased rate of illness.

Parents engaged in custody disputes may express concerns that their child is maltreated by the other parent. These concerns may include allegations of sexual abuse, which may require a referral to a child advocacy center (see Chapter 128).

Evaluation

The focus of the evaluation should be on the interviewing process. Determination of the full extent of the impact of the home factors on children's symptomatology may take several visits. It is not appropriate to pursue extensive laboratory tests without first adequately determining what changes are occurring within the household.

History

The medical evaluation of children experiencing a parental divorce should include a review of the medical history and a discussion with the child of factors of change (Questions Box). This may help open up a discussion that reveals that the parents are in the process of divorce or that the father has moved out of the household. Specific parental concerns related to child maltreatment should be noted in detail.

Questions

Divorce

- Is there anything different about the child's house now?
- Who lives in the house?
- How are things going between the parents?
- Has the child shown any regressive or aggressive behaviors?
- Has the child been eating and sleeping normally?
- How is the child doing in school?

Physical Examination

Any symptom or specific complaint, such as headache or abdominal pain, should also be addressed (see Chapters 112 and 116). Depression and the risk for suicide should also be evaluated (see Chapter 140). A complete physical examination is usually warranted because children who are experiencing stress may also develop stress-related medical problems. If there are concerns about the genital findings, a careful anogenital examination is indicated.

Laboratory Tests

Some simple baseline laboratory studies may be warranted, particularly in children who have complaints such as abdominal pain or enuresis. These tests may include a complete blood cell count or urinalysis.

Management

Management of children whose family is undergoing divorce is complex. In addition to treating any somatic complaints that may be related to the divorce, physicians play a key role in anticipatory guidance. Children need to understand that they didn't cause the divorce and that they will not be able to "cure" it. Physician involvement before parents actually separate helps. Initially, physicians should advise parents about how to talk to children and what to expect in terms of their reaction. It is important for parents to tell children that they are separating from one another and not from the children. As stated previously, parents undergoing a divorce are in so much turmoil that they themselves may not see their children's problems. In addition, their parenting skills may suffer, and routine procedures such as meals and bedtime may become disrupted, sporadic, and irregular.

Box 136-1 summarizes advice given to parents when talking with their children. **When, how, who,** and **what** to tell should be discussed. Generally, children should be told of impending divorce by both parents with support from the extended family. Unfortunately, studies report that 80% of preschoolers were told by one parent.

Box 136-1. Talking to Children About Divorce
Who
- Who tells? Both parents
- Who is told? Children, physicians, teachers, neighbors
When
- Before either parent leaves
- Age-dependent
- Older children: weeks ahead
- Younger children: days ahead
How
- Calmly, with emotional control
Where
- Privately, in the home
What
- Stress that children are not to blame; that the divorce is between parents, not between parents and children; it is the parents who cannot get along.
- Explain expected living arrangements.

When to tell depends on children's ages. Younger children should be told a few days before the actual separation. Older children should be told at least several weeks before. Practitioners should advise parents about **how** to tell. Displays of emotion are permissible. Parents should be encouraged to show their emotions, but not to the extent that they appear overwhelmed or uncontrollable.

Who to tell includes not only the children but also the neighbors and the school, so that the feeling of shame or secrecy is less. **What** to tell involves freeing the children of any blame for the divorce and answering their questions.

It is important for physicians not to become involved in custody disputes, but if they are asked to give an opinion, they should try to evaluate the parenting skills of both parents. In the past, custody was given to the mother in 90% of cases, but this is now decreasing. Questions that physicians should ask themselves when advising about custody include: What are the emotional ties between parents and children? Do children indicate a preference for one parent? Children may be overwhelmed by feelings of loyalty and be torn if asked to choose one parent over the other, which makes this a difficult problem. What is the capacity of each parent to provide emotional and physical support for children? It is important to consider a need for continuity, and it is vital to keep conditions as close as possible to the pre-divorce situation. Children should not have to move. Living arrangements need to be reassessed on a periodic basis.

Physicians should be aware of the factors that support joint custody. Joint custody tends to maintain a parent–child attachment, and children experience less of a sense of loss. They have more cognitive and social stimulation. Joint custody relieves the burden of single parenthood, and parents who have joint custody are less likely to use children as bargaining tools. Parents themselves are freer to enter into different relationships and are less emotionally dependent on their children. Although physicians should not become involved in monetary issues, concerns related to payment, insurance coverage, and cost of medical care are appropriate to discuss. Practitioners should consider involving noncustodial parents in children's health care. Such parents could be notified if medical problems occur.

Pediatricians may also be helpful in counseling noncustodial parents about interacting with children. Unfortunately contact with noncustodial parents may decrease rapidly following a divorce. While 25% of children have weekly visits with their noncustodial father, 20% of children see their father only several times a year or not at all. In general, visitation should reflect previous relationships as closely as possible. Noncustodial parents should be advised not to become camp counselors who focus on fun and games but to be influential figures who help the children meet the challenges of normal living, such as completing homework and doing chores and tasks. It is also important for noncustodial parents to be consistent. If a meeting is planned, the parents must show up. Although the parents are no longer married, they can still be co-parents rather than rivals. Noncustodial parents should be encouraged to participate in school and sports activities. Multiple modalities such as e-mail and texting can facilitate more frequent communication.

Custodial parents may attribute children's somatic complaints to poor care while under visitation with noncustodial parents. Allegations related to abuse, most often sexual abuse, may also arise. These allegations should be taken seriously. An appropriate medical and psychological evaluation is necessary (see Chapter 128). The most difficult situations involve allegations of sexual abuse of preverbal children, where conclusions may be contingent on the physical findings, which are usually inconclusive.

Issues related to parental dating and remarriage should be addressed at an early stage. Parents should be advised that pediatricians may be a resource in helping families readjust. Remarriage is often a difficult time for children because they experience feelings of rejection secondary to displacement by stepparents. Grandparents may also be a source of support.

The pediatrician can also serve as a resource for stepparents. Although stepparents do not have legal rights to consent for medical care of their stepchildren, they should become familiar with the children's medical history. Stepparents grow into their parenting role, and it takes 2 to 7 years for families to become blended. The pediatrician can help families adjust by recommending books or giving referrals to organizations such as the National Stepfamily Resource Center (www.stepfamilies.info).

Prognosis

The prognosis for children undergoing a parental divorce depends, in part, on the degree of dysfunction that existed in the family before separation and the ability of the children to communicate their concerns. Supportive intervention by family, friends, and physicians is key to facilitating the necessary adjustment. For adolescents, a positive belief about parental divorce is a major predictor of their adjustment. Family resilience and hardiness as well as family communication are associated with a good adjustment. Being a child of divorced and remarried parents has been likened to having dual citizenship. The experience is rewarding if the countries are not at war with one another.

CASE RESOLUTION

The case history reflects that functional somatic complaints are not uncommon, especially in school-aged children of divorced parents. The mother and her daughter should be advised about how stressful divorce is for children. A careful medical examination may reassure both the mother and child about the child's physical well-being. Issues related to custody, financial responsibility, and the need for consistency should all be addressed. In addition, the pediatrician should refer the family to outside agencies if necessary.

Selected References

Behrman RE. Children and divorce: overview and analysis. *Future Child.* 1994;4:4–14

Bryner CL. Children of divorce. *J Am Board Fam Pract.* 2001;14:178–183

Cohen GJ; American Academy of Pediatrics Committee on Psychosocial Aspects of Child and Family Health. Helping children and families deal with divorce and separation. *Pediatrics.* 2002;110:1019–1023

Dell ML. Divorce—are you ready to help? *Contemp Pediatr.* 1995;12:57–68

Emery RE, Coiro MJ. Divorce: consequences for children. *Pediatr Rev.* 1995;16:306–310

Hetherington EM. Divorce and the adjustment of children. *Pediatr Rev.* 2005;26:163–169

Shin SH, Kim MJ, Kim YH. Comparing adolescents' adjustment and family resilience in divorced families depending on the types of primary caregiver. *J Clin Nurs.* 2010;19:1695–1706

Storksen I, Roysamb E, Moum T, Tambs K. Adolescents with a childhood experience of parental divorce: a longitudinal study of mental health and adjustment. *J Adolesc.* 2005;28:725–739

Tomcikova Z, Madarasova Geckova A, Reijineveld SA, van Dijk JP. Parental divorce, adolescents' feelings toward parents and drunkenness in adolescents. *Eur Addict Res.* 2011;17:113–118

Velez CE, Wlchik SA, Tein JY, Sandler I. Protecting children from the consequences of divorce: a longitudinal study of parenting on children's coping processes. *Child Dev.* 2011;82;244–257

Books for Parents

Clapp G. *Divorce and New Beginnings: A Complete Guide to Recovery, Solo Parenting, Co-Parenting, and Stepfamilies.* Hoboken, NJ: John Wiley & Sons; 2000

Garon RJ. *Talking to Your Children about Separation and Divorce: A Handbook for Parents.* Columbia, MD: National Family Resiliency Center, Inc.; 1999

Books for Teens

Ricci I. *Mom's House, Dad's House for Kids: Feeling at Home in One Home or Two.* New York NY: Simon & Schuster; 2006

CHAPTER 137

School-Related Violence

Elizabeth A. Edgerton, MD, MPH

CASE STUDY

A mother brings her 9-year-old son, Alex, in complaining of recurrent abdominal pain. His pain has become so severe that Alex misses school frequently. He denies any vomiting or diarrhea. His weight has been stable over the last 6 months. Alex's mother reports that lately he seems more withdrawn and passive. He used to be engaged in his schoolwork but now with his frequent absences has lost interest in school. His mother says he is often anxious or nervous about new situations.

Questions

1. How does school-related violence affect children's health and well-being?
2. What is the relationship between bullying and adult criminal behavior?
3. What is cyberbullying?
4. What are strategies to address school-related violence?
5. What can pediatricians do to help address violence in the school, home, and communities?

Violence is defined as an act of aggression that can be **physical, sexual,** or **psychological** and is usually deliberate and intended to cause harm. Its form, level of severity, and frequency are impacted by biological, individual, clinical, intrapersonal, situational, and sociocultural factors. Categorization of violence is also dependent on the relationship of the perpetrator and victim, as well as their ages. Domestic or **intimate partner violence** occurs among individuals in an established relationship, **child abuse** predominantly occurs between an adult and a minor, and **bullying** is usually between peers. From a developmental perspective, bullying may be the earliest form of violence promulgated by children and can progress to intimate partner violence, **criminal delinquency, suicide,** or **homicide** in adolescence and adulthood. While violence may be considered a social issue, it impacts the physical and mental health of all of those involved. The primary care physician has unique opportunities to prevent violence and identify those potentially at risk.

Prevalence

Suicide and homicide represent the most lethal forms of violence. Suicide and homicide are responsible for approximately one-fourth of deaths among persons aged 10 to 24 years in the United States. Approximately 3 million youths are at risk for suicide, with 37% of at-risk individuals attempting to kill themselves (see Chapter 140). Suicide is the third leading cause of death among 15- to 24-year-olds, and over the last 20 years has increased 100% among 10- to 14-year-olds. It is estimated that approximately 12 youths die each day in the United States from suicide. Homicide is also increasing among children and adolescents. According to the Centers for Disease Control and Prevention, homicide is the fifth leading cause of death for youths 10 to 14 years of age and the second leading cause of death for 15- to 19-year-olds in the United States.

In 2007 emergency department data documented that more than 500,000 youth younger than 24 years were treated for injuries sustained due to violence. Nationwide surveys of high school students note that 33% report being in a physical fight one or more times in the 12 preceding months. An additional 17% reported carrying a weapon such as a gun, knife, or club on one or more of the 30 days preceding the survey. Furthermore, 6% of students reported not going to school on one or more days in the 30 days preceding the survey because they felt unsafe at school or on their way to and from school.

Those that admitted to being bullies in middle school had at least one criminal conviction by age 24 years, and 35% to 40% had 3 or more convictions by 24 years of age compared with 10% among control boys who were neither bullies nor victims as children. The aggressive antisocial behavior of bullying seems to contribute to future serious criminal behavior. Many of the recent killing sprees in the United States were committed by individuals who as children felt they were victimized. A review of 37 mass school shootings found more than two-thirds of perpetrators felt they had been persecuted, bullied, threatened, or attacked; often, they were acting out of revenge.

In a national survey of 6th- to 10th-grade students, approximately 30% reported moderate or frequent involvement in bullying; this could include being the bully, the victim, or both (known as the *bully-victim*). Those who reported being a bully or victim were more likely to carry weapons to school, as well as to be involved in frequent fights. Bullying itself is most common in the early school years. Initially, boys are more likely than girls to be involved in bullying. This gender gap decreases in middle and high school, as does the prevalence of bullying. Boys tend to participate in physical and verbal bullying, while girls use more subtle and indirect forms of bullying such as alienation or ostracizing.

Risk factors associated with violence are complex and involve the individual, family, peers, and community (Box 137-1). Demonstrated risk factors associated with violent behavior include exposure to violence as a witness or victim, childhood aggression and **antisocial behavior, substance abuse, depressed mood,** and **hyperactivity.** Protective factors include academic achievement and parent–family connectedness. Families that provide positive and consistent discipline and supervision can prevent involvement in violence.

Box 137-1. Risk Factors Associated With Violence

Individual Risk Factors[a]
- History of violent victimization or involvement
- Attention deficit, hyperactivity, or learning disorders
- History of early aggressive behavior
- Involvement with drugs, alcohol, or tobacco
- Low IQ
- Poor behavioral control
- Deficits in social, cognitive, or information-processing abilities
- High emotional distress
- History of treatment for emotional problems
- Antisocial beliefs and attitudes
- Exposure to violence and conflict in the family

Family Risk Factors
- Authoritarian childrearing attitudes
- Harsh, lax, or inconsistent disciplinary practices
- Low parental involvement
- Low emotional attachment to parents or caregivers
- Low parental education and income
- Parental substance abuse or criminality
- Poor family functioning
- Poor monitoring and supervision of children

Peer/School Risk Factors
- Association with delinquent peers
- Involvement in gangs
- Social rejection by peers
- Lack of involvement in conventional activities
- Poor academic performance
- Low commitment to school and school failure

Community Risk Factors
- Diminished economic opportunities
- High concentrations of poor residents
- High level of transience
- High level of family disruption
- Low levels of community participation
- Socially disorganized neighborhoods

[a] Adapted from the Centers for Disease Control and Prevention. Youth Violence Fact Sheet. www.cdc.gov/ncipc/factsheets/yvfacts.htm.

Bullying

Recently more attention and formal research regarding bullying is occurring in the United States. Tragic mass killing events, especially those at schools, coupled with reports of the perpetrators being victims or bullies during childhood, has raised the awareness of the seriousness of bullying as an early form of violence. Bullying has been extensively studied in Europe. Research, especially by Dr Olweus from Norway, demonstrates the serious consequences of this early form of aggression. Unfortunately, many parents, teachers, and health professionals still see bullying as a normal behavior of children.

Bullying is a type of aggression in which the intent of the behavior is to cause harm or disturb an individual. An imbalance of power exists with the more powerful attacking the less powerful. Opposed to what might be called "normal childhood conflicts," bullying occurs repeatedly over time. Bullying does not occur in isolation, but rather in an environment that supports the behavior. Participants include the bully, the victim, and the bystander. The bully is often an aggressive individual that uses violence to dominate others; he or she has little empathy for the victim. In contrast to common perception, bullies do not have poor self-esteem, but rather have a strong desire to control others. The victim may be more passive and anxious. This individual is often less secure than their peers and may be lonely, playing alone at school. When they are attacked by a bully, they usually withdraw rather than retaliate. A minority of youth may be classified as a bully-victim or a provocative victim. These individuals are both anxious and aggressive; while they are primarily victims of bullying, they may provoke the bully.

Bullying predominantly occurs in a school environment, during recess, at lunch, or on the way to or from school. Children often do not report bullying to adults for both fear of and retaliation by the bully and the concern of disbelief by the adult. Studies demonstrate that adults underestimate the prevalence of bullying events compared with student reports. Clinicians need to consider this when asking the parent or child about bullying.

Consequences of Bullying

Bullying impacts the physical and mental health of all of those involved. Fear and anxiety about the school environment is most common. This can progress to avoidance of school, low self-esteem, and depression. Children with chronic illness are more vulnerable because they may suffer worsened body image with frequent teasing. In adulthood, higher rates of depression and poor self-esteem are seen among individuals with a history of being bullied. Strong associations in adolescence and early adulthood have been made between bullying and suicide and murder. The child who was victimized may react later in life with self-destructive acts or lethal retaliation.

A prospective cohort study of children 9 to 11 years of age in the Netherlands found that victims of bullying had significantly higher chances of developing new psychosomatic and psychosocial problems compared with children who were not bullied. A larger proportion of victims had underlying depression and anxiety prior to being bullied but still suffered significant psychosomatic and psychological problems after being bullied. Common complaints included depression, anxiety, abdominal pain, sleeping problems, headache, feeling tense, bedwetting, feeling tired, and poor appetite. These complaints were present significantly more among children who had been victims of bullying.

Bystanders are also impacted because bullying distracts from the learning environment. Furthermore, they develop strategies to avoid being bullied that can include avoiding the restroom and staying home. One study reported that 1 in 5 secondary school children avoid restrooms out of fear at school. Another study stated that 7% of eighth graders stay home at least 1 day a month out of fear of other students.

Longitudinal studies report that bullies and bully-victims go on to more criminal activity than their counterparts. One study of Finnish boys reported 9% being bullies in childhood. These same individuals accounted for 37% of criminal activity in the study when the individuals reached adulthood. Bullies were more likely to commit occasional infractions while bully-victims were more likely to commit repeated offenses. Among bullies that participated in criminal activity, they were more likely to have underlying psychiatric symptoms. Other studies suggest that bullies have higher rates of conduct disorder.

In recent years there have been increasing reports of cyberbullying, where modern technology is used to pester, annoy, harass, and intimidate others, or to spread derogatory comments through chat rooms or other Internet sites. This represents yet another new problem related to computers (see Chapter 9).

Role of the Primary Care Physician

Childhood bullying is a complex abusive behavior with demonstrated serious consequences. Physicians are poised to identify at-risk individuals, screen for psychiatric comorbidities associated with bullying, counsel families, and advocate for school-based interventions. Because bullies or victims will not identify themselves as such, physicians need a systematic approach to screen for this early form of violence. Integrating screening during anticipatory guidance may be optimal for toddlers and school-aged children, while assessing risk factors at well and acute care visits may be needed for adolescents.

Multiple instruments have been used in a research setting for identifying bullying or associated internalizing or externalizing symptoms, but they have not been widely implemented in the primary care setting. Screening younger patients requires conversations with the child and family members. The American Academy of Pediatrics developed Connected Kids: Safe, Strong, Secure, which can be integrated into Bright Futures for well-child care visits. This preventive program focuses on discussing possible stressful developmental milestones that can lead to tension and on providing families with alternative approaches. When talking directly with adolescents, the use of the psychosocial interview **HEADDSSS** (*h*ome environment, *e*mployment and education, *a*ctivities, *d*iet, *d*rugs, *s*exual activity/sexuality, *s*uicide/depression, *s*afety) may be useful in

screening for high-risk behaviors and risk factors for violence (see Chapter 6).

When questioning a family about bullying, keep in mind that children will often not tell their parents that bullying occurred. When parents are told about bullying they may consider the situation as being normal behavior for young people and dismiss the event. Multiple forms of bullying exist. These include physical fights, verbal or cyber (text messaging or e-mail) harassment, and social isolation. Boys are more commonly involved in physical and verbal bullying while girls are more often involved in manipulative forms of bullying. As children become adolescents, intimate partner violence, suicide, and homicide are more likely consequences of bullying.

Prevention efforts need to focus on the individual, family, and community. In early childhood, parents can model for children appropriate social interaction, how to resolve conflict, and how to manage frustration and anger. School-wide bullying prevention programs are effective and should be advocated. The Olweus program focuses on adults at home and school showing positive interest in students, setting firm limits for unacceptable behavior, using consistent nonphysical or hostile consequences when rules are broken, and acting as positive role models to ultimately change the social and behavioral norms. For older children and adolescents, identifying psychiatric symptoms and providing the appropriate intervention may prevent more serious violent behavior. At the individual level, physicians and parents can counsel children who are bullies or victims regarding appropriate behaviors (Box 137-2).

Box 137-2. Physician's Role

- Be vigilant for signs and symptoms of bullying and other psychosocial trauma and distress in children and adolescents.
- Increase awareness of the social and mental health consequences of bullying and other aggressive behaviors.
- Screen for psychiatric comorbidities in at-risk youth, and provide appropriate referrals for treatment for affected youth.
- Counsel affected youth and their families on effective intervention programs and coping strategies.
- Advocate for family, school, and community programs and services for victims and perpetrators for bullying and other forms of violence and aggression.

In a randomized controlled study, Borowsky and colleagues demonstrated the effectiveness of identifying at-risk youth aged 7 to 5 years in a primary care setting and of providing a **family-level intervention** to reduce violent behavior and injuries among youth. Families that received the telephone-based intervention focusing on positive parenting reported decreased parent-reported bullying, physical fighting, fight-related injuries requiring medical care, and child-reported victimization by bullying.

The Maternal and Child Health Bureau in partnership with other federal agencies developed a resource kit on bullying, which is available online at www.stopbullyingnow.hrsa.gov. Online vignettes are directed at children in their preteen years and are geared toward helping the youth identify what role they might have in bullying and what appropriate behavior might allow them to better handle the situation. Printed resources are available for parents and teachers. For adolescents, the Centers for Disease Control and Prevention launched **Choose Respect,** a Web-based program on relationships available online at www.chooserespect.org. It provides tools for adolescents to identify healthy peer relationships and appropriate responses if they are concerned about intimate partner violence.

Physicians are a vital component of youth violence prevention (Box 137-3). Prevention begins early in the child's development by providing positive reinforcement of appropriate pro-social behavior. Bullying is an early form of aggression. In and of itself bullying may seem harmless, but longitudinal studies as well as analysis of mass school shootings demonstrate the large impact aggression early in life can have on the future well-being of children, adolescents, and adults. Successful interventions require cooperation by parents, teachers, students, and health professionals.

Box 137-3. Individual-Level Prevention Strategies

Advice for Victims of Bullying

- Resist reacting to the bully; hold your frustration and anger.
- Walk away from the situation; ignore the bullying.
- Avoid retaliation or bullying back.
- Tell an adult.
- Talk about the bullying event with your family.
- Use a buddy system at school and traveling to and from school.
- Develop friendships by joining social organizations.

Management of Bullies

- Reinforce that bullying is a serious problem.
- Set limits and provide consequences for acts of aggression.
- Emphasize tolerance for people's differences; everyone deserves respect.
- Determine whether friends are also involved in bullying; seek a group intervention.
- Provide positive reinforcement for appropriate behavior.
- Work closely with schoolteachers and staff regarding behavior modification.
- Emphasize that it's the "behavior" that is not acceptable.

CASE RESOLUTION

Victims of bullying often present with psychosomatic symptoms such as headache or abdominal pain. Once organic etiologies have been ruled out, further questioning should focus on psychosocial stresses. Alex's abdominal pain is worse in the morning before going to school. When asked specifically about bullying, Alex states that a few of his classmates tease him and rough him up each day on his way to school. In the last few weeks they are text messaging him about how they are going to haze him the next day. Alex has not told anyone about the experience because he thought he would be viewed as a coward. Alex shares that he would rather avoid going to school than face potential bullying.

The physician needs to assure Alex that it is not his fault that he is a victim of bullying. Prevention should include interventions at the individual, family, and school level. Alex should walk away from the conflict when possible and not feel uncomfortable about reporting the event to school staff. He may want to find a friend to walk to school with. His family needs to understand that bullying is not just a normal kid behavior. He should be encouraged to talk about bullying events and jointly identify solutions. The school should be notified about the event and encouraged to promote a non-bullying school environment.

Selected References

American Academy of Pediatrics Committee on Injury, Violence, and Poison Prevention. Policy statement: role of the pediatrician in youth violence prevention. *Pediatrics.* 2009;124;393–402

Borowsky IW, Mozayeny S, Stuenkel K, Ireland M. Effects of a primary care-based intervention on violent behavior and injury in children. *Pediatrics.* 2004;114:e392–e399

Boynton-Jarrett R, Ryan LM, Berkman LF, Wright RJ. Cumulative violence exposure and self-rated health: longitudinal study of adolescents in the United States. *Pediatrics.* 2008;122(5):961–970

Duke NN, Pettingell SL, McMorris BJ, Borowsky IW. Adolescent violence perpetration: associations with multiple types of adverse childhood experiences. *Pediatrics.* 2010;125(4):e778–e786

Fekkes M, Pijpers FIM, Fredriks AM, Vogels T, Verloove-Vanhorick SP. Do bullied children get ill, or do ill children get bullied? A prospective cohort study on the relationship between bullying and health-related symptoms. *Pediatrics.* 2006;117:1568–1574

Nansel T, Overpeck, M, Haynie DL, Ruan WJ, Scheidt PC. Relationships between bullying and violence among US youth. *Arch Pediatr Adolesc Med.* 2003;157:348–353

Reijntjes A, Kamphuis JH, Prinzie P, Telch MJ. Peer victimization and internalizing problems in children: a meta-analysis of longitudinal studies. *Child Abuse Negl.* 2010;34(4):244–252

Sourander A, Jensen P, Rönning JA, et al. Childhood bullies and victims and their risk of criminality in late adolescence: the Finnish From a Boy to a Man Study. *Arch Pediatr Adolesc Med.* 2007;161:546–552

Wang J, Iannotti RJ, Nansel TR. School bullying among adolescents in the United States: physical, verbal, relational, and cyber. *J Adolesc Health.* 2009;45(4):368–375

CHAPTER 138

Intimate Partner Violence

Sara T. Stewart, MD

CASE STUDY

A 6-year-old boy is brought in by his mother for an annual well-child visit. He sits quietly as his mother reports no significant medical history. His medical records reflect that at his last visit he was talkative, doing well in school, and enjoyed playing baseball. As you speak with his mother, she seems reticent and does not spontaneously offer information. You determine that the boy's school performance has declined significantly over the past year and that he no longer wants to play baseball.

On physical examination, the boy has linear ecchymoses over his buttocks, and you notice bilateral areas of bruising on his mother's upper arms. When you ask about the marks, she becomes tearful. You ask her if she would like to speak privately with you.

Questions

1. How often do child abuse and intimate partner violence (IPV) co-occur?
2. What are potential strategies to screen for IPV?
3. What are common clinical presentations of victims of IPV and children exposed to IPV?
4. What are the long-term consequences of IPV on children?
5. What are key factors to take into account when determining the degree and immediacy of danger to a victim of IPV?

Introduction

Intimate partner violence has been defined as a pattern of assaultive and coercive behaviors that may include repeated battering and injury, sexual assault, progressive social isolation, deprivation, and intimidation. It is perpetrated by an individual who is or was involved in an intimate relationship with an adult or adolescent, and whose intent is to establish control over the other partner. It is not only associated with negative physical and mental health outcomes for the victim but is also associated with negative mental health outcomes for children in the home. Childhood exposure to IPV is considered to have occurred when a child sees, hears, or observes the effects of verbal or physical assaults between partners. Intimate partner violence is also associated with the occurrence of child abuse in the home.

Epidemiology

Intimate partner violence affects both sexes and occurs in all ethnic, socioeconomic, sexual orientation, and religious groups. Approximately 2 to 4 million women and 500,000 to 1 million men report victimization annually in the United States. In 2005, 1,500 homicides were the result of IPV nationwide, and 78% of victims were female. While both men and women fall victim to IPV, there is increasing disparity between victimization rates with increased severity of physical assault, as women are more likely to sustain life-threatening injuries. The financial cost of IPV to society has been estimated at $8.3 billion, including medical and mental health costs as well as the indirect cost of lost productivity. In total, victims lose millions of days of paid work time annually.

While there is no uniform profile of either a victim or perpetrator of IPV, risk factors for victimization include a personal history of maltreatment as a child, adolescent or young adult age, disparity of status (educational, professional) between partners, and high level of dependence of one partner on another. Batterers have also been found to frequently have a history of emotional or physical maltreatment as a child, a history of substance abuse, very low levels of self-esteem, and difficulty identifying and expressing emotion.

Between 3 and 15 million children are exposed to IPV in their homes annually, and these children are at risk of victimization themselves. They are almost 5 times more likely than unexposed children to sustain physical abuse and 2.5 times more likely to be victims of sexual abuse.

Clinical Presentation

Adult victims of IPV may present for medical care for themselves, or may present for care of their children for issues related to the violence. Approximately one-third of victims injured in an assault by a partner seek medical care for their injuries. While these injuries vary in severity, skin injuries are most common. Injury can occur on any part of the body; however, injury to the head, neck, and face has been particularly associated with IPV.

Many victims present to primary care providers and to emergency departments, and only a fraction are correctly identified as suffering from IPV. A recent report noted that only 28% of abused women who sought care frequently (at least 7 times) were ever identified as victims of IPV. Barriers to diagnosis are both patient and provider based. Patients may not disclose the abuse due to fears of social, financial, or legal repercussions; concerns for safety based on prior threats from the abuser; feeling ashamed at being a victim; and inability to trust that others can help. They fail to appreciate that violence frequently escalates. Often they fear an investigation by child protective services and that they may lose custody of their children in the process. They may fabricate a story such as a fall to explain their injuries, thereby detracting the physician from further inquiry. Even in the absence of a story, physicians may avoid inquiring about the injuries, citing time constraints and lack of the knowledge to effectively respond if a disclosure is made.

Parents may also seek care for their children who manifest effects of the trauma, altered stress physiology, and disrupted caretaker attachment (Box 138-1). Children exposed to IPV are more likely than their peers to be anxious, fearful, and hypervigilant, and have difficulty with peer relationships. Adolescents are more likely to have school failure, substance abuse difficulties, high-risk sexual behaviors, and violent dating relationships. As they move to adulthood, these children are at higher risk for mental health disorders and substance abuse. In fact, the Adverse Childhood Experiences Study enumerates multiple negative overall physical and mental health consequences in adults exposed to IPV as children.

Box 138-1. Signs and Symptoms of Childhood Exposure to Intimate Partner Violence

- Depression
- Anxiety
- Somatization
- Attention-deficit/hyperactivity disorder
- Aggression
- Developmental delay
- Low self-esteem
- Hypervigilance
- Poor academic performance or truancy
- Antisocial or delinquent behaviors

Pathophysiology

The prevalent dynamic in relationships with IPV is the need for one partner to dominate or have power over the other. Often, this characteristic is interpreted as devotion early in a relationship, but an abuser eventually isolates the victim both socially and financially. Ultimately, the violence includes a physical and/or sexual component as well as a psychological one. The psychological component, which typically precedes any physical violence, includes threats, humiliation, and intimidation, and can be the most difficult to treat.

The cycle of violence between intimate partners is chronic and cyclical in nature with 3 phases. The first is the tension-building phase when the abuser uses verbal, emotional, and physical threats.

Next is the violent episode, which includes some combination of physical, sexual, emotional, and psychological assault. The final phase is the honeymoon phase, when the abuser apologizes and assures the victim that it will not happen again, and re-bonding occurs. These phases escalate over time, as the violence becomes more frequent and more severe and the honeymoon phase shortens. At least 50% of women who suffer sexual IPV report multiple rapes, and two-thirds of men and women with physical violence report multiple episodes of assault as well. The violence can also continue after the relationship has ended, and this most commonly manifests as stalking of the victim by the abuser. The violence also becomes intergenerational, as children exposed to IPV are at increased risk for victimization and perpetration of violence in their future intimate relationships.

There are particular circumstances that place IPV victims at even higher risk of harm. Threats from the perpetrator to harm or kill the victim or another person, the use of drugs or alcohol at the time of the violent episode, and the use of a weapon are all associated with an increased risk of injury. Approximately 4% to 8% of women report having experienced IPV during a pregnancy, though the reason for this increased incidence during this vulnerable period is unclear. It has been hypothesized that this is a time of increased stress as well as a time when a woman's attention may be diverted from her partner. Victims are also at increased risk of injury or death at the time they report the abuse or attempt to leave the relationship. In comparison to the systems in place for children, there are no protective service agencies with mandates to protect these adult victims and, as a result, disclosure of IPV may not occur unless the victim feels that she or he has a plan for escape.

Differential Diagnosis

Adult or adolescent victims of IPV often present with vague complaints, and abused women are 3 times more likely than non-abused women to present with gynecologic complaints, such as recurrent sexually transmitted infections, vaginal bleeding, or chronic pelvic pain. These victims may also present with nonspecific symptoms of sleeping difficulties, appetite changes, weight loss, chronic pain, or syncope. They are 3 times more likely to experience depression and 4 times more likely to experience post-traumatic stress disorder (PTSD) than non-abused women, and may present to their physician with symptoms of anxiety or following a suicide attempt. Other complaints reflect conditions associated with stress, such as irritable bowel syndrome, headaches, or temporomandibular joint disorder. Pregnant victims may present with vaginal bleeding, preterm labor, placental abruption, or fetal distress. The most common adverse birth outcome attributed to IPV during pregnancy is low birth weight of the infant.

The mental health manifestations of childhood exposure to IPV may vary depending on the developmental stage of the child; however, these children may present with developmental delay, low self-esteem, symptoms of PTSD and hypervigilance, poor academic performance or truancy, or antisocial behavior. Exposed children also have significantly more internalizing (depression, anxiety, somatization) and externalizing (attention-deficit/hyperactivity disorder, aggression) disorders than nonexposed children.

There is limited research on the short-term effects of IPV on the physical health of children. Some studies have shown a higher incidence of asthma, failure to thrive, and malnutrition. Children in the home may also sustain direct trauma, whether as the result of being held in a parent's arms during an episode of violence or as the result of an effort to intervene and protect a parent during a violent episode. The children may also be direct targets of the violence and present with head, skin, skeletal, or abdominal findings consistent with intentional trauma (see Chapter 127).

Evaluation

History

Many victims of IPV do not freely offer information about the violence occurring in their relationships, even if they present with overt injuries. Screening for IPV in medical settings is cited as the optimal approach and is an area of continued research. Proposed approaches in the primary care or emergency department environment have included both universal screening of all women and targeted screening of women with high-risk signs and risk factors. While there are proponents of each of these approaches, a US Preventative Services Task Force (USPSTF) statement in 2004 noted that there was insufficient evidence at that time to recommend for or against universal screening. Universal screening may detect increased numbers of cases of IPV and open the door to effective intervention, but the question remains as to whether there have ultimately been improved social, physical, or mental health outcomes with this approach. Critics of universal screening argue that forcing the issue before a woman is psychologically and logistically ready to leave the situation may put her at increased risk of harm and decreased likelihood of success. The universal screening approach has also not typically addressed the population of male victims of IPV. Supporters of universal screening decried the USPSTF for adversely affecting a program that was finally gaining some traction and being implemented in the medical community.

Alternatively, targeted screening is performed in some medical settings on patients who present with risk factors for IPV (Box 138-2). Studies have shown that self-administered, written screening tools are generally preferred by victims over verbal questioning. Such written screening tools have been validated for use in clinical settings and are available from the Centers for Disease Control and Prevention (CDC) at www.cdc.gov/NCIPC/pub-res/images/IPVandSVscreening.pdf.

Since IPV has been shown to have a direct effect on the health and well-being of children in the home, the pediatric medical setting is one potential site for IPV screening to occur. Targeted screening practices may focus on families of children with anxiety, depression, or somatization, or when child abuse is suspected. Surveys of mothers generally support IPV screening in the pediatric office setting. Two written sets of screening questions have been validated for use

---

Box 138-2. Risk Factors for Intimate Partner Violence

- History of childhood abuse
- Adolescent or young adult age
- Disparity in professional or educational status of partners
- Geographic or cultural isolation
- Dependency on partner due to chronic illness or disability
- Pregnancy
- Depression
- Anxiety
- Frequent physical injury
- Substance abuse
- Poor compliance with medical care

---

in the pediatric setting and are available through the CDC Web site noted previously. Sensitivity to whether children should witness discussions of positive screening questions is necessary, as older children may react to or repeat portions of an overheard conversation, ultimately placing the victim, their mother, at higher risk of harm.

Physical Examination

Caregiver Injuries

Although blunt trauma from a hand or fist is the most common scenario for the abused partner, IPV can result in injuries from either blunt force or penetrating trauma. Injury can occur on any part of a victim's body; however, studies have shown that trauma to the head, neck, and face is most specific for IPV as an etiology than other traumatic events. Findings may also include bruising of the bilateral upper arms from being grabbed and patterned injury from being hit with an object. Strangulation may result in bruising or abrasions on the neck, facial petechiae, or subconjunctival hemorrhage.

Child Injuries

Children in the home where IPV is occurring are at increased risk of physical abuse, and a complete unclothed physical examination should be performed to look for evidence of skin, head, skeletal, or abdominal trauma. Accidental injuries typically result in cutaneous bruises over bony prominences, such as knees and elbows, anterior shins, and the forehead. Unusual areas for accidental injury include the neck, ears, cheeks, medial thighs, and genital area. If physical abuse is suspected, additional radiographic imaging and an ophthalmology examination may be indicated (see Chapter 127).

Management

The response to any disclosure of IPV should be supportive and should focus on a safety assessment to determine the severity and the immediacy of danger (Box 138-3). This should include an assessment of the pattern of escalating violence, the availability of weapons to the abuser, and the comfort level of the victim to return home. More imminent danger necessitates the creation of an emergent safety plan, and social work colleagues or professionals from an IPV shelter,

- Is the violence escalating?
- How severe has the violence been in the past?
- Is the victim comfortable returning home?
- Is child abuse occurring?
- Are weapons available to the perpetrator?
- Does the perpetrator have substance abuse issues or a mental health disorder?
- Does the victim have a social support network?

hotline, or advocacy organization can assist with this. It is important to remain sensitive to the fact that leaving an abusive home is disruptive to the daily lives of the adult and child victims, and may be a difficult step to take.

If immediate safety is of less concern, a victim may opt to take more time in creating a safety plan for leaving. This may include things such as collecting money, car keys, house keys, and important documents; asking neighbors to contact police if violence is overheard in the home; establishing a code that the victim can use to communicate to others that violence is occurring and understanding what will be done if the code is used; and disarming or removing weapons from the home.

While all states require that medical providers report cases of suspected child abuse and neglect to child protective agencies, there is variability in the mandated reporting statutes for IPV and child exposure to IPV. State statutes fall into the following general categories with respect to IPV: requirement to report injuries caused by weapons, requirement to report injuries resulting from a crime, requirement to report IPV, and no mandatory reporting law. For those states with no mandatory reporting requirement, factors that may influence a provider's decision to report may include the potential for danger, the caregiver's ability to plan for safety, a victim's level of connection to family or community support, and the degree of suspicion that a child's exposure to IPV constitutes emotional abuse. Online resources such as www.endabuse.org can assist with the determination of local state laws regarding mandatory reporting of IPV. Any suspicion of child abuse should be reported to child protection authorities, regardless of whether IPV is being reported as well. If child abuse and IPV are co-occurring, it is important to note this in the child abuse report so that appropriate measures can be taken in the child protection response.

Prognosis

Direct victimization from IPV and childhood exposure to IPV are both associated with increased risk of adult morbidities. Women who have experienced interpersonal violence are at risk for depression, anxiety, and PTSD and are 15 times more likely to abuse alcohol and 9 times more likely to abuse drugs. Childhood exposure to IPV is associated with an increased risk of adult morbidities, including substance abuse disorders, obesity, physical inactivity, depression, and suicide attempts. This is of particular concern because of the limited availability of and often limited recognition of the importance of mental health resources in addressing the psychological impact of IPV.

For those women who do disclose the abuse and are referred to advocacy programs, preliminary data indicate that intensive programs may have a beneficial effect on reducing physical violence for several years. For other intervention strategies, the research is often limited and does not yet provide sound evidence of positive effects on physical, emotional, and quality of life outcomes. Further research is necessary to determine what components of the programs and what intensity and time frame of involvement are most beneficial in different clinical scenarios.

Although many IPV shelters and advocacy organizations have legal assistance available to victims, most victims do not obtain temporary restraining orders. Of those who do, approximately two-thirds have the orders violated by the abuser. Most cases are not prosecuted, and for those cases that do progress in the legal system, courts often struggle with how to address the IPV issues in the child custody and family treatment plans. While there are multiple models of treatment programs for perpetrators of IPV, there is evidence of only a small reduction in the likelihood of repeat violence. Further research is necessary to modify treatment approaches to reduce this recidivism.

Prevention

Prevention efforts may be primary, secondary, or tertiary. In this setting, primary prevention includes attempts to change social norms regarding violence and acts at the level of the individual, relationship, or community. Current efforts in that regard include attempts to break the generational cycle by studying and supporting resiliency factors in those who do not perpetuate violence after childhood exposure, the development of safe dating programs to reduce adolescent dating violence, the creation of peer empowerment programs for adolescents and young adults to enhance their ability to identify and intervene in IPV that they witness, and the development of family-based interventions to enhance nonviolent communication skills.

Secondary prevention includes early detection of IPV, and a significant amount of research is underway on screening practices in the medical setting. Tertiary prevention attempts to prevent death and disability in families where IPV occurs.

Sound research on IPV prevention is still a work in progress. Much of the current research has had methodological challenges, and many prevention strategies are not yet validated by sound evidence of benefit. Also, traditional thinking has been that most abusers are male and most victims are female, and prevention programs were built on this premise. Recent data, however, suggest that females also instigate IPV, so the subtleties of the patterns of violence of men versus women and how best to prevent them is a new area for growth and understanding.

CASE RESOLUTION

When alone with you, the mother reports that the boy's bruising occurred after her boyfriend hit him with a belt and that her marks occurred when the boyfriend was drunk and angry about the dinner she had prepared. She has contemplated leaving the relationship but is financially dependent on him, and pregnant with his child. He has threatened to harm her son if she leaves. She is currently afraid to return home but is not sure what to do.

You contact a social worker who assists in referring the mother and child to an IPV shelter and an IPV advocacy group. The social worker and the agencies work on an immediate safety plan while the mother and child wait in the office. As a mandated reporter of child abuse, you contact the child abuse hotline. The social worker assists you with the requirements in your state to report IPV or childhood exposure to IPV. The mother should be advised that a child abuse report was initiated, and the child protective authorities should also be made aware that IPV and child abuse are co-occurring in this family.

Selected References

Bair-Merritt MH. Intimate partner violence. *Pediatr Rev.* 2010;31:145–150

Basile KC, Hertz MF, Back SE. *Intimate Partner Violence and Sexual Violence Victimization Assessment Instruments for Use in Healthcare Settings: Version 1.* Atlanta, GA: Centers for Disease Control and Prevention, National Center for Injury Prevention and Control; 2007. www.cdc.gov/NCIPC/pub-res/images/IPVandSVscreening.pdf

Durborow N, Lizdas KC, O'Flaherty A, Marjavi A. *Compendium of State Statutes and Policies on Domestic Violence and Health Care.* San Francisco, CA: Family Violence Prevention Fund; 2010. www.endabuse.org/userfiles/file/HealthCare/Compendium%20Final.pdf

Felitti VJ, Anda RF, Nordenberg D, et al. Relationship of childhood abuse and household dysfunction to many of the leading causes of death in adults. The Adverse Childhood Experiences (ACE) Study. *Am J Prev Med.* 1998;14:245–258

Ramsay J, Carter Y, Davidson L, et al. Advocacy interventions to reduce or eliminate violence and promote the physical and psychosocial well-being of women who experience intimate partner abuse. *Cochrane Database Syst Rev.* 2009;(3):CD005043

Rhodes KV, Kothari CL, Dichter M, Cerulli C, Wiley J, Marcus S. Intimate partner violence identification and response: time for a change in strategy. *J Gen Intern Med.* 2011. Epub ahead of print

Thackeray JD, Hibbard R, Dowd MD; American Academy of Pediatrics Committee on Child Abuse and Neglect and Committee on Injury, Violence, and Poison Prevention. Clinical report—intimate partner violence: the role of the pediatrician. *Pediatrics.* 2010;125:1094–1100

Tjaden P, Thoennes N. *Extent, Nature, and Consequences of Intimate Partner Violence: Findings from the National Violence Against Women Survey.* Washington DC: National Institute of Justice, US Department of Justice; 2000. www.ncjrs.gov/pdffiles1/nij/181867.pdf

Toohey JS. Domestic violence and rape. *Med Clin North Am.* 2008;92:1239–1252

US Preventative Services Task Force. Screening for family and intimate partner violence: recommendation statement. *Ann Intern Med.* 2004;140:382–386

CHAPTER 139

Disaster Preparedness

Elizabeth A. Edgerton, MD, MPH

CASE STUDY

A family comes in for their children's well-child visit with their 9-month-old daughter who has complex congenital heart disease and their 7-year-old son. The mother is concerned after a recent tornado in the next town resulted in prolonged power outages and what the family might do in this situation. Their daughter needs daily breathing treatments and often requires oxygen at nighttime. She is on multiple medications and a special formula. All of her specialty doctors are at the children's hospital, which is more than an hour from their house. She is also concerned because her husband has a seizure disorder that requires medication. She asks whether the family should stay together in a disaster or separate to get her daughter to the children's hospital.

Questions

1. How should families prepare for disasters, particularly natural ones known to occur in their area?
2. What should be included in disaster preparedness kits? How should medications for all family members be included?
3. When should families consider getting a generator?
4. How can families notify the utility company that they need to be flagged for priority return of service during a power outage?
5. What is the role of the local hospital and emergency medical services provider when families have children with special health care and critical medical needs?
6. What should the pediatrician recommend to families about children's immunization records and important medical history?
7. How do you assess for the impact of traumatic events on children and their families?

Disaster preparedness is not a new concept in our society. We have always had natural disasters such as earthquakes and hurricanes. The potential of war or pandemic infections has been present for decades. In the past these threats were managed by the state and federal programs. With increasing population density, global warming, international trade, and terrorist threats, our view of disaster preparedness is broadening to include natural disaster; chemical, biological, and radioactive exposure; and emerging pandemic infections. Major disasters, including man-made events such as terrorist attacks in New York City and natural events such as hurricane Katrina, demonstrate the vulnerability of a community and the need for extensive local preparation for potential disasters. In both of these disasters, the community response in the first hours to days was vital to the well-being of others. While the state and federal systems are a vital component of disaster preparedness, communities may play a greater role than in the past.

Children are more vulnerable than adults during a disaster. Studies from refugee camps have found that children younger than 5 years had a higher mortality rate than the crude mortality rate of adults during the emergency situation. In the United States, children represent 30% to 85% of disaster victims and response teams often lack appropriate pediatric equipment or protocols for their care. Furthermore, children are reliant on others for food, shelter and, importantly, for psychological support. Their immune systems are often less mature; this puts them at greater risk of infection. Their unique nutritional needs put them at risk for malnutrition. Developmentally, they are at risk for acute and long-term psychological trauma from a disaster. The impact of being separated from their families can be devastating. Furthermore, children are at increased risk for exposure from chemical, biological, and radiation disasters due to their unique physiology. Infants and children have higher minute ventilation, resulting in increased inhalation of aerosolized agents. Their smaller height increases their exposure to high-vapor density agents, which are in higher concentrations closer to the ground. Infants' and children's skin is more permeable due to less keratinization; they also have a larger surface area to body mass ratio. As a result, exposed children receive a higher dose of transdermally absorbed toxins than adults exposed under identical circumstances.

A public health emergency occurs when the event exceeds the ability of community resources to provide routine care. This can be a result of any type of disaster. Preparedness experts suggest looking at public health emergencies from what is called an **all-hazards approach**. This approach focuses on the key elements that are needed to ensure that routine care can still be provided during a disaster. Specific case scenarios that occur rarely, such as chemical or radiation exposure, will require access to specialized resources that may be impractical to stockpile or are limited in availability. From a practical view, it is more effective to have the essential resources that are needed across all types of disasters. The primary care pediatrician plays a vital role in disaster preparedness on the local, regional, and national level, not only as a medical service provider but also as an advocate to the special needs of children.

Pediatrician's Role With Families

Pediatricians serve as a resource to families in preparation for disasters. Disaster preparedness can be incorporated into the primary care pediatrician's anticipatory guidance with families. The US Department of Homeland Security in collaboration with the American Academy of Pediatrics recommends families focus on 4 areas: a community evacuation plan, a family emergency response plan, disaster supply kit, and finally a maintenance of the emergency response plan. Pediatricians may need to assess a family's level of readiness for a disaster and then tailor their anticipatory guidance accordingly. It is important for families to realize that everyone is susceptible to some type of disaster whether natural, chemical, biological, or radiation. Pediatricians need to ensure families understand the importance of preparation as well as the special needs of children during a disaster. Families should prepare an emergency kit that provides up to 3 days of basic essentials, including food, water, and clothing. Families need to include formula and diapers for infants and any daily medications for all family members. Copies of immunization and general medical information can be useful as well as pictures of family members in case the family unit is separated. Parents need to be prepared to handle non-emergent problems because medical care may be limited to the seriously ill and injured. If a family needs acute medical care, children may have to be treated in adult facilities; alternatively, for the family unit to remain together, adults within the family may need to be treated in pediatric facilities. The more information families can provide about any medical conditions requiring attention, the easier it will be to receive appropriate care in a disaster.

Families of children with special needs are especially vulnerable following a disaster because access to routine medical care may not be available. Common supplies such as a feeding tube or catheters may be in short supply or unavailable during a disaster. Families should not only have a sufficient supply of medication, but a surplus of medical equipment and nutritional supplements if necessary. Families with a child on a ventilator or who is oxygen dependent should notify the local utilities to flag their address for priority status during power outages. These families would also benefit by notifying their local emergency medical services (EMS) and local hospital of their child's medical needs. The American Academy of Pediatrics (AAP) has **emergency information forms** that can be completed with the pediatrician and should be part of the emergency preparedness kit. Families can also contact the National Organization on Disability and Emergency Preparedness (www.nod.org) or Family Voices (www.familyvoices.org) for more detailed information regarding preparing for a disaster with a special needs child. Some communities have developed systems where posters are disseminated that are to be placed in the window specifying if any occupant may require special services from EMS should a disaster or terrorist attack occur.

After a disaster, children and adolescents may have chronic problems depending on the type of disaster. Such problems need to be addressed case by case. What is universal among all types of disasters is that there is a psychological impact on children. Multiple studies of various types of disasters demonstrate the increase in mental health symptoms among children and adolescents exposed to a disaster. This is true even if a family is not directly impacted by the disaster but is exposed to the event within the community, on the television, or via the Internet. Children may present with somatic complaints such as headaches and stomachaches, or may not want to participate in their normal activities. Long-term effects include depression, anxiety, aggression, and substance abuse. Age-appropriate discussions should be encouraged along with validation of the child's concerns while ensuring their individual safety. Post-traumatic stress disorder should be considered in patients with persistent symptoms that are not responding to family support. Families and health care providers can obtain further information through the AAP (www.aap.org) and the Substance Abuse and Mental Health Services Administration (www.samhsa.gov).

Pediatrician's Role in the Community

Pediatricians can participate in both the disaster preparedness planning as well as community surveillance to identify potential disasters. Many state and regional disaster preparedness plans are tailored for an adult population and may not consider the special needs of children. From an operational standpoint, it is more effective to have one plan that can take into consideration the needs of multiple vulnerable populations rather than have separate disaster preparedness plans for each population. Pediatricians can serve as consultants about local preparation, providing guidance about children's medical, nutritional, and psychological needs. For example, more staffing is required when caring for younger children, especially infants. Infants require formula and a sterile water supply, and young children require frequent meals. Ideally, children need to be with their caregiver, but if this is not possible then a child advocate needs to be with the child at all times. Children may not respond well to new environments and disaster protocols. The simple process of decontamination can be devastating to a young child without a parent. A child may have concerns about being sprayed with water or refuse to disrobe in front of strangers. This may impact the success of decontamination for children and adolescents. While adults may have similar issues, it is presumed they will comply with protocols; however, such compliance is less predictable in a pediatric population. Other issues may need to be addressed, such as providing for increased staffing in adult facilities caring for children, as well as the need for those facilities to stockpile pediatric supplies. Facilities also need to plan for children arriving without a caregiver and the need to establish an identification system allowing children to be reunited with their families. This was a significant problem for children displaced during hurricane Katrina. Refugee camps often use digital cameras to photograph children on arrival as a way to reunite families. Recommendations include photographing children in their original clothing.

Triage systems need to take into account physiological differences of children as well as their psychological response to strangers. They may not be able to communicate their complaint, and because their vital signs are normally different from those of adults, medical personnel accustomed to working with adults may misinterpret their findings, resulting in children being over-triaged (judged to be sicker than they are). Stockpiling of medications for biological, chemical, or radiation disasters needs to take into consideration dosing differences in children compared with adults. Suspensions of medications will need to be available in addition to pill forms. Furthermore, many of the recommended antidotes and treatments are not approved for use in the pediatric population. Policies regarding the risks and benefits of their use in disasters should be established.

Pediatricians can also assist schools in developing disaster preparedness plans should a disaster occur during the school day.

Pediatrician's Role in Disaster Surveillance and Management

Pediatricians function as key public health workers. Their knowledge and diligence aids in local and regional surveillance for potential chemical, biological, and radiation disasters. Families are more likely to seek care from their pediatrician than an emergency department for early symptoms during and after a disaster. Although it is beyond the scope of this chapter to provide details about signs and symptoms following every type of disaster, the following section highlights important concepts in identifying and treating patients with exposures to chemical and biological agents and radiation.

Chemical exposures usually result in immediate symptoms and require special protection for emergency personnel as well as decontamination for the victims. Nerve agents, the most toxic of chemical agents, inhibit the enzyme acetylcholinesterase, resulting in accumulation of acetylcholine and excessive cholinergic stimulation in smooth muscles, exocrine glands, skeletal muscle, and preganglionic fibers. Symptoms include increased salivation, lacrimation, urination, gastric distress, and emesis, referred to as the **SLUDGE toxidrome**. Vesicant exposure leads to irreversible damage to mucous membranes, skin, and the respiratory system that occurs within minutes of exposure, often without any antecedent symptoms. Agents include mustard and lewisite. Cyanide is another common chemical agent, known for its "bitter almond" taste. Agents other than nerve agents usually do not result in severe mortality but rather incapacitate the victim.

Biological agents include bacteria, viruses, and preformed toxins. These agents are easy to disperse and, thus, can affect large populations. Unlike chemical exposures, the onset of symptoms is delayed by hours to days, and symptoms are more difficult to distinguish from common ailments. Secondary transmission of the infection is also of concern. Management of biological disaster requires detailed surveillance and containment of exposed populations.

Although there are far too many biological agents to discuss in any detail in a brief chapter, a few of particular relevance for disaster planning are mentioned here. **Anthrax**, from *Bacillus anthracis*, is a gram-positive sporulating rod, which presents with severe influenza-like symptoms with a high case fatality rate. Fever and dyspnea associated with a widened mediastinum are common and may progress to shock. Ciprofloxacin and doxycycline are recommended for prophylaxis and treatment among adults, but ciprofloxacin is not approved by the US Food and Drug Administration (FDA) for children younger than 18 years and doxycycline is contraindicated in children younger than 8 years. Clinicians need to consider consulting with experts to assist in assessing the risks and benefits associated with using these medications. Among the viruses, variola, more commonly known as **small pox**, is of concern. After its global eradication in 1980, children were no longer immunized, leaving all children and most adults susceptible to the virus. Similar to varicella, it presents with vesicles with umbilicated centers but is associated with a higher mortality rate of 3% to 30% among non-immunized individuals. Exposure to **botulinum toxin,** one of the most potent toxins, results in cranial nerve disturbances, descending paralysis, and respiratory distress. **Ricin,** derived from the castor bean, is another potent toxin. Inhalation results in fever, cough, and pulmonary edema, often resulting in death within days. Ingestion presents with severe vomiting and diarrhea, resulting in hypovolemic shock. There is no antidote or treatment for these biological toxins. For a complete list of biological agents, presenting symptoms, and potential treatment and/or prophylaxis, clinicians should consult the Centers for Disease Control and Prevention (www.cdc.gov).

Radiation exposure may occur as a result of damage to a facility that contains nuclear material, detonation of a nuclear weapon, or dispersal of nuclear material by a radioactive dispersal device. Ionizing radiation, high-frequency energy, presents the greatest health risk. It causes chromosomal breaks in cells that can persist for years. There are 5 types of ionizing radiation that have specific characteristics, behaviors, and toxicities: alpha particles, beta particles, gamma rays, x-rays, and neutrons. Alpha particles have limited ability to penetrate, but when inhaled or ingested can cause damage to epithelial tissues. Beta particles usually are used in a medical setting or are a by-product of nuclear reactors, have greater penetration, and can cause skin damage as well as internal damage. Gamma rays and x-rays are part of the electromagnetic spectrum. Gamma rays are high-energy and cause significant damage. This type of radiation would be seen after a nuclear detonation or from radioactive materials. Much less common are neutrons, which can produce 10-fold more damage than gamma rays. Furthermore, exposure is classified as external, internal, whole body, and partial body. The effects of radiation can be directly on target tissue, or indirectly due to free radicals created by the radiation. Tissue sensitivity is based on the cell's rate of division and level of differentiation. The most sensitive to least is as follows: lymphoid>gastrointestinal>reproductive>dermal>bone marrow>nervous system. The severity of exposure is also dependent on the dose of radiation, type of radiation, and age of victim.

Radiation exposure is quantified by the amount of energy absorbed (the *rad*, for radiation absorbed dose) and the relative biological effectiveness of doses (RBE) based on the type of ionizing radiation. The rem is the product of the rad and RBE. Under the International System of Units, the rad and rem are being replaced by the gray (1 Gy = 100 rad) and sievert (1 Sv = 100 rem). Radiation exposure from common radiographic procedures can range from 0.00005 to 0.0001 Sv (5–10 mrem) for a chest radiograph and 0.05 Sv (5,000 mrem) for a computed tomography scan.

The symptoms associated with radiation exposure depend on the total exposure. Nausea and vomiting can present with exposures of 0.75 to 1.0 Gy, and lymphoid and bone marrow suppression with exposures of 3.0 to 6.0 Gy. The mean lethal dose, the radiation dose for which half of the population is expected to die within 60 days, is 4.0 Gy. Long-term effects of radiation include increased incidence of cancer and psychological distress. Evacuation is the ideal intervention to decrease exposure, but may not be feasible in highly populated areas. Seeking shelter can greatly decrease the level of exposure, with large cement structures providing the best protection. The use of potassium iodide is effective in exposures to radioactive iodine, which is associated with nuclear power facilities. It can be dispensed in a pill form, and home suspensions can be made for pediatric patients. Dosage is based on level of radiation exposure and the age of the patient. Clinicians should consult the FDA (www.fda.gov) or the Nuclear Regulatory Commission to determine the appropriate dosage of potassium iodide depending on the level of radiation exposure. For individuals seeking medical care, containment and decontamination are essential. Removal of clothing and washing the skin with warm water is very effective. Supportive medical care is essential in managing patients with radiation exposure. Radiation results in significant immune suppression, neutropenia, and lymphopenia, which last for weeks. Clinicians should be aggressive in managing infections and consider treatments to increase bone marrow regeneration.

In addition to caring for patients, the pediatrician needs to take into consideration the well-being of his or her family as well as that of the office staff. During a disaster, office staff may not be able to come to work. For those able to report to work, extra supplies of food and water need to be available in case they are not able to return to their homes. An office disaster plan should be implemented with emergency contacts and preparation for the staff's basic needs. Basic medical supplies should be available to care for patients during a disaster. Depending on the type and severity of the disaster, access to the office facility may be prohibited. Plans for backup of patient medical records should be implemented as well as alternative sites in which medical services can be delivered.

Clinicians need to review their medical liability policies regarding providing care in a disaster situation. Most policies only provide coverage of care that is provided in the office setting. Good Samaritan laws vary in each state regarding what level of protection is provided to the health care worker. The AAP recommends that during a disaster situation, pediatricians who volunteer do so under the auspices of an official disaster agency or recognized relief organization to ensure the greatest protection from liability.

Conclusion

Pediatricians have a vital role in pre-disaster, disaster, and post-disaster management. The essential components of disaster management are to provide for all basic human requirements, reduce an individual's vulnerability to disasters and, once a disaster has occurred, reduce the exposure risk. Pediatricians can educate and assist families in preparing for disasters. In addition, they can guide communities in their disaster preparedness planning to address and plan to accommodate the particular vulnerabilities of children. As with other health care providers, pediatricians also can contribute to the essential medical and public health workforce during a disaster. Pediatricians can access the most current guidelines and recommendations through multiple professional and governmental resources. It is imperative for the practitioner to have easy access to phone numbers and Web sites specific to pediatric disaster preparedness and response for the relevant local, state, and federal agencies.

CASE RESOLUTION

The family is relieved to discuss the importance of preparing for a disaster. They now have an idea of what is involved in disaster preparation (emergency kit with food, water, and medication) and feel less vulnerable. They will complete an emergency medical information form for the kit and call their local utility company to identify their house as a priority during a power failure. The mother shares with the pediatrician that her son has been sleeping less since the tornado and does not want to go to school because he is afraid of being away from the family. The pediatrician encourages the family to discuss his fears while ensuring his safety. Having the son participate in making the emergency kit and creating a family plan may help. A follow-up visit is scheduled to reassess his symptoms and decide if a further intervention is needed.

Selected References

American Academy of Pediatrics. Online resource for children in disasters. Children and Disaster. http://www.aap.org/disasters/. Accessed November 30, 2010

American Academy of Pediatrics. *Pediatric Terrorism and Disaster Preparedness: A Resource for Pediatricians.* Foltin GL, Schonfeld DJ, Shannon MW, eds. Rockville, MD: Agency for Healthcare Research and Quality; 2006. AHRQ Publication No. 06(07)-0056

American Academy of Pediatrics Committee on Pediatric Emergency Medicine, Committee on Medical Liability, and Task Force on Terrorism. The pediatrician and disaster preparedness. *Pediatrics.* 2006;117:560–565

Gausche-Hill M. Pediatric disaster preparedness: are we really prepared? *J Trauma.* 2009;67: S73–S76

Hagan JF; American Academy of Pediatrics Committee on Psychosocial Aspects of Child and Family Health and Task Force on Terrorism. Psychosocial implications of disaster or terrorism on children: a guide for the pediatrician. *Pediatrics.* 2005;116:787–795

Markenson D, Reynolds S; American Academy of Pediatrics Committee on Pediatric Emergency Medicine and Task Force on Terrorism. Technical report: the pediatrician and disaster preparedness. *Pediatrics.* 2006;117:e340–e362

Needle S. Pediatric private practice after hurricane Katrina: proposal for recovery. *Pediatrics.* 2008;122;836–842

Olympia RP, Rivera R, Heverley S, Anyanwu U, Gregorits M. Natural disasters and mass-casualty events affecting children and families: a description of emergency preparedness and the role of the primary care physician. *Clin Pediatr.* 2010;49:686–698

CHAPTER 140

Adolescent Depression and Suicide

Monica Sifuentes, MD, and Robin Steinberg-Epstein, MD

CASE STUDY

A 15-year-old girl is brought to your office by her mother with the chief complaint of easy fatigability. The mother is concerned because her daughter is always tired, although several other physicians have told her that the girl is healthy. The adolescent, who states no complaints or concerns, appears very shy. She is currently in the 10th grade, likes school, receives average grades, and speaks both English and Spanish. The mother, a single parent, moved to the United States from El Salvador approximately 2 years ago with her 2 daughters. They are currently living with relatives in a 2-bedroom apartment. The mother is employed as a housekeeper, and the patient and her sister help their mother clean homes on weekends. During the week they make dinner for the rest of the family as a means of contributing to the rent. When you speak to the girl alone, she acknowledges she has a few friends at school and adamantly denies any drug, alcohol, or tobacco use. She has never been sexually active and

reports no history of sexual or physical abuse. The girl's physical examination is entirely normal, although her affect appears somewhat flat.

Questions

1. What is the significance of nonspecific symptoms, such as fatigue, during adolescence?
2. What factors contribute to depression in adolescents?
3. What are the classic signs and symptoms of depression in adolescents?
4. What are some important historical points to cover when interviewing adolescents with suspected depression?
5. How is the risk of suicide assessed in adolescent patients?
6. How should suicidal behavior (ie, suicide attempts) be managed in adolescents?

Depression has been identified as one of the multiple risk factors that predispose adolescents to suicide. However, not all teenagers who try to take their own life are depressed and, conversely, not all depressed adolescents attempt suicide. This distinction is important to keep in mind when evaluating adolescents for either depression or suicidal behavior. Early identification of risk factors in the susceptible adolescent along with early intervention for those with depressive symptoms will hopefully benefit the teenager at risk for suicide and allow the primary care pediatrician to provide the first line of intervention for their adolescent patient experiencing emotional distress.

Epidemiology

Depression

The exact prevalence of depression in adolescents is difficult to determine because depression is both an illness and a symptom. However, it is considered one of the main psychiatric conditions affecting children, along with anxiety. Depressive symptoms have been reported in as many as 50% of girls and 40% of boys in the 14- to 15-year age group. The overall prevalence of depression as an illness is approximately 5%; mild depression is reported in 13% to 28%

of teens, moderate depression in 7%, and severe depression in 1.3%. Depression occurs more commonly in adolescents than in prepubertal children and is more frequent in females than males after puberty.

Several risk factors contribute to the development of depressive disorders in adolescents (Box 140-1). Certain psychiatric conditions also are associated with depression, including anxiety disorders, eating disorders, substance abuse, conduct disorders, and borderline personality disorders.

Suicide and Suicidal Behavior

Suicide is the third-leading cause of death in the United States in individuals 10 to 24 years of age; only motor vehicle crashes and homicides result in more deaths in young people. In 1960 the annual suicide rate in this age group was 5.2 per 100,000, and by 1990 it had more than doubled to the highest recorded level of 13.2 per 100,000. By 2007 the rate had decreased to 6.7 per 100,000 in part due to the use of selective serotonin reuptake inhibitor (SSRI) antidepressants, the first of which came out in 1990. This amounts to more than 4,000 completed suicides in adolescents 15 to 24 years old in 2007. It has been stated that for every suicide that is completed successfully, 50 to 100 suicides are attempted.

Box 140-1. Risk Factors Associated With Depressive Disorders in Adolescents

- Family history of psychiatric illness (eg, parent with an affective condition or another family member with a bipolar or recurrent unipolar disorder)
- Age at onset of depression in the affected parent (the earlier the age of onset, the greater the likelihood of depression in the children)
- Exposure to an unexpected suicide attempt/completion in the school or community
- History of environmental trauma (eg, sexual or physical abuse, loss of a loved one)
- Chronic illness
- Certain medications (eg, propranolol, phenobarbital, prednisone)

Box 140-2. Risk Factors Associated With Suicide in Adolescents

- History of a previous suicide attempt (most important)
- Male gender
- Preexisting psychiatric condition (depressive/bipolar disorder, conduct disorder post-traumatic stress disorder)
- Alcohol and illicit substance abuse or dependence
- Psychological characteristics such as aggression, impulsivity, and hopelessness or severe anger
- Family history of psychiatric disorders, especially depression, substance abuse, and suicidal behavior
- Family disruption or stressful life event, including violence, divorce, or the death of a loved one
- Impaired parent–child relationship
- Exposure to an unexpected suicide attempt/completion in the school or community
- Chronic debilitating illness
- Anxiety about sexual identity (homosexuality or bisexuality)
- History of physical/sexual abuse or exposure to violence
- Availability of firearms in the home
- Living outside the home (homelessness or in corrections facility or group home)

According to the 2006 Youth Risk Survey of the Centers for Disease Control and Prevention, 16.9% of all students in grades 9 to 12 nationwide had seriously considered attempting suicide during the previous 12 months. Approximately 13% of these students had made specific suicide plans, more than 50% of students with suicide plans reported attempting to take their lives, and 2.3% of the individuals who attempted suicide required medical attention. Rates also differ by race and ethnicity, with African American teenagers having lower suicide rates than white youth, and African American females having the lowest suicide rate of all adolescents. American Indian/Alaska Native males have the highest suicide rate among this age group.

Several risk factors associated with adolescent suicide have been identified (Box 140-2). Although adolescent females are more likely to attempt suicide than males (22% vs 12%), males are more likely to succeed (ratio of 4:1 boys to girls). This fact may result from the lethality of the methods, such as firearms or hanging, that males usually choose. While females are more likely to ingest pills, the role of firearms is increasing. The availability of firearms and alcohol, which varies from state to state, greatly contributes to the occurrence of suicide. Up to 45% of individuals who have committed suicide show some evidence of intoxication at the time of death. Although most suicide attempts are impulsive, studies have shown that adolescents often have communicated their suicidal intent or ideation to someone before the attempt. Fifty percent of adolescents who attempt suicide have sought medical care within the preceding month and 25% within the preceding week. In contrast, only one-third have received previous mental health care.

Clinical Presentation

Depressed or suicidal adolescents may visit physicians for a variety of clinical reasons, but rarely do they seek professional assistance for feeling "depressed." Adolescents have a difficult time accurately understanding their emotions. A depressed teen often presents as irritable, argumentative, or angry, rather than sad. They may exhibit diminished interest or pleasure in activities or relationships, changes in cognitive functioning (eg, concentration), sleep, appetite, or energy, which lead to impairments in multiple areas of daily living. They may also present with seemingly non-emergent complaints and a flat affect or with multiple somatic concerns and an anxious appearance. Additionally, the teen may have frequent visits to the primary care practitioner's office for acute conditions that on first glance seem unrelated, but later indicate possible substance abuse or a mood disorder. Some adolescents are accompanied by a family member or friend, which initially may make the teen reticent to discuss psychosocial issues with the provider. According to the *Diagnostic and Statistical Manual of Mental Disorders, Fourth Edition, Text Revision*, major depressive disorder (MDD) is diagnosed when at least 5 out of 9 listed symptoms or signs occur for at least 2 weeks. At least one symptom must be sadness or loss of interest for most of every day and there has to be a significant change in function. Changes can be manifested by poor academic performance, school attendance issues (including truancy and disruptive behaviors), and difficulties with peer and familial relationships (see Box 140-1).

Pathophysiology

The exact neurobiological etiology of depression remains elusive. It is believed to involve impaired serotonin and norepinephrine transmission in critical areas of the brain, most notably the frontal lobes. Like other complex psychiatric conditions, the etiology of depression seems to be multifactorial, with a strong genetic and psychosocial/environmental basis. The **genetic basis** of depression is suggested by statistics that indicate for instance that 25% of children who take their own lives have a family member or close relative that has committed suicide. Similarly, a family history of major depression is a significant risk factor for the development of depression in children. Studies suggest the incomplete penetrance of a dominant gene as a possible etiology for this finding. Regardless of the exact mechanism, genetic influences can increase the adolescent's vulnerability for depression. Specific **environmental events** can occur in an adolescent's life that may precipitate a depressive episode, such as the loss of a loved one or parental divorce. Other events such as physical or sexual abuse also can trigger depression in a susceptible teen. Major depressive disorder is diagnosed when the symptoms last for at least 2 weeks and there is a change in usual function.

Differential Diagnosis

The differential diagnosis of depression includes any condition that may alter the patient's cognition or affect. For example, if a disease alters the nutritional status and leads to malnourishment, this may alter affect and energy, which may resemble depression (Dx Box). Examples include cancer, tuberculosis, and eating disorders such as anorexia nervosa. Endocrine disorders such as hypothyroidism, hyperthyroidism, and Addison disease can mimic depression. Central nervous system (CNS) pathology, although rare, includes tumors, infections, postconcussive syndromes, and cerebrovascular accidents. Concomitant systemic illnesses such as systemic lupus erythematosus, diabetes mellitus, and AIDS can have CNS manifestations that may be mistaken for an isolated episode of depression. While the above diseases can occur, they pale in comparison to the prevalence and significant contribution of substance and alcohol abuse. Comorbid conditions such as early-onset bipolar disorder can present initially with depressive symptoms. In fact, 20% to 40% of children who have MDD eventually develop bipolar disorder. Children with autism often develop comorbid depression during adolescence as a manifestation of their isolation and poor coping skills. Other psychiatric diagnoses to consider include adjustment disorders, uncomplicated bereavement, separation anxiety, and dysthymia, which is more chronic and sometimes less severe than major depression. Lastly, side effects of both prescribed and over-the-counter medications may produce clinical symptoms consistent with depression and therefore should be considered in the differential diagnosis.

Evaluation

History

The assessment of an adolescent for depressive symptoms is an important part of any routine encounter, but the diagnosis of depression may be difficult to make after just one interview. At the initial visit, a complete psychosocial or **HEADDSSS** assessment (*h*ome, *e*mployment and *e*ducation, *a*ctivities, *d*iet, *d*rugs, *s*exual activity/sexuality, *s*uicide/depression, *s*afety) should be performed on all adolescents (see Chapter 5). The parent or guardian should be included during the first part of the interview to review their observations and concerns regarding their adolescent's behavior and mood. The teenager then should be interviewed alone, and a thorough history of recent feelings, behaviors, and attitudes should be obtained (Questions Box: Adolescent Depression). Mood changes should be noted; a labile affect can be a symptom of ongoing depression. Physicians should keep in mind that patients who are malnourished for any reason can have a depressed or seemingly flat affect. A full

Dx **Adolescent Depression**

SIG: E CAPS Mnemonic
S: Sleep changes
I: Interests—decreased interest in school or activities
G: Guilt, helpless, hopeless
E: Energy (decreased), fatigue
C: Concentration decreased
A: Appetite (increased or decreased)
P: Psychomotor agitation and retardation
S: Suicidal ideation

- Depressed or irritable mood
- Decreased interest in most daily activities, including school
- Significant weight changes
- Sleep problems
- Psychomotor agitation or retardation
- Low energy or fatigue
- Feelings of worthlessness or guilt
- Diminished ability to concentrate or think
- Preoccupation with death or suicide

Questions

Adolescent Depression

- Does the adolescent occasionally feel sad or "blue" and not understand why?
- Does the adolescent have unexplained crying spells?
- Does the adolescent feel "mad," "bored," or "grouchy"?
- Does the adolescent seem inappropriately jovial?
- Have there been any recent losses in the adolescent's life that may explain his or her feelings?
- Is the adolescent having trouble with concentration or memory?
- Does the adolescent have trouble falling asleep at night or have early morning awakening?
- Has the adolescent lost weight recently or shown any disinterest in food?
- Does the adolescent have feelings of hopelessness and have any desire to hurt himself or herself? Has the adolescent made any previous suicide attempts?
- Do the parents or siblings have a history of drug or alcohol use?
- Is there a family history of affective disorders? What has been their response to treatment?
- Is there a history of family violence?

psychiatric assessment also should be completed to obtain information about a possible comorbid condition. This includes features of psychosis, anxiety disorders, disruptive behaviors, and mania. However, severe depression can be accompanied by symptoms of psychosis. Information about a family history of psychiatric illness or substance abuse, including alcohol abuse, also should be reviewed with both the teenager as well as the parent/guardian.

To identify youth at risk for suicide, practitioners must inquire about specific areas of adolescents' lives including a history of sexual/physical abuse, violence, or neglect and current interpersonal conflicts. Almost all females with a history of sexual abuse develop suicidal ideation by age 15. Feelings of hopelessness, agitation, and impulsivity should be identified, along with frequent thoughts of suicide or death. It has been reported that having frequent thoughts of suicide is the best predictor of suicide attempts. Adolescents who are suspected of being at risk for suicide must be questioned directly about suicidal ideation, specifically whether they have a plan in mind and access to firearms, medications, or other means of suicide. Previous suicide attempts also need to be reviewed with the teenager because 35% to 45% of adolescents that complete suicide have a positive history of a previous attempt. Nonlethal suicide gestures or other methods of self-inflicted harm should never be taken lightly or minimized. As is recommended in other arenas, initial questions should be nonspecific and become more specific as the interview proceeds, especially if answers to the previous questions are positive (Questions Box: Adolescent Suicide).

Promises to maintain confidentiality with depressed adolescents who are considered at risk for suicide are discouraged because parental involvement is strongly advised. Precipitating and motivating factors for any previous suicide attempts should be determined prior to the development of a treatment plan. More importantly, the lethality of previous attempts must be evaluated.

Physical Examination

A thorough physical examination and a review of systems should be completed to rule out a chronic medical condition such as hypothyroidism, inflammatory bowel disease, lupus, or anemia, or an organic etiology for nonspecific complaints. If patients have a history of sexual abuse, assault, or sexual activity, a genital examination should be performed to evaluate for sexually transmitted infections. In most cases, the physical examination may be of little yield in the adolescent with a true affective disorder, but careful examination may reveal findings such as cut marks, track marks, skin picking, or loss of tooth enamel, any of which may be helpful in comorbid conditions such as substance abuse or eating disorders. A careful detailed neurologic examination, including a mental status examination looking at eye contact, rate of speech, spontaneity in conversation, thought content, affect, and processing, is essential in differentiating various psychiatric conditions such as bipolar disorder and schizophrenia.

Laboratory Tests

While no routine laboratory studies are regularly recommended, to rule out organic etiologies for depression one should consider thyroid, glucose, hemoglobin, or sodium abnormalities as contributing factors and test as indicated. Screening for substance abuse and for pregnancy in females is strongly advised. Obtaining screening laboratories may serve as baseline parameters if pharmacotherapy is indicated. A complete blood cell count with differential, glucose, electrolytes, blood urea nitrogen, creatinine, liver function tests,

---

Questions

Adolescent Suicide

- Is the adolescent on any prescribed medications (eg, phenobarbital)?
- Is the adolescent experiencing any psychiatric difficulties, social maladjustments, or family or environmental challenges (eg, recent parental divorce, school expulsion)?
- Does the adolescent have a history of symptoms of depression, conduct problems, or psychosis?
- How is the adolescent progressing in school?
- Does the adolescent have a history of substance abuse?
- Does the adolescent have any legal problems?
- Does the adolescent suffer any social isolation or have interpersonal conflicts with family or friends?
- Has the adolescent suffered any personal losses recently?
- Has there recently been a suicide in the school or community?
- Are there any family problems such as abuse or neglect?
- Has the adolescent ever thought that life was not worth living?
- Does the adolescent ever feel hopeless?
- Has the adolescent ever thought of hurting himself or herself?
- Does the adolescent have a previous history of suicide attempts?
- Does the adolescent presently have a plan for suicide?
- Does the adolescent have access to firearms, medications, or other means of suicide?

---

and thyroid function tests would be included. Psychometric testing may help rule out a concomitant learning disability or attention-deficit/hyperactivity disorder.

Imaging Studies

Radiographic imaging, such as computed tomography of the head or magnetic resonance imaging of the brain, would be indicated if the history of physical examination suggests a CNS process.

Management

Depression

Treatment for depression typically follows 1 of 3 paths: **psychotherapeutic, pharmacotherapy,** or a **combination**. Recent research conducted by the National Institute of Mental Health supports psychotherapeutic intervention for mild depression. The types of therapy shown to be most effective for adolescents with depression include cognitive behavioral therapy and interpersonal therapy for adolescents. For more severe depression, or depression with suicidal ideation, the current first-line medical treatment in the primary care setting involves the use of SSRIs. Pharmacotherapy may be used with the aforementioned talk therapies. It should be noted that not all therapists are trained in the delivery of these therapeutic methods and in many communities these interventions are not readily available. Prescribing SSRIs earlier in these instances may be necessary.

If depressive symptoms are associated with a specific adjustment disorder such as divorce, a recent move, or death, and if family, peers, or school factors are affected, **supportive counseling** is indicated. The duration and depth of counseling depends, in part, on how comfortable the primary care practitioner feels performing this task and how receptive the youth and his or her family are to this intervention. Identification of the specific problem, exploration of the teen's response to the problem, and development of a reasonable solution with the adolescent and the parents may be helpful to improve adherence to psychotherapy.

If family difficulties or dysfunction is the major issue, family members and the physician or counselor should meet to assess the magnitude of the problem and the motivation required to address it. Physicians should use this opportunity to educate both adolescents and families about the signs and symptoms of depression and the undeniable impact that depression has on school functioning, family and peer relationships, and social interactions. The need for individual cognitive-behavioral therapy as well as family therapy should be discussed as well as the effectiveness of psychiatric medication in the appropriate setting. Attention to parental mental health and to understanding the strategies necessary to manage the adolescent's irritability and isolation also are extremely important. Psychological referral should be initiated if patients require more prolonged or intensive psychotherapeutic treatment, the degree of depression seems to increase, suicidality becomes an issue and additional mental health consultation is needed, or a comorbid psychiatric condition is suspected.

Immediate **psychiatric consultation and referral** are indicated if adolescents have severe depressive features that interfere with daily functioning or if they are suicidal, homicidal, or psychotic. Ensuring the adolescent's safety is the priority. A mental health referral is also appropriate if supportive counseling by the primary care physician has been ineffective or when the depression is recurrent or chronic.

Psychiatric intervention generally includes **pharmacotherapy** in conjunction with psychotherapy because most cases of depression include psychological, social, and environmental components. Although much attention has been given to safety concerns regarding the use of antidepressant medications among children and adolescents, SSRIs are considered first-line medications for the treatment of moderate to severe depression in teenagers (see Chapter 114). Two SSRIs, fluoxetine (Prozac) and escitalopram (Lexapro), have been approved by the US Food and Drug Administration (FDA) for treating depression in adolescents. The side effects tend to be dose related, and most subside with time (1–2 weeks) or with a decrease in dosage. Common adverse effects include headache, abdominal pain, diarrhea, sleep changes, and jitteriness or agitation. Serious behavioral symptoms, such as aggression, hostility, and impulsivity, must be reviewed with a psychiatrist.

The black box warning for antidepressant medications was added by the FDA in 2004 stating that on rare occasions children and adolescents treated with these drugs are more likely to display suicidal behavior, but no increase in the risk of completed suicides was noted. This was based on a meta-analysis conducted by the FDA. Subsequently, physicians decreased their use of antidepressants,

which resulted in an increase in the rate of completed suicides. It now is generally accepted that although there may be a small risk of suicidal behavior, the benefits of prescribing antidepresssants outweigh the risks if patients are monitored. This caution should be put in context with the risks of untreated depression and discussed openly with the parent or guardian and the adolescent. Prior to starting the medication, informed consent must be obtained from the parent or guardian as well as assent from the teenager. Patients should be observed closely for worsening of symptoms, suicidality, or unusual changes in behavior. Families should be educated regarding the importance of close follow-up and immediate, open communication with the provider if these symptoms should occur. Initially, the adolescent should be seen or the family contacted frequently during the first 6 weeks. Improvements in vegetative functions such as sleep and appetite often can occur within the first 3 weeks. Family observations are initially more telling than self-observation. In fact, the last feature to improve often is the patient's self-report of mood. An adequate trial of SSRIs is reported to be at least 4 to 6 weeks. Frequent medication adjustments are not advised, and abruptly stopping SSRIs is not recommended due to withdrawal or flu-like symptoms. Stopping medication after several weeks should include a slow taper.

Suicide and Suicidal Behavior

Adolescents who are considered at risk for suicide must be asked directly at every visit if they are, in fact, suicidal and if they have a plan (Questions Box: Adolescent Suicide). Response to this inquiry determines whether adolescents will be treated on an inpatient or outpatient basis. In most cases, the adolescent with no previous suicide attempts, ambivalence regarding suicidal thoughts, no real intent to die, and a good family support system may be managed as an **outpatient.** In patients who deny current suicidal ideation, a written or verbal "no suicide" contract can be made between the physician or psychologist and the adolescent, although research does not support the conclusion that such contracts actively prevent suicide. Unwillingness to sign such a contract should raise alarming concern. The patient is asked to agree to contact the clinician, parent, or another responsible adult if he or she feels a suicidal urge or experiences suicidal intent. The precipitants for possible suicidality must be reviewed, and alternative methods for coping should be rehearsed with the teenager. In addition, all potential means of suicide, particularly firearms and toxic medications, must be removed from the home or place of residence. It is not enough to "secure" firearms; they must be removed. Referral to a therapist is recommended as soon as possible. Preferably, this should be arranged while adolescents are in the office, and they should be given a definite time and date for the appointment. Ideally, the therapist should meet with the family before the first appointment with the adolescent alone. Detoxification from drugs or alcohol, if necessary, also should be addressed.

Because all suicidal threats, gestures, or ideations by adolescents must be taken seriously, emergent psychiatric referral is required for most of these individuals. Adolescents judged to be at serious risk for suicide should be managed as **inpatients** and admitted to a pediatric or adolescent unit for 24 to 48 hours of observation. The purpose of this brief hospitalization is 3-fold: (1) to stabilize patients medically, if necessary; (2) to observe and evaluate patient–family dynamics; and (3) to impress on patients and families that the attempt has been recognized and taken seriously. Intervention requires the involvement of mental health professionals in addition to social services. Transfer to an inpatient psychiatric treatment center is indicated for those adolescents who are judged by mental health consultants to have serious suicidal intentions or an underlying psychiatric illness.

Prognosis

The risk of recurrence of major depression in adolescents who have recovered is substantial. One study reports that 5% of patients relapse within 6 months of recovery, 12% within 1 year, and an estimated 33% within 4 years. Higher rates of recurrence have been reported, however, with approximately 70% of teens with MDD experiencing another depressive episode within 5 years. In addition, youth who have a depressive disorder have a 4-fold risk of the same disorder as an adult. Prepubertal-onset depression is associated with an approximately 30% risk of developing future bipolar disorder or mania.

The risk of repeated suicidal behavior seems to be greatest within the first 3 months following the initial attempt. Reported reattempt rates are 6% to 15% in the first 1 to 3 years following the initial attempt.

CASE RESOLUTION

In the case history presented at the beginning of this chapter, the girl's symptoms may be indicative of depression because she has a flat affect and seems to be somewhat isolated (insufficient time for friends and just recently moved to the United States). She seems to be at low risk for suicide, however. The physician should nonetheless inquire about symptoms of depression and ask her directly about suicidality, and then make arrangements to follow the girl's condition closely. If depression is confirmed at future visits or if she becomes suicidal, both she and her family should be referred to a mental health professional for immediate consultation and intervention.

Selected References

Adler RS, Jellinek MS. After teen suicide: issues for pediatricians who are asked to consult to schools. *Pediatrics*. 1990;86:982–987

American Academy of Child and Adolescent Psychiatry. Practice parameter for the assessment and treatment of children and adolescents with suicidal behavior. *J Am Acad Child Adolesc Psychiatry*. 2001;40;24S–51S

Birmaher B, Brent D, Bernet W, et al Practice Parameter for the assessment and treatment of children and adolescents with depressive disorders. *J Am Acad Child Adolesc Psychiatry*. 2007;46:1503-1536

Bolfek A, Janowski JJ, Waslick B, Summergrad P. Adolescent psychopharmacology: drugs for mood disorders. *Adolesc Med Clin*. 2006;17:789–808

Borowsky IW, Ireland M, Resnick MD. Adolescent suicide attempts: risks and protectors. *Pediatrics*. 2001;107:485–493

Brookman RR, Sood AA. Disorders of mood and anxiety in adolescents. *Adolesc Med Clin*. 2006;17:79–95

Campbell AT. Consent, competence, and confidentiality related to psychiatric conditions in adolescent medicine practice. *Adolesc Med Clin*. 2006;17:25–47

Copelan R. Assessing the potential for violent behavior in children and adolescents. *Pediatr Rev*. 2006;27:e36–e41

Eaton DK, Kann L, Kinchen S, et al. Youth risk behavior surveillance—United States, 2005. *MMWR Surveill Summ*. 2006;55:1–108

Grossman DC, Mueller BA, Riedy C, et al. Gun storage practices and risk of youth suicide and unintentional firearm injuries. *JAMA*. 2005;293:707–714

Hammad TA, Laughren T, Racoosin J: Suicidality in Pediatric Patients treated with Antidepressant Drugs. *Arch Gen Psychiatry*. 2006;63:332-339

Hatcher-Kay C, King CA. Depression and suicide. *Pediatr Rev*. 2003;24:363–370

Jellinek MS, Snyder JB. Depression and suicide in children and adolescents. *Pediatr Rev*. 1998;19:255–264

Leslie LK, Newman TB, Chesney PJ, et al: The Food and Drug Administration's Deliberation on Antidepressants in Pediatric Patients. *Pediatrics*. 2005;116:195-201

Lewisohn PM, Clarke GN, Seeley JR, Rohde P. Major depression in community adolescents: age at onset, episode duration, and time to recurrence. *J Am Acad Child Adolesc Psychiatry*. 1994;33:809–818

March J, Silva S, Curry J, et al. Treatment for Adolescents with Depression Study (TADS): Longterm Effectiveness and Safety. *Arch Gen Psychiatry*. 2007;64 (10):1132-1143

Merikangas KR, HE JP, Burstein M, et al. Lifetime Prevalence of Mental Disorders in US Adolescent: Results from the National Comorbidity Survey Replication (NCS-A). *JAACAP*. 2010;49(10)980-989

Prager LM. Depression and suicide in children and adolescents. *Pediatr Rev*. 2009;30:199-206

Shain BN, American Academy of Pediatrics Committee on Adolescence. Suicide and suicide attempts in adolescents. *Pediatrics*. 2007;120:669–676

Slap GB, Vorters DF, Khalid N, Marqulies SR, Forke CM. Adolescent suicide attempters: do physicians recognize them? *J Adolesc Health*. 1992;13:286–292

Williams SB, O'Connor EA, Eder M, Whitlock EP. Screening for depression in children and adolescents in primary care settings: A systematic evidence review for the US Preventive Services Task Force. *Pediatrics*. 2009;123:e716-e735

Woods ER, Lin YG, Middleman A, Beckford P, Chase L, DuRant RH. The associations of suicide attempts in adolescents. *Pediatrics*. 1997;99:791–796

Chronic Diseases of Childhood and Adolescence

CHAPTER 141

Cancer in Children

Wendy Y. Tcheng, MD

CASE STUDY

A 10-year-old boy has a history of intermittent fevers of 102.2°F (39.0°C) for 1 month. For 2 days, he has experienced increasing shortness of breath with rapid respirations. His face is dusky and plethoric, and the veins in his neck are prominent. He has bilaterally enlarged cervical lymph nodes. The remainder of the examination is normal.

The blood cell count is normal, but the erythrocyte sedimentation rate is 110. A chest radiograph reveals a large mediastinal mass.

Questions

1. What signs and symptoms are associated with malignant conditions in children?
2. What oncological emergencies require immediate attention?
3. What factors correlate with the development of cancer in children?

Epidemiology

Childhood cancer is rare. Approximately 12,400 children and adolescents younger than 20 years are diagnosed with cancer each year in the United States. The likelihood of a child developing cancer before the age of 20 years is 1 in 300 for males and 1 in 333 for females. Cancer remains the leading disease-related cause of death in children younger than 15 years. The incidence is higher in children younger than 5 years and in children between the ages of 15 and 19 years. Acute leukemia is the most common childhood cancer, followed by brain tumors, lymphomas, neuroblastoma, Wilms tumor (nephroblastoma), and other less common pediatric solid tumors.

Environmental factors, genetic predisposition, and developmental processes may all play a role in influencing the cancer risk of a child. Case-control epidemiology studies looking for the causes of pediatric cancer have evaluated foods, prenatal exposures of parents and affected offspring, electromagnetic fields, radon, and various other environmental factors with no conclusive evidence of causality to date. Although many environmental factors are known to induce carcinogenesis, current evidence does not support a major causative role for exogenous factors in childhood cancer. Most childhood cancers result from aberrations in early developmental processes. Some known risk factors for selected childhood cancers include (1) *infectious agents* such as Epstein-Barr virus (B cell lymphomas [Burkitt], Hodgkin lymphoma, nasopharyngeal carcinoma), HIV (B cell lymphomas, Kaposi sarcoma, leiomyosarcoma), hepatitis B and C (hepatocellular carcinoma); (2) *ionizing radiation* (leukemia, osteosarcoma, brain tumors); (3) *chemotherapeutic agents* (leukemia, osteosarcoma); (4) *immunodeficiency* (non-Hodgkin lymphoma); and (5) *genetic conditions*. Approximately 4% to 10% of childhood cancer results from inherited genetic mutations that result in a cancer predisposition. Children with trisomy 21 syndrome have an increased risk of leukemia (both lymphoid and myeloid). Beckwith-Wiedeman syndrome is associated with an increased risk for hepatoblastoma and Wilms tumor. Inheritance of mutations in tumor suppressor genes such as the retinoblastoma gene or the p53 gene (Li-Fraumeni syndrome) predispose affected children in families with these mutations to particular malignancies at a greater frequency and an earlier age than in unaffected individuals.

Clinical Presentation (Table 141-1)

The signs and symptoms of childhood cancer are varied, often nonspecific at the start, and can mimic many common pediatric conditions. Acute lymphoblastic leukemia (ALL) is the most common childhood cancer, accounting for 80% of pediatric leukemia cases. Acute myeloid leukemia (AML) accounts for the remaining 15% to 20% of cases. Children with **acute leukemia** present with signs and symptoms that reflect leukemic infiltration of the bone marrow and extramedullary locations. Children commonly present with generalized bone pain and signs and symptoms related to pancytopenia (fever, fatigue, pallor, bleeding, bruising, and infections). Disseminated intravascular coagulation is characteristic of AML, especially acute promyelocytic leukemia. Leukemic infiltration of extramedullary sites can lead to hepatosplenomegaly, lymphadenopathy, chloromas, central nervous system (CNS) and, rarely, testicular involvement. Children with high white blood cell counts at presentation (leukocytosis) can present with signs and symptoms of leukostasis typically involving the lung or brain. Tumor lysis syndrome can occur, either spontaneously or with the initiation of chemotherapy. Tumor lysis syndrome occurs as a result of breakdown of leukemic blasts that results in the release of metabolic byproducts. It is characterized by a metabolic triad of hyperuricemia,

Table 141-1. Signs and Symptoms of Childhood Cancer		
Disease	*Symptoms*	*Signs*
Leukemia	Fatigue Bone pain Fever, infection Petechiae, purpura, bleeding Disseminated intravascular coagulation Superior vena cava (SVC) syndrome Headache Seizures Oliguria/anuria	Anemia Neutropenia Thrombocytopenia Lymphadenopathy Hepatosplenomegaly Mediastinal mass Petechiae, purpura Papilledema Cranial neuropathies Renal failure

Brain tumors	Supratentorial tumors
	    Seizures
	    Visual dysfunction
	    Unilateral motor dysfunction
	
	Infratentorial tumors
	    Deficits of balance
	    Difficulty breathing
	
	Increased intracranial pressure
	    Headache
	    Vomiting
	    Diplopia
	    Motor weakness
	    Loss of developmental milestones
		Upper motor neuron signs
		Marcus Gunn pupils
		Parinaud syndrome
		Diabetes insipidus
		Appendicular dysmetria
		Sixth nerve palsy
		Cranial neuropathies
		Horner syndrome
		Papilledema
		Systemic hypertension
		Sixth nerve palsy
		"Setting sun" sign
		Large head size

Lymphoma		

Non-Hodgkin	Supradiaphragmatic (lymphoblastic)
	    Respiratory difficulty, cough
	    SVC syndrome
	    Enlarged/enlarging lymph nodes
	
	Infradiaphragmatic (small, non-cleaved)
	    Abdominal obstruction
	    Intussusception
	    Abdominal distension
		Mediastinal mass +/− effusions
		Lymphadenopathy
		Abdominal mass
		Hepatosplenomegaly
		Obstructive jaundice

Hodgkin	Constitutional symptoms (fever, weight loss, pruritus)	Lymphadenopathy +/− matted nodes
Neuroblastoma	Abdominal mass Skin nodules Proptosis, "raccoon eyes" Nystagmus Diarrhea Spinal cord compression symptoms	Hypertension Hepatosplenomegaly Horner syndrome
Rhabdomyosarcoma	Related to primary site	

Table 141-1. Signs and Symptoms of Childhood Cancer, continued		
Disease	*Symptoms*	*Signs*
Lymphoma , continued		

Wilms tumor	Rapid development of abdominal swelling
	Painless hematuria
		Abdominal mass
		Hypertension
		Associated congenital anomalies
		    Aniridia
		    Hemihypertrophy
		    Urogenital anomalies

Ewing sarcoma	Painful swelling of bone Constitutional symptoms (fever, fatigue)	
Osteosarcoma	Painful swelling of bone	

hyperkalemia, and hyperphosphatemia, which places a child at risk for renal dysfunction or failure secondary to precipitation of urate or calcium phosphate crystals within the renal tubules. Involvement of the CNS by leukemia can result in signs of increased intracranial pressure (ICP) (ie, headache, vomiting, hypertension, seizures, cranial neuropathies).

T-cell ALL or T-cell lymphoblastic lymphoma can present with a large anterior mediastinal mass and symptoms related to compression of the mediastinal mass on the trachea and blockage of venous return and lymphatic drainage (superior vena cava [SVC] syndrome). Children with SVC syndrome can present with wheezing, dyspnea, dysphagia, plethora, and cyanosis. Pleural and/or pericardial effusions may also be present. Superior vena cava syndrome can rapidly progress and constitutes a true oncologic emergency that requires prompt intervention.

Lymphomas in children can be divided pathologically into either Hodgkin or non-Hodgkin lymphoma. Children with **Hodgkin lymphoma** typically have a prolonged history (often at least 2–3 months) of painless enlarging cervical or supraclavicular lymphadenopathy. Affected lymph nodes can be firm, immobile, rubbery, and non-tender. In two-thirds of cases, mediastinal adenopathy may be present resulting in cough or wheeze. Constitutional symptoms such as fatigue, pruritus, and anorexia can occur, as well as the classic "B" symptoms (ie, fever, night sweats, weight loss greater than 10% of body weight). **Non-Hodgkin lymphoma** can be distinguished as lymphoblastic or non-lymphoblastic. Children with **lymphoblastic lymphoma** often present with supradiaphragmatic disease and may have cervical or supraclavicular lymphadenopathy, sometimes in association with a mediastinal mass or SVC syndrome (as previously described for T-cell lymphoblastic lymphoma). Central nervous system disease in such children is associated with signs of increased ICP. Patients with **non-lymphoblastic lymphoma** of the Burkitt or non-Burkitt type often present with intra-abdominal disease that can manifest as intussusception, abdominal obstruction, hepatosplenomegaly, or obstructive jaundice. Children with sporadic Burkitt lymphoma can present with a rapidly enlarging abdominal mass associated with tumor lysis syndrome. Endemic Burkitt lymphoma (African) presents with facial or isolated jaw tumors. In addition, patients with lymphoma can manifest a number of paraneoplastic syndromes. These include idiopathic thrombocytopenic purpura, autoimmune hemolytic anemia, nephrotic syndrome, and peripheral neuropathies, which may be mediated by abnormal and lymphoma-driven humoral or cell-mediated processes. Children with lymphomas are also at risk for tumor lysis syndrome as described for leukemia. In general, patients may either have entirely normal blood cell counts or a mild anemia, but occasionally their bone marrow may be infiltrated, giving a clinical picture consistent with leukemia with anemia, thrombocytopenia, or neutropenia.

Children with **brain tumors** can present with diverse signs and symptoms, depending on the anatomical location of the tumor (infratentorial, supratentorial, or brain stem), age of the child (ie infants with open sutures), and presence and degree of increased ICP. Infratentorial tumors, which are more common in children, typically present with gaze palsies, cerebellar signs (especially truncal ataxia), dysmetria, or vomiting. Supratentorial tumors can cause seizures, upper motor neuron signs (ie, hemiparesis, asymmetrical hyperreflexia, clonus), sensory changes, behavioral changes, decreased school performance, and disorders of the midbrain (Parinaud syndrome—paralysis of upward gaze). Signs and symptoms of ICP are often in the forefront of complaints. Recurrent morning headaches, headaches that awaken the child at night, intense headaches, vomiting, lethargy, sun-downing (eyes deviating downward like a sun setting on the horizon), increasing head circumference and loss of developmental milestones in infants, and change in school performance in older children all warrant close evaluation.

Children with spinal cord involvement from a primary spinal tumor or a paraspinal tumor (neuroblastoma, Ewing sarcoma, leukemic chloroma) may present with persistent back pain, intense radicular pain, local bony tenderness of the affected vertebrae, abnormal reflexes, abnormal dermatomal sensory examination, weakness/evolving paralysis, and subtle symptoms of bowel or bladder dysfunction (constipation, difficulty urinating). Suspicion of a spinal cord compression is an oncologic emergency for which timely, appropriate consultation must be sought.

Neuroblastoma is a malignancy of sympathetic ganglionic cell origin and can arise anywhere along the sympathetic nervous system.

Most tumors arise in the abdomen (adrenal or paraspinal); additional sites include the neck, chest, and pelvis. At presentation, tumors may be localized, with or without regional lymph node extension, or disseminated involving bone, bone marrow, and liver. Children with localized disease are often asymptomatic and the tumor is detected when radiographic imaging is performed for other medical purposes. Children with disseminated disease are ill-appearing and may present with fever, bone pain, and irritability. Paraneoplastic syndromes may also be present at diagnosis with a variety of features such as opsomyoclonus/myoclonus/ataxia (random dysconjugate eye movements, myoclonic jerking), cerebellar ataxia, and diarrhea. Proptosis and hemorrhage due to metastases involving the periorbital region can result in periorbital swelling and ecchymoses ("raccoon eyes"). A cervical tumor may be associated with unilateral Horner syndrome (unilateral ptosis, myosis, and anhydrosis).

Nephroblastoma or **Wilms tumor,** which arises in the kidney, usually presents as a painless abdominal mass, often detected by a parent while bathing the child. Associated symptoms may include fever, abdominal pain, or hematuria. If there is abdominal trauma, these bulky masses can rupture and hemorrhage and a child may present with acute abdominal pain and swelling. On examination, children may have hypertension, stigmata of associated genetic syndromes (Beckwith Wiedeman syndrome, Denys-Drash syndrome), or other isolated congenital anomalies such as aniridia, hemihypertrophy, or hypospadias.

The **bone sarcomas** that occur in children include Ewing sarcoma, osteosarcoma, and other rarer sarcomas. These tumors are most common in adolescents and rarely seen in young children. Bone tumors can present with pain at the site of tumor, with or without an associated soft tissue mass. Osteosarcomas classically involve the metaphyseal portions of the long bones, with the distal femur and proximal tibia being the most frequently involved sites. Metastatic disease, if present (15%–20% of cases), primarily involves the lung, although other sites of bone can be involved. Ewing sarcomas that occur in bone, most commonly involve the flat bones of the axial skeleton. When affecting the long bones, they tend to arise in the diaphyseal region (unlike osteosarcoma). Twenty-five percent of cases will have metastatic disease at presentation involving lung, bone, or bone marrow. Children with Ewing sarcoma may also have associated constitutional symptoms such as low-grade fever, fatigue, and weight loss.

Rhabdomyosarcoma, a soft tissue sarcoma of childhood, presents with signs and symptoms dependent on the location of the primary tumor. Sites include the head, neck, chest, abdomen, genitourinary tract, or extremities. Less than 25% of children will present with metastatic disease, but when present can involve lymph nodes, lungs, bone marrow, and bone. Head and neck sarcomas commonly arise in parameningeal and orbital sites and can present with recurrent headache, vomiting, visual problems, and proptosis. Abdominal and pelvic primary tumors can present with a palpable abdominal mass, pain, constipation, urinary obstruction, or dysuria. Genitourinary tract tumors most often involve the bladder or prostate and can present with pain, constipation, and urinary obstruction. One classic presentation occurs in girls who present with a grape-like mass at the introitus and vaginal bleeding. This is due to tumor involving the vagina or uterus and is known as sarcoma botryiodes. Primary tumors involving an extremity present with swelling at the site of tumor that can be painful and tender on palpation.

Pathophysiology

Although the macroscopic causes of pediatric cancer are not well elucidated, significant research has been made in determining some of the cellular and subcellular events that either actively trigger or fail to prevent malignancy. Growth factors are responsible for stimulation of cellular proliferation, and growth factor receptors transduce this signal into the cell via cytoplasmic secondary messengers, which in turn transmit the signal to nuclear regulatory factors. These factors ultimately regulate transcription of new RNA and protein, resulting in the desired cellular response of either stimulation or inhibition of growth. Malignant cells have a genetic makeup that differs from the constitutional karyotype of the host. A series of mutations occurs in genes that regulate cell growth and differentiation resulting in dysregulation of cell growth, differentiation, and death. Oncogenes promote cell growth and tumor suppressor genes inhibit cell division. When there is inappropriate overexpression of a normal oncogene or underexpression of tumor suppressor genes, inappropriate cell growth and division occur resulting in a malignant transformation.

There are usually multiple genetic aberrations present that lead to malignant transformation of a cell. One of the most important tumor suppressor genes is *p53*. The *p53* gene encodes for a nuclear protein that is expressed in all cells of the body and serves to induce cell cycle arrest or apoptosis in response to DNA damage. Inactivation of *p53* has been identified in numerous cancers. An initial event can alter or knock out one allele of a *p53* gene pair, and a second event results in loss of heterozygosity for that genetic locus. Either an inherited abnormality of *p53* (Li-Fraumeni syndrome) or a serendipitous accident to *p53* can cause heterozygosity for that gene. If a second event knocks out complete function of *p53*, a DNA-damaged cell can escape the signal to arrest its growth or to undergo apoptosis. The result can be a malignant transformation that allows the abnormal cell to grow unchecked.

Cancer's threat to a living organism lies in its uncontrolled growth. By growing unchecked and invading, compressing, and metastasizing to vital organs, malignant cells threaten normal life functions and cause symptoms specific to the affected area of the body.

Differential Diagnosis

Cancer is rare and often challenging to diagnose in children. Many of the presenting symptoms can be nonspecific and easily attributed to more common childhood complaints. To add to the difficulty, a pediatric practice will on average see a case every 5 to 7 years.

The differential diagnoses for some of the common childhood complaints that may suggest an underlying malignancy will be discussed. **Lymphadenopathy** is a common pediatric complaint and is most frequently due to infections (see Chapter 85). Acute bacterial adenitis, usually involving the head and neck region, is typically associated with local signs of inflammation such as erythema, warmth, and tenderness. Cervical adenopathy due to viral illness is typically bilateral, and the lymph nodes are usually mobile, soft, and non-tender. Generalized lymphadenopathy or regional lymphadenopathy characterized by firm, matted, rubbery lymph nodes should raise the suspicion for an underlying malignancy. Lymphadenopathy that is persistent or progressive, despite empiric antibiotic therapy or resolution of infectious symptoms, also merits further evaluation for malignancy. Leukemia often presents with generalized lymphadenopathy, usually in association with hepatosplenomegaly and abnormal laboratory findings. Lymphoma typically presents with regional lymphadenopathy, often in the cervical or mediastinal region, in conjunction with other signs of systemic illness. Metastatic disease (neuroblastoma, rhabdomyosarcoma) may also present with regional lymphadenopathy. Nonmalignant causes of neck masses that can be mistaken for cervical lymphadenopathy include structural anomalies such as branchial cleft cysts or cystic hygromas (see Chapter 79).

Bone and joint pain are common complaints in children with acute leukemia, because of bone marrow involvement, and may be generalized. This presentation can be confused with various rheumatologic conditions. Localized bone pain is a common presentation for children with primary bone cancers (osteosarcoma, Ewing sarcoma) and is often attributed by the child or parents to some trauma. It is not unusual for the diagnosis to be delayed several months. Differential diagnosis includes infection (osteomyelitis), trauma, musculoskeletal conditions, and benign bone lesions.

Headache is a common complaint facing the general pediatrician, and few of these headaches are caused by intracranial brain tumors. When evaluating a child with headaches, signs to raise the index of suspicion for a brain tumor include persistent vomiting, recurrent morning headaches or headaches that awaken the child, worsening headaches, associated neurologic abnormalities, and visual changes (papilledema on examination). In infants, increasing head size, sundowning, and loss of acquired developmental milestones are red flags. The differential diagnosis for headaches in children is broad and includes infections (meningitis, sinusitis), migraines, hydrocephalus, hemorrhage, and seizures.

An **abdominal mass** in an infant or child is always concerning and merits an evaluation. The most common malignant causes for an abdominal mass in this age range include neuroblastoma, nephroblastoma (Wilms tumor), hepatoblastoma, non-Hodgkin lymphoma (ie, Burkitt lymphoma), sarcomas, and germ cell tumors. Massive hepatosplenomegaly due to leukemic or lymphomatous infiltration can also be palpated as an abdominal mass. Nonmalignant etiologies of an abdominal mass may include hepatomegaly or splenomegaly, renal cysts, hemangiomas, or constipation.

Pancytopenia or **single cytopenias** are always worrisome for a malignancy involving the bone marrow. Acute leukemia is the most common malignancy involving the bone marrow and can present with leukopenia, anemia, thrombocytopenia, or in combination. Any malignancy that can metastasize to the bone marrow (neuroblastoma, lymphoma, Ewing sarcoma, rhabdomyosarcoma) can also produce pancytopenia or depression of one of the cell lines due to replacement of the bone marrow. Pancytopenia can occur as a primary bone marrow failure syndrome, such as Fanconi anemia, or as an acquired aplastic anemia due to infections (post-hepatitis), drugs (chloramphenicol, anticonvulsants), radiation, or idiopathic causes. Transient mild depression of the cell lines (most often leukopenia or anemia) due to infectious causes is very common during childhood. Depression of 2 of the 3 bone marrow cell lines merits a closer evaluation.

Evaluation

History

The history should focus on the duration and evolution of symptoms as well as the presence or absence of constitutional symptoms (eg, anorexia, fever, night sweats, weight loss). The impact of the symptoms on daily activities (eg, school attendance, sports) should be determined and will clue the physician to the scope of the illness. Recent or persistent infections, medications, or unusual environmental exposures should also be ascertained (Questions Box). Relevant medical history should be considered. A previous cancer diagnosis would raise the index of suspicion for relapse or a secondary malignancy. Certain immunodeficiencies and genetic syndromes are associated with an increased risk for malignancy (eg, trisomy 21 syndrome and leukemia) and should also be considered. A family history of childhood cancers or genetic syndromes is also important.

> ## Questions
> ### Cancer
> - How long has the child had the symptoms?
> - Does the child have a family history of cancer?
> - Does the child have a history of constitutional symptoms (eg, fever, weight loss)?
> - Does the child have a history of recent onset of pallor, fever, bleeding, pain, swelling, hematuria, or malaise?
> - Has the child been attending school or participating in routine activities?
> - Has the child been exposed to any environmental toxins?

Physical Examination

A thorough physical examination is essential, with particular attention to symptomatic areas (see Table 141-1). In general, the lymph nodes should be carefully assessed for enlargement or malignant characteristics (firm, fixed, rubbery nodes) and the abdomen for organomegaly or masses. The skin should be evaluated for the presence of pallor, petechiae, or purpura that would suggest anemia or thrombocytopenia. A thorough search for signs of infection or persistent infection should be performed and, if present, may reflect bone marrow disease with neutropenia. Neurologic symptoms, including headache, vomiting, or focal complaints, warrant a full neurologic examination. Increased ICP may manifest as papilledema or sixth nerve palsy. In infants, increased ICP can manifest with a large head size, full fontanelles, or sun-downing. A complaint of back pain also merits a full neurologic examination with close attention to any signs of spinal cord compression, suggesting a possible spinal or paraspinal mass

Laboratory Tests (Table 141-2)

In a child with nonspecific or constitutional symptoms concerning for malignancy, it is reasonable to begin with a screening complete blood cell count (CBC), peripheral blood smear, and comprehensive chemistry panel (electrolytes, renal and liver function). If a malignancy is suspected, lactate dehydrogenase is useful as a nonspecific marker for increased cell turnover. If leukemia or lymphoma is suspected, evaluation for tumor lysis syndrome (by checking uric acid, potassium, phosphate, and calcium) should be performed. In addition, certain tumors secrete or synthesize characteristic markers and metabolites that are pathognomonic for their diagnosis. For example, elevated levels of the sympathetic neurotransmitter metabolites vanillylmandelic acid and homovanillic acid are found in the urine of individuals with neuroblastoma or pheochromocytoma. Tumor markers such as α-fetoprotein and β-human chorionic gonadotropin are characteristic of germ cell tumors. α-fetoprotein is a useful tumor marker for hepatoblastoma as well. Monitoring of these levels is useful as an indicator of response to therapy or relapse. Other laboratory values, such as ferritin or erythrocyte sedimentation rate, can be elevated and reflect an underlying systemic illness (see Table 141-2).

Imaging Studies

Radiographic studies are a necessity in the initial evaluation and staging of most childhood cancers. Once the diagnosis of malignancy has been confirmed, appropriate imaging studies to assess the local and metastatic spread of the disease should be performed before the initiation of therapy. The type of studies performed depends on the specific malignancy and its associated pattern of metastatic spread. Common studies performed include radiographs, computed tomography (CT), magnetic resonance imaging, and gallium or positron emission tomography (PET) scans. For leukemias and lymphomas, an initial chest radiograph is necessary to evaluate for a mediastinal mass (most commonly seen in T-cell leukemia/lymphoma). Additional imaging is typically not necessary for leukemia; however, lymphomas warrant further diagnostic imaging for staging (CT, gallium, or PET scans). Required imaging for evaluation of specific childhood cancers is provided in Table 141-2.

Pathology

Children with suspected malignancies should be referred to a children's cancer center where there are specialized pediatric oncologists, radiologists, surgeons, and pathologists who can work together to establish the best approach for diagnosis (biopsy or removal of tumor) and handling of tissue. Collection of fresh tissue at biopsy for specialized genetic tests and tumor banking is important and can contribute significantly to a complete pathologic diagnosis.

There are certain clinical scenarios where obtaining tissue for pathologic diagnosis is difficult. Children who present with a large mediastinal mass may be in respiratory distress (secondary to SVC syndrome), and at high risk during anesthesia. In this situation, coordinated efforts should be made to obtain pathology specimens in the least invasive manner, before the initiation of therapy. Diagnosis can often be made by less invasive procedures (CBC, peripheral blood flow cytometry, bone marrow aspirate/biopsy, pleurocentesis) that may require very minimal sedation. If therapy needs to be started, then biopsy should be performed as soon as clinically tolerated.

Management

If a diagnosis of cancer is suspected or confirmed in a child, then referral to a pediatric cancer center is important where appropriate diagnostic procedures, tissue handling, and treatment can be provided.

Diagnosing and treating childhood cancer requires a multidisciplinary team consisting of pediatric oncologists, surgeons, radiation oncologists, pathologists, and other pediatric subspecialists. In addition, supportive ancillary services such as social work, childlife, child psychology, pain service, palliative care programs, and religious support are important. When making a referral for a child with a suspected cancer, the referring physician should prepare the family with his or her suspicions and the likely workup that will ensue at the accepting center.

Because the management of specific childhood cancers is beyond the scope of this chapter, the discussion will focus on the general principles of pediatric oncologic management. The primary therapeutic modalities for the treatment of childhood cancer include **chemotherapy, surgery, radiation therapy,** and **stem cell transplantation.** Increasingly, as the molecular aberrations of cancer are becoming understood, cancer-targeted therapies are becoming more prevalent. Conventional, cytotoxic anticancer therapy is likened to a "shotgun" approach in which both cancer cells and normal cells are subject to toxicity. The effects of therapy on normal tissues and organs can manifest acutely (limiting dose) or in the long term (affecting quality of life). As more and more children are surviving childhood cancer, the late effects of therapy are increasingly evident, further emphasizing the need for risk-adapted therapy, cancer-targeted therapy, and a reduction of treatment-related toxicities.

Optimal outcome depends on several factors: correct pathologic diagnosis; careful medical management, including administration of chemotherapy and monitoring of side effects; precise customization of radiation fields if radiation therapy is necessary; optimal surgical resection, if indicated; and therapeutic ability and experience with administration of treatment to children. Centers that specialize in the treatment of pediatric cancer are experienced in the diagnosis and treatment of rare malignancies and are thus best equipped to treat affected children. In addition, the standard of care for children with cancer is treatment according to research study protocols from national collaborative research groups (Children's Oncology Group), available at most specialized pediatric cancer centers. Posttreatment

Table 141-2. Diagnostic Tests and Imaging Studies Used in the Evaluation of Childhood Cancer

Disease	Diagnostic Tests	Imaging Studies
Leukemia	Bone marrow aspirate and biopsy Cytogenetic analysis of bone marrow CBC with platelet count, differential PT, PTT, fibrinogen Serum electrolytes, Ca, PO4 BUN, creatinine, uric acid, LDH CSF cell count, cytology	Chest radiograph (look for mediastinal mass)

Brain tumors	None usually indicated except in case of suspected teratoma:
	    serum and CSF α-fetoprotein, β-human chorionic gonadotropin,
	    carcinoembryonic antigen
		MRI of brain with gadolinium
		MRI of spine for selected tumors

Lymphoma	Bone marrow aspirate and biopsy CSF cell count and cytology Serum LDH, electrolytes, Ca, PO4 ESR, ferritin	Gallium scan, PET scan CT of chest, abdomen, pelvis
Neuroblastoma	Serum ferritin CBC with platelet count Serum electrolytes, liver and renal panel Serum LDH Bone marrow aspirate and biopsy	CT or MRI of primary tumor site CT of chest, abdomen, pelvis (+/− head) with contrast Bone scan MIBG scan
Rhabdomyosarcoma	CBC with platelet count Liver and renal panel Bone marrow aspirate and biopsy CSF cell count and cytology (head and neck primary tumors only)	CT or MRI of primary tumor site CT of chest, abdomen, pelvis Bone scan
Nephroblastoma (Wilms tumor)	Urinalysis	CT of primary tumor site Ultrasound of inferior vena cava CT of chest Bone scan
Ewing sarcoma	ESR CBC with platelet count Bone marrow aspirate and biopsy Serum LDH	CT or MRI of primary tumor site CT of chest Bone scan
Osteosarcoma		MRI of primary tumor site CT of chest Bone scan

Abbreviations: BUN, blood urea nitrogen; Ca, calcium; CBC, complete blood cell count; CSF, cerebrospinal fluid; CT, computed tomography; ESR, erythrocyte sedimentation rate; LDH, lactate dehydrogenase; MIBG, metaiodobenzylguanidine; MRI, magnetic resonance imaging; PET, positron emission tomography; PO4, phosphate; PT, prothrombin time; PTT, partial thromboplastin time.

analysis of children treated on protocols at specialized pediatric cancer centers have 4-year disease-free survival rates that are significantly better than those of children treated outside this setting. Similarly, treatment of adolescents and young adults on protocols at specialized pediatric cancer centers yields better outcomes than those treated by oncologists who typically treat adults.

The placement of indwelling central venous catheters is standard in cancer therapy in pediatrics, making frequent venous access for both diagnostic and therapeutic purposes more easily tolerated by children. External catheters (Broviac, Hickman) or internal subcutaneous catheters (Port-a-Caths) are selected depending on the underlying diagnosis and intensity of therapy. All indwelling catheters are

at risk for infection, either from contamination of blood (line infections) or infections around the catheter site itself (tunnel infection). Most central line infections can be treated with intravenous (IV) antibiotic therapy; however, certain pathogens (fungi) are difficult to clear and require line removal. Central venous catheters may also be complicated with thromboses requiring local thrombolytic therapy.

In the interest of cost-containment and convenience as well as children's well-being, it is often more feasible for children to be closer to home between chemotherapy cycles. Primary care physicians should be familiar with the management of various infectious complications to which children undergoing cancer therapy are subject. Fever in children with neutropenia (absolute neutrophil count <500 cells/μL) requires a different therapeutic approach than fever in otherwise normal children. Until proven otherwise, children with fever and neutropenia (usually induced by chemotherapy, sometimes in combination with radiation therapy) must be assumed to have a serious bacterial infection. They should be treated accordingly, with hospitalization, IV antibiotics, thorough examination for site of infection, and careful hemodynamic monitoring. Initial treatment consists of antibiotic coverage for *Staphylococcus aureus,* gram-negative enteric organisms, and *Pseudomonas aeruginosa* (eg, cefepime with or without tobramycin, vancomycin). Additional coverage for anaerobic infection (eg, mucositis), viral infection (eg, herpes stomatitis, varicella), and other pathogens (eg, fungi) depends on the child's treatment history and clinical findings.

Prognosis

The prognosis for children with all forms of cancer has dramatically improved over the past 4 decades. Nearly 80% of children diagnosed with cancer can expect to be long-term survivors. Figure 141-1 shows the improvement in cure rates for ALL, the most common childhood cancer. This success is largely due to the efforts of national collaborative group science and treatment protocols. However, with increased survivorship, new concerns have arisen with respect to the long-term effects of treatment, the risks of secondary malignancies, and complex social and psychological issues. In a large study of childhood cancer survivors, adults treated for a childhood cancer in the 1970s and 1980s were 3 times more likely than their siblings to have developed a chronic health condition. Continued multidisciplinary surveillance of childhood cancer survivors through adulthood will help to optimize a favorable outcome.

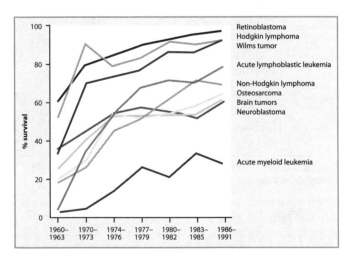

Figure 141-1. Five-year relative survival rates for specific cancers of children (0–14 years), 1973–2001. Data are from the Surveillance, Epidemiology, and End Results (SEER) program regions (9 areas). (From Pizzo PA, Poplack DG. *Principles and Practice of Pediatric Oncology.* **Philadelphia, PA: Lippincott Williams & Wilkins; 2006:5.)**

Selected References

Golden CB, Feusner JH. Malignant abdominal masses in children: quick guide to evaluation and diagnosis. *Pediatr Clin North Am.* 2002;49:1369–1392

Meck MM, Leary M, Sills RH. Late effects in survivors of childhood cancer. *Pediatr Rev.* 2007;27:257–263

Oeffinger KC, Nathan PC, Kremer L. Challenges after curative treatment for childhood cancer and long-term follow up of survivors. *Pediatr Clin North Am.* 2008;55:251–273

Park JR, Eggert A, Caron H. Neuroblastoma: biology, prognosis, and treatment. *Pediatr Clin North Am.* 2008;55:97–120

Poplack DG. Acute lymphoblastic leukemia. In: Pizzo PA, Poplack DG, eds. *Principles and Practice of Pediatric Oncology.* 5th ed. Philadelphia, PA: Lippincott Williams & Wilkins; 2006

Pui CH, Schrappe M, Ribeiro RC, Niemeyer CM. Childhood and adolescent lymphoid and myeloid leukemia. *Hematology Am Soc Hematol Educ Program.* 2004:118–145

Ries LAG, Smith MA, Gurney JG, et al, eds. *Cancer Incidence and Survival among Children and Adolescents: United States SEER Program 1975–1995, National Cancer Institute, SEER Program.* Bethesda, MD: National Institutes of Health; 1999. NIH Pub No 99-4649

Ullrich NJ, Pomeroy SL. Pediatric brain tumors. *Neurol Clin.* 2003;21:897–913

CHAPTER 142

Chronic Kidney Disease

Justine Bacchetta, MD, PhD; Walter Jimenez, MD; and Isidro B. Salusky, MD

CASE STUDY

During a consultation for diarrhea and dehydration the pediatrician notes that a 7-year-old boy has concomitant growth retardation. His parents report decrease in appetite as well as in physical activity level over the last few months associated with bedwetting, despite having been previously potty trained. His medical history is significant for multiple episodes of fever due to supposed ear infections during his first years of life and one episode of urinary tract infection without further studies. After hydration the physical examination reveals a pale and short patient (height 101 cm, <5th percentile) with blood pressure above 99th percentile for age, gender, and

height. Routine laboratory studies reveal anemia, a serum creatinine of 1.4 mg/dL, and 3+ proteinuria.

Questions
1. How do you estimate renal function in children?
2. What are the relevant questions to ask about medical and family history in children who present with **chronic kidney disease (CKD)**?
3. What additional diagnostic tests should be performed to determine the etiology of the kidney disease?
4. What are the approaches to the management of children with CKD?

Although the kidney is mainly responsible for excretion or "clearance" of waste products it also has a role in the synthesis and regulation of erythropoietin, renin, 1,25-dihydroxycholecalciferol, acid-base, electrolytes, and water. When the kidney is affected, regulation of multiple functions is disturbed. Currently **glomerular filtration rate (GFR)** is the best method to detect, evaluate, and manage CKD. The GFR varies according to gender, age, and body size and reflects the amount of plasma cleared by the kidney (Box 142-1). It can be challenging to evaluate GFR in children but the 2009 Schwartz formula has been shown to be accurate both in children with CKD and in children with normal renal function, thus allowing its easy use in clinical practice. Early recognition of children with CKD is important in order to prevent the complications associated with the progressive decline in renal function. The signs and symptoms of CKD in children are nonspecific; thus it is vital that the primary medical caretaker, usually the pediatrician or family practitioner, recognize the earliest signs and symptoms and institute proper medical care. Prompt referral to a pediatric nephrologist must be made, and follow-up consultations by both physicians should be performed regularly to optimize the management of these children.

Depending on the GFR, the physician can classify kidney function in 5 stages as defined by the National Kidney Foundation (Table 142-1). Stages 1 and 2 are defined with GFR of more than 90 mL/min/1.73 m² and 60 to 89 mL/min/1.73 m², respectively. The staging of CKD provides guidelines for the management of these patients because there are specific primary and comorbid conditions associated with the primary cause of renal failure as well as those that are associated with progression of CKD. Indeed, the reduction of some of those associated factors may reduce the risk factors for cardiovascular disease (CVD) and vascular calcifications. Particular importance should be placed on managing **growth, proteinuria, acidosis, anemia, hypertension,** and **metabolic bone disease** among others. Once GFR declines to 15 to 29 mL/min/1.73 m²

Box 142-1. How to Evaluate Glomerular Filtration Rate (GFR) in Children

1- Measuring the true GFR

Reference standard: inulin clearance, iothalamate, iohexol

Expensive, time-consuming

Not for everyday practice

2- Evaluating the GFR

A- Measured from a 24-hour urine collection

$$GFR = \frac{\text{Urine creatinine [mmol/L]} \times \text{Volume of urine [mL]}}{\text{Time of urine sampling [min]} \times \text{Plasma creatinine [mmol/L]}}$$

GFR (normalized for 1.73 m²) = Cl × 1.73/body surface area

B- Estimated by a spot blood (2009 Schwartz formula)

GFR = 0.413 Height (cm)/Plasma creatinine (mg/dL)

Table 142-1. Classification of Chronic Kidney Disease

Stage	Glomerular Filtration Rate (mL/min/1.73 m²)
1	≥90
2	60–89
3	30–59
4	15–29
5	≤15

(stage 4), patients and families should be prepared for **renal replacement therapy** and **renal transplantation. End-stage renal disease (ESRD) (or stage 5)** is defined as GFR less than 15 mL/min/1.73 m² or the need of **dialysis/transplant.** The staging of CKD is based on estimation of GFR but also additional factors are considered in the overall management of the patient, and the characteristics of the growth curve are very important in the assessment of the consequences of renal failure in childhood. All children with CKD should be referred early to pediatric nephrologists in order to carefully facilitate the future steps in the care of the patient and family. In adult patients with CKD, late referral is associated with increased rates of morbidity and mortality.

Epidemiology

The incidence of CKD in children is unknown. Current estimates are based on the number of children accepted for dialysis and renal transplantation; however, some children do not require dialysis or transplantation until adulthood. In 2008 the North American Pediatric Renal Transplant Cooperative Study (NAPRTCS) reported 7,037 patients with an estimated GFR 75 mL/min/1.73m² or less. The causes of CKD can be broadly categorized into 2 main groups: congenital and acquired. Congenital conditions such as **obstructive uropathy, aplasia/hypoplasia/dysplasia, reflux nephropathy,** and **prune belly syndrome** accounted for the majority (53%) and are summarized as CAKUT (congenital abnormalities of the kidney and urinary tract). Among the acquired conditions, **focal and segmental glomerulosclerosis** are the most prevalent diagnoses, accounting for 9%, with African Americans having a worse prognosis. Overall males are more often affected (64%), and 20% of children have entered the registry before the age of 2 years, 16% between 2 and 5 years, 32% between 6 and 12 years, 28% between 13 and 17 years, and 4% after the age of 17 years; however, time at entry into the registry does not strictly correspond to the age at time of CKD diagnosis.

Clinical and Biological Presentation

Children with CKD often present with no, or nonspecific, symptoms, and the abnormality is detected during routine health examinations or screening. For a small percentage of these patients, CKD is inadvertently discovered when they present with another illness such as diarrhea and dehydration. Patients may be referred to the physician because of **growth retardation, hypertension,** or **anemia** (Box 142.2). Frequently, a history of recurrent episodes of fever

Box 142-2. General Symptoms Associated With Chronic Kidney Disease
• Growth retardation/growth failure
• Anorexia
• Anemia
• Bone disease
• Metabolic acidosis
• Hypertension

without a source, or partially treated urinary tract infections (UTIs) secondary to undiagnosed vesicoureteral reflux, is uncovered. Children may also complain of vague generalized symptoms, including malaise, anorexia, and vomiting, which may be associated with advanced renal failure.

Metabolic and Water/Electrolyte Abnormalities

Children with congenital abnormalities such as obstructive uropathy and/or renal dysplasia may develop polyuria due to inability to concentrate urine, and salt wasting may become a prominent feature as well as polydipsia; in such a case, blood pressure is usually normal. A history of **bedwetting** may thus be a clue to CKD. In contrast, children with advanced CKD may have impaired sodium excretion leading to water retention and, consequently, fluid overload and secondary hypertension. **Hyperkalemia** is not an unusual component of CKD, and it becomes evident when the GFR falls below 10 mL/min/1.73 m². **Hypokalemia** is a less common problem and may be secondary to excessive diuretic use or a strict dietary restriction; it can also be the hallmark of a tubulo-interstitial disease (proximal tubulopathy) at the early stages of CKD.

Metabolic acidosis is mainly caused by the overall decrease in ammonia excretion from a reduced number of nephrons. Decreased excretion of titratable acid and bicarbonate wasting in cases of proximal renal tubular acidosis may play a role as well.

Glucose intolerance may occur in some children with CKD despite elevated insulin levels, independent of genetic diseases, which induce renal cysts and atypical diabetes mellitus (HNF1β mutations). The linear correlation between a decline in renal function and insulin resistance even at early stages of CKD has been shown in adults. More than 50% of children develop **hyperlipidemia** by the time they reach ESRD. The characteristic plasma lipid abnormality is a moderate **hypertriglyceridemia.** There is also a high prevalence of **hypercholesterolemia** and low levels of high-density lipids and albumin. These derangements have a role in the developing of CVD.

Growth Failure

Failure to thrive is the hallmark of CKD in children, and the degree of growth retardation varies according to the age of presentation. Indeed, because maximal growth occurs during the early years in life, children with congenital renal problems are the most affected. In the NAPRTCS study, height deficits were greatest for children younger than 5 years, with nearly 50% below the third percentile for age and gender. Growth failure develops early in the course of CKD and affects up to 35 % of this population; by the time of renal transplantation, most children present with severe short stature. Moreover, children with more severe degrees of affected renal function tended to have greater height deficits. Sexual development is often delayed in affected patients, as well as bone age. Uremia, anorexia, and frequent vomiting also explain the **protein and calorie malnutrition** frequently observed in the younger children; it requires an early and intensive management.

Mineral and Bone Disorders (MBD) associated With CKD (CKD-MBD)

The impact of CKD-MBD may be immediate (biological disequilibrium of calcium, phosphate, vitamin D and parathyroid hormone (PTH) or delayed (growth retardation, bone pain, fractures, bone deformities, extra-skeletal and vascular calcifications, increased morbidity and mortality). The development of CKD-MBD begins early in the course of CKD, and clinical manifestations include growth retardation and skeletal deformities such as **genu valgum, ulnar deviation of the hands, pes varus,** and **slipped capital femoral epiphyses.** As defined by the 2006 Kidney Disease: Improving Global Outcomes (KDIGO), the term renal osteodystrophy refers specifically to the different bone lesions as defined by bone histomorphometry. In contrast, the term CKD-MBD is used to define the clinical and biochemical abnormalities as well as the long-term consequences of alterations of bone and mineral metabolism associated with CKD. Thus, CKD-MBD is manifested by either one or a combination of the following abnormalities: (1) abnormalities of calcium, phosphorus, PTH, or vitamin D metabolism; (2) abnormalities in bone histology, linear growth, or strength; and (3) vascular or other soft tissue calcification.

Anemia

The anemia of CKD is normochromic and normocytic. Insufficient erythropoietin (EPO) production occurs when the GFR is less than 30 mL/min/1.73 m². Anemia is frequently accompanied by decreased serum iron levels, increased total iron binding capacity, and low reticulocyte counts. Dialysis patients are predisposed to develop bleeding tendencies because of platelet dysfunction and mechanical hemolysis.

Hypertension

The incidence of **hypertension** in children with CKD varies from 38% to 78%. Prolonged hypertension may accelerate deterioration of renal function. An acute rise in blood pressure usually results in seizures in children. Other manifestations include headache, epistaxis, congestive heart failure, nerve palsies and, not uncommonly, cerebral hemorrhage. Hypertension is frequently seen in children with CKD secondary to polycystic kidney disease or chronic glomerulonephritis.

Cardiac Dysfunction

In addition to the increased risk of vascular calcifications, **congestive heart failure** may be a prominent clinical finding associated with fluid overload, uncontrollable hypertension, severe anemia, or presence of uremic cardiomyopathy. Left ventricular hypertrophy diagnosed by echocardiographic assessment is present in 3 of 4 adults with CKD, with anemia and hypertension being the principal predisposing factors. Such findings are seen even in the pediatric population, with a prevalence of 10% to 20% in CKD stages 3 and 4.

Neurologic Dysfunction

Children with CKD may have **impaired neurodevelopment** related to the age of presentation. Memory deficits, lack of concentration, depression, and weakness may occur. Children younger than 5 years are more affected because significant brain growth and maturation occur during the early years of life. Children who are severely uremic may suffer from global developmental retardation and seizures. Unless neurodevelopmental delays are recognized promptly and early intervention is instituted, problems are most often progressive. Of note, some genetic diseases involving both cerebral and renal development may also play a role in the developmental delay.

Pathophysiology

The Global Final Pathway of the Reduction in the Nephron Number

Regardless of the type of initial injury to the kidney, glomerular hyperfiltration and tubulointerstitial damage are the final common pathways of glomerular destruction. Hyperfiltration occurs as a response by the residual glomeruli to compensate the loss of nephrons, as summarized on Figure 142-1. The reduced filtration results in increased production of **renin** and **angiotensin-converting enzyme (ACE)**. The resulting vasoconstriction of the efferent arteriole increases the hydrostatic pressure on the capillary wall, leading to a compensatory higher filtration rate per nephron but also to protein transit across the wall. Proteinuria recruits inflammatory cells and upregulates proinflammatory and profibrotic genes. Protein overload in the tubular cells stimulates their differentiation into myofibroblasts, thus favoring fibrosis. The inflammatory cascade activates at the same time as the complement cascade, leading

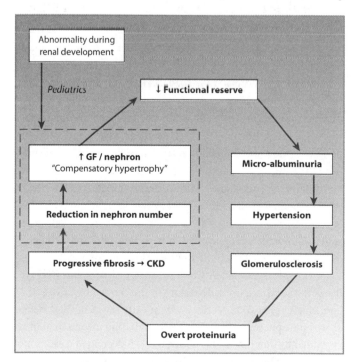

Figure 142-1. The consequences of the reduction in the nephron number. CKD, chronic kidney disease; GF, glomerular filtration.

to additional kidney damage. The interstitial fibrosis impairs oxygenation of the tubular cells; the chronic hypoxia then further activates the renin-angiotensin system. The activation of fibroblasts by hypoxia is another stimulus to the differentiation of the tubular cells. Reducing intraglomerular pressure, proteinuria, and the consequent tubulointerstitial fibrosis is the rationale for prescribing ACE inhibitors or angiotensin receptor blockers (ARBs) in order to slow the rate of progression of CKD, in addition to their anti-hypertensive properties.

Growth Failure

Multiple factors are involved in the pathogenesis of growth retardation in children with CKD, and the most predominant are deficient calorie and protein intake, decreased erythropoietin production, metabolic acidosis, decreased serum level of **insulin-like growth factor I**, peripheral resistance to growth hormone due to decreased levels of growth hormone–binding proteins and growth hormone receptors, renal osteodystrophy, hypogonadism, and drug toxicity (corticosteroids), further inducing major consequences for both physical and mental well-being in this population. A particularity of renal osteodystrophy in children is the alteration of the growth plate cartilage architecture, another possible detrimental element in the growth failure. Both adynamic bone lesions and severe hyperparathyroidism increase the severity of growth retardation, explaining that optimal target values for serum PTH should be related to the stage of CKD; in that setting the overuse of vitamin D analogs can also worsen the growth retardation. In CKD teenagers, the loss of the pulsatile release of the gonadotropin-releasing hormone also explains the delay and the shortening of the pubertal growth spurt, in association with a reduced growth velocity.

Mineral and Bone Disorders Associated With CKD (CKD-MBD)

The development of **renal osteodystrophy** is also multifactorial. The reduced renal mass results in a decreasing synthesis of 1,25-**dihydroxycholecalciferol**; therefore, the stimulus to absorb calcium from the gut decreases concomitantly. The resulting hypocalcemia and the lack of feedback by vitamin D on the parathyroid stimulate the production of PTH, facilitating the rapid mobilization of calcium and phosphorus from the skeleton, thus normalizing the serum calcium. In the early 2000s, another phosphaturic hormone of the bone kidney/axis (ie, the fibroblast growth factor 23, [FGF23]) was identified to play a key role in bone mineralization from rare genetic diseases such as hyphosphatemic rickets, autosomal-dominant hypophosphatemic rickets, and tumor-induced osteomalacia. FGF23 is both a phosphaturic factor and a suppressor of 1α-hydroxylase activity in the kidney, it also inhibits PTH synthesis in the parathyroid. Therefore in the context of CKD, FGF23 levels increase as GFR decreases, from early stages of CKD, before serum phosphate has become abnormal. This increase could be explained by different factors, such as (1) a decreased clearance of FGF23, (2) an increased synthesis by osteocytes, (3) a compensatory mechanism in an attempt to excrete the excess serum phosphate, or

(4) a response to the treatment with active vitamin D analogs. In CKD adult patients, serum FGF23 levels are positively correlated with serum phosphate and negatively with serum calcitriol and PTH. FGF23 may also provide prognostic information in CKD patients, mainly in terms of CKD progression, therapeutic response, and cardiovascular mortality: FGF23 is an independent predictor of CKD progression in adults, as well as a predictor of refractoriness to intravenous calcitriol therapy at 24 weeks and an independent risk factor for mortality in adults undergoing hemodialysis. One may thus hypothesize that a therapeutic reduction of FGF23 could have a clinical importance to delay the onset of secondary hyperparathyroidism, the onset of CKD-MBD, and may be the global morbi-mortality in CKD patients, but the question of whether FGF23 could exert both direct and systemic toxic effects will need further longitudinal studies. Very little data on FGF23 are available in children but some reference values have been proposed, and other authors have described a positive effect of FGF23 on bone mineralization in CKD children.

There is also skeletal resistance to PTH when CKD advances. The cycle is aggravated by an early alteration in the regulation of PTH gene transcription, a reduction in the calcium sensing receptor, and a progressive resistance to FGF23 in the parathyroid glands. **Hyperparathyroidism** and resulting high bone turnover produces fibrosis in bone, which is also called **osteitis fibrosa.** Hyperphosphatemia develops when the few remaining nephrons lose the ability to excrete the daily load of phosphorus from the diet; it is a late phenomenon, mainly in stages 4 and 5. The external administration of vitamin D and its derivatives can suppress such bone remodeling, but if not adequately monitored can result in low turnover bone disease (adynamic bone). In this later case, serum PTH and alkaline phosphatase levels are generally lower when compared with patients with secondary hyperparathyroidism. In the past, aluminum-containing phosphate binders were the main factors involved in the pathogenesis of osteomalacia and adynamic bone, but currently the use of large doses of calcium-based binders and active vitamin D sterols are implicated. The presence of abnormal calcium-phosphate metabolism and hyperparathyroidism, and increased FGF23 levels in association with other traditional risk factors as hypertension, hyperlipidemia, hyperhomocysteinemia, anemia, and oxidative stress are also associated with CVD, the leading cause of death in ESRD. In young adults with childhood-onset CKD, the prevalence of coronary artery calcification can be as high as 92% when evaluated by sequential computed tomography (CT) scan with electrocardiogram (ECG) gating.

Anemia

The anemia of CKD begins when the GFR falls below 30 mL/min/1.73 m^2 and is multifactorial: decreased EPO production, decreased red cell survival, bone marrow inhibition, iron deficiency, vitamin B$_{12}$ and folate deficiency, inflammation, antibodies directed against EPO, and osteitis fibrosa. In the past, aluminum toxicity also explained partly the anemia observed during CKD. Some patients can worsen their hemoglobin levels with blood loss during the hemodialysis sessions. In a similar manner as in the understanding of the CKD-MBD pathophysiology when the FGF23 was identified, a new hormone involved in the anemia in CKD has also been recently described. Indeed, hepcidin is a peptide hormone synthesized in the liver; the loss of hepcidin activity induces severe iron overload. In contrast, patients with increased hepcidin levels experience anemia. Hepcidin allows the internalization of ferroportin, the only cellular receptor of iron that exports iron from the intracellular to the extracellular compartment. Iron loading and inflammation increase while a treatment with EPO decreases hepcidin levels. In adults, there is an inverse relationship between GFR and hepcidin serum levels; in CKD children, ferritin and hepcidin levels are strongly correlated, as well as hepcidin and high-sensitivity C-reactive protein. Hepcidin could be a marker of EPO resistance and of the functional iron status; however, it is not used yet in clinical practice.

Differential Diagnosis

Instead of crafting a differential diagnosis, the main challenge for the physician initially will be to determine whether the renal impairment is acute or chronic and if chronic, its etiology. A variety of kidney problems, whether congenital, hereditary, acquired, or metabolic, may result in CKD. Although specific cures are not available for most of these renal conditions, it is essential to perform a complete diagnostic workup to determine the etiology of the renal problem. Such information may identify the presence of an inherited problem that may require genetic counseling and, in some cases, anticipation of problems associated with renal transplantation. Some renal diseases may in fact recur after renal transplantation (eg, focal segmental glomerulosclerosis or atypical hemolytic uremic syndrome); parents and children must be informed early about this possibility in preparation for future strategies for renal transplantation. The different etiologies of CKD, as well as their respective prevalence in the 2008 NAPRTCS registry, are summarized in Table 142-2.

It is also necessary to differentiate between acute and chronic renal failure at initial presentation because the therapeutic strategies may differ, and the long-term renal prognosis can be quite different. Patients with CKD present with retarded linear growth and signs of clinical and radiographic evidence of renal osteodystrophy. In advanced disease the renal ultrasound frequently reveals small, shrunken kidneys. The hereditary diseases most commonly encountered are hereditary nephritis (Alport syndrome or PAX2 nephropathy), branchio-oto-renal syndrome (BOR), and juvenile nephronophthisis. Acquired diseases such as chronic glomerulonephritis, membranoproliferative glomerulonephritis, and focal and segmental glomerulosclerosis, affect a large percentage of older children who progress to CKD. Anemia, hypertension, and fluid and electrolyte abnormalities are often associated with either chronic or acute renal failure.

Evaluation

A complete evaluation of children presenting with renal failure must be performed.

Table 142-2. Etiologies of Pediatric CKD (NAPRTCS 2008)		
	Disease	**Percentage**
CAKUT	Obstructive uropathy	20.7
	Aplasia/hypoplasia/dysplasia	17.3
	Reflux nephropathy	8.4
	Prune belly	2.7
Genetic diseases	Polycystic disease	4.0
	Cystinosis	1.5
	Oxalosis	0.1
	Drash syndrome	0.1
	Congenital nephrotic syndrome	1.1
	Medullary cystic disease	1.3
Glomerular diseases	FSGS	8.7
	Chronic GN	1.2
	MPGN type 1	1.1
	MPGN type 2	0.4
	IgA nephritis	0.9
	Henoch-Schönlein nephritis	0.6
	Idiopathic crescentic GN	0.7
	Membranous nephropathy	0.5
Systemic diseases	HUS	2.0
	SLE nephritis	1.6
	Wegener granulomatosis	0.4
	Other systemic immunologic	0.4
	Diabetic nephropathy	0.2
	Sickle cell nephropathy	0.2
Miscellaneous	Familial nephritis	1.6
	Pyelo/interstitial nephritis	1.4
	Renal infarct	2.2
	Wilms tumor	0.5
	Others	15.8
	Unknown	2.6

Abbreviations: CAKUT, congenital abnormalities of the kidney and urinary tract; CKD, chronic kidney disease; FSGS, focal segmental glomerulosclerosis; GN, glomerulonephritis; HUS, hemolytic uremic syndrome; IgA, immunoglobulin A; MPGN, membranoproliferative glomerulonephritis; NAPRTCS, North American Pediatric Renal Transplant Cooperative Study; SLE, systemic lupus erythematosus.

History

A thorough history must be obtained, including a complete and detailed family history that may provide some clues to the diagnosis of the patient's condition (Box 142-3).

Physical Examination

A complete physical examination is required. Height and weight must be measured accurately, and the result must be plotted in the

---

Box 142-3. Questions

- Does the child have
  — Abnormalities on prenatal ultrasound such as hydronephrosis or polyhydramnios/oligohydramnios?
  — A history of prolonged illness, pallor, weakness, vomiting, or loss of appetite?
  — Any history of headaches or visual or hearing problems?
  — Any history of hematuria, proteinuria (foamy or bubbling urine), urinary tract infections, or episodes of fever with unknown source?
  — Impaired growth or development compared with siblings and other children?
  — Any problems with micturition, such as dribbling or weak stream?
  — Polyuria or polydipsia?
  — Daytime or nighttime enuresis?

  If so, what was the age at presentation?

- Does any family member have
  — Any kidney diseases (including hematuria, proteinuria, kidney cysts, urinary tract infections) or have they undergone any urology surgery?
  — Need of dialysis or kidney transplantation?
  — History of ear/hearing or eye abnormalities?

---

same growth curve as in healthy children. The weight can be overestimated if fluid retention is present. Blood pressure, using the appropriate cuff size, must be taken by the primary physician. Blood pressure must be compared with 50th percentile for age, gender, and height (www.nhlbi.nih.gov). The presence of tachycardia, heart murmurs, or adventitious heart sounds that may indicate uncompensated anemia or cardiac or pericardial involvement must be noted. Gross eye examination should be performed, including fundal examination, to assess for evidence of chronic hypertension. In addition, macular abnormalities and hearing problems may provide clues to a heritable disease (eg, Alport syndrome). Any ear abnormalities (eg, preauricular pits or ear tags) accompanied by hearing deficits are usually associated with some form of renal disease (eg, BOR). Undescended testes may be evident in some children with urogenital problems.

Laboratory Tests

For the initial laboratory workup, complete blood cell count, electrolytes, blood urea nitrogen, creatinine, calcium, phosphorus, and urinalysis must be obtained (Figure 142-2). Glomerulonephritis usually presents with numerous red blood cells, white blood cells, proteinuria, and a variety of casts in the urine. In cases of proteinuria, if a 24-hour collection is impossible, quantified excretion should be estimated by a protein-creatinine ratio in a spot urine sample. A ratio greater than 0.2 is abnormal and is well correlated with urinary protein excretion greater than 4 mg/m²/hour in a 24-hour urine collection. In nephrotic syndrome, the proteinuria is usually greater than 40 mg/m²/hour. Immunologic studies including C_3, C_4, antinuclear antibody, and anti–double-stranded DNA, as well as a minimal infectious evaluation (hepatitis B and C), should be obtained if the

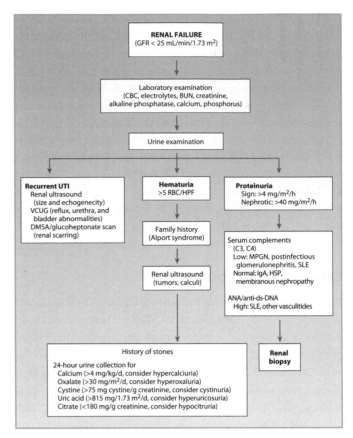

Figure 142-2. Initial diagnostic workup of a pediatric patient with chronic renal failure. ANA, antinuclear antibodies; ds, double-stranded; BUN, blood urea nitrogen; CBC, complete blood cell count; DMSA, dimercaptosuccinic acid; GFR, glomerular filtration rate; HPF, high-power field; HSP, Henoch-Schönlein purpura; IgA, immunoglobulin A; MPGN, membranoproliferative glomerulonephritis; RBC, red blood cell; SLE, systemic lupus erythematosus; UTI, urinary tract infection; VCUG, voiding cystourethrogram.

renal disease suggests the presence of an immune complex–mediated nephritis (eg, systemic lupus erythematosus, post-infectious glomerulonephritis, or membranoproliferative glomerulonephritis).

Imaging Studies

Ultrasound is by far one of the best radiographic tools in the assessment of patients with CKD. Renal ultrasound yields important information (eg, kidney size, echogenicity, presence of hydronephrosis, cysts or stones) that may help establish the diagnosis of the renal disease. The presence of small kidneys usually indicates chronic disease that may date back to fetal development. Increased echogenicity with normal kidney size indicates the presence of medical renal disease in more than 90% of cases.

A **voiding cystourethrogram** (VCUG) is indicated in patients with recurrent UTIs in order to diagnose vesicoureteral reflux and evaluate the anatomy of the upper urinary tract. The use of the spiral CT scan in the evaluation of patients with renal failure has increased over the last few years. This procedure requires relatively less time than the standard CT scan and can be used to evaluate the kidney parenchyma, and the upper and lower urinary tract.

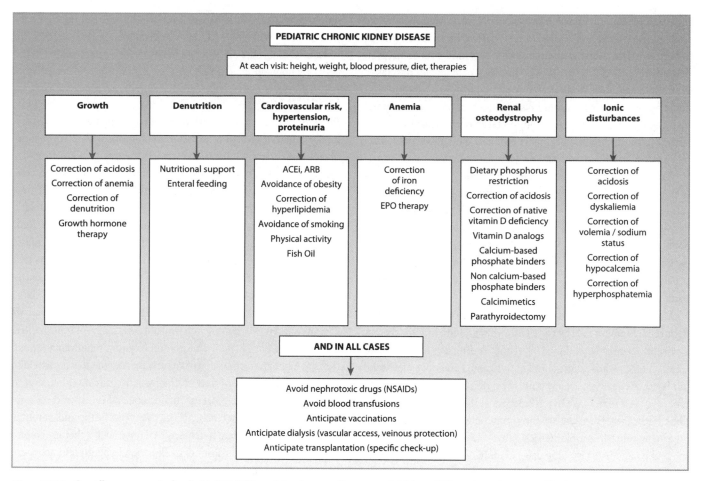

Figure 142-3. Overall management of pediatric CKD. ACEi, angiotensin converting enzyme inhibitors; ARB: angiotensin receptor blockers, sartans; EPO: erythropoetin; NSAIDs: non steroidal anti-inflammatory drugs.

Nuclear imaging of the kidneys has provided vital information in the workup of children with CKD. In general, nuclear studies are not routinely done unless specifically indicated. In some centers, the technetium (Tc)-99m-mercaptoacetyltriglycene is being used to evaluate the renal plasma flow, whereas Tc-99m-dimercaptosuccinic acid is currently done to assess renal parenchymal involvement in both acute pyelonephritis and recurrent UTIs. This nuclear imaging study provides an excellent image of the renal parenchyma, and is frequently used in the detection of renal scars in patients with recurrent UTIs. Significant renal parenchymal scars portend the development of hypertension later in life.

Management

The management of children with CKD has markedly improved over the last 2 decades and it is summarized in Figure 142-3. Newer modes of treatment and early intervention have made great improvements in the lifestyles and psychological well-being of affected children. These patients must be managed by a multidisciplinary team involving the primary care physician and nephrologists, nurses, social services, nutritionists, and psychologists. Such management includes the treatment of the primary disease and comorbid conditions, an optimization of growth, a slowing of the progression, a preservation of the residual renal function, a prevention of CKD-MBD

and CVD, as well as the preparation for renal replacement therapy and renal transplantation as CKD progresses. Available measures to retard the progression toward ESRD and cardiovascular mortality include strict control of hypertension; prevention of obesity; control of proteinuria with ACE inhibitors or ARB administration; control of serum calcium/phosphorus/PTH levels; and prompt control of infections, anemia, and hyperlipidemia.

Malnutrition; Metabolic and Water/Electrolyte Abnormalities

Dietary management remains an important and challenging part in the overall management of children with CKD. Frequently, these children are anorectic and require supplementation with fat, carbohydrates, and protein. Some patients, especially younger children, may require enteral feeding by nasogastric or gastrostomy tube in order to meet their daily nutritional requirements. A strict follow-up of nutritional status may therefore be performed at each visit, with a measurement of height and body weight; in children younger than 3 years, the cranial perimeter will also be measured and the brachial/cranial perimeter ratio will be calculated.

Children with CKD should receive the recommended daily allowance for protein and calories according to age and gender; adjustments need to be made depending on weight gain. Protein restriction is not advised; studies have shown that restriction of protein intake does not retard the progression of renal failure in these patients. In patients with hypertension, appropriate salt intake must be given but infants and children with congenitally obstructed, dysplastic kidneys or nephronophtisis often have polyuria, salt wasting, and acidosis, thus requiring a sodium supplementation and an adapted hydration. Sodium chloride or sodium bicarbonate must be administered to these children, and their required daily fluid intake may be higher to maintain normal intravascular volume.

Oral base therapy should be used to maintain a bicarbonate level in plasma above 22 mEq/L in order to facilitate skeletal growth, as recommended by the National Kidney Foundation Disease Outcome Quality Initiative guidelines since metabolic acidosis can have many deleterious effects (eg, worsening of bone disease and growth retardation, increased muscle wasting, decreased albumin synthesis, resistance to insulin, stimulation of inflammation, and eventually increased global mortality).

Most children with CKD do not become hyperkalemic unless their renal function falls below 10 mL/min/1.73 m². Initially dietary intervention may be sufficient, but this is difficult in infants and small children whose diet is limited to formula and only a few solid foods. Pharmacologic interventions (eg, diuretics, polystyrene sulfone) are used to manage **hyperkalemia** in these children. In situations where there is an acute rise in serum potassium level, emergent measures must be implemented (Box 142-4). Intravenous and inhaled β₂-agonists (eg, albuterol) acutely decrease serum potassium level by facilitating intracellular potassium uptake. If hyperkalemia is unresponsive to conservative medical measures, dialysis must be performed immediately. The use of a diuretic may be indicated in cases of fluid overload and hyperkalemia (potassium-sparing diuretics such as spironolactone should not be used). Diuretic therapy should not be used in patients with disturbed concentrating and diluting mechanisms because some of these children may have polyuria and develop dehydration on diuretic therapy.

There is increasing concern regarding the management of **lipid disturbances** due to their role in the progression of CKD. At present, no recommendations have been made about the use of lipid-lowering agents in children with hypercholesterolemia and

hypertriglyceridemia because of reported liver and muscle toxicity associated with some of these medications. Further studies are warranted to test the efficacy and safety of these medications in the pediatric population.

Growth failure

Recombinant human growth hormone therapy has improved the management of growth retardation in children with CKD; recombinant human growth hormone (rhGH) therapy should be rapidly discussed in children with a statural height below the 5th percentile: the 2009 KDIGO international guidelines recommend that CKD stage II-VD children and adolescents with related height deficits should be treated with rhGH when additional growth is desired, after first addressing malnutrition and biochemical abnormalities of CKD-MBD. Several studies have demonstrated a positive effect of rhGH on linear growth but with variable results according to CKD stage at the initiation of rhGH: In the NAPRTCS database, a catch-up growth after rhGH therapy was observed in 27% of children with chronic renal insufficiency, 25% of transplanted children, and only 11% of children undergoing renal replacement therapy, highlighting the need of an early management of growth failure in pediatric CKD. Moreover, the response during the first year correlates with final height. Growth hormone administration is continued until the patient reaches the 50th percentile for mid-parental height or renal transplant is achieved. Of note, such a therapy is contraindicated in case of history of malignancy, hyperglycemia, hyperinsulinemia, or significant scoliosis.

A recent retrospective multi-center US study noted the under-prescription of rhGH therapy in pediatric CKD patients and reported that more than half of short CKD children did not receive rhGH. The most common reasons were family refusal, secondary severe hyperparathyroidism, and noncompliance; however, in up to 25% of cases, no evident rationale was determined. Of note, waiting for an insurance company approval induced a significant delay in the initiation of rhGH therapy in 18% of patients. Access to rhGH therapy should be a high priority. Newer treatment modalities, targeting preferentially growth hormone resistance (such as recombinant IGF1, recombinant IGFBP3 or IGFBP displacers for example) are under investigation for the treatment of growth retardation in pediatric patients with CKD.

CKD-MBD

For the management of renal osteodystrophy, dietary phosphorus restriction is reinforced in children with CKD but is generally not well followed because of unpalatability of food. Moreover, hidden phosphate intakes in processed food are usually not taken into account but are important. As such, calcium-containing phosphate-binding medications have become an integral part in the management of these patients. Aluminum-containing phosphate-binding agents are infrequently used today because of the risk of aluminum toxicity and should be avoided as first-line therapies. If used, precautions must be taken in children who are concomitantly treated with citrate-containing medications (eg, sodium citrate) because citrate

---

Box 142-4. Treatment of Hyperkalemia
• Calcium gluconate, 0.5 mL/kg of 10% solution, or calcium chloride, 0.2 mL/kg of 10% solution (intravenous [IV])
• Sodium bicarbonate, 2 mEq/kg/dose (IV)
• Glucose-insulin solution, 0.5 g/kg glucose with 0.25 U of insulin per gram of glucose (IV, monitor serum glucose closely)
• Diuretics (loop diuretics; do not use potassium-sparing diuretics): furosemide, 1 mg/kg/dose (IV)
• Polystyrene sulfonate (Kayexalate), 1 g/kg/dose orally (if awake) or rectally (do not use in patients with any gastrointestinal problems or anomalies)
• Dialysis (if hyperkalemia persists despite the above measures)

enhances the absorption of aluminum and, thus, enhances the risk for aluminum intoxication. Recent developments in the understanding of the interaction between vitamin D, PTH, and the calcium-sensing receptor have led to novel treatment modalities for patients with CKD. Vitamin D, in the form of calcitriol, alfacalcidol, and doxercalciferol, has been used in the treatment of children with CKD. Earlier studies with vitamin D therapy demonstrated increases in linear growth in children with CKD; however, recent studies have not shown the same findings. In addition, concerns about a more rapid deterioration of renal function have also been raised in these patients. The 2010 Cochrane meta-analysis emphasized the lack of evidence-based long-term data for the management of pediatric CKD-MBD; however, bone disease (as assessed by changes in PTH levels) was improved by all vitamin D preparations, without consistent differences between routes of administration (eg, oral versus intraperitoneal calcitriol), frequencies of administration (eg, daily versus intermittent), or types of vitamin D preparations. Moreover, although fewer episodes of hypercalcemia occurred in patients receiving the non-calcium phosphate binder such as sevelamer, it was not possible to draw other conclusions since other biochemical parameters were not different. However, sevelamer hydrochloride therapy led to a safe utilization of active vitamin D sterols in a randomized trial in children undergoing peritoneal dialysis. In contrast, a recent prospective study has shown that sevelamer carbonate could be a safe and efficient phosphate binder with a better acid-base status in 24 pediatric dialysis patients. Such compounds have not been used in pediatric patients with CKD prior to dialysis; they should be used cautiously since their tolerance and efficacy in this pediatric population may be different than those observed in adults.

The use of large doses of calcium-based binders has been found to be associated with increased risk for vascular calcifications. To avoid these complications, certain biochemical markers including calcium, phosphorus, alkaline phosphatase, and PTH levels (intact assay, always in the same laboratory) must be followed closely in any child being treated with any vitamin D preparation and calcium-containing salts. The 2009 KDIGO guidelines recommend a serum PTH level within the normal range during CKD stage I–II, and between 2 to 9 times the upper normal levels of PTH in dialysis patients. Between 15 and 60 mL/min/1.73 m², the optimal level of PTH is not known; if PTH levels are above the normal range, serum calcium, phosphorus, and 25-OH vitamin D levels should be checked.

Last, 25-OH vitamin D deficiency should be regularly ruled out. Indeed, vitamin D deficiency seems to be more and more prevalent worldwide, due to several combined factors (eg, decreased sunlight exposure, relative scarcity of vitamin D in occidental diets, lack of supplementation in vitamin D due to the current underestimation for recommended daily intake, increased body fat mass in populations) and current data demonstrated that optimal levels should be above 30 ng/mL (ie, 75 nmol/L). Vitamin D deficiency is highly prevalent in pediatric patients across the spectrum of CKD (between 40% and 80% of children), resulting from several factors such as low dietary intake, chronic illness, skin changes, and sometimes urinary losses in proteinuric patients.

Anemia

The use of recombinant human EPO in the anemia associated with CKD has become a standard of treatment. The correction of anemia results in improved appetite, increased physical activity and, more importantly, avoidance of the risks associated with blood transfusion. Prior to the availability of EPO, most patients received frequent blood transfusions, increasing their risks of infection, transfusion reaction, and development of antibodies. The goal is to keep the hemoglobin between 11 to 12 g/dL. Iron stores are assessed by transferrin saturation and ferritin levels and should be maintained between 20% to 50%, and 200 to 800 ng/mL, respectively. With the description of the hepcidin pathway and the better understanding of the pathophysiology of anemia, new therapeutic modalities will probably be available in the future to improve the management of anemia during pediatric CKD, such as prolylhydroxylase inhibitors, EPO-receptor agonists (hematide), oxygen-carrier products, or GATA-inhibitors.

Arterial Hypertension

For chronic management, antihypertensive medications should be started in children if blood pressure levels are above age-matched controls and after failure of conservative therapy, such as dietary changes. Drugs currently used to treat hypertension in children with CKD include ACE inhibitors, diuretics, adrenergic blockers, peripheral vasodilators, and calcium channel blockers. As mentioned previously, treatment with ACE inhibitors has been shown to be beneficial in reducing the degree of proteinuria and, thus, decreasing the associated hyperfiltration and tubulointerstitial fibrosis associated with hyperfiltration. Caution must be exercised when ACE inhibitors are used in patients with a solitary kidney and in those with renal artery stenosis because these medications can acutely decrease kidney function and precipitate hyperkalemia in patients with renal failure. Sexually active adolescent females must be informed about the adverse effects of ACE inhibitors in pregnancy, including renal tubular dysgenesis in the fetus. Calcium channel blockers, especially nifedipine, have been used in cases of severe hypertension because of their rapid onset of action. However, great caution must be exercised because blood pressure may acutely decline in these patients. For patients with poor adherence to daily oral medications, clonidine is currently available in the form of transdermal patches. However, patients should be warned of rebound hypertension and central nervous system side effects if the patch is removed abruptly. Patients with long-standing hypertension must have regular ECGs to evaluate left ventricular hypertrophy, and serial ophthalmologic examinations to follow eye-ground changes. If hypertension is secondary to fluid overload and salt retention, aggressive fluid removal with diuretic therapy should be added. Pericarditis, however, is usually a manifestation of severe uremia and may require pericardiocentesis. In some instances, the lack of response to medical management may be used as an additional criterion for the initiation of dialysis therapy (Box 142-5).

Box 142-5. Indications for Initiation of Dialysis

Severe fluid overload
- Congestive heart failure
- Uncontrollable hypertension

Uremic neuropathy
- Paresthesia

Electrolyte abnormalities unresponsive to medical management
- Intractable metabolic acidosis
- Hyperkalemia

Pericarditis

Severe renal osteodystrophy
- Extra-skeletal calcification
- Severe skeletal deformities

Progressive malnutrition and severe growth retardation, especially in the first year of life

Severe anemia or bleeding diathesis

General Measures

In all cases, anticipation for dialysis and/or transplantation should be performed early in the course of CKD since it will be a life-long condition in these children, with probably both dialysis and transplantation periods, an early protection of the veins is required: Parents and nurses must be warned to avoid blood samples at the elbow, and to use the hand. Additionally, blood transfusions should be avoided as much as possible in order to avoid the development of hyper-immunization, potentially compromising a future transplant.

Children with CKD and their siblings and household contacts should receive all of the standard vaccines including varicella, influenza, and *Streptococcus pneumoniae*. Patients on immunosuppressive treatment due to glomerulonephritis or after transplant should not receive live-virus vaccines. Every attempt to administer live-virus vaccines such as measles, mumps, rubella, and varicella should be done before transplantation. Because children with CKD have a decreased ability to mount an immunologic response, repeated vaccination in order to induce protective serum antibody titers may be needed in dialyzed patients.

A review of all medications should be performed at every visit in order to adjust the dosages according to kidney function, detect possible adverse effects on the progression of the disease, and identify any drug interaction. Monitoring therapeutic dosage may be desirable when using antibiotics, anticonvulsants, digoxin, theophylline, and anticoagulants. In patients with reduced GFR, maintenance doses can be adjusted by increasing the interval between doses, reducing the individual dose, or both. Special care should be taken when using antibiotics such as aminoglycosides and vancomycin, as well as nonsteroidal anti-inflammatory drugs (NSAIDs), because of possible detrimental effects on residual kidney function, even in the early stages of CKD. Parents must be warned to avoid self-medication with NSAIDs.

Prognosis

The prognosis for children with CKD has changed in the last 2 decades. Options for dialysis (hemodialysis or peritoneal dialysis) and kidney transplantation (deceased or living-related donor) must be discussed prior to the occurrence of ESRD. Strategies such as pre-emptive transplantation (ie, transplantation before the need for dialysis) are probably preferred though may not be achievable because of the median time on the waiting list. Technical advances in dialysis allow the pediatric nephrologists to offer dialysis options to children of any age and have made long-term survival possible while children await renal transplantation.

Kidney transplantation is the ultimate treatment for children with CKD. Improvements in immunosuppressive medications and availability of other therapeutic strategies have considerably increased patient and graft survival after kidney transplantation. Full rehabilitation should be achieved after these children have undergone successful renal transplantation.

CASE RESOLUTION

The patient at the beginning of this chapter presents with a GFR of 30 mL/min/1.73 m² estimated by the 2009 Schwartz formula. The initial evaluation reveals hematocrit 28% (normal 36–48), a low serum bicarbonate (17 mEq/L, normal 22–26), hypocalcemia (8 mg/dL, normal 8.6–10), hyperphosphatemia (7 mg/dL, normal 2.7–4.5), and elevated PTH 700 pg/mL (normal 10–65). Diagnostic workup shows bilateral ureteral reflux on the VCUG. Small size and increased echogenicity of both kidneys are found on ultrasonography. Management of the primary disease is started with antibiotic prophylaxis to prevent further UTIs, and the patient is referred to pediatric urology. Measures to slow the progression to ESRD are initiated involving dietary intervention and treatment of comorbid conditions, including bicarbonate for metabolic acidosis, iron, and recombinant human EPO for anemia, and calcium carbonate as a phosphate binder/calcium supplement. The hypertension associated with proteinuria is best treated with an ACE inhibitor. Growth hormone will be considered once the acidosis, PTH, and anemia are corrected. Immunizations are up to date. An appointment with the pediatric nephrology team is scheduled.

Selected References

Boydstun II. Chronic kidney disease in adolescents. *Adolesc Med Clin.* 2005;16:185–199

Daschner M. Drug dosage in children with reduced renal function. *Pediatr Nephrol.* 2005;20:1675–1686

Geary, DF, Hodson, EM, Craig, JC. Interventions for bone disease in children with chronic kidney disease. *Cochrane Database Syst Rev.* 2010:CD008327

Hogg RJ, Furth S, Lemley KV, et al. National Kidney Foundation's Kidney Disease Outcomes Quality Initiative clinical practice guidelines for chronic kidney disease in children and adolescents: evaluation, classification, and stratification. *Pediatrics.* 2003;111:1416–1421

Juppner H, Wolf M, Salusky IB. FGF23: more than a regulator of renal phosphate handling? *J Bone Miner Res.* 2010 Epub

KDIGO. KDIGO clinical practice guideline for the diagnosis, evaluation, prevention, and treatment of chronic kidney disease-mineral and bone disorder (CKD-MBD). *Kidney Int.* 2009:S1–S130

Kuizon BD, Salusky IB. Growth retardation in children with chronic renal failure. *J Bone Miner Res.* 1999;14:1680–1690

Neuhaus TJ. Immunization in children with chronic renal failure: a practical approach. *Pediatr Nephrol.* 2004;19:1334–1339

Schwartz GJ, Munoz A, Schneider MF, et al. New equations to estimate GFR in children with CKD. *J Am Soc Nephrol.* 2009;20:629–637

Sedman A, Friedman A, Boineau F, Strife CF, Fine R. Nutritional management of the child with mild to moderate chronic renal failure. *J Pediatr.* 1996;129:S13–S18

Vimalachandra D, Hodson EM, Willis NS, Craig JC, Cowell C, Knight JF. Growth hormone for children with chronic kidney disease. *Cochrane Database Syst Rev.* 2006;(3):CD003264

CHAPTER 143

Diabetes Mellitus

Jennifer K. Yee, MD, and Catherine S. Mao, MD

CASE STUDY

A 7-year-old girl presents with a 3-week history of nocturnal polyuria. Her mother reports that her daughter seems to have lost weight in the past 2 months although she has had a good appetite. Laboratory tests reveal that the girl's serum sodium level is 130 mEq/L; potassium, 3.2 mEq/L; glucose, 324 mg/dL; and 1+ ketones. Urinalysis reveals specific gravity of 1.025 and moderate glucose and ketones. Her height and weight are slightly below normal for her age, and the remainder of her physical examination is unremarkable.

Questions

1. What is the pathophysiology of type 1 and type 2 diabetes?
2. What are diagnostic criteria for differentiating type 1 and type 2 diabetes?
3. What are the objectives of therapeutic interventions in children with diabetes?
4. What diagnostic evaluations are used in the ongoing management of diabetes?
5. What are the acute and chronic complications associated with diabetes?
6. What is the role of "tight glycemic control" in children and adolescents?

Diabetes mellitus is the second most common chronic illness after asthma among children in developed countries. Diabetes mellitus is a metabolic imbalance that results from insulin deficiency, impairment of insulin action, or both. Advancement in the knowledge about the pathophysiology supports the assessment that diabetes is a heterogeneous disease involving immunologic, environmental, and genetic factors. This has led to a categorization of diabetes based on its pathophysiology rather than the therapeutic intervention. Diabetes associated with absolute insulin deficiency and impaired beta cell function is called **type 1** (previously juvenile onset or insulin-dependent), and diabetes associated with insulin resistance as well as impaired beta cell function is called **type 2** (previously adult-onset or non–insulin-dependent).

Epidemiology

In the past more than 97% of children with diabetes presented with type 1 diabetes mellitus (DM1), with an overall incidence of 18 in 100,000 cases per year. Recently, 2 population-based studies showed a dramatic increase in the number of older children and adolescents presenting with type 2 diabetes mellitus (DM2). One study reviewed newly diagnosed cases of diabetes over a 12-year period and found that DM2 made up 4% of such cases before 1992 and 16% in 1994 in one Midwestern metropolitan area. Among adolescents, the relative incidence of DM2 increased from 3% to 10% before 1992 to 33% in 1994. By 1999 the proportion of diabetes in children and adolescents attributed to DM2 ranged from 8% to 45% depending on the geographic location. In addition, the populations affected by DM1 and DM2 seem to differ. Type 1 diabetes mellitus is seen equally among girls and boys, with the highest incidence among white youth. Type 2 diabetes mellitus is more prevalent among girls and has the highest incidence among African American, Mexican American, and Native American populations. The peak age of presentation for DM1 is between 5 and 15 years of age. Less is known about DM2 in children, but previous studies show a mean age of 13.8 years at presentation.

The SEARCH for Diabetes in Youth Study (SEARCH) is a population-based, observational study of physician diagnosed diabetes among youth younger than 20 years from 6 centers. The overall prevalence estimate for diabetes in children and adolescents was approximately 0.18%. Type 2 diabetes was found in all racial/ethnic groups but generally was less common than type 1, except in American Indian youth.

Clinical Presentation

Children can vary in their clinical presentation from being asymptomatic to having fulminate metabolic imbalance (Dx Box). Type 1 diabetes mellitus commonly presents with a classic triad of polydipsia, polyuria, and polyphagia. The most consistent presenting complaint is increased urinary frequency, manifested as nighttime polyuria or secondary enuresis. Alterations in appetite and thirst are most commonly recognized when disease onset occurs in the preschool years (probably because parents are most able to monitor eating and drinking behaviors during the first few years of life). Weight loss can be variable but is more common in DM1 than DM2. Diabetic ketoacidosis (DKA) occurs at the time of initial presentation in up to 45% in DM1 and 14% in DM2, and presents with vomiting,

Dx Diabetes Mellitus

- Symptoms (polydipsia, polyuria, and polyphagia) together with a random plasma glucose higher than 200 mg/dL
- Fasting blood glucose higher than 126 mg/dL (confirmed on a subsequent day)
- Oral glucose tolerance test with 2-hour peak plasma glucose higher than 200 mg/dL
- HbA1C ≥6.5%

polyuria, dehydration, and Kussmaul respirations. Children and adolescents with DM2 also report having the classic triad of symptoms, but are often identified through screening urinalysis. Type 2 diabetes mellitus is highly associated with obesity (body mass index ≥85th percentile [see Chapter 135]), acanthosis nigricans, and having a first-degree relative with DM2.

Pathophysiology

Patients with DM1 have an absolute insulin deficiency due to autoimmune destruction of the beta cells of the pancreas. The disease process is thought to be triggered by an environmental factor such as a virus or toxin in genetically susceptible individuals. The exposure occurs in early childhood, but disease progression can be variable. More than 90% of affected individuals carry either human leukocyte antigen (HLA) DR3 or DR4. Discordance of disease among twins supports the theory that DM1 involves an environmental exposure in genetically susceptible individuals. Twin studies show evidence of a preclinical autoimmune process, which also has predictive value in identifying susceptible individuals at risk for developing DM1. Immune changes include an increase in activated T-cells expressing HLA-DR, islet cell antibodies (ICA), insulin autoantibodies (IAA), and glutamic acid decarboxylase antibodies (GAD Ab) (Table 143-1).

Disordered immune function, in which some antigenic components of pancreatic islet cells are not recognized as self, seems to be the pathogenic mechanism for the development of DM1. It is generally believed that at least 90% of beta cell mass must be destroyed before problems with glycemic regulation are manifest. Endogenous insulin deficiency, occurring as a natural consequence of islet cell destruction, results in the inappropriate use of carbohydrate. Cellular uptake of glucose by liver, muscle, and adipose tissue is blocked. Synthesis of glycogen, protein, and fat is reduced, and a catabolic state marked by lipolysis, proteolysis, and ketone body formation ensues. Increased serum glucose and ketones present an overwhelming osmotic load to the kidneys, resulting in urinary losses of volume and cations (Na^+, K^+, NH_4).

The autoimmune phenomena described previously are not evident in DM2 as demonstrated by the absence of ICAs, IAA and GAD Ab. This disease, which is characterized by resistance to insulin, may assume different presentations in childhood. The more traditional form of DM2 presents in older children and adolescents and is highly associated with obesity and having a first-degree relative with DM2.

Immunologic Marker(s)	Risk of Developing DM1 (Within 5–8 y)
Islet cell antibodies (ICA)	25%–70%
Anti-glutemic acid decarboxylase antibodies	68% among siblings of DM1 proband and 50% in the general population
IA-2A	58% among siblings of DM1 proband and 43% in the general population
Insulin autoantibodies (IAA)	Variable (may not be specific to islet cell tissue)
Reduced first-phase insulin release	100%
ICA and IAA	90%
Human leukocyte antigen with index case	25%–30%

Table 143-1. Predictive Tests for Individuals Susceptible to Type 1 Diabetes Mellitus (DM1)[a]

[a] Individuals with first-degree relative with type 1 diabetes.

Differential Diagnosis

The diagnosis is usually straightforward given the symptomatology, except in children who present at a very young age. Although the onset of diabetes is rare before 1 year of age, the disease does occur but with nonspecific symptoms (eg, irritability, vomiting, tachypnea, and poor weight gain). When diabetes presents before 1 year of age, monogenic causes of diabetes needs to be considered. Chemotherapeutic agents (eg, L-asparaginase) and a variety of medications (eg, corticosteroids, diuretics, oral contraceptives, diphenylhydantoin, epinephrine) may induce glucose intolerance. Glycosuria without evidence of ketosis or elevated blood glucose occurs in certain renal conditions (eg, Fanconi syndrome, carbohydrate malabsorption syndromes, heavy metal intoxication). Transient hyperglycemia, with or without glycosuria, may occur in response to physiological stress (eg, burns, trauma, hyperosmolar dehydration). In most of these cases, glucose regulation returns to normal within several days.

Evaluation

Evaluation should focus both on the diagnosis of diabetes (hyperglycemia) and the category because DM1 or DM2 can have different treatment modalities and disease courses.

History

The history should focus both on classic symptomatology and whether there is a family history of diabetes. Up to 80% of youth with DM2 will report a positive family history of diabetes, compared with 20% of youth with DM1. In addition, exogenous causes of diabetes should be ruled out. Obtaining a history of viral infections or chemical exposures during early childhood may be useful (Questions Box).

Questions

Insulin-Dependent Diabetes Mellitus

- Is the child having increased urination (eg, nighttime urination, unusual bedwetting)?
- Is the child drinking or eating more than usual?
- Has the child experienced any weight loss?
- Has the child been taking or had access to any kind of medications (eg, corticosteroids, L-asparaginase, diuretics ["water pills"], birth control pills)?
- Are there any family members with diabetes (first- or second-degree relatives)?

Physical Examination

Growth parameters should be measured and plotted on standard growth curves. Obesity is present in 96% of DM2 youth, compared with 24% of DM1 youth. Even when obese, patients with diabetes may lose weight at the time of presentation. Youth with uncomplicated DM1 may have an unrevealing physical examination, while those with DM2 may have physical findings associated with obesity. One study demonstrated that 60% of adolescents with DM2 had acanthosis nigricans and 32% had hypertension at presentation. An intercurrent infection may trigger the symptomatology and should always be sought in cases of ketoacidosis. Children who present with ketoacidosis may have evidence of vomiting, dehydration, Kussmaul respirations and, in severe cases, altered mental status.

Laboratory Tests

Initial laboratory tests should include evaluation of the serum and urine for glucose and ketones. For patients presenting in DKA, evaluation should also include a full chemistry panel to assess for metabolic acidosis, hypokalemia, and serum osmolality. Once the diagnosis of diabetes is suspected, further testing can assist in categorizing the type of diabetes. Tests include insulin levels and C-peptide (a marker of insulin levels) levels. Both insulin and C-peptide levels are usually higher in patients with DM2 because they have insulin resistance rather than an absolute insulin deficiency. Insulin reserve can be measured by determining the basal and stimulated levels of C-peptide (>0.6 ng/mL basal level, >1.5 ng/mL 90 minutes after nutritional supplement such as Sustacal). In categorizing diabetes, it is important to note that some with DM1 can have insulin reserves up to 2 years after diagnosis.

Oral glucose tolerance tests may be necessary to confirm the diagnosis of diabetes in cases in which the onset of symptoms is not obvious. Two-hour postprandial values in excess of 200 mg/dL or fasting glucose of 126 mg/dL or higher are evidence of diabetes. The introduction of the intravenous glucose tolerance test with measurement of first-phase insulin release has allowed early diagnosis of individuals at risk for the disease prior to development of symptoms.

To assess children who are at risk for DM2, screening may be done every 2 years starting at age 10 years or at the onset of puberty (whichever comes first) and may be done using fasting plasma glucose (as recommended by the American Diabetes Association) and/or by oral glucose tolerance test (as recommended by the World Health Organization). The children who should be screened are those who meet criteria for obesity and have 2 or more of the following risk factors: family history of DM2 in first- or second-degree relatives, at-risk race/ethnicity (African American, Asian/Pacific Islander, Native American, Hispanic), or associated signs and symptoms of insulin resistance (acanthosis nigricans, dyslipidemia, hypertension, polycystic ovarian syndrome).

Management

Early diagnosis together with a comprehensive program of education and aggressive management are essential to prevent acute and long-term complications. Long-term objectives of therapeutic intervention in children with diabetes are (1) to facilitate normal physical growth and psychological and sexual maturation, (2) to promote normoglycemia through regulation of glucose metabolism, (3) to prevent acute complications (ie, hypoglycemia, ketoacidosis), (4) to prevent or delay long-term sequelae, and (5) to accommodate physiological changes that alter therapeutic needs (eg, exercise, adolescence, intercurrent illness).

Effective management requires a multidisciplinary team of professionals skilled in handling the myriad issues that arise for families and children with diabetes. Most clinics specializing in the care of children with diabetes include a nurse educator, dietitian, social worker, psychologist or counselor, and a pediatric endocrinologist. In settings where such special care centers are available, the primary care physician serves as a key adjunct, underscoring the importance of ongoing patient–family involvement in disease management and ensuring optimal growth, development, and nutrition. In the absence of special care centers, the primary care physician assumes responsibility for all aspects of management, including the treatment of acute complications, monitoring compliance and control, and surveillance for long-term complications.

Effective therapeutic intervention is based on individual needs for energy, insulin, and exercise. A number of factors, including physical growth, insulin requirement, glycemic control, and activity level, influence those needs and must be assessed on a regular basis. For DM1, insulin therapy is the mainstay of management, whereas DM2 therapeutic options include weight control through diet and exercise (see Chapter 135), oral hypoglycemic agents, and insulin. Oral hypoglycemic agents can lower blood glucose by increasing insulin secretion, increasing insulin sensitivity, decreasing hepatic glucose output, or decreasing nutrient absorption. These agents include sulfonylureas and other insulin secretogogues, metformin, thiazolidinediones, and acarbose. While DM2 may initially be managed with exogenous insulin, metformin is the oral agent prescribed most often for DM2 in children and adolescents. A newer class of medication acts by an incretin effect and increases glucose-dependent insulin secretion. These medications include exenatide (administered by injection) and a drug that inhibits dipeptidyl-peptidase-4, thereby prolonging the effect of endogenous insulin release after a meal. Similar to most drugs for the treatment of DM2, these newer drugs do not have a pediatric indication.

Insulin

The purpose of insulin therapy is to enable children to approach normoglycemia in response to adequate amounts of food, insulin, and exercise. The amount of daily insulin required is dependent on the child's age, weight, and development. On average for DM1, children younger than 5 years require 0.6 to 0.8 U/kg, children between 5 to 11 years of age require 0.75 to 0.9 U/kg, and 12- to 18-year-olds require 0.8 to 1.5 U/kg in a 24-hour period. Within 3 to 4 months of diagnosis, most individuals experience a partial remission, or "honeymoon" phase, during which time their insulin requirements decline dramatically. Conversely, illness, anxiety, and adolescence (ie, pubertal changes) may cause the insulin requirement to increase. Even under conditions of increased need, reported daily insulin dosages in excess of 2 U/kg of body weight should stimulate investigations into patient compliance.

A number of insulin regimens currently in use take advantage of the variable onset of action of the different insulin preparations (Table 143-2). The new insulin analogs are monomers of insulin rather than insulin aggregates. They provide a rapid onset and a shorter duration of action. This allows for easier adjustment of insulin dose depending on the child's appetite because the injection can be given immediately before the meal. Children with newly diagnosed diabetes should use semisynthetic or recombinant human insulin preparations to minimize the possibility of allergic reactions. Any change in insulin preparation should be undertaken cautiously and only under medical supervision because brands vary in strength, purity, and glycemic response.

Morning hyperglycemia may result from 1 of 2 phenomena, which must be distinguished because the appropriate therapeutic responses are opposite. The **dawn phenomenon** probably involves

a nocturnal surge of growth hormone, resulting in hyperglycemia that is present during the night (2:00–4:00 am) and is sustained until morning. The treatment involves increasing the evening dose of intermediate-acting insulin or moving the evening insulin to bedtime. In the **Somogyi phenomenon,** morning glucose is high as a physiological response to nighttime hypoglycemia. Treatment of this condition requires decreasing the evening intermediate-acting insulin or increasing the carbohydrate content of a bedtime snack.

Adolescents require special consideration. The sexual maturation process occurs in the setting of relative insulin resistance, other hormonal alterations, and a burden of developmental tasks, which make glycemic control problematic at best. Daily insulin requirements may increase to 1.5 to 2 U/kg during adolescence, but return to prepubertal levels at the end of the teenage years. Particular efforts must be made to ensure physical and psychological growth in the context of these special tasks. Dietary manipulation and consideration of alternative (usually more intensive) insulin and monitoring regimens is critical for successful glycemic control during this challenging period.

External infusion pumps are not widely used in young children because of the danger of mechanical malfunction (leading to hypoglycemia or hyperglycemia). Their use may be considered, however, in children with unstable diabetes or severe, chronic, intercurrent illness.

Glucose Monitoring

Self-monitoring of glycemic response through the in-home assessment of blood glucose levels is critical to effective therapy. The introduction of reflectance meters (glucometers) has obviated the need for inaccurate, visually read strips of glucose-sensitive paper. Patients who are taking insulin should measure glucose 3 to 7 times daily. Most endocrinologists advocate testing before each meal and at bedtime during the first year after diagnosis. Testing may also be done at 2:00 am to test for hypoglycemia or hyperglycemia. Depending on the age of the child, an acceptable range for glycemic control is 80 to 150 mg/dL. Additional short-acting insulin may be given to correct for high blood glucose. Patients also need to monitor their urine for ketones whenever their blood glucose readings exceed 240 mg/dL.

Glycosylated hemoglobin (HbA$_{1C}$) measurements reflect glucose control over the preceding 2 to 3 months. The normal value is 4% to 6% of total hemoglobin. Glycosylated hemoglobin values less than 7% are excellent, between 7% to 8% are good, between 8% to 10% are average, and more than 10% are poor. The Diabetes Control and Complications Trial studied the effect of different levels of glycemic control on the complications of diabetes. Although the study only included pediatric patients 13 years or older, the study did show that patients with "tight glycemic control" had lower HbA$_{1C}$ levels and fewer long-term complications than patients not tightly controlled. Adolescents with tight glycemic control had a greater risk of hypoglycemic events than the control group, a fact that must be taken into consideration in determining the ideal glycemic control for a child. In general, tight glycemic control is not recommended for children younger than 5 years; for older children, glycemic control should be individually tailored. Whenever children's routines undergo dramatic change, stepped-up home monitoring and medical

Table 143-2. Commonly Used Insulin Preparations[a]

Type	Onset of Action	Duration of Effect
Rapid-acting analogs Lispro, aspart, glulisine	Within 15 min	<5 h
Short-acting Regular	Within 30 min	5–8 h
Intermediate-acting (zinc or protamine) Neutral protamine Hagedorn	1.5–2.5 h	18–24 h
Long-acting Glargine Detemir	70 min 1.5–2.5 h	22–24 h 20–24 h

[a] Twice-daily injections: Two-thirds of the total daily dose before breakfast made up of intermediate- and short-acting insulin in 2:1 ratio. One-third before dinner made up of intermediate- and short-acting insulin in 1:1 ratio.

Basal bolus: Intermediate-/long-acting insulin at bedtime with regular insulin or short-acting insulin analog before each meal.

consultation are advisable. Caution should be used in interpreting HbA$_{1C}$ values in infants and others in whom fetal hemoglobin or other hemoglobin variants are present because these hemoglobin variants may falsely elevate or lower the value of HbA$_{1C}$. Although compliance with intensive regimens is an indisputable challenge (particularly as responsibility for management shifts from parent to child), increasing evidence underscores the importance of tight glycemic control.

Nutrition

The timing, amount, and types of foods eaten for meals and snacks should be relatively consistent from one day to the next to match the relative constancy of the exogenous insulin. Daily caloric requirements should be distributed in the following way: carbohydrate, 50% to 55% (<10% in the form of sucrose); protein, 20% to 25%; and fat, 25% to 30% (6%–8% polyunsaturated, <10% saturated). The distribution of these calories should be approximately 25% for breakfast, 25% for lunch, 30% for dinner, and 20% for snacks. Snacks are an important part of the nutrition regimen for children with diabetes. Most nutritionists recommend 3 snacks for young children (between meals and at bedtime) and 2 for older children. Some investigators promote the ingestion of cornstarch at bedtime as a means of stabilizing the serum glucose. Dietary discipline is a tremendous challenge for many children. Introducing one change at a time may make such dietary manipulations more acceptable over the long run. In addition, establishing healthy eating habits requires availability of healthy choices in the child's environment. Cooperation from the school and home enhances the likelihood of a child developing healthy eating practices.

Carbohydrate counting is an important part of matching insulin requirements to nutritional intake. For patients on multiple daily insulin injection schedules, there is flexibility in tailoring each dose of insulin based on the carbohydrate content of each meal or snack. For patients on twice-daily insulin injection regimens, consistent carbohydrate content of the meals and snacks is important in maintaining blood glucose levels. Learning carbohydrate counting takes time for the patient and families, and they need ongoing nutrition support to become familiar and comfortable with how different foods affect their blood glucose levels.

Exercise

Exercise contributes to glucose control by facilitating the use of glucose without the assistance of insulin. If not carefully undertaken on a regular basis, exercise can precipitate acute hypoglycemia. Physical activity enhances the body's sensitivity to insulin and can even decrease the daily insulin requirement. Thoughtful planning of exercise involves compensatory changes in food intake and insulin doses. For example, extra energy intake at bedtime may offset the nighttime hypoglycemia that accompanies late afternoon exercise. Seasonal physical activities may necessitate an adjustment in the insulin regimen at certain times of the year.

Education

The role of education is pivotal to the successful management of diabetes in childhood and throughout life. During childhood, educational efforts must be focused on the entire family unit. Affected children must be involved as early as possible and in ways that are developmentally appropriate. The process should involve the early introduction of basic survival information, such as insulin therapy and management of complications. This can be followed by more detailed information, including strategies to reduce long-term sequelae.

Prognosis

Diabetic ketoacidosis is the major cause of morbidity and mortality in children and adolescents, followed by **hypoglycemia.** Clinical signs of hypoglycemia in older children include shakiness, blurred vision, and dysarthria. Concerns about the neurodevelopmental impact of hypoglycemia in young children have led to the recommendation of more liberal glycemic control in early onset disease. Diabetic ketoacidosis, precipitated by an intercurrent infection or poor compliance, is a metabolic derangement that always requires urgent medical attention and often necessitates hospitalization. Replacement of fluids, attention to electrolyte abnormalities, and insulin therapy are the mainstays of treatment in the face of this complication.

There has been an increase in the number of pediatric patients presenting with hyperglycemic hyperosmolar syndrome (HHS). Since the treatment of HHS is different from DKA, the clinician needs to be aware of this entity. In fact the treatment for children with HHS may be different than the treatment of this disorder in adults.

Long-term complications include **proliferative retinopathy, nephropathy, peripheral and autonomic neurologic impairment,** and **early onset of cardiovascular disease.** Ophthalmologic evaluation, overnight urine protein measurement, and a detailed neurologic examination should occur once or twice each year depending on the duration of disease. Intensive therapeutic intervention results in significant reduction in retinopathy, nephropathy, and cardiac and peripheral vascular disease. Preliminary evidence warrants consideration of such therapy with the expectation of benefit in long-term outcomes.

CASE RESOLUTION

The girl in the opening case history is admitted to the hospital to help determine appropriate insulin dosing. She and her family require ongoing education. Careful management is necessary to optimize normal growth and development as well as delay or prevent long-term sequelae.

Selected References

Fagot-Campagna A, Saaddine JB, Engelgau MM. Is testing children for type 2 diabetes a lost battle? *Diabetes Care.* 2000;23:1442–1443

Fellar LA, Schrader K, Nansel TR. Healthy eating practices: perceptions, facilitators, and barriers among youth with diabetes. *Diabetes Educ.* 2007;33:671–679

Hannon TS, Gunfor N, Arslanian S. Type 2 diabetes in children and adolescents: a review for the primary care provider. *Pediatr Ann.* 2006;35:880–887

Kaufman FR. Type 2 diabetes in children and youth. *Endocrinol Metab Clin North Am.* 2005;34:659–676

Leslie RDG, Elliott RB. Early environmental events as a cause of IDDM: evidence and implications. *Diabetes.* 1994;43:843–850

Libman I, Arslanian S. Prevention and treatment of type 2 diabetes in youth. *Horm Res.* 2007;67:22–34

Mohamadi A, Clark LM, Lipkin PH, Mahone EM, Wodka EL, Plotnick LP. Medical and developmental impact of transition from subcutaneous insulin to oral glyburide in a 15-yr-old boy with neonatal diabetes mellitus and intermediate DEND syndrome: extending the age of KCNJ11 mutation testing in neonatal DM. *Pediatric Diabetes.* 2010; 11:203–207

Pinhas-Hamiel O, Zeitler P. Acute and chronic complications of type 2 diabetes mellitus in children and adolescents. *Lancet.* 2007;369:1823–1831

Pinhas-Hamiel O, Zeitler P. The global spread of type 2 diabetes mellitus in children and adolescents. *J Pediatr.* 2005;146:693–700

Report of the Expert Committee on the Diagnosis and Classification of Diabetes Mellitus. *Diabetes Care.* 1997;20:1183–1197

Scott CR, Smith JM, Cradock MM, Pihoker C. Characteristics of youth-onset noninsulin-dependent diabetes mellitus and insulin-dependent diabetes mellitus at diagnosis. *Pediatrics.* 1997;100:84–91

SEARCH for Diabetes in Youth Study Group. the burden of diabetes mellitus among US youth: prevalence estimates from the SEARCH for Diabetes in Youth Study. *Pediatrics.* 2006;118:1510–1518

Siljander HT, Veijola R, Reunanen A, Virtanen SM, Akerblom HK, Knip M. Prediction of type 1 diabetes among siblings of affected children and in the general population. *Diabetologia.* 2007;50:2272–2275

Silverstein J, Klingensmith G, Copeland K, et al. Care of children and adolescents with type 1 diabetes: a statement of the American Diabetes Association. *Diabetes Care.* 2005;28:186–212

Tamborlane WV, Ahern J. Implications and results of the diabetes control and complications trial. *Pediatr Clin North Am.* 1997;44:285–300

Tamborlane WV, Bonfig W, Boland E. Recent advances in treatment of youth with type 1 diabetes: better care through technology. *Diabet Med.* 2001;18:864–870

Zeitler P, Haqq A, Rosenbloom A, Glaser N for the Drugs and Therapeutics Committee of the Lawson Wilkins Pediatric Endocrine Society. Hyperglycemic hyperosmolar syndrome in children: pathophysiological considerations and suggested guidelines for treatment. *J Pediatr.* 2011;158:9–14

CHAPTER 144

Juvenile Idiopathic Arthritis/ Collagen Vascular Disease

Elizabeth A. Edgerton, MD, MPH

CASE STUDY

A 4-year-old girl is evaluated for pain in the legs and arms for 4 months' duration. Symptoms began with pain and swelling in the left elbow. Initially she was diagnosed with a bad sprain and was treated with a course of nonsteroidal anti-inflammatory drugs. The elbow improved, but it still caused occasional discomfort. About 2 months ago, the child was evaluated for painful knees and was diagnosed with growing pains. She has had no history of trauma, fevers, or rashes, but her activity level has decreased since the symptoms began. The mother has noted swelling in all 3 of the joints at one time or another but reports no redness. On physical examination the vital signs are normal. Both knees are swollen but not erythematous. Her range of motion in the knees and elbow is decreased.

Questions

1. What findings are indicative of juvenile idiopathic arthritis (JIA)?
2. How can the clinical history and laboratory evaluation assist in determining the subtype of juvenile idiopathic arthritis?
3. What are the long-term outcomes for patients with juvenile idiopathic arthritis?
4. What similar clinical findings are present in other collagen vascular diseases?
5. What types of agents are used in the treatment of juvenile idiopathic arthritis?

Collagen is a protein that represents 30% of the body's protein and is glue-like, shaping the structure of tendons, bones, and connective tissues. Malfunctioning of the immune system can affect these structures and result in what is termed *collagen vascular disease*. Diseases categorized as collagen vascular diseases include JIA, systemic lupus erythematosus (SLE), dermatomyositis (DM), and scleroderma (SD). While primarily known as collagen vascular diseases, they are also considered a subset of connective tissue disorders with a prominent immune component referred to as diffuse connective tissue diseases. They are also included in the category of secondary vasculitides.

An abnormal autoimmune reaction is common to all of these disorders, and it is not until specific vascular damage within an organ system occurs that more characteristic symptoms allow for diagnosis. Furthermore, the prevalence of these disorders is difficult to determine since their symptoms may overlap and no diagnostic gold standard exists. Each disease, though, has characteristic clinical presentations and serologic findings that guide in diagnosis. Treatment usually requires the use of anti-inflammatory and immunosuppressive therapy. Morbidity and mortality are dependent on the level and duration of inflammation, the target organs affected, and secondary complications that may arise from treatment.

Epidemiology

In JIA the predominant symptom is chronic arthritis that presents in children younger than 16 years. Juvenile idiopathic arthritis is the most common pediatric rheumatologic disease and one of the more common chronic diseases of childhood. The estimated worldwide incidence is 0.8 to 22 per 100,000 and the prevalence is 7 to 400 per 100,000 children. It is most prevalent among non-Hispanic whites. The International League of Associations for Rheumatology (ILAR) system is used for classification of the disease. Based on presenting symptoms, serology, age, gender, race, and/or ethnicity, the disease is divided into the following subtypes: oligoarthritis, polyarthritis, systemic, enthesitis-related, and psoriatic arthritis in decreasing frequency. Clinically, symptoms may change over time leading to a reclassification of a patient's subtype of JIA.

The incidence of SLE varies greatly by gender and ethnicity, with females and Hispanics, African Americans, Native Americans, and individuals from Southeast and South Asia most commonly affected. For individuals with onset before the age of 19 years, the incidence is approximately 6 to 18.9 per 100,000 among white females, 20 to 30 per 100,000 among African Americans females, and 16 to 36.7 per 100,000 among Puerto Rican females. The male-female ratio varies from 1:4 to 1:7 depending on the ethnicity of the cohort. Five- and 10-year survival rates have improved to as high as 100% and 86%, respectively, among pediatric patients. Survival is impacted by organ involvement, with those with renal and central nervous system (CNS) involvement fairing worse.

The incidence of juvenile DM (JDM) is 2.5 to 4.1 per million among children younger than 17 years. It is predominantly seen in white, non-Hispanic individuals (65%). Median age of presentation is 7 years of age, with girls affected more often. The clinical presentation and course of JDM is less severe than of adult-onset DM.

Overall, the annual incidence of systemic SD is 0.45 to 1.9 per 100,000 with a prevalence of 15 to 24 per 100,000. Scleroderma is very rare in childhood, with fewer than 10% of all patients younger than 20 years. While the adult-onset disease has a strong female predominance, gender and age specifics have not been identified in the juvenile form. Localized SD is 10-fold more common than systemic SD based on data from rheumatology referrals. Few epidemiological studies exist, but the overall prevalence of localized SD is estimated to be 1 in 100,000.

Clinical Presentation

Collagen vascular diseases may present with a variety of symptoms including joint pain or swelling, skin rashes, kidney disease, or neuropsychiatric problems depending on the specific disorder.

Differential Diagnosis

The differential diagnosis of collagen vascular diseases includes JIA, SLE, DM, and SD.

Dx Juvenile Idiopathic Arthritis

- Systemic: arthritis with daily fevers, rash, and general malaise
- Oligoarthritis: arthritis affecting 1 to 4 joints in the first 6 months
- Polyarthritis: arthritis affecting more than 5 joints in the first 6 months
- Enthesitis-related: arthritis and/or enthesitis and presence of human leukocyte antigen-B27
- Psoriatic: arthritis and psoriasis or arthritis and dactylitis, nail abnormalities, and family history of psoriasis

Juvenile Idiopathic Arthritis

The diagnosis of JIA is based on the clinical symptoms during the first 6 months following presentation (Dx Box).

The ILAR system of classification defines the following subtypes: systemic, oligoarthritis (persistent and extended) polyarthritis rheumatoid factor positive and negative, enthesitis-related arthritis, psoriatic arthritis, and other. Each subtype has varying clinical symptoms and long-term complications.

The **systemic form** is present in 10% to 20% of patients with JIA and is associated with the greatest morbidity and mortality. This subtype lacks gender, age, or human leukocyte antigen association seen among other subtypes. It is characterized by fever, rash, lymphadenopathy, hepatosplenomegaly, and serositis. The arthritis may present with or separate from these other symptoms. Classically the fever peaks twice a day and is associated with an evanescent rash that consists of discrete salmon-colored macules seen predominantly on the trunk and proximal extremities. The arthritis is polyarticular, affecting both large and small joints, and is present within the first 6 months of symptoms.

Up to 37% of patients develop chronic disease with destructive arthritis while the others may experience disease remission. Predictors of poor prognosis are age younger than 6 years at diagnosis, disease duration of more than 5 years, and persistence of systemic symptoms requiring treatment. Overall mortality is 0.3% in North America. A rare but life-threatening complication is macrophage activation syndrome. Patients present with hepatosplenomegaly, lymphadenopathy, and purpura and may progress to multiorgan failure. Sedimentation rate is low in macrophage activation syndrome in contrast to elevated during a disease exacerbation. Treatment involves steroids and immunosuppressive therapy. Triggers to macrophage activation syndrome include viral infections and addition or change in medications such as nonsteroidal anti-inflammatory drugs, sulfasalazine, and etanercept.

Oligoarticular JIA is the most common form. Arthritis is present in fewer than 5 joints during the first 6 months of disease. Often the large joints of the lower extremities are affected, and children may present with single joint involvement. Oligoarticular JIA is divided into persistent and extended forms, the latter associated with more severe disease course. Extended oligoarticular JIA can only be diagnosed after the first 6 months of symptoms in which patients suffer involvement of greater than 5 joints. Individuals, especially girls, who are antinuclear antibody (ANA)–positive have an increased risk of uveitis (asymptomatic). The American Academy of Pediatrics suggests frequent screening examinations because the uveitis can result in significant ophthalmologic morbidity. Among individuals with persistent oligoarticular JIA, 75% report remission of disease while only 12% of those with extended subtype report remission, with the remaining continuing to suffer symptoms into adulthood.

Polyarticular JIA presents with involvement of 5 or more joints during the first 6 months of disease. Rheumatoid factor (RF) negative disease is the more common subtype and tends to present in early childhood while RF positive disease presents later. Rheumatoid factor positive patients are often adolescent girls with symmetrical small joint disease and characteristic subcutaneous nodules. The arthritis is erosive and results in boutonniere deformities (proximal interphalangeal joint flexion and distal interphalangeal joint hyperextension) and swan-neck deformities (proximal interphalangeal joint hyperextension and distal interphalangeal joint flexion). Uveitis is present in approximately 10% of patients.

Enthesitis-related arthritis is characterized by inflammation where tendons insert at the bone. It usually affects the axial and peripheral skeleton. This subtype includes patients with ankylosing spondylitis and reactive arthritis associated with inflammatory bowel disease. Ankylosing spondylitis generally affects boys aged 8 years or older. This subtype is RF and ANA negative. Extra-articular symptoms include anterior uveitis, which is acute and painful in contrast to uveitis seen in oligoarticular and polyarticular arthritis, which is more insidious in onset.

Psoriatic JIA occurs in patients with chronic arthritis and psoriasis or those who meet 2 of the following criteria: dactylitis, nail pitting or onycholysis, and family history of psoriasis. Peak onset is in middle childhood. The arthritis, which is asymmetrical, may present before the psoriatic rash, making the diagnosis difficult. Up to 17% of patients will have asymptomatic uveitis and require routine slit-lamp examinations for diagnosis.

Systemic Lupus Erythematosus

Diagnosis of SLE is based on both clinical and laboratory findings and exclusion of other autoimmune diseases. Most patients have at least 4 of 11 of the American College of Rheumatology Classification Criteria for SLE. Criteria can be present over any period together or in isolation. Median age of presentation among pediatric patients is approximately 12 years of age. Patients usually present with constitutional symptoms such as fever, fatigue, weight loss, and systemic inflammation as demonstrated by lymphadenopathy and hepatosplenomegaly. The most common organs affected are skin and musculoskeletal and renal systems and their level of involvement directs treatment decisions.

A predominant feature of SLE is the rash. **Mucocutaneous involvement** includes classical malar rash or butterfly rash that spares the nasolabial folds, photosensitivity, and discoid rash. Approximately 10% to 30% of patients will have painless oral and nasal ulcers. Most patients also have some level of **musculoskeletal involvement** that includes arthritis, arthralgia, or tenosynovitis. The arthritis is usually a symmetrical polyarthritis affecting both small and large joints. In contrast to JIA, this arthritis is usually non-erosive as demonstrated radiographically, but clinically appears more painful. Musculoskeletal pain can be secondary to treatment resulting in what is called pain amplification syndrome attributed to glucocorticoid therapy.

Neuropsychiatric manifestations affect 20% to 70% of patients with SLE. This variation is due to the difficulty of diagnosing the often vague and varied symptoms. Headache is the most common symptom and can be isolated or be part of a constellation of other neurologic symptoms. Headaches that are refractory to treatment may be secondary to active CNS vasculitis, increased intracranial pressure, or cerebral vein thrombosis. Elevated levels of lupus anticoagulant (LAC) are usually present with cerebral vein thrombosis and are an indication for emergent imaging. Psychosis manifested by visual and tactile hallucinations may be present in 30% to 50% of patients. Psychotic symptoms will usually present with other neurologic symptoms. Imaging studies of the CNS provide little assistance in diagnosis. When psychosis is in isolation, secondary effects of glucocorticoids need to be considered. More difficult to delineate is cognitive impairment, which may present as a broad range of symptoms ranging from confusion and difficulty concentrating to coma. Other less common neurologic symptoms include seizures, movement disorders including chorea, and cranial nerve abnormalities.

Lupus nephritis is present in 29% to 80% of patients, with most presenting during the first year of diagnosis. In contrast, less than 10% of patients suffer from renal vasculitis. Prognosis for patients is based on the histologic classification of nephritis as established by the World Health Organization using renal biopsy (class I–V). Unfortunately, clinical markers (proteinuria, hematuria, creatinine level) may not correspond to histologic classifications, but when renal function is impaired patients have class III or IV disease. Hypertension is common along with lupus nephritis and, when present with peripheral edema, carries a worse prognosis. Overall survival for patients with renal involvement has improved. The 5-year survival for class IV is 88% to 93% and 10-year survival of 85%.

Hematologic manifestations including anemia, thrombocytopenia, and leukopenia may be present in 50% to 75% of patients. Patients have a normochromic normocytic anemia typical of anemia of chronic disease. Of patients who are Coombs positive, only 10% suffer significant hemolysis. Thrombocytopenia is present in 15% of patients. Patients with chronic autoimmune idiopathic thrombocytopenic purpura (AITP) with ANAs have a greater risk of developing SLE, as do patients with Evan syndrome (AITP and Coombs positive anemia). Leukopenia is thought to represent a general marker of disease activity.

Cardiac manifestations of SLE most often affect the pericardium. Patients suffering from pericarditis complain of chest pain exacerbated by positional changes. Up to 50% of patients have Libman-Sacks endocarditis, which results in sterile verrucous vegetations, putting them at risk for subacute bacterial endocarditis. The major cardiac mortality associated with SLE is premature arthrosclerosis; this is attributed to the chronic inflammation.

Pleuropulmonary disease is seen in 25% to 75% of patients with SLE. Again the variation in prevalence is due to the lack of specificity of symptoms. Pleuritic chest pain secondary to effusion can be a presenting symptom. Abnormal pulmonary function tests are common among asymptomatic patients. Patients can suffer acute respiratory failure secondary to SLE or opportunistic infection. **Gastrointestinal (GI) symptoms** are difficult to distinguish from the disease process versus adverse side effects of treatment. Abdominal pain can be secondary to peritoneal inflammation (serositis), vasculitis, pancreatitis, malabsorption, pseudo-obstruction, paralytic ileus, or direct bowel involvement (enteritis). **Endocrine abnormalities** can also be the result of the disease process or adverse effects of treatment. Hypothyroidism is associated with the presence of antithyroid antibodies while diabetes is secondary to steroid use. Delayed puberty and menstrual abnormalities are a consequence of chronic disease. Female patients managed with cyclophosphamide can suffer secondary ovarian failure.

Serologic presence of **ANA** is universal among patients with SLE. These include anti-DNA (60%–70%), anti-RNA–binding proteins (70%–90%), anti-U1RNP and anti-SM antibodies (40%–50%). Anti-Ro and La antibodies (30%) are seen less frequently.

Anticardiolipin (50%) and LAC (20%) are the most common antiphospholipid antibodies. The greatest risk of thrombosis is associated with LAC rather than with the other antiphospholipid antibodies.

Inflammatory Myopathies

Inflammatory myopathies are rare conditions in pediatrics but are discussed here because their symptoms overlap with other collagen vascular diseases. **Juvenile DM** is the most common myopathy presenting with rash and muscle weakness. It is a vasculopathy resulting from intimal proliferation of small blood vessels. Skin and muscle are the primary systems affected, but the vasculopathy can target any organ. **Juvenile polymyositis** is an idiopathic myositis without the dermatologic manifestations.

Patients present with proximal muscle weakness of the shoulders, hips, neck flexors, and abdominal musculature. Muscle tenderness and inflammation are less common. Patients can have both positive Gower (using one's hands to go from a supine to a standing position) and Trendelenburg (see Chapter 100) signs. Muscle weakness may also present with swallowing difficulties. When arthritis is present it is mild, transient, and non-erosive. As with other autoimmune diseases, fever, malaise, anorexia, and weight loss can be associated with disease activity.

Further diagnostic evaluation is essential in confirming the diagnosis of JDM. Muscle biopsy may show necrosis, atrophy, or inflammatory exudates. Electromyogram may or may not be abnormal. Evaluation of muscle enzymes often shows an elevated creatinine phosphokinase, aldolase, and/or lactate dehydrogenase.

The clinical course is varied, and multiple organ systems can be affected. Patients develop dystrophic calcinosis on the extremities. Although a characteristic finding of DM, it is usually not present at the time of diagnosis. Lipodystrophy, a progressive and symmetrical loss of subcutaneous fat, affects approximately 14% to 25% of patients. Patients may suffer esophageal dysmotility and malabsorption. Vasculopathy of the GI tract may result in pain, bleeding, or perforation. One-third of patients may have respiratory weakness during their disease course, primarily following an asymptomatic restrictive pattern. Up to 78% of patients have decreased ventilatory capacity. Although rare, patients are at increased risk of aspiration secondary to pharyngeal muscle weakness and to pneumonia secondary to immunosuppressive therapy.

Rash is critical for the diagnosis of DM and can occur prior to or after the presentation of muscle weakness. The heliotrope eyelid rash and Gottron papules are pathognomonic for DM. Eyelid or facial edema may be present with the rash, which may also have a malar component that includes nasolabial folds, in contrast to systemic lupus. Gottron papules or collodion patches are flat-topped, violaceous or red papules that can be scaly. They are seen predominantly on the extremities (extensor aspect of knuckles, elbows, knees, and medial malleoli). Nail bed changes demonstrating vasculopathy are also present. Neurologic symptoms are rare, but may present as generalized tonic-clonic seizures. Unlike adult-onset DM, malignancy is uncommon in juvenile DM.

Scleroderma

Juvenile SD is characterized by the presence of hard skin before age 16. Localized SD involves only the skin and related tissues while systemic SD is a multisystem autoimmune disorder.

In **systemic SD,** skin, musculoskeletal system, GI tract, lungs, and heart are the organs most commonly affected. While the skin and musculoskeletal systems are the most common among pediatric cases, disease complications of the cardiopulmonary system are associated with the greatest mortality.

The diagnosis of systemic SD is based on the presence of major criteria that include sclerosis and/or induration, sclerodactyly, or Raynaud phenomenon in addition to minor criteria of the targeted organ systems. Diagnosis is often delayed due to the slow onset of disease and the initial subtlety of symptoms. Characteristic presentation starts with Raynaud phenomenon with associated tightening, thinning, and atrophy of the skin overlying the hands and face. Cutaneous changes start with edema, followed by induration and finally sclerosis. The skin becomes tightened by contractures and atrophy, giving the appearance of being hard, waxy, and tight. There may be either hypopigmentation or hyperpigmentation, and deposits of calcium may appear in the subcutaneous skin.

Musculoskeletal symptoms are the next most common symptom among patients and usually occur near the onset of disease. Arthralgias are usually mild and transient. Patients may suffer joint contractures over the proximal interphalangeal joints and elbows. Muscle inflammation occurs in approximately 38% of pediatric cases.

Up to 40% of patients will eventually have upper GI involvement. Dysphasia is caused by esophageal dysmotility or gastroesophageal reflux. Half of patients suffer small bowel involvement. Functional tests demonstrate GI abnormalities even among asymptomatic patients. Similarly, patients may have pulmonary involvement as demonstrated by abnormal function but initially appear asymptomatic. As the disease progresses, patients develop dry, hacking cough with dyspnea on exertion. A rare but severe complication is interstitial pulmonary fibrosis. Cardiac involvement is less common but is the primary cause of morbidity. Cardiac fibrosis leads to conduction defects, arrhythmias, and impaired ventricular function. Aggressive immunosuppressive therapy is required when the cardiomyopathy is severe.

As with many of the collagen vascular diseases, patients will have ANA (80%). Approximately 20% to 30% of patients have Scl-70 (anti-topoisomerase I), in contrast to adult onset in which only 7% of patients have this antibody. Approximately 25% of pediatric patients will have blood indices consistent with the normocytic normochromic anemia of chronic disease.

Localized Scleroderma

Similar to systemic SD, **localized SD** is secondary to abnormalities of fibroblast regulation, collagen production, and autoimmune regulation. Localized SD predominantly affects the skin and only occasionally involves other organs. Localized SD is divided into 5 subtypes: plaque morphea, generalized morphea, bullous morphea, linear SD, and deep morphea. **Morphea** are areas of indurated, waxy skin with an ivory center and violaceous halo and are most commonly found on the trunk. When they become confluent they are classified as generalized morphea. **Linear SD** is the most common form of localized SD among children and adolescents. One or more linear streaks are present on the extremities. These cutaneous changes can extend into the subcutaneous tissue and muscle leading to significant deformities. Linear lesions on the face or head are referred to as *coup de saber* SD. Deep morphea involves subcutaneous morphea, eosinophilic fasciitis, and morphea profunda, in which the entire skin is thickened and feels bound down. This form is the least common and considered the most disabling.

The presence of extra-cutaneous involvement in cases of localized SD raises the controversial issue of whether localized SD can transition to systemic SD. Approximately 25% of patients with juvenile localized SD have extra-cutaneous involvement, most commonly articular. Diagnosis is based on clinical presentation and skin biopsy. Antinuclear antibodies and antihistone antibodies may be present. Approximately 13% of patients will have anticardiolipin antibodies, but unlike SLE their presence is not associated with thrombosis. Cosmetic appearance is often the focus of disease management. Systemic treatment is reserved primarily for subtypes with significant disability such as linear SD and deep morphea.

Pathophysiology

Autoimmune diseases result from an alteration in the selection, regulation, or death of T-cells or B-cells, which results in an abnormal response to a particular antigen. Genetic factors increase an individual's vulnerability but are not sufficient for disease expression. It is the interplay of environmental triggers and genetic susceptibility that leads to clinical manifestations. In JIA, the T-cell arm of the cell-dependent inflammation is best understood. It supports many of the clinical and biochemical factors into the subtypes of JIA. T cells are dependent on the major histocompatibility complex (MHC) to recognize an antigen. Human leukocyte antigen types that have been classically associated with certain subtypes of JIA play a role in the presentation of a specific antigen. Studies of synovial fluid in JIA patients demonstrate specific families, or cohorts, of T-cells depending on the subtype of JIA. Furthermore, each subtype of JIA has a specific T-cell response with key inflammatory mediators and secondary effects. Current theory suggests that JIA is linked to an antigen-specific response in the synovial fluid. Systemic lupus erythematosus is characterized by abnormal autoantibody production against nucleic acids, especially double-stranded DNA. The T-cell and B-cell receptor-signaling pathways may be abnormal, as well as have an abnormal clearance of self-antigens, resulting in autoactivation of lymphocytes. In SD, autoantibodies target topoisomerase, centromeric proteins, and RNA polymerases, resulting in dysregulated fibroblast activation. Over-expression of MHC I is a major component of inflammatory myopathies. Local injury of vessels and muscles results from complement-mediated immune response and soluble adhesion molecules.

The molecular understanding of JIA has increased greatly, providing insight to the disease process and leading to a new classification system for the disease. Juvenile idiopathic arthritis is the result of an inflammatory process in the synovial fluid of a joint. The inflammatory process consists of an innate inflammatory phase and a cell-dependent phase. Initially there is an egress of cells and proteins from the bloodstream. The inflammation progresses with migration of neutrophils and monocytes to the location of tissue injury. Cell-dependent inflammation involves both T-cells and B-cells. T-cells are dependent on MHC to recognize an antigen. Furthermore, each subtype of JIA has a specific T-cell response with key inflammatory mediators and secondary effects. While B-cells are known to play a role in the pathogenesis of JIA based on their presence in synovial fluid, their specific mechanisms of action are only hypothesized.

Evaluation

History

The history should clearly delineate the duration and the extent of the symptoms (Questions Box). Has there been joint involvement and, if so, which joints? Do the joints ache and are there also visible changes such as swelling and erythema? Are the symptoms more pronounced at specific times of the day, such as in the morning on arising? Has the patient experienced weakness? If so, which muscle groups are most affected? Has the patient had a rash? What is the nature and location of the rash? What other symptoms are present, such as headache, fever, fatigue, and weight loss?

> ## Questions
>
> ### Juvenile Idiopathic Arthritis/Collagen Vascular Disease
>
> - Has the child ever had any swelling, warmth, or redness of joints?
> - Does the child have difficulty walking or running? If so, does it occur at any particular time of the day?
> - Has the family noticed any type of skin rash or skin changes?
> - Has the child had any eye complaints?
> - Has the child had any recent illnesses such as gastroenteritis?
> - Has the child traveled recently or been bitten by a tick?

Physical Examination

Patients should undergo a complete physical examination that includes a full assessment of the skin, all joints, flexibility of the spine, the strength of the muscles, and a neuropsychiatric assessment. Lymphadenopathy should be noted as well as the presence of organomegaly. Patients suspected of having JIA should also undergo a slit lamp examination of the eyes.

Laboratory Tests

In general laboratory testing includes a complete blood cell count, erythrocyte sedimentation rate, C-reactive protein, urinalysis, and other studies as determined by the differential diagnosis. Evaluation of patients for JIA includes rheumatoid factor, ANAs, and complement. Patients suspected of having SLE should have an anti-DNA, anti-RNA–binding protein, anti-U1RNP and anti-SM antibodies, and complement analyzed. Electrocardiograms and echocardiograms are appropriate in patients with SLE suspected of having cardiac involvement. Patients suspected of inflammatory myopathies should have creatine phosphokinase, aldolase, and lactate dehydrogenase levels and possibly myositis specific antibodies. Electromyogram and muscle biopsy may also be undertaken to complete the evaluation.

Imaging Studies

Magnetic resonance imaging is playing a larger role in the diagnosis and management of JIA and JDM. For SLE patients with neuropsychiatric symptoms, computed tomography scans and magnetic resonance imaging are rarely abnormal.

Management

The management of collagen vascular diseases varies with the specific condition.

Juvenile Idiopathic Arthritis

The objective of treatment for JIA is to control pain and inflammation while preserving function and normal growth, development, and well-being. Physical and occupational therapy are essential to maintain function. Medications used for the treatment of JIA include nonsteroidal anti-inflammatory drugs (NSAIDs), disease-modifying antirheumatic drugs (DMARDs), and tumor necrosis factor inhibiting agents. Corticosteroids are reserved for patients with serious systemic manifestations and are not considered ideal for long-term use in JIA secondary to the side effects. Most patients respond to the various NSAIDS, although the time to respond may vary greatly. Only nonspecific cyclooxygenase inhibitors are approved for pediatric use. Individuals with persistent joint disease require DMARDs, with methotrexate being the most common. Clinical improvement may not be seen for 1 to 6 months, but eventually 70% of patients will respond. A recent controlled trial demonstrating early use of DMARDs was associated with improved long-term prognosis measured by improved health status and decrease use of DMARDs long term, suggesting that treating JIA early with DMARDs may be of benefit. The study also highlighted the poor compliance with medications. Gastrointestinal disturbances are the most commonly seen side effects, with hepatotoxicity being rare. Sulfasalazine is another DMARD that is especially effective in patients with enthesitis-related JIA. Etanercept is a biological agent that is a tumor necrosis factor receptor antagonist reserved for patients not responding to methotrexate.

Systemic Lupus Erythematosus

A multidisciplinary team is essential to care for patients with SLE. Specific therapies are tailored to the symptoms, severity, and level of response. Initial treatment of musculoskeletal symptoms, primarily arthritis, is with NSAIDs combined with an antimalarial drug such as hydroxychloroquine. Resistant symptoms may require steroids or methotrexate. Treatment of neuropsychiatric manifestations is based on symptoms and severity. These include steroids, immunosuppressive medications (azathioprine or cyclophosphamide), antiepileptics, and antidepressants. The treatment of renal manifestations is based on the histologic classification of renal involvement. Medications include steroids and immunosuppressive agents and may also include angiotensin-converting enzyme inhibitors to decrease proteinuria. In practice, patients at risk for thrombosis may be treated with low-dose aspirin, although not all studies support the efficacy.

Complications of treatment with glucocorticoid steroids include avascular necrosis of the femoral head, affecting approximately 10% of patients. Furthermore, patients are at increased risk for osteoporosis due to low calcium and vitamin D intake and diminished physical activity. A severe complication of SLE is antiphospholipid antibody syndrome with severe microangiopathic thrombolytic changes, resulting in thrombosis to multiple organs. It is primarily associated with elevated antibody levels of lupus anticoagulant. It can occur anywhere in the body and can be difficult to recognize. Although antiphospholipid antibodies can be present in patients with JIA, DM antiphospholipid antibody syndrome is rare.

Dermatomyositis

Methotrexate is the primary medication for treatment of DM. Corticosteroids are often used when initiating treatment due to the slow onset of clinical improvement with methotrexate. Methylprednisolone pulses, immunoglobulin intravenous, and cyclophosphamide are reserved for nonresponsive cases or severe exacerbations.

Systemic Scleroderma

As with other collagen vascular disease, the treatment of systemic SD focuses on optimal function and control of inflammation. Many of the medications used in SD lack rigorous evaluations regarding efficacy. Immunosuppressive agents that are often used include methotrexate, mycophenolate, and cyclophosphamide in severe cases. Glucosteroids are primarily effective for the inflammatory phase of muscle involvement or edematous phase of cutaneous disease. Vasodilator agents, especially calcium channel blockers, are used for symptomatic relief of Raynaud phenomenon. Few studies exist on the long-term survival of patients with juvenile systemic sclerosis. Clinically, as the skin tightens and contractures progress, the disease becomes extremely disabling. Cardiac, renal, and pulmonary disease progressions are most often responsible for premature death. The extent of sclerosis may be a prognostic factor.

Prognosis

Making the diagnosis of a collagen vascular disease requires a thorough history and physical examination, as well as a broad differential diagnosis. While there is no gold standard for diagnosing these diseases, each type has characteristic symptoms and laboratory findings as well as specific ages for presentation. Consultation with rheumatologists, neurologists, nephrologists, and infectious disease specialists may be required to assist in the final diagnosis.

Likewise, the care of a child with a collagen vascular disease also requires a multidisciplinary approach involving a primary care physician, rheumatologist, and subspecialists with expertise in affected target organs. The role for the primary care physician is to ensure optimal function of the patient as well as prevention of long-term disease and treatment sequelae. Because many of the agents used to manage collagen vascular disease have significant side effects, it is vital for the primary care physician to be well versed with a patient's medication regimen. Patients with collagen vascular disease often suffer from growth failure either from the disease process or its treatment. Ensuring appropriate diet and physical activity is vital. Supplementation with calcium and vitamin D is beneficial to prevent osteoporosis. Periodic ophthalmologic screening is essential for patients with uveitis. In the long term, patients with collagen vascular disease are at a higher risk for cardiovascular disease (CVD) secondary to chronic inflammation. They may require annual cardiovascular risk assessments that include lipid profiles. While pediatric patients often don't have other CVD risk factors, it is important to ensure healthy behaviors. Individuals that have suffered thrombolytic events or are at high risk for thrombosis may benefit from low-dose aspirin prophylaxis. As with any patient with a chronic disease, maintaining a feasible quality of life is essential. Disease management for patients suffering from collagen vascular disease is a balance of optimal function, minimal complications, and improved quality of life.

CASE RESOLUTION

The young girl in the case scenario has a presentation consistent with oligoarthritic JIA based on the number of involved joints (3 joints) and her age (between 1 and 5 years). She has a number of laboratory studies including a complete blood cell count, erythrocyte sedimentation rate, RF, and ANA. Her ANA is positive. She is referred to a pediatric ophthalmologist for an eye examination to determine if she has uveitis. She is also referred to a pediatric rheumatologist for assistance in managing her disease and a physical therapist to address her limitation of motion.

Selected References

Allen E, Farewell VT, Isenberg DA, Gordon C. A statistical analysis of the interrelationships between disease activity in different systems in systemic lupus erythematosus. *Rheumatology (Oxford)*. 2006;45:308–313

Amital H, Szekanecz Z, Szücs G, et al. Serum concentrations of 25-OH vitamin D in patients with systemic lupus erythematosus (SLE) are inversely related to disease activity: is it time to routinely supplement patients with SLE with vitamin D? *Ann Rheum Dis*. 2010;69(6):1155–1157

Benseler SM, Silverman ED. Systemic lupus erythematosus. *Pediatr Clin North Am*. 2005;52:443–467

Cassidy J, Kivlin J, Lindsley C, Nocton J; American Academy of Pediatrics Section on Rheumatology and Section on Ophthalmology. Ophthalmologic examinations in children with juvenile rheumatoid arthritis. *Pediatrics*. 2006;117:1843–1845

Christen-Zaech S, Hakim MD, Afsar FS, Paller AS. Pediatric morphea (localized scleroderma): review of 136 patients. *J Am Acad Dermatol*. 2008;59(3):385–396

Feldman BM, Rider LG, Reed AM, Pachman LM. Juvenile dermatomyositis and other idiopathic inflammatory myopathies of childhood. *Lancet*. 2008;371(9631):2201–2212

LeBovidge JS, Lavigne JV, Donenberg GR, Miller ML. Psychological adjustment of children and adolescents with chronic arthritis: a meta-analytic review. *J Pediatr Psychol*. 2003;28:29–39

Riise ØR, Handeland KS, Cvancarova M, et al. Incidence and characteristics of arthritis in Norwegian children: a population-based study. *Pediatrics*. 2008;121(2):e299–e306

Smith JA, Mackensen F, Sen HN, et al. Epidemiology and course of disease in childhood uveitis. *Ophthalmology*. 2009;116(8):1544–1551

Tseng CE, Buyon JP, Kim M, et al. The effect of moderate-dose corticosteroids in preventing severe flares in patients with serologically active, but clinically stable, systemic lupus erythematosus: findings of a prospective, randomized, double-blind, placebo-controlled trial. *Arthritis Rheum*. 2006;54:3623–3632

van Rossum MA, van Soesbergen RM, Boers M, et al. Long-term outcome of juvenile idiopathic arthritis following a placebo-controlled trial: sustained benefits of early sulfasalazine treatment. *Ann Rheum Dis*. 2007;66(11):1518–1524

Vastert SJ, Kuis W, Grom AA. Systemic JIA: new developments in the understanding of the pathophysiology and therapy. *Best Pract Res Clin Rheumatol*. 2009;23(5):655–664

Wedderburn LR, Rider LG. Juvenile dermatomyositis: new developments in pathogenesis, assessment and treatment. *Best Pract Res Clin Rheumatol*. 2009t;23(5):665–678

Weiss JE, Howite NT. Juvenile idiopathic arthritis. *Pediatr Clin North Am*. 2005;52:413–442

Zulian F. Systemic sclerosis and localized scleroderma in childhood. *Rheum Dis Clin North Am*. 2008;34(1):239–255

CHAPTER 145

Nephrotic Syndrome

Elaine S. Kamil, MD

CASE STUDY

A 2-year-old boy is brought to the office because of abdominal distention. He has just recovered from a runny nose that lasted a week, with no fever or change in activity. His mother complains that his eyelids were very swollen that morning, and she says that his thighs look "fat." She has noticed that he has fewer wet diapers. He has always been a healthy child, and his immunizations are up to date. The family has a history of asthma and allergic rhinitis. Physical examination shows an active 2-year-old boy. Head and neck examination is clear, except for a few shotty anterior cervical lymph nodes and some minimal periorbital edema. Chest examination reveals some decreased breath sounds at the bases. The abdomen is moderately distended; bowel sounds are active and a fluid wave is detectable. There is 2+ pitting edema of the lower legs, extending up to the knees. The urine has a specific gravity of 1.030; pH 6; 4+ protein; and trace, nonhemolyzed blood. Microscopic examination shows 4 to 6 red blood cells per high-power field and 10 to 20 hyaline and fine granular casts per low-power field.

Questions

1. What is the differential diagnosis of edema and ascites in previously healthy young children?
2. What criteria are used to determine if children with nephrotic syndrome require hospitalization or can be managed as outpatients?
3. What laboratory evaluation and therapy are instituted initially?
4. What are the important issues to address in parent education?
5. What is the prognosis of young children with nephrotic syndrome?

Although nephrotic syndrome is not a common childhood disease, every pediatrician can expect to care for 1 to 3 nephrotic children at some time. Nephrotic syndrome may have serious or even fatal complications, and the disease tends to follow a chronic, relapsing course. Thus it is important for the pediatrician to become familiar with the signs and symptoms of the disease and with the most current treatment modalities aimed at keeping affected children healthy and active.

Nephrotic syndrome occurs when an individual excretes a sufficient quantity of plasma proteins, primarily albumin, in the urine to cause hypoalbuminemia. Substantial urinary protein losses, hypercholesterolemia, and hypoalbuminemia characterize nephrotic syndrome. The condition is usually accompanied by obvious edema, but occasionally edema is not clinically detectable (Dx Box).

In children, proteinuria of more than 40 mg/m^2/hour (>50 mg/kg in 24 hours) is considered nephrotic range proteinuria. (In adult-sized patients, proteinuria of more than 3.5 g in 24 hours is associated with nephrotic syndrome.) Collection of a 24-hour urine sample is cumbersome in children, and the urinary total protein/creatinine ratio (U TP/CR) done on a random urine sample, preferably a first morning urine, is a useful alternative. Whereas a ratio greater than 3.5 is considered nephrotic range proteinuria in adults with normal renal function, a ratio greater than 1.0 is considered diagnostic in children (see Chapter 94). Twenty-four–hour urine protein losses (g/m^2/day) in children can be estimated by multiplying the U TP/CR by 0.63.

Epidemiology

Minimal change disease (MCD) is the most common form of nephrotic syndrome in childhood. The annual prevalence of new cases of nephrotic syndrome is 2 in 100,000 to 3 in 100,000 children in the population younger than 16 years. The cumulative prevalence of this chronic disease is 16 in 100,000. Ninety percent of childhood cases are not associated with any systemic disease, and two-thirds of cases of childhood nephrotic syndrome present before age 5 years. The ratio of boys to girls in young children with nephrotic syndrome is 2:1. By late adolescence, both sexes are equally affected.

Clinical Presentation

The typical child presenting with nephrotic syndrome is a preschool-aged boy who is brought to the physician because he appears swollen to the parents. Some children are active and relatively asymptomatic despite the edema, whereas others may be very uncomfortable, with

---

Dx Nephrotic Syndrome

- Heavy proteinuria (>40 mg/m^2/hour or 50 mg/kg/24 hours in children)
- Hypoalbuminemia
- Hypercholesterolemia
- Edema

markedly swollen eyelids, abdominal discomfort, scrotal or labial edema, and even respiratory compromise. Usually children have a history of preceding infection, most typically an upper respiratory infection (URI). Occasionally children develop diarrhea secondary to edema of the bowel wall.

Occasionally children with nephrosis are critically ill due to peritonitis, bacteremia, or (rarely) a major thrombotic episode. Because their immune state is compromised, rapid evaluation and treatment of children with these complications of nephrotic syndrome are essential for survival. The primary peritonitis associated with nephrotic syndrome may be confused with an acute abdomen, such as may be seen with appendicitis. Some children who are experiencing a severe relapse have hypotensive symptoms secondary to intravascular volume depletion.

Pathophysiology

The exact cause of MCD and focal segmental glomerulosclerosis (FSGS) is not known. Although this is controversial, many nephrologists believe that FSGS may result from severe, treatment-resistant MCD. The best current theory postulates that some stimulus (usually infectious) causes a clone of lymphocytes or monocytes to proliferate and produce one or more cytokines that are toxic to the glomerular epithelial cells (podocytes), cells that maintain the glomerular basement membranes. The cytokine induces a reduction in the net negative charge across the glomerular basement membrane. The constituents of this membrane and of the chemicals coating the glomerular epithelial and endothelial cells normally bear a net negative charge. The presence of these negatively charged chemicals creates a charge-selective barrier to filtration. This barrier plays a significant role in the ultrafiltration of macromolecules present in the plasma, enhancing the filtration of molecules bearing a positive electrical charge and retarding the filtration of molecules bearing a negative electrical charge. During episodes of relapse, patients with MCD show a breakdown in the normal charge-selective barrier to filtration, often resulting in massive proteinuria. Kidney biopsies from patients with nephrotic syndrome demonstrate a net reduction in anionic sites during periods of relapse. In addition, some children have mutations in podocyte proteins such as nephrin and podocin that lead to nephrotic syndrome. Children presenting with nephrosis before 1 year of age have a high likelihood of having a genetic mutation causing nephrotic syndrome, and any child with steroid resistant nephrotic syndrome should also be screened for such genetic mutations.

Evidence indicating that the proteinuria in the MCD or FSGS patient may be due to some soluble factor is 3-fold. (1) Some patients who develop end-stage renal disease from idiopathic nephrotic syndrome (particularly FSGS) have experienced a relapse of the nephrotic syndrome with massive proteinuria immediately after transplantation of a normal kidney. (2) Infusion of peripheral blood mononuclear cell products from nephrotic children induces albuminuria in rats. (3) Removal of serum proteins by adsorption to a protein A Sepharose column has led to remission of proteinuria in some patients who have experienced a recurrence of nephrotic syndrome after transplantation. The remission of the proteinuria after treatment with immunosuppressive medication provides further evidence that the nephrotic syndrome is mediated in some way by the immune system.

Normal adults are able to synthesize 12 g of albumin per day in the liver, and adults with nephrotic syndrome may synthesize 14 g of albumin per day. Therefore, the **hypoproteinemia** characteristic of nephrotic syndrome cannot be explained completely by measured amounts of urinary protein losses (about 3.5 g/day). The difference between the hepatic synthetic capacity for albumin and the measured urinary losses can be explained by protein catabolism in the kidney. Renal tubular epithelial cells reabsorb filtered plasma proteins and catabolize them to amino acids, which then reenter the amino acid pool of the body. Thus the magnitude of losses of plasma proteins at the glomerular level is far greater than the amount measured in a 24-hour urine sample.

The **hypoalbuminemia** seen in nephrotic syndrome is a result of the massive proteinuria, and the **hypercholesterolemia** occurs as a consequence of the hypoalbuminemia. The hyperlipidemia is partially the result of a generalized increase in hepatic protein synthesis that also involves the overproduction of lipoproteins. In addition, less lipid is transported into the adipose tissue, because the activity of lipoprotein lipase is reduced in adipose tissue during active nephrotic syndrome. Hyperlipidemia is most pronounced in children with MCD. Serum albumin and serum cholesterol are generally inversely correlated. The hyperlipidemia is the last biochemical abnormality to clear after the child achieves remission from an episode of nephrotic syndrome.

Differential Diagnosis

Nephrotic syndrome is considered either primary or secondary. Primary nephrotic syndrome is not associated with a systemic disease. Secondary nephrotic syndrome is a feature of a systemic disease such as anaphylactoid purpura, immunoglobulin (Ig) A nephropathy or systemic lupus erythematosus (SLE). Most children with nephrotic syndrome have the primary form of the disease.

Children with primary nephrotic syndrome are also classified according to their response to steroid therapy. Affected individuals may be categorized as steroid-sensitive, steroid-dependent, or steroid-resistant. Typically, children who are steroid-sensitive and remain so have MCD although, strictly speaking, a renal biopsy must be performed before the diagnosis of MCD is made. Sensitivity to or dependence on corticosteroids is a critical factor in determining a child's prognosis.

Nephrotic syndrome is also classified by the appearance of the glomeruli on renal biopsy. A summary of the histologic lesions causing nephrotic syndrome appears in Table 145-1. About 95% of young children with nephrotic syndrome have MCD. In these children, light microscopy shows normal-appearing glomeruli. Immunofluorescent microscopy is generally negative but may show some mesangial IgM deposits, and electron microscopy simply shows foot process

Table 145-1. Distribution of Histologic Type by Age of Onset in Children With Nephrotic Syndrome

Age (y)	MCD[a]	FSGS	MN	MPGN	Other GN
1–4	95%	3%	2%	—	—
4–8	75%	15%	1%	7%	2%
8–16	52%	15%	2%	25%	6%

Abbreviations: FSGS, focal segmental glomerulosclerosis; MCD, minimal change disease; MN, membranous nephropathy; MPGN, membranoproliferative glomerulonephritis; other GN, other forms of glomerulonephritis.

[a] MCD remains the dominant histologic type through mid-adolescence but becomes relatively less important in later childhood and adolescence.

effacement of the podocytes. In individuals with FSGS, light microscopy may show enlarged glomeruli and glomeruli with segments of sclerosis. Immunofluorescence may reveal some IgM and complement in the sclerotic segments, and electron microscopy shows areas of foot process effacement of podocytes. Biopsies performed later in the disease course show some totally sclerotic glomeruli, areas of interstitial fibrosis, and atrophy. Several recent series have noted an apparent increase in the incidence of FSGS among nephrotic children.

Other primary renal diseases that can cause nephrotic syndrome in children include membranous nephropathy, membranoproliferative glomerulonephritis, IgA nephropathy and other forms of chronic glomerulonephritis, congenital nephrotic syndrome, and diffuse mesangial proliferative glomerulonephritis. Chronic hepatitis B infection may cause membranous nephropathy or membranoproliferative glomerulonephritis. In endemic areas the incidence of hepatitis B associated membranous nephropathy has been reduced since the implementation of universal hepatitis B vaccination programs. Rarely, post-streptococcal acute glomerulonephritis and other forms of postinfectious acute glomerulonephritis may also cause nephrotic syndrome. With the exception of congenital nephrotic syndrome, all of these diseases show (1) the presence of immune deposits in the glomerular mesangial regions or along the glomerular basement membrane and (2) some element of cellular proliferation, which may be severe. In these disease states, the presence of nephrotic syndrome is indicative of marked injury to the glomerular capillary wall. Infants with congenital nephrotic syndrome, Finnish type, have a mutation of the gene encoding the nephrin molecule, a podocyte protein with a large extracellular domain that is an integral part of the glomerular slit diaphragm. These infants have massive proteinuria beginning in utero and have severe nephrotic syndrome presenting in the first month of life.

Because of the varying distribution of edema fluid at presentation, nephrotic syndrome may be confused with sinusitis or an allergic reaction (periorbital edema), obesity (ascites), or an abdominal mass (ascites). Other causes of generalized edema, such as congestive heart failure or liver disease, can be easily excluded.

Evaluation

History

The clinical evaluation should include a careful history (Questions Box).

Questions

Nephrotic Syndrome

- Has the child recently had any infections, such as pharyngitis or an upper respiratory infection?
- Are the child's eyelids swollen? Do they look more or less puffy at certain times during the day, especially on awakening or after crying?
- Does the child have a history of rashes characteristic of diseases that are associated with nephrotic syndrome?
- Is there a history of fever, oliguria, or abdominal pain?
- Is there a family history of nephrotic syndrome or kidney disease?
- Is the child playful and active, or is the edema so significant that movement is uncomfortable?
- Are the ascites and pleural effusions so severe that some respiratory compromise is evident?

Physical Examination

A complete physical examination is necessary. Blood pressure should be monitored because hypertension or hypotension may occur. The extent of the peripheral and central edema, including swelling of the eyelids, should be assessed. The physician should obtain a reliable, overall impression of the child's level of comfort and activity. The examination should also include a careful search for infection, particularly life-threatening infections such as pneumonia or peritonitis. Examination of the head and neck should focus on signs of recent infection such as otitis media. The presence of dullness to percussion at the bases of the thorax is consistent with large pleural effusions. Ascites may be minimal or massive. With severe ascites, scrotal or labial edema may occur. If the child has a history of abdominal pain, a careful check for signs of peritoneal irritation should be made. The skin should be inspected for infection and rashes.

Laboratory Tests

The laboratory evaluation of children with nephrotic syndrome begins with a urinalysis. The dipstick shows 3+ or 4+ protein, although a dilute urine may be only 2+. Microscopic hematuria may be present in up to 25% of children with MCD. The presence of associated glycosuria in a nephrotic child who is not on steroid therapy raises a concern for FSGS. Careful microscopic examination of the urine is necessary. Casts are seen frequently because urinary proteins precipitate in the tubules. The casts are hyaline, fine, and coarse granular. White blood cell (WBC) casts are sometimes seen because some children with nephrotic syndrome may also have increased amounts of leukocytes in their urine. Large amounts of red blood cells (RBCs) and RBC casts are not seen in uncomplicated MCD and, if present, indicate another cause for the nephrotic syndrome. If RBC casts are seen together with substantial hematuria, an antistreptolysin-O titer should be added to the preliminary evaluation. A random U TP/CR should be done to determine whether children have nephrotic range proteinuria.

If the urine shows only proteinuria, with perhaps some microscopic hematuria, blood tests should include a complete blood cell count (CBC), serum creatinine and blood urea nitrogen (BUN), electrolytes, serum calcium, serum albumin, cholesterol, complement component 3 (C3), and antinuclear antibody (ANA). The CBC may show a high hematocrit from hemoconcentration because many children experience volume contraction as a complication of hypoproteinemia. Children may also have very high platelet counts (sometimes >1 million/μL). The BUN and creatinine help assess renal function. A hyperchloremic metabolic acidosis is sometimes seen. The serum albumin and cholesterol are required to differentiate nephrotic syndrome from other edematous states. A low level of C3 is associated with other renal diseases such as membranoproliferative glomerulonephritis, acute postinfectious glomerulonephritis, and SLE. The ANA is useful in screening for SLE and other collagen vascular diseases. Hepatitis B serology is helpful in children who come from a population at risk for hepatitis B infection, such as recent immigrants from Southeast Asia or children of intravenous (IV) drug abusers. Although not part of the routine laboratory evaluation, measurement of quantitative Ig often shows low IgG levels and elevated IgM levels. The febrile child should also have blood and urine cultures, and if there are signs of peritoneal irritation, a culture of peritoneal fluid. Though not part of the routine evaluation, if there is a family history of thrombotic events, a thrombophilia evaluation should be considered because of the association between renal vein thrombosis and nephrotic syndrome, particularly in adults.

Imaging Studies

Chest radiographs help assess the severity of pleural effusions in children with marked ascites and respiratory compromise.

Management

Hospitalization

The decision to admit a child with nephrotic syndrome to the hospital is determined by the child's functional status. All children with severe edema compromising ambulation or respiration should be admitted. Other indications for admission include unstable vital signs, fever, marked oliguria, and severe hemoconcentration (hematocrit >48%–50%).

Most children with nephrotic syndrome are hospitalized for control of edema or treatment of a complication such as infection. The management of children in relapse is aimed at minimizing edema and preventing complications until the disease can be controlled

with immunosuppressive therapy. Intake, output, and weight need to be closely monitored. Blood pressure should be followed, although hypertension is not common. If children have a fever (temperature: >100.7°F [38.2°C]), blood and urine cultures should be obtained and antibiotics started pending culture results. If signs of peritoneal inflammation are evident, paracentesis should also be performed to obtain samples of the ascites fluid for Gram stain, cell count, and culture. Broad-spectrum antibiotics should be given to cover respiratory pathogens, especially pneumococcus, and enteric pathogens. All children who are newly diagnosed with nephrotic syndrome should have a purified protein derivative test because immunosuppression associated with steroid therapy may facilitate reactivation of tuberculosis infection.

Intravenous albumin (25%) should be used selectively because albumin infusions are expensive, and the infused albumin is excreted very rapidly in the urine. Infusions are indicated in children with marked ascites, scrotal or labial edema, or significant pleural effusions. They are also helpful in maintaining blood pressure and renal perfusion in septic children with nephrotic syndrome. The usual dose is 1 g/kg, up to 25 g, infused over 2 to 4 hours, with close monitoring of blood pressure. Furosemide (1 mg/kg intravenously) is usually administered post-infusion. The albumin infusions may be repeated every 12 to 24 hours as necessary. If children with oliguria fail to increase their urine output after the first or second albumin infusion, they need to be evaluated immediately for the presence of acute renal failure (see Chapter 67). The albumin-induced mobilization of edema fluid in nephrotic children with acute tubular necrosis can precipitate pulmonary edema.

Children with nephrotic syndrome have an increased tendency to thromboembolic phenomenon. Increased risk factors for this complication include loss of antithrombin 3 in the urine, age 12 years or older, the existence of a central line, and secondary causes of nephrotic syndrome such as SLE.

Supportive Therapy

Diet

Because sodium plays a key role in edema formation, children with nephrotic syndrome should be placed on a no-added-salt diet that limits dietary sodium to 2 or 3 g/day. Technically, sodium restriction is indicated only during times of relapse, but a constant no-added-salt diet helps entire families maintain a consistent regimen. In general, fluid restriction is not necessary except in unusual circumstances (eg, a steroid-resistant patient with persistent edema). Although earlier teachings recommended the use of high-protein diets, newer research has shown that these diets may actually increase urinary protein losses.

Activity

In the past, children with nephrotic syndrome were treated with bed rest because the supine position somewhat reduces urinary protein losses. No evidence shows that bed rest has a significant impact on children's clinical state, however. Therefore, most pediatric nephrologists recommend that children be allowed full activity. Boys with marked scrotal edema may be more comfortable resting in bed while diuresis is being initiated. Children with nephrotic syndrome should not be isolated from other children and should be allowed to attend school.

Diuretics

Diuretics are often helpful in children in relapse, particularly in children with steroid-resistant disease. Serum potassium levels, as well as clinical signs of intravascular volume, should be monitored. If children have moderate intravascular volume contraction, the injudicious use of diuretics could precipitate hypotension and increase the risk of thrombosis and acute tubular necrosis. The most commonly used diuretic is furosemide (1–2 mg/kg per dose given orally or intravenously). Spironolactone is sometimes added to the diuretic regimen for its potassium-sparing effect.

Long-term Management

The goal of long-term management is induction and maintenance of remission from active nephrotic syndrome. At the same time, the side effects of medications should be minimized. Spontaneous remission may eventually occur in children with MCD, but the 70% historical mortality rate makes waiting for a spontaneous remission unacceptable. Remissions are induced and maintained with the use of immunosuppressive medications. Figure 145-1 summarizes an

Table 145-2. Treatment Options in Childhood Nephrotic Syndrome		
Medication	**Dose**	**Length of Therapy**
Prednisone	60 mg/m²/d	Varies
Cyclophosphamide	2–3 mg/kg/d (cumulative dose <200 mg/kg)	12 weeks
Chlorambucil	0.15–0.2 mg/kg/d (cumulative dose ≤8.2 mg/kg)	8 weeks
Cyclosporine	3 mg/kg every 12 h, monitor levels	Varies
Levamisolea	2.5 mg/kg every other day	Varies
Mycophenolate mofetil	20 mg/kg every 12 h	Varies
Tacrolimus	0.1mg/kg every 12 h, monitor levels	Varies

ᵃ Levamisole is no longer recommended for childhood nephrotic syndrome in the United States.

approach to the overall management of nephrotic syndrome with these agents. A list of commonly used medications and dosages appears in Table 145-2.

Corticosteroids and Alkylating Agents

More than 90% of children with primary nephrotic syndrome respond to corticosteroid therapy. Steroids are, therefore, both diagnostic and therapeutic because failure to respond to steroids can be a marker for disease other than MCD or for a genetic cause of nephrotic syndrome. Even so, some children with MCD are steroid-resistant at some time in their disease. Steroids can be started in children who are newly diagnosed with nephrotic syndrome if they have no signs of systemic disease, no more than microscopic hematuria, a normal C3 (or results pending), and normal renal function. Acute infection should be managed with specific antimicrobial therapy to avoid infection-related steroid resistance.

Prednisone is usually started at 60 mg/m²/day. It can either be given once a day, in the morning, or divided into 2 or 3 daily doses. If first episodes of nephrotic syndrome are treated with a prolonged course of corticosteroids (60 mg/m²/day for 6 weeks followed by 40 mg/m²/48 hours for an additional 6 weeks), the children are subsequently less likely to follow a frequently relapsing course. Newly diagnosed children younger than 4 years are less likely to experience frequent relapses if their every-other-day steroids are tapered off over a 6-month period. Proteinuria resolves within 2 weeks in many children with MCD and by 4 weeks in more than 90%. Serum albumin normalizes soon after proteinuria clears, but hypercholesterolemia may take many weeks to return to normal.

The pediatrician can easily manage steroid-sensitive children, but children with more difficult nephrotic syndrome should be managed in conjunction with the pediatric nephrologist. Children with relapses are treated with daily prednisone (60 mg/m²) until the urine is protein-free for 3 days. This regimen is followed by 4 weeks of 40 mg/m² every other morning. An increased incidence of side effects

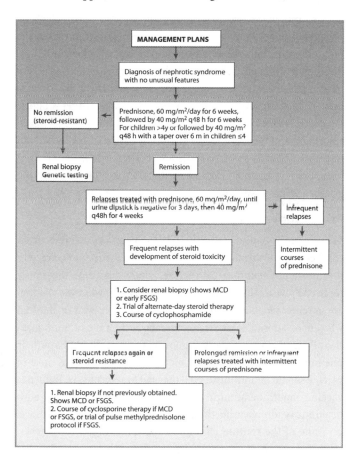

Figure 145–1. Management of nephrotic syndrome in children. FSGS, focal segmental glomerulosclerosis; MCD, minimal change disease; q, every.

(eg, cushingoid appearance, hypertension, obesity, glucose intolerance, cataracts, osteopenia, decreased growth rate) occurs when children require frequent courses of prednisone therapy. In frequently relapsing children, a chronic course of alternate-day steroid therapy may eliminate relapses and reduce steroid toxicity. Usually prednisone 60 mg/m^2 is given every other morning initially. The dose is then gradually tapered over several months to the lowest dose that keeps the child in remission. A recent study has found that children on chronic low-dose alternate-day therapy are less likely to experience a relapse following a URI if they receive daily prednisone at their stable prednisone dose for 7 days during the illness.

If alternate-day steroid therapy fails to maintain remission, cyclophosphamide or chlorambucil is administered. Either of these alkylating agents may induce long-lasting remission, which persists for years in children with steroid-dependent or frequently relapsing nephrotic syndrome. Either agent is started while children are on steroid therapy, and the steroids are gradually tapered during the course of treatment with the alkylating agent. In the past a diagnostic renal biopsy was routine prior to starting an alkylating agent. Many pediatric nephrologists now consider such therapy in steroid-sensitive or steroid-dependent children without a biopsy, however, provided that renal function is normal. Initially a daily dose of cyclophosphamide (2 mg/kg) was recommended for 8 weeks. However, a 12-week course is more likely to induce prolonged remission and still be safe.

Potential toxicities of cyclophosphamide include bone marrow suppression with increased risk of infection, alopecia, hemorrhagic cystitis, gonadal toxicity, and possibly a small but indeterminately increased risk of developing a malignancy at some time. Complete blood cell counts should be monitored weekly, and parents should be cautioned about the increased risk of overwhelming varicella infections in children who have not yet had a varicella infection or immunization. The cyclophosphamide dose should be withheld if the WBC count falls below 4,000/μL and restarted when the WBC returns to or exceeds 4,000/μL. Alopecia and hemorrhagic cystitis are rare when the recommended dose is used. A 12-week course of cyclophosphamide (2 mg/kg/day) does not seem to increase the risk of infertility, but longer courses are associated with oligospermia, aspermia, and ovarian dysfunction. Postpubertal individuals may be at greater risk for gonadal toxicity than prepubertal children.

When steroid-sensitive or steroid-dependent children have failed to achieve prolonged remission after cyclophosphamide therapy, a diagnostic renal biopsy should be performed. Renal biopsy is indicated early in the course of illness for steroid-resistant children. If FSGS is identified on biopsy, treatment may involve a prolonged course of IV methylprednisolone therapy, cyclosporine, or tacrolimus. Therapeutic options for children with MCD who continue to be steroid-dependent after a course of cyclophosphamide include treatment with mycophenolate mofetil, cyclosporine, tacrolimus, or levamisole. Although cyclosporine is more likely to induce prolonged remission, it only maintains remission while being administered. Children trade steroid dependence for cyclosporine dependence. Nevertheless, for children with steroid toxicity, a 6- to 12-month course of cyclosporine allows resolution of the adverse effects of steroids and is generally well tolerated when administered by an experienced physician. Side effects such as hirsutism and gingival hyperplasia are frequent at the onset of therapy. These effects regress as the dose is decreased or the drug is discontinued, however. Hypertension is not uncommon. The most common metabolic abnormality seen with cyclosporine use is hypomagnesemia. Long-term therapy may lead to significant nephrotoxicity and, rarely, patients experience liver toxicity. Tacrolimus, like cyclosporine, is a calcineurin inhibitor. It has a similar toxicity profile to cyclosporine, but it does not cause gingival hyperplasia or hirsutism.

Because of potential toxicity, cyclosporine and tacrolimus should only be prescribed by a physician familiar with the drug. Dosing requirements may change with remission and relapse, and the family and physician should be aware of several drug interactions. Any medication interfering with the cytochrome P-450 enzyme system in the liver, such as erythromycin, greatly increases cyclosporine levels and should be used only under extraordinary circumstances. Diarrhea may increase tacrolimus blood levels to a toxic range. Children who require prolonged treatment with cyclosporine or tacrolimus should have follow-up kidney biopsies performed after a year or two of therapy to assess for any nephrotoxicity.

Nephrotic children who fail to achieve a good remission with immunosuppressive therapy are given supportive therapy with angiotensin-converting enzyme inhibitors or angiotensin blockers, which reduce proteinuria and have also been shown to reduce the progression of glomerulosclerosis. These medications are also first-line therapy for nephrotic children who develop hypertension. There have been some promising preliminary results with the use of rituximab in children with difficult nephrotic syndrome. Other supportive measures for children with persistent edema include sodium restriction and the chronic use of diuretics. Genetic testing should be performed early in steroid resistant children, and further immunosuppressive therapy should be withheld until the results of the genetic testing is available.

Immunization Issues

Because of the unusual susceptibility to pneumococcal infections, children with nephrotic syndrome older than 2 years should receive the 23-valent pneumococcal vaccine, even if they have previously received Prevnar. The vaccine is best administered while the children are in remission, but it produces protective titers even in children who are on alternate-day steroid therapy at the time of immunization. Patients on multiple immunosuppressives should have their pneumococcal antibody titers measured, and a second dose of vaccine should be administered if they fail to seroconvert. Influenza vaccine should be administered each autumn to children with nephrotic syndrome using the age-appropriate schedule and dosage.

Some of the routine childhood immunizations (diphtheria-tetanus-pertussis, *Haemophilus influenzae* type b, hepatitis B, poliovirus vaccine inactivated) should be administered by the usual schedule but while children are in remission, if possible (see Chapter 32). Some controversy exists concerning the use of live virus vaccines in children who require long-term immunosuppressive therapy. No vaccines should be administered if children are currently being treated with an alkylating agent. The measles-mumps-rubella vaccine could potentially cause a relapse. Based on the limited data on the use of varicella vaccine in nephrotic children, it is probably safe to administer varicella vaccine while the children are in remission and not on immunosuppressive medications.

Parent Education

Because nephrotic syndrome follows a chronic, relapsing course, parent education is essential for effective long-term management. Parents need to be instructed about using urinary dipsticks (Albustix) to monitor protein excretion. Generally urine dipsticks should be used daily during periods of active relapse and when medication is being tapered. Otherwise, the dipstick should be checked whenever children have infections, including URIs; whenever they look "puffy"; and weekly when asymptomatic.

Weight should also be monitored, especially during relapse. Children should be weighed each morning when they awaken. Urine output should be measured in more difficult cases. As parents become more familiar with the nephrotic syndrome, they may become partners with the physician about medication changes. Parents should also contact the physician about "danger signs" such as fever (temperature: >100.7°F [38.2°C]), significant abdominal pain, or exposure to varicella. If children do not have protective antibodies against varicella and if they are taking any immunosuppressive medication (including prednisone), the varicella-zoster Ig should be administered within 72 hours of exposure to varicella. If varicella infection develops, IV acyclovir should be instituted.

Prognosis

In the pre-antibiotic era, nephrotic syndrome was frequently fatal, usually because of overwhelming infection. After the introduction of antibiotics, the mortality rate fell. The use of corticosteroids has led to a further reduction in mortality. Currently the mortality rate is about 5%, almost exclusively due to infections from encapsulated organisms or from thrombosis. The greatest risk of death in children with nephrotic syndrome (approaching 50% over 20 years in some series) is among the children with resistance to corticosteroid therapy.

The long-term outlook for most children with nephrotic syndrome is favorable, particularly for steroid-sensitive patients. Relapses often disappear by the completion of puberty. Occasionally individuals continue to have relapses into adulthood. Approximately 20% of children with steroid-sensitive MCD still experience relapses 15 years after the onset of their disease. Disease recurrence is highly unlikely if 8 years pass without a relapse. Less than 10% of initially steroid-sensitive children with nephrotic syndrome develop end-stage renal disease. This occurs almost exclusively in children with FSGS. Focal segmental glomerulosclerosis may recur after kidney transplants, particularly in young children with aggressive FSGS.

Selected References

Bayazit AK, Noyan A, Cengiz N, Anarat A. Mycophenolate mofetil in the children with multidrug-resistant nephrotic syndrome. *Clin Nephrol.* 2004;61:25–29

Benoit G, Machuca E, Antignac C. Hereditary nephrotic syndrome: a systematic approach for genetic testing and a review of the associated podocyte gene mutations. *Pediatr Nephrol.* 2010;25:1621–1632

Bernard DB. Extrarenal complications of the nephrotic syndrome. *Kidney Int.* 1988;33:1184–1202

Eddy AA, Schnaper HW. The nephrotic syndrome: from the simple to the complex. *Semin Nephrol.* 1998;18:304–316

Filler G. Treatment of nephrotic syndrome in children and controlled trials. *Nephrol Dial Transplant.* 2003;18(suppl 6):vi75–vi78

Guan N, Ding J, Zhang J, et al. Expression of nephrin, podocin, α-actinin, and WT-1 in children with nephrotic syndrome. *Pediatr Nephrol.* 2003;18:1121–1127

Gulati S, Sharma AP, Sharma RK. Changing trends in histopathology in childhood nephrotic syndrome. *Am J Kidney Dis.* 1999;34:646–650

Hodson E, Willis N, Craig J. Corticosteroid therapy for nephrotic syndrome in children. *Cochrane Database Syst Rev.* 2007;(4):CD001533

Hodson EM. Willis NS. Craig JC. Interventions for idiopathic steroid-resistant nephrotic syndrome in children. [Review] Update of Cochrane Database of Systematic Reviews. 2006;(2):CD003594. *Cochrane Database Syst Rev.* 2010;(11):CD003594

Kerlin BA, Blatt NB, Fuh B, et al. Epidemiology and risk factors for thromboembolic complications of childhood nephrotic syndrome: a Midwest Pediatric Nephrology Consortium (MWPNC) Study. *J Pediatr.* 2009;155:105–110

Lewis MA, Baildom EM, Davis N, Houston IB, Postlethwaite RJ. Nephrotic syndrome: from toddlers to twenties. *Lancet.* 1989;1:255–259

Loeffler K, Gowrishankar M, Yiu V. Tacrolimus therapy in pediatric patients with treatment-resistant nephrotic syndrome. *Pediatr Nephrol.* 2004;19:281–287

Mendoza SA, Reznik VM, Griswold WR, Krensky AM, Yorgin PD, Tune BM. Treatment of steroid-resistant focal segmental glomerulosclerosis with pulse methylprednisolone and alkylating agents. *Pediatr Nephrol.* 1990;4:303–307

Minimal change nephrotic syndrome in children: deaths during the first 5 to 15 years' observation. Report of the International Study of Kidney Disease in Children. *Pediatrics.* 1984;73:497–501

Quien RM, Kaiser BA, Deforest A, et al. Response to the varicella vaccine in children with nephrotic syndrome. *J Pediatr.* 1997;131:688–690

Vester U, Kranz B, Zimmerman S. Cyclophosphamide in steroid-sensitive nephrotic syndrome: outcome and outlook. *Pediatr Nephrol.* 2003;18:661–664

CHAPTER 146

Seizures and Epilepsy

Kenneth R. Huff, MD

CASE STUDY

A 6-year-old boy is evaluated for unusual episodic behaviors. The previous week his mother was awakened by the boy's brother and found her son lying in bed unresponsive and drooling, with his head and eyes averted to the right, his right arm slightly raised, and his body stiff. His face was jerking intermittently. When the paramedics arrived, the boy's posturing and movements had stopped. After the event he could speak but was somewhat incoherent. He was taken to the local emergency department, where his examination and mental status were normal. Screening blood and urine tests were normal, and he was discharged, with instructions to see his pediatrician for further recommendations.

His father remembers 2 or 3 other episodes of a somewhat different nature in the past month. These occurred as the boy was being put to bed. They involved some body stiffening and facial grimacing, with the mouth slightly open and the tongue twisted and deviated to one side. The child could not speak but appeared to be trying to talk. The episodes lasted 20 to 30 seconds. Afterward the boy was his usual self and could tell his father what had been said to him.

The child has had no intercurrent illnesses or abnormal behavior apart from these "spells," and he has lost no abilities. A paternal cousin and grandfather had seizures during childhood but "grew out of them." The examination is completely normal.

Questions

1. How likely is it that the episodic behavior represents a seizure?
2. What historical data about an event support the diagnosis of a seizure disorder?
3. How does the electroencephalogram (EEG) help in classifying the type of seizure disorder?
4. What rationale should be used to formulate short-term and long-term treatment plans?

Seizures are a common medical problem in children. Diagnosing an episode that does not contain generalized convulsing movements as a seizure is sometimes problematic, however. Seizures are defined as episodic, stereotypical behavior syndromes of abrupt onset with loss of voluntary control by the patient, resulting in loss of responsiveness and rarely provoked by external stimuli. Frequently the occurrence of this behavior correlates with interictal brain electrical discharges on EEG, and the behavioral ictus (seizures) should match temporally with a period of electrical hypersynchrony if it occurs during the EEG recording.

A detailed history of the nature of the episodic behavior from an eyewitness is paramount, both in making the diagnosis of a seizure disorder and in elucidating the type of seizure problem. The EEG is most often an adjunct to diagnosis. It is abnormal in many individuals who do not have clinical seizures and it may be normal interictally in many patients with clinical seizures because of its sampling limitations. Special techniques can sometimes help alleviate these limitations.

The type of seizure problem is important information in devising the management plan. Seizures can simply be classified as primary generalized seizures (involving the whole cerebrum from the outset) or partial seizures. However, some partial seizures can secondarily generalize, thereby clinically mimicking primary generalized seizures after their onset. Distinguishing these entities illustrates the importance of eyewitness information. Many treatment options are available, but the therapeutic plan must be individualized to the child's seizure type or clinical syndrome to optimize seizure control and minimize side effects. With appropriate treatment, most children with seizure disorders are not handicapped scholastically or socially and can enjoy normal lives.

Epidemiology

About 0.5% to 1.0% of all children experience at least one afebrile seizure. Recurrent seizures can occur as a component of a static encephalopathy after brain malformation or dysgenesis, encephalitis or meningitis, metabolic disorder, hypoxic-ischemic injury, or severe head trauma. Such secondary or symptomatic seizures make up approximately one-third of childhood epilepsies. The remaining two-thirds of epileptic seizures occur presumably as part of a genetic epileptic syndrome. As genetic knowledge increases, eventually it may no longer be true that most often seizures occur in children without any known cause or association.

Clinical Presentation

Children present with a history given by observers of an episode of abrupt onset characterized by a loss of ability to respond to external stimuli (Dx Box). The child themselves may experience various

Dx Seizures

- Abrupt loss of responsiveness
- Rhythmic clonic movements
- Sustained changes in posture or tone
- Simple automatic movements
- Staring without change in tone
- Simultaneous change in cerebral electrical activity (repetitive discharges)

difficult to describe sensory phenomena (aura) before losing consciousness. Observers then see convulsive muscle activity following which the patient may be sleepy. With some seizures, observers may note only an akinetic or staring spell, but with others, dramatic, rhythmic spasms of the face, extremities, or torso. Major motor seizures are frequently also associated with systemic autonomic changes, including changes in skin vascular supply causing color change, sweating, saliva production, and loss of sphincter control. Most seizure episodes are neither provoked nor attenuated by environmental factors (except for the provocative factors of fever, intercurrent illness, and sleep deprivation). Between episodes, children's general physical and neurologic examination may be entirely normal.

Pathophysiology

A seizure represents a sudden, synchronous depolarizing change in the electrical activity of a network of neurons that becomes widely propagated over the cortex, affecting awareness, responsiveness to external stimuli, and motor control. The propagation may be enhanced by defects in cell ion channels. Partial seizure disorders may result from a focal cortical lesion, such as a glial scar or dysplasia caused by a remote insult (eg, an infarct), or dysgenesis or primary cortical dysplasia that disrupts the electrical circuitry. The focal abnormality could also contain hamartomatous immature cells and synaptic properties; and allow for periodic, abnormal transmission of impulses.

Exactly what initiates the synchronous depolarization of the neurons and the widespread network propagation is not well understood. Several physiological mechanisms, including neuronal circuitry, membrane ion channel abnormalities, neurotransmitter production metabolism or uptake, and perhaps glial support mechanisms are probably involved. An understanding of the mechanism involved in familial epilepsy syndromes awaits the definition of relevant genes, their expression and product functions, and the effects of variability in base pair sequence and transcription on membrane polarization, synaptic function, and circuitry physiology. An example is cryptogenic West syndrome (infantile spasms), an "interneuronopathy," which has been associated with several genes including *LIS1, DCX,* and *ARX* (sometimes resulting in lissencephaly), which are important in GABAergic inhibitory interneuron development. Another example is the neuronal voltage-gated sodium channel alpha subunit type 1 gene, which is mutated in the mild phenotype of "generalized

epilepsy with febrile convulsions plus" and also mutated but in different regions of the gene sequence in the much worse phenotype of severe myoclonic epilepsy of infancy.

Seizure Types

Seizures can be simply classified as either **primary generalized seizures,** which include grand mal, generalized tonic-clonic convulsions, and petit mal (absence) seizures (so named because of the child's complete loss of awareness at the outset of the episode), or **partial seizures,** which include focal motor, psychomotor, and other partial disorders (Box 146-1). The examples presented here should not be considered an exhaustive list of seizure syndromes but some of the more important types encountered in practice.

Box 146-1. Classification of Epileptic Seizures

Partial seizures (seizures beginning locally)
- Elementary symptoms: focal seizures
- Complex symptoms: psychomotor seizures
- Partial seizures evolving secondarily to generalized seizures

Generalized seizures (bilaterally symmetrical; onset not local)
- Absence seizures (petit mal): typical and atypical
- Tonic-clonic seizures
- Tonic seizures
- Myoclonic seizures (minor motor)
- Atonic seizures (drop attacks)
- Infantile spasms

Unclassified seizures (includes neonatal "subtle" seizures)

Most seizures in older children result from a partial seizure disorder. **Psychomotor seizures** are partial seizures that are usually preceded by a sensory aura or sometimes emotional behavioral manifestations, and have a wide range of ictal behaviors, including focal clonic jerking, aversive or asymmetrical hypertonic posturing, and more complex stereotypic fumbling or fingering behaviors. The seizures may be followed by postictal confusion or drowsiness. In some instances, children have partial sensory awareness but are unable to respond during seizures. In other cases, however, they are completely unconscious. The initial partial motor manifestations may not be seen by the observer before the movements rapidly generalize. Partial seizures are more often associated with focal brain pathologic processes, including traumatic lesions, infarcts, malformations, infections (eg, viral encephalitis or cerebral cysticercosis), and hippocampal sclerosis. These etiologies each may have a characteristic appearance on magnetic resonance imaging (MRI), although in many cases the etiology is not visible on MRI.

Benign epilepsy syndromes occur in children with normal developmental history, respond well to therapy, and remit without sequelae. **Rolandic seizures** are a relatively common partial seizure syndrome that sometimes is familial and has a good prognosis for resolving by adolescence. These episodes commonly occur when children are falling asleep or awakening. Sensory auras precede the motor manifestations, which involve the tongue, mouth, or face and which can sometimes generalize to the rest of the body. The clinical syndrome is accompanied by a characteristic focal EEG discharge over the central temporal region of the scalp. Other benign syndromes include **benign familial infantile seizures, benign infantile seizures with mild gastroenteritis,** and **Panayiotopoulos syndrome,** which is characterized by paroxysmal autonomic dysfunctions such as vomiting and other gastrointestinal (GI) motility problems, pallor, mydriasis, and cardiorespiratory and thermoregulatory abnormalities (lasting up to 30 minutes) ending often in generalized convulsing and largely occurring in sleep.

An **absence seizure** may sometimes be difficult to distinguish from a partial seizure (Table 146-1). The absence spell is a brief (2–15 seconds) loss of consciousness without loss of tone. Staring into space and minor movements such as lip smacking or semi-purposeful-appearing movements of the hands are often the only observed behaviors. There is no postictal period. Because absence seizures occur multiple times a day and children are often unaware of them, parents may dismiss the subtle behavior change as selective attention or daydreaming; however, these seizures may adversely affect learning and carry a risk of injury. Hyperventilation, a useful diagnostic test that can be performed in the office, may provoke absence seizures. The EEG is generally confirmatory and may also distinguish classic petit mal seizures with 3-per-second spike-wave discharges from variant syndromes. The classic petit mal is more often familial with dominant inheritance, age-specific occurrence between 4 and 16 years, and sensitivity to ethosuximide treatment; whereas the atypical variant has a poorer prognosis for early resolution and is more resistant to anticonvulsant therapy.

A number of age-related seizure syndromes exist, perhaps related to maturational events in brain circuitry. Although the appearance of these syndromes is stereotypical, in most cases the prognosis depends on the etiologic diagnosis.

Neonatal seizures may be tonic, focal clonic, or multifocal clonic. The seizure problem is less often primary, and a vigorous search for an etiology of the seizure is more often successful than with older children. Problems commonly leading to neonatal seizures include hemorrhage (germinal matrix in the premature infant or subarachnoid from birth trauma in older neonates); hypoxic-ischemic damage from asphyxia; infections producing postnatal sepsis/meningitis or prenatal encephalitis; birth trauma; drug withdrawal in the infant of a substance-abusing mother; metabolic problems including hypoglycemia, hypocalcemia, or hypomagnesemia in the infant of a diabetic mother; amino or organic acidopathies occurring a few days after feedings have begun; and congenital brain malformations.

Infantile spasms are an age-related seizure syndrome with typical movements of flexion contraction of the trunk with the head bowed or sudden raising of the arms sometimes accompanied by a cry. These behaviors occur stereotypically several times in succession in a series. This syndrome occurs in infants between 3 months and 2 years of age. Another perhaps related but rarer syndrome of serial spasms, **Ohtahara syndrome,** occurs at a younger neonatal age and is associated with structural brain abnormalities and characterized by a different EEG pattern, but carries a similar ominous prognosis for impaired intellectual development. A third syndrome in older children that is also associated with a different but characteristic EEG pattern, **Lennox-Gastaut syndrome,** has the same poor prognosis for seizure control and cognitive development but produces several different behavioral seizure types, including tonic, absence, and drop attacks. Different types of brain lesions in these age groups (including focal lesions) can result in the same generalized seizure syndromes. Examples include tuberous sclerosis; neonatal ischemia, hemorrhage, or meningitis; and major central nervous system (CNS) malformations. These disorders most often coexist with moderate to severe learning disability or mental retardation.

Differential Diagnosis

Seizures are distinguished from non-epileptic paroxysmal disorders on the basis of history. The circumstances of place and time as well as details about the symptoms and nature of the behavior are important pieces of data. The syncopal episode is also frequently situational, unlike a seizure. It occurs when children are in hot or stuffy environments; when they have been standing in one place for a long time; or when they see or experience a painful event such as an injection or phlebotomy. Boys may experience micturition syncope standing in the bathroom shortly after arising in early morning. **Syncope** is often preceded by symptoms of lightheadedness, nausea, tinnitus, and eventually a gradual darkening of vision sometimes without total loss of auditory perception.

Breath-holding spells are characterized by apnea and loss of responsiveness accompanied by either cyanosis or pallid skin color. Breath-holding spells are also situational. Infants or children are often upset or crying just before such spells. They may be frightened by a seemingly minor injury or angry after a toy is taken away or they

	Table 146-1. Partial Complex Versus Absence Seizures	
Characteristic	**Partial Complex**	**Absence**
Aura	Frequent	None
Loss of consciousness	Sometimes partial	Complete
Motor movements	Sometimes complex	Blinking or none
Postictal state	Frequent	None
Duration	>30 seconds	<15 seconds
Frequency	Few per month to few per day	Many per hour or day
Hyperventilation provoked	No	Yes
Electroencephalogram findings	Variably localized discharge or normal	3/s spike-wave generalized
Prognosis past adolescence	Frequently persists	Rarely occurs

are disciplined. Children may then throw themselves backward and stiffen while closing their glottis in expiration, and they may even have a few clonic jerks after losing consciousness (see Chapter 49).

Selective attention is frequently mistaken for absence seizures. This behavior often occurs when children are involved in relative passive activities (eg, watching television, playing a video game, or daydreaming) and do not respond to verbal stimuli such as hearing their own name called. Generally, the attention lapses do not occur during talking or eating; seizures will occur, however, even during these activities.

Epileptic seizures must also be differentiated from **pseudoseizures,** which actually occur most often in patients who have true seizures. Such episodes may resemble true seizures accurately, the psychodynamics of secondary gain or other motivation for the behavior may not be readily apparent, the "need" for attention may be legitimate, and the finding that the standard EEG is normal does not exclude a true seizure and thus is not helpful. Pseudoseizures should be suspected in children who may have witnessed seizures in relatives or close friends, who have seizures that consistently recur in the same situations, whose seizure frequency is not decreased with therapeutic levels of anticonvulsants, and whose seizures appear "suggestible." Diagnosis can often be supported in complicated cases by simultaneous video EEG monitoring, which will show a lack of correlation of electrical abnormalities with the behavior in question. Postictal serum prolactin level also may be normal, and psychological assessment may detect underlying emotional problems related to prior trauma (eg, sexual abuse or other major psychological trauma). The prognosis of pseudoseizures in children generally is better than in adults and relates to the more acute psychosocial genesis of the problem in most children.

Paroxysmal events in sleep may also be a challenge for accurate diagnosis because the motor behaviors of non–rapid eye movement sleep or other **parasomnias** may mimic nocturnal frontal lobe epileptic seizures. Video EEG polysomnography will also help distinguish these, as the former will not be associated with ictal discharges. Infantile gastroesophageal reflux (Sandifer syndrome) may look like brief epileptic tonic spasms, but should have a consistent temporal relationship to feeding. Benign paroxysmal vertigo occurs in the infant or toddler and presages migraine later in childhood but does not cause loss of responsiveness.

Evaluation (Box 146-2)

History

The history should determine the exact events surrounding the seizure episode. A detailed history of the nature of the behavior from an eyewitness is extremely important (Questions Box). The physician must determine whether children experienced any loss of their normal level of responsiveness. Most often this change in mental status is abrupt, although a warning behavior or aura that lasts for a few seconds may precede complete loss of responsiveness. The warning behavior or aura may be a cry, an expression of fear or anxiety, or

---

> **Box 146-2. Initial Evaluation of Seizure Patients**
>
> - Eyewitness account of the episode
> - Description of children's own experiences before, during, and after the episode if they are articulate enough
> - History from caregiver concerning remote injuries to the nervous system, progressive neurologic symptoms, or intercurrent illness
> - Careful neurologic examination looking for signs of cerebral hemisphere lateralization
> - Brain imaging study when a partial seizure is observed, a crescendo history of neurologic symptoms is obtained, focal neurologic signs are found on interictal examination, or the postictal encephalopathy persists too long
> - Waking and sleep electroencephalogram with hyperventilation

---

> **Questions**
>
> **Seizures**
>
> - Where was the child and what was he or she doing when the episode began?
> - Did the child experience a loss of responsiveness?
> - Did the child show any warning behavior or aura (eg, a cry, a facial expression of fear, irritability)?
> - Did any part of the child's body become stiff? Was any shaking or jerking apparent?
> - What did the child's eyes do and was saliva produced at the mouth?
> - Did the child's skin change color?
> - Did the child experience a loss of sphincter control?
> - How long did the episode last?
> - Has the child been well recently?
> - Did the child have a complicated birth, head trauma, meningitis, or other previous brain damage?
> - Have episodes of a similar nature occurred previously? If so, when did they begin and how frequently do they occur?
> - Has the child's development and school experience progressed normally?
> - Does the child have any relatives who have had seizures?

---

nonspecific irritability. If children are articulate, they may be able to describe a discrete sensory phenomenon or relate a less distinct or even indescribable sensation.

A change in muscle tone and activity is frequently associated with the abrupt change in mental status unless the spell is an absence seizure. Most often, the tone is increased with general extensor posturing, more focal hypertonicity, or more complex torsion or "aversive" upper-body posturing. The patient may fall if not supported. Rhythmic jerking or clonic movements (focal or general), including the trunk, limbs, face, and eyes, may occur concomitantly. Respirations may involve gagging sounds, rhythmic grunting, or nearly imperceptible movements. Swallowing may not occur, so that saliva pools or forms bubbles at the lips. Autonomic changes including skin color change (circumoral cyanosis), increased pulse, and loss of sphincter control frequently occur with major motor spells. The ictal period generally lasts 30 seconds to 2 minutes, although observers frequently overestimate this time. Postictal periods of sleepiness or lethargy may occur. Their length is often correlated with the length or intensity of the seizure.

Children and those around them are often unaware of the occurrence of absence seizures. Often an observant teacher brings the child's problem to a physician's attention. During a spell, a child has no change in tone or clonic movements and may have only subtle facial or hand movements. The episode lasts only a few seconds, and there are no preictal or postictal behaviors.

Historical information can also help determine potential etiologies of the seizure problem. A known distant brain insult or a hereditary disposition may be related to the cause. A progressive loss of skills indicates a need for a degenerative disease investigation.

Physical Examination

Children should be examined carefully for focal neurologic signs, particularly cerebral hemisphere-related asymmetries in strength, tone, or tendon reflexes. The examination should include a developmental assessment and mental status examination. The physician should look for signs of potential genetic problems, such as dysmorphic features or organ malformations, which often correlate with cerebral dysgenesis; abnormal skin pigmentation or vessels, suggesting a neurocutaneous disorder; and organomegaly or bony abnormalities, indicating the possibility of a storage disorder. Children who are old enough to cooperate should be asked to hyperventilate, which might provoke an absence spell if the history is suggestive of this type of seizure.

Laboratory Tests

An EEG should be requested to help with the diagnosis of the type of seizure disorder. In children with partial seizure disorders, the interictal discharge is helpful in localizing the initial site of abnormal electrical activity. A sleep record is often essential for observing any abnormalities. If a normal waking EEG is obtained and seizures continue to recur, it is sometimes useful to help ensure sleep during the record by prior sleep deprivation carried out by the parents or caretaker. Special techniques (eg, prolonged monitoring with telemetry or special anatomical electrode placements) can sometimes help overcome the standard EEG limitations of sample time and inaccessible areas of cerebral cortex. It should be noted, however, that even the standard EEG is rarely normal in petit mal disorders.

Historical information can frequently guide the need for metabolic tests. A blood sugar determination should be done acutely, but electrolytes are rarely abnormal in older children who have been well prior to the seizure. Neonates and infants with recurrent unexplained seizures should have metabolic screening including organic acid and amino acid levels and a diagnostic/therapeutic trial of pyridoxine. Tissue biopsy histologic analysis and specific assays may be indicated when physical signs suggest possible storage or other metabolic etiologies.

Imaging Studies

Magnetic resonance imaging scans are particularly helpful if a progression in neurologic symptoms or signs has occurred, if there is a history of prior neurologic insult, if an asymmetry of strength or tone is noted on examination, or if signs of dysgenesis are present in other parts of the body. Even in the absence of these factors, partial or focal seizures have a higher yield of abnormal imaging results than do febrile seizures or petit mal disorders, which have a low yield. Acutely, intravenous contrast should generally be given because loss of focal blood-brain barrier with an inflammatory or neoplastic lesion can help with diagnosing the cause of the seizure. Children with recurrent or resistant seizures should have an MRI scan, particularly when surgical treatment is under consideration. Coronal MRI scans can detect mesial temporal sclerosis, a lesion in the hippocampus seen in chronic temporal lobe epilepsy, and 20% of these will have had febrile seizures. Helpful additional modalities in studying surgical candidates include ictal positron emission tomography (PET) using fluorodeoxyglucose, interictal PET using α-methyl-L-tryptophan, single photon emission computerized tomography, functional MRI, and magnetoencephalography. These studies help define the nature of damaged or epileptic cortex and differentiate it from normal cortex.

Management

When there has been an episode of abrupt loss of consciousness or tone with a potential for recurrence, families need to be cautioned about the risks of drowning, falls from high places, and accidents with operating machinery including vehicles. Anticonvulsants are the mainstay of management of seizure disorders (Table 146-2). At the same time the clinician must realize seizures and antiepileptic drugs affect brain development and could have long-term consequences, such as altered cognition and epilepsy susceptibility. (This observation may be especially true in the case of neonatal seizures where the seizures themselves may contribute to adverse outcomes; the standard treatment of phenobarbital has been shown in some long-term treatment models to be inhibitory of learning.) Anticonvulsants are prescribed if the risk of recurrence of seizures, particularly prolonged seizures, is significant based on seizure classification and individual factors. A known structural lesion or the EEG may also suggest a higher recurrence risk. The choice of anticonvulsant depends on age, gender, neurologic diagnosis, seizure type or epilepsy syndrome, other conditions or medications, and social factors. The doses and combination of anticonvulsants prescribed for children depend on a balance of seizure resistance, risk of recurrence, and potential toxicity of medication. The initial goal is control with a single medication and as little toxicity as possible.

Oxcarbazepine and carbamazepine are often recommended for partial seizures. Toxicity is generally mild or nonexistent; adverse effects include GI upset, dizziness, and headache. Carbamazepine has been known to aggravate idiopathic generalized and myoclonic epilepsies, however. Phenytoin is also effective for partial types of seizures, and it can be given intravenously for status epilepticus. Phenobarbital

Table 146-2. Drugs Useful for Treating Seizures

Seizure Type	Dose	Toxic Symptoms/Side Effects
Partial Seizures		
Carbamazepine	Approx 15 mg/kg/d	Gastrointestinal distress, headache
Phenytoin	4–8 mg/kg/d	Ataxia, nystagmus, bone changes
Primidone	12–25 mg/kg/d	Drowsiness, ataxia
Oxcarbazepine	30 mg/kg/d	Drowsiness
Lamotrigine	4–7 mg/kg/d	Dizziness, sedation, rash (Stevens-Johnson syndrome)
Gabapentin	4–8 mg/kg/d	Somnolence, ataxia
Vigabatrin	15–50 mg/kg/d	Drowsiness, visual field defects
Topiramate	6–10 mg/kg/d	Weight loss, sedation, speech disturbance
Zonisamide	4–6 mg/kg/d	Sedation
Levetiracetam	10–60 mg/kg/d	Behavior or personality change
Rufinamide	10–45 mg/kg/d	Sedation, headache
Lacosamide	1.5–6mg/kg/d	Dizziness, ataxia, caution with cardiac disease
Neonatal Seizures		
Phenobarbital	5–6 mg/kg/d	Lethargy, irritability, osteopenia
Topiramate	6–10 mg/kg/d	Sedation
Generalized Seizures		
Valproic acid	20–60 mg/kg/d	Tremors, hair loss, thrombocytopenia, weight gain
Felbamate	45 mg/kg/d	Insomnia, anorexia, bone marrow aplasia
Topiramate	6–10 mg/kg/d	Weight loss, sedation, speech disturbance
Clorazepate	0.1–0.4 mg/kg/d	Drowsiness
Clonazepam	0.15 mg/kg/d	Drowsiness, ataxia
Absence Seizures		
Ethosuximide	30 mg/kg/d	Nausea, hiccups
Valproic acid	20–60 mg/kg/d	Tremors, hair loss, thrombocytopenia, weight gain
Infantile Spasms		
Adrenocorticotropic hormone	40 U/m^2	Increased appetite, irritability, acne
Valproic acid	20–60 mg/kg/d	Tremors, hair loss, thrombocytopenia, weight gain
Vigabatrin	15–50 mg/kg/d	Drowsiness, visual field defects

is effective in neonatal seizures but may have deleterious effects on behavior and learning in older children. Ethosuximide is used for petit mal seizures. Valproic acid is used for more common atypical petit mal and other seizure disorders resistant to other anticonvulsants. It should not be used in a woman who might conceive because of an increased risk of fetal neural tube defects, however. Felbamate is also effective in many difficult to treat epilepsy syndromes, although a small incidence of irreversible severe bone marrow suppression and liver toxicity has limited its use. Other anticonvulsants including gabapentin, lamotrigine, vigabatrin, topiramate, zonisamide, and levetiracetam have proven effective. Gabapentin and levetiracetam are useful as adjunctive agents because of their lack of interaction with other anticonvulsants. Lamotrigine is useful in both partial and primary generalized seizure disorders. Vigabatrin is useful in infantile spasms when caused by tuberous sclerosis. Topiramate is effective in partial seizures, generalized seizures, and Lennox-Gastaut syndrome. Rufinamide, newly marketed, is also effective in the latter syndrome particularly. Zonisamide and levetiracetam are effective in both partial and generalized seizure disorders, and lacosamide, another new medication, is also effective in partial disorders. The latter 2 medications can also be used intravenously.

Periodic monitoring of efficacy and side effects is essential in children who take medication daily on a long-term basis. A log of seizure frequency helps assess medication efficacy. Gastrointestinal and neurologic symptoms (sedation and ataxia) are the most common side effects. The perception of symptoms being related to the medication as well as the actual presence of side effects or toxicity both contribute to the complex issue of compliance. Serum drug levels are useful in monitoring compliance, dosage, and the likelihood that symptoms are the result of drug side effects. Organ toxicity (bone marrow, liver, and pancreas) must be considered and monitored with many medications. Hypersensitivity reactions and Stevens-Johnson syndrome usually, but do not always, occur within 2 months of beginning the medication. Drug interactions can be important and can include the liver cytochrome P450-inducing potential of barbiturates and the potential of other medications, such as erythromycin, to inhibit other liver detoxification systems, such as that involved with carbamazepine metabolism, which produce acutely high levels and clinical toxicity. The recent onset of educational problems in a child with epilepsy deserves aggressive evaluation, both for determining a common etiology to the underlying seizure condition and alternatively for assessing medication toxicity or long-term effects.

Non-medication therapeutic options are also available for refractory cases. The ketogenic diet has success in about 50% of cases but requires considerable knowledge and commitment. The vagal nerve stimulator delivers a regular electrical stimulus afferently to the CNS and also allows for an abortive intervention by the caretaker with an external magnet. It is also effective in about 50% of cases, and when this occurs less medication may be used, allowing a better overall quality of life. Intracranial surgery for epilepsy in childhood must sometimes be considered. Children with seizure-associated syndromes including Sturge-Weber syndrome, Rasmussen encephalitis, catastrophic seizure disorders of early childhood such as infantile spasms related to a localized zone of epileptogenic cerebral tissue, and hamartomatous cortex–producing seizures have benefitted the most often, but patients with refractory partial seizure disorders, including temporal lobe epilepsy, may also be candidates for surgical extirpation. Extensive pre-surgical imaging and physiological monitoring are necessary for resective surgery candidates.

Prognosis

In general, approximately two-thirds of children who have experienced a tendency for seizure recurrence have a good prognosis for prevention of further recurrence and little or no problem with side effects of medication. They can lead normal lives without handicap. The etiologic diagnosis is the most important prognostic factor. The type of epilepsy, EEG findings, child's age, difficulty of initial seizure control, and time since the last seizure are also important. Some seizure types have intrinsically poor prognoses. For example, infantile spasms are prognostically ominous because even in the absence of a metabolic diagnosis, children frequently suffer temporary brain growth and developmental arrest unless the seizures are controlled with medication. About 10% to 25% of children, most often those with generalized symptomatic epilepsies, frequent seizures, high anticonvulsant use, and early onset of epilepsy, show some intellectual decline. Partial complex disorders and the atypical variant

of petit mal disorders sometimes have a poorer prognosis for early resolution and may be more resistant to treatment with anticonvulsants. However, some of the seizure syndromes with a familial tendency such as Rolandic seizures and typical petit mal seizures have a relatively good prognosis for both control by medication and ultimate complete resolution.

The individualized decision to discontinue medication is often complex. The prognosis for recurrence of seizures, the parents' and children's reactions to seizures and to the prospect of their recurrence, and social factors such as school participation may all contribute to the decision. Children and parents must be aware that none of the prognostic factors, whether considered individually or in combination, is an absolute predictor of seizure recurrence or non-recurrence in a given child.

CASE RESOLUTION

The boy described in the case history at the beginning of the chapter had a generalized seizure when he was taken to the emergency department. The previous episodes recalled by the father had characteristics of partial seizures. The tonic-clonic seizure was probably a secondary generalized rather than a primary generalized seizure. The possibility of Rolandic seizures is suggested by the circumstances of the prior episodes, drowsiness, "facial" or "oral" symptomatology, and the family history. This diagnosis was confirmed by EEG. Oxcarbazepine was prescribed. The boy experienced no side effects or seizure recurrences and was successfully able to discontinue the medication 3 years later.

Selected References

Camfield P, Camfield C. Pediatric epilepsy: an overview. In: Swaiman K, Ashwal S, Ferriero D, eds. *Pediatric Neurology: Principals and Practice.* 4th ed. Philadelphia, PA: Elsevier; 2006

Clancy R. The newborn drug development initiative workshop: summary proceedings from the neurology group on neonatal seizures. *Clin Ther.* 2006;28:1342–1352

Faught E. Epilepsy case studies. *Neurol Clin.* 2006;24:291–307

Glauser T, Ben-Menachem E, Bourgeois B, et al. ILAE treatment guidelines: evidence-based analysis of antiepileptic drug efficacy and effectiveness as initial monotherapy for epileptic seizures and syndromes. *Epilepsia.* 2006;47:1094–1120

Kato M. A new paradigm for West syndrome based on molecular and cell biology. *Epilepsy Res.* 2006;70(suppl 1):S87–S95

Koh S, Menkes J, Sankar R, Wu J. Paroxysmal disorders. In: Menkes J, Sarnat H, Maria B, eds. *Child Neurology.* 7th ed. Philadelphia, PA: Lippincott, Williams & Wilkins; 2006

Marsh ED, Brooks-Kayal AR, Proter BE. Seizures and antiepileptic drugs: does exposure alter normal brain development? *Epilepsia.* 2006;47:1999–2010

CHAPTER 147

Pediatric Palliative Care: Principles and Practice

Rick Goldstein, MD

CASE STUDY

Jason is a 17-year-old boy with spastic quadriplegia, severe global developmental delays, a seizure disorder, cortical blindness, and dystonia. Since leaving the neonatal intensive care unit (NICU) at 3 months of age, he has lived in a skilled nursing facility and spends weekends at home with his family. He was born after 24 weeks' gestation and had a turbulent NICU course. During that hospitalization, in accord with his neonatologists, he was treated for comfort and extubated due to his severe respiratory failure, but managed to survive and breathe independently. Once beyond the newborn period, his medical course was fairly stable, notable for episodic respiratory decompensations requiring hospitalization and numerous orthopedic procedures. In the past 2 years, however, he has spent substantially more time in the intensive care unit due to increasing

respiratory fragility. With so much time spent in the hospital and so little time when he is comfortable "at home," his parents have begun questioning whether the intensive medical care he has been receiving translates into a quality of life and whether they should begin to limit efforts at resuscitation. They do not know what it would mean to place limitations on his care and, whatever their choices, they do not want Jason to suffer.

Questions

1. What is palliative care?
2. What is involved in the practice of palliative care?
3. How do children understand death? How does their understanding vary with their age?
4. What role does a primary care pediatrician play in the palliative care of her patients?

During the typical career of a primary care pediatrician, only a few patients die. Many more patients will develop complex medical conditions, sometimes life-threatening, generally requiring high levels of management. Caring for these patients can be among the most challenging yet rewarding experiences a pediatrician may have. Close, long-standing relationships with a family make it apparent how the impact of the illness on the child and family goes beyond biomedical issues, and many feel called to respond to the suffering that occurs. These children especially benefit from a medical home providing care that is accessible, continuous, comprehensive, family-centered, coordinated, and compassionate, led by an invested primary care pediatrician empathetic of their experience.

Even with the best of intentions, the care of these patients can accentuate changes in modern medical care. There can be a divide between the goals of subspecialty-based care provided in hospitals and those of the generalist care in the community. The increasing use of new medical technologies in the home setting can leave primary care pediatricians uncertain even as they are asked to sign the orders for home care. There can be uncertainty about whether unexpected symptoms can be managed quickly, effectively, and authoritatively in the community setting. Continuity of care can be challenging with

prolonged hospitalizations. And lastly, there is the matter of case ownership: Who is "in charge" and who will help the family and patient not only with the illness, but in accord with their hopes and wishes for their child?

A new subspecialty, pediatric palliative care, addresses many of the central concerns in the care of these children. It builds on an important cornerstone from hospice care, namely, acceptance of the fact that some children do die, and the circumstances of their death can be improved with specialized expertise directed toward improving the process and relieving pain and suffering. In all cases, it exists to help children and their families live as well as possible in the face of complex, life-threatening illness. The developing expertise of this subspecialty supports and augments the important work that emanates from the patient's medical home. Palliative care also deals with more complex cases that require enhanced care and coordination, and can assist the primary providers when they need help, or when most patient care is hospital-based. Far from signifying an abandonment of hope, palliative care practitioners work with families to redefine hope in a realistic way, and clarify what the family may need to align the treatment decisions with the child and family's vision of what is best.

The Scope of Pediatric Palliative Care

Each year more than 50,000 children in the United States will die and 10 times that number will cope with life-threatening conditions. In 2008, 55% of deaths of children younger than 19 years occurred in children younger than 1 year, with 20.1% of those infant deaths attributed to congenital malformations, deformations, and chromosomal abnormalities; 16.9% to short gestation and low birth weight; 8.2% to sudden infant death syndrome; 6.2% to newborns affected by maternal complications of pregnancy; and 4.6% to unintentional injuries. For older children, aged 1 to 19 years, the leading causes of death were unintentional injuries (38.8%); homicide (12.4%); malignant neoplasms (8.6%); suicide (8.0%); and congenital malformations, deformations, and chromosomal abnormalities (4.7%). Approximately 47% of US children die outside of a hospital.

Research by Feudtner and others has increased our understanding of children with complex chronic conditions (CCC) in the United States. These children are estimated to make up one-fifth of all pediatric deaths. Complex chronic conditions have been defined as medical conditions that can be reasonably expected to last at least 12 months (unless death intervenes) and that involve either several different organ systems or one organ system severely enough to require specialty pediatric care and probably some period of hospitalization in a tertiary center. The leading categories of CCCs leading to death are cardiovascular (22.2%), malignancy (21.4%), congenital/genetic (19.4%), neuromuscular (18.1%), and respiratory (9.3%). Increasingly, these children are dying at home, perhaps due to longer survival, the migration of advanced medical technology into the home, and shifting attitudes about what is better care, with a greater focus on quality of life among children with life-threatening conditions. Many studies indicate that, overall, home is the preferred site of ongoing care for children with life-threatening illnesses, regardless of their condition.

The American Academy of Pediatrics (AAP) endorses an integrated model of palliative and curative treatment where components of palliative care are offered at diagnosis and continued throughout the course of illness, whether the outcome is cure or death. The prevailing view is that the palliative care "approach should be instituted when diagnosis, intervention, and treatment are not limited to a disease process, but rather become instrumental for improving the quality of life, maintaining the dignity, and ameliorating the suffering of seriously ill or dying children in ways that are appropriate to their upbringing, culture, and community." (See selected references, Himelstein.) Palliative care is often incorrectly equated with hospice care, a program of coordinated services offering comfort-centered care at the end of life in the home or community setting. While there is a shared philosophy and an overlap of many of the priorities of care, palliative care should not be considered only at the end of life, nor is it exclusive of curative care. Changes in hospice benefits for children, reviewed later, further blur the distinction.

Palliative care should be considered in 4 categories of illness: conditions for which curative treatment is possible but may fail (eg, cancer with a poor prognosis); conditions requiring intensive long-term treatment aimed at maintaining the quality of life (eg, cystic fibrosis or advanced muscular dystrophy); progressive conditions in which treatment is exclusively palliative after diagnosis (eg, progressive metabolic disorders); and conditions involving severe, nonprogressive disability, causing extreme vulnerability to health complications (eg, holoprosencephaly or other severe brain malformations) (Box 147-1).

Box 147-1. Conditions Appropriate for Pediatric Palliative Care[a,b]

Conditions for which curative treatment is possible but may fail
- Advanced or progressive cancer or cancer with a poor prognosis
- Complex and severe congenital or acquired heart disease

Conditions requiring intensive long-term treatment aimed at maintaining the quality of life
- HIV infection
- Cystic fibrosis
- Severe gastrointestinal disorders or malformations, such as gastroschisis
- Severe epidermolysis bullosa
- Severe immunodeficiencies
- Renal failure in cases in which dialysis, transplantation, or both are not available or indicated
- Chronic or severe respiratory failure
- Muscular dystrophy

Progressive conditions in which treatment is exclusively palliative after diagnosis
- Progressive metabolic disorders
- Certain chromosomal abnormalities, such as trisomy 13 or trisomy 18
- Severe forms of osteogenesis imperfecta

Conditions involving severe, nonprogressive disability, causing extreme vulnerability to health complications
- Severe cerebral palsy with recurrent infection or difficult-to-control symptoms
- Extreme prematurity
- Severe neurologic sequelae of infectious disease
- Hypoxic or anoxic brain injury
- Holoprosencephaly or other severe brain malformations

[a] Reprinted with permission from Himelstein BP, et al. Pediatric palliative care. *N Engl J Med.* 2004;350:1752–1762
[b] Premature death is likely or expected with many of these conditions.

In addition, there is an emerging role for palliative care in the NICU. At this point, it is unclear whether, from a palliative care perspective, the needs of newborns and their families in NICUs are fully addressed. Neonatologists certainly have expertise dealing with the medical needs of critically ill children and the care-related concerns of their families. The pace of the NICU and the absence of a primary care practitioner no doubt have some impact on the priorities of care. A palliative care approach emphasizes critical communication, symptom management, and assistance with shared decision-making and articulating goals. Alternatively, pediatric deaths due to sudden unexplained infant death and traumatic injuries, intentional and unintentional, occur largely outside of medical settings. First responders and emergency medicine clinicians would benefit from palliative care guidance about symptom management in the face of imminent death and decision-making related to resuscitation.

Not every dying child requires the involvement of pediatric palliative care specialists. Realistically, primary care pediatricians provide essential contributions to the care of these children. Most children with life-threatening illnesses lead lives and receive at least some of their care in the community setting. There may be differences in the willingness of primary care practitioners to become involved or in the ability of practices to manage the complexities of care, but the primary care pediatrician can be the central coordinating figure in the medical care offered these children.

Efforts to enhance the quality of life for these children require a willingness to address biomedical, psychological, sociocultural, and spiritual matters. Families need guidance in navigating the administrative, financial, and coping challenges placed on them. Importantly, there is a fundamental need to promote the sense of a lived life of value and identity, in contrast to a life determined by the course of illness alone. These needs are best served when an interdisciplinary team attends to the unique needs of each child. Such a team may have a pediatrician leader, but benefits from involvement by nursing, social work, psychosocial clinicians, and pastoral care. Subspecialists are often involved, with varying relationships with the family. There may be a hospice program or a community-based palliative care program. The care of children additionally may involve representatives from the school, child life, and practitioners of functional therapies, whether occupational therapy, physical therapy, and speech therapy, or massage, hippotherapy, and Feldenkrais. Strong communication and reliable continuity within the team are essential to success.

Pain and symptom management for chronically ill or dying children is a foundation of quality of life and a core concern of pediatric palliative care. When the parents of children dying from cancer were asked about symptoms, 89% reported that their children suffered "a lot" or "a great deal" from at least one symptom as they were dying. Other research has found that parents list emotional distress, fatigue, nutritional concerns, and pain as troubling areas at the end of life. While the medical focus is on pain, there also is concern about symptoms such as dyspnea, nausea and vomiting, constipation, secretions, fatigue, anorexia, pruritis, sleep issues, anxiety, and anorexia. A full discussion of pain and symptom management can be found in Chapter 12.

Prognosis, Disclosure, Decision-making

The care of these children is marked by periods of intense uncertainty and fearful realities. Helping families determine the goals of care, appropriate treatment choices, and all aspects of planning for the child's life is facilitated when they understand their child's prognosis. To accomplish this, careful and thoughtful communication is of paramount importance. Yet research has found that many parents feel they receive confusing, inadequate, or uncaring communication related to prognosis and treatment. They are expected to reach decisions with a different understanding of medical details than their children's health care professionals. Such decisions are especially difficult in a setting of misunderstanding, disagreement or, worse, lack of trust.

Most illness has prognostic uncertainty. Despite this, parents benefit from direct communication about the disease severity, and the timeline for progression and potentially death. This is a difficult task, not only because imparting bad news is an uncomfortable and complex task, but also the exact prognosis is truly uncertain. Studies of prognosis have found that physicians are accurate only 20% of the time and tend to be overly optimistic. While more experienced clinicians tend to have less error, there is also a correlation between the length of a relationship with a patient and a lowered likelihood that the prognosis will be correct. Parents nonetheless seek a clear disclosure. They interpret hidden or minimal information as their doctor withholding frightening information. Alternatively, parents who receive more elements of prognostic disclosure are more likely to report communication-related hope, even when the likelihood of cure is low. The benefits of honest communication about the prognosis exceed the hazards.

When parents and some children ask about prognosis, they are asking about both the time remaining and the pace of expected decline. Three typical trajectories for progressive chronic illness have been described in adults and are informative for pediatric patients as well (Figure 147-1). The first is a pattern of illness with a modest impact on function during most of its course followed by a precipitous decline near the time of death. Cancer death classically fits this pattern, and cancer research has led to models where timelines can be discussed with some accuracy. An implication for care with this trajectory is that there is life to live even in the face of imminent death and also that when decline comes, there has been time to review the priorities of care before circumstances at the end of life.

The second trajectory is one of long-term limitations with intermittent serious episodes. Cystic fibrosis and severe disability following prematurity are 2 examples of this trajectory. Although there is slow, steady decline that can generally be discussed with some clarity, there are unpredictable decompensations that often bring the child close to death, and which will affect the overall rate of decline. A predicted timeline to death can only be described in general terms. These patients sometimes survive their decompensations after seeming, to all appearances, beyond recovery. This can make it very difficult to talk about placing limitations on resuscitation, even when quality of life is extremely compromised. The third trajectory, described as prolonged dwindling, can apply to children with severe metabolic abnormalities, trisomy 13 or 18, or severe brain abnormalities. It is a life of ever-diminishing function. The families tend to become quite "medicalized" and organize their lives around the child's care. A key challenge in these cases is to help the family articulate what they see as giving the child's life meaning, and helping them evaluate interventions in terms of their goals, not simply whether they are possible.

Uncomfortable as it is, anticipating death and addressing it clearly and frankly allows families, and some patients, to make choices about the time remaining. The early recognition of a poor prognosis predicts

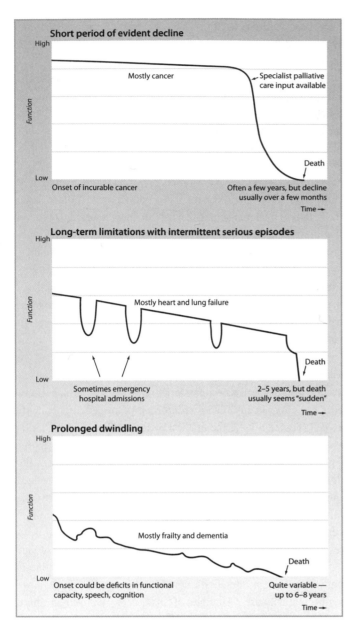

Figure 147-1. Typical illness trajectories for people with progressive chronic illness. (Modified with permission from Lynn J, Adamson DM. *Living Well at the End of Life. Adapting Health Care to Serious Chronic Illness in Old Age.* Washington, DC: Rand Health; 2003.)

an earlier do not resuscitate (DNR) order, less use of disease-directed therapies in the last months of life, and a greater chance of incorporating the child's comfort as a goal. It allows a narrative to evolve of who this child was and the terms under which he lived. It allows for some sense of control and expression of values in overwhelming circumstances. Mack and Wolfe have nicely outlined an approach to communicating with children and families once prognosis has been shared and palliative care is under consideration (Table 147-1).

The Burden of Suffering and the Power of Hope

It is indeed surprising that the topics of suffering and hope can seem, at first glance, to be nontechnical and not properly "medical." It is hard to imagine how concepts so central to the call to heal can seem

peripheral. This is rooted in the bias that matters of the body are appropriate areas of treatment whereas matters of the mind and soul are left to other subspecialties or areas outside of medicine.

Disease and its treatment can cause physical distress, but suffering is much larger and more complex. Cassel defines suffering as "the state of severe distress associated with events that threaten the intactness of a person." When a child or parent worries "what will happen..." or their complaints seem greater than their physical basis, they may be reflecting the suffering that comes from a threat to any of the multiple aspects of personhood—"the lived past, the family's lived past, culture and society, roles, the instrumental dimension, associations and relationships, the body, the unconscious mind, the political being, the secret life, the perceived future, and the transcendent dimension." In caring for patients with life-threatening illness, understanding all aspects of suffering is critical to effective care, and reflection and understanding are prerequisite to a healing presence. Pain and symptom management are foundational, but the relief of suffering requires helping a child and family struggle with issues of meaning and transcendence.

Hope involves expectations or belief in a worthy future. It carries a sense of trust and reliance. Life-threatening illness makes it complicated to know what to hope for, trust in, or rely on. Medical particulars aside, as Cassell has written, "the imperative to tell the truth seems an insufficient guide to what you should tell patients." It is not that truth or the best understanding should be withheld, but rather it should be communicated with the goal of reducing uncertainty and providing a basis for action. Hope can be sustained when a meaningful way forward is elucidated even in the face of dismal diagnosis.

Barriers to Palliative Care

Parenting a child with chronic and potentially terminal illnesses can be frightening, confusing, frustrating, and exhausting. While a decision to involve palliative care practitioners is in no sense a decision to stop working strenuously for their child's life, it is crucial that palliative care is introduced with a sensitivity to this misinterpretation. If palliative care is viewed by the parents or child as an act of abandonment or disloyalty, the benefits of the consultation may not be forthcoming. Parents should be advised that a growing body of research has demonstrated that involvement of palliative care strategies leads not only to an improved quality of life for extremely ill patients even as their illness progresses, but also longer survival. Palliative care offers much more than "doing nothing and letting the disease take its toll."

One of the greatest obstacles to palliative care and hospice has been a reimbursement model based on the Medicare Hospice Benefit, which required patients in hospice to forego curative care and gear care toward survival of 6 months or less. Parents, understandably, find it very hard to give up curative efforts for their children. They appreciate a quality of life in a developing though ill child that is different than in a dying geriatric patient. Because hospice was associated with the elderly, parents felt a disincentive against selection of hospice insurance as a benefit. While certain states offer palliative care programs to remedy this, the Patient Protection and Affordable

Table 147-1. Communicating With Children and Families About Integrating Palliative Care	
Beginning the conversation	• What is your understanding of what is ahead for your child? • Would it be helpful to talk about how his or her disease may affect him or her in the months and years ahead? • As you think about what is ahead for your child, what would you like to talk about with me? • What information can I give you that would be helpful to you?
Introducing the possibility of death	• I am hoping that we will be able to control the disease, but I am worried that this time we may not be successful. • Although we do not know for certain what will happen for your child, I do not expect that your child will live a long and healthy life; most children with this disease eventually die because of the disease. • I have been noticing that your child seems to be sick more and more often. I have been hoping that we would be able to make him or her better, but I am worried that his or her illness has become more difficult to control and that soon we will not be able to help him or her to get over these illnesses. If that is the case, he or she could die of his or her disease.
Eliciting goals of care	• As you think about your child's illness, what are your hopes? • As you think about your child's illness, what are your worries? • As you think about your child's illness, what is most important to you right now? • You mentioned that what is most important to you is that your child be cured of his or her disease. I am hoping for that too. But I would also like to know more about your hopes and goals for your child's care if the time comes when a cure is not possible.
Introducing palliation	• Although I hope that we can control your child's disease for as long as possible, at the same time I am hoping that he or she feels as good as possible each day. • Although it is unlikely that this treatment will cure your child's disease, it may help him or her to feel better, and possibly to live longer.
Talking about what to expect	• Would it be helpful to talk about what to expect as your child's illness gets worse? • Although we cannot predict exactly what will happen to your child, most children with this disease eventually have [difficulty breathing]. If that happens to your child, our goal will be to help him or her feel as comfortable as possible. We can use medications to help control his or her discomfort.
Talking to children	• What are you looking forward to most of all? • Is there anything that is worrying you or making you feel afraid? • Is there anything about how you are feeling that is making you feel worried or afraid?

a From Mack JW, Wolfe J. Early integration of pediatric palliative care: for some children, palliative care starts at diagnosis. *Curr Opin Pediatr.* 2006;18:10–14, with permission from Wolters Kluwer Health.

Care Act of 2010 removed the prohibition against curative treatment as a hospice benefit by or on behalf of a Medicaid or Children's Health Insurance Program–eligible child. States are not required to provide hospice services, although this is increasingly the norm, but where hospice services are provided, concurrent curative treatment must be offered. Despite these changes, eligibility still requires a physician to certify the child as likely to die in the next 6 months.

A Child's Understanding of Death

Ultimately, death is a singular transcendent experience, likely beyond the understanding of the living. But parents want to know what their children can understand as they go through the process. Caregivers, too, wonder what a child knows as they try to anticipate needs or reckon with enigmatic statements from them. Most would agree that a child's suffering due to avoidance of discussions of their fears about their condition and death is especially tragic and counterproductive.

The pediatrician should communicate with children about what is happening to them, while respecting the cultural and personal preferences of the family. A developmental understanding of children's concepts of health and illness can help frame the discussion with children, or serve to advise parents in their discussions. The child's concept of death reflected in the medical literature has changed very little from that extrapolated from Piaget's work in cognitive development and is based on the stages of sensorimotor, preoperational, concrete operations, and formal operations.

Up to 2 years of age (sensorimotor), there is probably no concept of death per se. Death is understood and responded to as a separation. Grief relates to the loss of an attachment figure and is expressed through protest and difficulty attaching to other adults. The degree of difficulty dealing with the loss depends on the availability of other nurturing adults who have cared for the child and with whom the child has had a good previous attachment.

Once they are 3 years of age, children can recognize death as a changed state. In the preoperational stage (ages 3–5 years), however, they cannot understand the meaning of a severe illness nor the finality and universality of death. Limited language abilities can give the appearance of little insight, and moods or behavior can be the means of expression. Bad things happen for an immediately identifiable reason, and death may be viewed as punishment. For instance, if a child's newborn sibling suddenly dies and the child had previously wished them to have died or gone back to where he or she came from, they may feel their wish was the cause of the death. Children this age can feel overwhelmed when confronted with the strong emotional reactions of their parents at the time of loss.

Ages 6 to 11 years (school age) are considered the late preoperational to concrete operational stages of cognitive development. In this age range, the finality of death comes to be understood. Eight-year-olds are aware of personal mortality, and work by Hinds has found that children as young as 10 years are able to speak about their experiences and decisions at the end of life. Magical thinking gives way to a need for detailed information to gain a sense of control. Older children in this range will often feel a need to control their emotions by compartmentalizing and intellectualizing.

The developmental stage of adolescents (>12 years old) is considered formal operations. The concept of death includes universality and finality, and they can understand personal mortality. Adolescents handle death issues at an abstract or philosophical level and can be realistic. They may seem closed off to information and resist frank discussions with undercurrents of deep emotion, and rely on anger or disdain. Communication with peers, perhaps involving social networking technologies, can be more open, although critically ill children are sensitive about not burdening their friends, just as they often feel their friends are unable to fully comprehend their situation. Adolescents can discuss withholding of treatments. Their personal goals should be understood, respected, and discussed on their own terms.

A child's cognitive limitations will obviously have an impact on their understanding. Another matter is how illness has affected their development—it is observed that chronically ill children may possess a precocious and advanced understanding of certain things, for instance the details of their illness or the way to address their symptoms, while simultaneously being less mature in other developmental areas.

Parents can struggle with whether they should talk with their child about their imminent death. While research supports a bias toward speaking frankly to dying children, each individual case presents its own complexities based on the child's age, cognitive development, disease, timeline of disease, and parental psychological state. In a study by Kreicsberg of parental disclosure to children with impending cancer death, no parent who talked with their child about their death regretted doing so and, of those who did not speak frankly about imminent death, 27% regretted not having done so. Among those who did not talk with their child about death, parents who sensed their child was aware of imminent death, parents of older children, and mothers more than fathers were more likely to feel regretful.

Primary Care at the End of Life: Normal and Extraordinary

There is no disputing the important role that primary care pediatricians can play in the care of children with life-threatening illness. The medical home is even more beneficial to these children. A constant, continuous physician who understands the child and his family holistically can contribute profoundly to their care. Because caring for these children is a rare experience in general practice, the complexities of care can be daunting. There is a need to understand an appropriate role and develop a supportive structure for the primary care pediatricians in a way that supports best practice.

Primary care is provided outside of the hospital and "at home." Families and children may develop strong feelings about returning to the hospital, having spent difficult times there. They may feel relief in not having to deal with the logistical, seemingly less personal, hurdles of hospital-based care. Care provided in the normal setting of primary care tends to be more tolerable.

General pediatric care under the guidance of the primary care physician also can be an important affirmation of the normal and can contribute to quality of life. For the patient, routine health care visits, vaccinations, and developmental assessments are important because the rationale for this care is not their disease but the positive and ordinary characteristics of childhood. The focus on development, education and learning, social engagement, play, and involvement with family and community affirms the whole child and the importance of his life. The primary care pediatrician is often seen as a trusted advisor who understands the family and child in the normal context, and thus "knows" them best. He is the child's doctor without qualification.

A trusted primary care pediatrician also has a role in complex disease management. The primary care pediatrician is in the best position to assess the family's level of understanding and address any gaps. Importantly, he can help families understand complex medical information, terminology (medical jargon), or other specific medical details. An involved primary care practitioner also can help the medical team better understand the patient and family perspective. They can ease the adjustment between home and hospital and help ensure a more seamless transition in either direction. In order for the pediatrician to have relevant involvement in crucial developments, there must be a timely sharing of information between all members of the team, generalist, and specialist. Ideally the primary care physician should participate in hospital rounds on the patient and in team meetings. This is especially important for meetings with the family where goals of care and medical decision-making are the focus. Fostering collaboration between the primary care physician and the palliative care specialist is essential (Box 147-2).

When a child is facing the end of life at home, the primary care physician has additional opportunities to facilitate things for the child and family. The primary care physician works with the hospice

---

Box 147-2. Fundamental Elements of Successful Collaboration Between Primary Care and Palliative Care[a]

- Timely sharing of information
- Mutual inclusion in clarifying goals of care and medical decision-making
- Coordinated designation of responsibilities
- Explicit review of case management and social work needs
- Technical backstopping for pain and symptom management
- Trusted, timely collaboration and assistance with urgent symptom management issues

[a] Adapted from Steinhorn D, Goldstein R, Orloff S. Relationships with the community: palliative care and beyond. In: Wolfe J, Hinds P, Sourkes B. *Textbook of Interdisciplinary Pediatric Palliative Care.* Philadelphia, PA: Saunders; 2011.

team to continuously fine-tune approaches to pain and symptoms. Their greater availability and sense of the family are important assets. Primary care pediatricians can also play a central role in delineating resuscitation orders.

Research finds that parents consider end-of-life decisions to be the most difficult treatment decisions they face. It is not unusual for them to operate in a way that continues to seek a cure even as they accept the inevitability of death, and these decisions reveal the tensions of holding both views. It is not surprising that DNR orders are frequently instituted near the time of death. Paradoxically the child may spend less time at home as the parents still expect efforts toward an impossible cure. The proper timing to introduce these issues is early in the course of the child's illness, not in the midst of crisis or very late in the patient's course. Thoughtful conversation with a trusted primary care pediatrician who has a broad perspective on the medical details as well as the family identity and values is invaluable.

Most important is to help the family determine realistic goals for their child. This is facilitated by a frank discussion of whether resuscitation efforts support their goals or not. A powerful guide for these discussions is the document *Five Wishes*, or for younger children up to approximately age 11, *My Wishes*, distributed by Aging With Dignity. These are guided conversations that approach advance directives, and the *Five Wishes* document is legally recognized in 42 states (Box 147-3). Simply addressing "DNR orders" is inadequate. Another important contribution that differs in each state are comfort care forms and physician orders for life-sustaining treatment. These are DNR orders that are not particular to the inpatient setting. For instance, emergency medical technicians in the field must resuscitate a child found in cardiac or respiratory failure unless orders exist to refrain. Once a family has come to the difficult decision to limit interventions, it is important to advocate for their wishes in all potential settings.

Case coordination should explicitly address outpatient management and clarify the responsibilities of the primary care team as well of each of the subspecialists. The potential for this collaboration to improve the care offered by all of the members of the child's medical team is enormous.

Loss and After

The loss of a child or sibling changes life forever. It begins a process of bereavement, the psychological and spiritual accommodation to death on the part of the child and the child's family, and grief, the emotional response caused by the loss. Grief can cause pain, distress, and physical and emotional suffering but, except in cases of prolongation, is a normal adaptive human response, not a disease. Anticipatory grief begins with the awareness of impending loss or death in parents and in children with sufficient awareness and cognitive development. Palliative care attends to the grief reaction before and following death. Assessing the coping resources and vulnerabilities of the affected family system before death takes place is central to the palliative care approach.

Box 147-3. My Wishes and Five Wishes[a]

My Wishes (for children up to approximately 11 years)
- How I want people to treat me
- How comfortable I want to be
- What I want my loved ones to know
- What I want my doctors and nurses to know

Five Wishes
- The person I want to make care decisions for me when I can't
- The kind of medical treatment I want or don't want
- How comfortable I want to be
- How I want people to treat me
- What I want my loved ones to know

[a] Reprinted with permission from Aging with Dignity. Available at http://www.agingwithdignity.org.

Parental grief is more intense and sustained than other types of grief. Parents may never completely accept the loss of their child. Most parents work through their grief, though studies have found that more than one-fourth had not worked through their grief in 4 to 9 years after the loss of the child. Research suggests that parents who share their problems with others during the child's illness, who have had access to psychological support during the last month of their child's life, and who have had closure sessions with the attending staff are more likely to resolve their grief.

Surviving siblings are also burdened. The AAP recommends that primary care pediatricians reach out to children and families at the time of loss, evaluate their bereavement to understand the personal meaning of their loss and their process of mourning, and monitor their process, especially in the year following a death. There is a further role of explaining to parents how surviving children are managing their loss, and that children often reexamine the meaning of loss in their lives during each developmental period. When necessary, referrals to skilled mental health professionals should be offered.

Those involved in the care of children and families should appreciate how meaningful simple things like condolence letters and attendance at funerals or memorial services are to families. Notes remembering the anniversary of the deceased child's birthday, or helping the family think about developing the child's legacy or a remembrance also contribute to an improved bereavement. Helping bereaved children safely remember their deceased siblings and appreciating their success as they integrate the loss can be a powerful part of a health care visit.

CASE RESOLUTION

The hospital-based palliative care team arranges to meet with the parents. During their conversations, they help the parents articulate what gives Jason's life meaning, what happiness and unhappiness are for him, and what is a hopeful versus a hopeless existence. The parents decide they would still opt for intubation and respiratory interventions should he become compromised by an acute, likely reversible issue but could not imagine that a further deterioration of his condition after the need for cardiac resuscitation would prove consistent with their goals. Therefore, a limitation is placed on cardiac resuscitation. With their permission, the palliative care team speaks with personnel at the skilled nursing facility, their primary care pediatrician, and the palliative care team at the community hospital where Jason would be taken if ill. Documents are prepared and shared for use in all of the settings. The palliative care team continues to meet with Jason and his family for each hospital admission and has made visits to his nursing facility to help the staff.

Selected References

Aging With Dignity. Five Wishes. www.agingwithdignity.org

American Academy of Pediatrics Committee on Bioethics and Committee on Hospital Care. Palliative care for children. *Pediatrics. 2000;*106:351–357

American Academy of Pediatrics Committee on Psychosocial Aspects of Child and Family Health. The pediatrician and childhood bereavement. *Pediatrics.* 1992;89:516–518

Cassel EJ. The nature of suffering and the goals of medicine. *N Engl J Med.* 1982;306:639–645

Feudtner C, Feinstein JA, Satchell M, Zhao H, Kang IT. Shifting place of death among children with complex chronic conditions in the United States, 1989–2003. *JAMA.* 2007;297:2725–2732

Himelstein BP, Hilden JM, Boldt AM, Weissman D. Pediatric palliative care. *N Engl J Med.* 2004;350:1752–1762

Hinds PS, Drew D, Oakes LL, et al. End-of-life preferences of pediatric patients with cancer. *J Clin Oncol.* 2005;23:9146–9154

Kreicsberg UC, Lanne P, Onelov E, Wolfe J. Parental grief after losing a child to cancer: impact of professional and social support on long-term outcomes. *J Clin Oncol.* 2007;25:3307-3312.

Mack JW, Wolfe J, Cook EF, Grier HE, Cleary PD, Weeks JC. Hope and prognostic disclosure. *J Clin Oncol.* 2007;25:5636–5642

Mack JW, Wolfe J. Early integration of pediatric palliative care: for some children, palliative care starts at diagnosis. *Curr Opin Pediatr.* 2006;18:10–14

Mathews TJ, Minino AM, Osterman MJ, Strobino DM, Guyer B. Annual summary of vital statistics: 2008. *Pediatrics.* 2011;127:146–157

Murray SA, Kendall M, Boyd K, Sheikh A. Illness trajectories and palliative care. *BMJ.* 2005;330:1007–1011

Wolfe J, Grier HE, Klar N, et al. Symptoms and suffering at the end of life in children with cancer. *N Engl J Med.* 2000;342:326–333

Index